THIRD EDITION

Psychosocial Occupational Therapy

AN EVOLVING PRACTICE

Elizabeth Cara, PhD, OTR/L, MFT
Professor, Occupational Therapy
San Jose State University
San Jose, California

Anne MacRae, PhD, OTR/L, BCMH, FAOTA
Professor, Occupational Therapy
San Jose State University
San Jose, California

Occupational Therapist and Project Consultant
Trinity County Behavioral Health Service
Weaverville, California

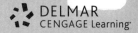

DELMAR
CENGAGE Learning

Australia • Brazil • Japan • Korea • Mexico • Singapore • Spain • United Kingdom • United States

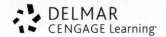
DELMAR
CENGAGE Learning·

Psychosocial Occupational Therapy: An Evolving Practice, 3rd Edition
Elizabeth Cara, PhD, OTR/L, MFT and
Anne MacRae, PhD, OTR/L, BCMH, FAOTA

Vice President, Careers and Computing:
Dave Garza.

Director of Learning Solutions:
Matthew Kane

Associate Acquisitions Editor:
Christina Gifford

Managing Editor: Marah Bellegarde

Senior Product Manager: Laura J. Wood

Editorial Assistant: Anthony Souza

Vice President, Marketing:
Jennifer Ann Baker

Marketing Director: Wendy E. Mapstone

Senior Marketing Manager: Nancy Bradshaw

Marketing Coordinator: Piper Huntington

Production Manager: Andrew Crouth

Content Project Manager: Anne Sherman

Senior Art Director: David Arsenault

Library of Congress Control Number: 2011934187

ISBN-13: 978-1-111-31830-7

ISBN-10: 1-111-31830-1

Delmar
5 Maxwell Drive
Clifton Park, NY 12065-2919
USA

Cengage Learning is a leading provider of customized learning solutions with office locations around the globe, including Singapore, the United Kingdom, Australia, Mexico, Brazil, and Japan. Locate your local office at: **international .cengage.com/region**

Cengage Learning products are represented in Canada by Nelson Education, Ltd.

To learn more about Delmar, visit **www.cengage.com/delmar**

Purchase any of our products at your local college store or at our preferred online store **www.cengagebrain.com**

Printed in the United States of America
2 3 4 5 6 7 14

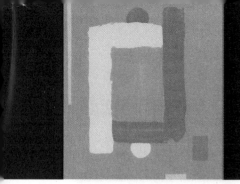

CONTENTS

Preface to the Third Edition • ix
Acknowledgments • xix
About the Authors • xxi
Contributors to the Third Edition • xxiii

PART I

Understanding the Person in Context • 1

Chapter 1
Recovery Perspectives • 3

Carol Underwood and Anne MacRae

Introduction • 4

Section One: Personal Perspective • 4
Mental Illness—What It Feels Like • 6
Recovery—What Is It? • 7
Is Recovery a Realistic Goal? • 10
Peer Interventions and Recovery-Oriented
    Support • 11

Section Two: Professional Perspective • 16
Definitions and Scope of Recovery • 16
Impact of the Recovery Movement • 19
The Changing Role of Mental Health Professionals • 19
The Role of Occupational Therapy
    in a Recovery Paradigm • 22
Summary • 24

Chapter 2
Environmental and Cultural Considerations • 28

Anne MacRae and Tiffany (Debra) Boggis

Introduction • 29
Environment • 29

Culture • 41
Summary • 57

Chapter 3
A Context for Mental Health Research in
Occupational Therapy • 61

Pamela Richardson and Madeleine Duncan

Introduction • 62
Why Do Research? The Burden of Mental
    Illness • 63
Evidence-Based Practice • 64
Research Priorities in Mental Health • 66
Research Priorities in Mental Health
    Occupational Therapy • 69
Thinking in Research • 74
Methodological Positions • 85
Research Examples: Learning from Others • 87
The Way Forward • 90
Summary • 92

PART II

Theoretical Concepts • 97

Chapter 4
The History and Philosophy of Psychosocial
Occupational Therapy • 99

Kathleen Barker Schwartz

Introduction • 100
Treatment of the Insane Before the Twentieth
    Century • 100
The Founding of Occupational Therapy • 103

Treatment of Mental Illness in the Twentieth
Century • 111

The Evolution of Psychosocial Occupational
Therapy • 113

Summary • 122

Chapter 5
Psychological Theories and Their
Treatment Methods in Mental Health
Practice • 128

Lynne Andonian, Elizabeth Cara, and Anne MacRae

Introduction • 129

Humanistic Perspective • 130

Biological Perspective • 136

Psychodynamic Perspective • 144

Behavioral Perspective • 150

Cognitive Perspective • 153

Summary • 157

PART III

Diagnosis and Dysfunction • 165

Chapter 6
Diagnosis and Psychopathology • 166

Anne MacRae

Introduction • 167

Clinical Terminology • 167

Diagnosis • 168

Psychopathology • 175

Psychiatric Intervention in the Era of
Recovery • 183

Summary • 188

Chapter 7
Schizophrenia • 192

Anne MacRae and Lynne Andonian

Introduction • 193

Myths and Misconceptions • 193

Etiology of Schizophrenia • 196

Diagnosis of Schizophrenia • 198

Positive Symptoms • 199

Negative Symptoms • 203

Prognosis • 204

Collaborative Treatment • 206

Occupational Therapy Intervention • 210

Summary • 214

Chapter 8
Mood Disorders • 221

Elizabeth Cara

Introduction • 222

Diagnostic Criteria • 222

Causes, Occurrence, and Theories of Mood
Disorders • 226

Clinical Picture • 231

Common Evaluation and Management • 233

Occupational Therapy Treatment and
Intervention • 238

Summary • 251

Chapter 9
Anxiety Disorders • 258

Elizabeth Cara

Introduction • 259

Encountering People with Anxiety Disorders:
Settings • 260

Description of Anxiety Disorders • 261

Impact on Daily Functioning • 263

DSM-IV-TR Descriptions of Anxiety • 265

General Treatment Strategies • 269

Occupational Therapy and Self-Management
Techniques • 277

Assessment • 278

Treatment Interventions • 280

Goals • 298

Treatment • 299

Summary • 302

Chapter 10
Personality Disorders • 308

Elizabeth Cara

Introduction • 309

The Personality Continuum and Etiology of
Personality Disorders • 311

The *DSM-IV-TR* Personality Disorders • 314

Interdisciplinary Assessment and Treatment • 323

Occupational Therapy Treatment
Interventions • 328

Summary • 334

PART IV

Mental Health Across the Lifespan • 341

Chapter 11

Mental Health of Infants: Attachment Through the Lifespan • 343

Elizabeth Cara and Elise Holloway

Introduction • 344

History of Attachment • 345

What Is Attachment Exactly? • 348

Phases of Attachment • 349

Internal Working Models • 350

Categories of Attachment: Evidence-Base of Attachment • 351

The Patterns of Attachment • 354

Cross-Cultural Studies • 356

Attachment and Affect Regulation • 357

Attachment and Abuse and Neglect • 359

Clinical Programs That Focus on Attachment • 364

Occupational Therapy Treatment Guided by Programs that Promote Attachment • 366

Summary • 378

Chapter 12

Mental Health of Children • 384

William L. Lambert

Introduction • 385

DSM-IV-TR Diagnoses • 386

Helpful Concepts for Treating Children • 393

Child Settings and Programs • 402

Implementing Programming for Children • 405

Examples of Emerging Areas of Practice • 416

Summary, Current Trends, and Recommendations • 420

Chapter 13

Mental Health of Adolescents • 427

William L. Lambert and Elizabeth Carley

Introduction • 428

Etiology of Adolescent Mental Health or Illness • 429

Disorders, Diagnoses, and Presenting Problems • 431

Bullying and School Violence • 442

Helpful Concepts for Treating Adolescents • 444

Adolescent Settings and Programs • 450

Implementing Programs • 459

Evaluation • 460

Intervention • 461

Summary • 468

Chapter 14

Mental Health of the Older Adult • 473

Anne MacRae and Jerilyn (Gigi) Smith

Introduction • 474

The Demographics of Aging • 474

Psychiatric Diagnosis • 475

Mental Health Assessment • 482

Occupational Therapy Intervention • 486

Summary • 496

PART V

Mental Health with Physical Disorders • 501

Chapter 15

Psychosocial Issues in Physical Disability • 502

Heidi McHugh Pendleton and Winifred Schultz-Krohn

Introduction • 503

Occupational Therapy and the International Classification of Functioning • 504

Cultural and Societal Factors • 505

Concept of Self • 507

Models of Adapting to Physical Disability • 510

Life Satisfaction and Quality of Life • 517

Specific Psychosocial Issues with Select Disabilities • 519

Summary • 534

Chapter 16

The Cognitive, Behavioral, and Psychosocial Sequelae of Brain Injury • 541

Shawn Phipps

Introduction • 542

Diagnosis and Etiology • 543

Prognosis for Recovery • 544

Premorbid Psychosocial Factors • 547

Occupational Therapy Evaluation and Intervention • 550

Cognitive Sequelae Following Brain Injury • 557

Behavioral Sequelae Following Brain Injury • 560

Psychosocial Sequelae Following Brain Injury • 564

Summary • 567

Chapter 17
Managing Pain in Occupational Therapy: Integrating the Model of Human Occupation and the Intentional Relationship Model • 573

Renee R. Taylor and Chia-Wei Fan

Introduction • 574
Acute Versus Chronic Pain • 574
Examples of Disorders Involving Chronic Pain • 576
Assessing Pain: An Occupational Therapy Perspective • 579
Applying the Model of Human Occupation in Treatment • 582
Effective Use of Self: The Intentional Relationship Model • 587
Areas of Related Knowledge: The Unique Role of the Occupational Therapist • 592
Summary • 593

PART VI
Occupational Therapy Intervention in Mental Health • 597

Chapter 18
Assessment, Evaluation, and Outcome Measurement • 600

Alison Laver-Fawcett

Introduction • 601
An Overview of Assessment • 601
Key Concepts in Assessment and Evaluation • 603
The Assessment Process • 615
Considering the Different Purposes of Assessment • 625
Summary • 636

Chapter 19
The Use of Psychosocial Methods and Interpersonal Strategies in Mental Health • 643

Elizabeth Cara and Pamela R.R. Stephenson

Introduction • 644
Interpersonal Strategies • 645
Occupational Therapy Methods • 652
Summary • 667

Chapter 20
Groups • 671

Elizabeth Cara

Introduction • 672

What Makes a Group a Group? • 672
Advantages and Limitations of Groups • 673
Overview of Group Therapy • 674
Occupational Therapy Groups • 692
Starting a Group • 699
The Group Protocol • 701
Documentation and Outcome • 703
Summary • 709

PART VII
Specialized Roles for Occupational Therapy in Mental Health • 713

Chapter 21
Occupational Therapy in Criminal Justice • 715

John A. White, Crystal Dieleman Grass, Toby Ballou Hamilton, and Sandra L. Rogers

Introduction • 716
Overview of Criminal Justice System: Stages of Offender Involvement • 718
Scope of Criminal Justice • 719
Health Care in the Criminal Justice System • 721
Mental Health in Criminal Justice and Corrections: U.S. and International Perspectives • 722
Occupational Therapy in Criminal Justice • 724
Occupational Justice and Injustice • 725
Evaluation, Assessment, and Intervention • 726
Occupation-Based Self-Determination (OBSD) • 727
Therapeutic Competencies • 730
Sexuality in Forensic and Correctional Settings • 742
Occupational Therapy Interventions in Criminal Justice and Evidence for Practice • 744
Prisonization and Errors in Critical Thinking • 754
Criminal Thinking • 758
Crime as Occupation: Stages of the Criminal Career • 761
An Occupational Perspective of Crime • 762
Reentry to the Community • 763
Summary • 765

Chapter 22
Psychosocial Occupational Therapy in the School Setting • 774

Sue Ann Folker and Sara L. Woodward

Introduction • 775

Inclusion and Participation in the School Community:
An Occupational Justice Perspective • 777
Participation and Psychosocial Well-Being • 779
School-Based Occupational Therapy:
A Community-Based Practice • 781
Actions to Address Psychosocial Issues in the School
Setting • 801
Summary • 803

Chapter 23
Vocational Programming • 809
Eileen S. Auerbach

Introduction • 810
History of Work Programming in Occupational
Therapy • 810
Expanding Roles of Occupational Therapists • 814
Knowing Your Customers—New Alliances • 814
Implementation of Occupational Therapy
Services • 815
Summary • 835

Chapter 24
Substance Abuse and Occupational Therapy • 840
Steve Hoppes, Helen R. Bryce, and Suzanne M. Peloquin

Introduction • 841
Use, Abuse, and Dependence • 842
Treatment Approaches • 844
Rationale for Inclusion of Occupational
Therapy • 849
Occupation-Based Intervention Programming in
Recovery Programs • 849
Occupational Therapy at the Alcohol and Drug Abuse
Center • 861
Advice • 869
Summary • 869

Chapter 25
Occupational Therapy in the Military: Working with Service Members in Combat and at Home • 876
Robinette J. Amaker, Anne Pas Burke, Cecilia Najera, and Mary Vining Radomski

Introduction • 877
Working in the Field • 878
Rehabilitation of Traumatic Brain Injury • 889
Treating Warriors at Home: Acute Stress
Reactions • 898
Summary • 913

Chapter 26
Fieldwork Supervision in the Mental Health Setting • 920
Patricia Crist and Elizabeth Cara

Introduction • 921
Role of the Fieldwork Educator or Supervisor in
Mental Health • 923
Transformative Learning • 926
Dimensions of Fieldwork Education and
Supervision • 929
Clinical Reasoning and Reflection • 932
Theoretical Foundations of Supervision • 932
Practical Models and Methods of Supervision • 934
Situational Supervision • 943
Coaching During Supervision • 948
Maximizing Learning—Benefiting from
Supervision • 952
Trends and Recommendations • 953
Summary • 957

Glossary • 963
Index • 975

PREFACE TO THE THIRD EDITION

INTRODUCTION

The subtitle of this text is now called *"An Evolving Practice"* to best capture the dramatic and rapid transformation of mental health services. *Evolving practice* presents the case that occupational therapy can regain and strengthen our role in mental health services by not only adapting to this transformation but also becoming proactive leaders in a new paradigm. This text is designed to prepare occupational therapy students, as well as entry level through advanced practitioners, to meet this challenge. Our intent is to also provide occupational therapists with the background and language to be able to educate others regarding the unique focus and skills that occupational therapy brings to mental health practice.

The mental health services transformation is largely being spurred by the world-wide recovery movement, which is discussed throughout this book and is especially captured in the perspectives described in the opening chapter. Occupational therapy has a history of using a strength-based focus, that is, they target an individual's strengths (not problem areas), with practical skill development, and recognition of personal motivation and goals, within the realities of an environmental and cultural context. These are all professional traits that are not only consistent with the beliefs and values of recovery-oriented individuals but can also be the basis for effective collaboration. However, current practice still exists within a medical model of mental health conditions and so also dictates that mental health professionals be versed in not only a social model of practice, but also in the medical orientation of mental illness, through knowledge of psychopathology, diagnosis, and treatment from broad theoretical principles and models. The chapters in this book deftly cover this wide range of knowledge needed for occupational therapy expertise in this area. It remains to be seen how mental health care will merge the medical and social perspectives, as there are massive changes occurring in how mental illness is viewed, the relationship between physical and mental illness, what the diagnostic process will be, and how services will be delivered. It is our position that the well-prepared occupational therapist is uniquely qualified to be a key constituent in the future mental health care arena.

CONCEPTUAL APPROACH TO TEXT DEVELOPMENT

The psychosocial core of occupational therapy in all practice areas is firmly rooted in our history and has recently been the subject of much scholarly discourse (Ikiugu, 2010). We strongly support this initiative and have strived to incorporate this broad psychosocial perspective that is encouraged in all editions of this text. However, we are concerned that the term "psychosocial" has recently taken on varied and sometimes vague meanings. This in turn might have the unintended consequence of undermining the value and need for occupational therapists to have a strong presence in the delivery of mental health services. Although the term *psychosocial* is used in the title and throughout the chapters of this text, our conceptualization of psychosocial occupational therapy includes the specific expertise needed to work with people with mental illness. Indeed, it is our position that without a recognized and vibrant mental health practice, our claim to have a "psychosocial core" will not remain credible. Moreover, the need for a substantial knowledge base about mental illness is not limited to practice in designated mental health agencies as there is a growing awareness of the interrelationship between physical and mental health and recognition of the high incidence of comorbidity of physical and mental disorders (Druss & Reisinger Walker, 2011).

It was a conscious decision to not use one conceptual model or frame of reference for this text as it is our belief that occupational therapists need to be versed in a variety of well established as well as emerging schools of thought for practice. The individual chapter authors discuss a range of models and how they are situationally applied in specific practice arenas and contexts. The use of terms to designate the person or persons receiving services also varies within these chapters. We advocate for the use of "person first" and non-discriminating language. But for the sake of clarity, terms such as *client, patient, consumer, person with lived experience of mental illness*, or with a particular diagnosis are used as they relate to the context and relationship.

A guiding strategy in the development of this text was to insure that the varied practices presented are all clearly in the domain of occupational therapy and represent the values, beliefs, skills, and unique occupation-based perspective of the profession. The second edition of the Occupational Therapy Practice Framework (AOTA, 2008) is the primary document cited in many chapters to meet this goal. However, additional sources representing global occupational therapy are also cited. Among them are several documents published by the World Federation of Occupational Therapists (WFOT) as well as Great Britain's College of Occupational Therapists (COT) document titled *Occupational Therapy Defined as a Complex Intervention* (Creek, 2003).

In the development of this text we strived to expand the global voice of occupational therapy. We are very pleased to have five new international authors in this edition whose occupational therapy training from outside of the United States enriches us all. These authors are Madeleine Duncan (South Africa), Chia-Wei Fan (Taiwan), Alison Laver-Fawcett (United Kingdom), Pamela Stephenson (Northern Ireland), and

Crystal Dieleman Grass (Canada). Although the majority of authors in this text are from the United States, each chapter is based on a review of all international literature available. While the practical examples provided in the chapters may be rooted in the author's home environment, readers are encouraged to adapt the authors' presentations to their own cultural, political, and geographical settings. Many of the chapters utilized an occupational justice perspective to not only facilitate this need for situational adaptation but to also recognize the role of occupational therapy in reducing disparity and injustices in their home communities.

ORGANIZATION OF THE TEXT

The book is divided into parts on understanding the person in context, theoretical concepts, diagnosis and dysfunction, mental health across the lifespan, mental health with physical disorders, occupational therapy intervention, and specialized roles for occupational therapy in mental health.

Each part includes a brief explanation of the chapters that are contained in that part. Each chapter follows the same format found in the second edition, which includes key terms, case illustrations, summaries, review questions, and references. The section formerly titled "Suggested Reading" has now been expanded to include media and Internet sites and is now titled "Suggested Resources." The key terms aid the reader in quickly understanding the main ideas in the chapter as well as alerting him or her to the language of mental health and psychiatry. The case illustrations have been universally praised by students, academics, and practitioners for making the ideas come alive and, more important, assisting the reader in understanding the lives of people with mental illness and practice outside of the textbook. End-of-chapter summaries integrate the information in each chapter as well as aid the reader in remembering what is important, or what are the "take home" points. Review questions provide the same assistance as the summaries, but in a much deeper way. If the reader thinks about and answers the questions, she or he will be assured that everything that the chapter has to offer has been learned. For students the questions may serve as an assessment of how much they have learned from each chapter while for clinicians the questions may offer an expanded way of thinking about their practice. The extensive references and suggested resources not only tell the reader where to go for additional current information on each topic, but together they offer the latest research concerning each topic and suggest how the research has been applied in practice.

NEW AND SIGNIFICANTLY REVISED IN THIS EDITION

Part I of the text, "Understanding the Person in Context," includes three chapters that set the stage for the remainder of the book by addressing the changing dynamics of mental health intervention with a recovery perspective, and the cultural, personal, and temporal contexts of the individual within a physical and social environment. Understanding the person in context, and the relationship of environment to mental health is not only the basis for psychosocial occupational therapy intervention, but is also critical for advancing the knowledge base of the profession through meaningful research.

In the first chapter, "Recovery Perspectives," Carol Underwood and Anne MacRae describe the evolution of the recovery movement through the personal perspectives or narratives of people who have this lived experience as well as a critical review of the professional perspective on the concept of recovery. This chapter provides a qualitative overview through the powerful voices of those who live with mental illness and recovery and those who work in the recovery movement. The chapter also discusses the controversies regarding the term *recovery*, the growing evidence of recovery from mental illness, and the challenges for mental health professionals in instituting service delivery changes in the era of recovery. The goal of the chapter is to explore recovery perspectives and to help the mental health practitioner forge collaborative partnerships that facilitate recovery.

In Chapter 2, "Environmental and Cultural Considerations," Anne MacRae and Tiffany Boggis address the concepts of environment and culture. As in the first two editions of this text, the emphasis is on how these contexts specifically relate to occupational performance of people with mental illness but the concerns discussed in this chapter are applicable to occupational therapy in all settings with all populations. The chapter is revised to reflect the updated literature on the concepts of culture and environment. This includes an occupational justice perspective and the utilization of culturally sensitive instruments such as the Kawa Model (Iwama, 2006).

In Chapter 3, "A Context for Mental Health Research in Occupational Therapy," Pamela Richardson and Madeleine Duncan discuss mental health research in occupational therapy that is not designed to teach the mechanics of research but is focused on the significance of understanding the life experiences of the individual, and the interconnectedness of social and political realities with individuals and communities. This interconnectedness is in keeping with current trends in occupational therapy that emphasize occupational justice and global perspectives. Readers are encouraged to use this chapter as a background to analyze the research presented in the subsequent chapters.

Part II, "Theoretical Concepts," includes two chapters that focus on the theoretical underpinnings of psychosocial occupational therapy, and the history and thinking of the founders, and the underpinnings of all psychology and psychiatric fields. Kathleen Barker Schwartz, in Chapter 4, "The History and Philosophy of Psychosocial Occupational Therapy," like in the second edition, follows the beginning of occupational therapy with explicating the ideas and thinking of the founders and societal events to describe the evolution of occupational therapy. This chapter, unlike the previous edition, follows occupational therapy to the present moment in keeping with the vast array of research, practice, and policy emphasizing occupation.

Lynne Andonian, Elizabeth Cara, and Anne MacRae authored Chapter 5, "Psychological Theories and Their Treatment Methods in Mental Health Practice." As previously, this chapter elucidates the interdisciplinary ways in which psychological and psychiatric theories have influenced all areas of mental health, including occupational therapy. A significant change in this edition is the truncation of psychological concepts that are now part of everyday lexicon, because these ideas are now covered in most introductory or abnormal psychology texts. As well and perhaps more important, contemporary ideas have supplanted the archaic ones. Like the previous edition, they discuss how occupational therapy applies these ideas.

Part III, "Diagnosis and Dysfunction," includes four chapters that discuss the psychopathology and diagnostic process and the *DSM* disorders. This section presented interesting choices because the process of diagnosis will be significantly different with the new edition of the DSM-5 expected to be published shortly after this edition. Therefore, in the opening chapter of this part, Chapter 6, "Diagnosis and Psychopathology," Anne MacRae discusses the anticipated changes to the *DSM* and further alignment with the World Health Organization's (WHO) *International Classification of Diseases* (*ICD*) and the *International Classification of Function* (*ICF*). The diagnostic process and the identification of symptoms are being significantly influenced by recovery perspectives that includes an emphasis on wellness rather than illness, as well as the shared information now available through technology. These influences and trends are very consistent with the philosophy of occupational therapy and can pave the way for the proactive occupational therapist to have a leadership role in this changing arena.

Anne MacRae and Lynne Andonian authored Chapter 7, "Schizophrenia," and Elizabeth Cara authored Chapter 8, "Mood Disorders," Chapter 9, "Anxiety Disorders," and Chapter 10, "Personality Disorders." They updated all chapters with the most recent evidence and incorporated current thinking and progress in treatment for these conditions. In addition, they discuss ideas in the *International Classification of Disease (ICD-10)* that will inform material about psychopathology and these conditions and did their best to incorporate expected changes in the DSM-5. Although changes in diagnostic concepts are coming, the contemporary information in these chapters is useful for evaluation and treatment, and specific occupational therapy interventions.

Part IV, "Mental Health Across the Lifespan," represents a conceptual difference from the second edition by including all ages across the lifespan. New to this edition, Chapter 11, "Mental Health of Infants: Attachment Through the Lifespan," is authored by Elizabeth Cara and Elise Holloway who both have extensive knowledge and experience in infant mental health. This chapter, discussing attachment through the lifespan, sets the context for the following chapters because attachment problems can influence people at any stage of life. Also, the theory of attachment has influenced both research and practice in psychotherapy and psychosocial approaches for all age groups. At the same time, occupational therapy practice has expanded in infant intervention and pediatrics and the American Occupational Therapy Association (AOTA) has made children and adolescents a special focus of practice. Therefore, thorough knowledge of attachment ideas should be part of all occupational therapists' repertoire of skills and expertise.

William Lambert authored Chapter 12, "Mental Health of Children," and, with Elizabeth Carley, authored Chapter 13, "Mental Health of Adolescents." These chapters are significantly changed following AOTA's adoption of the president's new freedom committee (Fleming Cottrell, 2007). The children and adolescent chapters provide individual, group, and systems interventions that are contemporary and innovative. They also focus on current societal conditions that are more prevalent for those age groups including family and societal violence, suicide, substance abuse, self-mutilation, and eating disorders to name a few.

Anne MacRae and Gigi Smith authored the final chapter in this section, "The Mental Health of Older Adults." As the population ages, changes in health care affect treatment for the older adult. Thus, as in the other chapters in this section, innovative and contemporary practice, individual, group, and systems, are presented. These chapters capture the problems and conditions that can occur throughout one's life but are more prevalent at certain times in one's life.

Part V includes three chapters that address psychosocial concerns across a spectrum of conditions, including a broad look at physical disability of various etiologies, brain injury, and chronic pain. Clients with dysfunction related to these conditions may or may not be seen in traditional "mental health" settings. Unfortunately, the psychosocial, cognitive, and behavioral issues discussed in these chapters are too often under-recognized or inadequately treated, yet they have been repeatedly reported to have significant impact on an individual's functional outcome with intervention.

Heidi McHugh Pendleton and Winifred Schultz-Krohn authored Chapter 15, "Psychosocial Issues in Physical Disability," and Shawn Phipps authored Chapter 16, "The Cognitive, Behavioral, and Psychosocial Sequelae of Brain Injury." As in the other chapters in this edition these have been thoroughly researched and updated and present current evidence and progress in evaluation and treatment.

Renee R. Taylor and Chia-Wei Fan authored the third chapter in this section, Chapter 17, "Managing Pain in Occupational Therapy: Integrating the Model of Human Occupation and the Intentional Relationship Model." Although a chapter on pain was included in the previous edition, this chapter is essentially a new one with its focus on the use of the Human Occupation Model and the Intentional Relationship Model for treating pain. It is fitting that these chapters are included in a psychosocial text because the authors of these chapters advocate for an occupation-based approach that addresses the various psychosocial issues through assessment and intervention regardless of treatment setting.

Part VI addresses occupational therapy intervention. Although many of the chapters throughout this text address assessment and intervention for various conditions, this section presents the process of assessment and the general and broad methods that are used in all treatment. In Chapter 18, "Assessment, Evaluation, and Outcome Measurement," Alison Laver-Fawcett presents a thorough description of all aspects of the assessment process and highlights its importance in the overall occupational therapy process. Although some individual instruments are discussed, the focus is on the meaning, process, and procedures of assessment and readers are urged to refer to this chapter in order to better understand the evaluation and assessment presentations throughout the text. In a significant departure from the earlier editions, this new chapter presents an international understanding of the assessment process, both from within occupational therapy, and in health disciplines in general. Although the terminology used in this chapter is consistent with the most common usage throughout the world, readers are cautioned that there may be discrepancies in how the terms are defined in one's local professional governing body and these sources should also be consulted. These discrepancies in the regional use of terminology, point to the professions' need to further refine our uniform terminology to reflect not only a global understanding within occupational therapy but also to provide for greater consistency across disciplines.

Elizabeth Cara and Pamela Stephenson authored Chapter 19, "The Use of Psychosocial Methods and Interpersonal Strategies in Mental Health." In keeping with current trends regarding the therapeutic use of self, a change is that it focuses more specifically in the context of the therapeutic relationship and repairing relationships as well as the traditional occupational therapy processes of clinical reasoning and activity analysis. Both chapters follow and elucidate various sections of the Occupational Therapy Practice Framework (AOTA, 2008).

Chapter 20, "Groups," by Elizabeth Cara focuses on group interventions, how to design, start, implement, and lead groups for individuals with various levels of function and conditions. A change is that it also includes group treatment for large communities, such as clubs, or psychosocial rehabilitation programs and those following the recovery model. This compact chapter should be all one needs to pursue group treatment in contemporary mental health and other settings.

The final section of this text is Part VII, "Specialized Roles for Occupational Therapy in Mental Health," and includes new and significantly revised chapters. Just as occupational therapists treat psychiatric conditions, lifespan issues, and psychosocial consequences of physical disorders, they also intervene with psychiatric conditions within various organizational structures and through systematic treatment approaches. John White, Crystal Dieleman Grass, Toby Ballou Hamilton, and Sandra Rogers authored Chapter 21, which considers psychosocial occupational therapy for those with mental illness or psychosocial distress who are incarcerated within prison systems—institutions that house an alarmingly growing population with a myriad of occupational dysfunctions. A criminal justice chapter was included in the previous editions, but this current chapter is situated within an occupational justice and international perspective.

It details treatment not just in psychiatric forensic settings but also in larger systems and also discusses more contemporary and innovative intervention programs.

Sue Folker and Sara Woodward authored a new chapter to this edition, Chapter 22, "Psychosocial Occupational Therapy in the School Setting," to address the complex social, environmental, and behavioral problems seen in schools and the need for significant attention to be paid to school children with mental health issues. This chapter addresses the occupational justice issues found in the organizational structure of schools as well as suggestions for individual and group intervention.

Eileen Auerbach, the author of Chapter 23, "Vocational Programming," thoroughly updated it with the latest references, and Steve Hoppes, Helen Bryce, and Suzanne Peloquin provide a new perspective in Chapter 24, "Substance Abuse and Occupational Therapy." The chapter thoroughly reviews the scope of the abuse and addiction problem, as well as the major approaches in the treatment of substance abuse. The chapter also presents how the occupational therapy perspective is beneficial to individual clients as it enriches and enhances the effectiveness of a team approach. Many practical suggestions for OT interventions with this population are included along with the "real life" experiences of both the advanced OT practitioners and OT students working in substance abuse programs.

Robinette J. Amaker, Anne Pas Burke, Cecilia Najera, and Mary Radomski authored a new Chapter 25, "Occupational Therapy in the Military: Working with Service Members in Combat and at Home." These service members and OT practitioners working with service members present a very compelling portrayal of life for service members in combat zones and in treatment at home. They also give us a vivid portrait of important occupational therapy interventions for a population that occupational therapists will see more often in all settings. As with all wars (perhaps ironically and sadly), new treatment techniques will benefit the field, specifically, in the present wars, interventions for comorbid traumatic brain injuries and post-traumatic stress syndrome, as well as the best of disaster responses. Although the occupational therapists who authored this chapter represent and serve the U.S. military, the devastation of war is seen throughout the world, and health intervention, which may be needed for decades after the initial injury or trauma, is too often forgotten.

Patricia Crist and Elizabeth Cara substantially revised Chapter 26, "Fieldwork Supervision in the Mental Health Setting." Specific sections discuss supervision targeted toward mental health; however, updated information on dimensions, transformational supervision, and coaching, to name a few, can and should be used in all settings. This chapter will be particularly helpful to new fieldwork supervisors and experienced ones alike. Also, students will benefit from information targeted to what they should know, how to behave, and questions to ask that will enhance their experience and ensure a smooth transition. All of the chapters in this part are filled with creative and innovative programming ideas for these far reaching and much needed services. This chapter should significantly aid the fieldwork supervisor in mental health practice settings. The editors have both developed and been involved in mental health fieldwork. They have also been fieldwork educators and academic fieldwork educators. In addition, Dr. Cara has created a group fieldwork 1 academic class using online technology. Thus, both of the editors urge mental health practitioners to expand their fieldwork programs to include more students and they urge educators and academic programs to maintain existing mental health fieldwork sites and to go further to advance mental health practice by developing new and innovative mental health fieldwork sites.

INSTRUCTOR COMPANION WEBSITE

The companion website contains additional resources to aid in the teaching of coursework related to this topic. Content includes slides created in Microsoft PowerPoint® to accompany each chapter, guided responses for the end of chapter review questions, and learning activities.

Instructors can access the website via login.cengage.com. Follow the instructions for creating a Faculty Account or contact your sales representative to obtain access.

ISBN-13: 978-1-1113-1831-4

PROFESSIONAL AND STUDENT COMPANION WEBSITE

Many of the forms and worksheets provided in the textbook are available in printable and editable formats along with a master list of useful websites organized by topic. To access these materials:

1. GO TO: http://www.cengagebrain.com
2. ENTER author, title or ISBN in the **Find your Textbook or Materials** search box, CLICK on **Find** button.
3. At the Product page, CLICK the **Access Now** button.

SUMMARY

As we did in the first edition, we sincerely believe that working in mental health and with psychosocial concepts is interesting, exciting, and satisfying work, and we hope that students and practitioners will continue to benefit from this practice based text. We also hope that students, academics, and practitioners will continue to send us their comments. Enjoy the adventure!

Anne MacRae, PhD, OTR/L, BCMH, FAOTA
amacrae@sjsu.edu

Elizabeth Cara, PhD, OTR/L, MFT
elizabeth.cara@sjsu.edu

REFERENCES

American Occupational Therapy Association (AOTA). (2008). Occupational therapy practice framework: Domain and process (2nd ed.) *American Journal of Occupational Therapy, 62,* 625–683.

Creek, J. (2003). *Occupational therapy defined as a complex intervention.* London: College of Occupational Therapists.

Druss, B., & Reisinger Walker, E. (2011). *The Synthesis Project: Mental disorders and medical comorbidity.* Princeton, NJ: Robert Wood Johnson Foundation. Retrieved from http://www.rwjf.org/files/research/71883.mentalhealth.report.pdf

Fleming Cottrell, R. (2007), The New Freedom Initiative—Transforming mental health care: Will OT be at the table? *Occupational Therapy in Mental Health, 23*(2), 1–24. Retrieved from doi: 10.1300/J004v23n02_01

Ikiugu, M. (2010). The new occupational therapy paradigm: Implications for integration of the psychosocial core of occupational therapy in all clinical specialties. *Occupational Therapy in Mental Health, 26*(4), 343–353.

Iwama, M. K. (2006). *The Kawa model: Culturally relevant occupational therapy.* Edinburgh: Elsevier.

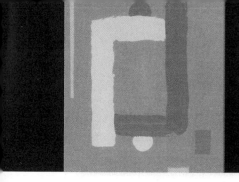

ACKNOWLEDGMENTS

REVIEWERS

Diane R. Anderson, PhD, MPH, OTR/L
Assistant Professor
Department Chair
The College of St. Scholastica
Duluth, MN

Patricia A. Donovan, EdD, MSOT, OTR/L
Assistant Professor
Department of Occupational Therapy
Worcester State University
Worcester, MA

Tamera Keiter Humbert, DEd, OTR/L
Associate Professor
Elizabethtown College
Elizabethtown, PA

Eleanor Anne (Ellie) Raffen, MA, OTR
Associate Clinical Professor
School of Occupational Therapy
Texas Woman's University
Denton, TX

Peter Talty, MS, OTR/L
Professor of Occupational Therapy
Keuka College
Keuka Park, NY

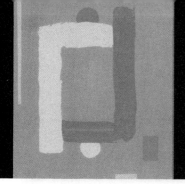

ABOUT THE AUTHORS

Elizabeth Cara received her Certificate of Proficiency in occupational therapy from the University of Pennsylvania. She also holds a Bachelor of Arts degree in History from Santa Clara University, a Master of Arts degree in Clinical Psychology from John F. Kennedy University, and a PhD in Clinical Psychology from the Fielding Graduate University. For the last 20 years, she has been a Professor of Occupational Therapy, teaching various topics at the undergraduate and graduate levels. Dr. Cara's clinical experience is in mental health with all ages and settings. Her scholarly interests include psychobiography, clinical supervision and fieldwork training, infant and family mental health, group dynamics, leadership and intervention, interpersonal communication and clinical skills, and contemporary psychoanalytic relationship psychotherapy. She is the co-creator of a successful vocational program, Community Vocational Enterprises, in San Francisco, California.

Anne MacRae received her Bachelors of Arts degree in education from Antioch College, Yellow Springs, Ohio, and her Masters degree in occupational therapy from San Jose State University. She also has a Doctorate in Human Science from Saybrook Institute, San Francisco. Dr. MacRae is a professor at San Jose State University in California. In addition to teaching, she also supervised the campus-based psychosocial occupational therapy clinic for 20 years. Her other clinical experience includes inpatient acute psychiatry, partial hospitalization programs, and home health care. She is also a recipient of multiple Fulbright Fellowships and engages in international consultation about occupational therapy and mental health care. Her current research and scholarly interests include cultural diversity, phenomenology, occupational justice, recovery perspectives, environmental issues in intervention, community mental health, and functional deficits of psychiatric symptoms. Dr. MacRae is currently on a pre-retirement tract from the university, which provides a reduced role at the university and therefore she is able to pursue additional personal and professional opportunities.

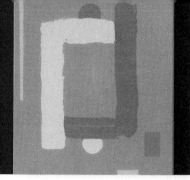

CONTRIBUTORS TO THE THIRD EDITION

Robinette J. Amaker, PhD, OTR/L, CHT, FAOTA
Colonel, U.S. Army
Joint Base
San Antonio, TX

Lynne Andonian, PhD, OTR/L
Assistant Professor, Occupational
   Therapy
San Jose State University
San Jose, CA

Eileen S. Auerbach, MS, OTR/L
Retired from Mission Assertive
   Community Treatment Center
   (Mission ACT) 2008

Tiffany (Debra) Boggis, MBA, OTR/L
Associate Professor, Occupational Therapy
Pacific University
Hillsboro, OR

Helen R. Bryce, MA, OTR/L
Adjunct Assistant Professor, Rehabilitation
   Sciences
University of Oklahoma
   Health Sciences Center
Tulsa, OK

Anne Pas Burke, EdD, OTR/L, FAOTA
Supervisory Occupational Therapist
Director, Therapeutic Programming

Inpatient Psychiatry Service
Clinical Instructor: OTR's and COTA's
Walter Reed Army Medical Center
Washington, DC

Elizabeth Carley, OTD, OTR/L
Occupational Therapist
Aggression Replacement Training Program
   Coordinator
Occupational Therapy Training Program
   (OTTP)
Torrance, CA

Patricia Crist, PhD, OTR, PC, FAOTA
Professor
Department of Occupational Therapy
John G. Rangos, Sr., School of Health
   Sciences
Duquesne University
Pittsburgh, PA

Madeleine Duncan, MScOT, DPhil (Psych)
Senior Lecturer, Occupational Therapy
University of Cape Town
Cape Town, South Africa

Sue Ann Folker, MS, OTR/L
Occupational Therapist
Federal Way Public Schools
Federal Way, WA

Crystal Dieleman Grass, PhD, OT Reg(NS)
Assistant Professor, Occupational Therapy
Dalhousie University
Halifax, Nova Scotia, Canada

Toby Ballou Hamilton, PhD, MPH, OTR/L
Assistant Professor, Occupational Therapy
University of Oklahoma Health Sciences Center
Oklahoma City, OK

Elise Holloway, MPH, OTR/L
Occupational Therapist
Huntington Memorial Hospital
Pasadena, CA and
Eastern Los Angeles Regional Center
Alhambra, CA

Steve Hoppes, PhD, OTR/L
Associate Professor, Rehabilitation Science
University of Oklahoma Health Sciences Center
Tulsa, OK

William L. Lambert, MS, OTR/L
Faculty Specialist
Department of Occupational and Physical Therapy
The University of Scranton
Scranton, PA

Alison Laver-Fawcett, PhD, DipCOT, OT(C), PCAP
Head of Program, Full-time BHSc (Hons) Occupational Therapy
York St. John University
North Yorkshire, United Kingdom

Cecilia Najera, MOT, OTR, CPT, SP
Occupational Therapist
Occupational Therapy Services
Brooke Army Medical Center
Ft. Sam Houston, TX

Suzanne M. Peloquin, PhD, OTR, FAOTA
Professor, Occupational Therapy
University of Texas Medical Branch at Galveston, TX and
Alcohol and Drug Abuse Center for Women
Galveston, TX

Heidi McHugh Pendleton, PhD, OTR/L, FAOTA
Professor and Chair, Occupational Therapy
San Jose State University
San Jose, CA

Shawn Phipps, PhD, OTR/L, FAOTA
President, Occupational Therapy Association of California
Chief Strategic Development Officer
Rancho Los Amigos National Rehabilitation Center
Rancho Los Amigos, CA

Mary Vining Radomski, PhD, OTR/L, FAOTA
Sister Kenny Research Center
Minneapolis, MN

Pamela Richardson, PhD, OTR/L, FAOTA
Professor, Occupational Therapy
San Jose State University
San Jose, CA

Sandra L. Rogers, PhD, OTR/L
Associate Professor, Occupational
Therapy
Pacific University
Hillsboro, OR

**Kathleen Barker Schwartz, EdD,
OTR/L, FAOTA**
Professor Emeritus, Occupational
Therapy
San Jose State University
San Jose, CA

**Winifred Schultz-Krohn PhD,
OTR/L, BCP, FAOTA**
Professor, Occupational Therapy
San Jose State University
San Jose, CA

Jerilyn (Gigi) Smith, MS, OTR/L
Assistant Professor, Occupational
Therapy
San Jose State University
San Jose, CA

Pamela R.R. Stephenson, MS, OTR/L
Augusta County Public Schools
Fishersville, VA

Renee R. Taylor, MA, Ph.D.
Professor, Occupational Therapy
University of Illinois
Chicago, IL

Carol Underwood
Peer Specialist
Trinity County Behavioral Health
Service
Weaverville, CA

Chia-Wei Fan, MS, OTC
PhD Student of Kinesiology, Human
Nutrition and Rehabilitation
Sciences
University of Illinois
Chicago, IL

John A. White, PhD, OTR/L
Professor and Director, Occupational
Therapy
Pacific University
Hillsboro, OR

**Sara L. Woodward, MEd, MOT,
OTR/L**
Supervisor of Special Education
Clover Park School District
Lakewood, WA

Understanding the Person in Context

The three chapters included in Part I set the stage for the remainder of the book by addressing the changing dynamics of mental health intervention with a recovery perspective and the cultural, personal, and temporal contexts of the individual within a physical and social environment. Understanding the person in context, and the relationship of environment to mental health is not only the basis for psychosocial occupational therapy intervention, it is also critical for advancing the knowledge base of the profession through meaningful research.

The first chapter describes the evolution of the recovery movement starting with the presentation of mental illness through the voices of people who have this lived experience. A professional perspective on the concept of recovery is also presented. The differences between the concept of personal recovery and clinical recovery are discussed along with some of the challenges in providing authentic, recovery-oriented mental health services. The goal of the chapter is to not only explore the differences in recovery perspectives but also help the mental health practitioner forge truly collaborative partnerships to foster recovery.

The second chapter addresses several different contexts through the concepts of environment and culture. The emphasis is on how these contexts specifically relate to occupational performance of people with mental illness. However, the psychosocial concerns discussed in this chapter are applicable to occupational therapy in all settings with all populations.

The third chapter provides a context for mental health research in occupational therapy by focusing on the significance of understanding not only the life experiences of the individual but also the interconnectedness of social and political realities with individuals and communities. Although this chapter is not designed to teach the mechanics of conducting research, it does help frame the questions one needs to ask to engage in meaningful research studies and understand the significance of research studies in the fast-changing mental health arena. Readers are encouraged to use the concepts described in this chapter to analyze all of the research presented in the subsequent chapters.

Chapter 1

Recovery Perspectives

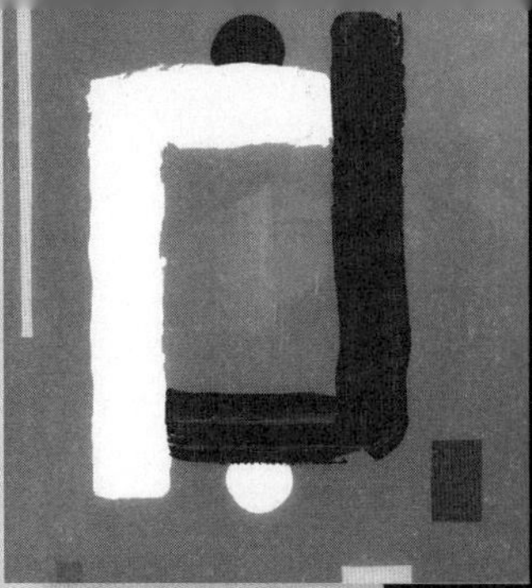

Carol Underwood
Anne MacRae, PhD, OTR/L, BCMH, FAOTA

KEY TERMS

advocacy
board and care
electroconvulsive therapy (ECT)
institutionalized
lived experience
paradigm shift
recovery model

CHAPTER OUTLINE

Introduction
Section One: Personal Perspective
Mental Illness—What It Feels Like
Recovery—What Is It?
 Is Recovery a Realistic Goal?
Peer Interventions and Recovery-Oriented Support
 The Role of Community and Family
 Peer Counseling and Teaching
 Wellness Recovery Action Plan (WRAP)
Section Two: Professional Perspective
Definitions and Scope of Recovery
 Research and Evidence
Impact of the Recovery Movement
The Changing Role of Mental Health Professionals
 Resistance and Concerns
 Developing Collaborative Relationships
The Role of Occupational Therapy in a Recovery Paradigm
Summary

INTRODUCTION

The purpose of this chapter is to help students, educators, and practitioners understand the **lived experience** of people with mental illness, the goal and principles of recovery, and the role of the occupational therapist and other mental health professionals, within the context of recovery. In the first section, Carol Underwood shares not only her personal experience, but also the stories of many others in her community who participated in focus groups and interviews throughout Northern California. The Case Illustrations are based on the personal stories shared with Carol Underwood, so these and the participant quotes in the figures are not representative of the full range of how mental illness may manifest, and do not address the contextual and political realities of other geographical areas. Nevertheless, the message of these personal stories is remarkably similar to personal stories being voiced throughout the world, and it is the authors position that these voices of people with lived experience of mental illness can best inform practice.

In the second section, Anne MacRae discusses the controversy regarding the term *recovery* as well as the mounting evidence for recovery as a realistic goal, and its impact on mental health service delivery. The changing roles of all mental health professionals including the concerns regarding a recovery perspective that are voiced by professionals are also discussed. Occupational therapy's role in recovery is presented together with a challenge for the profession to revitalize mental health occupational therapy by demonstrating an alignment with recovery principles. The focus groups and interviews conducted by Carol Underwood are the source of the quotes and case illustrations presented in this section.

SECTION ONE: PERSONAL PERSPECTIVE

Carol Underwood

It is my hope that by presenting the thoughts, feelings, experiences, and suggestions of people with mental illness a truly collaborative partnership for recovery can emerge. In order for that to happen, there must be open communication and understanding. So, I begin by sharing my own personal journey.

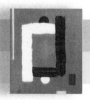

CASE ILLUSTRATION

Carol's Story

I am left-handed, so that is supposed to mean I am in my right mind, correct? Well, maybe now, but that wasn't always the case!

My story begins with the onset of a 30-plus year mental illness. I was first diagnosed with schizoaffective disorder at the age of 21, at which time I began a journey filled with terror, confusion, humiliation, and most of all . . . self-loathing.

For probably the first 20 years I had no understanding of my disease and was never given any real assistance in understanding why these things were happening to me. During the course of my mental illness I spent most of my time in acute-care, locked psychiatric hospitals or long-term **board and care** facilities, although there were brief periods of time when I was able to live on my own and hold down jobs.

I experienced auditory hallucinations, mainly the voice of my deceased mother telling me what a horrible person I was and how I had no right to exist. I went through extremely severe bouts of depression, often with suicidal thoughts and plans (in great detail). I only made two real attempts at ending my life; other times they were "fake" attempts that occurred when I didn't know any other way of asking for help.

Early on I began burning myself with cigarettes and curling irons—they temporarily took away my mother's haunting voice, but later they became a habit, and a way to get myself "5150'd" (a 72-hour hold in a locked psychiatric unit) when I felt incapable of handling the real world. Psychiatric hospitals became a place of safety, peace, and security. I became totally **institutionalized**.

Various treatments were tried over the years; many different psychiatric medications, group therapy, individual therapy, and three series of **electroconvulsive therapy (ECT)** each consisting of 12 treatments. Nothing was effective. Everyone who knew me in any capacity assumed that I would always have a mental illness, and would basically always be under the care of a psychiatrist and would always need medication. Did I ever show them!

Discussion

Everyone has a theory on how I regained my mental health. I myself belief that it was a true miracle of God, but I don't discount the role of neuroscience research in understanding mental illness and in developing effective treatments. I have now been employed by a county behavioral health department for close to 5 years, am taking leadership roles within the mental health system, and have began an 18-month program to complete my Bachelor of Arts in psychology. I own my home, and enjoy my two dogs and one cat, am active in my church and community, and lead a whole and healthy life. My story of recovery is only one of many stories of regaining mental, spiritual, and physical health that are becoming voiced more in today's realm of mental health. Although my success story is one that I am grateful to be alive to tell, the road to recovery varies tremendously from one person to the next.

MENTAL ILLNESS—WHAT IT FEELS LIKE

Each person with a mental illness experiences it in his or her own unique way. The symptoms may be relatively minor or they may be so overpowering that they totally obstruct the person's ability to take care of himself or herself. Figure 1-1 is a sample of descriptions and experiences of mental illness. These quotes demonstrate not only how the symptoms of mental illness affect someone's ability to function, but also how one's living environment and societal stigma can be ongoing challenges on the road to recovery. The main themes that seem to stand out in the hearts and minds of people suffering from these debilitating illnesses are despair, darkness, helplessness, and loneliness. However, as dire as these feelings may be, dramatic and life-changing recovery is possible.

It is also important to acknowledge that the effects of mental illness are not limited to the individual but also affect entire families. In many cases, family members are not involved with developing a care plan with the client and treatment team due to financial and legal constraints of the mental health service. Unfortunately a common result is family members who are confused and anxious about the relative's difficulties and therefore cannot provide the much-needed support.

- I suffered a lot of losses. Growing up I was different. I was told I was retarded. When I did grow up, because of what I was told, I made bad choices. It was hard for me to take care of myself. I stopped living.
- I was a child, a loony child! I couldn't have children because I was a child myself.
- I put all my eggs in the wrong basket, and they all broke.
- I grew up in a family of alcoholics. There was a lot of fighting. I don't really know how I handled it. It was hard mentally to watch my brothers destroy themselves, and I would get really depressed. After my husband died, I was so depressed I wasn't sure I wanted to live anymore.
- I have not been diagnosed with a mental illness, but I've got some problems. I have always watched the way people act and try to be like them. I'm an alcoholic, so I guess that is a mental illness.
- It feels sad, scary, like I'll never be happy. I'm always worrying. I feel so helpless, and like I'll never get well. It feels like hell.
- I don't know how to talk about it. I feel intimidated and ashamed. I'm sort of secretive. It's hard to share how I feel.
- It was all about everything being hard. It was all black, not light. I couldn't even imagine that light existed.
- Sometimes I don't know if I'll make it to tomorrow. It's a lonely place to be. I get so depressed about being depressed.
- I feel like such a failure. I'm always crying, I don't have any money, and I feel so guilty that I can't be "normal" like everyone else.

FIGURE 1-1. What It Is Like to Have a Mental Illness

CASE ILLUSTRATION

A Family Member Speaks of His Confusion, Fear, and Anger

I knew my sister was sick because our parents told me. When I heard the news, it made absolutely no sense to me. I heard that she was in hospitals, board and care homes, had ECT. I had no idea what that was about—I just remember movies that showed horrible convulsions and the patients, eyes rolling back and drooling all over themselves. I had conjured up so many images on how she would act, what she would look like, how I would handle it, what it would be like, what I would say to her. How could she do this to her family? Why did she have to be my sister? After about two or three years, I started reading books, articles, magazines, and anything on mental illness that would help me understand what was happening to her. Although I became well informed, it took much longer for me to be able to talk about it with her. I was so afraid I would say the wrong thing, or look at her funny, something that would send her over the edge. After several years, I began to be more comfortable talking with her. I realized that she was still my sister, I still loved her, and that there was more to her than her illness. I also had to get over being embarrassed about it. It has been a long rocky road for me and other family members, but today we can discuss it more openly and sometimes even talk to her about how it made us feel. There is still some discomfort, but on the whole, the lines of communication are opening up. I really hope I can reach out to the community on behalf of her and others with illnesses like hers. I just want to tell them not to run from their sister or brother, or mother or father, just to love them, and tell them that you love them over and over again.

Discussion

The stigma and disruption of mental illness have far-reaching consequences. But as difficult as it can be for both the person with mental illness and members of his or her family to come to grips with the situation, it is possible to learn and grow in the relationship. This family member took great initiative to learn about mental illness, but other people may not have the resources or knowledge to do so. Outreach, support, and information sources are vital services for family members.

RECOVERY—WHAT IS IT?

Survivors of mental illness first advocated the concept of recovery in the literature. Of particular impact was Patricia Deegan's "Recovery: The lived experience of rehabilitation" (1988) and Esso Leete's "How I perceive and manage my illness" (1989). It was these and many other personal stories that prompted scholars and researchers in the early 1990s to seriously consider using this concept as a basis for mental health treatment. One of the first scholars to write about recovery from mental illness was Professor William Anthony of Boston University. Although there are many scholarly interpretations and critiques of recovery (discussed in Section Two of this chapter), Anthony's early definition captures the key elements of the principle of recovery as it is used today.

> Recovery is described as a deeply personal, unique process of changing one's attitudes, values, feelings, goals, skills, and/or roles. It is a way of living a satisfying, hopeful, and contributing life even with limitations caused by illness. Recovery involves the development of new meaning and purpose in one's life as one grows beyond the catastrophic effects of mental illness. (Anthony, 1993, p. 11)

Although the message of recovery is one of hope and optimism, new ideas often gain momentum as a reaction to pain, frustration, anger, and injustices. In order to move forward, the pain of the past must be acknowledged. The following case illustration, based on reports in a focus group and interview, highlights some of the negative interactions in clinical settings and how this spurred one person to explore alternatives.

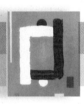

CASE ILLUSTRATION

Jennifer—A Missed Opportunity

After two years of battling depression, Jennifer sought professional help and was prescribed an antidepressant and two other medications. Within a month, she began experiencing severe side effects and her symptoms of depression were not being alleviated. She continued to take various medications as prescribed, but also started looking into alternative treatment methods. When she broached these subjects with her therapist, she was given only negative feedback. Jennifer started looking into, and actually started, a self-help group with some friends. She became a member of the local mental health board, and believed that she could have an impact on the therapeutic community.

Twelve years later, Jennifer is now in remission and identifies herself as a recovered mental health patient. She continues to take two psychotropic medications, and is part of the recovery-oriented community. In looking back, Jennifer believes that if she had thought that the mental health practitioners who worked with her had shown any real interest in her own research and thoughts on her recovery, she quite possibly could have benefited from the earlier attempts at treatment.

Discussion

The word "recovery" is now spoken with enthusiasm and guarded optimism. However, it is important for all mental health professionals to be aware that the people they serve may have endured years of negative attitudes regarding their prognosis, which in turn not only affected their road to recovery but also their ability to trust and work collaboratively with professionals.

A key in sustaining the recovery movement as a positive force is the emergence of leaders who have the lived experience of mental illness, and are willing to talk about their past. These leaders have not only been successful with their own recovery but are also inspirational to others in the recovery process by being positive role models. They also play a major role in educating the community and influencing the political process related to mental health services. Figure 1-2 features one of the outstanding leaders of the recovery movement in the state of California.

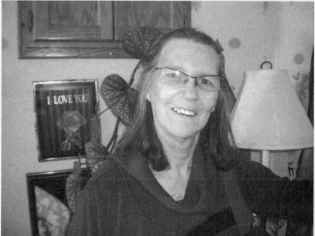

© Cengage Learning 2013

Joyce has dealt with mental illness for her entire life, undiagnosed until early adulthood. Once Joyce began receiving services she soon recognized the need for community outreach and the need for education. She began attending every mental health–related meeting possible, including the mental health board, the county Board of Supervisors, senior center meetings, and any meeting she knew of where she could not only gain information herself, but where she could make her voice heard. She realized that stigma was high and the acceptance of people with mental illness in the community had not yet occurred.

(Continues)

Joyce became involved with National Alliance for the Mentally Ill (NAMI), as well as the California Network of Mental Health Clients (CNMHC), where she was elected to the various offices, and became a part of several committees on a statewide level that allowed her to participate in and have a vote in the policies that affect mental health clients throughout the state. She is the co-founder of the California Association of Local Mental Health Boards and Commissions (CALMHB/C) and is presently a contract employee in her county behavioral health agency acting in the capacity of Patients Rights Advocate. She continues to play an active role on committees such as Mental Health Services Oversight and Accountability Commission and a host of other committees and councils.

Joyce continues to manage her wellness recovery process with the aid of the team she helped create, who support her all-round health needs. She states: "While I am very passionate about getting care when needed, the key to my success is the right type of care within the right time frame." She is an assertive and persistent angel for the needs of those who deal with mental illnesses, and she believes that people with mental illness, families, caregivers, friends, and providers must work together to build a team that models the values of recovery oriented services.

Achieving her goals with collaborative team efforts is a dream that Joyce continues to accomplish on a daily basis and she is valued for her knowledge of local and state systems, as well as for the caring and compassionate attention she pays to all who are fortunate enough to know her. She has gone from homeless to a homeowner, from being unemployed to being an employee in a position she loves, and is passionate about affirming the client voice and ensuring that the community continues to grow in understanding and acceptance of people with mental health challenges.

FIGURE 1-2. Joyce Ott—A Recognized Leader

© Cengage Learning 2013

IS RECOVERY A REALISTIC GOAL?

Do all people with mental illnesses want to recover? Do people know they can recover? Is it really possible for everyone to recover? These are the questions that are asked by people with mental illness, by their families and friends, and by mental health professionals. The answer goes back to the definition of recovery as a deeply personal and unique process. Not everyone will regain full function, skills, or participation in their community. However, the message of hope in the **recovery model** is that everyone can strive to find meaning and purpose in their lives.

People who have a long-standing mental illness must look at what it could mean for them if and when they were to recover. Often just thinking about taking back responsibility of one's own life is enough of a deterrent to prevent them from going forward, and it could even cause a relapse. Family, friends, and practitioners, as well as the individual, must be aware that recovery can look insurmountable after having

CASE ILLUSTRATION

Cassie's Worldview of Her Mental Illness

Cassie is a 59-year-old woman who has no intention of ever being off medications or of ever being able to do any kind of paid work. She feels that she will be dependent on others in most life situations during her remaining years. Professionals and family have told Cassie that she will always have a mental illness and she firmly believes it to be a fact.

Discussion

There are many reasons why Cassie is not motivated to change her situation. It is possible that even with medication, Cassie continues to have severe symptoms that impede her ability to initiate change. However, it is also likely that the long duration of her illness has essentially "institutionalized" her into a comfortable routine. In every therapeutic encounter, it is also important to take into consideration the cultural and religious values and beliefs of the individual. It is possible that Cassie's worldview dictates acceptance of one's fate and her beliefs must be respected. It might be tempting to push Cassie out of her comfort zone toward greater independence, but perhaps a more effective approach would be to help Cassie identify and strengthen the parts of her daily routine that provide structure and purpose to her life. This approach is still very much in the spirit of recovery. As Cassie explores the quality and meaning of her life, it is likely that her sense of competence and control will strengthen, paving the way for additional changes if she chooses.

been protected and sheltered. Figure 1-3 consists of participant quotes regarding their fears and attitudes about recovery.

PEER INTERVENTIONS AND RECOVERY-ORIENTED SUPPORT

Although many people in the recovery process utilize and value professional mental health services, intervention within the recovery perspective is not limited to clinical treatment. Peer support, self-help groups, information sharing, peer teaching, and role modeling, as well as community and family support, are all important components of recovery. As shown in the previously presented case illustration of Jennifer, some people are drawn to nonclinical approaches because of past negative experiences with traditional mental health services. However, clinical and nonclinical interventions are not incompatible as long as there is respect for people's choices.

- I don't think I'll ever recover to the point that I can totally take care of myself, and I'm not sure I can or want to.
- If I get better, people will expect more of me.
- It almost seems impossible to forget about my mental illness. It's been such a part of me for so long.
- I've been told for so long that I will never recover and will always need meds and therapy. Is it even possible to be whole and healthy again?
- If I recover, does that mean I have to work?
- Recovery sounds good. It would be nice to feel good again. I don't know anyone who really works with recovery-based therapy. I'm sure they're around. Where do I look?
- Man, I'll bet that word means a lot of different things to a lot of different people. To me it sounds like a burden. I don't like feeling depressed and seeing things, but I'm not sure I could do everything I would have to if I were totally sane. It's overwhelming to me.

FIGURE 1-3. Fear of Recovery

© Cengage Learning 2013

CASE ILLUSTRATION

Maria—Conquering Fear of Recovery

Maria was headed toward mental, spiritual, and physical health, but didn't know what to do with it. She had been in and out of hospitals for most of her adult life and resided mainly in board and care facilities. Now Maria was regaining her mental health, and she knew that very soon her life would be headed in a different direction. There were so many questions and concerns: Where would she go? Could she ever work again? Was she going to relapse? What would people think about her? What would she think about herself? She was terrified, but knew that at that point there was no turning back. Her mental health was being restored, and she had to welcome it, and move forward. Her heart raced, she had nightmares, she had great anxiety, and fear

overwhelmed her. Was recovery really happening? Would it last? Her overwhelming thought was "I want to take back control of my life, but the idea scares the hell out of me!"

Discussion

This case illustration is a common scenario when a person recovering from a long mental illness is faced with a new life, a new adventure. Although the prospect of being freed from the grips of mental illness is enticing, it brings with it great skepticism and much anxiety. All people who reach this point have a difficult choice to make, and many times people don't even realize that it is truly a choice. It is scary and the thought of striking out on one's own can be completely devastating. Mental health professionals can help the recovery process by validating the emotions being experienced while at the same time helping the individual identify manageable and realistic short-term goals to reach the larger goal of full recovery.

The Role of Community and Family

The recovery process is driven by the desires, choices, and motivations of the individual. However successful recovery, which includes regaining meaningful roles and social participation, is also dependent on support from all aspects of the community. The most immediate community is often family members who can be a valuable social support for the person with mental illness. Figure 1-4 contains comments by focus group participants reflecting on family involvement in their recovery.

Empathy from family members can be overwhelmingly comforting and often makes the difference between stability and relapse. It can be a far more difficult road for individuals with mental illness who are estranged or isolated from family. For these individuals, developing surrogate family with healthy friendships and meaningful roles in the community can be an enormous advantage in the recovery process. Mental health drop-in or wellness centers often provide the environment for developing such surrogate families through peer support, opportunities for socialization and activities, shared meals, and group celebrations of cultural and community events.

Peer Counseling and Teaching

Many recovery-oriented mental health agencies are now hiring people with a history of mental illness to provide varying degrees of peer counseling and teaching, as well as outreach to the community. The Trinity County Behavioral Health Service (TCBHS) in California where I work hires peer counselors as part of the Milestones Outreach Support Team (MOST). The members of this team are introduced in Figure 1-5. We are people with lived experience of mental illness who can provide **advocacy** and support through a paid position in which we in turn are also provided support and training. We actively participate in the planning and implementation of Milestones Wellness Center programs and are taking a lead role, in collaboration with the occupational therapist, in a recently funded innovation project providing services to residents temporarily living in a local board and care facility for respite.

Peer teaching takes many forms, from one-to-one instructions and providing informational literature, to running groups. I personally co-teach a leadership class, and I am a certified Wellness Recovery Action Plan (WRAP) facilitator and do WRAP groups (described in the subsequent heading). In addition I have also received training and teach the Psychosocial Rehabilitation programs that were developed by the University of California at Los Angeles (UCLA).

- My family is totally behind me. Sometimes I have to watch out that my brother doesn't beat someone up for saying the wrong thing. He's very protective of me.
- Mom has always been there for me, maybe a little bit too much sometimes. It seems like she's smothering me a lot of the time.
- When I was first diagnosed with major depression, my family was afraid to talk about it to me. If I said anything, they sort of started talking about something else.
- The best thing my parents did when I told them I had a mental illness was to go out and learn as much as they could about my diagnosis and the medications I was taking. They also helped find a good psychiatrist and therapist, and they did research on self-help groups and things like that. I think they knew more about my illness than I did!
- It's too bad there isn't a family support group where I live. I think that would help them and also me in the long run. They need support too.
- I had no family near me when I was at my worst. I was sort of glad, because I would have been embarrassed and they wouldn't have known how to act. I did send them brochures and literature on my diagnosis, but they never responded or even mentioned that they had received them. I don't know if they read them or not.
- My entire family has been my biggest supports and advocates. They read up on everything, but didn't go overboard with their knowledge. They helped me make it ok to be around company, they went with me places when I was afraid to go alone, but they didn't smother me. They were awesome. They still are.

FIGURE 1-4. The Role of Family in Recovery

© Cengage Learning 2013

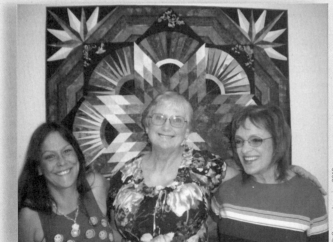

© Cengage Learning 2013

Boe Anna: I did not have a dramatic breakdown but I did have altered life situations, attitudes, and behaviors. The behavioral health agency in my county has been a blessing to me starting with the first group I attended. I had been sent to a state hospital for a competency evaluation concerning a court case. Upon my return I joined a cognitive-behavioral group offered by the agency. This group opened a new door for me and it is one that I believe should be available to all clients. My connection to behavioral health helped me get my job at the agency and the Milestones Wellness Center, a job I dearly love and which was a goal for me. I have grown in areas that I previously had no experience in, such as computer skills, and I have mastered other skills that I have been able to use in both positions I hold at the behavioral health agency. I am humbled by the variety and humongous challenges that many of the people that I am privileged to serve, have met and overcome. I greatly respect and admire them. These people are very important to me. They are my people and they are my friends. God has blessed me and I want to be able to pass on His blessings. To have a job in which I am paid to do that is amazing and wonderful to me. In all honesty, the income is one of the things that enables me to survive and it has built my self-esteem, but the other aspects of the job are equally important to me.

Roslynn: For me, working at Milestones is an honor. I have been through a lot during my lifetime, including depression, lowered self-esteem, and emotional and physical abuse. My personal life experiences, the joys and sorrows I have felt during my recovery process, and the opportunity to work with the other MOST members, have allowed me to use skills and techniques in my work with participants at the center and in respite. I value what I have learned through my experiences and I know that I am contributing my own unique talents to MOST. Being able to help others is healing in its own rewarding way, inside and out. I love my job!

Carol: It's so cool to be thought of as a positive role model, and to actually believe that I am one! It's been a long, mainly uphill climb for me, but now that it's behind me, I am so thrilled to be where I am, not only as a MOST member, but as a true contributor to people's recovery. I can't believe it—when I first came back to behavioral health in a healthy frame of mind (for the most part!) I started out shredding papers. I was a volunteer just begging for a chance to be useful. Since then, I have done various jobs for behavioral health and am now a peer specialist at our wellness center, where I have taken on a role in developing and implementing many programs. I am also involved with community outreach, and I have the opportunity to speak with truly influential people about the recovery model. I am close to completing my B.A. in psychology, and I am writing a chapter in a textbook. What more can I ask for?! I have been so blessed in so many ways! What I want most in this life is to assist people with mental health challenges to blossom and become the happiest, healthiest people they can be. I want them to realize just how valuable they really are. It's all about the journey. I am so grateful for the journey I am on.

FIGURE 1-5. The Milestones Outreach Support Team (MOST)
© Cengage Learning 2013

It is beyond the scope of this chapter to mention all of the possible intervention strategies for people with mental illness. However, there is one intervention (WRAP) that can be used by certified peers or professionals, that is particularly well aligned with the recovery model and deserves further discussion.

Wellness Recovery Action Plan (WRAP)

The Wellness Recovery Action Plan (WRAP) is a system that was developed by and for people who want to be active participants in gaining and retaining their personal health. A facilitator who has completed the certification course in WRAP facilitation guides the process. According to Copeland (2002):

> The Wellness Recovery Action Program is a structured system for monitoring uncomfortable and distressing symptoms, and, through planned responses, reducing, modifying, or eliminating those symptoms. It also included plans for responses from others when your symptoms have made it impossible for you to continue to make decisions, take care of yourself, and keep yourself safe. (p. 3)

There are several key elements of WRAP and the reader is encouraged to explore the website and other material provided in the Suggested Resources at the end of this chapter. However, readers are especially encouraged to review the WRAP Crisis Plan as this document, completed by an individual with mental illness as part of the WRAP process, is the directive that will guide treatment in the event that the individual is not capable of making informed decisions when in a crisis (see Chapter 6 for further discussion).

Although WRAP is only one of many paths one can take to assist in the recovery process, it has proved to be a valuable tool, not only with mental health issues but also with children, teenagers, veterans, elders, people with chronic pain, and people with a variety of other life-inhibiting circumstances. As one WRAP participant summarized: "WRAP is all about you personally, you know that there are so many things that you can do, that you can make a whopping difference in your life. You know that when you do the plan, you are competent and know what works and what does not work."

SECTION TWO: PROFESSIONAL PERSPECTIVE

Anne MacRae, PhD, OTR/L, BCMH, FAOTA

DEFINITIONS AND SCOPE OF RECOVERY

Since Anthony's original published definition in 1993, there have been many definitions of "recovery" in the literature. For example, in 2004, the Substance Abuse and Mental Health Service Administration (SAMHSA) together with other federal agencies developed a National Consensus Statement, which states: "Mental health recovery is a journey of healing and transformation enabling a person with a mental health problem to live a meaningful life in a community of his or her choice while striving to achieve his or her full potential." In addition to this definition, SAMHSA added 10 components of recovery, which are depicted in Figure 1-6.

Both Anthony's and SAMHSA's definitions focus on what recovery may mean to the person with mental illness. However, a myriad of other definitions found in the literature focus more on clinical outcomes. Many authors agree that a duality has developed in defining recovery. Slade (2009) terms this "personal" versus "clinical"

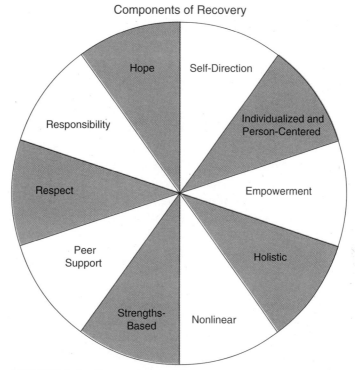

FIGURE 1-6. Components of Recovery

Data from the National Consensus Statement on Mental Health Recovery Substance Abuse & Mental Health Services Administration Rockville, MD 20857 Publication Number (SMA) 05-4129

recovery; Rodgers et al. (2007) discusses "process" versus "outcome" in recovery, and Davidson and Roe (2007) suggest that clarity is needed in defining "recovery from versus recovery" in mental illness. This chapter primarily focuses on personal recovery, however the authors agree with Slade (2009) that for many people, clinical recovery and treatment are a part of their personal recovery. This duality of definitions is especially significant when addressing the need for evidence-based practice and the nature and types of research proposed and funded.

Research and Evidence

Perhaps the most significant research on clinical recovery was the multiple longitudinal studies of people with schizophrenia, conducted between the mid 1970s through the late 1990s with some studies ongoing (Liberman & Kopelowicz, 2005; Davidson & Roe, 2007; Slade, 2009). These studies concluded that approximately 45% to 70% of people with schizophrenia experience a partial to complete remission of symptoms (see Chapter 7 for further discussion). The widely variable outcomes reported is due to a lack of consensus as to what constitutes recovery; some studies include elements of personal recovery and others conflict on how to measure remission of symptoms. Nevertheless, these studies had a profound influence on professional perceptions and attitudes, hence leading to the development of recovery-oriented clinical practice. Prior to these studies, schizophrenia was viewed as either a progressively deteriorating condition or, at best, a condition marked by cyclical exacerbations and remissions. These studies have also raised a number of questions that have not as yet been adequately answered by research. Is poor recovery due to the nature of the disorder, inadequate clinical treatment, or functional deficits associated with long periods of social isolation, stigma, and lack of living skills development? Clinical trials of new medications have significant financial support from the pharmaceutical industry and may indeed provide some new and useful treatments. However, funding for research addressing various elements of personal recovery is limited.

A research agenda and gathering evidence within the personal recovery framework are problematic for a number of reasons. First, it stands to reason that if mental health professionals are going to study personal recovery outcomes, then it must be done in collaboration with people in recovery. Collaborative and participatory research are typically qualitative or mixed method designs that often do not meet the hierarchical and empirical criteria that many scholarly journals require for publication (see Chapter 3 for further discussion on research). Furthermore, within the personal recovery framework, there is debate on the value of measuring outcomes as they are seen by some recovery advocates as dehumanizing and impersonal (Browne, 2006). Inherent in the recovery perspective is the concept that desired outcomes are individually determined, but traditional outcome measures used in research are meant to be applied with all people identified within a particular population (Dickens, 2009). While there are certainly ways to individualize outcome measures (see Chapter 18), the large-scale, population-based, outcome studies are the most professionally valued and hence most frequently published. Clearly a rethinking of both research priorities and valued methodologies is in order. "If we are to embrace outcome measures, let's measure things that are relevant to the new culture" (Browne, 2006, p. 153).

Occupational therapists are in an ideal position to engage in research on personal recovery because the types of specific outcomes measured in occupational therapy are often individual in nature. For example, Kirsh and Cockburn (2009) suggest that the use of the Canadian Occupational Performance Measure (COPM) is a useful tool in recovery-oriented intervention and research as it "is designed to foster partnership between clients and practitioners and it encourages identification of occupationally-focused issues and goals. This instrument promotes an agenda of participation, resumption of life roles, and inclusion in environments of choice" (p. 171).

Even when population level outcomes are explored, the goals and desired outcomes most frequently identified as important and valued within the personal recovery perspective, such as having a quality of life and being a productive and accepted member of the community, are consistent with the domain and practice of occupational therapy. Examples of occupational therapy interventions and research that focus on these recovery-oriented goals can be found throughout this book.

IMPACT OF THE RECOVERY MOVEMENT

The recovery movement is best viewed as a fundamental change in attitude and beliefs; a **paradigm shift** that is having profound effects on intervention, program development, funding, research and service delivery. Many countries, including the United Kingdom, Canada, New Zealand, Australia, and the United States, have adopted recovery as the core principle and each country has its unique "blueprint" for recovery-oriented mental health service provision. In the United States, the document that provides the vision statement and operational framework for mental health agencies to develop recovery-based interventions is titled, *Achieving the Promise: Transforming Mental Health Care in America* (New Freedom Commission on Mental Health, 2003). However, we are far from institutionalizing this vision in all mental health service delivery. There is a tendency to oversimplify new ideas and adopt the language of recovery but not the intent. Recovery concepts cannot simply be an "add on" to existing services, supports, or systems (Davidson, Tondora, & O'Connell, 2007). It requires a complete rethinking of the role of mental health professionals and how services are delivered.

THE CHANGING ROLE OF MENTAL HEALTH PROFESSIONALS

Mental health care professionals who are attempting to realign their practices with a recovery orientation face continued challenges in clarifying and communicating their roles, preserving their professional identities and livelihoods, and reexamining their training and biases. In order for this transition to be authentic, there must be an honest appraisal of the concerns voiced by professionals.

Resistance and Concerns

Some of the professional resistance to recovery as a guiding principle of practice is rooted in the confusion regarding definitions previously discussed. For example, Lal (2010) states that there are "concerns about the application of the recovery concept cross culturally, across the lifespan, and at different levels of service delivery" (p. 82). Remington and Shammi (2005) express a concern that the case for recovery is overstated, which may be setting unrealistic expectations. While these are legitimate areas to critically analyze, when a personal recovery perspective is applied, it is the individual, not a mental health care practitioner, who defines the meaning of recovery within a personal worldview that incorporates culture, context, and motivation.

Yet another often-voiced concern regarding adoption of a recovery approach is the lack of support required to make such a transition. A variety of professional organizations, government offices, and nonprofit agencies provide a wealth of material related to recovery-oriented practice through workshops, printed material, webinars, and Internet informational sites (see Suggested Resources). However, budget constraints have limited the amount of agency and employer support for mental health professionals to avail themselves of these resources and often the onus for professional development and continuing education falls on the busy clinician. In order for recovery-oriented intervention to move from rhetoric to universal practice, it is essential that adequate time, money, and other resources be allotted for education and training purposes, as well as program development.

Obstacles to accepting a recovery-oriented approach also include professional biases and fears that may only diminish with time, education, creative problem solving, and strong leadership. One of the professional concerns reported by Davidson et al. (2006) is a common belief that "recovery approaches devalue the role of professional intervention" (p. 642). The value that an individual places on professional intervention is not absolute, but rather is dependent on the individual's situational and contextual experience with such intervention. However, there is no doubt that the role of the professional changes within a recovery approach and perhaps the most difficult part for professionals in embracing recovery is the need to give up control and their privileged position in the health care arena. While trained professionals do have specific expertise, the goal is to share that expertise with the client for their recovery, not to impose or dictate the course of intervention. Recovery is based on the concept that individuals do know what is best for them; however, it also must be acknowledged that an individual's symptoms may result in poor decisions due to impulsivity and denial as well as a lack of judgment, confidence, or reality orientation. These situations are especially difficult for caring clinicians, as they may want to protect the individual from damaging consequences of poor decisions. However, as long as a decision is not harmful to oneself or others, everyone has the right to make mistakes. Indeed it is through making mistakes that true learning occurs. Recovery is a process as well as an outcome, and for those outcomes to be effective and timely, the process must begin with the very first professional contact regardless of the severity of the individual's symptoms. It is the mental health professional's responsibility to work with the individual to learn self-management for reducing symptoms, but ultimately the choice of action is the individual's.

Developing Collaborative Relationships

Mental health professionals are prepared with a wealth of knowledge and techniques that can facilitate recovery. However, that knowledge is only helpful if the recipient of services understands and values its significance in his or her life.

CASE ILLUSTRATION

Veronica Finds Effective Collaboration

Veronica had been in therapy for years but never felt that it really helped. She saw therapy as something you were supposed to do if you had a mental illness. After several years she was assigned a new therapist who changed everything. The first question that her therapist asked her was: "Do you think you can recover from your mental illness and do you want to?" Veronica was quite perplexed by the new experience, but was able to respond with a polite "yes, I think so." The therapist then asked Veronica what she thought were the four most important achievements she wanted to accomplish during her therapy, and then they together set a length of time that they thought it would take to accomplish these goals. The goals were written and prioritized, and the date of 18 months from the initial session was set for the accomplishment of the goals. The individual therapy was intense and focused throughout every session. Obviously there were twists and turns in the therapeutic process, and the road was often rough, but both therapist and client pressed ahead and the goals were achieved. After 16.5 months, Veronica told her therapist that she believed she had accomplished all she could, and that the next session would be her last. The therapist respected her decision and during the last session, they said farewell, both realizing that all the work they had done was paying off and they were both pleased with the outcome.

Discussion

Veronica had never before experienced goal-oriented therapy and the sense of competency and accomplishment that goes with it. The success of this intervention was partially due to the development of a true collaboration based on respect. In an era when all health care professionals are under tremendous pressure to demonstrate positive outcomes in limited time, it is especially important to recognize that focused and goal-oriented intervention, conducted in partnership with the client, is both effective and efficient.

The above Case Illustration exemplifies that collaboration and mutual understanding between the mental health therapist and an individual can facilitate recovery.

The most important skill in collaborative work is the willingness to truly listen, and in order to do so, the clinician needs mastery of a full range of professional therapeutic techniques (see Chapter 19). Figure 1-7 contains advice from people with lived experience of mental illness regarding therapeutic interactions.

What doesn't work	What does work
■ Assuming and telling me what is wrong with me	■ Having my Dr. and therapist listen to me and value what I have to say
■ Not listening to me	■ Working with my treatment team, and being considered the center of the team
■ Not being told about my medication	■ Letting me talk and ask questions
■ Not feeling valued or validated	■ Being helped to see that there really is a light at the end of the tunnel
■ Being given a dismal forecast of what my life will be like with a mental illness	■ A positive, cheerful attitude
■ Not being respected	■ Being given options about my treatment, talking about them, and deciding for myself what direction I want to take.
■ Being condescending and placating toward me	
■ Thinking they know better than I do what will help me.	■ Feeling like I am in control, in charge, and that they know I can do it
■ Being treated as if I'm very fragile	

FIGURE 1-7. What Doesn't Work and What Does

© Cengage Learning 2013

THE ROLE OF OCCUPATIONAL THERAPY IN A RECOVERY PARADIGM

Much has been written about the underrepresentation of occupational therapy in the mental health system, particularly in the United States. It is of course an ironic situation considering that our early history was primarily devoted to mental health (see Chapter 4 for further discussion). The reasons for the decreased presence of occupational therapy in mental health are complex and varied and cannot be adequately addressed in the confines of this chapter. Nevertheless, the recovery paradigm offers occupational therapy an opportunity for revitalizing this branch of our profession. There is a natural alignment with the principles of occupational therapy and the principles of recovery (Merryman & Riegel, 2007; Rebeiro Gruhl, 2005). The profession has always analyzed and incorporated the strengths of clients in their treatment plans and has focused treatment on meaningful and practical goals, broken down into achievable, success-oriented steps. Recent literature, which is cited throughout this book, has paid special attention to incorporate the client's perspective in assessment, intervention, program planning, and research. "Occupational Therapy services are delivered in collaborative partnerships with the expressed needs of the client being central to the process" (World Federation of Occupational Therapists, 2010). There has also been a noticeable increase in the occupational therapy literature on the role of both personal and societal advocacy.

However, the profession of occupational therapy has not always demonstrated the ability to either advocate for further inclusion in mental health treatment or to recognize and align ourselves with important trends (Cotrell, 2007; Dowling & Hutchinson, 2008). In an effort to not repeat mistakes of the past, various occupational therapy organizations have published position statements defining the role of occupational therapy in mental health care and are attempting to widely disseminate this information to the public and to policy makers. One example is the document titled, *Specialized Knowledge and Skills in Mental Health Promotion, Prevention, and Intervention in Occupational Therapy Practice"* developed by the Commission on Practice (COP) of the American Occupational Therapy Association (AOTA) (2010).

Although dissemination of information and political advocacy by organizational representatives is crucial to the survival of occupational therapy, it is still up to individual occupational therapists to continue advocating for our place in recovery-oriented mental health services and develop relationships with consumer organizations—the heart of the recovery movement. The first step is for occupational therapy practitioners to be well versed in the recovery literature authored by occupational therapists. An extensive bibliography, which includes position statements as well as examples of programs, interventions, and research, is included in the Suggested Resources. However, given that occupational therapy has always struggled to articulate our practice, it is also crucial to engage in outreach and program development that can demonstrate our effectiveness.

I developed one such demonstration project in a rural behavioral health agency that had never before had occupational therapy on staff. The idea was to introduce occupational therapy to the agency by launching a pilot OT internship program. Funding for my supervision time, as well as an intern stipend, and program development time was provided by the recovery-oriented California Mental Health Services Act (MHSA). The following case illustration exemplifies the agency and the consumer response to this newly introduced program.

CASE ILLUSTRATION

Perspective on the Value of Occupational Therapy

These two girls came to Milestones (Wellness Center) and started putting all this stuff on the table. They were friendly but I didn't know why they were even there! By the end of the summer, all the materials they had put on the table made sense to me and I figured out how they could help me. There were things I could actually do with my hands that were so helpful to me and they included using my heart and mind. They taught me so much about myself, and ways to look at my life and the circumstances I was dealing with. They explained things to me in a way that made me really understand what was going on with me. They also showed me new and different ways to handle life situations. It was an approach that I had never before been aware of and a way to approach my problems that really worked. I loved those OT interns! I hope they come back!

Discussion

The participants at this Wellness Center, as well as the professional staff of the county agency, were unfamiliar with what occupational therapy had to offer. Yet the interns and OT supervisor of this pilot program were wholeheartedly welcomed and supported. The OT approach was seen as "refreshing" and "energizing" and very much in agreement with recovery principles. The interns provided individual and group services throughout the county, not only at the county's two Wellness Centers, but also at the senior center, the juvenile hall, the behavioral health clinic, and in people's homes. Partially due to the vocal advocacy of the consumer participants, the county Behavioral Health Service decided to not only renew the OT internship program but also funded a part-time OT position for direct services and consultation.

Successful demonstrations such as shown in the previous Case Illustration can create additional opportunities for occupational therapists to reclaim our psychosocial heritage. Our most important allies in this endeavor are the people with the lived experience of mental illness. If they understand and value the interventions provided by occupational therapy, they can be strong supporters in advocating for the inclusion of OT in services. A question and challenge posed to me by my co-author, Carol, is: "Why aren't occupational therapists more visible in the mental health community?" It is a question that the profession must continue to address. Further collaboration between people with mental illness and occupational therapists would be a win-win—advancing the recovery movement and benefiting both individuals and communities.

SUMMARY

Although there remains much work to be done to see the vision of recovery fully realized, this new paradigm is an exciting development in all mental health services including occupational therapy. An important key for professionals working with a recovery orientation is to form true collaborative relationships with the people they serve, which entails listening to and respecting their experiences. They are the ones who know their stories, who know what has worked, who know themselves. The pain of the past and the hope for the future must be honored to support recovery. Indeed, if there is one word to summarize the power of the recovery model it is *HOPE*.

REVIEW QUESTIONS

1. What is the role of a peer specialist in providing mental health services?
2. What is the difference between personal recovery and clinical recovery?
3. What kinds of research and outcomes are most suited to a recovery-oriented practice?

4. How would you pursue developing a collaboration with a client?
5. How are occupational therapy principles similar to recovery principles?
6. What steps can be taken by occupational therapists to increase our visibility and practice in recovery-oriented mental health services?

REFERENCES

Anthony, W. (1993). Recovery from mental illness: The guiding vision of the mental health service system in the 1990s. *Psychosocial Rehabilitation Journal, 16*(4), 11–13.

Browne, G. (2006). Outcome measures: Do they fit with a recovery model? *International Journal of Mental Health Nursing, 15*, 153–154.

Commission on Practice (COP). (2010). *Specialized Knowledge and Skills in Mental Health Promotion, Prevention, and Intervention in Occupational Therapy Practice.* Rockville, MD: American Occupational Therapy Association (AOTA).

Copeland, M. E. (2002). *Wellness Recovery Action Plan.* West Dummerston, VT: Peach Press.

Cotrell, R. (2007). The new freedom initiative—transforming mental health care: Will OT be at the table? *Occupational Therapy in Mental Health, 23*, 1–25.

Davidson, L., O'Connell, M., Tondora, J., Styron, T., & Kangas, K. (2006). The top ten concerns about recovery encountered in mental health system transformation. *Psychiatric Services, 57*(5), 640–645.

Davidson, L., & Roe, D. (2007). Recovery from versus recovery in serious mental illness: One strategy for lessening confusion plaguing recovery. *Journal of Mental Health, 16(*4), 459–470.

Davidson, L., Tondora, J., & O'Connell, M. (2007). Creating a recovery-oriented system of behavioral health care: Moving from concept to reality. *Psychiatric Rehabilitation Journal, 31*(1), 23–31.

Deegan, P. (1988). Recovery: The lived experience of rehabilitation. *Psychiatric Rehabilitation Journal, 11*, 11–19.

Dickens, D. (2009). Mental health outcome measures in the age of recovery-based services. *British Journal of Nursing, 18*(15), 940–943.

Dowling, H., & Hutchinson, A. (2008). Occupational therapy—Its contribution to social inclusion and recovery. *A Life In the Day, 12*(3), 11–14.

Kirsh, B., & Cockburn, L. (2009). The Canadian Occupational Performance Measure: A tool for recovery-based practice. *Psychiatric Rehabilitation Journal, 32*(3), 171–176.

Lal, S. (2010). Prescribing recovery as the new mantra for mental health: Does one prescription serve all? *Canadian Journal of Occupational Therapy, 77*, 82–89.

Leete, E. (1989). How I perceive and manage my illness. *Schizophrenia Bulletin, 15*(2), 197–200.

Liberman, R., & Kopelowicz, A. (2005). Recovery from schizophrenia: A concept in search of research. *Psychiatric Services, 56*(6), 735–742.

Merryman, M. B., & Riegel, S. K. (2007). The recovery process and people with serious mental illness living in the community: an occupational therapy perspective. *Occupational Therapy in Mental Health, 23*, 51–73.

National consensus statement on mental health recovery. (2006). Rockville, MD: Substance Abuse & Mental Health Services Administration (SAMHSA). Publication number (SMA) 05-4129.

New Freedom Commission on Mental Health. (2003). *Achieving the promise: Transforming mental health care in America.* Washington, DC: Author.

Rebeiro Gruhl, K. (2005). Reflections on the recovery paradigm: Should occupational therapists be interested? *Canadian Journal of Occupational Therapy, 72*(2), 96–102.

Remington, G., & Shammi, C. (2005). Overstating the case about recovery? *Psychiatric Services, 56*(8), 1022.

Slade, M. (2009). *Personal recovery and mental illness: A guide for mental health professionals.* Cambridge: Cambridge University Press.

World Federation of Occupational Therapists. (2010). Update—Position statement: *Consumer interface with occupational therapy.* Author, 1–3.

SUGGESTED RESOURCES

Occupational Therapy Articles Related to Recovery

Asmundsdottir, E. E. (2009). Creation of new services: Collaboration between mental health consumers and occupational therapists. *Occupational Therapy in Mental Health, 25*(2), 115–126.

Bellamy, C. (2007). Making recovery a habit: Supportive socialization dimensions and recovery from mental illness. *OTJR: Occupation, Participation and Health, 27*(Suppl1), 79S.

Blank, A., & Hayward, M. (2009). The role of work in recovery. *British Journal of Occupational Therapy, 72*(7), 324–326.

Cotrell, R. (2007). The new freedom initiative–transforming mental health care: Will OT be at the table? *Occupational Therapy in Mental Health, 23*, 1–25.

Dowling, H., & Hutchinson, A. (2008). Occupational therapy–Its contribution to social inclusion and recovery. *A Life In the Day, 12*(3), 11–14.

Gibson, R., D'Amico, M., Jaffe, L., & Arbesman, M. (2011). Occupational therapy interventions for recovery in the areas of community integration and normative life roles for adults with serious mental illness: A systematic review. *American Journal of Occupational Therapy, 65*(3), 247–256.

Kirsh, B., & Cockburn, L. (2009) The Canadian Occupational Performance Measure: A tool for recovery-based practice. *Psychiatric Rehabilitation Journal, 32*(3), 171–176.

Lal, S. (2010). Prescribing recovery as the new mantra for mental health: Does one prescription serve all? *Canadian Journal of Occupational Therapy, 77*, 82–89.

LeBoutillier, C., & Croucher, A. (2010). Social inclusion and mental health. *British Journal of Occupational Therapy, 73*(3), 136–139.

Lloyd, C., Tse, S., & Bassett, H. (2004) Mental health recovery and occupational therapy in Australia and New Zealand. *International Journal of Therapy and Rehabilitation, 11*(2), 64–70.

Lloyd, C., Tse, S., & Deane, F. (2006). Community participation and social inclusion: How practitioners can make a difference. *Australian e-Journal for the Advancement of Mental Health (AeJAMH), 5*(3), 1–10.

McKay, E. (2010). 'Rip that book up, I've changed': Unveiling the experiences of women living with and surviving enduring mental illness. *British Journal of Occupational Therapy, 73(3),* 96–105.

Merryman, M. B., & Riegel, S. K. (2007). The recovery process and people with serious mental illness living in the community: An occupational therapy perspective. *Occupational Therapy in Mental Health, 23*, 51–73.

Rebeiro Gruhl, K. (2005). Reflections on the recovery paradigm: Should occupational therapists be interested? *Canadian Journal of Occupational Therapy, 72*(2), 96–102.

Rodgers, M. L., Norell, D. M., Roll, J. M., & Dyck, D. G. (2007). An overview of mental health recovery. *Primary Psychiatry, 14*(12), 76–85.

Russell, A., & Lloyd, C. (2004). Partnerships in mental health: Addressing barriers to social inclusion. *International Journal of Therapy and Rehabilitation, 11*(6), 267–273.

Sutton, D. (2010). Recovery as the re-fabrication of everyday life: Exploring the meaning of doing for people recovering from mental illness. *New Zealand Journal of Occupational Therapy, 57*(1), 41.

Swarbrick, M. (2009). A wellness and recovery model for state psychiatric hospitals. Historical perspective—From institution to community. *Occupational Therapy in Mental Health, 25,* 343–351.

Swarbrick, M., & Ellis, J. (2009). Peer-operated self-help centers. *Occupational Therapy in Mental Health, 25,* 239–251.

Swarbrick, M., Schmidt, L., & Pratt, (2009). Consumer-operated self-help centers: Environment, empowerment, and satisfaction. *Journal of Psychosocial Nursing, 47*(7), 41–47.

Woodside, H., Schell, L., & Allison-Hedges, J. (2006). Listening for recovery: The vocational success of people living with mental illness. *Canadian Journal of Occupational Therapy, 73*(1), 36–43.

Wright, C., & Rebeiro, K. (2003). Exploration of a single case in a consumer-governed mental health organization. *Occupational Therapy in Mental Health, 19,* 19–32.

Young, J., & Passmore, A. (2007). What is the occupational therapy role in enabling mental health consumer participation in volunteer work? *Australian Occupational Therapy Journal, 54*(1), 66–69.

RECOVERY WEBSITES

SAMHSA Sites

There are many websites and links that can be found through the main website:

http://www.samhsa.gov

Listed here are some recommendations of SAMHSA recovery-oriented websites:

Partners for Recovery	http://www.partnersforrecovery.samhsa.gov
Recovery Month	http://www.recoverymonth.gov
Resource Center to Promote Acceptance, Dignity, and Social Inclusion Associated with Mental Health	http://www.promoteacceptance.samhsa.gov
What a difference a friend makes	http://www.whatadifference.samhsa.gov/

Nonprofit Organizations

Included here are only national sites for the United States. You are encouraged to explore the many sites from your country, region, state, or county.

U.S. Psychiatric Rehabilitation Association	http://www.uspra.org
Depression and Bipolar Support Alliance (DBSA):	http://www.dbsalliance.org
Facing Us (stories of recovery)	http://www.facingus.org
Mental Health America	http://www.mentalhealthamerica.net
National Alliance on Mental Illness (NAMI)	http://www.nami.org
National Empowerment Center	http://www.power2u.org
Schizophrenia.com	http://www.schizophrenia.com

Other Sites of Interest

Boston University Center for Psychiatric Rehabilitation	http://www.bu.edu/cpr
Internet Mental Health	http://www.mentalhealth.com
Mental Health Recovery and WRAP	http://www.mentalhealthrecovery.com

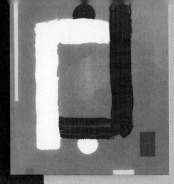

Chapter 2

Environmental and Cultural Considerations

Anne MacRae, PhD, OTR/L, BCMH, FAOTA
Tiffany (Debra) Boggis, MBA, OTR/L

KEY TERMS

allopathic

ayurvedic

culture-bound syndrome

Feng-Shui

Intercultural Development
  Continuum (IDC)

KAWA Model

least restrictive environment

monochronic (M-time)

moxibustion

occupational justice

polychronic (P-time)

polyculturalism

proxemics

TM/CAM

universal design

CHAPTER OUTLINE

Introduction
Environment
    The Natural and Built Environment
    Occupational Therapy Conceptual Models
    Environmental Assessment and Intervention
    Environmental Analysis and Adaptation
    Mental Health Treatment Environments
    The Institutional and Clinic Environment
    The Community and Home Environment
Culture
    Culture and Health Care
    Culture and Mental Health
    Cultural Identification
    Culturally Appropriate Language

    Communication
    Values and Social Relationships
    Time Sense
    Culturally Competent OT Practice
Summary

INTRODUCTION

The second edition of the Occupational Therapy Practice Framework (OTPF) refers to the environment as being either physical or social, and further delineates context as being cultural, personal, temporal, or virtual (AOTA, 2008). However, the OTPF recognizes that these terms are often used interchangeably and are interrelated conditions. According to the International Classification of Function (ICF), contextual factors "represent the complete background of an individual's life and living. They include environmental factors and personal factors that may have an effect on the individual with a health condition" (WHO, 2001, p. 16). This chapter is organized using the concepts of environment and culture, while recognizing that these concepts are interrelated with all of the contextual areas outlined by the American Occupational Therapy Association (AOTA) and the World Health Organization (WHO). Environmental and cultural considerations have unique implications for mental health as occupational therapy practitioners work together with their clients toward the goal of personal recovery.

ENVIRONMENT

The role of environment in health is of critical importance in all of the health care disciplines and is discussed in both clinical and theoretical terms throughout the scholarly literature. Recently, environmental considerations for health have also been a focus for many non–health-related disciplines, such as architecture, as well as becoming a prominent theme in the popular literature. Although occupational therapists have always been and will continue to be involved in adapting existing environments, there is now a trend toward **universal design**, which "is defined as the design of products and environments to be usable by all people, to the greatest extent possible, without adaptation or specialized design" (Christophersen, 2002, p. 13). The benefits of universal design are in its ultimate cost-effectiveness and reduction of stigma often associated with adapted environments for people with disabilities (Joines, 2009). Occupational therapists are urged to increase their awareness and use of universal design, as it "contributes to health and well-being by enabling engagement in self-care, productivity, and leisure (Canadian Association of Occupational Therapists, 2009, p. 1). The move toward universal design has gained momentum throughout the world in the past decade but nowhere is it more evident than in Norway, where the Norwegian State Housing Bank has created incentives and projects geared toward the inclusion of universal design in the curricula of "architects, planners, designers, engineers, occupational therapists and craftsmen" (Christophersen, 2002, p. 7).

Well-developed universal design concepts, particularly the principles of "simple and intuitive use," "perceptible information," and "tolerance for error," are not limited to the physical needs of individuals but also take into account the personal, social, emotional, and cognitive contexts of the inhabitants (Joines, 2009). For example, appliances with unfamiliar or complicated components may add to the confusion or agitation of a client, which ultimately will affect her or his ability to function in the environment. Clients with poor judgment, impulsivity, or memory deficits may also experience burns, electrical shock, or trauma through interaction with poorly designed elements in the built environment.

Although universal design can improve quality of life and reduce stigma, the occupational therapist must balance these considerations with individual client preferences when making recommendations. The personal meaning of objects or the emotional attachment to part of the environment may take precedence in any decision to change the environment. In other words, the personal and cultural contexts must always be considered.

Interest in such philosophies as **Feng-Shui**, a Chinese art form that is concerned with how energies of the environment interact with individuals and their dwellings, has greatly increased as people strive to attain an emotional and spiritual balance in fast-paced and stressful environments (Wong, 1996). Although it is a specific cultural practice, Feng-Shui and universal design both propose simplifying the environment. This is in direct contrast to the often-cluttered and chaotic physical environments in which people with mental illness may live. Social, particularly economic, realities may limit the ability to create an optimal environment, but even small changes may assist people with mental illness in feeling more calm, safe, and organized.

The Natural and Built Environment

Universal design primarily refers to the built environment (created by human beings). Experiencing the natural environment, however, has widespread appeal and is seen by many people as a critical element of mental health. A walk on the beach, in a park, or in woodlands may provide relaxation and stress reduction as well as a mechanism for the development of healthy hobbies and leisure pursuits. For some individuals, the natural environment is crucial in establishing a meditative or reflective state of mind. As elements of nature seem to be particularly important in developing a healthful environment, there has been an increased interest in combining the natural world with the built environment. For example, the role of gardens and animals in a balanced environment is the topic of many studies related to health care (Barker & Dawson, 1998; Cole & Gawlinski, 2000; Perrins-Margalis, Rugletic, Schepis, Stepanski, & Walsh, 2000). However, people in developed countries, especially children and young adults, are increasingly alienated from nature through reliance on electronic media for recreation and communication. There is a growing concern that this "nature deficit" may be linked to reported rises in such disorders as attention deficit and depression (Louv, 2005).

Animals and plants are often used by occupational therapists to facilitate nurturing and a sense of connectedness as well as help develop the roles and responsibilities of daily living. A case study by Zimolag and Krupa (2010) suggests that pet ownership can enable community reintegration by fostering a sense of belonging and acceptance. Hammon, Kellegrew, and Jaffe (2000) concluded that pet ownership can be a meaningful and significant occupation and studies on the use of animals in conjunction with occupational therapy have demonstrated improved social interaction among clients (Fick, 1993; Roenke & Mulligan, 1998). Indeed in 1936, Anna Freud recognized the importance of animals, plants, and things in people's lives in her seminal work on the mechanisms of defense. Additionally, other cultures, notably Greek and Japanese, caring for animals and plants is a function of being human (Cara, n.d.; Young-Bruehl, & Bethelard, 2000). Figure 2-1 is an example of the potential calming and nurturing effects of interaction with an animal.

However, animals and plants should not be viewed as a panacea for all dysfunction nor are they a replacement for comprehensive occupational therapy. Plants and animals may provide a mechanism for achieving or enhancing therapeutic outcomes, but occupational therapists must use their clinical judgment and skill in activity and environmental analysis to determine the specific uses, benefits, and risks for particular clients. Included in such an analysis is the determination of personal and cultural attitudes, as well as the risk of infection, injury, or allergic reactions.

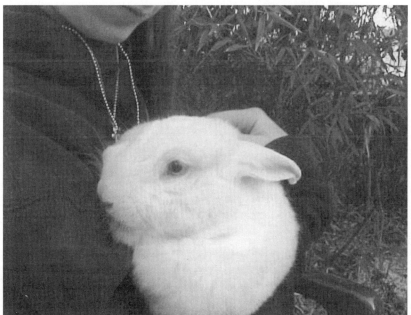

© Cengage Learning 2013

FIGURE 2-1. The Soft Fur of a Rabbit Providing Comfort

Occupational Therapy Conceptual Models

"A unique concept within client-centered occupational therapy is the acknowledgment that clients are not divorced from the environments and community in which they live, work and play" (Law & Mills, 1998, p. 15). That occupation occurs in a context appears to be obvious, and it has always been embedded in the thinking of occupational therapy. However, in recent years renewed emphasis on the role of the environment has been found in the occupational therapy literature, especially with the development of conceptual and practice models in occupational therapy that specifically address the role of the environment in occupational performance and that can be used to promote overall mental and physical well-being. These models include a plethora of ecological/environmental frameworks as well as the Model of Human Occupation (MOHO) and the Canadian Model of Occupational Performance (CMOP). The **KAWA Model** (Iwama, 2006a) also provides an excellent metaphoric and culturally sensitive framework for understanding the relationship between an individual and the social and physical environment. It can be used not only as a conceptual model but also as an evaluation and starting point of intervention in collaboration with the client. Figure 2-2 depicts the elements of the model and their meaning.

The river is a metaphor for one's life from birth to death. The water represents one's life energy or flow. Various life circumstances (rocks), one's assets and liabilities (driftwood), and the social and physical environment (river walls and floor) influence the volume and ease of the flow. The role of the therapist is to enhance life flow.

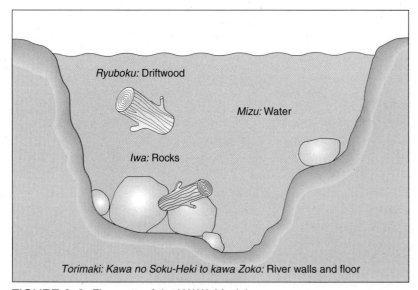

FIGURE 2-2. Elements of the KAWA Model

Reprinted from Iwama, M.K. (2006a). *The Kawa model: culturally relevant occupational therapy.* Figure 7.2, p. 144. Copyright Elsevier (2006). Reprinted with permission.

An overarching conceptualization of the environment that can be used with other models is the **occupational justice** perspective. At the very heart of this perspective is an understanding of the relationship between a person and society and the interrelatedness of all aspects of humanity, both individual and community. Furthermore, an occupational justice perspective is not limited to observing and understanding the environment, but rather focuses on the actions required to empower individuals and communities to create or facilitate positive change in their environments (Standnyk, Townsend, & Wilcock, 2010). This occupational justice perspective is particularly useful when addressing the sociocultural environment, as it is the lack of inclusiveness that many people with mental illness experience that is most damaging to potential recovery. Lloyd, Tse, and Deane (2006) propose four key strategies to improve social inclusiveness for people with mental illness. These are: Addressing attitudes and beliefs; promoting employment opportunities; supporting families and community, and addressing housing, finances, and transport and access issues. Occupational therapists who were primarily trained in a medical model of practice may not be comfortable with the level of advocacy, political awareness, and community involvement that is inherent in an occupational justice perspective. However, this perspective is an example of how occupational therapists are "reclaiming our heritage," which is the title of Schwartz's Eleanor Clark Slagle lecture, in which she states that the reformers of the early twentieth century held "strong views about democracy and social justice . . . In particular, the reform movements involving arts and crafts, moral treatment, scientific management, and women's suffrage would have a significant and direct influence on the founders of the profession of occupational therapy" (Schwartz, 2009, p. 682).

Environmental Assessment and Intervention

The most obvious environmental role of the occupational therapist is related to architectural barriers and adapting the physical environment for increased accessibility. Occupational therapists also address the cognitive and sensory components of occupational performance through such tools as the Allen Cognitive levels screening assessment (ACL) (Allen et al., 2007) to determine what kind of structure and environmental cues are needed to engage the client in task completion and Brown and Dunn's (2002) Adolescent/Adult Sensory Profile Assessment to determine with the client the optimum environment for her or his sensory processing preferences. Recent studies have demonstrated that there may be an association between certain mental health conditions, such as depression and anxiety, and sensory overresponsiveness. Kinnealey, Patten Koenig, and Smith (2011) state that people who are overresponsive to environmental stimuli "describe their daily experience as irritating, overwhelming, disorganizing, and distracting. They spend an inordinate amount of time coping with their responses to environmental stimuli, a situation that leaves them feeling exhausted and frequently isolated" (p. 320). Such experiences have an obvious impact on one's ability to engage in occupation; therefore, sensory sensitivity should be identified as early as possible in assessment and addressed in all recommended environmental adaptations.

Occupational therapists have made important contributions to the understanding and evaluation of the physical, cognitive, and sensory aspects of the environment that affect occupational performance. Attention to the influence of the larger sociocultural context, inclusive of political-economic factors, on the occupational engagement of communities and populations is emerging. The pADL (political activities of daily living reasoning tool) (Pollard, Kronenberg, & Sakallariou, 2008) and the Participatory Occupational Justice Framework (Whiteford & Townsend, 2011) offer conceptual frameworks and tools to guide the therapist in the assessment and analysis of environments that account for the interests and goals of multifaceted societal entities. Wilcock (2006, pp. 222–243) describes an occupation-focused eco-sustainable community development (OESCD) approach to assessment and intervention to promote policies and community-wide action that support participation in ecologically sustainable occupations. Further research needs to be done on addressing the environment in its totality. Specifically, studies are needed that focus on the interrelatedness of the social and physical environments, with the cultural, personal, temporal, and virtual contexts, and the role of occupational therapists in enabling occupation within these environments and contexts.

Environmental Analysis and Adaptation

Occupational therapists tend to be creative problem solvers and be action (doing) oriented. They also are highly trained in observation and occupational analysis. In addition, occupational therapy philosophy is consistent with client-centered practice and a recovery perspective. This constellation of traits makes occupational therapists the ideal collaborative partner to analyze and adapt environments with a client to facilitate the recovery process. Table 2-1 provides examples of specific observations within each context and environment as defined by the OTPF as well as recommendations for adaptation. This table represents an individual client, however, a "client" may also be a family, population, or organization (AOTA, 2008). The format presented in this table can easily be used with a variety of populations and settings. For example, the format of this table was used as the basis for an occupational therapy consultation with the staffs of a recently opened board and care home and a wellness drop in center.

Mental Health Treatment Environments

Mental health occupational therapy is provided in a wide variety of treatment settings. Among the most common are inpatient hospitals with both locked and unlocked units, outpatient clinics, day treatment or the broad array of psychosocial rehabilitation and clubhouse programs, and partial hospitalization programs. In addition, occupational therapists are developing mental health programs in home health care, vocational and community programs, jails and prisons, homeless shelters, and private practices. Many of these sites are discussed in chapters throughout this book, and, although divergent in appearance, they are all appropriate venues for occupational

TABLE 2-1. Environmental Analysis and Adaptation

Context and Environment	Examples of Analysis (Observations)	Examples of Adaptation (Interventions)
Cultural	Bare walls with stains and cracks. No evidence of artifacts. that represent a cultural identity or diversity.	Plan with client(s) additions of art or other artifacts that represent a specific cultural group and/or demonstrate sensitivity to potential diversity. Provide opportunities for multi-model cultural expression—space for celebrations and rituals.
Personal	Apartment shows little personal representation with the exception of collection of cookbooks. Grooming and hygiene items are minimal and/or outdated.	Organize cookbooks for increased display and accessibility. Consider with client(s) adding other items that represent personal investment. (i.e., decorations and space/equipment for hobbies). Create grooming kit with client(s) to be stored on bathroom shelf.
Temporal	Previous tenants left child-size table/chairs. Cartoon sheets used as curtain. Prior year calendar on corner wall.	Relevant, meaningful, and age appropriate, artwork, decorations, and furniture. Addition of current calendar and large display clock in prominent site. Seasonal displays as appropriate and desired.
Virtual	No computer or gaming console visible.	Computer access as well as training and supervision as needed to ensure personal safety.
Physical	Several pieces of furniture are poor ergonomic fit. Underutilized outside space. Light blocked by outside ivy growth. Poor ventilation.	Adapt furniture heights. Consider with client(s) increased use of natural objects (e.g., plants) and outside furniture. Adequate light for tasks via additional lamps and trimming garden growth (adjustable window covers needed for privacy). Instruct client(s) on use of existing vents and fans. Consider asking landlord for security screen door. Practice communication skills as needed.
Social	Limited space for interaction. No observed incorporation of social roles and routines.	Change furniture placement to facilitate interaction. Support the development of meaningful roles as well as healthy social routines and habits. Provide cueing as needed.

therapy services. It is common practice in mental health to attempt to treat a client in the **least restrictive environment**, meaning the environment with the optimum balance of individual freedoms and supervision for the client to function. However, as discussed throughout this chapter, there are many variables in the optimum environment for function; restrictions are simply among them.

Regardless of the treatment setting, and in many cases despite some of the limitations of the treatment setting, occupational therapists place great importance on the environment in the occupational therapy (OT) process. This has been documented since the early writings of the profession. In 1954, Wade and Franciscus stated the following:

> An orderly, well-kept, attractive unit is good mental hygiene in itself and is important for the morale of patient and therapist alike. It gives to the patient a feeling of order and direction rather than one of chaos and indirection. All supplies and equipment should have a given place in which to be kept when not in use, and the therapist must assume the responsibility of seeing that each item is returned to its proper place, not merely pushed aside in a heap on a shelf until it is impossible to locate desired items as they are needed. In addition, a working area need not be drab and depressing, for with ingenuity, some inexpensive material and paint, any room can be made inviting and attractive, and many patients would enjoy working on a project, taking pride in the end result. These latter considerations are an important part of the therapist's responsibility in creating a therapeutic atmosphere. (Wade & Franciscus, 1954, p. 83)

The atmosphere created in a clinic or other institutional setting is indeed important to the overall safety, health, and comfort of clients. However, as recovery-oriented practice and other health care trends move occupational therapists more into the homes and communities of clients, therapists must use their considerable skill in adaptation of various environments and their creativity to problem solve and compensate for the immutable limitations of any given environment.

The Institutional and Clinic Environment

There has been extensive documentation on the particularly negative effects of institutional environments (Chou, Lu, & Chang, 2001; Topf, 2000) where the expense, space limitations, and the necessity of medical procedures as well as security limit the amount of environmental adaptation that is actually possible. However, within these environments, a separate space (clinic) is usually designated for OT that can be therapeutically altered to enhance function and comfort. Indeed, hospitalized clients often view the OT clinic as an oasis (Cara, 1992).

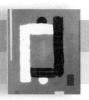

CASE ILLUSTRATION

Mrs. Vigar—The Safety and Comfort of the OT Clinic

Mrs. Vigar is a 57-year-old housewife diagnosed with major depression and hospitalized in a locked psychiatric unit because of severe suicidal ideation. Initially, Mrs. Vigar refused to leave her room, even though she was quite agitated by the noise of her roommate and the proximity to the nurses' station. The occupational therapist was able to coax her out of her room for a short visit to the OT clinic for a cup of tea. The following day, the therapist once again escorted Mrs. Vigar to the clinic and invited her to look at the artwork on the walls and engaged her in the task of watering the plants. Mrs. Vigar attended clinic regularly thereafter, sometimes engaging in clinic activity, other times simply observing.

However, she never missed a session and the nursing staff reported that she was less agitated during and after OT.

Discussion

The OT clinic environment was arranged to provide a sense of comfort, familiarity, and safety as well as a balance of sensory stimulation. This had a direct impact on Mrs. Vigar's sense of control and symptom reduction.

An OT clinic should be a warm, inviting, and safe place. All aspects of the individual client's humanity should be recognized and acknowledged. What may seem like trivial details on the surface can greatly affect the overall "feel" of the clinic. For example, it is optimum if fresh water is available at all times in the clinic. This is a gesture of courtesy, and a desire to have clients in the clinic feel comfortable. It is also an acknowledgment of the problems of dehydration and "dry mouth" commonly found in people on medication. It is, therefore, a tool to educate clients about symptom and side effect management, as well as role-modeling healthy nutritional habits.

Determining the level of sensory stimulation in the clinic can be difficult, especially regarding auditory stimulation. People have very different thresholds of tolerance to sound. For some individuals, it is necessary to have a quiet room for them to engage in any task. It is especially important for the therapist to provide a quiet place for some clients to retreat to if other clients are engaging in a particularly noisy activity. On the other hand, sound (as in music), if used judiciously, can enhance the therapeutic effect of an activity and the clinic environment. "Music can facilitate mood changes, alter states of awareness, modify one's consciousness and increase affective response. Music can be effectively used to shift a person's attention, soothe agitation and as an aid with visualization techniques" (MacRae, 1992, p. 275).

The visual representations found in a clinic ideally are pleasant and calming but most important, they should have some personal meaning for the clients. For example, Figure 2-3 shows the mandala quilt that is displayed in the San Jose State University (SJSU) Occupational Therapy Clinic. Each individual square of this quilt consists of the expressive artwork of a client or an OT student enrolled

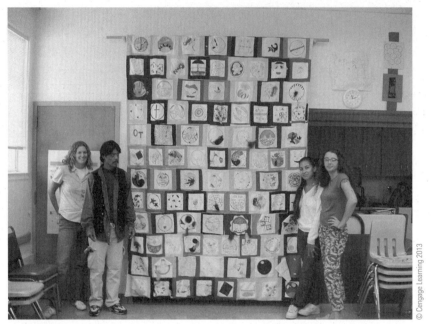

© Cengage Learning 2013

FIGURE 2-3. Group Quilt Project at San Jose State University

in the campus clinic course. Returning clients often look for their contribution and new clients have not only enjoyed its aesthetics but also have become motivated by its presence to contribute to other long-term projects for the clinic environment.

There are many advantages to creating a therapeutic environment within an institutional or clinical setting. It may be especially important for acute care where the primary goal is stabilization, but it is also important for any client who has experienced repeated failures in life and needs to develop a sense of mastery and competency. However, there are also several drawbacks to the clinical environment. The client's home and community environment may be substantially different than the created OT clinic; therefore, functional assessment may not be reliable. Performance that occurs in the controlled clinical environment may not carry over to "real-world" situations or be indicative of a client's actual performance in a community environment (Hoppes, Davis, & Thompson, 2003). A study conducted by Jacobshagen (1990) concluded that interruption in activity performance significantly decreased both the satisfaction with and performance of the activity. A well-ordered clinic may limit interruptions but the living situations of many clients remain chaotic. Assessments conducted in a clinical environment often represent the clients' potential for community functioning, but may not represent actual performance.

CASE ILLUSTRATION

Uyen—Performance in Community

Uyen is a 24-year-old woman with a 4-month-old baby. Her parents expressed concern about her ability to care for the child and took her to a psychiatrist. She was diagnosed as having obsessive compulsive disorder and was referred to a community treatment program. Several functional assessments were completed to document her skills and abilities. Treatment initially consisted of role-playing various living skills for the purpose of providing practice in managing her anxiety. The occupational therapist felt that she was ready to try these skills in the community and accompanied her on a trip to the store. Uyen was able to negotiate the market effectively until she arrived at the checkout counter, where she dropped her intended purchases and ran from the building. She later told the therapist that the man at the counter scratched under his arm and she "knew" that the germs would be given to her and her baby and make them sick.

Discussion

While Uyen was successful in carrying out simulated living skills in the safety of the clinical environment with a therapist whom she trusted, it is not possible to account for the behavior of all individuals or the levels of stimulation in the community at large. In order to master the necessary living skills needed for parenting, Uyen will need further intervention in the community with the goal of developing coping skills for environments that she cannot change.

Health care institutions encounter growing numbers of clients from diverse ethnic and cultural backgrounds. In response, the U.S. Department of Health and Human Services' Office of Minority Health (2001) developed the *National Standards for Culturally and Linguistically Appropriate Services in Health Care* (CLAS). Though primarily directed at the institutional level, therapists are encouraged to use the 14 standards to adapt their practice environments to be more culturally accessible. To facilitate Cultural Competent Care (Standards 1–3), therapists can continually increase personal knowledge of the impact of culture on health and intervention in addition to specific knowledge about the communities being served. Adaptations to clinic space and waiting areas may be possible to accommodate for multiple family members to be involved in the client's care. Scheduling service at nontraditional times can facilitate a client's ability to attend and participate in therapy. The Organizational Cultural Competence Assessment Profile (U.S. Department of Health and Human Services, Health Resources and Services Administration, 2002) offers a starting point to informally assess the Organizational Supports for Cultural Competence (Standards 8–14).

The therapist can advocate for and assist in the creation of a culturally competent organizational environment to meet the diverse needs of their clients.

The Community and Home Environment

Ideally, a therapist can continue to follow a client into a different environment or at the very least be in communication with the therapist who will follow the client in the community. Skills learned in a clinic require practice in the community and can best be integrated by feedback, encouragement, and modification from the occupational therapist. For example, a young man with a goal of productive employment may have developed a resume, problem-solved job-seeking strategies with the clinic-based OT, and even role-played various interview strategies. Nevertheless, he may experience failure in his first community attempt. Follow-up in the community is essential for successful completion of goals, and without the support of a community-based therapist, an initial failure may persuade the client not to try again.

There is a growing body of evidence that social disparity is a major determinant of overall poor health, including psychosocial dysfunction and mental illness (Sapolsky, 2005). A study conducted by Nelson, Hall, and Walsh-Bowers (1998) showed "that the number of living companions, housing concerns, and having a private room all significantly predicted different dimensions of community adaptation" (p. 57). As critical as the physical and sensory environment is to overall functioning, the community-based occupational therapist must also look at the many complex realities of community living, including such variables as social stratification and poverty (Blais, 1997; Hartery & Gahagan, 1998). For example, students in the SJSU clinic frequently address the issue of money management in their treatment plans. While it is true that the poor judgment and impulsivity found in many psychiatric disorders may lead to poor money management skills, students are often surprised to discover how limited the financial entitlements, if they exist at all, are for their clients. Money management implies that the individual has funds to actually manage. Even taking into account the often limited budgets of clients, skills learned in the clinic do not account for the many community variables of budgeting, including the greatly increased opportunities for careless spending and the vulnerability of many clients to financial exploitation.

Another variable in the community is the level of comfort the client feels. Unfortunately, stigma and violence against people with mental illness are very real phenomena (Hunter-Jenkins & Carpenter-Song, 2009; Maniglio, 2009). Therefore, fears voiced by mental health clients in the community are often based on actual negative experiences, not on paranoid delusions, and have a significant impact on independent living. For example, fear of harm or ridicule is often a major factor in clients' poor performances in negotiating public transportation. In a secondary analysis of several research studies, Rebeiro (2001) explored how the environment influenced the participants' occupational performance. Her findings validated the devastating effects of stigma, as participants voiced the need for acceptance, belonging, and safety.

Occupational therapists have vital roles to play in both clinical and institutional environments as well as in the community. They understand the limitations of any environment and creatively problem-solve to either change the environment or assist the client in developing coping strategies to negotiate the environment.

CULTURE

Culture is a conscious and unconscious internal process of identification with overt manifestations of traditions, beliefs, and values, often involving the use of objects, which create meaning and guide human beings in organizing their lives. It is probably obvious that this definition reflects the values of an occupational therapist. But all definitions of culture reflect the specific situation and environment being addressed. "There is no single definition of culture, and all too often definitions omit salient aspects of culture or are too general to have any real meaning" (Spector, 2009, p. 9). The OTPF defines the context of culture as "customs, beliefs, activity patterns, behavior standards, and expectations accepted by the society of which the client is a member" (AOTA, 2008, p. 645). The definition also incorporates an occupational justice perspective by including "ethnicity and values as well as political aspects, such as laws that affect access to resources and affirm personal rights. Also includes opportunities for education, employment, and economic support" (AOTA, 2008, p. 645). Although the AOTA definition provides parameters for culturally responsive care (Muñoz, 2007), it lacks an explanation of the purpose of culture, which is to create meaning, develop or enhance personal as well as role identity, and provide structure and organization to our daily lives. The World Federation of Occupational Therapy (WFOT, 2010) states "every person is unique in the way they combine the dynamic interplay between cultural, social, psychological, biological, financial, political and spiritual elements in their personal occupational performance and participation in society" (para. 5). WFOT's set of *Guiding Principles on Diversity and Culture* provides a resource for practitioners, educators, and researchers to discuss and explore strategies for culturally competent and inclusive practice (Kinébanian & Stomph, 2009).

Every profession comes with inherent biases, as does the profession of occupational therapy. The culturally competent therapist must take care to recognize the cultural biases inherent in the theory, philosophy, and models of occupational therapy practice. Therapists are encouraged to be acutely aware of one's own cultural identity and that of the unique people whom they serve in order to discern the appropriateness and applicability of the documented ideals of the profession (Watson, 2006). The word *occupation*, itself, may have a negative connotation to a client that has experienced life under the occupation of an oppressive governmental regime. The seven core values embraced by the AOTA (2010) include *altruism, equality, freedom, justice, dignity, truth,* and *prudence.* These values may not be interpreted in the same way by all cultures. The profession of occupational therapy historically derives its philosophy grounded in Western thought embracing social norms of individualism, autonomy, independence, self-determination, and notions of mastery over nature and the environment. Other cultures may embrace alternative values of collectivism, interdependence, hierarchy, and multiple truths, balance with nature and less emphasis on "doing." Western values are reflected in the Canadian Model of Occupational Performance and the Model of Human Occupation, among others, that focus on the individual as the central agent to effect change in the environment and occupational performance (Iwama, 2005). The Kawa Model (Iwama, 2006a) arose from a Japanese or Eastern social context that focuses on the harmony between the individual and the collective wider environment. Identification of an optimal model to guide the occupational therapy process with any given client is not dependent on the country where services are provided or the client's country of origin. The Kawa Model has been used successfully in various contexts including a mental health setting in the United Kingdom with clients of Caucasian and Asian backgrounds (Lim, 2006) and in Canada with a client of Guatemalan origin (Iwama, 2006b). It is the responsibility of the therapist to determine which model, or adaptation thereof, is the best fit given the cultural identity and cultural contexts relevant to the client.

Culture and Health Care

There has been much recent effort devoted to understanding health and illness in a cultural context and to research the role of traditional medicine as well as complementary and alternative medicine (**TM/CAM**) in providing adequate health care for the world's population. The literature is inconsistent in the use of the terms *traditional, alternative,* and *complementary*; therefore, some definitions are in order. Traditional medicine simply means the tradition or approach that is primarily used within one's culture. In the dominant culture of the United States, **allopathic** or Western medicine is traditional (also called the medical model), whereas in India, the traditional medical system is **ayurvedic**. This ancient health care system (approximately 4,000 years old) is primarily based on using elements of nature, including diet and herbs (Spector, 2009), and is frequently used in occupational therapy in the form of yoga (Mailoo, 2007).

Alternative practices are health care techniques and approaches that are not typically viewed as compatible with Western medicine but may or may not be viable health care options (*instead of* Western medicine). Complementary health care practices are those that can be used in conjunction with Western medicine but fall outside of the traditional domain of the allopathic system. Whether a particular practice should be considered alternative or complementary often depends on the attitudes and knowledge of the health care provider and the client rather than on any inherent quality of the practice. It is becoming more common to find physicians and other health care providers willing to work in conjunction with an alternative/complementary practitioner and, perhaps most important, willing to work with their clients, the consumers, for health promotion and awareness. This pluralistic wellness model is both client-oriented and holistic. Consumers and health professionals alike are beginning to nurture this trend.

There are several alternative and complementary practices that have become so popular they are now considered somewhat mainstream. These include chiropractic, acupuncture, homeopathy, various bodywork, movement, and massage techniques, as well as the use of diet and herbs. Some of these practices have ancient cultural histories while others are more recent. As our population changes, the mixture of these beliefs becomes profound. Given that the majority of people throughout the world now use some form of nonallopathic treatment either in isolation or in conjunction with Western medicine (WHO, 2008), occupational therapists are likely to encounter unfamiliar practices in their work and may misinterpret their observations. For example, **moxibustion** and cupping are healing rituals based on the traditional Chinese medicine principles of heat and cold. These techniques as well as the Vietnamese ritual of coining, or rubbing the body with a coin for the treatment of colds and flu, tend to leave marks on the body that have been misconstrued as evidence of abuse. Although these practices, like many others, can be potentially dangerous if administered incorrectly, they have been in use for a very long time and there is ample evidence that when properly administered, such techniques do no permanent harm and may have positive psychological as well as physical effects. In order for occupational therapists to provide the optimal interventions for their clients, it is imperative that clinicians continue to expand their knowledge base of TM/CAM and to determine its importance in the individual client's life.

People in Western society tend to be either very skeptical of TM/CAM or uncritically embracing of nonallopathic approaches. The WHO is addressing this gap through the WHO TM/CAM strategy document (WHO, 2002), which aims to assist countries to develop national policies for evaluation and regulation of TM/CAM practices, create an evidence base, determine the safety of practices, and ensure the affordability and availability of TM/CAM throughout the world.

Culture and Mental Health

Cultural awareness is necessary for the delivery of all quality health care, but it has particular significance for the mental health field because of the very nature of practice. Concepts of normal and abnormal behavior are the basis for psychiatric diagnosis. Normality, however, can differ cross-culturally. What is normal to one can be abnormal to another. Since the concept of normality is undoubtedly value laden, the issue of culture must be addressed not only in the treatment process but in the evaluation and diagnostic process as well. There have been efforts to identify manifestations of mental illness unique to a particular cultural group. For example, *ataque de nervios*, which is a sense of being out of control, where the person may exhibit verbal or physical aggression, uncontrollable crying, shouting, and sometimes fainting, and dissociative experiences. This condition is commonly recognized among the Caribbean Latino population as well as other Latino groups around the world. Another **culture-bound syndrome** is *Shenjing shuairuo*. This condition, found in China and among other traditional Chinese populations, is characterized by fatigue and irritability as well as various physical complaints including headaches and stomachaches. Individuals who experience either of these culture-bound syndromes may or may not also meet the existing psychiatric criteria for an anxiety or mood disorder. However, the conditions are unique and it cannot be assumed that they are synonymous with the Western view of psychopathology. Whether or not a clinician acknowledges these syndromes as distinct conditions, it is important to understand the perspective of the client, as he or she may use these terms to explain his or her experiences.

Cultural Identification

One common method of cultural identification is race or ethnicity. This is partially because there are usually easily recognized and observable features. Although ethnicity can certainly be a part of culture, it is not synonymous with culture. Identification of culture with ethnicity alone does not represent the many interrelated facets of culture such as gender, socioeconomics, age, and geographic location. Cultural identity may also be linked to chosen or inherent lifestyles based on personal choice, disability, or sexual orientation; thus, care must be taken to not assume that an individual will always represent or agree with all aspects of a designated ethnic culture. One of the hallmark traits of culture is that it is dynamic and so are the individuals within a culture.

In our complex society, influenced by many events, some people may feel "cultureless," while others identify themselves as members of several cultures (i.e., African American, gay, Christian, occupational therapist, etc.). This **polyculturalism** gives rise to a situation where some people feel cultural conflicts within themselves, let alone with their various communities in which they must interact. The clinical significance of either a lack of cultural identity or a conflicted cultural identity is profound. Stress, guilt, poor self-esteem and self-concept, and lack of support are all contributing factors to poor health. For example, a woman who has immigrated to the United States from a traditional Islamic culture may want to be a part of the working and social world of American women but feels conflicted about her role. She may also lose the emotional support of her family for choices they view as rebellious. Another example is a young man from a fundamentalist Christian family coming to grips with an emerging homosexual identity. For some individuals, acknowledging an identity as a gay man would mean a conscious rejection of familial or religious culture. Unless other support networks are available, the individual may feel cultureless or disconnected from any group. For others, especially those who continue to cherish some parts of their cultural upbringing, there are unresolved conflicts regarding morals, lifestyle, and acceptance that can lead to guilt, shame, and poor self-esteem.

As society becomes more polycultural, there must be greater sophistication in how cultures are identified. The first question is often why we need cultural identification at all. It is clear that the concept of culture, especially as it pertains to race or ethnicity, has often been used to marginalize and stereotype certain groups of people, and several erroneous conclusions have been drawn from research on ethnicity. However, simply choosing not to recognize differences in people is a form of cultural blindness (Cross, Bazron, Dennis, & Isaacs, 1989). In a more naive era than the present, many well-meaning people felt that "everybody is the same" and we shouldn't even acknowledge the differences. Unfortunately, what this often meant was "I will accept you looking different if you think and act like me." Cultural blindness today takes many forms, including some public officials who are supporting the dismantlement of equalization policies such as affirmative action legislation. Even in the scholarly literature, there are suggestions that the concept and definitions of "multiculturalism" are too limited and need to be broadened to include a global multinational, post-ethnic perspective. While such melding and equalization may someday become reality, it seems that we have a long way to go in embracing the world's diversity. As long as racism and discrimination exist, a concerted effort to understand, not ignore, differences is needed.

Culturally Appropriate Language

The literature and teachings regarding culturally appropriate language tend to agree that terms used to denote cultural groups or practices must be sensitive and devoid of negative connotations. Of course, terms that are used in a derogatory and mean-spirited way are offensive and unacceptable; however, the designation of which terms they might be is more difficult than one might think. There are geographical, generational, situational, and personal differences in one's choice of terms. For example, depending on a person's age and where she or he grew up, one might identify themself as Negro/Black/African American/or Person of Color. Another example is how to designate people who speak Spanish as their primary language or people who originate from Spanish-speaking countries. In the eastern United States, the term *Hispanic* is most commonly used (geographical difference), whereas in the West, the term *Latino* or *Latina* (gender difference) is more common. To further complicate these identifications, some people who originate from the countries so designated may have no European (Spanish) background at all and are members of the indigenous populations of Mexico, Central America, or South America. Another scenario is that people may be the ancestors of Africans or American slaves (as is the case in several of the Spanish-speaking Caribbean islands). Still another example, in Canada the preferred term for indigenous people is *First Nation*. To some people the designation of "tribal" is considered archaic and offensive. However, in many parts of the United States, the word *tribal* is used with pride (regional difference). There are still "tribal" councils

that have political authority on reservations and "tribal" ceremonies that are conducted, sometimes for members of the group only, other times for the larger community. The designation *Indian* to mean Native Americans (rather than East Indian)
is usually considered to be derogatory (at least by Caucasians!). However, the term is
used frequently by tribal political activists. Some tribal members report that the term
Native American is an artificial distinction coined to assuage the guilt of white liber-
als (personal difference). There is also quite a bit of debate going on among American
Indian groups about the value of being identified only by one's tribe or nation (i.e.,
Mohawk, Pomo, etc.). Although this is probably more precise and acknowledges the
differences between the groups, it can also weaken their unity when addressing political and social issues (situational difference).

Culturally sensitive or what is commonly called "politically correct," or PC, terminology is an attempt to eliminate or reduce bias and stereotypes. However, it does
nothing to solve the underlying problem of why stigma developed in the first place.
Attitudinal differences may not be significantly affected by a change in terminology.
Sometimes the concern about not offending anyone becomes so complicated that
conversation simply shuts down. That is the worst possible scenario for culturally
competent health care. Figure 2-4 lists guidelines for cross-cultural communication
that can be used in any clinical or community environment.

Communication

Both nonverbal and verbal communication can vary in style and this is at least partially culturally determined. In the northeastern United States, there is a strong value
placed on direct, assertive communication. Sometimes this value is taken to the point

There are times when using a cultural or ethnic term is necessary for the preciseness of a
particular topic in conversation. However, sometimes the use of qualifiers is its own form
of bias. In a client-centered practice it is important to not define a person by a label (Black,
Latino, etc.).

Make an attempt to identify a person as she or he wants to be identified, keeping in mind
the generational, geographic, situational, and personal differences affecting choice of terms.
(Don't make assumptions—ask!)

Be sensitive to different cultural standards of speech, including rate of speech (fast or
slow), acceptable volume, use of silence, appropriate response time, and order of speakers
(amount of deference, acceptance of interruptions, or simultaneous multiple speakers).

Be aware of use of time and acknowledgment of relationships. Clients may need to establish a social relationship prior to a professional relationship, which may not be viewed as
"productive" time by the therapist.

Be aware of posture and body language. Familiarize yourself with culturally acceptable use
of eye contact, proximity of speakers, and hand gestures.

FIGURE 2-4. Guidelines for Cross-Cultural Communication

© Cengage Learning 2013

where all other styles of communication are considered to be pathologic. However, there are many cultures where either aggressive or passive communication styles are the norm and "American"-style communication either is not respected or is considered offensive. Clinicians must sometimes adjust their style to the client's and adjust their expectations of the client. This becomes particularly difficult when the demands of the environment do not match the cultural background of the individual.

CASE ILLUSTRATION

The Passivity of Oi Ling

Oi Ling is a 19-year-old college student being treated for major depression in an interdisciplinary outpatient treatment program. One of the regular weekly groups is on the topic of assertive communication. The social worker and the occupational therapist who co-lead the group encourage her to speak up and coach her in both nonverbal and verbal techniques for assertive communication. The clinical documentation reflects little change in Oi Ling's demeanor or affect.

Discussion

While passivity may be a symptom of depression, many cultures value silence and expect people, especially women, to be quiet and deferential, particularly to their elders. It is up to the team and Oi Ling together to decide whether this group is appropriate for her. If her home or community environment does not value assertive "Westernized" style of communication, there is little benefit to be derived from participation in this group and it is very unlikely that any meaningful change would occur. The social worker and occupational therapist should avoid pathologizing behavior that is acceptable in the context of the client's life.

On the other hand, if Oi Ling needs to function within a school, work, or community environment that expects assertiveness, then an open discussion about the topic should be pursued. The leaders of an assertive communication group need to assess the relevance of the topic in all clients' lives and help them identify what, if any, benefits would be gained from participating in the group. If Oi Ling sees the lack of assertiveness as a problem in her daily life, then participation is appropriate. However, the group leaders need to be aware that Oi Ling may be experiencing polyculturalism, living in two cultural worlds, and may need to develop further strategies for dealing with inherent conflicts.

Communication is often thought of merely in terms of language. Although this is a critical component of communication, it is not the sum total, nor in many cases is it even the most important or reliable means of communication. Nonverbal communication, including body language and gestures, often carries more meaning and is more readily understandable. But this is assuming that one knows the meaning of the nonverbal communication for a particular culture. Even when people are competent linguists, misunderstandings can and do occur because of poorly understood nonverbal communication.

Occupational therapists by tradition are "doers" and do not overly rely on verbal communication. However, all clinicians require practice in both using and accurately reading nonverbal messages as well as understanding the context of verbal language. Table 2-2 provides several clinical examples highlighting the linguistic challenges between a therapist and a client.

Obviously, people who do not share a common language or dialect will have serious limitations in communication. It is certainly in the best interest of the professional to be fluent in more than one language. (In large, culturally diverse urban areas, linguistic ability often becomes a factor in hiring policies.) However, it is not sufficient to simply know the words or the grammar because all language occurs within a cultural context. This leads to a practice dilemma for monolingual therapists. Words are often used interchangeably but they are really very different. A translator is able to provide the words as closely rendered in English as possible, often leaving out the words that cannot be translated. An interpreter takes into account the cultural meanings of the words and applies them to the concepts of the other language. Many health care providers prefer translation, because it allows the professional to interpret the meaning within the health care context. There is always a concern that the interpreter will inadvertently withhold valuable information because of widely different cultural contexts and values. However, literal translations often fall very short of providing the occupational therapist with the whole story. In a profession that prides itself on client-centeredness, which implies hearing the client's story, translation alone is usually insufficient. Taking the time to learn other languages may be more than individual occupational therapists can realistically be expected to do. However, occupational therapists should strive to become cultural interpreters themselves or learn to work closely with interpreters and translators so as not to miss the nuances of the languages encountered. Additionally, the therapist can collaborate with these specialists and the organization within which the therapy service resides to ensure linguistic access to written home therapy programs, educational materials, survey instruments, and signage to the clinic area in languages and terminology that is responsive to the clients' culture and literacy level. It should not be assumed that all clients are literate even in their native language. Use of demonstration and visual representations may be viable methods to incorporate into therapeutic interventions.

TABLE 2-2. Communication in Context

Clients	Example	Comment
Individuals who are monolingual are often treated in settings that do not routinely use their primary language.	A Spanish-speaking person being treated in an English-speaking clinic.	The use of translators/interpreters is highly recommended but cannot take the place of direct clinician interaction with the client for building rapport; therefore, nonverbal communication is essential.
Individuals who may be bi-or multi-lingual may be treated in a setting that does not routinely use their primary language.	A Cantonese-speaking person known to have learned English as an adult and uses English when needed in routine community tasks.	During times of stress, such as might occur during interactions with any authority figures (i.e., health care providers or police), it is typical for an individual to revert to the use of primary language and have difficulty with recently acquired language.
Individuals may speak the same primary language as the health care provider but use a colloquial form of the language not shared by the clinician.	An African American urban youth may have difficulty explaining personal experiences in terms understandable to the clinician and may resent the expectation to use "standard" English.	It is NOT acceptable for the clinician to attempt to use the colloquial form of the language if it is not part of her or his cultural identity. Rather than building rapport, this attempt will more likely be seen as ridicule.
Individuals may have limited or nonexistent language usage secondary to a perceived social climate.	Situations that may induce fear, suspicion, or paranoia such as a recent arrest, political refugee status, or other concerns for personal safety.	Clinicians need to take care not to overpathologize behavior that in fact may be appropriate to the context.

© Cengage Learning 2013

CASE ILLUSTRATION

The OT and Cultural Interpretation

Mary is an American occupational therapist working in Central America. She knows some Spanish but not the indigenous dialect spoken here. Several of her clients insist on calling her "Doctor." Each time she feels an ethical responsibility to correct him or her, stating, "No, I'm the OT, not the doctor." The clients look puzzled but drop the subject.

Discussion

It could be that the clients don't know the role of the various health professionals, but more likely the problem lies in the literal translation of the language. In most countries throughout the world, there is a word or words for "healer" that often gets translated as "doctor." The culture may not have the rigid regulations (years of schooling, licenses, etc.) that Americans assume entitles one to be called "Doctor," but they do understand and respect the role of healers. These individuals would not feel comfortable using their native word for healer (curandera, santeria, shaman) because clearly the OT is not one of them.

Values and Social Relationships

Closely tied to communication is the process of relationship development, the values and attitudes regarding relationships, and the concept of social space. How one interacts with others is largely environmentally and culturally determined. Embedded in one's culture are beliefs and attitudes regarding spirituality, family structure, gender roles, and health care. All of these affect relationships, choice of activity, and preferred environment.

Proxemics, a term coined by E. T. Hall (1966), is an aspect of culture that refers to people's use and comfort with personal and social space. For example, in some cultures it is acceptable and expected to touch frequently and to stand very close together in a conversation. However, in other cultures, this closeness would feel intrusive. Therapists must be aware of the cultural value of proxemics in their clients and adjust their interactions accordingly. It may not be possible to have advanced knowledge of this particular cultural trait, but an occupational therapist with strong observation skills will take cues from the client and adapt to his or her sense of proximity. In mental health service, this becomes difficult because there are many space-related behaviors that are part of psychopathology. For example, someone who is experiencing paranoia or who has sensory processing problems may not want to have anyone near, let alone touching, her or him. Conversely, a person with a brain injury or psychotic disorder may lose sense of personal boundaries and act impulsively with touch. He or she will often not be able to pick up the subtle social cues that the behavior is inappropriate or is uncomfortable for another person. Each situation is unique, but the OT who has an understanding of cultural traits such as proxemics will be less likely to over-pathologize behavior simply because it is different from his or her own.

Cultural values regarding relationships and space vary tremendously and must be taken into account when planning any aspect of intervention. For example, grooming in European-American culture is considered a private activity usually undertaken in the morning time in one's bedroom or bathroom. But in some cultures, such as among Latina women, grooming can be a very social activity, where helping each other with hair styles and makeup is considered highly desirable (Dillard et al., 1992). It is the responsibility of occupational therapists to educate themselves about the particular values and relationship styles of the cultural groups who may be the recipients of OT services. The degree of privacy is only one of several important values that must be considered in OT practice. Table 2-3 lists other common cultural values and provides examples and suggestions for the clinician.

TABLE 2-3. Cultural Values

Cultural Value	Comments and Suggestions
Formality	Specific knowledge of a particular culture's value of formality will help clinicians decide how to introduce themselves, plan for treatment, address the client, and explain their role. For example, in some societies it is expected to arrange appointments with another family member and be granted permission to proceed, while in others the informality of arriving without notice is perfectly acceptable. Some cultures expect the use of formal titles, while others would see this type of communication as cold and distant.
Individuality	The emphasis in American culture and health care is to meet the needs of the individual. However, many cultures around the world value the needs and health of the family, or even the whole community, above the individual. When planning treatment, the OT should be cognizant of who else, besides the individual client, should be involved. It may include immediate or extended family as well as other members of the community.
Independence	Independence is highly valued in Western, particularly dominant American, culture. It is also highly emphasized within the professional culture of occupational therapy. However, in many cultures, care giving is a strong and noble value and there is no shame in having to be cared for. For some cultures, wanting a client to be independent is seen as selfish because family members would not be taking their expected responsibility to care for the person.
Locus of Control	Many people around the world believe that what happens to them is out of their control. Either a greater spiritual power is in control or "things just happen." People with an external locus of control may not be willing to make a large investment (emotionally, financially, or otherwise) to change the course of their health. Occupational therapists tend to hold the value of internal locus of control and usually attempt to "empower" their clients to take both responsibility and control of their lives. The downside of this approach is that clients may feel guilt, shame, denial, or personal responsibility for their illness.
Authority	Respect for authority is common in many cultures. As occupational therapy moves more toward a client-centered approach, it is important to consider that many clients expect the therapist to be the expert and to know what's best for them. They may not feel comfortable in expressing their personal goals.

© Cengage Learning 2013

Time Sense

Although the importance of temporality has long been recognized in the OT literature, it must be acknowledged that particularly in the profession's early writings, the view of temporality was firmly embedded in Western society's concept of time. This view of temporality does not take into account the vastly different time sense or perception that is partially mediated in individuals by their culture. Some cultures value a future orientation, while others are firmly grounded in the present or past.

People in poverty tend to have a present sense of time, meaning that the day-to-day issues or crises must take priority over future plans; therefore, goal setting may be difficult or unrealistic for a person who may not know where the next meal is coming from. Since health care providers will typically be in a higher socioeconomic bracket than many of their clients, it is critical that an awareness of the effects of poverty on time sense be developed. This increased awareness will help occupational therapists negotiate realistic and manageable goals for their clients in poverty.

Hall (1976) suggests that the perception of time is not an inborn trait but rather determined by the culture or society. He classified time sense as being either **monochronic (M-time)** or **polychronic (P-time)**. M-time societies view time as linear and rely on implicit or explicit scheduling. People in M-time societies also tend to view time as a commodity, as a thing that can be saved or lost, spent or wasted, or squandered or managed (Peloquin, 1991). However, P-time cultures do not share the same time values. P-time tends to be cyclical and unscheduled, typically a natural rhythm where several things can happen at once and is not controlled by human beings.

Treating a client with a different time sense is one of the most frustrating aspects of working cross-culturally. Part of the frustration stems from not being aware that different time senses even exist. A culturally competent therapist first determines if the client's time sense is culturally different than what would be expected in the treatment setting or dominant culture. Otherwise, it is possible to erroneously assume a pathology or dysfunction that does not exist within the individual's cultural world.

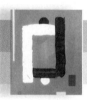

CASE ILLUSTRATION

Mr. Maliu's Perception of Time

Mr. Maliu recently arrived in the United States from a small village in Samoa. He now lives with his brother's family, who arranged for his migration because they felt that he could receive better care in the United States for his long-standing mental illness. His brother arranged for an initial evaluation at a county mental health office that also operates a day treatment center on site. Mr. Maliu arrived two hours late for his initial appointment and was asked to reschedule for another time. He was considerably late for the second appointment as well; however, the interviewing team, consisting of a psychiatrist, a social worker, and an occupational therapist, was able to accommodate him. He was accepted into the program but told that he would have to arrive on time to remain in the treatment group. He immediately established a pattern of late arrival to the group. Therefore, the treatment team is considering discharging him and referring him to outreach case management only. The conclusion of the treatment team is that he is perhaps too ill to benefit from the program at this time. Furthermore, his behavior is disruptive to the rest of the group.

Discussion

Time-related behaviors such as those displayed by Mr. Maliu may be due to symptoms of serious mental illness such as disorganization, disorientation, or avolition. However, care must be taken to avoid pathologizing behaviors that may be culturally appropriate. First and foremost, an understanding of the meaning of time to the client is essential to determine if Mr. Maliu's behavior is related to his illness or not. If it is determined that his time sense is consistent with his cultural background and lifestyle, the treatment team has several options. It may indeed be in the client's and the group's best interest for him to receive individual treatment or case management initially. However, another approach would be to involve the family in a discussion of the norms, expectations, and benefits of group participation. If the client and his family saw the group treatment as desirable, then strategies, such as telephone reminders and schedules or pairing him with a travel partner from the group, could be developed to help Mr. Maliu adapt to the environment's expected time sense. Still another option open to the team is to simply let Mr. Maliu attend the program with late arrival. Often clients are more tolerant of flexible time schedules than professionals and his late arrival may not be as disruptive as the team assumes.

In order for occupational therapists to provide culturally competent treatment to a diverse population it is essential that the profession's beliefs about time be explored. Occupational therapy originally developed in an M-time society. Specifically, the middle- and upper-class values of the northeastern United States at the turn of the century greatly affected the development of occupational therapy as a profession. However, in today's multicultural environment and with the growth of the profession around the world, occupational therapists must adapt to include, or at least recognize, the values of other societies. There are many implications for treatment when the therapist has a different time sense than the person receiving services. The trends toward managed care and increased productivity in the workplace have placed a high value on a minute increment therapy model, in which quantity of therapy minutes is equated with quality of intervention. This trend must somehow be reconciled with the trends toward incorporating multicultural and individual client perspectives and needs.

Culturally Competent OT Practice

Guidelines for culturally competent occupational therapy began to emerge in the literature in the early 1990s (Dillard et al., 1992) and continue to be a topic of discussion in the current literature (Balcazar, Suarez-Balcazar, & Taylor-Ritzler, 2009). Occupational therapy educators and researchers around the globe are becoming increasingly interested in the cultural competency development of occupational therapists (Cherry et al., 2009; Cheung, Shah, & Muncer, 2002; Murden et al., 2008; Rasmussen,

Lloyd, & Wielandt, 2005). Although several definitions of cultural competence have been introduced, all of them go beyond the simple acquisition of knowledge and skills to discuss the necessity for interpersonal skills and attitudes such as self-reflection, flexibility, acceptance of differences, and lifelong learning. The ability to understand different cultural values and viewpoints and integrate these into thera-peutic interventions is necessary for the client to have a meaningful occupational therapy experience.

The development of cultural competency is a dynamic process that occurs throughout one's lifespan. Hammer (2009) describes the **Intercultural Development Continuum (IDC)**, adapted from Bennett's (1993) origi-nal formulation of the Developmental Model of Intercultural Sensitivity. The IDC provides a developmental continuum to understand how people tend to think and feel about diversity, progressing from a lesser to a more complex perception and experience of cultural differences. Five specific orientations that range from monocultural to more intercultural or global mindsets are described. Those who have a more intercultural mindset have a greater capability to respond effectively to cultural differences. The first two orientations are monocultural in nature and include *denial*, defined as an indifference to or ignorance of cultural difference, and *polarization*, characterized by either a negative evaluation of cultures differ-ent than one's own (i.e., defense) or a perception that other cultures are better than one's own (i.e., reversal). *Minimization* is a transitional phase in which there is recognition of superficial differences such as food and dress preferences, while similarities of human beings are emphasized. The final two orientations are inter-cultural in nature. An intercultural mindset includes the *acceptance* stage at which point difference is recognized and appreciated. The final stage, *adaptation,* is char-acterized by the development of empathy to take on another's point of view and ability to adapt behaviors to accommodate for the differences. Figure 2-5 depicts the stages of the IDC. Students enrolled in an occupational therapy educational program in the United States, as measured by the *Intercultural Developmental Inventory* (Hammer, Bennett, & Wiseman 2003; Hammer, 2009), were found to have an overall developmental orientation in minimization yet tended to perceive them-selves as having an acceptance orientation.

Gaining an understanding and appreciation of commonalities between ones culture and that of others is helpful to avoid negatively judging cultures in terms of "us" and "them," indicative of a monocultural perspective. It allows for toler-ance of other cultures, characteristic of a minimization worldview. Development of an in-depth understanding of how one's own culture differs from other cultures as well as alternative culture-specific knowledge lays the foundation for accep-tance and fosters the ability to make ethical judgments that take into consider-ation other cultural values as well as one's own. A more thorough recognition and

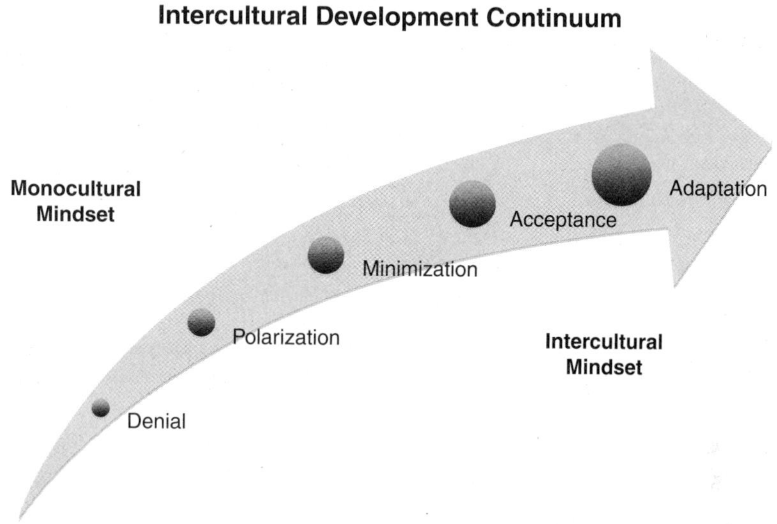

Intercultural Development Continuum

FIGURE 2-5. The Intercultural Development Continuum
© 2010, Mitchell R. Hammer, Ph.D., IDI, LLC. Used with permission by author.

appreciation of cultural differences pave the way to shift cultural perspectives and to adapt intervention in consideration of cultural differences, characteristic of an adaptation orientation.

As world demographics continue to shift toward a diverse society and occupational therapy strives to be increasingly client-centered, it is necessary that every occupational therapist develop a myriad of interventions that can acknowledge, honor, and address the complex cultural backgrounds of clients. Choices of occupations, including styles and approaches to activities of daily living, work habits, hobbies, and recreation, as well as the practice of rituals and traditions are all representative of one's culture and must be individually tailored to the client or client group. Throughout this book the illustrations and examples are designed to represent the diversity of occupational therapy clients. An aware occupational therapist creatively addresses culture in treatment; however, culturally appropriate assessment provides different challenges.

The cultural sensitivity of standardized assessments continues to be a controversial subject and many formal evaluation tools have such significant bias that their use with culturally diverse populations is questionable. Even the informal tools and interview protocols commonly used in occupational therapy rarely adequately address the cultural background of the client. Table 2-4 provides a format for a culturally based interview and observation. This structure allows the therapist to understand the client's values and beliefs as well as cultural style, in addition to the personal meaning of the individual's culture.

TABLE 2-4. Cross-Cultural Initial Interview and Observation

Name: _____

Setting (Context): _____

Cultural Identity	Observations
Where were you born?	Apparent cultural identity (features, dress, icons, etc.)
How long have you lived here?	
Do you identify with a specific culture? (or do you feel more like a part of the culture in which you live or a different culture?)	
Do you identify with a specific religion?	

Communication	Observations
What is your preferred language?	Use of Silence:
	Appropriate ___ Not Appropriate ___
	Comments:
If you have something important to discuss with your family, how would you approach them?	Use of Nonverbal Communication (e.g., hand movement, eye movement, entire body movement, gestures, expression, stances, etc.):
	Comments:
	Style of Communication: Passive ____
	Assertive ____ Aggressive ____
	Comments:

Time Sense	Observations
Do you use a device to tell time? (e.g., a watch, phone, computer, etc.)	Arriving at scheduled appointment
Do you use a schedule or date book? (electronic or paper)	Early_____ On time _____
Do you usually arrive early, late, or right on time to planned events?	Late _____
Is that pattern typical in your family or community?	Comments:

Social and Spatial Organization	Observations
What are some activities you enjoy? (or What are your hobbies? or What do you like to do during your free time?)	Touch (e.g., startles or withdraws when touched, accepts touch/ touches others with or without difficulty):
What are your roles? (or What is your role (or obligations) in your family/community?)	Degree of comfort with space/distance in conversations:

Health/Locus of Control	
What is good health to you?	
Is there anything in your heritage/background that affects your approach to being well/healthy?	
What do you think is going to make you or keep you well? (or What is going to keep you from getting well?)	

SUMMARY:

© Anne MacRae, PhD, OTR/L, BCMH, FAOTA. Adapted from Giger and Davidhizar's Transcultural Assessment Model (Giger & Davidhizar, 1999).

SUMMARY

Occupational therapy intervention occurs within both environmental and cultural contexts. Occupational therapists must continually broaden their skills in these areas to provide competent services in a client-centered tradition. Furthermore, the unique focus on occupation within these contexts makes the occupational therapist a key member of the treatment team and also opens the possibility for a role as consultant or program developer. Mental health is directly affected by both the environmental and cultural contexts of individual clients. All members of a treatment team, including the occupational therapist, must understand the impact of these contexts on client function.

REVIEW QUESTIONS

1. How does environment affect assessment?
2. Why is it important for occupational therapists to be familiar with TM/CAM?
3. How does cultural competence affect OT assessment and intervention?

REFERENCES

Allen, C. K., Austin, S. L., David, S. K., Earhart, C. A., McCraith, D. B., & Riska-Williams, L. (2007). *Allen Cognitive Level Screen 5 (ACLS-5), Large Allen Cognitive Level Screen 5 (LACLS-5).* Camarillo, CA: ACLS and LACLS Committee.

American Occupational Therapy Association. (2008). Occupational therapy practice framework: Domain and process (2nd edition). *American Journal of Occupational Therapy, 62,* 625–683.

American Occupational Therapy Association. (2010). Occupational therapy code of ethics and ethics standards (2010). *American Journal of Occupational Therapy, 64,* 151–160.

Balcazar, F. E., Suarez-Balcazar, Y., & Taylor-Ritzler, T. (2009). Cultural competence: Development of a conceptual framework. *Disability and Rehabilitation, 31*(14), 1153–1160.

Barker, S. B., & Dawson, K. S. (1998). The effects of animal-assisted therapy on anxiety ratings of hospitalized psychiatric patients. *Psychiatric Services, 49*(6), 797–801.

Bennett, M. J. (1993). Towards ethnorelatism: A developmental model of intercultural sensitivity. In R. M. Paige (Ed.), *Education for the intercultural experience* (pp. 21–72). Yarmouth, ME: Intercultural Press.

Blais, L. (1997). The issue of mental health in the context of poverty [French]. *Canadian Journal of Community Mental Health, 16*(1), 5–22.

Brown, C., & Dunn, W. (2002) *Adolescent/Adult Sensory Profile.* San Antonio, TX: Pearson.

Canadian Association of Occupational Therapists. (2009). *Position statement: Universal design and occupational therapy.* Ottawa: CAOT.

Cara, E. (1992). Neutralizing the narcissistic style: Narcissism, self-psychology and occupational therapy, *Occupational Therapy in Health Care,* 8, 2–3, 135–156.

Cara, E. (n.d.). Dian Fossey's Motivations: An example of Two Psychoanalytic Concepts—Lack of Cherishment and Altruistic Surrender. Unpublished Manuscript.

Cherry, K., Kitchens, K., Nicholson, C., Soden, I., Tomkiewicz, J., Kedia, M., & Shah, S. (2009). Cultural awareness and competency of graduate entry-level OT students. *Education Special Interest Section Quarterly, 19,* 1–4.

Cheung Y., Shah S., & Muncer S. (2002). An exploratory investigation of undergraduate students' perceptions of cultural awareness. *British Journal of Occupational Therapy, 65,* 543–550.

Chou, K., Lu, R., & Chang, M. (2001). Assaultive behavior by psychiatric in-patients and its related factors. *Journal of Nursing Research, 9*(5), 139–51.

Christophersen, J. (2002). *Universal design: 17 ways of thinking and teaching.* Oslo: Husbanken.

Cole, K. M., & Gawlinski, A. (2000). Animal-assisted therapy: The human-animal bond. *AACN Clinical Issues, 11*(1), 139–149.

Cross T., Bazron, B., Dennis, K., & Isaacs, M. (1989). *Towards a culturally competent system of care, Volume I*. Washington, D.C.: Georgetown University Child Development Center, CASSP Technical Assistance Center.

Dillard, M., Andonian, L., Flores, O., Lai, L., MacRae, A., & Shakir, M. (1992). Culturally competent occupational therapy in a diversely populated mental health setting. *American Journal of Occupational Therapy, 46*, 721–726.

Fick, K. M. (1993). The influence of an animal on social interactions of nursing home residents in a group setting. *American Journal of Occupational Therapy, 47*(6), 529–534.

Freud, A. (1936/1974). *The ego and the mechanisms of defense*. New York: International Universities Press.

Giger, J. N., & Davidhizar, R. E. (1999). *Transcultural nursing* (3rd ed.). St. Louis, MO: Mosby.

Hall, E. T. (1966). *The hidden dimension*. Garden City, NY: Doubleday.

Hall, E. T. (1976). *Beyond culture*. Garden City, NY: Anchor/Doubleday.

Hammer, M. R., Bennett, M. J., & Wiseman, R. (2003). Measuring intercultural sensitivity: The intercultural development inventory. *International Journal of Intercultural Relations, 27*, 421–443.

Hammer, M. R. (2009). The Intercultural Development Inventory. In M. A. Moodian (Ed.), *Contemporary leadership and intercultural competence* (pp. 203–217). Thousand Oaks, CA: Sage.

Hammon, A., Kellegrew, D., & Jaffe, D. (2000). The experience of pet ownership as meaningful occupation. *Canadian Journal of Occupational Therapy, 6*, 271–278.

Hartery, T., & Gahagan, T. (1998). Social stratification and social class. In D. Jones et al. (Eds.), *Sociology and occupational therapy*. Edinburgh: Churchill Livingstone.

Hoppes, S., Davis, L. A., & Thompson, D. (2003). Environmental effects on the assessment of people with dementia: A pilot study. *American Journal of Occupational Therapy, 57*(4), 396–402.

Hunter-Jenkins, J., & Carpenter-Song, E. (2009). Awareness of stigma among persons with schizophrenia. *Journal of Nervous and Mental Disease, 19*(7), 520–529.

Iwama, M. K. (2005). Situated meaning: An issue of culture, inclusion, and occupational therapy. In F. Kronenberg, S. Simó Algagdo, & N. Pollard (Eds.), *Occupational therapy without borders* (pp. 127–139). Edinburgh: Elsevier Churchill Livingstone.

Iwama, M. K. (2006a). *The Kawa model: Culturally relevant occupational therapy*. Edinburgh: Elsevier.

Iwama, M. K. (2006b). The Kawa model as a window into client occupational therapy contexts: The case of Pedro Mendez. In M. Iwama (Ed.), *The Kawa model: Culturally relevant occupational therapy* (pp. 180–184). Edinburgh: Elsevier.

Jacobshagen, I. (1990). The effect of interruption of activity on affect. *Occupational Therapy in Mental Health, 10*(2).

Joines, S. (2009). Enhancing quality of life through universal design. *NeuroRehabilitation, 25*, 155–167.

Kinébanian, A., & Stomph, M. (2009). *Guiding principles on diversity and culture*. World Federation of Occupational Therapy (WFOT). Retrieved from http://www.wfot.org

Kinnealey, M., Patten Koenig, K., & Smith, S. (2011). Relationships between sensory modulation and social supports and health-related quality of life. *American Journal of Occupational Therapy, 65*, 320–327.

Law, M., & Mills, L. (1998). Client centered occupational therapy. In M. Law (Ed.), *Client centered occupational therapy*. Thorofare, NJ: Slack.

Lim, K. H. (2006). The Kawa model in mental health contexts: Two cases from the UK. In M. Iwama, *The Kawa model: Culturally relevant occupational therapy* (pp. 197–205). Edinburgh: Elsevier.

Lloyd, C., Tse, S., & Deane, F. (2006). Community participation and social inclusion: How practitioners can make a difference. *Australian E-Journal for Advancement of Mental Health, 5*(3). Retrieved from http://www.auseinet.com/journal/vol5iss3/lloyd.pdf

Louv, R. (2005). *Last child in the woods: Saving our children from nature deficit disorder*. Chapel Hill, NC: Algonquin Books of North Carolina.

MacRae, A. (1992). The issue is: Should music be used therapeutically by occupational therapists? *American Journal of Occupational Therapy, 46*, 275–277.

Mailoo, V. J. (2007). The ayurvedic model of human occupation. *Asian Journal of Occupational Therapy, 6*(1), 1–13.

Maniglio, R. (2009). Severe mental illness and criminal victimization: A systematic review. *Acta Psychiatrica Scandinavica, 119*, 180–191.

Muñoz, J. P. (2007). Culturally responsive care in occupational therapy. *Occupational Therapy International, 14*(4), 256–280.

Murden, R., Norman, A., Ross, J., Sturdivant, E., Kedia, M., & Shah, S. (2008). Occupational therapy students' perceptions of their cultural awareness and competency. *Occupational Therapy International, 15*, 191–203.

Nelson, G., Hall, G. B., & Walsh-Bowers, R. (1998). The relationship between housing characteristics, emotional well-being and the personal empowerment of psychiatric consumer/survivors. *Community Mental Health Journal, 34*(1), 57–59.

Pollard, N., Kronenberg, F., & Sakellariou, D. (2008). A political practice of occupational therapy. In N. Pollard, D. Sakellariou, & F. Kroneberg (Eds.), *A political practice of occupational therapy* (pp. 3–19.) Edinburgh: Elsevier.

Peloquin, S. (1991). Time as commodity: Reflections and implications. *American Journal of Occupational Therapy, 45*(2), 147–154.

Perrins-Margalis, N., Rugletic, J., Schepis, N., Stepanski, H., & Walsh, M. (2000). The immediate effects of a group-based horticulture experience on the quality of life of persons with chronic mental illness. *Occupational Therapy in Mental Health, 16*(1), 15–32.

Rasmussen, T. M., Lloyd, C., & Wielandt, T. (2005). Cultural awareness among Queensland undergraduate occupational therapy students. *Australian Occupational Therapy Journal, 52*, 302–310.

Rebeiro, K. (2001). Enabling occupation: The importance of an affirming environment. *Canadian Journal of Occupational Therapy, 68*(2), 80–89.

Roenke, L., & Mulligan, S. (1998). The therapeutic value of the human-animal connection. *Occupational Therapy in Health Care, 11*(2), 27–43.

Sapolsky, R. (2005). Sick of poverty: New studies suggest that the stress of being poor has a staggeringly harmful influence on health. *Scientific American, 293*(6), 92–99.

Schwartz, K. (2009). Reclaiming our heritage: Connecting the founding vision to the centennial vision. *American Journal of Occupational Therapy, 63*(6), 681–690.

Spector, R. (2009). *Cultural diversity in health and illness* (7th ed.). Upper Saddle River, NJ: Pearson.

Standnyk, R., Townsend, E. & Wilcock, A. (2010). Occupational justice. In C. Christiansen & E. Townsend (Eds.), *Introduction to occupation: The art and science of living* (pp. 329–358). Upper Saddle River, NJ: Pearson.

Topf, M. (2000). Hospital noise pollution: An environmental stress model to guide research and clinical interventions. *Journal of Advanced Nursing, 31*(31), 520–528.

U.S. Department of Health and Human Services, Office of Minority Health. (2001, March). *National standards for culturally and linguistically appropriate services in health care: Final report.* Washington, DC. Retrieved from http://minorityhealth.hhs.gov/templates/browse.aspx?lvl=2&lvlID=15

U.S. Department of Health and Human Services, Health Resources and Services Administration. (2002). *Indicators of cultural competence in health care delivery organizations: An organizational cultural competence assessment profile.* Retrieved from http://www.hrsa.gov/culturalcompetence/healthdlvr.pdf

Wade, B., & Franciscus, M. L. (1954). Occupational therapy for the mentally ill. In H. Willard & C. Spackman (Eds.), *Principles of occupational therapy* (2nd ed.). Philadelphia: Lippincott.

Watson, R. (2006). Being before doing: The cultural identity (essence) of occupational therapy. *Australian Occupational Therapy Journal, 53*(3), 151–158.

Wilcock, A. (2006). *An occupational perspective of health* (2nd ed.). Thorofare, NJ: Slack.

Whiteford, G., & Townsend, E. (2011). Participatory occupational justice framework (POJF 2010): Enabling occupational participation and inclusion. In F. Kronenberg, N. Pollard, & D. Sakellariou (Eds.), *Occupational therapies without borders (Vol. 2): Towards an ecology of occupation-based practices* (pp. 65–84). Edinburgh: Elsevier.

Wong, E. (1996). *Feng-Shui: The ancient wisdom of harmonious living for modern times.* Boston: Shambhala.

World Federation of Occupational Therapy (WFOT). (2010). *Position statement on diversity and culture*. WFOT. Retrieved from http://www.wfot.org

World Health Organization (WHO). (2001). *International classification of functioning, disability and health (ICF)*. WHO. Retrieved from http://www.who.int/classifications/icf/en/

World Health Organization (WHO). (2002). Press Release WHO/38 (2002, May 16). *Who launches the first global strategy on traditional and alternative medicine*. WHO. Retrieved from http://www.who.int/en/

World Health Organization (WHO). (2008). Fact Sheet No. 134 (2008, December). *Traditional Medicine*. WHO. Retrieved from http://www.who.int/mediacentre/factsheets/fs134/en/

Young-Bruehl, E. and F. Bethelard (2000). *Cherishment: A psychology of the heart*. New York: Simon and Schuster.

Zimolag, U. & Krupa, T. (2010). The occupation of pet ownership as an enabler of community integration in serious mental illness: A single exploratory case study. *Occupational Therapy in Mental Health, 26*, 176–196.

SUGGESTED RESOURCES

Black, R. M., & Wells, S. A. (2007). *Culture occupation: A model of empowerment in occupational therapy*. Bethesda, MD: AOTA Press.

Cooper Marcus, C., & Barnes, M. (1999). *Healing gardens: Therapeutic benefits and design recommendations*. Indianapolis: Wiley.

Cross Cultural Communication. Retrieved from http://www.pbs.org/ampu/crosscult.html

Cultural Competence by the U.S. Dept. of Health and Human Services. Retrieved from http://www.hrsa.gov/culturalcompetence/

Fadiman, A. (1997). *The spirit catches you and you fall down: A Hmong child, her American doctors, and the collision of two cultures*. New York: Noonday.

Fearing, V., & Clark, J. (2000). *Individuals in context: A practical guide to client-centered practice*. Thorofare, NJ: Slack.

Friedman, S., & Wachs, T. (1999). *Measuring environment across the life span: Emerging methods and concepts*. Washington, DC: American Psychological Association.

Howarth, A., & Jones, D. (1999). Transcultural occupational therapy in the United Kingdom: Concepts and research. *British Journal of Occupational Therapy, 62*(10), 451–458.

Leavitt, R. (2010). *Cultural competence: A lifelong journey to cultural proficiency*. Thorofare, NJ: SLACK Inc.

Letts, L., Rigby, P., & Stewart, D. (2003). *Using environments to enable occupational performance*. Bethesda, MD: American Occupational Therapy Association.

Linde, P. R. (2002). *Of spirits and madness: An American psychiatrist in Africa*. New York: McGraw Hill.

Louv, R. (2005). *Last child in the woods: Saving our children from nature deficit disorder*. Chapel Hill, NC: Algonquin Books of North Carolina.

National Center for Complementary and Alternative Medicine (NIH). Retrieved from http://nccam.nih.gov/

National Center for Cultural Competence. Retrieved from http://www11.georgetown.edu/research/gucchd/nccc/

Pomerinke, K., Crawford, J., & Smith, D. (2003*). Therapy pets: The animal human healing partnership*: Amherst, NY: Prometheus.

Purnell, L., & Paulanka, B. (1998). *Transcultural health care*. Philadelphia: F. A. Davis.

The Kawa Model. Retrieved from http://www.kawamodel.com/

Watson, R. (2006). Being before doing: The cultural identity (essence) of occupational therapy. *Australian Occupational Therapy Journal, 53*(3), 151–158.

Well, S. (1997). *Horticulture therapy and the older adult population*. Binghamton, NY: Haworth.

Chapter 3

A Context for Mental Health Research in Occupational Therapy

Pamela Richardson, PhD, OTR/L, FAOTA
Madeleine Duncan, MScOT, DPhil (Psych)

KEY TERMS

Critically Appraised Topics (CATs)
DALYs
Delphi Study
epistemology
evidence-based practice

meta-analyses
ontology
systematic reviews
translational research/science

CHAPTER OUTLINE

Introduction
Why Do Research? The Burden of Mental Illness
Evidence-Based Practice
Research Priorities in Mental Health
 Mapping Mental Health Resources
 Identifying Grand Challenges
 Developing Interventions
 Using Translational Science
 Building Partnerships
Research Priorities in Mental Health Occupational Therapy
 Cost Benefit: Effectiveness and Efficacy
 Comprehensive Research Scope
 Role Emergent Research Areas
 Research Orientation
Thinking in Research
 Ways of Thinking

      Questioning Conventions
      Checking Assumptions
      Valuing Research Integrity
Methodological Positions
      Fit for Purpose
      Numbers and Experience
Research Examples: Learning From Others
The Way Forward
      Making Local-Global Research Links
      Considering a Human Scale Research Agenda
Summary

INTRODUCTION

Research refers to the diligent and systematic inquiry or investigation into a subject in order to discover facts or principles. Why include a chapter on research in a book dedicated to clinical practice? The simple answer is that research evidence provides a foundation for occupational therapy interventions. Occupational therapists who read, evaluate, and selectively apply the available evidence are able to offer service users access to current best practice. The results of individual studies and multistudy analyses help clinicians to better understand the conditions under which mental health may be achieved, to clarify the needs of persons with mental health disorders, to align interventions with empirical evidence, to more effectively evaluate outcomes, to advocate with clients, and to lobby for occupational therapy services.

A less obvious but potentially more important answer is that the state of research, specifically, how much research is available and what topics are being researched with whom, and how, informs occupational therapy clinicians and researchers about priorities and values within occupational therapy, in interdisciplinary mental health practice, and in society as a whole. Addressing mental health research in a book written to guide clinical practice tells therapists what questions are deemed to be important by those requesting and conducting research, and how occupational therapy researchers may perceive that those questions should be answered. It affirms for clinicians that their daily work is a form of research because it entails a process of discovering facts and applying principles that bring about change in people's lives. As evidence-based practitioners, occupational therapy clinicians are also research consumers. They are in the best position to determine which questions, viewpoints, or issues are not receiving attention in the research literature and what questions need to be answered that would build a solid evidence base for occupational therapy mental health practice. External drivers such as funders, policy makers, and research consortiums, however, tend to determine what research is conducted and its impact. The identification of research agendas, the allocation of research funding, and the interpretation and dissemination of research results tend to happen beyond the sphere of clinicians.

Being informed about the factors that influence the way external drivers operate and what information they need will help clinicians locate their practice as part of the research landscape.

The goal of this chapter is to describe the landscape within which the production and application of research in occupational therapy mental health practice occur. It argues that critical academic reflection lies at the heart of contextually relevant research. An exploration of the broader aspects of inquiry such as ways of thinking about the world within which practice unfolds will point readers toward the pre-conditions for innovative and socially engaged mental health occupational therapy research. Since each chapter in this book contains discussions of research evidence related to the specific topic, this chapter will not repeat these discussions. Various research methodologies are described in the body of occupational therapy research as well as other research literature and will not be addressed in this chapter (see the Suggested Resources at the end of the chapter). The aim is rather to guide the reader toward critical reflection about the value of research evidence and about the ideologies that inform what and how research is conducted. As the authors of this chapter we represent two distinct contexts: Silicon Valley, California, and the Western Cape of South Africa. We present our specific contextual challenges and experiences in the individual case discussions and reflections. Located in high and low income countries, the differences between our contexts are considerable, yet the core issues of socially responsible research in mental health are remarkably similar. We hope to illustrate how a global perspective in mental health research can be enacted by occupational therapists.

WHY DO RESEARCH? THE BURDEN OF MENTAL ILLNESS

Mental health research and program development has been a low priority relative to other types of health concerns in high and low income countries (Miller, 2006; Mitlin, 2005). However, the burden of disability created by mental health disorders is substantial and research is needed to identify ways of alleviating the impact of mental illness on society. Mental illness accounts for 12.3% of the global burden of disease and is estimated to rise to 15% by the year 2020 (World Health Organization [WHO], 2001). The WHO measures the total burden of disability in units called disability-adjusted life years (**DALYs**), representing the total number of years lost to illness, disability, or premature death within a given population. Neuropsychiatric disorders are the leading contributor to DALYs in North America, representing 28% of the total. This burden of disability is twice that of cardiovascular disease and cancer combined (National Institute of Mental Health [NIMH], n.d.[a]). Worldwide, depression is the third largest contributor to the total burden of disability, and it is the largest contributor in high income countries (WHO, 2008).

The burden of mental illness in low income countries is also substantial (Sharan et al., 2009). Miller (2006, p. 461), discussing the global incidence of mental illness, reports that "the majority of the world's 450 million people who suffer from neuropsychiatric disorders live in developing countries and that fewer than 10% of these people have access to treatment." Cross national surveys have shown that common mental disorders are about twice as frequent among the poor as among the rich in Brazil, Chile, India, and Zimbabwe (WHO, 2001). Poverty deprives humans of the essential opportunities and choices needed for individual, household, and community well-being and creates disabling social conditions, which may precipitate the onset of mental illness (Lund, Breen, Flisher, et al., 2007; Patel & Kleinman, 2003). Clearly the links between poverty and mental health warrant serious research attention. Baingagan (cited in Miller, p. 461), a Ugandan psychiatrist advising the WHO on mental health issues, warns that many officials and policy makers do not have enough evidence to recommend investments in mental health services in poorer countries. He suggests that ". . . convincing skeptics will require demonstrating the economic costs of untreated illness more clearly and countering the persistent view that a person with a mental disorder will never function at a normal level . . . [W]hen we show that people with neuropsychiatric disorders can be productive, then we will have greater interest." Occupational therapy, as a role player in public mental health systems concerned with human productivity through occupation, is in a position to contribute the kind of evidence that is being asked for by policy makers. A socially oriented research focus aimed at "meeting societal needs for health and well-being" (American Occupational Therapy Association, 2007, p. 614) will make this possible.

EVIDENCE-BASED PRACTICE

A socially oriented research focus will generate a different and wider evidence base for mental health occupational therapy practice—one that considers not only the clinical dimensions of mental disorders and therapeutic interventions but also the social conditions that precipitate and perpetuate mental illness such as the cultural, political, and economic influences on life course development. **Evidence-based practice** has been defined as the process of integrating critically appraised research evidence with the clinician's expertise and the values of the client (Sackett, Straus, Richardson, Rosenberg, & Haynes, 2000). In part, the process of evidence-based practice involves a systematic evaluation of the quality of research evidence. The widely used hierarchy of evidence used in the practice of medicine employs a five-point scale to rank the strength of evidence from various research designs, and guidelines for its use in occupational therapy have been discussed (Gutman, 2008; Lieberman & Scheer, 2002). However, the limitations of the five-point hierarchy of evidence have also been discussed within occupational therapy, as it fails to recognize the active engagement of the client in the intervention process and the diversity of evidence and knowledge brought by the client and therapist to the intervention context (Lee & Miller, 2003).

The neglect of qualitative research as evidence and the lack of attention to the role of professional reasoning in evidence-based practice have also been criticized (Rappolt, 2003). Tickle-Degnan and Bedell (2003) propose a heterarchal approach to evaluating evidence that uses flexible clinical reasoning based on analysis of a wide variety of research evidence integrated with other forms of knowledge and information.

The previous commentaries highlight that the less-discussed aspects of evidence-based practice—the therapist's practice experience; the client's preferences, beliefs, and needs; and the contextual factors that influence mental well-being—are also essential components of evidence-based practice. The less-discussed and critically important aspects of evidence-based practice pertain to the importance and value of gathering information from citizens including mental health service consumers about the social conditions that promote mental and physical well-being and those that precipitate, predispose, and perpetuate mental ill-being and illness. The need for additional research on beliefs, experiences, and perceptions of different populations is also implied (Richardson & MacRae, 2011; Rose, 2008).

The number and variety of evidence-based resources, in particular the quantity of reviews of multiple studies, such as **Critically Appraised Topics (CATs)**, **systematic reviews**, and **meta-analyses** are increasing. These reviews of multiple experimental studies typically address efficacy of interventions. Evidence for occupational science is also growing. As a multidisciplinary research discipline created by occupational therapy pioneers in North America in the 1980s to study humans as occupational beings (Clark, Parham, Carlson, et al., 1991), occupational science is advancing the profession's epistemological foundations for understanding human occupation in context. Table 3-1 contains web-based resources for evidence-based practice in mental health.

TABLE 3-1. Web-Based Resources for Evidence-Based Practice in Mental Health

Resource	Description
American Occupational Therapy Association: http://www.aota.org/ebp.aspx	Evidence-based practice resources for AOTA members.
Campbell Collaboration: http://www.campbellcollaboration.org	International research network that produces systematic reviews of the effects of social interventions in the areas of education, crime and justice, and social welfare.
Centre for Reviews and Dissemination, York University, UK: http://www.crd.york.ac.uk/CRDWeb/	Abstracts of systematic reviews of health and social care interventions and details of Cochrane reviews and protocols.
Cochrane Collaboration: http://www.cochrane.org	International network providing independent systematic reviews of health care interventions published online in the Cochrane Library.
Directory of Open Access Journals: http://www.doaj.org	International directory of open access online journals, including journals in health care and social sciences.

(Continues)

TABLE 3-1. Continued

Resource	Description
Google Scholar: http://scholar.google.com	Online searching and access to a broad range of scholarly journals.
Highwire Press: http://highwire.stanford.edu	Digital publisher of journals, reference works, books, and proceedings.
International Alliance for Child and Adolescent Mental Health and Schools: http://www.intercamhs.org/index.html	An international alliance that aims to promote the mental health and well-being of children and young people. The site contains numerous evidence-based resources.
National Registry of Evidence-Based Programs & Practices: http://www.nrepp.samhsa.gov	U.S. database of mental health and substance abuse interventions reviewed and rated by experts.
Occupational Therapy Critically Appraised Topics: http://www.otcats.com	Australian site with critically appraised topics on occupational therapy interventions; links to other evidence-based practice sites.
OT Evidence: http://www.otevidence.info	Canadian web portal to resources and information to support evidence-based practice in occupational therapy.
OT Seeker: http://www.otseeker.com	International database of abstracts of systematic reviews and randomized controlled trials relevant to occupational therapy.
Psychological Database for Brain Impairment Treatment Efficiency: http://www.psycbite.com	International database of studies of cognitive, behavioral, and other treatments for psychological issues occurring due to acquired brain impairment (ABI), rated for methodological quality.
PubMed Central: http://www.pubmedcentral.nih.gov	U.S. National Institutes of Health (NIH) free digital archive of biomedical and life sciences journal literature.
Research Centre for Occupation and Mental Health, York St. John University, UK: http://w3.yorksj.ac.uk/research/research-centres/rcomh.aspx	International research center with the mission to develop world class research in occupation and mental health to influence best practice.
Substance Abuse and Mental Health Services Administration (SAMHSA): http://www.samhsa.gov	U.S. site with a variety of resources for professionals, consumers, and the public.
U.S. Department of Veterans Affairs Center of Excellence on Implementing Evidence Based Practice (CIEBP): http://www.ciebp.research.va.gov/CIEBP/index.asp	U.S. site with information on sponsored research projects aimed at improving health care service delivery.
World Health Organization (WHO) Mental Health Evidence and Research: http://www.who.int/mental_health/evidence/en/	WHO site with information on WHO programs to increase the information and evidence base on mental health in order to strengthen mental health care systems.

RESEARCH PRIORITIES IN MENTAL HEALTH

In this section we review the research priorities identified by selected international and national bodies with the aim of highlighting the broader landscape within which mental health occupational therapy research is located. It points researchers in mental health occupational therapy to the kinds of information that they may contribute toward positioning the profession as a service resource for at-risk populations. For clinicians, this informs about current and emerging initiatives in research and how these research initiatives may influence best practice (Gutman, 2008). Current international and national research priorities reflect the need to understand the nature of mental health disorders and how these disorders affect people's lives and health status including the functioning of communities. Since disparities in access to mental health care are also widespread due to financial barriers, stigma, lack of coordinated and culturally appropriate systems of care, and lack of awareness, research initiatives also emphasize the development and provision of effective mental health services.

Mapping Mental Health Resources

Aiming to reduce the burden of mental disorders and to promote mental health as an important focus for government action, WHO has established initiatives to close the gap between identified mental health needs and available services worldwide. Specific projects include mapping mental health resources throughout the world, development of an instrument to collect information on the mental health systems of countries and regions, and generating resources and an evidence base for mental health intervention and psychosocial support in emergencies, including refugees, internally displaced persons, disaster survivors, and terrorism-, war-, or genocide-exposed populations (WHO, n.d.).

Identifying Grand Challenges

Led by the U. S. National Institute of Mental Health (NIMH) and the Global Alliance for Chronic Disease, in collaboration with other international partners, the Grand Challenges in Global Mental Health Initiative (GMHI) was launched in 2010 (GMHI, 2010). The aim of GMHI was to identify, through a **Delphi study** with expert respondents from across the globe, the top 10 challenges shaping the future of global mental health research. A grand challenge is a specific barrier that, if removed, would help to improve the lives of those affected by mental, neuropsychiatric, and substance use disorders. The goal of identifying these challenges is to ultimately develop interventions that, if successfully implemented, would have a high likelihood of feasibility for scaling up and impact (GMHI, 2010).

Although the outcome of the GMHI Delphi study was not yet available at the time of going to print, its value for occupational therapy mental health clinicians and researchers is the identification of nodal areas of action by the profession. It is likely that the identified top 10 challenges for global mental health research will generate dedicated funding from multiple sources as well as opportunities for interagency, interdisciplinary, and cross-national research collaborations. By designing studies that are aligned with or nested within the larger jigsaw puzzle of global-national knowledge and evidence construction, occupational therapy researchers are more likely to attract research partners, secure funding, and, in the longer term, make a contribution to social change.

Developing Interventions

In the United States, the NIMH has identified four strategic research priorities: (1) promote discovery in the brain and behavioral sciences to fuel research on the causes of mental disorders; (2) chart mental illness trajectories to determine when, where, and how to intervene; (3) develop new and better interventions that incorporate the diverse needs and circumstances of people with mental illnesses; and (4) strengthen the public health impact of NIMH-supported research (NIMH, n.d.[b]). These research priorities address a broad range of initiatives, from basic science research investigating the biological determinants of behavior, to the effects of mental health disorders on communities. The priorities also acknowledge how factors such as age, gender, culture, ethnicity, and geographic location can impact individuals' experience of mental health disorders and responsiveness to various intervention approaches. The NIMH research priorities extend over the life span, and in addition to the areas traditionally addressed in mental health practice they encompass other areas where occupational therapists are actively engaged, including infant mental health, school mental health, autism spectrum disorders, traumatic brain injury, domestic violence, substance abuse, homelessness, dementia, and Alzheimer's disease. These priorities illustrate the broad range of intrapersonal and contextual influences on mental health and the variety of contexts where intervention and research occur.

Using Translational Science

The developing field of translational developmental neuroscience has evolved from basic, translational, and clinical neuroscience, where research suggests that mental health disorders are trajectory-based and begin early in life. The NIMH recommends research collaboration between disciplines to improve the ability to identify individuals at risk for developing mental health disorders (National Advisory Mental Health Council's Workgroup, n.d.). The NIMH has also proposed increasing the amount of stakeholder input into development of clinical trials, increasing the number of community-focused interventions, and expanding the representation of historically underrepresented populations in clinical research (National Advisory Mental Health Council's Workgroup on Clinical Trials, n.d.). These research priorities confirm the contribution that investigations into the biological and clinical dimensions of performance component impairments and occupational performance dysfunction can make in interrupting the trajectory of mental illness.

Building Partnerships

The broad range of research priorities discussed here share some commonalities. These include the need for rigorous and well-designed intervention studies, improving assessment and measurement, longitudinal and descriptive studies, individualization and generalization of interventions, and collaborative involvement of various stakeholders, including individuals with mental health disorders, and families, clinicians, and local communities in the design and implementation of research. Such a broad scope of investigation will require the collaboration of scholars from various disciplines, thus placing occupational therapy research in an interdisciplinary context and hinting at the benefits of nesting the profession as a contributor to and stakeholder in national and international research consortiums.

RESEARCH PRIORITIES IN MENTAL HEALTH OCCUPATIONAL THERAPY

In this section we consider some of the national mental health research priorities, which have been identified by professional bodies. We then make some suggestions for broadening the scope of mental health research in occupational therapy by using the Complete State Model of Mental Health as a point of reference. This model, shown in Figure 3-1, presents both the subjective experiences of wellness with the presence of (illness) symptoms. This holistic, person-centered view of the experience of mental illness is not only consistent with a recovery perspective (discussed in Chapter 1), but also aligns with the occupational therapy perspective of understanding context, meaning and inclusion, as well as capitalizing on an individual's strengths to improve overall function.

Cost Benefit: Effectiveness and Efficacy

The American Occupational Therapy Association (AOTA) and American Occupational Therapy Foundation (AOTF) have identified people with mental disorders as one of six priority populations for intervention research (AOTA/AOTF, 2009). Priorities of intervention research include client-centered (individualized) interventions, occupation focused interventions, and basic research exploring the experience of disability for individuals and their families. "Recognizing that the science of occupational therapy practice is in its infancy, the priority is broadly defined to include preliminary work leading to efficacy (research under tightly controlled conditions) or effectiveness (research under real-world conditions) trials, that is, it includes "proof of concept" studies of interventions (including quantitative, qualitative, and mixed methodologies); pilot, feasibility studies of interventions; and, single-subject intervention studies" (AOTA/AOTF, p. 2). While the need for more research in occupational therapy in

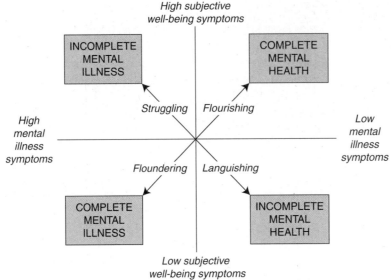

FIGURE 3-1. The Complete State of Mental Health
© Cengage Learning 2013

general is widely acknowledged, there has been concern expressed regarding the limited amount of research being conducted in the area of mental health (D'Amico, Jaffe, & Gibson, 2010). These authors contend that the viability of mental health practice in occupational therapy in the United States is dependent on producing evidence of the efficacy of our interventions.

Addressing the AOTA's Centennial Vision, D'Amico et al. (2010) ask occupational therapists to assume responsibility for defining occupational therapy in mental health and for demonstrating its effectiveness through research. They identify occupational therapy intervention effectiveness and efficacy as two major research gaps that warrant specific attention because these are the areas that "reimbursement sources and policy makers look at for allocating funds" (p. 668). Similar calls for research action aimed at affirming the cost-saving benefits of occupational therapy in mental health have gone out in Great Britain (Craik et al., 1998). The establishment of the Research Centre for Occupation and Mental Health (RCOMH) at York St. John University in 2010 (see Table 3-1) opens up the possibilities of nesting the profession within national and global mental health investigations. Acting as an international bridge for multisite research collaboration, the RCOMH aims to build evidence for occupational therapy intervention in core domains of mental health practice with a particular focus on occupation. A research agenda for mental health occupational therapy in South Africa has not yet been recommended by the Occupational Therapy Association of South Africa. Examples of research-led practice however include social transformation through occupation (Watson & Swartz,

2004); community-based psychosocial rehabilitation (Alers & Crouch, 2010); and the dynamic intersections between poverty, psychiatric disability, and occupation (Duncan & Watson, 2010).

Comprehensive Research Scope

A comprehensive scope of research priorities includes studies that focus on the promotion of mental health: the prevention of mental illness, the treatment of mental illness, and the rehabilitation of persons with psychiatric disability. Research may strengthen the medical model of health and disability with its emphasis on treatment and rehabilitation (e.g., Chan, Cardoso, & Chronister, 2009) or it may explore the social model of disability with its emphasis on the politics of difference, oppression, and marginalization (e.g., Barnes & Mercer, 2004). More importantly a comprehensive research agenda situates mental health at the center of individual and community well-being and therefore a pivotal dimension of research across the life span and across domains of practice including physical health, education, work, child learning and development, active aging, and community development.

The Complete State Model of Mental Health (Slade, 2009) provides a comprehensive schematic representation of potential domains of mental health research in occupational therapy. It represents mental health as a multidimensional phenomenon that interacts along two intersecting continuums: high and low subjective symptoms of well-being and high and low symptoms of mental illness. Situated in one of four quadrants, mental health status may be described as either floundering, struggling, languishing, or flourishing depending on the interaction between emotional, psychological, and social subjective well-being and the objective presence of high to low (or no) symptoms of mental illness (see Figure 3.1). With a particular focus on the study of occupational engagement and participation, the goal of mental health research in occupational therapy is twofold: to contribute to the body of knowledge in each of the four quadrants and toward understanding the systematic processes that predispose, precipitate, and perpetuate progressive or regressive transitions of mental health between the quadrants. The five categories for occupational therapy research (i.e., assessment/measurement, intervention, basic, translational, and health service) identified by the Occupational Therapy Research Agenda (AOTA/AOTF, 2009) can be applied within each quadrant and to answer research questions associated with the dynamic interactions between the two axes.

Role Emergent Research Areas

A comprehensive scope of research priorities moves mental health occupational therapy research beyond the individual clinical domain concerned with the treatment of psychiatric disorders into role-emerging practice domains concerned with public mental health and community development. A broader research landscape will require engagement with socioeconomic, sociocultural, political, and other theories concerned with the way society (as opposed to the individual) functions. Delivering the Eleanor Clarke Slagle lecture, Hasselkus (2006, p. 635) alerted occupational therapists to the impact of "cultural tendencies and invisible social forces" on occupation. Referring to Kronenberg et al. (2005) and Watson and Swartz (2004), she stated that:

> The writers of these texts are challenging us therapists as well as the occupational therapy profession more broadly to expand beyond the western ideologies of individualism and independence: beyond the medical model; beyond the traditional categories of work, leisure and self-maintenance. The aim is to reorientate occupational therapy away from its overwhelming focus at only the individual level and toward the social forces that affect whole communities and populations, so that we may act as catalysts for social transformation. (p. 635)

Defining, describing, and investigating new population-oriented research areas will enhance the potential and the realm of what occupational therapists might do to advance social transformation. A focus on social change will "extend the role and function of occupational therapy into community activities aimed to promote occupational engagement and participation of the total population and to prevent secondary conditions among those already living with disabling conditions. This (*role emergent*) area, also, is in its infancy in occupational therapy and requires efficacy and effectiveness studies, but may require a more population-based approach to methodology" (AOTA/AOTF, 2009, p. 2; italics added). Much research is still needed to address the gaps in our knowledge and evidence base for population- and community-oriented occupational therapy mental health practice. In examining occupational therapy interventions, the AOTA and AOTF (2009) propose that priority is given to interventions that are client centered, occupation based, theory driven, and activity focused. Some of the assumptions on which occupational therapy theories are based may need to be questioned and reframed for community action aimed at social transformation. For example, can population-based approaches be client centered (a construct that is informed by Western values of individualism)? Is occupation a universally understood and valued construct in multicultural communities? In which ways do structural and systemic forces influence what people are able to do every day? Some of these and other questions are being addressed in the growing body of occupational therapy literature, which provides examples of innovative work being done within and beyond traditional practice contexts (Pollard, Kronenberg, & Sakellariou, 2008; Kronenberg, Pollard, & Sakellariou, 2011). Irrespective of where individual clinicians, researchers, and research consortia position themselves within the research landscape, every piece of diligent and systematic inquiry matters because it contributes to the evidence base of the profession. There are benefits for research that focuses on the individual and on the societal level. Changes that are prompted through social intervention can impact opportunities at the individual level while individuals, in turn, can influence their communities and make a contribution to society.

Research Orientation

How could these suggested research priorities affect daily occupational therapy practice in the vast array of places where mental health occupational therapists work? Whether clinicians are doing formal research (i.e., a funded and ethics approved study) or are research consumers (i.e., evidence-based practitioners), they are ideally positioned to use research methodologies to document and publish their practice and, in so doing, contribute to the growing body of professional knowledge. We identify some implications and make recommendations for promoting a research orientation to everyday practice:

- Practice is constantly evolving and there may be little direct evidence to support specific interventions or limited opportunity to do formal, funded on-site research in the clinical practice environment. Continuing professional development paves the way for a research orientation to practice (Alsop, 2000). Clinicians could build a substantive body of locally relevant professional knowledge by articulating the theoretical approaches and reasoning processes that guide their actions and by documenting the specific interventions provided and the outcomes achieved.

- A commitment to staying up to date on chosen interventions and regularly communicating with colleagues regarding emerging research and client progress will hone critical thinking skills that form the basis of interpretive inquiry. Response to clinical intervention is individual; therefore learning as much as possible from and about individual clients will ensure that occupational therapists discover fresh insights into the factors that exacerbate or mitigate mental distress and gain understanding about the implications these factors have for the occupational human in context. This kind of learning is a valid form of inquiry, especially if discoveries and insights are systematically documented.

- The identification of assessment models, methods, and procedures that attend to both individual and contextual factors will go a long way toward creating a valid and reliable baseline for the documentation of practice-based inquiries (e.g., see Law, Baum, & Dunn, 2005; Rush, First, & Blacker, 2008). With society as a key site for occupation-based interventions, assessments and screening tools that identify the conditions that precipitate and perpetuate psychiatric disability are also indicated (e.g., see Miller & Bell, 2002).

- Collaboration is a key component of emerging research—with clients, families, colleagues, and communities. The collaborative focus speaks to the complexity of mental health disorders and the need for all stakeholders to contribute their specific knowledge and skill to intervention initiatives that address the broad range of factors that create and sustain these disorders. By developing collaborative inquiry relationships with a range of pertinent stakeholders, occupational therapists will create a platform for multifaceted knowledge construction and for applying the occupational core of the profession within a variety of contexts. To do so will create additional benefits such as making occupational therapy known to a wider funding and research audience while marketing occupational therapy as a contributing component of public mental health programs and services.

THINKING IN RESEARCH

In the preceding section we discussed mental health occupational therapy research priorities including international research agendas and role-emerging practice areas. Identifying the focus of occupational therapy research usually emanates from two key questions: What do occupational therapists perceive current research needs in mental health practice to be, and which methodological approaches best facilitate the exploration of these needs? There are many ways of answering these questions as the preceding section of the chapter illustrates. We suggest the inclusion of a reflective step before engaging with these two important strategic questions. Our suggestion is based on the conceptual implications of embracing a comprehensive scope of research and of engaging in socially transformative, population-based practice. Taken-for-granted ideas in occupational therapy may need to be reconsidered as emerging domains of practice and inquiry open up. Assuming that population-based practice and research involves "business as usual" (i.e., the translocation of clinical intervention methods and clinical reasoning from clinical to social settings) will be to miss the point of transformation. A distinctly different reasoning process is indicated, one that consciously foregrounds social dynamics and processes of power and the politics of participation. In this section we discuss how all research action is informed by an ideological position and argue that best practice occupational therapy mental health research in emergent settings will be promoted with critical, reflexive, and ethical thinking.

Ways of Thinking

All research is framed, whether consciously or unconsciously, within a paradigm, which may be defined as a network of coherent ideas about the nature of the world. A paradigm consists of a number of building blocks that enable the researcher to clarify his or her ideological position in relation to a set of questions about how reality is understood. A paradigm provides a broad coherent framework of perceptions, understandings, and beliefs within which theories and practices operate. The network of coherent ideas within a paradigm comes from three interconnected building blocks: ontology, epistemology, and methodology. Figure 3-2 depicts the building blocks within a research paradigm. **Ontology** is concerned with being in the world and reflects worldviews including claims and assumptions about the nature of reality. It asks and answers questions such as: "How do you look at reality?" and "What's out there to know?" **Epistemology** is concerned with the origin, nature, methods, and limits of knowledge. It captures the image of social reality upon which theory, concepts, constructs, and models are based and seeks to answer questions such as: "What can we know?" and "How can we know?" Methodology provides the coherent structure for systematic and rigorous inquiry. Consisting of principles that guide how research action should unfold, methodology answers the question: "How can we go about acquiring knowledge?" Once this question is

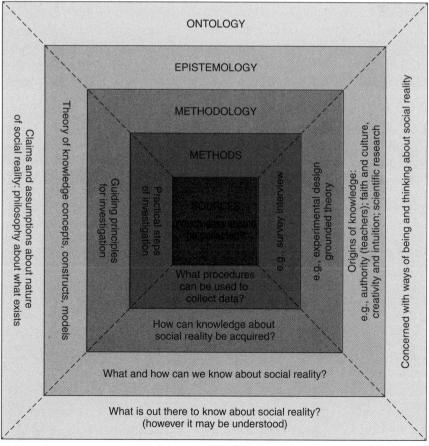

FIGURE 3-2. The Building Blocks of the Research Design
© Cengage Learning 2013

answered, the most suitable methods and sources for gathering information (data) can be identified by asking the following questions: "What procedures can be used to collect information (e.g., surveys, interviews, assessment instruments)" and "Which data can we collect (e.g., which people or materials such as documents will provide the information we are looking for)?"

Table 3-2 provides an example of two research paradigms. A qualitative research paradigm is concerned with understanding the views of informants. It unfolds in natural settings and builds a complex, holistic picture, formed with words, of a social or human problem (Cresswell, 1994). Alternatively, a quantitative study, consistent with the quantitative paradigm, is an inquiry into a social or human problem, based on testing a theory composed of variables, measured with numbers, and analyzed with statistical procedures, in order to determine whether the predictive generalizations of the theory hold true (Creswell, 1994).

In thinking about the design of a study, it is important to remember that some research may require a moral-political orientation on the part of the researcher. Such a thinking position sees research as a mechanism for effecting social change and not primarily as a mechanism for gathering information. There are ideological positions, which inform how the questions about design may be approached. The identification of a research problem and the purpose of the

TABLE 3-2. Examples of Research Paradigms

	Quantitative	Qualitative
Ontology	Scientific materialism (nature of reality can be objectified)	Scientific constructivism (nature of reality is constantly changing)
Epistemology	Positivism (theories describe laws and causal relationships within reality)	Relativism (theories describe multi-constructed realities)
Methodology	Deductive reasoning that focuses on objective, measurable, and observable proof	Inductive reasoning that focuses on subjective and non-deterministic understanding of social reality
	'Truth' about social reality can be reliably and validly determined by breaking the whole down into units for measurement	Plausible patterns of 'truths' emerge by considering the complexity of the whole
Methods	Focus on numbers (mathematical and statistical)	Focus on words, ideas, and concepts
	e.g., epidemiological surveys; randomized control trials, descriptive statistics	e.g., grounded theory, case studies, ethnography
Sources	Statistically significant sample sizes within populations	Single or multiple cases

study may reflect the values of the profession and be influenced by prevailing sociopolitical ideologies. For example, following the demise of apartheid in South Africa in 1994, the National Health Service adopted the primary health care approach as the fundamental guiding philosophy for policy development and implementation. As a signatory of the Declaration of Alma Ata (WHO, 1978), the South African government is committed to positioning health as a fundamental human right and to addressing the gross inequality in the health status of previously politically oppressed people. Primary health care is "essential health care based on practical, scientifically sound and socially acceptable methods and technology made accessible to individuals and families through their full participation and at a cost that the community and country can afford to maintain at every stage of their development in the spirit of self reliance and self-determination" (WHO, p. 1). What primary health care in effect entails is an ideological reorientation from health care as biomedical intervention to health care as social development. Aligning occupational therapy practice and research with the primary health care approach has presented the profession in South Africa with an array of moral-political challenges not least its contribution to the alleviation of a range of human poverties associated with a racist social history (Watson & Swartz, 2004). The paradigmatic reorientation of occupational therapy is still unfolding. It has not been easy because public mental health occupational therapy services were historically based on the medical model, located in psychiatric institutions and guided by Eurocentric ontology and epistemology. By recognizing the role that research can play in effecting social change, occupational therapy research in the public health sector is being guided by the political and philosophical tenets of the Declaration of Alma Ata and other policy drivers such as the Universal Declaration of Human Rights (United Nations, 1948).

In the United States, mental health services have historically resided within both the social and medical models of health. Social movements such as the moral treatment movement in the nineteenth century and the deinstitutionalization movement of the twentieth century were driven by beliefs that people with mental health disorders deserved respectful treatment and social inclusion (see Chapter 4 for further discussion). In practice, however, funding sources have been the primary driver of the availability and access to services. As a result, the most consistent and available source of funding for both clinical services and research has been through the medical establishment. To some extent this has dictated where and how occupational therapy services are provided. With roots in the progressive treatment movement, the core values and practices of occupational therapy align most readily with socially based mental health services. However, variable and inconsistent funding for community-based social programs as well as a strong alignment with the medical model has shifted American occupational therapy mental health intervention into primarily medically based services narrowly focused on acute intervention and symptom alleviation. Occupational therapy has not found a clear and identifiable role in community-based mental health practice, which has impacted its visibility and therefore availability of funding for intervention and research. A current challenge for American occupational therapists engaged in research and intervention in mental health is how to recapture the social vision of the founders and expand the scope of intervention to align with national and international research priorities for broader and more contextually focused services. Clear documentation of a broad range of outcomes of community-based interventions and of the specific contribution of occupational therapy to these outcomes will enhance the evidence base of the profession and contribute to interdisciplinary best practices. Different but equally pressing moral-political challenges face the profession in other social contexts and each country will have a range of policy drivers, which guide how research action is framed. Figure 3-3 illustrates some of the peripheral factors that may need to be thought about before designing a study. Peripheral to the research paradigm, these and other factors influence the direction that a study may take, the

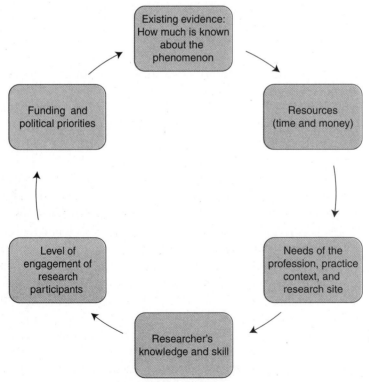

FIGURE 3-3. Peripheral Factors in Research Design
© Cengage Learning 2013

paradigm best suited to its purposes, and the impact that it may have in meeting identified research priorities.

Questioning Conventions

While the nature of the research problem determines the methodology best suited to achieving the research purpose and answering the related research questions, the ideological debate (i.e., about paradigm, ontology, epistemology, and methodology) is a place where researchers "think through what is going on in the discipline" and where we elaborate theoretical work that will enable us to take some distance from occupational therapy and "produce a different kind of knowledge in a different way" (Parker, 2005, p. 1). Is our research task to legitimize the way we have come to do things in mental health occupational therapy or the way occupational therapists think about the world and people with mental health concerns or is our professional task to keep in mind the sociopolitical impetus and effects of our work? A focus on finding out what is wrong with people and with determining the efficacy of occupational therapy interventions used to put things right so that funding is attracted, which ensures people are served better in the short term (and in so doing affirm the profession's role in mental health and psychiatry), must be balanced with a focus on research agendas that may have greater impact on society and demonstrate the transformative value of occupational therapy in the longer term. In short, what motivates a research agenda? Is it the survival of the profession by proving its cost benefits within the medical model or social change by using our collective research power to understand and address the occupational implications of social conditions (e.g., poverty, homelessness, gender oppression, and violence), which precipitate and perpetuate mental ill-being? The research landscape described earlier in this chapter accommodates both these and other research agendas. Irrespective of where the research agenda is located, the socially responsible task of the investigator or researcher as change agent is to become aware of ideological and attitudinal barriers that may curtail the effective engagement with the people they seek to learn with and from during the research endeavor by questioning conventional ways of thinking and practicing, for example, automatically slipping into diagnostic, "fix-it" or "do-something" mode in a community setting. Socially transformative research will require reflexive engagement with issues of power, position, and privilege (Nabudere, 2006). The conventions of therapeutic practice may have to be bracketed so that conventions suited to a particular community and its social development objectives are privileged. Richardson and MacRae (2011) suggest that occupational therapists who engage in research that can contribute to social change will possess a wide range of content and process knowledge, as well as interpersonal and performance skills. Knowing how to apply a reflexive research stance is a useful performance skill with inter- and intraper-sonal benefits within the research context. Reflexivity is "a way of working with subjectivity in such a way that we are able to break out of the self-referential circle that characterizes most academic work" (Parker, 2005, p. 25). Figures 3-4 and 3-5 describe two researchers' thought processes in integrating these skills and knowl-edge in developing a reflexive research stance and in conducting practice-based action research.

Checking Assumptions

Professional theories come to have meaning and are perceived to work because they are repeated so many times. Assumptions about what is considered "true" are trans-mitted so effectively that they acquire the status of common sense and are then used to frame the standpoint from which occupational therapy researchers seek to prove the efficacy of their interventions. Occupational therapists are, as Hammell (2009) suggests, vividly invested in our own conventional rhetoric. Perceived to be "true," theories about human occupation and occupational performance are formed by the very practices through which they are known. This does not mean we should reject the "regimes of truth" (Parker, 2005, p. 3) on which occupational therapy epistemology is grounded. What it does mean is that we recognize that no standpoint is truly objec-tive and value-free and that a radical, reflexive research agenda will help occupational therapy researchers interrogate the sociopolitical implications of self-referential rhetoric. Research that enables the free and critical interchange of divergent stand-points rather than the impositions of fixed standards is likely to have a greater impact in effecting social change. In short, the ways in which we produce and disseminate knowledge are as important as the things we think we have discovered or need to investigate.

Hammell (2009) challenges the beliefs and assumptions inherent in occupa-tional therapy and unmasks some of the taken-for-granted interpretations we make about the human experience. For example:

- Occupation and meaning are not universally linked. Choice, control, mastery, and self-efficacy are not outcomes that may be valued when gender, ability, caste, class, ethnicity, religion, and other features of diversity are considered. If the goal is to demonstrate the mental health benefits of participation in "meaningful" occupation, then the research endeavor must span all forms of evidence including those that emanate from the perspectives of people on the margins of society. The construct "meaningful" is, for example, infused with assumptions about what people value and how they spend their time. As Parker (2005) reminds us, knowledge is always different for the powerful than it is for the oppressed.

CONTEXT: This is an excerpt from a research journal kept during a longitudinal, mixed method research project that investigated the relationship between chronic poverty, psychiatric disability, and occupation (PDO) in peri-urban informal settlements in Cape Town, South Africa, where the majority of the population are *isiXhosa*-speaking people. Informal settlements typically consist of dwellings constructed from corrugated iron, plastic sheeting, and cardboard serviced by communal toilets and taps.

EXCERPT: *As an outsider my search for a vestige of truth about the complex human relations and occupational practices of individuals living with serious and enduring mental health problems in the context of structural and chronic poverty has been, for me, a constant disjunction between the demands for a scholarly implementation of Western constructions of methodology on the one hand and on the other hand, a commitment to let informants speak for themselves through the creation of ideas and statements about their lived experiences. This commitment is in fact an impossible task because, irrespective of my post-structuralist intentions, I remain psychologically bound by modernist perspectives about the rational, self-reflexive 'individual' who is able to give an unmediated account of themselves and 'voice' to their subjective experiences. Alldred and Gillies (2002) refer to this subject/object split as "the impossibility of escaping understandings through which we are ourselves formed" (p. 147). The ideal of emancipating the 'Other' through the outcome of scientific research "is as much a reflection of ideology as it is of academic training" (Smith, 1999, p. 2). It would be naïve to assume that I could embody the ideals of implementing decolonising research methodology or be a representative of the 'ways of knowing and being' of people who inhabit a world completely outside my frame of reference. At stake was research as a site of struggle between the hegemony and ways of knowing of a Western 'knowledgeable expert'; 'able bodied', bi-lingual (English and Afrikaans), middle class White women and the interests, experiences and ways of resisting by the 'Other': black African, isiXhosa-speaking, mentally ill individuals and their chronically poor households living on the margins of an inequitable (South African) society. This demography matches that of mental health practitioners and service users in South Africa, making cultural difference a constant site of contestation between different worldviews (Swartz, 1998). My articulation of difference here is intricately embedded in racialized, class and gendered discourses which Foucault (1972) [Foucault, 1980] argues are the consequences of Western experiences under imperialism. He suggests that race, gender, class and ability distinctions and hierarchies are so deeply encoded in Western languages, cultural archives and research paradigms that the West itself (and by inference myself and I) cannot discern its tacit 'rules of practice' because it operates within and through such rules and therefore takes them for granted. According to Smith (1999) Western theories and rules of research "are underpinned by a cultural system of classification and representation, by views of human nature, human morality and virtue, by conceptions of time and space, by conceptions of gender and race. Ideas about these things help determine what counts as real" (p. 44). How could I discover, as an outsider, what the research participants counted as 'real' when I was bound not only by the rules of systematized knowledge that scientific and academic debate in the West*

(Continues)

FIGURE 3-4. Outsider-Insider: Rationale for a Reflexive Research Stance: Madeleine Duncan

requires but also by a cultural 'force-field that unconsciously screens out competing and oppositional discourses' (Smith, 1999, p. 47). How could I, for example, minimise the possibility that my observations and interpretations would inadvertently resonate with views about the occupational human based on Western notions of time, space and subjectivity? The challenge was to use methodology that would enable me to think about what things mean, why things happen and about the different ways in which the world can be understood in order to contribute to social change. In short, how could I come to know responsibly?

STEPS: Knowing responsibly is an attitude of knowing that you don't know and being willing to unlearn what you think you know. Parker (2005) proposes four dimensions that, if interrogated regularly throughout the research process, will promote socially transformative research: first person confessions (i.e., being transparent about personal assumptions and biases, etc.), second person social positions (acknowledging how social features of difference such as gender and race influence thought and action), third person theorizing (i.e., adopting a critical perspective of taken for granted ideas), and a fourth dimension of crafting a report that foregrounds instances of disjunction (i.e., writing about things that were difficult or that make us uncomfortable).

FIGURE 3-4. Outsider-Insider: Rationale for a Reflexive Research Stance: Madeleine Duncan (*continued*)

CONTEXT: Hired as an occupational therapy consultant in a new residential program aimed at preparing young adults with Asperger's syndrome for success in college and independent living, I was asked to teach a class in sensory integration and to design and monitor individual sensory diets for the students. While research evidence documents the effects of sensory processing disorders on children with autism spectrum disorders, I had little research or clinical evidence to guide me in knowing how sensory processing affects the lives of adults with these disorders and how best to address it with these students. I began by blending didactic presentation of sensory integration concepts with experiential sensory activities, with mixed success. I found that while an understanding of one's sensory processing provided some benefit, many students also experienced depression, anxiety, attention deficit, or executive function disorder, which combined to make success in their daily occupations elusive. I questioned whether a focus on sensory processing was the best way to approach the broad range of challenges they experienced.

STEPS: I reflected on the occupational core of the students' lives, asking myself what I could do to help them have more success and satisfaction with their current occupations while preparing them for success in future occupations. In both group and individual sessions I asked them about their daily routines and listened carefully to their answers. This informal data collection revealed two key themes: Students were overwhelmed by their daily schedules, and they felt powerless in making decisions about their present and future occupations. Many of them actively resisted participating in various aspects of their program. Discussions with staff and parents uncovered concerns regarding students' ability to make responsible decisions and to meet participation expectations for the program. How could I respect everyone's valid concerns while creating opportunities for students develop a sense of ownership and competence in managing their lives? I read about and attended workshops on executive function disorder and motivation. I reflected on this information and the importance of self-generated action to motivation and growth. Finally, I reflected that an inadvertent message I may have been sending to the students was that they needed to be "fixed." I refocused the class on self-management and coping strategies, reminding the students that this was in the service of enabling them to be able to do the things they needed and wanted to do every day. Use of sensory strategies was still a part of the class, but it was blended with mindfulness practice and specific strategies to deal with anxiety and feelings of being overwhelmed. The concepts of awareness and acceptance, central to mindfulness practice, became the theme for the class. Students' specific areas of knowledge and interest were woven into class activities. A group of students whose preference was to avoid social sharing and resist behavioral change slowly began to challenge themselves in these areas and their internal self-direction began to grow. This process is reflective of Schön's (1995) epistemology of a new form of scholarship; a culture of inquiry about practice that involves negotiating personal and social meanings rather than focusing on measurement of outcomes (McNiff & Whitehead, 2006).

FIGURE 3-5. Action Research Transforming Practice: Pamela Richardson
© Cengage Learning 2013

- Entrenched in occupational therapy models is the categorization of occupation into what Hammell (2009) refers to as the privileged triad of self-care, work, and play. She points out that the assumption that so-called "balance of occupation" is essential for well-being will be difficult to defend in some contexts where leisure and work are not culturally divisible. The individualism promulgated by this privileged triad differs from the indivisible use of time in collectivist societies.

- The assumption that a positive relationship exists between occupation and health warrants particular mention. This assumption has little research evidence to support it. The definitions of both health and occupation are contestable, and need to be further explored with people who have had different experiences with and perspectives on these constructs. Figure 3-6 illustrates a researcher's process of checking assumptions with regard to a different way of understanding.

Valuing Research Integrity

Thinking about research ethics should not end once "ethics approval" has been granted by an ethics review board because "this can obscure the need to continually reflect on the ethical implications of researching people's lives" (Miller & Bell, 2002, p. 54). Research ethics are fraught with ambiguity, conflicting interests, fine lines, judgment calls, and awkward decisions (Duncan & Watson, 2010). Social inquirers can be blithely unaware, simply uncaring, or reflectively deliberate in thinking through the ways in which their everyday treatment of others (research participants) is intimately linked to wider social forces (Parker, 2005). Morality in research cannot be separated from the politics of power which, according to Parker (2005),

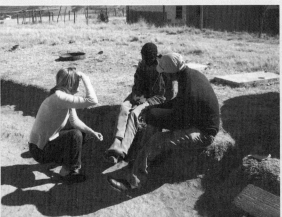

During a research trip investigating the dynamic relationship between chronic poverty, disability, and human occupation in a remote rural region of South Africa, we met a mute and unkempt young man wandering around a local village. We traced a relative who told us that he was doing well at school until he become mentally ill after the unexpected death of his parents two years previously. He was unable to apply for a disability grant because he did not have a birth certificate. The household did not know about mental health care at the local primary health care clinic and relied on traditional healers for advice.

Swartz (1998) reminds us that it is a cultural construction to consider mental health a health as opposed to social, political, or cultural issue. He states that "diagnosis in African indigenous healing may be better understood as related to theories of causation of illness rather than simply to taxonomies" (for example, *DSM-IV-R* diagnostic categories). African ideas about causation of illness (and by inference impairments and disability emanating from such illness) relate to a range of influences in the natural, social, personal, spiritual, and political realms. Cultural explanations for any illness and eventual diagnosis usually rest on four key questions: "Which sickness is it? How has it happened? Who or what produced it? and Why did it occur at this moment in this individual?" (Swartz). These questions may, in African healing systems, be answered through the intervention of traditional healers, ancestors, and shades. "Traditional beliefs permeate every aspect of African life, there is little distinction between secular and sacred, material and spiritual. Where you meet the African, there you will find his religion: in a field harvesting maize; at a funeral ceremony; in the market place. Far from being confined to a church or mosque once a week on a Friday or Sunday, the traditional African's religion embraces his whole environment: his entire time on earth and beyond" (Holland, 2001, p. xiv).

Occupation, considered from this perspective, cannot be categorized into self-care, work, or leisure; categories that assume time use is linked to individual preference and choice. In this context, occupation is shaped by structural poverty (dysfunctional governance, lack of infrastructure such as electricity, potable water, schools, jobs, etc.) and informed by a community of beings (ancestors and shades) that operate within different realms of reality and time.

FIGURE 3-6. Checking Assumptions: A Different Way of Understanding

means attending to the political issues that straddle the gap between anticipation and reflection. He suggests that the moral imperatives for ethics is, first, *transparency* about what transpires between the means and ends of the research process, second, *representation* of "others" using language that has been carefully considered for its political consequences, and, third, using *reflexivity* as a way of managing the subjectivity of the researcher and the dialectical (contradictory and mutually implicative) relationship between the researcher and the researched. Ethical processes and principles such as informed consent, confidentiality, beneficence, and anonymity become a series of moral choices that have to be made in the moment during every research encounter. Research integrity can be practiced through the simple edicts proposed by Silverman (2010): do no harm, do not cheat, respect difference, and withhold judgment.

METHODOLOGICAL POSITIONS

In the preceding section we discussed various aspects of research that warrant thinking about how to promote socially transformative professional action: paradigms, conventions, assumptions, and ethics. In this section we briefly discuss the notion of "truth" and argue that methodology is ultimately about whether the research results, findings or outcomes are accountable to the audiences involved.

Fit for Purpose

No single methodological approach, whether quantitative, qualitative, or mixed, is superior to another in developing health care knowledge. Each methodological approach is selected to fit a particular purpose. If the goal of mental health research is to predict or control factors that influence mental health problems a post-positive quantitative approach may be appropriate. Critical theory approaches are beneficial to understand mental health experiences where the aim is emancipation in circumstances of oppression. Pragmatism is an alternative approach that can be used when research problems do not align exclusively with a single paradigm. Multiple research methodologies and approaches are needed to develop the holistic knowledge necessary to answer the array of research priorities alluded to earlier in this chapter. Goodness of fit is facilitated by recognizing the strengths and limitations of different methodologies.

What, for example, may the implications be for mental health occupational therapists as social scientists of positioning their research, and by inference their art and science, external to the workings of power and politics? Does a knowable "occupational being" exist and is it possible to be discover "objective," universal intervention processes that guarantee positive outcomes when applied under controlled circumstances? Does the "correct" method or choice of instrument really produce a guarantee of "truth" and whose "truth" is being discovered, described, or reinforced?

Smith (1999, p. 47), writing about colonizing research and its impact on indigenous peoples, calls the mind trained by Western notions of reality a "force-field that unconsciously screens out competing and oppositional discourses." She argues that Western theories and rules of research "are underpinned by a cultural system of classification and representation, by views of human nature, human morality and virtue, by conceptions of time and space, by conceptions of gender and race. Ideas about these things help determine what counts as real" (p. 44). Herein lies the paradox of science: on the one hand it seduces us with the promise of progress and on the other hand it reduces our commitment to the affirmation of human diversity.

Numbers and Experience

The knowledge industry, toward which most research is geared, is expansive and overwhelming. An electronic database search using terms such as "rating scale," "child [or other focus] psychiatry," and "functioning" is likely to yield an astonishing number and range of standardized instruments. Handbooks also abound that provide occupational therapists with an array of tools for measuring change and establishing the efficacy of intervention (Baer & Blais, 2010; Hemphill, 2008; Law et al., 2005; McDowell, 2006; Rush et al., 2008). There is, however, no evidence showing any available scale to be a "gold standard" yardstick for demonstrating treatment efficacy or discovering an absolute truth about any human condition including mental illness. Too little is known about the real world reliability and predictive validity of measures to allow them to replace the judgement of experienced clinicians (Baer & Blais).

Statistical knowledge is open to change and reinterpretation despite the belief that numbers can provide an absolute, unchanging "truth," which can be discovered through sound and rigorous study. The hypothetic-deductive model of science stands in contrast to the social constructionist version of "truth" as being multiple and constantly in flux (Macleod, 2004). Statistics, as representations of the world, reflect material that has been identified and measured; material that has been infused with choices made by the investigator about the way the world should be divided up. The mathematical theories of representation that support statistics are themselves the product of certain sets of social circumstances and political agendas (e.g., the idea of "normal distribution" contains assumptions about the human qualities being described and the notions of validity and reliability are based on assumptions about the importance of consistency and rationality) (Parker, 2005). In short, the basic assumptions of positivist research should be challenged because, by couching its processes and procedures in universalizing, "apolitical" scientific terms, it serves as a legitimating tool for exclusionary or discriminatory practices (Macleod).

Treatment (i.e., clinical intervention) in occupational therapy is directed as much at symptom reduction as it is at improved functioning, returning the person to valued life roles and a host of other outcomes related to occupational performance, well-being, and quality of life. To obtain a valid assessment of treatment efficacy, all of these areas might need to be assessed and the time frame might need to be measured in months and even years. Although short-term functional improvements may be favored by those paying for care, the most necessary and meaningful changes may be harder (and take longer) to measure (Baer & Blais, 2010). The choice of efficacy measures is therefore very difficult because occupational therapy is contextually and relationally embedded. Therefore, "meaningful variables" for measurement should highlight clinical, social, and structural effects. In short, research on the outcomes of intervention needs to attend as much to the context in which knowledge is produced as it does to the relationship between the researcher and the researched and to changes effected within (and by) the person participating in an occupational therapy process.

RESEARCH EXAMPLES: LEARNING FROM OTHERS

In this section we present examples of how research can be conducted and applied in a variety of contexts (Figures 3-7 through 3-9). The common characteristic of these vignettes is the emphasis on collaboration for social change. Each vignette is followed by a set of questions that will enable an integration of material covered in the chapter.

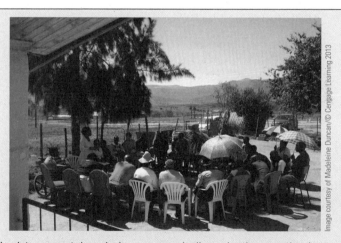

Image courtesy of Madeleine Duncan/© Cengage Learning 2013

CONTEXT: This picture was taken during a research dissemination meeting in a rural African village. Entry into the community occurred with permission from tribal elders to visit households with a disabled member including persons with mental illness. The community health workers who accompanied the research team in this area did not have any training in mental health and community members held traditional beliefs

(Continues)

FIGURE 3-7. Locating Knowledge Construction
© Cengage Learning 2013

about the causes of mental illness. An action research approach was adopted with the aim of generating social awareness about the rights of psychiatrically disabled people.

APPROACH: Action research combines the process of social reform with investigation. Conscious that all forms of research involve power, it puts social change on the agenda irrespective of the methodology being used. Action research is not a method but an approach to investigation that transforms research into a prefigurative political practice aimed at learning about both the freedom of movement to create progressive social forms and about the constraints that the present order imposes (Kagan & Burton, 2000; Parker, 2005). Methods and topics emerge during action research; ideas and processes are discovered and adapted as coresearchers determine the issues that are of relevance to them. A growing tradition of participatory action research exists among occupational therapists across the globe paving the way for increased critical engagement with the politics of development practice as an alternative research domain for occupational therapists and occupational scientists (Kronenberg, Pollard, & Sakellariou, 2011; Watson & Swartz, 2004).

QUESTIONS:

- What contribution could action research make in addressing the burden of mental illness in high and low income countries?

- Considering the comprehensive scope of mental health occupational therapy research, which quadrant of the Comprehensive State Model of Mental Health (Slade, 2009) would this scenario fit into and why?

- Which mental health occupational therapy conventions and assumptions may need to be revisited before commencing research in this context?

FIGURE 3-7. Locating Knowledge Construction (*continued*)

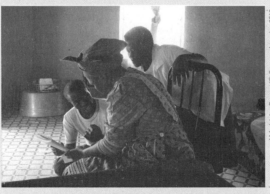

Image courtesy of Madeleine Duncan/© Cengage Learning 2013

CONTEXT: Here a researcher (kneeling) is talking to the mother of a mentally ill child in a remote rural village. As a research participant she contributed valuable information on the needs of persons with mental illness in underresourced contexts. In reciprocation, the researcher is explaining the role of medication in recovery. A community rehabilitation worker listens attentively, gathering information for dissemination to other people in the community.

APPROACH: Research is inextricably linked to politics. Its processes, relationships, ideological content, and theoretical approaches are all implicated by the distribution of power linked to wider social forces. Irrespective of whether these forces are managed statistically or through methodological and ethical rigor, a critical analysis of the patterns of privilege, the relation between the powerful and the powerless, the structural position through which certain people have access to resources and others do not, the contradictory and mutual implicative (dialectical) quality of knowledge that is shared between the researcher and the researched all present contradictory and contestable versions of truth (Parker, 2005). Research as a moral-political activity must attend to the relationships through which knowledge is produced and what we do with what we have found. Action research is not about producing knowledge but about the explicating way that knowledge is produced and about being clear about who the knowledge is for (Macleod, 2004). Smith (1999, p. 10), in discussing the politics of colonizing research, suggests that the questions to be asked by communities and activists who are approached by social researchers should include: "Whose research is it? Who owns it? Whose interests does it serve? Who will benefit from it? Who has designed its questions and framed its scope? Who will carry it out? Who will write it up? How will its results be disseminated?"

QUESTIONS:

- In what ways may evidence-based practice promote the effectiveness of psychoeducation as a strategy in psychosocial rehabilitation?

- What ethics are involved with the dissemination of research findings?

- What methodologies could be considered to gather information about the needs of persons with mental illness in under resourced contexts?

FIGURE 3-8. Psychoeducation as Research Reciprocity
© Cengage Learning 2013

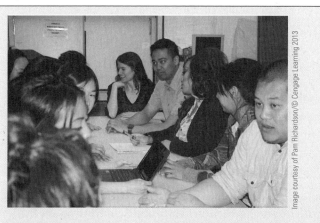

Image courtesy of Pam Richardson/© Cengage Learning 2013

(Continues)

FIGURE 3-9. A Participatory Research Approach to Program Development
© Cengage Learning 2013

CONTEXT: Here a group of occupational therapy graduate students meets with college students who are former foster youth to select topics for independent living skills (ILS) workshops that will be designed and taught collaboratively.

APPROACH: The idea for the workshops arose from an inquiry into the experiences, outcomes, and needs of young people who had "aged out" of the foster care system upon reaching the age of 18. This research took the form of a comprehensive review of the literature on the outcomes of former foster youth, collection of data on the characteristics of ILS programs in the region, and a focus group study with former foster youth exploring their experiences in receiving ILS services. The findings of our small local studies were in line with larger research studies in identifying systemic problems in the design and pedagogy of ILS programs and in the appropriateness and availability of the programs for young people in foster care. Based on these findings we identified a group of former foster youth who had experienced success since aging out of foster care (i.e., had been admitted to a four-year university) who could help us to identify ILS topics that would benefit them and also educate us as to the best way to conduct the workshops. The three workshop topics identified by the student participants (driver's license and car care, healthy shopping and cooking on a college budget, and planning a trip) represented living skills that were meaningful and immediately useful to them. Through the teaching process the workshop modules were collaboratively refined into informational packages that were put onto a website we developed for this purpose. Ongoing work will result in the development of additional modules and teaching methods, with long-term goals of adapting modules for ILS programs for adolescents currently in foster care. Former foster youth will take a leadership role in developing and teaching modules.

QUESTIONS:

- How did this method of program development influence the participation of the former foster youth in this program?

- What is the role of the occupational therapist in a participatory program development model?

- How should program outcomes be selected and measured?

FIGURE 3-9. A Participatory Research Approach to Program Development (*continued*)

THE WAY FORWARD

Having provided some research scenarios to introduce the idea of critical thinking in research, we now draw the chapter to a close by proposing that implementation science and human scale development provide two directions for the way forward.

Making Local-Global Research Links

The new field of global mental health involves a large body of cross-cultural research concerned with improving mental health and achieving equity in mental health for all people worldwide. A core focus in global mental health is related to both reducing the overall burden of health conditions (i.e., effectiveness) and reducing and, ultimately, eliminating health inequalities within and between countries. In addition, the term "global" refers to global influences on mental health (e.g., cross-national factors such as climate change or macroeconomic policies). The responsibility for improving global mental health transcends national borders, class, race, gender, ethnicity, and culture; its promotion requires collective action based on global partnerships.

Premised on the twin principles of scientific evidence and human rights, global mental health aims to reduce the disparity in provision of services for persons living with mental disorders in rich and poor countries. Low and middle income countries are home to more than 80% of the global population but demand less than 20% of the share of available mental health resources (Patel & Prince, 2010). There are also many underserved populations in high and middle income countries where packages of care have already been identified but little is known about how these need be delivered. Much attention needs to be directed to the implementation science. It is at this junction that occupational therapists are likely to make their greatest contribution to knowledge economy in mental health. The identified international research priorities are likely to take a long time to implement, document, and disseminate as sources of evidence for clinicians. Prioritizing some meta-ethnographies and systematic or integrated reviews of what mental health occupational therapists currently know will inform practice in the short term. Recent systematic reviews of interventions for employment and education (Arbesman & Logsdon, 2011) and recovery in the areas of community integration and normative life roles (Gibson, D'Amico, Jaffe, & Arbesman, 2011) for adults with serious mental illness have found positive outcomes of occupational therapy interventions.

Large treatment effects are achieved with the sustained implementation of appropriate drug and psychological intervention. As a coalition of individuals and institutions committed to closing the inequity gap, global mental health initiatives will apply **translational research/science** to make the advances in the neurosciences and social sciences accessible in the global mental health context. Particular attention must be paid to the effective interaction between professional and nonprofessionals.

Considering a Human Scale Research Agenda

We have argued that coalescing our research efforts toward the transformation of society and toward addressing the human conditions that create mental illness and compromise well-being will require coherence between a range of unifying frameworks for local, national, and international action. We propose that occupational therapists concerned with population-focused research consider the perspectives of human scale development because it assumes a direct and participatory democracy with the emphasis on civil society to nurture a form of development based on fundamental human needs. It emphasizes the role of social actors, of social participation, and local communities.

Arising from the discipline of economics but encompassing a transdisciplinary perspective, Human Scale Development (Max-Neef, Elizalde, & Hopenhayn, 1989) simultaneously takes a large-scale view of social structures and of the impacts of these structures on individuals (see Chapter 5). It proposes an approach to development that is driven by a focus on basic human needs rather than the production and distribution of commodities. The paradigm identifies a matrix of human needs and satisfiers (Max-Neef, 1991). Human needs are both individual and collective, and the influence of societal values and practices is foundational. The key question asked by this paradigm is to what extent can people influence their environmental structures that affect their opportunities? This paradigm of Human Scale Development expands on the Complete State Model of Mental Health discussed earlier (Slade, 2009) by contextualizing the subjective symptoms of well-being and mental illness. Together they provide a framework for inquiry into the intrapersonal and societal drivers of mental health as well as the structure and focus of intervention efforts.

SUMMARY

The burden of mental health disorders on the health and well-being of individuals, communities, and societies around the world is enormous. The scope and complexity of mental health challenges require occupational therapists to be informed about the causes and effects of mental health disorders at many different levels. The traditional individual-focused approach to research and practice in occupational therapy is not adequate to address contemporary global problems in mental health, nor can it be expected to be the sole way to advance the knowledge base in occupational therapy. A contextual focus is required, which includes understanding how problems are defined and conceptualized at local, national, and international levels and identifying collaborative methods to investigate and address these problems. At the individual level, this entails an understanding of the social, cultural, and political contexts that influence the ability of individuals to engage with and create change and opportunity within their environments. Population-based research and practice is one way that occupational therapists can address problems of health disparities, access to care, and institutional, cultural, and societal barriers to health and wellness. This necessitates taking a reflexive and collaborative approach, actively engaging individuals, communities, families, and other professionals as equal participants. While this may appear to be an overwhelming charge, the examples we present in this chapter illustrate how occupational therapists can engage at a local level, taking a broad-based awareness of context into the specific contexts of individuals and groups and creating a foundation for change. We have also presented examples of resources that are increasingly available to support occupational therapists who are taking a broader focus in their practice.

REVIEW QUESTIONS

1. What are the mental health research priorities of the WHO and the NIMH? How do the research priorities of AOTA/AOTF (or other professional bodies in other countries) align with these priorities?

2. When conducting research in mental health, why is it important to consider the social, cultural, and political contexts?
3. What are the major differences between the quantitative and the qualitative research paradigms?

REFERENCES

Alers, V., & Crouch, R. (2010). *Occupational therapy: An African perspective.* Johannesburg: Sarah Shorten Publishers.

Alldred, P. & Gillies, V. (2002). Eliciting research accounts: Re/producing modern subjects? In M. Mauthner, M. Birch, J. Jessop, & T. Miller (Eds.), *Ethics in qualitative research* (pp. 146–165). London: Sage Publications.

Alsop, A. (2000). *Continuing professional development: A guide for therapists.* Oxford: Blackwell Science.

American Occupational Therapy Association [AOTA]. (2007). AOTA's centennial vision and executive summary. *American Journal of Occupational Therapy, 61*, 613–614.

American Occupational Therapy Association/American Occupational Therapy Foundation [AOTA/AOTF]. (2009). *Occupational therapy research agenda.* Retrieved from http://www.aota.org/DocumentVault/Research/45008.aspx

Arbesman, M., & Logsdon, D. W. (2011). Occupational therapy interventions for employment and education for adults with serious mental illness: A systematic review. *American Journal of Occupational Therapy, 65*, 238–246.

Baer, L., & Blais, M. A. (Eds.) (2010). *Handbook of clinical rating scales and assessment in psychiatry and mental health.* New York: Humana Press.

Barnes, C., & Mercer, G. (2004). *Implications of the social model of disability: Theory and research.* Leeds: The Disability Press.

Chan, F., Cardoso, E.D.S., & Chronister, J. A. (2009) *Understanding psychosocial adjustment to chronic illness and disability: A handbook for evidence based practice in rehabilitation.* New York: Springer Publishing Company.

Clark, F., Parham, D., Carlson, M., Frank, G., Jackson, J., Pierce, D. et al. (1991). Occupational science: Academic innovation in the service of occupational therapy's future. *American Journal of Occupational Therapy, 45*(4), 300–310.

Craik, C., Austin, C., Chacksfield, J. D., Richards, G., & Schell, D. (1998). College of Occupational Therapy Position Paper on the way ahead for research, education and practice in mental health. *British Journal of Occupational Therapy, 61*(9), 390–392.

D'Amico, M., Jaffe, L., & Gibson, R. W. (2010). Centennial Vision—Mental health evidence in the American Journal of Occupational Therapy. *American Journal of Occupational Therapy, 64*, 660–669.

Duncan, M., & Watson, R. (2009). *The occupational dimensions of poverty and disability.* Working Paper 14, Institute for Land and Agrarian Studies (PLAAS). University of Western Cape. Retrieved from http://www.plaas.org.za/pubs/wp

Duncan, M., & Watson, R. (2010). Taking a stance: Socially responsible ethics and informed consent. In M. Saven-Baden & C. Taylor (Eds.), *New approaches in qualitative research: Wisdom and uncertainty.* London. Routledge Francis and Taylor Group.

Foucault, M. (1980). *Power/knowledge: selected interviews and other writings: 1972–1977.* Brighton, UK: Harvester Press.

Gibson, R. W., D'Amico, M., Jaffe, L., & Arbesman, M. (2011). Occupational therapy interventions for recovery in the areas of community integration and normative life roles for adults with serious mental illness: A systematic review. *American Journal of Occupational Therapy, 65*, 247–256.

Grand Challenges in Global Mental Health Initiative. (2010). *What are the grand challenges in global mental health?* Retrieved from http://grandchallengesgmh.nimh.nih.gov/

Gutman, S. (2008). Research priorities of the profession. *American Journal of Occupational Therapy, 62*(5), 499–501.

Hammell, K. W. (2009). Sacred texts: A skeptical exploration of the assumptions underpinning theories of occupation. *Canadian Journal of Occupational Therapy, 76*(1), 6–13.

Hasselkus, B. (2006). The world of everyday occupation: Real people, real lives. *American Journal of Occupational Therapy, 60*(6), 627–640.

Hemphill, B. J. (2008). *Assessments in occupational therapy mental health: An integrative approach.* Thorofare, NJ: Slack Inc.

Holland, H. (2001). *African magic: Traditional ideas that heal a continent.* London: Penguin Putnam Inc.

Kagan, C., & Burton, M. (2000). Prefigurative action research: An alternative basis for critical psychology? *Annual Review of Critical Psychology, 2,* 73–87.

Kronenberg, F., Pollard, N., & Sakellariou, D. (Eds.) (2005). *Occupational therapy without borders: Learning from the spirit of survivors.* London: Elsevier.

Kronenberg, F., Pollard, N., & Sakellariou, D. (Eds.) (2011). *Occupational therapies without borders: Towards an ecology of occupation-based practices.* London: Elsevier.

Law, M., Baum, C., & Dunn, W. (2005). *Measuring occupational performance: Supporting best practice in occupational therapy.* Thorofare NJ: Slack Inc.

Lee, C. J., & Miller, L. T. (2003). Evidence-Based Practice Forum—The process of evidence-based clinical decision making in occupational therapy. *American Journal of Occupational Therapy, 57,* 473–477.

Lieberman, D., & Scheer, J. (2002). AOTA's Evidence-Based Literature Review Project: An overview. *American Journal of Occupational Therapy, 56,* 344–349.

Lund, C., Breen A., Flisher, A., Swartz, L., Joska., J., Corrigall, J., et al. (2007). Mental health and poverty: A systematic review of the research in low and middle income countries. *The Journal of Mental Health Policy and Economics,* 10, Supplement 1, S26–S27.

Macleod, C. (2004). Writing into action: The critical research endeavour. In D. Hook (Ed.). *Critical psychology.* Cape Town: University of Cape Town Press. pp. 523–539.

Max-Neef, M. (1991). *Human scale development: Conception, application, and further reflections.* New York: Apex Press.

Max-Neef, M., Elizalde, A., & Hopenhayn, M. (1989). *Human scale development: Development dialogue.* Uppsala, Sweden: Dag Hammarskjöld Foundation.

McDowell, I. (2006). *A guide to rating scales and questionnaires.* Oxford, England: Oxford University Press.

McNiff, J., & Whitehead, J. (2006). *All you need to know about action research.* London: Sage Publications.

Miller, G. (2006). The unseen: Mental illness's global toll. *Science, 311,* 458–461. Retrieved from http://www.sciencemag.org

Miller, T., & Bell, B. (2002). Consenting to what? Issues of access, gate-keeping and 'informed' consent. In M. Mauthner, M. Birch, J. Jessop, & T. Miller (Eds.). *Ethics in qualitative research.* (pp. 53–69). London: Sage Publications.

Mitlin, D. (2005). Chronic poverty in urban areas. *Environment and Urbanisation, 17*(2), 3–10.

Nabudere, D. W. (2006). Development theories, knowledge production and emancipatory practice. In V. Padayachee (Ed.), *The development decade? Economic and social change in South Africa, 1994–2004* (pp. 13–32). Cape Town: Human Sciences Research Council Press.

National Advisory Mental Health Council's Workgroup. (n.d.). *Transformative neurodevelopmental research in mental illness.* Retrieved from http://www.nimh.nih.gov/about/advisory-boards-and-groups/namhc/neurodevelopment_workgroup_report.pdf

National Advisory Mental Health Council's Workgroup on Clinical Trials. (n.d.). *Treatment research in mental illness: Improving the nation's public mental health care through NIMH funded interventions research.* Retrieved from http://www.nimh.nih.gov/about/advisory-boards-and-groups/namhc/reports/interventions-research.pdf

National Institute of Mental Health. (n.d.[a]). *Leading categories of diseases/disorders.* Retrieved from http://www.nimh.nih.gov/statistics/2LEAD_CAT.shtml

National Institute of Mental Health. (n.d.[b]). *NIMH strategic research priorities.* Retrieved from http://www.nimh.nih.gov/research-funding/research-priorities/index.shtml

Parker, I. (2005). *Qualitative psychology: Introducing radical research.* Maidenhead, UK: Open University Press.

Patel, V., & Kleinman, A. (2003). Poverty and common mental health disorders in developing countries. *Bulletin of the World Health Organisation, 81*(8), 609–615.

Patel, V., & Prince, M. (2010). Global mental health. *Journal of the American Medical Association, 303*(19), 1976–1977.

Rappolt, S. (2003). Evidence-Based Practice Forum—The role of professional expertise in evidence-based occupational therapy. *American Journal of Occupational Therapy, 57,* 589–593.

Richardson, P. K., & MacRae, A. (2011). An occupational justice research perspective. In F. Kronenberg, N. Pollard, & D. Sakellariou (Eds). *Occupational therapies without borders: Towards an ecology of occupation-based practices* (Vol. 2, pp. 339–348). London: Elsevier.

Rose, D. (2008). Commentary: Madness strikes back. *Journal of Community Applied Social Psychology, 18,* 638–644.

Rush, A. J., First, M. B., & Blacker, D. (2008). *Handbook of psychiatric measures.* Washington, DC: American Psychiatric Publishers.

Sackett, D. L., Straus, S. E., Richardson, W. S., Rosenberg, W. M., & Haynes, R. B. (2000). *Evidence-based medicine: How to practice and teach EBM* (2nd ed.). Edinburgh: Churchill Livingstone.

Schön, D. (1995, November–December). Knowing-in-action: The new scholarship requires a new epistemology. *Change,* 27–34.

Sharan, P., Gallo, C., Gureje, O., Lamberte, E., Mari, J. J., Mazzotti, G., et al. (2009). Mental health research priorities in low- and middle-income countries of Africa, Asia, Latin America and the Caribbean. *British Journal of Psychiatry, 295,* 354–363.

Silverman, D. (2010). *Doing qualitative research: a practical handbook (3rd edition).* London: Sage.

Slade, M. (2009). *Personal recovery and mental illness: A guide for mental health professionals.* Cambridge: Cambridge University Press.

Smith, L. T. (1999). *Decolonising methodologies: Research and indigenous peoples.* London: Zed Books.

Swartz, L. (1998). *Culture and mental health: A Southern African view.* Cape Town: Oxford University Press.

Tickle-Degnan, L., & Bedell, G. (2003). Evidence-Based Practice Forum—Heterarchy and hierarchy: A critical appraisal of the "levels of evidence" as a tool for clinical decision-making. *American Journal of Occupational Therapy, 57,* 234–237.

United Nations. (1948). *The universal declaration of human rights.* Retrieved from http://www.un.org/en/documents/udhr/index/shtml

Watson, R., & Swartz, L. (2004). *Transformation through occupation: Human occupation in context.* London: Whurr Publishers.

World Health Organization. (1978). *Declaration of Alma Ata.* International Conference on Primary Health Care, Alma Ata, USSR, 6-12 September. Retrieved from www.who.int/hpr/NPH/docs/declaration_almaata.pdf

World Health Organization. (2001). *The world health report 2001: Mental health: New understanding, new hope.* Retrieved from http://www.who-int/whr/2001/en

World Health Organization. (2008). *The global burden of disease: 2004 update.* Geneva, Switzerland: WHO Press. Retrieved from http://www.who.int/healthinfo/global_burden_disease/GBD_report_2004update_full.pdf

World Health Organization. (n.d.). *Mental health evidence and research.* Retrieved from http://www.who.int/mental_health/evidence/en/

SUGGESTED RESOURCES

Carpenter, C., & Suto, M. (2008). *Qualitative research for occupational and physical therapists: A practical guide.* Oxford: Blackwell Publishing.

Denzin, N., & Lincoln, Y. S. (2008). *Strategies of qualitative inquiry.* Thousand Oaks: Sage Publications.

Department of Health and Human Services. (1999). *Mental health: A report of the Surgeon General.* Retrieved from http://www.surgeongeneral.gov/library/mentalhealth/home.html

Doucet, S, A., Letourneau, N. L., & Stoppard, J. M. (2010). Contemporary paradigms for research related to women's mental health. *Health Care for Women International. 31*, 296–312.

Duncan, M. (2009). *Human occupation in the context of chronic poverty and psychiatric disability.* Unpublished doctoral dissertation, Department of Psychology, Faculty of Arts and Social Sciences, University of Stellenbosch. Retrieved from http://scholar.sun.ac.za

Goodley, J., & Lawthom, R. (Eds.) (2006). *Disability and psychology: Critical introductions and reflections.* New York: Palgrave MacMillan.

Gostin, L. O., & Gable, L. (2008). *Global mental health: Changing norms, constant rights.* Wayne State University Law School Legal Studies Research Paper Series No. 08-26. Retrieved from http://ssrn.com/abstract=1242163

Hammell, K. W., & Carpenter, C. (2004). *Qualitative research in evidence-based rehabilitation.* Edinburgh: Churchill Livingstone.

Hermann, H., & Swartz, L. (2007). Promotion of mental health in poorly resourced countries. *The Lancet, 370* (9594), 1195–1197.

Hood, S., Mayall, B., & Oliver. S. (Eds.) (1999). *Critical issues in social research: Power and prejudice.* Buckingham, UK: Open University Press.

Kaplan, D. (2004). *Sage handbook of quantitative methods for the social sciences.* Thousand Oaks: Sage Publications.

Kielhofner, G. (2006). The aim of research: Philosophical foundations of scientific inquiry. In G. Kielhofner, *Research in occupational therapy: Methods of inquiry for enhancing practice.* Philadelphia: F.A. Davis.

Mahaffey, L., & MHSIS Standing Committee. (2009). Incorporating evidence in mental health practice. Articles from the AOTA mental health annotated bibliography project. *Mental Health Special Interest Section Quarterly, 32*(3), 1–4.

Patel, V. (2003). *Where there is no psychiatrist: A mental healthcare manual.* Glasgow: Gaskell.

Pollard, N., Sakellariou, D., & Kronenberg, F. (2008). *A political practice of occupational therapy.* London: Elsevier.

Tomlinson, M., Rudan, I., Saxena, S., Swartz, L., Tsai, A. C., & Patel, V. (2009). Priorities for global mental health research. *Bulletin of the World Health Organization, 87,* 438–446.

Van Niekerk, L. (2005). Occupational science and its relevance to occupational therapy. In R. Crouch & V. Alers (Eds.), *Occupational therapy in psychiatry and mental health* (pp. 62–73). London: Whurr Publishers.

Watson, R., & Buchanan, H. (2005). Making our practice evidence-based. *South African Journal of Occupational Therapy, 35*(3), 14–19.

Watson, R., & Duncan, E. M. (2010). The 'right' to occupational participation in the presence of chronic poverty. *WFOT Bulletin, 62,* 26–32.

Whiteford, G., & Townsend, E. (2011). Participatory occupational justice framework (POJF2010): Enabling occupational participation and inclusion. In F. Kronenberg, N. Pollard, & D. Sakellariou (Eds.), *Occupational therapies without borders: Towards an ecology of occupation-based practices* (Vol. 2, pp. 65–84). London: Elsevier.

Theoretical Concepts

Part II includes two chapters that focus on the theoretical underpinnings of psychosocial occupational therapy, both what is unique to OT and what guides it in the fields of psychology and psychiatry. Chapter 4, like in the second edition, follows the beginning of occupational therapy, explicating the ideas and thinking of the founders and societal events to describe the evolution of occupational therapy. The focus on occupation is the cornerstone of our profession and occupations are chronicled throughout the decades of occupational therapy. Certainly the last two decades have seen a vast array of research, practice, and policy emphasizing occupation.

Chapter 5, which was titled "Theories of Mental Health and Illness," has changed to "Psychological Theories and Their Treatment Methods in Mental Health Practice." As previously, this chapter elucidates the interdisciplinary ways in which psychological and psychiatric theories have influenced all areas of mental health, including occupational therapy. In this edition, exposition of concepts that are now part of everyday lexicon, such as egotist, fixation, collective consciousness, or behavior modification in all psychological theories, has been truncated because the editors acting on suggestions from reviewers agreed that these ideas are now covered in most introductory or abnormal psychology texts. As well, contemporary ideas have supplanted the archaic ones and the editors believed that these more contemporary concepts needed to be understood by occupational therapists. Like the previous edition, the unique ways in which occupational therapy is influenced by and applies these ideas are discussed in the chapter. As in the previous edition, unique occupational therapy models that drive research, evaluation, and practice do not appear in this part.

There are many detailed texts and articles regarding various occupational therapy models. Rather than superficially discussing them, we have left it to the chapter authors to discuss which occupational therapy models and ideas guide their interventions. Readers are encouraged to access primary materials to learn more about specific models.

Chapter 4

The History and Philosophy of Psychosocial Occupational Therapy

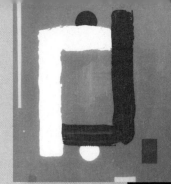

Kathleen Barker Schwartz, EdD, OTR/L, FAOTA

KEY TERMS

curative occupations

electroconvulsive therapy (ECT)

habit training

lobotomy

moral treatment

neurasthenia

psychoanalysis

psychobiological

CHAPTER OUTLINE

Introduction

Treatment of the Insane Before the Twentieth Century

The Founding of Occupational Therapy

    William Rush Dunton: Moral Treatment, Crafts, and Science

    Adolph Meyer: Psychobiology, Occupation, and Habits

    Eleanor Clarke Slagle: Curative Occupations and Habit Training

    Herbert James Hall: Neurasthenia and Work Therapy

Treatment of Mental Illness in the Twentieth Century

The Evolution of Psychosocial Occupational Therapy

    The 1920s and 1930s

    The 1940s and 1950s

    The 1960s and 1970s

    The 1980s and 1990s

Summary

INTRODUCTION

In order to understand psychosocial occupational therapy fully, it is necessary to know how practice has evolved from its inception to today. The history of psychosocial occupational therapy is rich in ideas, events, and people who have helped to shape its development. The purpose of this chapter is to provide a history of psychosocial occupational therapy with an emphasis on the field's philosophical underpinnings, including the values and ideas upon which the profession was founded, and to describe how these ideas changed over time. Thus, this chapter provides the broader context from which to understand how contemporary practice has been influenced by earlier events, people, and ideas.

TREATMENT OF THE INSANE BEFORE THE TWENTIETH CENTURY

Prior to the twentieth century, care of the insane (the term *mental illness* is modern terminology) took place primarily at home or in asylums. For example, in France in 1860, the situation was described as follows:

> In our rural areas, where people are still imbued with absurd prejudices, public opinion sees having madness in the family as shameful and will not send the person to an asylum. This is the principal reason that motivates our peasants to keep poor afflicted individuals at home. If the insane person is peaceful, people generally let him run loose. But if he becomes raging or troublesome, he's chained down in a corner of the stable or an isolated room, where his food is brought to him daily. (Caradec, 1860, as quoted in Shorter, 1997, p. 11)

In England if people were not kept at home they might be sent to workhouses or poorhouses, and the situation in the United States was similar to that in Europe. In rural Massachusetts in 1840, social reformer Dorothea Dix noted finding a woman in a cage in Lincoln, a man chained in a stall in Medford, and four women in animal pens in Barnstable (Dix, 1971/1943, pp. 5–7). In addition, she visited almshouses such as the one in Danvers, where she came upon a woman beating on the bars of a cage, "the unwashed frame invested with fragments of unclean garments, the air so extremely offensive, though ventilation was afforded to all sides save one, that it was not possible to remain beyond a few moments" (p. 6). Before 1800 there were only two hospitals in the United States that admitted the insane: Pennsylvania Hospital, established in 1752 by the Religious Society of Friends, and New York Hospital, which had a separate psychiatric building that was called the Lunatic Asylum.

Asylums, which had existed in Europe since the Middle Ages, were frequently referred to as madhouses and, for obvious reasons, were regarded as places to be avoided. That began to change with the introduction of a new approach in the nineteenth century that became known as **moral treatment**. Phillipe Pinel of France is commonly recognized as its initiator, although efforts were under way in all of Europe and England to create new-style asylums based on moral treatment philosophy. Moral treatment was humanitarian and therapeutic. Pinel's philosophy was a humanistic one characterized by kindness and respect, in which clients would be treated with dignity and optimism in place of the previous view of persons with mental illness as dangerous and incurable. The asylums for moral treatment were designed around the belief that orderly routines and occupations would have a therapeutic effect on clients. Pinel (1809) advocated a carefully planned treatment approach based on the use of "occupational activities of different kinds according to individual taste; physical exercise, beautiful scenery, and from time to time soft and melodious music" (p. 260).

What began in Europe ultimately came to the United States, where several private institutions were created under the moral treatment philosophy. They included McLean Asylum in Massachusetts, Hartford Retreat in Connecticut, Friends Hospital in Pennsylvania, and Sheppard Enoch Pratt Asylum in Maryland. Public asylums using the moral treatment approach were also established, with one of the most prominent founded in Worcester, Massachusetts. These facilities were impressively equipped with a variety of craft rooms, gardens, and recreational areas designed to provide clients with an active schedule of productive, creative, and recreational occupations. Figures 4-1 and 4-2 show samples of the occupational therapy environment where clients engaged

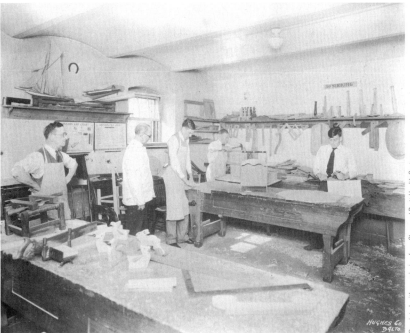

Reprinted with permission from Sheppard Pratt Health System

FIGURE 4-1. Furniture Making at Sheppard Enoch Pratt Asylum

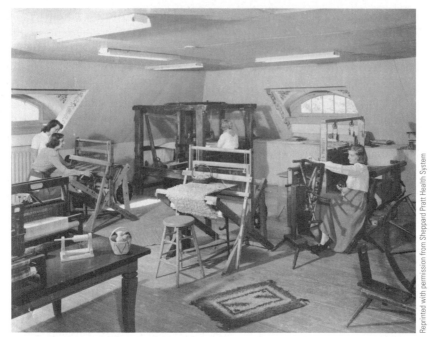

Reprinted with permission from Sheppard Pratt Health System

FIGURE 4-2. Textiles at Sheppard Enoch Pratt Asylum

in furniture making and repair as well as textile creation at Sheppard Enoch Pratt Asylum (now Sheppard Pratt Health Systems). Another such program, Gardner State Colony in Massachusetts, also provides a typical example of the rich occupation base of treatment: the clients were largely responsible for the development of 1,500 acres of productive farmlands that yielded 142,526 quarts of milk and 2,000 dozen eggs (Occupational Treatment of Patients in State Hospitals, 1914, p. 302). Inside the facility there was a carpenter shop, furniture factory, machine shop, shoemaking department, and rug weaving department (p. 304). "But it is not all work at Gardner. The patients have a good time . . . [with] tennis, golf . . . reading and entertainment. They have their orchestra and have musicals frequently. They have an excellent library, bowling and billiard rooms, and on the whole it is not such a terrible thing to be insane if one can be sure of the happy, even passage of one's life at a place like Gardner" (p. 305).

In a way, the success of the asylums based on moral treatment ultimately led to their demise. Once asylums gained a good reputation, people were willing to be admitted to them. After a while there were more people than could be accommodated with the available resources. Ultimately, the asylums did not have the funding to support the increasing numbers of individuals needing care. This resulted in overcrowded conditions and understaffing (Rothman, 1971). Moreover, by the beginning of the twentieth century, there was a shift in the view of mental illness away from the beliefs of moral treatment that centered on the importance of the therapeutic environment to the view that the science of brain pathology would provide the information that would ultimately lead to a cure.

THE FOUNDING OF OCCUPATIONAL THERAPY

The National Society for the Promotion of Occupational Therapy (NSPOT, later to be renamed the American Occupational Therapy Association [AOTA]) was founded in 1917. Occupational therapy was unique in that its founders came from a wealth of backgrounds and professions, which included psychiatry, medicine, architecture, settlement house work, nursing, education, and vocational rehabilitation. Although at the time occupational therapy was not divided into specialty areas, there were several people who were particularly instrumental in articulating the ideas that would provide the foundation for psychosocial occupational therapy. They were William Rush Dunton, Jr., Adolph Meyer, Eleanor Clarke Slagle, and Herbert James Hall. We will examine their backgrounds, work, and ideas in order to understand the significance of their contributions. As we do so, we will also introduce any relevant ideas in psychiatry or society at large that may have influenced their thinking.

William Rush Dunton: Moral Treatment, Crafts, and Science

At the founding meeting of NSPOT, Dunton (1917) presented a paper in which he traced the philosophical roots of occupational therapy to the moral treatment movement of the 1800s. At the time Dunton was a psychiatrist and supervisor of occupation classes at the prestigious Sheppard-Pratt Hospital in Towson, Maryland. He had received his medical training at the University of Pennsylvania, and began his career as an assistant physician at Sheppard Asylum (as it was then called) in 1895. Although Dunton initially worked in the laboratory, he became frustrated by the lack of progress and began to work directly with clients on the clinical wards. Dunton was introduced to the concept of therapeutic occupations by Edward Brush, MD, the superintendent of Sheppard. In 1902 a separate building for occupation classes was created, and Dunton took responsibility for overseeing client occupations, which included leatherwork, weaving, art, metalwork, bookbinding, electrical repair work, and printing (Fields, 1911). Dunton's ideas about occupational therapy can be found in a published outline of lectures (AOTA, 1925), of which he was primary author. These guidelines exemplified the principles of moral treatment in their focus on productive employment in occupation based on each client's capabilities and interests, and "carried on by encouragement, not criticism" (AOTA, p. 279).

Dunton was a craftsman himself, and firmly believed in the therapeutic value of crafts. His interest in crafts was supported by the proliferation of arts and crafts societies in the United States in the early 1900s. The arts and crafts movement originally began in England in the late 1800s with John Ruskin and William Morris, who were disturbed by the negative effects that industrialization and bureaucracy were having on British society. They proposed a return to a simpler way of life in which objects were handcrafted. They argued that handcrafted goods were natural, honest, and pleasing whereas manufactured goods were neither aesthetic nor moral because the worker who produced them was treated like an extension of the machine (Levine, 1987). In the United States craftsmanship offered to the middle class the promise of a return to a life that was slower-paced and grounded in familiar values, and was therefore very attractive (Boris, 1984). Crafts were also taught at settlement houses such as Hull House as a way to help immigrants assimilate into their new culture and to offer them an opportunity to learn a potential skill (Addams, 1911).

Dunton and his colleagues took the arts and crafts movement one step further: They applied the concept of engagement in crafts to the treatment of children and adults with emotional disabilities. "Handcrafts have a special therapeutic value as they afford occupation that combines the elements of play and recreation with work and accomplishment. They give a concrete return and provide a stimulus to mental activity and muscular exercise at the same time, and afford an opportunity for creation and self-expression" (Johnson, 1920, p. 69). Particularly in the treatment of the mentally ill, crafts became the chief occupation of choice.

One approach to using crafts in occupational therapy was to divide the clients and the crafts by levels of function and complexity. Haas (1924) proposed three "classes" of clients and three levels of crafts. The first group could not be entrusted to work with tools, so it was recommended that they engage in "preliminary" crafts that required modest tool use, such as basketry, weaving, brush making, and chair caning. The second group were those who could be trusted with tools but were at times confused as to their use. Crafts that were more structured and required less technical skill were recommended for these individuals, such as cement work, bookbinding, and printing. The third group was the highest-functioning and consisted of individuals who could use tools and were interested in the crafts. For them, the more complex and artistic crafts were recommended, including metal work, jewelry, carpentry, and pottery.

The challenge to occupational therapists using crafts was to plan the treatment so that it combined a therapeutic process with a satisfying outcome. It was commonly acknowledged that craft work must be of value and interest to the client. "With adults one thing above all is essential, that the work be important . . . Therefore all products should be useful, at least, as well made as is possible, and in some instances should be artistically beautiful" (Haas, 1924, p. 416). At the same time, "therapeutic value should not be lost sight of. Care should be taken not to discourage one who, after an effort, produces a very poor piece of work. The important thing is the therapeutic satisfaction it has given him. For him it is and should be an achievement" (Haas, 1924, p. 416). Most therapists tried to solve the process versus product issue by creating a balance so that clients engaged in crafts that were of interest to them and matched their abilities.

Dunton (1928) was a proponent of making the use of crafts "scientific" in order to justify occupational therapy practice within the medical community. In this case, the science consisted of elaborate activity analyses in which the mental processes (i.e., interest, concentration, initiative) were described, along with the physical requirements (i.e., ankle flexion, controllable posture, good eye-hand coordination); gradation of the activity was determined (from simple to complex, and slow to rapid); and a description was provided of those clients who would be best served by this particular craft (Analysis of Crafts, 1928). There was debate, however, about whether such a classification system was wise or feasible. "There seems to be a feeling that before it can be admitted to the rank of a therapeutic science the kinds of work to be used in occupational therapy must be labeled and arranged like the bottles on the pharmacist's shelves to be administered each for its specific disease. How far is such a definite classification possible or desirable?" (Humphrey, 1922, p. 554). In particular, there was concern about the use of a classification system when it came to the treatment of those with mental illness.

> Along physical lines the classification is comparatively simple . . . and work can be selected according to the required movements. Knotting gives finger movements, weaving gives arm and body development . . . jigsaws furnish foot and leg exercises . . . But where the mental effect upon the patient is the primary end, our whole problem takes on a different aspect. As soon as we get away from the physical standpoint, we at once realize that there is not firm basis for a rigid classification. The demand is not for the exercise of a group of muscles, but the reorganization of a personality. (p. 554)

This debate highlights the conflicting ideals underlying the use of arts and crafts in occupational therapy. A rigid ("scientific") classification of crafts and matching diseases goes against the humanistic, individualistic approach of moral treatment. Humphrey (1922) argued that in the treatment of mental illness, the occupational therapist should be free to choose any craft that might be helpful, regardless of its classification, as long at it was suited to the client's interest, intellectual capability, and disability. On the other hand, as a physician, Dunton (1928) was well aware of the need for occupational therapy to establish itself within the medical community as a health profession with a basis in science. The best way for occupational therapists to have their work recognized as a legitimate therapeutic endeavor was to be able to document its efficacy scientifically.

Adolph Meyer: Psychobiology, Occupation, and Habits

As one of the leading psychiatrists of the early twentieth century, Meyer was well aware of science and its importance in the treatment of people with mental illness. However, Meyer was concerned that scientific thinking could be reductionistic and mechanistic: "The great mistake of an overambitious science has been the desire to study [human beings] altogether as a mere sum of the parts, if possible of atoms . . . and as a machine, detached, by itself" (Meyer, 1948/1921, p. 3). In contrast, Meyer argued that nurture and nature were both important. He proposed **psychobiological** as an approach, which considered an individual's performance and occupational history, in addition to biological and neurological data. "We take up a survey of functions of the person beginning with the full-fledged performances and achievements and attempt to give an idea of the individual; the personal care, the jobs and hobbies . . . family, sociability, public life, education, religious activity, etc . . . [all] interests and ambitions, one's perceptive life (sensual and esthetic gratification) dreaming, thinking, acting" (Meyer, 1948/1934, p. 319).

Meyer earned his MD in Zurich in 1892 and immigrated to the United States to study neurology. At the time there was no recognized specialty examination in psychiatry, so practitioners called themselves by various titles: alienist, psychiatrist, psychologist, neurologist, pathologist, or internist. Meyer's first appointments were as a researcher. Ultimately, he tired of pathology and decided that the study of psychiatry was best done at the bedside. He was appointed professor of psychiatry at Johns Hopkins in 1910, where he came to know both Dunton and Slagle.

Meyer was a supporter of occupational therapy, and in response to Dunton's request, he published his thoughts in a paper entitled "The Philosophy of Occupation Therapy" in 1922. In this paper he conceptualized mental illness as "problems of living, and not merely diseases of a structural and toxic nature on the one hand or of a final lasting constitutional disorder on the other" (Meyer, 1922a, p. 4). He emphasized the importance of viewing each individual from a holistic and temporal perspective, and of balancing work and rest: "Our body is not merely so many pounds of flesh and bone figuring as a machine, with an abstract mind or soul added to it. It is throughout a living organism pulsating with its rhythm of rest and activity . . . Our conception of man is that of an organism that maintains and balances itself in the world of reality and actuality by . . . acting its time in harmony with its own nature and the nature about it" (p. 5).

Meyer proposed engagement in occupation as a way to address the problems of living. "Our role consists in giving opportunities rather than prescriptions. There must be opportunities to work, opportunities to do and plan and create, and to learn to use material" (Meyer, 1922a, p. 7). One important aspect of occupation was habits. "It will be our duty to define in actual cases what sets of habits we find interwoven and with what effect. This directs the attention to the investigation of matters which are open to influence in education, and to a more rational management of dementia praecox [an early term for schizophrenia], as well as many other mental disorders" (Meyer, 1948/1905, p. 181). Meyer proposed that "habit disorder is to be treated by habit training" (p. 180). As the director of the Phipps Clinic at Johns Hopkins Hospital, Meyer was in an excellent position to see that his ideas on **habit training** were implemented. He recruited Eleanor Clarke Slagle to direct the first Occupational Therapy Program.

Eleanor Clarke Slagle: Curative Occupations and Habit Training

At a retirement dinner in Slagle's honor, Harriet Robeson (1937) characterized Slagle as a "pioneer by nature, with a searching mind and a keen interest in social problems and their psychological aspects" (p. 3). Slagle brought to the new profession of occupational therapy her dedication to social reform in mental hygiene. She first became acquainted with the concept of therapeutic occupations when she took a course in **curative occupations** conducted at Hull House in 1911. The course was designed to educate "institution attendants in occupations for the insane" (Taylor, 1909, quoted in Quiroga, 1995, p. 42). Later, in 1912, Slagle was recruited by Meyer and came to Phipps clinic to oversee the new Department of Occupational Therapy.

One of her contributions was the creation and implementation of a habit training program, based on Meyer's focus on habits. According to Meyer (1948/1922b, p. 486), "the first point is development of habits which can be thoroughly satisfied in harmony with the environment and with ample opportunity for satisfaction . . . There must be habits of work for which there is a market and call, habits of care of oneself in keeping with the probable opportunities, habits of recreation easily enough dovetailed with life, habits of melioristic self-culture—social, educational, civil and religious habits and contacts."

Habit training required the health practitioner to "make distinctions of various types of habit disorganization, to study the working of the various sets of activities and habits in the patient, determine their relative value by accurate observation . . . and shape our therapeutic measures in accord with these principles" (Meyer, 1948/1905, p. 181).

Slagle designed a habit training program for a group of the most profoundly ill clients, who were diagnosed as having dementia praecox. "To visualize the picture more clearly, let us consider a group of sixteen untidy, destructive, assaultive, abusive and rapidly deteriorating young women" (Slagle, 1924, p. 100). Slagle structured the program so that the clients followed a strict schedule of self-care, physical activities, occupation classes, and meals. At the end of a year, she judged their progress as quite successful. "This group are entirely retrained in decent habits of living and are now being trained in carefully graded tasks" (p. 100).

Stimulated by Meyer and Slagle's example, habit training programs were introduced at other mental health facilities. Wilson (1929), chief occupational therapist at Brooklyn State Hospital, New York, described the program she supervised as a "progressive schedule through which the patient is carried to the highest level of adjustment possible to that particular individual" (p. 189). She vividly portrays the extent of the mental disorders they attempted to address through habit training.

> The regressed mental patient has been unable to adjust at an adult level of existence, but has slipped back to a lower level at which he feels comfortable, content and safe. This level may be so low that he leads a practically

vegetative existence. He may not feed, dress or undress himself and frequently wets and soils bed and clothing; in fact he does nothing for himself, and is a great economic burden to those charged with his care. He is often mute, stuperous, and resistive. (p. 190)

The habit training program was the most successful treatment approach for these severely involved clients, Wilson argued, because it provided "intensive care and re-education." However, she noted that this intensive care made it possible to treat only a small, select group of individuals. (She recommended that the ratio of clients to employees be no more than 10:1.) Thus, similar to moral treatment, the habit training programs could be overwhelmed by the large number of clients requiring services alongside the inadequate staffing and resources.

Herbert James Hall: Neurasthenia and Work Therapy

At the turn of the twentieth century it was much more comforting for clients to suffer from "nerves" than insanity. For this reason many more people identified themselves as needing relief from nervous disorders than from mental illness. In Europe, people went to spas and sanitariums, which employed psychiatrists to oversee the therapeutic regimen that commonly included rest, diet, and water therapy. Psychiatrists in the United States coined the term **neurasthenia** to refer to nervous conditions such as hysteria, hypochondria, depression, compulsive behavior, and anxiety. The typical treatment was the same as in Europe—the rest cure—and was equally expensive.

Herbert Hall did not believe that rest was the answer; instead, he advocated work as the remedy. "Probably every practitioner of medicine has felt that if he could get his weary and irritable neurasthenic to care for something outside his own little circle of troubles, to work perhaps at some absorbing occupation, a cure would be accomplished. It is, no doubt, normal and right for a man to be busy; or unoccupied for any length of time, his nervous energies turn in upon themselves and are likely to create mental confusion and depression" (Hall, 1913, p. 5). Hall designed a treatment regimen that began with a few days of rest, followed by a program in which the hours of rest were gradually decreased and the hours of work increased "until the day is full of interest and self-forgetfulness . . . The progression leads to the shop and depends upon the work there, to fix and render permanent the improvement" (pp. 9–10).

His pioneering work brought him to the attention of Dunton and Slagle, and Hall became an early spokesperson and leader within occupational therapy. Hall graduated from Harvard University Medical School in 1895, where he did an internship at Massachusetts General Hospital. Like all doctors at the time, he had no special training in psychiatry, and therefore gained his knowledge in his practice treating individuals with neurasthenia. In an article on what he called the "high-grade neurasthenic," Hall (1921) described his clients as people "who go from one physician to another, who are sometimes cured by Christian Science or Chiropracty, by a tonic or a few weeks at a sanatorium and unfortunately also, they are the patients who often do not get well or reach a level of efficiency and comfort which they or we may fairly call health" (p. 232).

Hall founded the Devereux Workshops in order to implement his ideas about the value of work as a remedy. He ran an announcement that read: "Through the generosity and understanding of a friend of Occupational Therapy, it has become possible to establish at Marblehead, Massachusetts, a small experimental station for the study of problems of invalid occupations" (Research in Occupational Therapy, n.d.). He went on to say that the workshop would be staffed by designers and craftsmen who would help "in the development of new occupations which will be elastic enough to meet the varied requirements of invalids and which will, at the same time result in really valuable products." Ultimately, one of the popular occupations that evolved was toy making. Hall describes how "this shop or laboratory, as it may be called, has supplied its toys to more than seventy-five different hospitals scattered all over the country . . . The wooden toy stands very high among the crafts available for the handicapped" (Hall, 1922, p. 63).

Hall's workshop emphasized engagement in craftwork that was not only intrinsically valuable but also commercially viable:

> Surely here is a brave and practical way of looking at the problem of occupations for the handicapped. Every man who can be made fit must be reinstated in his old trade. Those who cannot compete with able-bodied labor may nevertheless resume their own trades under special and favored conditions. Those who cannot go back to their original work may find remunerative employment in their own homes or in especially devised handicapped workshops. Why is this not a sensible model for all handicapped industries in our own country? If the little shops, the hospital industries can be made self-supporting, well and good; if not, they have served a larger purpose. (Hall, 1917, p. 384)

Besides his clients with neurasthenia, Hall was concerned with the many wounded soldiers who were returning after World War I. Hall likened the "shell shock" that the soldiers suffered to the neurasthenia of his clients. Hall, along with his colleagues, justified the creation of the new profession of occupational therapy by emphasizing its potential to enable clients to return to useful, productive lives. It was this aspect of the new profession that most captured the imagination of the public (Ambrosi & Schwartz, 1995). This was in part due to society's preoccupation with what would happen to the soldiers who had suffered psychological or physical injury as a result of World War I. This concern is reflected in the platforms of both major political parties in the 1924 elections, in which they cite as one of their goals the restoration of the veteran with disability to a position of social usefulness (Full text, 1924; Text of platform, 1924). It was also in keeping with the values of American society during the Progressive era, which emphasized economic self-sufficiency, social contribution, and the Protestant work ethic (Wiebe, 1967).

Thus, occupational therapy promoted itself as the profession that would restore persons with mental and physical disabilities to full economic and social usefulness. Slagle (1923) described occupational therapy as an evolutionary process in which individuals make "a complete change in their whole relationship to life . . . from the position of a liability to that of an asset" (p. 57). Dunton asserted that occupation teachers could play an important role in the instruction of veterans in crafts that could help them earn a living (Seek Occupations for War Cripples, 1917). Thomas Kidner and George Barton, two of the profession's founders, created environments that would foster the abilities of clients to return to satisfying, remunerative work. Kidner (1925), former vocational secretary of the Canadian Military Hospitals Commission, developed the "pre-industrial shop" to promote "re-adjustment to normal living by affording opportunity for the development of habits of industry that have been impaired by disease or injury" (p. 188). Barton created Consolation House in an effort to "get away from institutional life" to one where the individual "could be happy, get well, and become self-supporting" (Newton, 1917).

The Arequipa Sanatorium in Marin, California, addressed the problem of "remunerative permanent occupation" by teaching the women clients to make pottery. "As originally planned, it was not intended to do more than provide an interesting occupation during the tedious convalescence from depression and disease and possibly [make] enough profit to contribute to the support of the patient. But the unexpected development of latent talent, as well as the impossibility in many cases of returning to the old employment, led to a consideration of possible connection with the working world and permanent remunerative occupation in the future" (Brown, 1917, p. 394). Brown, who was the medical director, noted that of the 66 clients who learned pottery making, "twenty-four have made good" (p. 395), meaning that they were able to be discharged and to live on their earnings independently. Arequipa pottery came to be highly valued, and some of the craftswomen, with the support of wealthy patrons, went on to become acclaimed artists.

It was not uncommon for state mental hospitals and private asylums to have clients perform work around the institutions as part of their "occupational" therapy. Thus, clients were given the opportunity to "earn something toward the support of their families" (Hospital Will Restore the Industrial Wounded, 1923, p. 3). The reason the New York State Hospital Commission recommended the hiring of occupational therapists was so that they could train clients with mental illness for a useful activity (Hard Times Cause Record in Insane, 1922). Hall (1917) wholeheartedly agreed with this approach. He wrote that his experience with therapeutic occupations led him to conclude that "the more useful the work, the better its therapeutic effect; and conversely, the more trivial and valueless the product of the work, the less effective" (p. 383).

Thus, the work of the founders provided the basis for the underlying tenets of psychosocial occupational therapy practice. The roots are founded in the humanistic philosophy of moral treatment, which provided engagement in occupations and a regularity of schedule as the focus of the treatment for the mentally ill. Engagement in occupation is at the center of the therapeutic process. Occupations provide a way to address the holistic needs of the individual and to help create a balance of work, play, and rest. Habit training is proposed as a way to decrease negative habits by instilling a healthy regimen of daily activities. Arts and crafts are advocated to arouse interest, promote good work habits, and increase skills. Engagement in work is promoted as a way to motivate and reinvigorate individuals, and to develop new skills that will ultimately enable people to return to socially productive lives.

TREATMENT OF MENTAL ILLNESS IN THE TWENTIETH CENTURY

The twentieth century was a time of great experimentation in the treatment of mental illness. Since no one thus far had discovered a cure for mental illness, any and all theories, modalities, and approaches that might work were tried. The century began under the influence of Emil Kraepelin (1883), a German psychiatrist, who revolutionized the psychiatric world by proposing the classification of symptoms into major psychiatric disease entities, such as manic-depressive illness and dementia praecox. He based his findings on the careful, systematic study of a large number of his clients over time. These studies revealed that the diagnoses presented with different symptoms and the courses of the diseases were different as well. Although his classifications were a precursor to the *Diagnostic and Statistical Manual of Mental Disorders* (*DSM*), Kraepelin's motivation was not to pigeon-hole people into a diagnosis. Rather, as a clinician, he wanted to understand and be able to help families understand the probable course over time of their loved one's disease. In the United States his constructs were adopted by psychiatrists such as Meyer. Indeed, Meyer's ideas about habit training were specifically directed at the treatment of clients with dementia praecox.

However, even with a better understanding of the various disease entities and knowledge of their probable clinical course, practitioners were still uncertain as to what treatments would be most effective. **Psychoanalysis** offered a new theory and a new hope for an effective treatment. Sigmund Freud, the founder of psychoanalysis, proposed that psychological problems arose as a result of unconscious conflicts over past events, especially of a sexual nature (Gay, 1989). Treatment consisted of the client spending considerable time with the therapist, examining past events and possible feelings that they evoked. Thus, the psychoanalytic process emphasized the importance of the doctor-client relationship. Freud's approach spread from Vienna to the rest of Europe, and ultimately to the United States, where it became a pervasive force in psychiatry from 1930 through the 1970s. Although psychoanalysis was originally directed toward individuals with neurosis, American psychiatrists such as Meyer and Harry Stack Sullivan proposed it could be used with clients with serious mental illness. Thus, many of the private hospitals that had originally been founded under the moral treatment model, including Phipps Clinic and Sheppard and Enoch Pratt Hospital, added psychoanalysis to their treatment approach.

At the same time that psychoanalysis was spreading, alternative approaches were being tried in an attempt to address the many clients who were stagnating in the state mental institutions, as asylums had come to be called. "Walking through the wards, one would see the schizophrenics who spent their entire day in assumed statuesque postures . . . or in rocking rhythmically and tirelessly backwards and forwards" (Rollin, 1990, p. 191). Drugs, including morphine, phenobarbital, and chloral hydrate, were used to try to diminish symptoms. **Electroconvulsive therapy (ECT)** was first introduced in the United States at the New York Psychiatric Institute in 1940. Although some clients developed fractures as a result of their movements during the convulsions, as well as a myriad of other side effects, for many clients it made a profound change in their condition. By 1959, ECT had become the treatment of choice for major depression (Shorter, 1997). Psychosurgery was practiced in the United States from 1936 to 1954 in the form of the lobotomy. In the **lobotomy**, part of the brain's frontal lobe was excised, making clients much calmer and less threatening but also depriving them of judgment and social skills. By 1951, no fewer than 18,608 individuals had undergone psychosurgery (Grob, 1991).

At the same time in England, the concept of the therapeutic community was introduced as an alternative to psychoanalysis, drugs, physical modalities, and surgery. It built upon the ideas from moral treatment about respect for the client and the belief that the environment was a significant influence in the therapeutic process. It added a new dimension in advocating that the client should have autonomy and a voice in determining how the therapeutic community would be run. Joshua Bierer introduced the concept of milieu or therapeutic community therapy in London in the late 1930s. Bierer (1980), a psychotherapist who fled Vienna for London during World War II, proposed that psychotherapy groups be run by the clients. In order to provide a suitable environment for the groups to meet, Bierer also established one of the first psychiatric day hospitals. Thus, a therapeutic community was created where clients could run their group sessions, and where they could also receive counseling, occupational therapy, and other supportive services. The idea of the therapeutic community became so popular in the United States that by 1960 almost all mental health facilities claimed to use this approach. Shorter (1997) argues that the American version of the therapeutic community was significantly different from the English, in that the necessary resources to make it successful were never provided and it was not fully embraced by psychiatrists who remained enamored with psychoanalysis.

By mid-century, despite all these therapeutic innovations, mental hospitals still contained many seriously ill people who could not benefit from any of the therapeutic approaches or modalities. That situation began to change in 1954 when chlorpromazine was introduced in the United States. Clinical trials revealed that this drug calmed agitated clients and ameliorated the severe behaviors associated with psychosis (Rollin, 1990). Thus began the era of psychopharmacology, which has since seen the development of many sophisticated antipsychotics, antimanics, and antidepressants. There is little doubt that the introduction of these drugs represented a significant step forward for the many people who would have been lifelong inmates in institutions. Many of them could now lead relatively normal lives in the community. The drugs, however, did come at a price. One problem was the side effects, particularly of the early drugs. The most tragic consequence was an unintended one: as the numbers of clients in the state and county institutions decreased substantially, these institutions were closed. In theory, discharged clients were to be supported by resources in the community, thus linking the deinstitutionalization movement to the community mental health movement. In practice, the funding was paltry or nonexistent and many clients were left to fend for themselves on the streets (Torrey, 1988).

THE EVOLUTION OF PSYCHOSOCIAL OCCUPATIONAL THERAPY

The history of mental health treatment in the twentieth century provides a backdrop from which to view the evolution of psychosocial occupational therapy. It is important to remember that the profession did not develop in a vacuum, and in fact responded to changes in mental health treatment by coming up with its own innovative version of treatment, which blended work in occupations and activities with new ideas about treatment of the mentally ill. This portion of the chapter examines the ideas, approaches, and treatments that most influenced psychosocial practice during the decades that followed the profession's founding.

The 1920s and 1930s

From the founding years through the 1930s, psychosocial occupational therapy practice remained focused on improving clients through their engagement in occupations. "The therapist, through stimulating the patient to engage in certain activities, aims to awaken interest, develop concentration, restore coordination, revive hope, inspire confidence, and give satisfaction through personal achievement" (Haas, 1931, p. 244). Practice took place primarily in the state hospitals, where occupational therapy was responsible for overseeing the environment in which the occupations occurred. Clients worked throughout the hospital, including the laundry, the shops, the sewing room, and the farm (Patterson, 1931). On the ward clients were engaged in habit training and crafts (Fagley, 1931). Physical activities were also deemed important, such as walks, dances, baseball, and fishing trips. At the time therapy was still very much influenced by a humanistic philosophy: "Our patients are people, like you and me, to whom something has happened, and as a result [they] are unable to make satisfactory adjustments to life . . . and must be treated accordingly" (Stevenson, 1931, p. 85).

The 1940s and 1950s

During these decades psychosocial practice shifted in response to the establishment of the psychoanalytic perspective as a part of occupational therapy's treatment rationale. This does not mean that occupational therapy abandoned its belief in the importance of adaptation and the environment. "Persons suffering from mental disease are generally ill as a result of an accumulation of unsuccessful efforts on the part of the individual to adjust to the environment" (Wade, 1947, p. 83). The psychoanalytic perspective was simply added to the occupational therapy treatment rationale. In the first edition of the Willard and Spackman text, Wade (1947) describes occupational therapy as a "supplement" to psychoanalysis. "In the type of treatment, consisting primarily of psychotherapy using the psychoanalytic approach, occupational therapy functions as indirect therapy. It provides a socially acceptable means of sublimation for the conscious expression of the instinctual urges of the patient" (p. 104).

By the late 1950s the psychoanalytic object relations approach had become a recognized rationale to treat persons with schizophrenia (AOTA, 1959). Its major proponents were Fidler (1958) and Azima and Azima (1959). Gail Fidler (1958) argued that the primary goal of treatment was ego integration and maturation: "The development of a realistic self concept and ego strength can occur for the schizophrenic only to the extent that his primitive narcissistic needs are gratified" (p. 10). Fidler (1957) recommended that occupational therapy activities use objects and object relations as the primary treatment method. "Activities used as treatment provide an almost unique situation in which the patient as an active participant can deal with his actions as well as his feelings and thoughts" (p. 8). Crafts were advocated as an excellent medium in that they offered the opportunity for creative expression and affective display (Smith, Barrow, & Whitney, 1959). For example, clay was commonly used with "regressed patients, on the assumption that unstructured manipulation . . . is at once an easy and satisfying anal activity" (p. 21). Occupational therapists were also urged to use art (Friedman, 1952) and music (Reese, 1952) as occupations that would encourage expression of feelings.

However, Fidler (1957) envisioned a much larger significance for occupational therapy than simply enabling the client to experience certain feelings as she or he hammered a copper tray. "Occupational therapy provides the patient with a laboratory for living, a situation in which he can learn and practice new skills in living, experiment in a give and take relationship with others, utilize insights gained in psychotherapy, and learn and test more effective means of communication" (p. 8). Hand in hand with providing a "laboratory for living" was the therapist's own ability to influence the interaction. This came to be termed "the therapeutic use of self" and was formally recognized as an important therapeutic tool by the profession (AOTA, 1959).

Indeed, Huntting (1953) argued that the occupational therapist should put as much thought into how she or he related to the client as to the choice of activity.

Near the end of the 1950s, occupational therapists began to document the effects of thorazine and serpasil on clients with major psychoses (Elkins & Van Vlack, 1957). The changes seen in clients were quite substantial: They became much more relaxed and organized, and were able to participate more fully in occupational therapy activities (Clauer & Wise, 1958). However, it was also noted that at high doses of thorazine clients showed signs of incoordination and Parkinson-like symptoms. Occupational therapists also treated clients who underwent ECT or lobotomies. "Occupational therapists must be alert to the anxiety and dread of shock therapy by the patients and try to alleviate it through their interest in activity" (Elkins & Van Vlack, 1957, p. 269). The focus of treatment after the ECT was to prevent relapse (Clauer & Wise, 1958). Occupational therapists who treated clients with lobotomies were urged to use graded activities to decrease their confusion and regression (Shalik, 1955).

The 1960s and 1970s

These decades were a time of great concern with the role of psychosocial occupational therapy. One way to view this crisis was to see it within the larger context of the field of mental health. Shimota (1965), a psychologist, suggested in an address to occupational therapists that their questions were similar to those raised by other mental health professionals who were questioning the effectiveness of current approaches to treatment. Many of these questions concerned the effectiveness and appropriateness of psychoanalysis, particularly in the treatment of schizophrenia. Questions were also raised by psychiatrists such as Szasz (1960), who proposed that mental illness was a myth—a social construct. At the root of these questions, he believed, was a concern for "the ineffectiveness of current forms of treatment. If one method does not work, we have to find a new one but, had it worked, we'd be quite satisfied with it" (p. 80).

Woodside (1971), in a paper ostensibly about the history of occupational therapy, situated the problem within the profession itself. "Psychiatric occupational therapy could cease to exist because other professions are rapidly absorbing our body of knowledge, they appear to the public to be offering the same services that we offer, and they are selling their programs to other professionals and the public more effectively than we are" (p. 229). As an occupational therapist Woodside was discouraged when she saw nurses, psychologists, social workers, vocational counselors, and recreation, music, art, dance, and activity therapists doing aspects of occupational therapy. "*Their* 'therapy' looks very similar to ours and I wonder if we can adequately explain our uniqueness to those concerned with the rising costs of medical care and the overlapping of professional services" (pp. 229–230). Psychosocial occupational therapy was floundering, Woodside argued, because it was unable to articulate its uniqueness and to fight for its services. "I suggest that occupational therapy is gradually losing its professional role in psychiatric care because we have always been unsure of our unique professional responsibilities . . . and have not fought to maintain the boundaries of our services to patients, but have repeatedly capitulated to more established and more verbal professions" (p. 230). Woodside ended her address with a warning and a challenge to all psychosocial occupational therapists: "Society may lose a profession with a vibrant history and the potential for a healthy future. What are you doing to prevent this?" (p. 230).

In answer to Woodside's question, innovative ideas were being offered within psychosocial occupational therapy. Howe and Dippy (1968) proposed that the next site for practice should be the new, comprehensive community mental health centers funded by the federal government as well as the psychiatric day hospitals that were becoming increasingly popular. This idea built on the growing recognition within the profession that the best environment for psychosocial occupational therapy was the community. "If the fundamental principles of occupational therapy are carefully examined, the idea emerges that the most meaningful place to carry out such treatment would be in the home and in the community. The most natural social context in which to treat a patient would be with the family or people with whom he lives" (Watanabe, 1967, p. 353). Bockoven (1971) urged occupational therapy practitioners to set up services in the community based on moral treatment. He said, "It is the occupational therapist's inborn respect for the realities of life, for the real tasks of living, and for the time it takes the individual to develop his modes of coping with his tasks, that leads me to urge haste on the profession . . . to assert its leadership in fashioning the design of human service programs. . . . Don't drop dead, take over instead!" (p. 224).

Sandra Watanabe (1967) argued that community treatment enabled the occupational therapist to focus on the "life tasks of the patient—his education and work, avocational and social interests, and all activities of daily living, including self care, housekeeping and child-rearing" (p. 354). In particular, she emphasized the importance of treatment based on a knowledge of the habits and patterns the individual had adopted. She proposed that the primary treatment modalities were to be found in the client's home: making a cup of tea, doing financial planning, developing child care techniques, practicing vocational skills, or initiating a hobby. She de-emphasized crafts except where they were contextually appropriate: "the most realistic tasks and objects would be the life tasks and personal objects of the individual" (p. 353). The ultimate advantage of treatment in the community, she argued, was that it promoted occupational therapy treatment that was client-centered. "When the consultation is patient-centered, we direct our attention to general case management, with a life task focus [on] the activities of daily living, motivational techniques and enriching activities" (p. 355).

Another important idea was the activity or task-oriented group led by the occupational therapist, as a complement to the psychotherapy group. Shannon and Snortum (1965) argued that the occupational therapist was in a perfect position to initiate activity groups where clients could have an opportunity to learn and practice

new skills. "While intensive group psychotherapy is useful as a point of origin for verbal insights, patients require assistance in converting verbal insights into new behavior. By working in a group of limited size, the patient could be provided with a more
closely supervised opportunity for practicing rudimentary social skills and could
receive needed feedback from actual experience" (p. 345). They urged therapists to
think beyond their traditional beliefs about their work: "Traditionally the responsibility for group psychotherapy in psychiatric hospitals has rested with the psychiatrist,
psychologist or the social worker. The failure of the occupational therapist to become
actively involved in this area may be attributed to the belief that group work is not the
occupational therapist's responsibility" (p. 344).

Fidler (1969) envisioned the task-oriented group as one context in which her
"laboratory for living" could take place. "The nature of the occupational therapy setting which expects active involvement in doing, provides a microcosm for life-work
situations which can be seen and explored as they occur rather than in retrospect"
(p. 69). She proposed that the intent of the task-oriented group was to provide a shared
work experience where the relationship between "feeling, thinking and behavior, their
impact on others and on task accomplishment, and productivity can be viewed and
explored" (p. 45). She defined a task as any activity or process directed toward creating a service or end product. Examples included publishing a newspaper, cooking,
gardening, and planning an outing. A primary goal of the groups was to promote
problem solving: "Responsibility for selecting and accomplishing a task provides opportunity for the group to explore problem-solving and decision-making skills, [and]
to have concrete evidence of their ability to function" (p. 45). Even though the group
might take place in an institution, the task-oriented group, as Fidler defined it, more
closely resembled living in the community, and thereby provided practice in learning
those skills needed for community adjustment.

In response to questions raised at the University of Southern California as to
whether psychosocial occupational therapy practice should remain a legitimate part
of the university curriculum, Mary Reilly (1966) set up a model occupational therapy
program. Reilly observed that there was little theory or research to substantiate its
effectiveness. The model program had several key components. One was that clients
would graduate from classes in the Department of Occupational Therapy to employment in various departments of the hospital and then to work in the community. Thus,
the program was set up on a developmental model that assumed that old behaviors
could be reconstituted and new behaviors could be learned. It also emphasized the
importance of work in an individual's life. A second principle was that the program
was focused on developing the individual's capacity for self-direction and decision
making. This was based on the belief that therapy needed to go beyond simply guiding and directing, by giving the client sufficient autonomy to take responsibility for
his or her own decisions. Otherwise, Reilly felt that treatment just perpetuated social
disability. The third principle focused on the importance of providing normal living

experiences that were performed at natural times. Thus, each client had a structured schedule that more or less corresponded to the "natural social order of daily living" (p. 63). This principle drew on Meyer's ideas regarding habits, routine, temporal adaptation, and balance of work and play. For these ideas Reilly credits Meyer and urges a recommitment to his principles. We can see in this program the foundation for a theoretical model that Reilly and her colleagues would call Occupational Behavior and ultimately would become the Model of Human Occupation (Kielhofner, 2002).

The 1980s and 1990s

The final two decades of the twentieth century brought significant changes to occupational therapy psychosocial practice. A critical area for psychosocial practice was the development and refinement of theoretical models and assessments. Kielhofner introduced A Model of Human Occupation (MOHO) (1985, 1995), which provided a theoretical model that addressed "the motivation for occupation, the patterning of occupational behavior into routines and lifestyles, the nature of skilled performance, and the influence of environment on occupational behavior" (Kielhofner, 1997, p. 187). Although designed to be used with all client populations, it provides a particularly strong model for psychosocial practice in its focus on occupation, habits and routines, and motivation. In addition, several assessments based on MOHO were developed. For example, the Occupational Performance History Interview (OPHI) was an instrument "designed to gather an accurate and clinically useful history of an individual's work, play, and self-care performance" (Kielhofner & Henry, 1988, p. 489) for adolescents and adults. Another valuable theoretical approach was created by Dunn, Brown, and McGuigan (1994), who proposed the Ecology of Human Performance framework to provide "a structure for thinking about context as a key variable in assessment and intervention planning" (p. 595). They argued that, "contextual factors such as the physical qualities of an environment, the cultural background of a person, or the effect of friendships on performance are often missing from assessment tools typically used in occupational therapy" (p. 595). A client-centered approach to assessment is embodied in the Canadian Occupational Performance Measure (COPM), "an outcome measure designed to be used by occupational therapists to assess client outcome in the areas of self-care, productivity, and leisure" (Pollock, 1993, p. 299). This assessment is an obvious fit with psychosocial practice in its focus on therapist-client interaction. Indeed, these three approaches—focused on occupation, context, and client-centered practice—reflect what became the major tenets of the Occupational Therapy Practice Framework (OTPF), published by the AOTA in 2002 and revised in 2008.

Building on Fidler's "laboratory for living," a major focus of psychosocial rehabilitation was training in life skills (Hayes & Halford, 1993). This included training in social skills, independent living skills, prevocational skills, stress management, and assertion. In addition to life skills training, new arenas for psychosocial practice were proposed.

Schindler (1988) explored the role of psychosocial occupational therapy in helping people cope with AIDS—a relatively new phenomenon at that time. She argued, "With all of the physical, psychosocial, and cognitive aspects of the AIDS illness, working with the AIDS population can be a vital role for [psychosocial] occupational therapy" (p. 512). Sholle-Martin and Alessi (1990) defined child psychiatry as an emerging area of practice for psychosocial practitioners. They proposed an approach based on MOHO, which they suggested could provide practitioners with a way to assess the child's volitional, habituation, performance, and environmental dimensions (p. 873). Fike (1990), in a special issue on multiple personality disorder proposed that "Occupational therapy can serve as a stabilizing force for patients with multiple personality disorder" (p. 1006) by providing developmental play, role management, daily living skills training, and prevocational support.

Issues of gender and cultural sensitivity arose during these decades. Nahmias and Froehlich (1993) argued for the importance of addressing women's mental health issues: "In the past two decades, mental health professionals have been active in reversing issues of sexism in clinical practice. Occupational therapists, however, have been slow to integrate the psychological developmental theories for women . . . Occupational therapy's domain of concern—work, leisure, and self-maintenance—is compatible with the needs of women, as is our emphasis on collaboration and caring in the patient-therapist relationship" (p. 40). Dillard et al. (1992) identified the importance of cultural competence in psychosocial practice, and proposed an innovative multicultural model consisting of special focus programs. They emphasized that, "The key to success of such programs is a culturally competent professional staff" (p. 721). Furthermore, they asserted, "all [occupational] therapists have a responsibility to develop cultural competence by being open to inspection of their own culture and developing an interest and knowledge base about other cultures" (p. 725).

As exemplified by MOHO, this period marked the beginning of a return to occupation for the profession, both in concept and terminology. As Nelson expressed it in his 1996 Slagle lecture, the profession should use the term *occupation*, not the "A" word (Nelson, 1997, p. 549). He argued, "We are called occupational therapists, and the essence of our profession is the use of occupation as a therapeutic method. The term *activity* [italics added] denotes motion, for example, volcanic activity . . . not occupation that is replete with meaning and purpose" (p. 549). Thus, after almost a century, the profession returned to using the term *occupation*, which was first coined by the founders in 1917. More than a word, it gave occupational therapists in contemporary practice an organizing principle around which they could communicate with other professionals, and conceptualize their assessments and interventions. It should be noted, however, that although psychosocial occupational therapists were among those therapists who used the word *activity* prior to the 1990s, they of all the specialties adhered most closely to the founding value of engagement in occupations through arts and crafts, work, and habit training.

Psychosocial therapists also adhered most closely to the humanistic principles of moral treatment, even when they worked in the medical model of inpatient psychiatric hospitals. However, unlike physical disabilities practice—where the humanistic approach was dwarfed by the scientific reductionism of the medical model—practitioners in psychosocial practice faced a difference challenge. It became clear in the 1980s and 1990s that scientific advances in the psychotropic drugs drastically reduced the length of inpatient stay, and reduced the need for occupational therapy. It should be noted that occupational therapists were not alone. In his history of psychiatry, Shorter (1997) writes, "In two hundred years' time, psychiatrists had progressed from being the healers of the therapeutic asylum to serving as gatekeepers for Prozac. Psychiatric illness had passed from a feared sign of bad blood—a genetic curse—to . . . a treatable condition not essentially different from any other medical problem. . . . Indeed, so much like other medical illnesses had disorders of the mind become that the uncomfortable question arose, who needed psychiatrists?" (p. 325). In terms of occupational therapy, the figures speak for themselves: In 1973, 13.8% of all occupational therapists worked in an inpatient psychiatric setting. In 1990, the number had declined to 4.6% (AOTA, 2006).

The advent of effective pharmacological treatment is not the only factor that has contributed to a decline in the number of psychosocial occupational therapists.

Theoretically, the loss of inpatient opportunities should have been offset by an increase in community mental health services due to the deinstitutionalization that began in the 1970s. Indeed community treatment is a much better fit with the services that occupational therapists can provide (Baum & Law, 1998). However, by the 1980s, it became apparent that deinstitutionalization was a failure (Mollica, 1983). Sufficient funding was never provided to hire the necessary mental health professionals; community mental health centers were never built; residential homes were scarce and thus those with mental illness returned home to be cared for by their families, or were shifted from state institutions to nursing homes, or joined the ranks of the homeless. Unfortunately, Bockoven's vision of a Consolation House on every block did not come to pass. However, this shift from inpatient care did provide impetus for a model shift from a medical to a social one that focuses on the power of individuals with mental illness to direct and participate in their own recovery. This has ultimately developed into what is known today as the Recovery Movement (Swarbrick, 2009) that has as its fundamental concepts a holistic, individualized, and person-centered approach, one very much in keeping with the founder's original vision.

Another challenge to psychosocial therapists is managed mental health care. VanLeit (1995) describes it this way: "The topic of managed care has stimulated much emotional discussion among occupational therapists. When therapists get together, our talk turns to short lengths of stay, the impossibility of providing effective treatment, the hassles of paperwork and bureaucracy, and the seeming loss of control over professional decision making. Anger, frustration, loss, and grief are the dominant feelings about a changing mental health care system that we no longer recognize" (p. 428). Trickey and Kennedy (1995) did a survey of the agencies in South Carolina with mental health units in order to examine why only a small percentage of therapists in their state worked in mental health. They found that salary demands, turnover, lack of available applicants, and ability to generate revenue, were among the reasons facilities did not hire occupational therapists (p. 452). This sobering picture of psychosocial practice is balanced by some positive factors. Cottrell (1990) found that despite the concerns voiced in the literature about psychosocial practice, she found a high level of perceived competence in psychosocial therapists she surveyed: ". . . ninety percent of the 95 respondents perceived their ability to adapt their role to a changing practice and mental health system as good or excellent" (p. 122). She emphasized that it was important to nurture those who chose the field, and to support their development through continuing education and professional activities. In the previously discussed article on managed care, Van Leit proposed that, "At its best, managed care may actually support innovations and diversity of treatment approaches as long as empirical evidence supports the effectiveness of these approaches. It is even possible that mental health and substance abuse practices and outcomes may be improved (p. 433). She argues that occupational therapists need to be "visible, proactive and accountable in the process of defining and developing a cost-effective continuum of programs and services that emphasizes the community over inpatient settings, identifies effective methods to measure outcomes, and develops clinically reasonable and flexible guidelines and protocols" (p. 433). Friedland and Renwick (1993) argued that the perception that psychosocial occupational therapy practice is declining can lead to a self-fulfilling prophecy. They proposed that therapists needed to get more involved in prevention and health promotion. "We should be involved in developing appropriate environments for housing the homeless . . . in facilitating adaptation in daily tasks for new immigrants . . . and in reducing stress and increasing well-being of persons in work and school environments" (p. 470). Finally, in her article about the state of mental health practice, Bonder (1987) poses these questions: "Is occupational therapy in mental health in the midst of an insoluble crisis, or can therapists follow psychologists' example and use this occasion to expand their realm of influence? Can changes in practice be developed in a positive direction, or will occupational therapy in mental health disappear? Can mental health occupational therapists move into new areas of practice, such as employee assistance programs, boarding homes, and community centers, or will they remain bound to the existing arenas of inpatient practice?" (p. 498). Her answer is to argue that although change brings uncertainty it can also bring opportunity. She quotes Duhl (1982), who asserts, "mental health practitioners can influence the new paradigms that emerge by the ways they choose to work with their patients and in their communities. Thus, through our visions, we can create the future" (p. 693).

SUMMARY

This chapter has traced the history of psychosocial occupational therapy through the 1990s. The rest of the book will discuss contemporary issues and the most recent changes in practice. In looking back, one way to see the psychosocial occupational therapy of today is to view it as an amalgam of past best practices. In viewing the last 90 years we can identify many ideas that have been retained, albeit in a somewhat different form, and other approaches that have been dropped. In part this is due to the fact that mental health practice has changed, and so occupational therapy treatment has changed along with it. For example, psychoanalysis no longer provides the predominant framework for treatment that it did in the 1940s and 1950s. But occupational therapists still retain the notion of the importance of meaning in occupation, which one could argue was derived from the focus on the symbolic nature of the projective activities.

At times the founding concepts of occupational therapy were de-emphasized, as new approaches and techniques were introduced. However, by the end of the twentieth century there was a reemphasis on the founding ideas, as psychosocial occupational therapy practice appears to have returned to its roots. Today we see practice that is still grounded in the humanistic philosophy of moral treatment, "the conception that occupational therapy is based first and foremost upon respect for human individuality and on a fundamental perception of the individual's needs to engage in creative activity" (Bockoven, 1971, p. 223).

The central concept of occupational therapy is the same as that articulated by the founders: engagement in valued occupations (Law, 2002). Occupations continue to provide a way to help create a balance of work, play, and rest (Kielhofner, 2002). Habits are seen as integral to optimal performance in both personal and instrumental activities of daily living (AOTA, 2008). Arts and crafts remain a viable medium for motivating, promoting good work habits, and increasing skills. Vocational occupations help to develop new skills and productive habits that can sustain independent living in the community.

In addition to the founding concepts, innovations from the 1960s have also been incorporated into today's practice. More psychosocial treatment today is done in groups and conducted in the community. Treatment is client-centered and focused on providing functional living skills (Melville, Baltic, Bettcher, & Nelson, 2002). Drug management has become a critical aspect of treatment for most clients, and this has allowed many to live in the community with the support of occupational therapy services. Thus, contemporary psychosocial practice consists of some of the best ideas of the past reformulated into models and treatments that also reflect today's beliefs regarding mental illness.

As this book demonstrates, psychosocial occupational therapists today are actively engaged in many aspects of practice. However, the declining numbers of therapists who choose to work in mental health suggests, there is a need for vigilance and innovation. Conflicts remain over which mental health professional should provide which service. The need to justify services to third-party payers is critical, and occupational therapists must continue developing their role in all community aspects of treatment. The need for evidence-based research continues, as does the need to support the practice of mental health in educational programs. A recent analysis of mental health research published in the *American Journal of Occupational Therapy* concluded that evidence-based research was sparse and that the level of evidence was weak (D'Amico, Jaffe, & Gibson, 2010). They recommended that more research be conducted in the United States, and that clinicians, researchers, and educators collaborate on generating research questions and the best methods for data collection and analysis. Furthermore, they recognized that research is not done in a vacuum: "Any expectation for future research in the mental health practice arena must be linked with the policies of occupational therapy practice and education and individual behavior. We cannot expect therapists to practice in mental health without concerted efforts to recruit and train people interested in the practice area. Our educational programs cannot erode, dilute, or disparage mental health education and must strengthen the research training of our students" (p. 668).

In summary, psychosocial occupational therapists must continue to clearly articulate what occupational therapy can contribute to an individual's mental health, and how its services can be effective. Or, as our founder Eleanor Clarke Slagle (1923) expressed it, we need to better define occupational therapy's role in the evolutionary process in which an individual makes the change from a position of liability to asset. It is hoped that this history will help psychosocial occupational therapists understand their rich past as well as future promise.

REVIEW QUESTIONS

1. How are the contributions of the founders exemplified in current psychosocial occupational therapy practice?
2. What values have endured from the founding of occupational therapy to the present?
3. Describe six innovations introduced by occupational therapy leaders in the 1950s and 1960s that contribute to practice today.

REFERENCES

Addams, J. (1911). *Twenty years at Hull House*. New York: Macmillan.

Ambrosi, E., & Schwartz, K. B. (1995). The profession's image, 1917–1925: Occupational therapy as represented in the media. *American Journal of Occupational Therapy, 49*, 715–719.

American Occupational Therapy Association. (1925). An outline of lectures on occupational therapy to medical students and physicians. *Occupational Therapy and Rehabilitation, 4*(4), 277–292.

American Occupational Therapy Association. (1959). The schizophrenic patient. In AOTA (Ed.), *The objectives and functions of occupational therapy* (pp. 130–136). Dubuque, IA: Wm. C. Brown.

American Occupational Therapy Association. (2006). Workforce and Compensation Report.

American Occupational Therapy Association. (2008). Occupational therapy practice framework: Domain and process (2nd edition). *American Journal of Occupational Therapy, 62* 625–683.

Analysis of Crafts. (1928). Continuation of the Report of the Committee on Installations and Advice. *Occupational Therapy and Rehabilitation, 7*, 417–420.

Azima, H., & Azima, F. (1959). Outline of a dynamic theory of occupational therapy. *American Journal of Occupational Therapy, 13*, 215–221.

Baum, C., & Law, M. (1998). Community health: A responsibility, an opportunity, and a fit for occupational therapy. *American Journal of Occupational Therapy, 52*, 7–10.

Bierer, J. (1980). From psychiatry to social and community psychiatry. *International Journal of Social Psychiatry, 26*, 77–79.

Bockoven, J. S. (1971). Legacy of moral treatment: 1800's to 1910. *American Journal of Occupational Therapy, 25*(5), 223–225.

Bonder, B. (1987). Occupational therapy in mental health: Crisis or opportunity? *American Journal of Occupational Therapy, 41*, 495–499.

Boris, E. (1984). *Art and labor: John Ruskin, William Morris, and the craftsman ideal in America 1876–1915.* Philadelphia: Temple University Press.

Brown, P. K. (1917). The potteries of Arequipa Sanatorium. *Modern Hospital, 8*(6), 394–396.

Caradec, L. (1860). Topographie medico-hygienique du departement du Finiestere. In E. Shorter (Ed.). (1997), *A history of psychiatry* (p. 11). New York: Wiley.

Clauer, C., & Wise, K. (1958). Tranquilizing drug effects on the schizophrenic patient in occupational therapy. *American Journal of Occupational Therapy, 12*, 69–73.

Cottrell, R. F. (1990). Perceived competence among occupational therapists in mental health. *American Journal of Occupational Therapy, 44*, 118–124.

D'Amico, M., Jaffe, L., & Gibson, R. (2010). Mental health evidence in the *American Journal of Occupational Therapy. American Journal of Occupational Therapy, 64*, 660–669.

Dillard, M., Andonian, L., Flores, O., Lai, L., MacRae, A., & Shakir, M. (1992). Culturally competent occupational therapy in a diversely populated mental health setting. *American Journal of Occupational Therapy, 46*, 721–726.

Dix, D. (1971/1943). *Report to the legislature of Massachusetts.* New York: Arno, pp. 5–7.

Duhl, L. J. (1982). New paradigms for mental health. *Hospital and Community Psychiatry, 33*, 693.

Dunn, W., Brown, C., & McGuigan, A. (1994). The ecology of human performance: A framework for considering the effect of context. *American Journal of Occupational Therapy, 48*, 595–607.

Dunton, W. R. (1917). History of occupational therapy. *Modern Hospital, 8*(6), 380–382.

Dunton, W. R. (1928). The three "R's" of occupational therapy. *Occupational Therapy and Rehabilitation, 7*, 345–348.

Elkins, H., & Van Vlack, N. (1957). Changes in occupational therapy due to the tranquilizing drugs. *American Journal of Occupational Therapy, 111*, 269–272.

Fagley, R. C. (1931). The value of occupational therapy in treatment of mental cases. *Occupational Therapy and Rehabilitation, 10*, 291–298.

Fidler, G. S. (1957). The role of occupational therapy in a multi-discipline approach to psychiatric illness. *American Journal of Occupational Therapy, 11*, 8–35.

Fidler, G. S. (1958). Some unique contributions of occupational therapy in treatment of the schizophrenic. *American Journal of Occupational Therapy, 12*, 9–12.

Fidler, G. S. (1969). The task-oriented group as a context for treatment. *American Journal of Occupational Therapy, 23*, 43–48.

Fields, G. E. (1911). The effect of occupation upon the individual. *American Journal of Insanity, 8*, 103–109.

Fike, M. L. (1990). Considerations and techniques in the treatment of persons with multiple personality disorder. *American Journal of Occupational Therapy, 44,* 999–1007.

Friedland, J., & Renwick, R. M. (1993). The issue is: Psychosocial occupational therapy: Time to cast off the gloom and doom. *American Journal of Occupational Therapy, 47,* 467–471.

Friedman, I. (1952). Art therapy, an aid to reintegrative processes. *American Journal of Occupational Therapy, 6,* 64–65.

Full text of the Republican platform as reported to the convention last night. (1924, June 12). *New York Times,* p. 4.

Gay, P. (1989). *The Freud reader.* New York: Norton.

Grob, G. (1991). *From asylum to community: Mental health policy in modern America.* Princeton, NJ: Princeton University Press.

Haas, L. J. (1924). The men's occupational therapy work at Bloomingdale Hospital. *Modern Hospital, 22*(4), 410, 420.

Haas, L. J. (1931). Precision in presenting occupational therapy to the mentally and nervously ill. *Occupational Therapy and Rehabilitation, 10,* 241–249.

Hall, H. (1913). *The systematic use of work as a remedy in neurasthenia and allied conditions.* Boston: W. M. Leonard.

Hall, H. (1917). Remunerative occupations for the handicapped. *Modern Hospital, 8*(6), 383–386.

Hall, H. (1921). The high-grade neurasthenic. *Boston Medical and Surgical Journal, 185*(8), 232–235.

Hall, H. (1922). Occupational therapy in 1921. *Modern Hospital, 18*(1), 61–63.

Hard Times Cause Record in Insane. (1922, January 2). *New York Times,* p. 12.

Hayes, R., & Halford, W. K. (1993). Generalization of occupational therapy effects in psychiatric rehabilitation. *American Journal of Occupational Therapy, 47,* 161–167.

Hospital Will Restore the Industrial Wounded. (1923, July 8). *New York Times,* p. 3.

Howe, M., & Dippy, K. (1968). The role of occupational therapy in community mental health. *American Journal of Occupational Therapy, 22,* 521–524.

Humphrey, E. F. (1922). Classifying therapeutic occupations from the standpoint of mental patients. *Modern Hospital, 18*(6), 554–556.

Huntting, I. (1953). The importance of interaction between patient and occupational therapist. *American Journal of Occupational Therapy, 7,* 107–109.

Johnson, S. C. (1920). Instruction in handicrafts and design for hospital patients. *Modern Hospital, 15,* 69–75.

Kidner, T. B. (1925). The hospital pre-industrial shop. *Occupational Therapy and Rehabilitation, 4*(3), 187–194.

Kielhofner, G. (1985). A model of human occupation (1st ed.). Baltimore: Williams and Wilkins.

Kielhofner, G. (1995). A model of human occupation (2nd ed.). Baltimore: Williams and Wilkins.

Kielhofner, G. (1997). Conceptual foundations of occupational therapy (2nd ed). Philadelphia: F.A. Davis.

Kielhofner, G. (2002). *Model of human occupation* (3rd ed.). Philadelphia: Lippincott Williams & Wilkins.

Kielhofner, G., & Henry, A. (1988). Development and investigation of the Occupational Performance History Interview. *American Journal of Occupational Therapy, 42,* 489–498.

Kraepelin, E. (1883). *Compendium der psychiatrie.* Leipzig: Abel.

Law, M. (2002). Participation in the occupations of everyday life. *American Journal of Occupational Therapy, 56,* 640–649.

Levine, R. E. (1987). The influence of the arts-and-crafts movement on the professional status of occupational therapy. *American Journal of Occupational Therapy, 41*(4), 248–254.

Melville, L., Baltic, T., Bettcher, T., & Nelson, D. (2002). Patients' perspectives on the self-identified goals assessment. *American Journal of Occupational Therapy, 56,* 650–659.

Meyer, A. (1948/1905). The role of habit-disorganizations: Paper for the New York Psychiatrical Society. In A. Lief (Ed.), *The commonsense psychiatry of Dr. Adolph Meyer: Fifty-two selected papers* (pp. 178–183). New York: McGraw Hill.

Meyer, A. (1948/1921). The contributions of psychiatry to the understanding of life problems: An address at the celebration of the 100th anniversary of Bloomingdale Hospital. In A. Lief (Ed.), *The commonsense psychiatry of Dr. Adolph Meyer: Fifty-two selected papers* (pp. 1–15). New York: McGraw Hill.

Meyer, A. (1922a). The philosophy of occupation therapy. *Archives of Occupational Therapy, 1*, 1–10.

Meyer, A. (1948/1922b). Normal and abnormal repression: Address to the Progressive Education Association. In A. Lief (Ed.), *The commonsense psychiatry of Dr. Adolph Meyer: Fifty-two selected papers* (pp. 479–490). New York: McGraw Hill.

Meyer, A. (1948/1934). The birth and development of the mental hygiene movement. In A. Lief (Ed.), *The commonsense psychiatry of Dr. Adolph Meyer: Fifty-two selected papers* (pp. 312–319). New York: McGraw Hill.

Mollica, R. F. (1983). From asylum to community: The threatened disintegration of public policy. *New England Journal of Medicine, 308*, 367–372.

Nahmias, R., & Froehlich, J. (1993). Women's mental health: Implications for occupational therapy. *American Journal of Occupational Therapy, 47*, 35–41.

Nelson, D. L. (1997). 1996 Eleanor Clarke Slagle Lecture: Why the profession of occupational therapy will flourish in the 21st century. *American Journal of Occupational Therapy, 51*, 11–24.

Newton, I. (1917). Consolation House. Archives of the Wilma L. West Library, Bethesda, MD: American Occupational Therapy Association.

Occupational Treatment of Patients in State Hospitals. (1914). *Modern Hospital, 2*(4), 302–305.

Patterson, W. L. (1931). Occupational therapy in a state hospital for the insane. *Occupational Therapy and Rehabilitation, 10*, 281–289.

Pinel, P. (1809). *Traite medico-philosophique sur l'alientation mentale* (2nd ed.). Paris: J. A. Brosson.

Pollock, N. (1993). Client-centered assessment. *American Journal of Occupational Therapy, 47*, 298–301.

Reese, M. R. (1952). Music as occupational therapy for psychiatric patients. *American Journal of Occupational Therapy, 6*, 14–49.

Reilly, M. (1966). A psychiatric occupational therapy program as a teaching model. *American Journal of Occupational Therapy, 20*, 61–67.

Research in Occupational Therapy: An Announcement. (n.d.). Archives of the Wilma L. West Library, Bethesda, MD: American Occupational Therapy Association.

Robeson, H. (1937). A testimonial to Eleanor Clarke Slagle. Twenty-first Annual Meeting of the American Occupational Therapy Association, September 14. Archives of the Wilma L. West Library, Bethesda, MD: American Occupational Therapy Association.

Rollin, H. R. (1990). The dark before the dawn. *Journal of Psychopharmacology, 4*, 109–114.

Rothman, D. J. (1971). *The discovery of the asylum*. Boston: Little, Brown.

Seek Occupations for War Cripples. (1917, September 4). *New York Times*, p. 20.

Schindler, V. (1988). Psychosocial occupational therapy intervention with AIDS patients. *American Journal of Occupational Therapy, 42*, 507–512.

Shalik, H. (1955). Refining the use of occupational therapy with the lobotomized patient. *American Journal of Occupational Therapy, 9*, 118–120.

Shannon, P., & Snortum, J. (1965). An activity group's role in intensive psychotherapy. *American Journal of Occupational Therapy, 19*, 344–347.

Shimota, H. (1965). Psychiatric occupational therapy. *American Journal of Occupational Therapy, 19,* 79–82.

Sholle-Martin, S., & Alessi, N. (1990). Formulating a role for occupational therapy in child psychiatry: A clinical application. *American Journal of Occupational Therapy, 44,* 871–882.

Shorter, E. (1997). *A history of psychiatry.* New York: Wiley.

Slagle, E. C. (1923). Report of the secretary-treasurer. *Archives of Occupational Therapy, 1,* 49–59.

Slagle, E. C. (1924). A year's development of occupational therapy in New York state hospitals. *Modern Hospital, 22,* 98–104.

Smith, P., Barrow, H., & Whitney, J. (1959). Psychological attributes of occupational therapy crafts. *American Journal of Occupational Therapy, 12,* 16–26.

Stevenson, G. H. (1931). The healing influence of work and play in a mental hospital. *Occupational Therapy and Rehabilitation, 11,* 85–89.

Swarbrick, M. (2009). Historical perspective—From institution to community. *Occupational Therapy in Mental Health, 25,* 201–223.

Szasz, T. S. (1960). *The myth of mental illness.* New York: Harper & Row.

Taylor, G. (1909, June). Letter from Graham Taylor to Governor Charles Deneen. In V. Quiroga (1995), *Occupational therapy: The first 30 years* (p. 42). Bethesda, MD: American Occupational Therapy Association.

Text of platform as presented to the Democratic National Convention. (1924, June 29). *New York Times,* p. 4.

Torrey, E. F. (1988). *Nowhere to go: The tragic odyssey of the homeless mentally ill.* New York: Harper & Row.

Trickey, B. A., & Kennedy, D. B. (1995). Use of occupational therapists in mental health settings in North Carolina. *American Journal of Occupational Therapy, 49,* 452–455.

VanLeit, B. (1995). Managed mental health care: Reflections in a time of turmoil. *American Journal of Occupational Therapy, 50,* 428–434.

Wade, B. (1947). Occupational therapy for patients with mental disease. In H. Willard & C. Spackman (Eds.), *Principles of occupational therapy* (pp. 81–111). Philadelphia: Lippincott.

Watanabe, S. G. (1967). The developing role of occupational therapy in a psychiatric home service. *American Journal of Occupational Therapy, 21,* 353–356.

Wiebe, R. H. (1967). *The search for order, 1877–1920.* New York: Hill & Wang.

Wilson, S. C. (1929). Habit training for mental cases. *Occupational Therapy and Rehabilitation, 8*(3), 189–197.

Woodside, H. (1971). The development of occupational therapy 1910–1929. *American Journal of Occupational Therapy, 25*(5), 226–230.

SUGGESTED RESOURCES

Hasselkus, B. R. (2002). *The meaning of everyday occupation.* Thorofare, NJ: Slack.

Fidler, G., & Fidler, J. (1954). *Introduction to psychiatric occupational therapy.* New York: Macmillan.

Fidler, G., & Fidler, J. (1963). *Occupational therapy, a communication process in psychiatry.* New York: Macmillan.

Lief, A. (Ed.). (1947). *The commonsense psychiatry of Dr. Adolph Meyer: Fifty-two selected papers.* New York: McGraw-Hill.

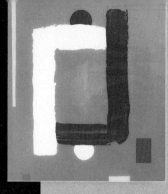

Chapter 5

Psychological Theories and Their Treatment Methods in Mental Health Practice

Lynne Andonian, PhD, OTR/L
Elizabeth Cara, PhD, OTR/L, MFT
Anne MacRae, PhD, OTR/L, BCMH, FAOTA

KEY TERMS

applied behavioral analysis (ABA)

biopsychosocial focus

brain plasticity

cognitive-behavioral therapy (CBT)

dialectical behavioral therapy (DBT)

eclectic

milieu treatment

positive regard

psychopharmacology

CHAPTER OUTLINE

Introduction
Humanistic Perspective
    Development of the Perspective
    The Social Context of Humanism
    Applications in Occupational Therapy
Biological Perspective
    The Brain
    Causal Factors of Psychopathology
    Applications in Occupational Therapy
Psychodynamic Perspective
    Psychoanalytic Concepts
    Neo-Freudian Theories
    Contemporary Psychodynamic Theories
    Applications in Occupational Therapy
Behavioral Perspective
    Applied Behavioral Analysis
    Applications in Occupational Therapy

Cognitive Perspective
    Expectations
    Appraisals
    Attributions
    Beliefs
    Applications in Occupational Therapy
Summary

INTRODUCTION

As discussed in Chapter 1, there has been a paradigm shift toward the concept of recovery as the driving force of mental health intervention. However, under the umbrella of recovery, it is generally understood, from a professional point of view, that a comprehensive understanding of a client, including relevant biological, psychological, and sociocultural factors, creates more effective and meaningful treatments. This greater understanding, including what is meaningful and motivating to her or him, is likely to enhance treatment compliance, thereby facilitating more positive outcomes. It is in this process of developing an understanding of the individual clients and their needs that an appreciation for multiple theories of mental illness becomes critical. Among the more prominent theoretical perspectives are the humanistic, biological, psychodynamic, behavioral, and cognitive. Each perspective represents a unique set of basic assumptions about psychological disorder, including relevant etiological factors and appropriate treatment strategies. In order to familiarize the reader with these theoretical perspectives, the major concepts of each will be presented independently. Although presented separately, it is not our intention to convey that these perspectives are necessarily incompatible. In order to gain a comprehensive understanding of the client, an integration of concepts from the varied perspectives is most useful. After all, no single one exists that is capable of explaining all psychopathology and mental health. Attending to the complex array of biological, intrapsychic, and interpersonal factors that may be creating and/or maintaining mental dysfunction allows for a comprehensive **biopsychosocial focus** understanding of the individual client. This, in turn, will foster the development of more individualized and effective treatment protocols.

Most contemporary therapists use an **eclectic** approach, employing ideas and techniques from a variety of perspectives in order to understand and treat effectively a client's presenting problems (Birkholtz & Blair, 2001; Ikiugu, Smallfield, & Condit, 2009; Yancosek, & Howell, 2010).) An eclectic approach means that an individual chooses the best of each and synthesizes the features into an overall approach. While eclectic approaches and attempts at theoretical integration have become quite popular, their success is variable (Patterson, 1989) and their use continues in the treatment of eating disorders (Henderson, 1999), the psychosocial aspects of pain management (Birkholtz & Blair, 2001), and the management of depression (Hudson, 2009). Although their success is variable, it seems reasonable to expect that practitioners who are eclectic in their orientation will have more tools available to them to address complex mental health needs.

HUMANISTIC PERSPECTIVE

The humanistic perspective emphasizes the value, worth, and potential of the individual, with a focus on the integrity of the client–therapist relationship. This model of psychological functioning offers a philosophy and an approach to dealing with clients in psychological distress to which all practitioners, regardless of theoretical orientation, should attend. With its primary focus on broad dimensions of an individual's life experience, the humanistic view is generally more encompassing than the other perspectives, which attend to rather specific aspects of human functioning such as physiological processes, unconscious conflicts, learned behaviors, and cognitive processes. For example, humanism pays careful attention to the individual's concept of self as well as personal values. Because of their global perspective, humanistic theories are often seen as more than simply explanations of psychological adjustment and personality development. In fact, they are often viewed as philosophies of life.

Development of the Perspective

The basic tenets of humanistic psychology arose in the early twentieth century as an alternative to the two prominent theoretical models of the time: the psychodynamic and behavioral paradigms. Humanistic principles, however, were evident prior to the development of the formal field of humanistic psychology. For example, early humanistic philosophies are evident in the work of G. Stanley Hall and William James, both of whom stressed the unique characteristics of human beings. In addition, the bridge between theoretical humanism and clinical practice was first seen in the early 1800s by Samuel Tuke, an English Quaker. Tuke developed a program, known appropriately as "moral treatment," stressing the humane treatment of the mentally ill. Prior to this time, clients with psychiatric illnesses were locked up in asylums, where they were provided with basic necessities (i.e., food, water, and shelter), but essentially removed from the community at large. Moral treatment encouraged active involvement in the care and upkeep of the asylum, as well as participation in selected self-care and leisure activities, which included woodworking, gardening, and sewing. Tuke found that engagement in daily tasks had a positive, reality-orienting effect on the psychiatric clients with whom he worked. As described by Schwartz in the previous chapter, moral treatment is quite consistent with the principles and practice of occupational therapy. Underlying Tuke's treatment principles is the basis of a humanistic treatment approach: the ability to look beyond the psychiatric disease, unconscious conflicts, and environmental precursors of behavior and toward the inherent worth of each individual.

The popularity of humanistic approaches in clinical practice waxed and waned, but the theoretical principles continued to be expounded, especially in Europe, where humanistic principles were closely tied to existential philosophy. The sociocultural trends of the 1950s and 1960s contributed to the reemergence of humanistic principles and practices in psychology. Humanists stressed that behaviorism and psychodynamic theory were too reductionist, with the former focusing on environmental stimuli and resulting observable behavior and the latter focusing on human behavior as being primarily sexually driven (Reilly, 1962). Both Abraham Maslow (1968) and Carl Rogers (1951) proposed more global and healthy perspectives of human functioning than these other paradigms, and both held as basic the belief that individuals were innately good and driven to achieve self-actualization (i.e., realize their potential as whole and self-contained beings).

Maslow defined a pyramidal hierarchy representing five levels of needs. The lower levels of the pyramid comprise "deficiency," or survival-based, needs (i.e., physiological needs, safety needs, the need to be loved, and the need to belong to a social group). As one moves up the hierarchy, needs become less survival driven and more focused on the components of happiness and personal success. Among these higher-level needs, or "meta-needs," is the need for esteem. Self-actualization, the point at which a person has realized fully his or her potential, lies at the peak of the pyramid. According to Maslow (1968), a person is only able to concentrate on and meet higher-level needs after lower-level needs have been met. Although Maslow's hierarchy of needs remains a valuable conceptualization, there is ongoing controversy about the rigidity of the "one-way linear trend—an ascent from lower to higher levels" (Rowan, 1999, p. 125). Hierarchical models tend to oversimplify the many factors, both internal and external, that influence human behavior and therefore do not account for the sometimes cyclical, rather than linear, progression through identified stages. A more recent model of human needs that is highly contextual and nonlinear is called *Human Scale Development* (1991) by Chilean economist, environmentalist, and professor Manfred Max-Neef. The matrix of "needs and satisfiers" that are part of this model succinctly describes the individual's fundamental human needs and how they are connected to society at large. This matrix is presented in Figure 5-1.

Carl Rogers was heavily influenced by Maslow's hierarchy of needs. He, too, felt the motivating drive of humans was to achieve a state of self-actualization. He believed that it is only through the process of trying to achieve self-actualization that an individual develops an increasingly differentiated self-concept. Reflecting on Maslow's need hierarchy, Rogers proposed that human beings have a basic need for **positive regard**, especially from parents and significant others in their lives. Rogers conceptualized positive regard as a freely provided and unconditional liking for another person as an individual, without demands or expectations on that person's behavior. When this

Fundamental Human Needs	Being (qualities)	Having (things)	Doing (actions)	Interacting (settings)
SUBSISTENCE	Physical and mental health, equilibrium, sense of humor, adaptability	Food, shelter, work	Feed, procreate, rest, work	Living environment, social setting
PROTECTION	Care, adaptability, autonomy, equilibrium, solidarity	Insurance systems, savings, social security, health systems rights, family, work	Co-operate, prevent, plan, take care of, cure, help	Living space, social environment, dwelling
AFFECTION	Self-esteem, solidarity, respect, tolerance, generosity, passion, determination, sensuality, sense of humor	Friendships, family, partnerships, relationships with nature	Make love, caress, express emotions, share, take care of, appreciate	Privacy, intimacy, home, space of togetherness
UNDERSTANDING	Critical conscience, receptiveness, curiosity, astonishment, discipline, intuition, rationality	Literature, teachers, method, educational policies, communication policies	Investigate, study, experiment, educate, analyze, meditate	Settings of formative interaction, schools, universities, academies, groups, communities, family
PARTICIPATION	Adaptability, receptiveness, solidarity, determination, dedication, respect, passion, sense of humor	Rights, responsibilities, duties, privileges, work	Become affiliated, cooperate, dissent, obey, interact, agree on, express opinions	Settings of participative interaction, parties, associations, churches, neighborhoods, family
IDLENESS	Curiosity, receptiveness, imagination, recklessness, sense of humor, tranquility, sensuality	Games, spectacles, clubs, parties, peace of mind	Day-dream, brood, dream, recall old times, give way to fantasies, remember, relax, have fun, play	Privacy, intimacy, spaces of closeness, free time, surroundings, landscapes
CREATION	Passion, determination, intuition, imagination, boldness, rationality, autonomy, inventiveness, curiosity	Abilities, skills, method, work	Work, invent, build, design, compose, interpret	Productive and feedback settings, workshops, cultural groups, audiences, spaces for expression, temporal freedom
IDENTITY	Sense of belonging, consistency, differentiation, self-esteem, assertiveness	Symbols, language, religion, habits, customs, reference groups, sexuality, values, norms, historical memory, work	Commit oneself, integrate oneself, confront, decide on, recognize oneself, get to know oneself, actualize oneself, grow	Social rhythms, everyday settings, settings which one belongs to, maturation stages
FREEDOM	Autonomy, self-esteem, determination, passion, assertiveness, open-mindedness, boldness, rebelliousness, tolerance	Equal rights	Dissent, choose, be different from, run risks, develop awareness, commit oneself, disobey	Temporal/spatial plasticity (anywhere)

FIGURE 5-1. Matrix of Needs and Satisfiers

Adapted from Max-Neef, M. (1991). *Human Scale Development: Conception, Application and Further Reflections.* Reprinted with permission from the author.

regard is provided unconditionally to developing children, they will grow up in a better position to realize self-actualization. More often than not, however, children are not raised with unconditional positive regard. Instead, they are taught that positive regard is, in fact, conditional; that is, certain behaviors, thoughts, and emotions valued by the caregiver (typically the parent) are required in order to receive positive regard. What results is a set of conditions of worth, which impacts the child's subsequent behaviors.

That is, in an effort to receive positive regard, the child begins to behave in a manner consistent with the conditions and expectations set forth by the caregiver rather than his or her own desires and needs. As a result, the child's need to self-actualize may be in direct competition with his or her need to receive positive regard from the caregiver. The adoption of the standards and values of others may inhibit self-actualization, especially if the standards are very restrictive. It is the discrepancy between one's experience (shaped by conditions of worth) and one's self-concept that creates psychological abnormality. In order to maintain the integrity of the self-concept, discrepant experiences are distorted and denied. The self-concept itself becomes distorted over time as it begins to internalize the conditions of worth set forth by others.

Rogers (1942, 1951, 1961) applied humanistic principles to create client-centered therapy, a nondirective therapeutic approach focused on helping individuals realize their potential by creating a safe, supportive environment to promote self-enhancement. Characteristics present in this nonjudgmental environment include empathy, unconditional positive genuineness, and regard. *Empathy* refers to experiencing the world from the client's perspective. This is accomplished through the use of active listening and reflecting techniques in which the therapist communicates an understanding and acceptance of the client. *Genuineness* involves responding to the client as a human and not just as a therapist. It also requires that therapists stay in touch with their own feelings and be able to communicate them to the client in an effective, appropriate manner. Finally, an environment of *unconditional positive regard* should be created so that clients feel comfortable and secure when engaging in the change process. That is, clients should not feel judged in this environment; they should feel valued and accepted regardless of their thoughts, behaviors, and emotions (Farber & Doolin, 2011).

Although notably more existential than humanistic, the beliefs of Victor Frankl (1967, 1972), a survivor of the Nazi concentration camps, represent another strong influence in this phenomenological domain. Frankl disagreed with Rogers and Maslow that the motivating drive toward fulfillment in life is self-actualization. Instead, he postulated that there was a basic drive toward meaning in life and, therefore, that psychiatric disturbances arose from an inability to find meaning in life. This parallels the thinking in occupational therapy, as the significance of the personal meaning of occupation has been well documented in the literature and today the search for meaning is a pivotal principle of occupational science (Larson, Wood, & Clark, 2003). Also, the emphasis on client-centered practice (Law, 1998; Sumsion & Lencucha, 2007) and on the acknowledgment of spirituality as a fundamental orientation that provides inspiration, personal meaning, and motivation (American Occupational Therapy Association [AOTA], 2008) have contributed to the recognition of the essential need for and the driving force of meaning. However, Frankl's interpretation of meaning was not limited to the meaning of doing that is often implicit in the occupational therapy literature.

Frankl, along with other existentialists, asserted that there was an anxiety, shared by all humans, that resulted from the knowledge that death, or "nonbeing," is a known outcome of being. It was Frankl's belief that some people resolve this anxiety by finding meaning in their lives. *Meaning* represents different things to different people. It does not have to represent actions toward a specific goal, but it may represent the freedom to take responsibility for an attitude or belief, even if unspoken. Frankl argued that meaning could also be found through the ability to believe in one's inherent worthiness. Accordingly, a person could create meaning or purpose in life simply through the act of taking the responsibility to believe a certain way.

It is the humanist perspective in both psychology and occupational therapy that provides the focus on the whole human being and acknowledges the interconnectedness of the mind, body, and spirit, as well as with the community at large. There are other shared philosophical tenets of humanistic psychology and occupational therapy that are quite striking. Early humanistic psychologists, especially Abraham Maslow, recognized the quality of human adaptation (Rowan, 2004), which is also a cornerstone of occupational therapy (Schultz, 2009).

The Social Context of Humanism

"Too often do we think of ourselves as just individuals, separated from one another, whereas we are connected and what we do affects the whole world" (Tutu, 2011, p. ix). One criticism of psychological perspectives is that they do not adequately address the individual in context. However, it is the humanistic perspective that facilitated the development of human rights philosophies, as well as social justice. Even in the early writings of humanistic philosophers, there was an implicit and explicit understanding that personal meaning was tied to a feeling of belonging, and that self-worth was at least in part determined by one's sense of value, respect, and responsibility in the community. Also, as previously mentioned, models expressing basic human needs, such as Max-Neef's *Human Scale Development* (1991) show a clear link between the health and growth of the individual and the community. Occupational therapy has always acknowledged the role of environment in human behavior, but the recent literature certainly shows that the profession has reconnected to the social context of humanism through extensive publications on OT's role with human rights and dignity (Kronenberg, Simo Algado, & Pollard, 2005; Kronenberg, Pollard, & Sakellariou, 2011); the many applications of occupational justice (Townsend, 2003; Townsend & Wilcock, 2004); and the emphasis on social inclusion (Le Boutillier & Croucher, 2010; Russell & Lloyd, 2004).

Applications in Occupational Therapy

Applications of the theories of Rogers, Maslow, and Frankl have been extended into the arena of occupational therapy practice through the integration of humanistic and existential principles into prominent occupational therapy models. Moreover, as noted by Mosey (1980), the philosophical basis of occupational therapy appears to be grounded in humanistic and existential principles. As previously stated, inherent in the occupational therapy theory base is the belief that individuals find meaning through occupation (Fidler & Fidler, 1978).

The most obvious application of humanistic principles in occupational therapy is the emphasis on client centeredness, which is found in guiding documents such as the Occupational Therapy Practice Framework (OTPF) (AOTA, 2008). Occupational therapists are taught to see each client as an individual with unique qualities. The client-centered occupational therapy approach requires that the client be allowed, even encouraged, to share their perspective of their occupational performance, and to collaborate with the occupational therapist on personally meaningful goal setting. This approach reflects a significant shift in perspective by clients and service providers by embracing a strengths-based and self-determination focused approach to recovery through tools and skills implemented and administered by clients themselves (Hodges, Hardiman, & Segal, 2004). Self-help groups, sometimes called mutual help groups, have been found to be beneficial for people with chronic mental illness, depression/anxiety, and bereavement issues; thus these are important client-centered–based resources for clients (Pistrang, Barker, & Humphreys, 2010). In a genuine client-centered practice, occupational therapists must be careful not to apply these concepts superficially and strive to truly collaborate with clients and respect their choices. For example, in a study conducted by Richard and Knis-Matthews (2010), they found a "client/therapist disconnect in goal setting and the need to continue to examine client-centered practices in mental health settings" (p. 51).

In today's managed care environment, insurance companies are often perceived as defining which services are covered, thus dictating a structure within which goals must be chosen. However, occupational therapists can, and should, define treatment priorities within this structure according to client needs and desires, and also be involved with systemic advocacy for change in mental health delivery. Benjamin (2011) also suggests networking with colleagues for support and to discuss potential ethical dilemmas brought about by these tensions. But he concludes that "the core ingredients of empathy, authenticity, and realness . . . are apparently being practiced with partial success through the cleverness, flexibility, and humaneness of mental health workers despite the enormous obstacles against this kind of humanistic practice" (pp. 82–83).

Humanistic principles reinforce the notion that no matter how well conceived the therapeutic protocol, the treatment outcome depends on both the client's capacities and his or her choice to utilize them (Law, 1998; Sumsion, & Lencucha, 2007; Yerxa, 1967). This basic concept highlights perhaps the most salient contribution of humanistic theory—the importance of the individual client in determining his or her own outcomes. This concept is also in complete accord with the tenets of recovery. Humanistic theories remind therapists that "man, through the use of his hands can influence the state of his own health" (Reilly, 1962, p. 6). Approaching therapy with this dictum in mind encourages therapists to assume a more nondirective approach with the clients they treat (see also Chapter 19, "The Use of Psychosocial Methods and Interpersonal Strategies in Mental Health"). Taking such an approach with a client who has become disabled allows him or her to gain a better understanding of his or her own areas of interest and determine the extent to which his or her own cultural and spiritual identity will impact treatment priorities. Empowering a client to take an active role in the healing process may be the first step toward helping him or her to reestablish meaning in life and therefore the will to live.

Occupational therapists can strive to involve clients as much as possible in designing as well as participating in programs and in advocating for additional services (Dressler & MacRae, 1998). As Yerxa eloquently states, "I believe our broad purpose is to produce a reality-orienting influence upon the client's perceptions of his physical environment and self" (1967, p. 5).

In summary, the client-centered principles of the humanistic model are very useful in establishing rapport and trust between client and therapist. This is a significant predictor of treatment outcome in all disciplines, including occupational therapy. The practicing occupational therapist, therefore, would be well served by employing humanistic principles as part of the therapeutic process. Being nonjudgmental and genuine toward clients and understanding their perspective or frame of reference (i.e., providing empathy) may be critical to the change process (see Chapter 19, "The Use of Psychosocial Methods and Interpersonal Strategies in Mental Health"). In general, therapists should make every effort to create a nonjudgmental environment in which the vulnerable client feels safe in expressing himself or herself and in learning new, and relearning old, skills, as well as expanding their roles and connection to the community.

BIOLOGICAL PERSPECTIVE

The biological perspective has sought to understand the physiological mechanisms underlying behavior. This knowledge allows us to understand the behavior of clients from a biological or medical perspective. According to this model, symptoms of psychological disorder are caused by underlying biological factors. Included among these causal factors may be viral infections, neuroanatomical defects, biochemical (i.e., neurotransmitter and hormonal) imbalances, and genetic predispositions. While other perspectives propose theories regarding the nature of thinking, learning, feeling, and perceiving, this branch attempts to identify the physiological mechanisms underlying brain pathology, although new research indicates that the brain's structure and function are a "result of the transaction among genetic, physiological, and experiential influences" (Cozolino & Siegel, 2009, p. 619).

Although biological factors were long considered as possible determinants of abnormal behavior, it was not convincingly demonstrated that mental illness had an organic basis until syphilis was identified as the cause of a constellation of psychological symptoms, including delusions of grandeur as well as paralysis. From this key discovery, scientists began to speculate about the causal factors of other mental disorders, stimulating revived interest in biological explanations of psychopathology. This perspective views abnormal behavior as an illness caused by malfunctioning parts of the organism, primarily the brain, yet specific illnesses have not been consistently localized to specific brain regions—rather a complex of interrelated factors are being identified (Gershon & Rieder, 1992; Ovsiew, 2009; Rosenzweig, Leiman, & Breedlove, 2001). Therefore, a brief overview of brain structure and function is presented next.

The Brain

The brain is made up of billions of neurons and many more support cells, called glia. Groups of neurons form brain regions, such as the hindbrain, midbrain, and forebrain; further differentiation is noted within each region and is shown in Figure 5-2. For example, the hindbrain is comprised of the medulla, pons, cerebellum, and reticular activating system; it is connected to the spinal cord. The forebrain consists of the cerebrum (i.e., the two cerebral hemispheres), thalamus, and hypothalamus. The midbrain coordinates communication between the forebrain and hindbrain regions.

Within the forebrain, the cerebrum is further differentiated into the cerebral cortex, corpus callosum (which connects the two brain hemispheres), basal ganglia, and amygdala. The cerebral cortex has four distinct regions: the frontal, parietal, temporal, and occipital lobes, as is shown in Figure 5-3. The frontal lobe is located near

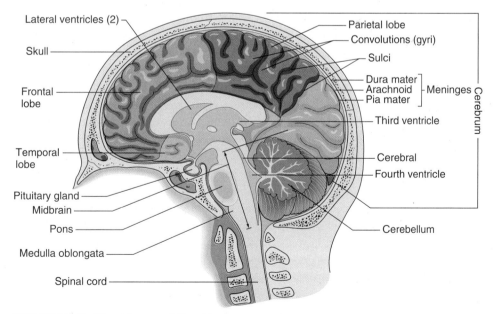

FIGURE 5-2. Structures of the Brain
© Cengage Learning 2013

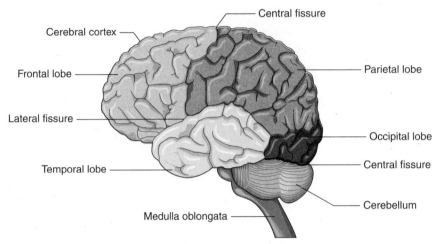

FIGURE 5-3. The Four Lobes of the Cerebral Cortex
© Cengage Learning 2013

the front of the brain and contains the motor cortex. The parietal lobe contains the somatosensory cortex. The temporal lobes are located on the sides of the brain and contain the auditory cortex, and the occipital lobe, at the back of the brain, contains the visual cortex. Finally, the limbic system is located at the base of the forebrain and includes portions of the thalamus, hypothalamus, and amygdala.

Each of these brain regions and subregions is comprised of neurons responsible for specific brain functions. The medulla controls heart rate, respiration, and gastrointestinal function. The pons is involved in sleeping, waking, and dreaming; it is also a pathway for motor information traveling from the cerebral hemispheres to the cerebellum. The cerebellum receives and processes information from peripheral sensory structures (i.e., hair cells of the inner ear, joint receptors, and muscle spindles). It also is responsible for processing feedback from the motor centers of the cortex (e.g., the coordination of head/eye movements, force and timing when reaching for an object, etc.). The reticular activating system screens incoming information and stimulates other brain regions whose pathways pass through the pons and medulla; it is thought to be primarily responsible for the mediation of states of arousal.

In the forebrain, the thalamus is important in processing and relaying information between other regions of the central nervous system and the cerebral cortex. Specifically, it directs incoming sensory information from the visual, auditory, and somatosensory systems to the correct locations within the cerebral cortex. The cerebral cortex is primarily responsible for sensory processing, motor control, and higher mental functions, such as learning, memory, planning, and judgment. The hypothalamus helps regulate body temperature, hunger/satiety, thirst, and the sex drive. It also controls the release of hormones by the pituitary and modulates feelings of pleasure and aggression. The amygdala is involved in the coordination of the autonomic nervous system and the endocrine system, as well as emotional states.

Similar to other brain regions, each of the lobes of the cerebral cortex has specific brain functions. The frontal lobe is involved in higher mental functions such as thinking and planning, as well as in the control of the body muscles. The parietal lobe processes information about pain, pressure, and body temperature. The temporal lobes are involved in memory, perception, and language processing, and the occipital lobe is responsible for visual processing. Although specific locations within the brain are not tied to specific disorders, recent research has indicated brain regions/structures, such as the limbic system and hippocampus, as being associated with anxiety disorders, schizophrenia, and depression (DiCicco-Bloom & Falluel-Morel, 2009; Drevets & Charney, 2009; Ovsiew, 2009; Stan, Lesselyong, & Ghose, 2009).

Causal Factors of Psychopathology

Psychopathology can be caused by any number of physiological dysfunctions. Included among the possible physiological causes of psychopathology are infections, such as syphilis. Anatomical aberrations may also be present. That is, the size or shape of certain brain regions may be abnormal, thereby creating abnormal behavior. For example, Huntington's disease, which presents with violent emotional outbursts, memory and other cognitive difficulties, delusions, suicidal thinking, and involuntary body movements, has been traced to a loss of neurons in the brain area called the basal ganglia. Conversely, elevated neuronal density has been found in the prefrontal cortex of people with schizophrenia and this combined with changes in the neurons themselves (i.e., smaller neurons and fewer dendritic spines) may impair synaptic connectivity between cells (Stan, Lesselyong, & Ghose, 2009).

However, infections and brain structure defects are not the only determinants of abnormal behavior. It may also be that neurons are not communicating effectively with one another due to improperly functioning neurotransmitter substances and systems or physical changes in the neurons themselves. Hormonal imbalances may also contribute to aberrant behavior. In addition, genetic factors may also be operating in the manifestation of a psychological disorder.

Biochemical Factors

Biochemical factors, including neurotransmitter dysfunction and hormonal imbalances, have been implicated as possible causal factors in many psychological disorders. Several of the neurotransmitter substances receiving particular attention in psychopathology research are serotonin, dopamine, gamma-aminobutyric acid (GABA), glutamate, and norepinephrine (Coyle, 2009). An electrical impulse is received by a neuron's dendrites (located at one end of a neuron) and then travels down its axon (a long fiber) to the axon's terminus, where it stimulates the release across the synapse of tiny packets of neurotransmitter substances in chemical form. These substances cross the synapse and bind to receptors (actually proteins) on the dendrites of the next neuron. Depending on the nature of the neurotransmitter substance, this binding either stimulates or inhibits the firing of the next neuron. In either case, neurotransmitter substances are essential to effective communication between the neurons.

Many different types of neurotransmitter substances have been discovered in the brain. It has also been discovered that different types of neurotransmitters serve different brain regions; that is, each neuron uses only certain kinds of neurotransmitters (Barondes, 1993). Neurotransmitter problems may include:

(a) excessive or insufficient amounts of neurotransmitter substances in the synapse

(b) too few receptor sites on the postsynaptic membrane

(c) the presence or absence of other chemicals that interfere with neural transmission

(d) the interrelationships between different neurotransmitter systems (environmental factors such as stress can also inhibit neural transmission)

Neurological studies have indicated that abnormalities in the activity of different neurotransmitters may be associated with different mental disorders. Dopamine regulation has been the leading neurological hypothesis for the etiology of schizophrenia, yet there hasn't been evidence of dopamine dysfunction in postmortem studies of people with schizophrenia (Stan, Lesselyong, & Ghose, 2009). Norepinephrine is thought to play a major role in the development of depression and serotonin has been linked with both schizophrenia and mood disorders. Recent studies suggest that other neurotransmitters such as glutamate and aminobutyric acid (GABA) may play a significant role in the pathophysiology of schizophrenia, bipolar disorder, major depression, and anxiety disorders (Coyle, 2009). Decreased levels of GABA have been found in people with major depression while increased levels of GABA are noted in people with panic disorder (Coyle, 2009).

Increased knowledge of biochemistry, specifically the role of neurotransmitters, has led the way to the development of the most widely used form of intervention, which is **psychopharmacology**. However, dependence on biological theory alone is insufficient for successful pharmacological treatment: "Issues that are still awaiting further clarification include the following: How do we assess patients' beliefs and expectations related to psychotropic treatment? How do we minimize the communication gaps between patients and clinicians who are often from divergent sociocultural backgrounds?" (Lin, Smith, & Ortiz, 2001, p. 523). Medication is not the panacea once hoped for. Nevertheless, it is an important component of many treatment plans and often stabilizes the client sufficiently for other forms of therapy to be effective. Knowledge of brain function continues to grow and, as a result, a plethora of new drugs have been developed that not only are more effective in reducing symptoms but often do so with fewer "side" effects (all drugs have effects specific to individuals so perhaps the term " side effects" is misleading). Increased understanding of the special regions of the brain, the mechanisms surrounding neural connectivity, and the functions of the neurotransmitters has certainly furthered our understanding of the biological basis of behavior. Even with the advancement of imaging technology and its use in neuroimaging (Schneider, Backes, & Mathiak, 2009), our knowledge of the physiological factors present in psychopathology is by no means complete due to the profound complexity of the human brain (Grebb & Carlsson, 2009).

Hormonal Factors

In an effort to develop a more comprehensive biological understanding of abnormal behavior, another biochemical system, the endocrine system, has become the subject of investigation. Unlike the neural connections, this system communicates by means of the circulatory system. The hypothalamus regulates endocrine system functioning in one of two ways: (1) by releasing hormones directly into the bloodstream, and (2) by emitting hormone release factors, which stimulate the anterior pituitary gland to release the appropriate hormone into the bloodstream. In both cases, hormones circulate throughout the body until they bind to target receptors. Similar to the mechanisms of neurotransmitters, the target receptors are selective for the particular hormones with which they bind.

One frequently studied hormone is adrenocorticotropin (ACTH). The target receptor site of ACTH is the adrenal gland. When ACTH binds to the adrenal gland, it causes steroid hormones to be released. One of these is cortisol, which serves to elevate blood sugar and increase metabolism. When a person is under significant stress, the hypothalamus stimulates the pituitary gland to secrete large amounts of cortisol. Some people with depression, anxiety disorders (Tyrka et al., 2008), and borderline personality disorder (Wingenfeld, Spitzer, Rullkötter, & Löwe, 2009) have documented increased secretion of cortisol related to increased sensitivity to stressors and hyperactivity of the hypothalamic–pituitary–adrenal (HPA) axis.

Genetic Factors in Psychopathology

Many theorists who follow the biological perspective believe that inherited vulnerabilities mediate psychological disorders. Certain personality traits, temperamental styles, and specific disorders may have a genetic component (Bouchard, Lykken, McGue, Segal, & Tellegen, 1990). In fact, researchers and clinicians have long noted that certain disorders tend to run in families. The COMT gene has been linked with risk for schizophrenia and anxiety disorders. The amygdala and its role in mediating fear responses have been found to be related to anxiety disorders; genetic variants appear to influence the responsiveness of the fear circuit (Domschke & Dannlowski, 2010).

In an effort to study the genetic influence on psychopathology, researchers have utilized studies of twins, family pedigrees, adoptions, and risk. These research methodologies attempt to tease out the unique genetic contributions to psychopathology from the vast array of influential biological and environmental factors present. In many cases, a unique genetic contribution proves elusive to the investigator. In such cases, it appears likely that a combination of factors is essential to the manifestation of psychopathology. Thus, multiple interacting genes coupled with psychological risk factors may be required for psychological disorders to manifest themselves. While genes may influence brain development, they are less clearly related to specific mental illnesses at this time; the same gene pattern may manifest as schizophrenia in one person, as bipolar disorder in another, and as attention deficit hyperactivity disorder in another; thus different outcomes are possible depending on the genetic, environmental, and stress related contexts, which is sometimes referred to as the diathesis-stress model (Insel & Wang, 2010).

Twins are frequently studied in the effort to learn more about the genetic influences on psychopathology. There are two types of twins, monozygotic (identical) and dizygotic (fraternal). While identical twins share all the same genes, fraternal twins have an average of only half their genes in common. Twin studies often help to tease out genetic contributions to psychology because twins are typically raised in the same environment, thus controlling external influences to a large degree. Several studies show that bipolar disorder is much more heritable than major depression (Fears, Mathews, & Freimer, 2009). Research on several disorders, such as schizophrenia, autism, and bipolar disorder, has demonstrated that identical twins are more likely to share the same disorder than dizygotic twins. Interestingly, physical differences alone do not account for the appearance of a given disorder. For example, neuroimaging indicates that the hippocampus in people with schizophrenia may be significantly (about 5%) smaller, yet monozygotic twins who both have a smaller hippocampus may not both develop schizophrenia thus hippocampal size may be a "biological marker of genetic susceptibility" (DiCicco-Bloom & Falluel-Morel, 2009, p. 61).

Adoption studies help to further delineate the roles of nature and nurture in the development of psychopathology. One type of adoption study is to compare adopted children to their adoptive and biological parents. Another, perhaps stronger, methodology is to study twins who have been adopted by different families and therefore reared apart. Studies such as these have demonstrated that numerous personality traits, such as IQ, alcohol and drug use, crime and conduct problems, depressiveness, danger seeking, and neuroticism, are strongly related in identical twins and related, but to a much lesser degree, in fraternal twins (Beaver et al., 2009; Bouchard et al., 1990; Brant et al., 2009; Foroud, Edenberg, & Crabbe, 2010; Shane, Nicolaou, Cherkas, & Spector, 2010).

Brain Plasticity

Newer evidence indicates that the brain is much more changeable than formerly considered. This **brain plasticity**, "the ability of the nervous system to change" indicates that neurons grow and change throughout the lifespan in reaction to new experiences through the growth of new neurons and the dendritic branching of existing neurons to connect with other neurons (Cozolino & Siegel, 2009, p. 620). Cozolino and Siegel (2009) state, "If everything humans experience is represented within neural networks, then psychopathology of all kinds, from the mildest symptoms to the most severe psychosis, must be represented within and among neural networks" (p. 620). Most likely, then, the biological field will continue to produce many new ideas regarding psychopathology and functioning and occupational performance that will influence occupational therapy treatment in mental health.

Applications in Occupational Therapy

The biological perspective provides much useful information to the occupational therapist working with clients who have mental illness. An understanding of the biological basis of the disorder can guide clinicians in the formulation of appropriate treatment plans. For example, understanding the biological basis of schizophrenia allows a clinician to appreciate the importance of medication management in the treatment of symptoms. Thus, working with a client to develop a medication routine or schedule may be a treatment priority. Furthermore, family members and caretakers may find some relief in understanding the biological basis of the disorder and eliminate self-blame on their part.

The biological perspective may underlie sensory modulation approaches as well. Preliminary research linking neuroscience and deficits in sensory modulation resulting in behavioral disturbance are being explored (Lane, Lynn, & Reynolds, 2010). Sensory modulation approaches are being used in occupational therapy practice with people with mental health conditions as a tool to manage behavior. In this approach, clients' sensory sensitivities and needs are assessed and then addressed. The idea is that some of the behavior that people engage in reflects attempts to modulate their sensory input. There have been positive results in reducing aggressive behavior to self and others through sensory modulation techniques. Sensory inputs may be self-administered so clients become agents of their own behavioral change in relation to their sensory needs (Champagne, 2006; Champagne, Koomar, & Olson, 2010). (See Chapters 7, 9, 10, 11, 12, and 20 for more information about these approaches that can be categorized under the rubric of sensory interventions with a sensory approach.) In summary, the biological perspective continues to develop through ongoing advances in knowledge related to the interrelationships between the brain, the body, and experiences. Due to recent scientific advances such as magnetic resonance imaging (MRI), magnetoencephalography (MEG), positron emission tomography (PET) scanning, and computerized tomography (CT) scanning, scientists are now able to study the brain and its processes more closely. These technological breakthroughs, along with the tremendous advances in the use of pharmacological treatments to ameliorate psychological disorders, have enabled clinicians to develop a better understanding of the physiological mechanisms underlying aberrant behavior. Occupational therapy treatment targeting new skills or routines may influence the neuronal pathways and brain plasticity as new learning may result in changes to neurons and connections between neurons (Cozolino & Siegel, 2009).

The enhanced appreciation for the role of biology facilitates the work of all service providers, including occupational therapists, who work directly with clients with psychological disorders. Biological factors, however, are not the only determinants of psychological disturbance; psychological factors, such as unconscious conflicts, learning histories, and cognitive processes, may also be etiologically significant. The perspectives described in the remainder of this chapter attempt to explain psychopathology in terms of these psychological factors.

PSYCHODYNAMIC PERSPECTIVE

The psychodynamic perspective primarily focuses on the emotional and personality development of the individual and emphasizes early childhood experiences as formative. According to psychodynamic theorists, both normal and abnormal behaviors are largely determined by unconscious psychological forces and internal processes. It is the interaction among these forces that creates behavior, thoughts, and emotions. Abnormal behavior results when these dynamic forces come in conflict (defined as intrapsychic conflict). (See Table 5-1 for definitions of classical psychoanalytic terms.) Psychodynamic theorists assume a deterministic view of behavior. That is, all behavior can be seen as the product of forces beyond the immediate awareness and control of the individual. Although patterns of behavior are viewed as having their origins in early childhood, they may not emerge until adulthood.

The most prominent of the psychodynamic theories was developed by the Viennese neurologist Sigmund Freud in the early twentieth century. His interest in hypnosis as a form of treatment for hysterical illnesses (i.e., physical ailments with no apparent medical explanation) and his early work with the neurologist Jean Charcot and the physician Josef Breuer ultimately led to the formulation of his theory of psychoanalysis, which was the first truly psychological theory of normal and abnormal behavior. This theory postulates that unconscious factors are responsible, not only for hysterical illnesses, but for all psychological functioning, both normal and abnormal. Treatment involves the use of free association, hypnosis, dream analysis, and the interpretation of resistances and transference (i.e., the process by which the client comes to attribute characteristics of important figures from childhood to the therapist) in order to help unconscious conflicts become conscious. Once available to consciousness, psychological conflicts can be worked through and resolved.

Psychoanalytic Concepts

Psychoanalytic theory represents a set of elaborate assumptions about human behavior that are quite complex and, due to their abstractness, often difficult to comprehend. However, many early psychoanalytic concepts including structures of the mind, ego defense mechanisms, levels of consciousness, and psychosexual developmental stages (Freud, 1923/1976; Sadock & Sadock, 2003) have become ingrained in the American culture. For example, people use terms that emerged from psychoanalysis in everyday descriptive conversation. You may hear ideas such as egomaniacs, anally retentive, denial, suppression, or unconscious to describe people, personality traits, or behavior. Additionally, it seems that the idea of an "oedipal complex" is known by many. The colloquial cultural terms do not fully describe psychoanalytic theory's complex ideas, although they do indicate that psychoanalytic ideas are alive and well

TABLE 5-1. Classical Psychoanalytic Terms

Id—The innate structure of the mind that represents an individual's instinctual needs, drives, and impulses. The id was viewed by Freud to be the primary motivating force in personality. The id strives for immediate and constant gratification according to seeking what is pleasurable.

Ego—Represents the rational aspect of the mind that conforms to society or civilizations demands. The ego involves planning, reasoning, remembering, evaluating, and decision-making processes. That is, the ego determines whether it is safe or dangerous to express an impulse by considering the factors present in reality. The ego experiences anxiety and/or guilt when the id presses to make its desires conscious or get them gratified.

Superego—Is comprised of two components, the conscience and the ego ideal. It is the conscience that reminds us that certain behaviors, thoughts, and emotions are acceptable or unacceptable. The ego ideal represents the person we are striving to become; it incorporates all the values and standards of our caregivers.

Defense Mechanisms—In an effort to control unacceptable id impulses and reduce the anxiety and/or guilt they arouse, the ego develops unconscious coping responses, called ego defense mechanisms by Anna Freud (1936/1974), to protect the self. Defense mechanisms are unconscious methods generated by the ego to protect itself from anxiety and guilt related to unacceptable id impulses. (See Table 5-2 for definitions of the ego defense mechanisms.)

Conscious—Contains elements of the mind that are easily accessed and a person is aware of.

Unconscious—Contains elements, such as instincts or drives, that actively seek to become conscious but may be viewed as unacceptable for expression by the ego (creating anxiety) or by the superego (creating guilt) and, therefore, prevented from being expressed consciously. A large portion of mental activity is unconscious, meaning that it occurs outside a person's normal awareness and is not readily accessible.

Psychosexual Stages—A theory of development based on sexuality, included stages called oral, anal, phallic, and genital referring to parts of the body on which an infant focused for gratification. Adjustment depended on moving through the stages. Maladjustment meant a "fixation" or being stuck in one of the stages.

NOTE: An important idea is that much of one's mental life occurs unconsciously. This particular idea that there is a level of life that is unconscious was a revelation in Freud's time and the concept of the unconscious and its effect on everyday thinking continues to be discussed, even in the era of biological science.

TABLE 5-2. Ego Defense Mechanisms

Mechanism	Description
Repression	Preventing unacceptable impulses or desires from becoming conscious
Denial	A primitive or early defense mechanism by which a person disavows or refuses to acknowledge the external source of anxiety
Projection	Attributing personally unacceptable impulses or desires to the external world
Displacement	Shifting repressed desires and impulses from a dangerous object to one that is more safe and acceptable
Reaction Formation	Adopting behavior that is in direct opposition to one's unacceptable impulses or desires
Intellectualization	Repressing of the emotional components of one's experience, but not the informational components
Regression	Retreating to an earlier, more immature developmental stage in response to anxiety
Identification	Adopting the values and feelings of a person who causes anxiety in an attempt to increase self-worth
Sublimation	Expressing sexual and aggressive impulses in a socially acceptable manner

NOTE: You may recognize most of the defense mechanisms because they have been assumed by the culture and become everyday terms.

© Cengage Learning 2013

and psychology has taken hold in some way in our modern culture. Also, Freud's original concepts have evolved in modern, contemporary practice so that they do not have quite the same meaning in contemporary practice.

Neo-Freudian Theories

Freudian theory has been altered over the years by many theorists who believe strongly in the power of the unconscious and intrapsychic conflict but who disagree with other aspects of Freud's theory. Carl Jung developed analytical psychology, which combined Freudian and humanistic theories. Compared to Freud, he believed the unconscious to be more positive, creative, and spiritual, and he de-emphasized the role of sexuality as a motivator of behavior. He also believed that in addition to the personal unconscious, there exists a collective unconscious, which represents all the experiences of all people over the centuries.

Other theorists attended to psychosocial aspects of personality development. Alfred Adler, for example, believed that human beings were motivated more by social needs than sexual drives. According to Adler's theoretical notions, children's goals evolve from selfish to more social over the course of development. Harry Stack Sullivan similarly emphasized the importance of interpersonal relationships in personality development on the grounds that one's developing personality cannot be separated from one's social context. He also stressed that human beings have a basic need for security, as we live in a potentially hostile world. The concept of security and the importance of social relationships in achieving security were also addressed by Karen Horney, who believed that childhood relationships were most critical in determining security and adjustment later in life. The experience of anxiety, according to her theoretical notions, was due primarily to social (i.e., interpersonal) factors rather than factors that were biological or sexual. Finally, Erik Erikson conceptualized a life span theory of psychosocial development in which he emphasized the relationship between individuals and the social context in which they live their lives. Erikson also stressed the impact of this changing relationship on personality development from infancy through old age, a developmental theory familiar to occupational therapists. Each of these stages is characterized by a specific developmental challenge, or crisis, whose resolution affects how the individual deals with subsequent stages.

Although the neo-Freudian's ideas developed separately and apart from original Freudian concepts, these newer ideas about the creative and collective unconscious, the need for security, the influence of the social environment, lifespan development, and interpersonal relationships in turn later influenced and enriched psychoanalytic ideas.

Contemporary Psychodynamic Theories

Contemporary psychodynamic theories currently stress the importance of one's social environment in individual development. Psychoanalytic theory is now considered by many a two-person theory instead of the one-person theory it previously was. That is, psychoanalytic theories now recognize that change takes place in the presence of another person, and we can no longer think that change takes place in an individual alone. Presence does not imply only physical presence but also includes mental representations that are derived from concrete interactions and that are formed in an individual's mind. These two-person concepts have given rise to two theoretical developments in psychotherapy and research. In both theoretical developments, the primary relationship, usually with a mother, but also with whoever is the significant caregiver, is considered the basis for later personality development.

Psychoanalysts who first believed in these two-person concepts were called object-relationists. They believed that the first object in an infant's life, one's mother, shaped the infant's world and that the infant's development could not be separated from their environment. Accordingly, they focused on how the infant was primarily merged, then separated and became autonomous from one's mother and developed relationships with other objects, or people in their environment.

Those who follow attachment, or relational psychoanalysis believe that the primary relationship particularly shapes how people represent their self or others in their minds (Bowlby, 1988a, 1988b; Bretherton, 1990a, 1990b; Cassidy & Shaver,

2008; Seligman, 1994; Sroufe & Waters, 1977; Zeanah & Anders, 1987). These self or other representations then guide people's interactions throughout their lives. These later ideas about relationship and primary caregiver evolved from the British school of psychoanalysis, the object relationists, and from the British psychiatrist John Bowlby's ideas about attachment (Bowlby, 1988a, 1988b; Bretherton, 1992; Cassidy & Shaver, 2008).

Object relations was an important evolution of psychoanalytic theory because it focused on early development and acknowledged the influence of the caregiver on an infant. This was the first theory that discussed the idea that one's mental and emotional development could not be separated from the environment and objects (other people, primarily the first object, the mother) in the infant's environment. A period of developmental stages was posited based on the infant's relationship, first thought to be merged and then evolving through different stages to separation and autonomy from, its caregiver. An individual's mental life as influenced by the relationship became the focus of development.

Currently, object relations and attachment theory ideas influence a wide range of psychotherapy practice (Stern et al., 1998), child development (Sroufe, 1998; Stern, 1985), and theories of research and practice. In another development, psychotherapeutic approaches recognize the importance of early relationships in organizing psychic structure, or one's psychological self (Sroufe & Waters, 1977) and self-regulation. These approaches focus on how intersubjectivity, a shared subjective experience, influences relationships (Beebe, 2003) and therapy (Stern, 2003; Stolorow, 1994; Stolorow, Atwood, & Branchaft, 1994) and on how early relationships may affect one's later actions, primarily through forms of guilt (Weiss, 1993).

In addition, specific research and programs of psychotherapy have borrowed from Freudian and neo-Freudian ideas. For example, programs for people with borderline personality disorder follow Freud's (Gabbard, 2001) and Harry Stack Sullivan's (Benjamin & Pugh, 2001) theories with modifications and additions.

Applications in Occupational Therapy

Gail S. Fidler has been credited as being the first occupational therapist to use a psychodynamic approach in treatment (Hopkins, 1988). She encouraged the study and use of projective techniques to guide the interpretation of nonverbal communication displayed by the clients within her activity groups (Fidler & Fidler, 1954). Based on object relations theory, Fidler believed a person's relationships with objects in the environment to be integral to the development of the ego. Because occupational therapy used activities requiring clients to interact with both human and nonhuman objects, she felt it was a rich medium through which clients could reveal both feelings and needs and through which the therapist could ascertain unconscious conflicts and the strength of clients' ego defense mechanisms (Miller, Seig, Ludwig, Shortridge, & Van Deusen, 1988).

Fidler's work led to explorations into the meaning of activities (Fidler & Velde, 1999) and their associated action processes and objects including "the potential of activities in their own right to represent, reflect, and infer social, cultural, and personal meanings and to communicate and call into play certain physical, affective, and cognitive responses" (p. xi). Her perspective acknowledged the importance of an unconscious inner life to "open the door to a fuller understanding of how one level influences processes at another" (p. 13).

Anne Cronin Mosey was heavily influenced by Gail Fidler and also described psychiatric function from a psychodynamic frame of reference. She believed that "occupational therapy attempted to bring . . . unconscious content to consciousness and integrate it with conscious content" (Hopkins, 1988, p. 29). Since that time, other occupational therapists have written about the use of projective tests within the realm of occupational therapy but generally have cautioned that the interpretation of an activity in this way requires additional education and collaboration with psychologists and/or psychiatrists. Although, asking clients to describe and interpret their own projective work (e.g., paintings, ceramic work, collage) is a helpful technique to generate perhaps what is considered unconscious or preconscious ideas while practicing within occupational therapy's typical knowledge base. Generally, such authors suggest that a therapist can learn about a client's self-esteem, the presence of underlying conflicts (i.e., control or expression of anger), the ability to relate to the therapist, and the use of ego defense mechanisms through such activities as making tile mosaics, drawings, clay sculpture, and magazine collages (Griffiths & Corr, 2007; Sheffer & Harlock, 1980). The therapist would also use such information to learn about what is meaningful to the individual and what and how occupations are satisfying (Banks & Blair, 1997; Mackenzie & Beecraft, 2004). This information would then inform both individual and group intervention strategies. Finally, understanding of the defense mechanisms can aid occupational therapists in intervention approaches that use therapeutic use of self (See Chapter 19, "The Use of Psychosocial Methods and Interpersonal Strategies in Mental Health" for more information on therapeutic use of self and therapists approaches and techniques.)

In summary, psychodynamic theory has had a profound impact on Western culture. Its influence can be seen in our educational system, literature, the arts, and, of course, all the mental health professions. In particular, a knowledge of psychodynamic concepts can assist the occupational therapist in becoming sensitive to intrapsychic factors (e.g., psychological factors not immediately accessible to consciousness) and early childhood experiences impacting an individual client's functioning. An awareness of defense mechanisms and maladaptive coping mechanisms may also prove to be clinically useful for the occupational therapist. Moreover, a self-reflective, "analytical" way of thinking about the self as therapist stems from the psychoanalytical model. Assessing such factors may facilitate the therapy process as well as the development of more effective treatment plans for clients. Such thinking also supports the therapeutic use of self as defined by the OTPF (AOTA, 2008; see also, Taylor, 2008).

BEHAVIORAL PERSPECTIVE

Many concepts of the behavioral perspective, much like the psychodynamic perspective, have become imbedded in popular culture and are taken for granted as truisms. Techniques to change or teach specific behaviors are an integral part of parenting in Western society, as well as the basis of many learning principles found in both formal and informal education in schools, places of employment, and in criminal justice systems. However, Behaviorism as a branch of psychology is only traced back to 1913, when John Watson, using the work of Ivan Pavlov on conditional reflexes, presented a model of stimulus–response behaviorism (Chaney, 2010; Moore, 2010). B. F. Skinner, perhaps the most recognized name in the development of behavioral psychology, refined the work of Watson and others (Skinner, 1938, 1953) and is primarily responsible for the terminology that is still used in behavioral interventions today. Table 5-3 defines commonly used terms in behaviorism.

Scientifically, behaviorism is historically linked to the rise of "positivism," which is the research perspective that assumes that scientific knowledge can only come from studying and measuring directly observable phenomenon (Moore, 2010). This linkage to positivism has lead to strong criticism of a behavioral approach in both scientific research and therapeutic intervention, as other schools of thought better reflect the complexity of the human experience (Kielhofner, 2006). (See Chapter 3 for further discussion of research perspectives.)

The therapeutic interventions based strictly on behaviorism are no longer widely used in adult mental health treatment, except with clients who display moderate to severe behavioral disturbances. Another situational use of behavioral techniques is in the event of an acute hospitalization or other dramatic contextual change where people may have to learn or relearn socially acceptable behavior in order to benefit from other forms of therapeutic intervention. For example, inpatient hospital settings, using a **milieu treatment** approach, generally have "rules" expecting or encouraging clients to attend groups and to eat meals in a common dayroom. This is to provide practice in interacting with others and in managing symptoms in a social environment.

The treatment approach that is most consistent with the theoretical and philosophical basis of behaviorism is **applied behavioral analysis (ABA)**, which is discussed in the next paragraphs. The development of **cognitive-behavioral therapy (CBT)** and **dialectical behavioral therapy (DBT)** (discussed in subsequent section on Applications in Occupational Therapy) were certainly

TABLE 5-3. Commonly Used Terms in Behavioral Interventions

Classical Conditioning—A process developed by Ivan Pavlov of learning by temporal association. For example, noticing that dogs salivated by the presence of food (an unconditioned response), he then paired another stimulus (a bell) with the food. Soon, dogs did not need the food to salivate but salivated just with the presence of the bell (termed a *conditioned response*).

Shaping—Proposed by Skinner (1938, 1953, 1971), involves reinforcing a person for closer and closer approximations of a target behavior. Initially, only a simple response is required. The criteria for reinforcement are then gradually made more stringent in an attempt to elicit more complex or refined target behaviors (Becker, 1985).

Chaining—Proposed by Skinner (1938, 1953, 1971), chaining refers to a method of reinforcement involving the linking of component skills to teach a more complex behavior. This procedure involves reinforcing in a particular sequence simple behaviors that are already in the individual's repertoire in an effort to teach more complex skills (Deitz, 1985a, 1985b). Chaining can be accomplished in either a forward or backward format (Schreibman. 1985).

Positive and negative reinforcement—Behavior followed by a positive consequence (i.e., reward) will result in an increase in that behavior and behavior followed by a negative consequence (i.e., punishment) will result in a decrease in that behavior.

Operant Conditioning—Proposed by Edwin Thorndike (1898) who concluded that when a response is followed by a positive event it is more likely to be repeated; conversely, if a response is followed by a negative event it is likely to cease.

Unconditioned response (UCR)—A response that is reliably produced by a desired stimulus (food in the above example) without prior training (Gormezano, Prokasy, & Thompson, 1987).

Conditioned response (CR)—A response elicited by a conditioned stimulus (bell in the above example) alone, that is, without the presentation of the unconditioned stimulus (food in the above example).

Principle of reinforcement—Proposed by B. F. Skinner (1938, 1953, 1971) that behavior can be modified by its consequences. Reinforcement is the primary mechanism for learning and for explaining human behavior.

Extinction of behaviors—Refers to the decline in rate of a target behavior and ultimate elimination of that behavior. For example, in the case of phobias, if you can create an acceptable stimulus (such as relaxation) and pair it with the presentation of a feared stimulus (such as snakes), the anxiety that results from the fears will ultimately be eliminated or extinguished.

Modeling—Proposed by Albert Bandura (1977, 1997, 1986) that learning occurs through observation and imitation of the behaviors of others and that persons can learn by observing the consequences that people receive for their behaviors.

© Cengage Learning 2013

influenced by behaviorism, and therefore included in this section. However, it should be noted that these forms of therapy are a blend of theoretic principles and not purely based on a behavioral perspective.

Applied Behavioral Analysis

ABA is a systematic model that strives to objectively measure, evaluate and influence socially important human behavior (Baer, Wolf, & Risley, 1968). It is extensively used with people having intellectual and developmental disabilities (Hassiotis et al., 2009; Luiselli, Bass, & Whitcomb, 2010;) as well as in geriatric settings that serve people with dementia (Molinari & Edelstein, 2011). While ABA is generally considered to be highly successful with these populations, there is some criticism of the quality of the research supporting this premise (Coyne, Thombs, & Hagedoorn, 2010). One reported benefit of using ABA is a decrease in the use of pharmaceutical agents in controlling behavior (Molinari & Edelstein, 2011). This has special significance for children as the long-term developmental effects of many pharmaceuticals is unknown. Also, given the potential side effects of many medications, particularly with the older adult, further research and development of the role of ABA in reducing or eliminating the use of medication as behavioral management is a priority.

Applications in Occupational Therapy

The basic principle of behaviorism is that all behavior is learned. This is not consistent with the philosophy and practice of occupational therapy, which acknowledges that behavior can be influenced by a wide array of factors, such as interaction with the environment and sensory modulation, in addition to learning. Nevertheless, occupational therapists as well as other health care providers do commonly incorporate some behavioral principles, such as reinforcement and reward, especially when working in long-term care facilities for people with mental illness as well as school-based occupational therapy practices with children with behavior issues.

Because behavioral strategies are relatively concrete and do not require complex verbal, cognitive, or psychosocial abilities, they can be used effectively with these populations. In addition, attending to a client's learning history, including reinforcement contingencies that influence behavior, can be very useful to the practicing occupational therapist when designing treatment protocols and may facilitate more positive outcomes for clients. Occupational therapists working with adults may also assist clients in determining which reinforcers may be motivating or helpful for them (clients) and facilitate the integration of these reinforcers into clients' daily or weekly routines.

CBT, which merges elements of both behavioral and cognitive perspectives, is now widely used in occupational therapy as well as in other mental health disciplines. For example, Strong (1998) showed positive results using this approach in occupational therapy for pain management. Giles (1985) also advocates using a behavioral perspective as well as CBT within an occupational therapy framework. This approach has shown to be successful with various populations, including those with eating disorders such as anorexia nervosa and bulimia, people with traumatic brain injury (Giles, Ridley, Dill, & Frye, 1997), substance abuse (Stoffel & Moyers, 2004), autism (Lim, Kattapuram, & Lian, 2007), as well as addressing occupational performance deficits common to mental health conditions such as difficulty sleeping (Green, Hicks, Weekes, & Wilson, 2005), interaction skills (Lim, Kattapuram, & Lian, 2007), or challenges with emotional regulation (Tang, 2001).

DBT is a popular intervention method with some outcomes-related research that has emerged within cognitive-behavioral approaches and is used with people with borderline personality disorder or other disorders in which there is impusive and self-injurious behavior such as self-cutting (Linehan et al., 2002; Moro, 2007). (See Chapter 10, "Personality Disorders" for more information about DBT and Chapter 8, "Mood Disorders" and Chapter 9, "Anxiety Disorders" for more information about CBT.)

COGNITIVE PERSPECTIVE

Although interest in cognitive processes has a long history, a clinical model of their significance in psychopathology only began to emerge in response to traditional behavioral notions that rejected the mediating influence of mental processes on abnormal behavior. Proponents of the cognitive perspective, therefore, believe that behavior is influenced by factors other than observable environmental stimuli and the responses they elicit. These theorists argue strongly that what people think, believe, expect, remember, and attend to influences how they behave (O'Leary & Wilson, 1987). Specifically, dysfunctional cognitive processes are thought to produce psychological disorder. Furthermore, altering a person's cognitions (i.e., making him or her more functional and adaptive) can ameliorate psychological difficulties. Although the behaviorists, such as Skinner (1971), acknowledged that mental life existed, they denied the causal role of cognitions in behavior. Cognitive psychologists, on the other hand, view cognitions as primary causal agents in psychopathology, and therefore, as priority targets in treatment.

Cognitive psychologists take issue with the basic stimulus–response conditioning theories of behaviorists, which they find far too passive and simplistic. These theorists believe that the learner actively interprets novel information relative to previously acquired information, which they refer to as a schema (Neisser, 1976).

The application of cognitive psychology concepts and principles to the understanding and treatment of psychopathology is popular, especially when combined with behavioral approaches in CBT and occupational therapy (Hudson, 2009; Stoffel & Moyers, 2004; Tang, 2001). The focus of related treatments generally is to alter cognitions and cognitive processes in order to facilitate behavioral and emotional changes. The general term for this treatment approach is *cognitive restructuring*. Several prominent professionals in the field have proposed cognitive theories of psychopathology that bear mentioning. Notable figures include Albert Bandura, Aaron Beck, and Albert Ellis. For the purposes of therapy, cognitive processes can be divided into those that are short term and those that are long term. Short-term processes, including expectations, appraisals, and attributions, are processes of which we either are or can become aware through practice. On the other hand, long-term processes, including beliefs, are generally not readily available to consciousness.

Expectations

Expectations refer to cognitions that anticipate future events. In his seminal work on modeling and observational learning, Albert Bandura assessed the impact of expectations on the performance of learned behaviors. Bandura demonstrated that individuals learn behavior, not only by receiving reinforcement directly for the expression of that behavior, but also by observing others receiving reinforcement for the same behavior. As a result of this evidence for vicarious learning, Bandura hypothesized that learning must involve expectations in addition to operant conditioning principles (Bandura, 1977, 1978; Bandura & Walters, 1959). According to Bandura's theory, two types of expectations are relevant to behavior change: an outcome expectation and an efficacy expectation. An outcome expectation is a person's belief that a given behavior will lead to a desired outcome, while an efficacy expectation is the person's belief that he or she can, in fact, perform the behavior necessary to produce the desired outcome despite obstacles. Both are critical to understanding the mechanisms underlying the acquisition and application of learned behavior. In fact, it has been shown that individuals may learn that a specific behavior will result in a desired outcome but, because they do not believe they have the capacity to perform the target behavior, it nonetheless fails to be produced. As a result, some desired outcomes do not occur (Bandura, 1977, 1978; Bandura & Adams, 1977).

Appraisals

Human beings are constantly evaluating events occurring in their everyday lives. Sometimes these appraisals are evident. Other times, these evaluative processes are not conscious, but rather automatic, most likely due to a lifetime of practice. In his cognitive explanations for psychopathology, Aaron Beck (1976) emphasizes automatic thoughts as causal agents of psychological disorder; in fact, he argues that emotion states are always preceded by related thought processes. In therapy, the individual is taught to slow down and become aware of relevant negative automatic thoughts so that they may then be restructured (Froján-Parga, Calero-Elvira, & Montaño-Fidalgo, 2011; Kipper, 2002).

Beck is primarily interested in cognitive processes related to depression (Beck, 1967, 1976; Beck, Rush, Shaw, & Emery, 1979), but his theoretical concepts have also been successfully applied to other psychological conditions, including personality and anxiety disorders (Hope, Burns, Hayes, Herbert, & Warner, 2010). Specifically, Beck noted that individuals with depression tend to distort their realities by engaging in dysfunctional thought processes. Beck's cognitive therapy of depression is primarily concerned with altering negative thoughts about one's self, the world, and the future and with correcting general misinterpretations of life events that individuals with depression typically possess. The pattern of negative thinking described by Beck is called the "cognitive triad," which refers to negative self-evaluation, a pessimistic view of the world, and a sense of hopelessness regarding future outcomes. These thoughts reflect the drawing of false conclusions by selectively attending to isolated aspects of a situation (selective abstraction), the exaggerating of the importance of negative events (magnification), and the generalizing of the significance of isolated events for one's life (overgeneralization). These pervasive negative thoughts represent primary treatment targets in Beck's cognitive therapy for depression. The goal of therapy, therefore, is to help the client monitor and systematically refute illogical and negative self-statements.

Mindfulness or mindfulness-based cognitive therapy is used by occupational therapists to address everyday appraisals and how they relate to managing stress, depression, and cultivating a healthy lifestyle. Mindfulness-based approaches have been found useful in the treatment of obsessive-compulsive disorder, generalized anxiety, and borderline personality disorder and in the prevention of relapse for depression and substance abuse (Cozolino & Siegel, 2009). According to Hudson (2009), mindfulness "allows an individual to first take ownership and have awareness and acceptance of a situation in order for change to take place" (p. 82) through fostering present-moment awareness and being during activities. Mindfulness activities may include meditation, poetry, diaphragmatic breathing, physical activity such as walking, and lifestyle adjustments to address healthy living (Hudson, 2009). (See also Chapters 8, 9, and 10.)

Attributions

Attributions are an individual's beliefs about cause-and-effect relationships. For example, an individual might make internal or external attributions (Rotter, 1966), stable or unstable attributions (Van Vliet, 2009), or global or specific attributions (Abramson, Seligman, & Teasdale, 1978; Seligman, 1994; Van Vliet, 2009); the specific array of attributions made determines differential behavioral outcomes. Internal attributions emphasize the causal role of intrapersonal variables, while external attributions focus on the role of the environment or other factors out of the individual's personal control. Stable attributions are those that are persistent over time, whereas unstable attributions are considered transient. Finally, global attributions emphasize the persistence of behavior across tasks, while specific attributions relate to one's understanding that a certain behavior is specific to a certain task. Occupational therapists using a cognitive approach may help clients make more rational and adaptive attributions to support the individual's roles and routines. Motivational interviewing is a highly empathetic and nonconfrontational therapeutic communication style used by clinicians including occupational therapists to help clients explore attributions and resolve ambivalence toward change (Stoffel & Moyers, 2004).

Beliefs

Albert Ellis (1962) argues that irrational beliefs, instilled in us over the course of our lives by parents and society, are at the root of psychological disorder. In addition to being maladaptive in and of themselves, these beliefs are also presumed to shape short-term, dysfunctional expectations, appraisals, and attributions. Specifically, maladaptive behaviors and emotions are due to false assumptions (e.g., illogical "shoulds" and "musts") that individuals make about their behavior and the world. As defined by Ellis, six such assumptions are as follows:

1. Adult human beings must be loved and approved by all significant others.
2. In order to be worthy, one should be competent, adequate, and successful in all possible respects.
3. It is catastrophic when things are not the way one would like them to be.
4. Unhappiness is externally caused, and one has little or no control over negative events.
5. Past history is the critical determinant of present behavior, and events that strongly affect one's life will continue to do so.
6. There is always a perfect solution to one's problems, and it is catastrophic if that ideal solution is not found (Ellis, 1962).

Ellis's rational emotive therapy (RET) actively confronts and challenges these assumptions or false beliefs and attempts to replace them with those that are more rational and, hence, more adaptive to an individual's functioning.

Applications in Occupational Therapy

The cognitive perspective is clearly among the more prominent in contemporary thinking. Its focus on cognitive processes that mediate behavior has proved to be a very rich area for empirical study. In addition, the inclusion of cognitive components in psychological assessment and intervention has resulted in more comprehensive and effective treatment outcomes for many clients. By attending to dysfunctional appraisals, expectancies, attributions, and beliefs, therapists may be better able to help clients recognize how their own cognitive processes relate to their mood, thus facilitating behavioral and emotional changes in their clients.

Many of the life skills workbook activities used by occupational therapists are examples of how occupational therapists apply cognitive therapy (see Suggested Resources). Also, one aspect of activity gradation uses a cognitive perspective to simplify and structure a task, and the cognitive disabilities model (Allen, 1985) uses a cognitive perspective to analyze and treat the needs of individuals to support participation in contexts and physical and social environments (AOTA, 2008).

SUMMARY

The broad perspectives discussed in this chapter contribute to occupational therapy's underlying philosophy and also contribute to the tools and strategies used in occupational therapy treatment. These theoretical concepts (as well as the philosophical tenets described in Chapter 3) provide the basis of psychosocial occupational therapy. This is essential knowledge not only for use in mental health settings, but also for all occupational therapy practice in order to address the psychosocial needs of clients. Kielhofner (1997) described a fundamental paradigm of occupational therapy, in which the major themes "affirm the value of occupation and emphasize a client-centered practice and respect for the subjective perspectives of clients and patients. These themes also affirm that therapy is a process of active engagement and empowerment that must be guided by a balance of art and science" (p. 88). The OTPF (2008) reaffirms this paradigm by stating that "engagement in occupation to support participation in context is the focus and targeted end objective of occupational therapy intervention" (p. 611).

Since every client is unique, intervention plans must be personalized in order to ensure that the goals of treatment are those that are most meaningful to the particular client. To understand clients' behavior, it is imperative that occupational therapists have a comprehensive understanding of the biological, intrapsychic, and interpersonal factors mediating that behavior. For example, it is essential to have an understanding of the clients' level of cognitive and perceptual functioning, their ability to process sensory input and produce motor output, their cultural belief system, personality factors that were present prior to injury or disease onset, and valued life roles. Only then can a therapist establish and carry out a treatment plan that is meaningful to the particular client. Psychological theory and research provides many of the tools necessary to develop effective treatment plans. Although the theoretical concepts presented here from the biological, psychodynamic, behavioral, cognitive, and humanistic perspectives are distinct in their understanding and treatment of psychological disorders, they are not necessarily incompatible. In fact, the eclectic integration of concepts should provide the practicing clinician with a better understanding of the biopsychosocial factors influencing behaviors, thoughts, and emotions. Theoretical integration should also allow for the development of individualized treatment plans that are both more comprehensive and more effective.

REVIEW QUESTIONS

1. Describe the benefits and disadvantages to using an eclectic approach to therapy.
2. How is a humanistic perspective related to occupational justice and social inclusion?
3. Explain Manfred Max-Neef's matrix of "needs and satisfiers" and its relevance to occupational therapy.

4. What are the differences between classical psychoanalytic concepts (Freudian) and contemporary psychoanalytic concepts?
5. Which client groups are most likely to benefit from behavioral interventions?

REFERENCES

Abramson, L. Y., Seligman, M. E. P., & Teasdale, J. (1978). Learned helplessness in humans: Critique and reformulation. *Journal of Abnormal Psychology, 87*, 49–74.

Allen, C. (1985). *Occupational therapy for psychiatric diseases: Measurement and management of cognitive disabilities*. Boston: Little, Brown.

American Occupational Therapy Association. (2008). Occupational therapy practice framework: Domain and process. 2nd ed. *American Journal of Occupational Therapy, 62*(6), 625–683.

Baer, D. M., Wolf, M. M., & Risley, T. R. (1968). Some current dimensions of applied behavior analysis. *Journal of Applied Behavior Analysis, 1*, 91–94.

Bandura, A. (1977). *Social learning theory*. Englewood Cliffs, NJ: Prentice-Hall.

Bandura, A. (1978). The self system in reciprocal determinism. *American Psychologist, 37*, 122–147.

Bandura, A. (1986). *Social foundations of thought and action: A social cognitive theory*. Englewood Cliffs, NJ: Prentice-Hall.

Bandura, A. (1997). *Self efficacy: The exercise of control*. New York: Freeman.

Bandura, A., & Adams, N. E. (1977). Analysis of self-efficacy theory of behavioral changes. *Cognitive Theory and Research, 1*, 287–310.

Bandura, A., & Walters, R. H. (1959). *Adolescent aggression: A Study of the influence of child-training practices and family interrelationships*. Oxford, England: Ronald.

Banks, E., & Blair, S. (1997). The contribution of occupational therapy within the context of the psychodynamic approach for older clients who have mental health problems. *Health Care in Later Life, 2*(2), 85–92.

Barondes, S. H. (1993). *Molecules and mental illness*. New York: Scientific American.

Beaver, K. M., Shutt, J., Boutwell, B. B., Ratchford, M., Roberts, K., & Barnes, J. C. (2009). Genetic and environmental influences on levels of self-control and delinquent peer affiliation: Results from a longitudinal sample of adolescent twins. *Criminal Justice and Behavior, 36*(1), 41–60.

Beck, A. T. (1967). *Depression: Clinical, experimental, and theoretical aspects*. New York: Harper & Row.

Beck, A. T. (1976). *Cognitive therapy and the emotional disorders*. New York: International Universities Press.

Beck, A. T., Rush, A. J., Shaw, B. F., & Emery, G. (1979). *Cognitive therapy of depression*. New York: Guilford.

Becker, R. E. (1985). *Shaping*. In A. S. Bellack & M. Hersen (Eds.), *Dictionary of behavior therapy techniques* (p. 205). New York: Pergamon.

Beebe, B. (2003). *Forms of intersubjectivity in infant research and their implications for adult treatment*. Paper presented at the New Developments in Attachment Theory: Applications to Clinical Practice, Los Angeles, CA.

Benjamin, E. (2011). Humanistic psychology and the mental health worker. *Journal of Humanistic Psychology, 51*, 82–111.

Benjamin, L. S., & Pugh, C. (2001). *Using interpersonal theory to select effective treat*ment interventions. In W. J. Livesley (Ed.), *Handbook of personality disorders: Theory, research and treatment* (pp. 414–436). New York: Guilford.

Birkholtz, M., & Blair, S. (2001). Chronic pain—the need for an eclectic approach: 1. *British Journal of Therapy & Rehabilitation, 8*(2), 68–73.

Bouchard, T. J., Lykken, D. T., McGue, M., Segal, N. L., & Tellegen, A. (1990). Sources of human psychological differences: The Minnesota study of twins reared apart. *Science, 250*, 223–228.

Bowlby, J. (1988a). Developmental psychiatry comes of age. *American Journal of Psychiatry, 145*(1), 1–10.

Bowlby, J. (1988b). *A Secure Base: Parent-child attachment and healthy human development* (Ch. 2, pp. 20–38). New York: Basic Books.

Brant, A. M., Haberstick, B. C., Corley, R. P., Wadsworth, S. J., DeFries, J. C., & Hewitt, J. K. (2009). The developmental etiology of high IQ. *Behavior Genetics, 39*(4), 393–405.

Bretherton, I. (1990a). Communication patterns, internal working models, and the intergenerational transmission of attachment relationships. *Infant Mental Health Journal, 11*(3), 237–252.

Bretherton, I. (1990b). Open communication and internal working models: Their role in the development of attachment relations. In R. A. Thompson (Ed.), *Nebraska Symposium on Motivation: Vol. 36. Socioemotional development* (pp. 59–113). Lincoln: University of Nebraska Press.

Bretherton, I. (1992). The origins of attachment theory: John Bowlby and Mary Ainsworth. *Developmental Psychology, 28*(5), 759–775.

Cassidy, J., & Shaver, P. (Eds.). (2008). *Handbook of attachment: Theory, research, and clinical applications*. New York: Guilford.

Champagne, T. (2006). Creating sensory rooms: Environmental enhancements for acute inpatient mental health settings. *Mental Health Special Interest Section Quarterly, 29*(4), 1–4.

Champagne, T., Koomar, J., & Olson, L. (2010). Sensory processing evaluation and intervention in mental health. *OT Practice, 15*(5), CE-1–8.

Chaney, S. (2010). Historical keyword: Behaviour. *Lancet, 376*, 1893.

Coyle, J. T. (2009). Amino acid neurotransmitters. In B. J. Sadock, V. A. Sadock, & P. Ruiz (Eds.), *Kaplan and Sadock's comprehensive textbook of psychiatry* (9th ed.). Philadelphia: Lippincott Williams & Wilkins.

Coyne, J., Thombs, B., & Hagedoorn, M. (2010). Ain't necessarily so: Review and critique of recent meta-analyses of behavioral medicine interventions in *Health Psychology. Health Psychology, 29*(2), 107–116.

Cozolino, L. J., & Siegel, D. J. (2009). Contributions of the psychological sciences. In B. J. Sadock, V. A. Sadock, & P. Ruiz (Eds.), *Kaplan and Sadock's comprehensive textbook of psychiatry* (9th ed.). Philadelphia: Lippincott Williams & Wilkins.

Deitz, D. E. D. (1985a). Chaining. In A. S. Bellack & M. Hersen (Eds.), *Dictionary of behavior therapy techniques* (p. 53). New York: Pergamon.

Deitz, D. E. D. (1985b). Forward chaining. In A. S. Bellack & M. Hersen (Eds.), *Dictionary of behavior therapy techniques* (p. 131). New York: Pergamon.

DiCicco-Bloom, E., & Falluel-Morel, A. (2009). Neural development and neurogenesis. In B. J. Sadock, V. A. Sadock, & P. Ruiz (Eds.), *Kaplan and Sadock's comprehensive textbook of psychiatry* (9th ed.). Philadelphia: Lippincott Williams & Wilkins.

Domschke, K., & Dannlowski, U. (2010). Imaging genetics of anxiety disorders. *NeuroImage, 53*(3), 822–831.

Dressler, J., & MacRae, A. (1998). Advocacy, partnerships, and client centered practice. *Occupational Therapy in Mental Health, 14*(1/2), 35–43.

Drevets, W. C., & Charney, D. S. (2009). Neuroimaging and the neuroanatomical circuits implicated in anxiety, fear, and stressed-induced circuitry disorders. In B. J. Sadock, V. A. Sadock, & P. Ruiz (Eds.), *Kaplan and Sadock's comprehensive textbook of psychiatry* (9th ed.). Philadelphia: Lippincott Williams & Wilkins.

Ellis, A. (1962). *Reason and emotion in psychotherapy*. New York: Lyle Stuart.

Farber, B. A., & Doolin, E. M. (2011). Positive regard. *Psychotherapy, 48*(1), 58–64.

Fears, S. C., Mathews, C. A., & Freimer, N. B. (2009). Genetic linkage analysis of psychiatric disorders. In B. J. Sadock, V. A. Sadock, & P. Ruiz (Eds.), *Kaplan and Sadock's comprehensive textbook of psychiatry* (9th ed.). Philadelphia: Lippincott Williams & Wilkins.

Fidler, G. S., & Fidler, J. W. (1954). *Introduction to psychiatric occupational therapy.* New York: Macmillan.

Fidler, G. S., & Fidler, J. W. (1978). Doing and becoming: Purposeful action and self-actualization. *American Journal of Occupational Therapy, 32,* 305.

Fidler, G., & Velde, B. P. (1999). *Activities: Reality and symbol.* Thorofare, NJ: Slack.

Foroud, T., Edenberg, H. J., & Crabbe, J. C. (2010). Genetic research: Who is at risk for alcoholism? *Alcohol Research & Health, 33*(1/2), 64–75.

Frankl, V. E. (1967). *Psychotherapy and existential papers on logotherapy.* New York: Square.

Frankl, V. E. (1972). *The doctor and the soul.* New York: Knopf.

Freud, A. (1936/1974). *The ego and the mechanisms of defense.* New York:International Universities Press.

Freud, S. (1976). *The ego and the id.* In J. Strachey (Ed. & Trans.), *The complete psychological works* (Vol. 19). New York: Norton. (Original work published 1923).

Froján-Parga, M., Calero-Elvira, A., & Montaño-Fidalgo, M. (2011). Study of the Socratic method during cognitive restructuring. *Clinical Psychology & Psychotherapy, 18*(2), 110–123.

Gabbard, G. O. (2001). Psychoanalysis and psychoanalytic psychotherapy. In W. J. Livesley (Ed.), *Handbook of personality disorders: Theory, research and treatment* (pp. 359–376). New York: Guilford.

Gershon, E. S., & Rieder, R. O. (1992). Major disorders of the brain. *Scientific American, 267,* 127–133.

Giles, G. M. (1985). Anorexia and bulimia: An activity oriented approach. *American Journal of Occupational Therapy, 39,* 510–517.

Giles, G. M., Ridley, J. E., Dill, A., & Frye, S. (1997). A consecutive series of adults with brain injury treated with a dressing retraining program. *American Journal of Occupational Therapy, 51,* 256–266.

Gormezano, I., Prokasy, W., & Thompson, R. (1987). *Classical conditioning* (3rd ed.). Hillsdale, NJ: Erlbaum.

Grebb, J. A., & Carlsson, A. (2009). Introduction and considerations for a brain-based diagnostic system in psychiatry. In B. J. Sadock, V. A. Sadock, & P. Ruiz (Eds.), *Kaplan and Sadock's comprehensive textbook of psychiatry* (9th ed.). Philadelphia: Lippincott Williams & Wilkins.

Green, A., Hicks, J., Weekes, R., & Wilson, S. (2005). A cognitive-behavioural group intervention for people with chronic insomnia: An initial evaluation. *British Journal of Occupational Therapy, 68*(11), 518–522.

Griffiths, S., & Corr, S. (2007). The use of creative activities with people with mental health problems: A survey of occupational therapists. *British Journal of Occupational Therapy, 70*(3), 107–114.

Hassiotis, A., Robotham, D., Canagasabey, A., Romeo, R., Langridge, D., Blizard, R., Murad, S., & King, M. (2009). Randomized, single-blind, controlled trial of a specialist behavior therapy team for challenging behavior in adults with intellectual disabilities. *American Journal of Psychiatry, 166,* 1278–1285.

Henderson, S. (1999). Frames of reference utilized in the rehabilitation of individuals with eating disorders. *Canadian Journal of Occupational Therapy, 66*(1), 43–51.

Hodges, J. Q., Hardiman, E. R., & Segal, S. P. (2004). Predictors of hope among members of mental health self-help agencies. *Social Work in Mental Health, 2*(1), 1–16.

Hope, D. A., Burns, J. A., Hayes, S. A., Herbert, J. D., & Warner, M. D. (2010). Automatic thoughts and cognitive restructuring in cognitive behavioral group therapy for social anxiety disorder. *Cognitive Therapy and Research, 34*(1), 1–12.

Hopkins, H. L. (1988). A historical perspective on occupational therapy. In H. L. Hopkins & D. H. Smith (Eds.), *Willard and Spackman's occupational therapy* (7th ed., pp. 16–37). Philadelphia: Lippincott.

Hudson, F. (2009). Mindfulness based cognitive therapy (MBCT) and occupational therapy in mental health. *Mental Health Occupational Therapy, 14*(2), 82–83.

Ikiugu, M., Smallfield, S., & Condit, C. (2009). A framework for combining theoretical conceptual practice models in occupational therapy practice. *Canadian Journal of Occupational Therapy, 76*(3), 162–170.

Insel, T. R., & Wang, P. S. (2010). Rethinking mental illness. *Journal of the American Medical Association, 303*(19), 1970–1971.

Kielhofner, G. (1997). *Conceptual foundations of occupational therapy*. Philadelphia: F. A. Davis.

Kielhofner, G. (2006). The aim of research: Philosophical foundations of scientific inquiry. In G. Kielhofner (Ed.), *Research in occupational therapy: methods of inquiry for enhancing practice*. Philadelphia: F. A. Davis.

Kipper, D. A. (2002). The cognitive double: Integrating cognitive and action techniques. *Journal of Group Psychotherapy, Psychodrama & Sociometry, 55*(2-3), 93–106.

Kronenberg, F., Simo Algado, S., & Pollard, N. (Eds.). (2005). *Occupational therapy without borders: Learning from the spirit of survivors*. London: Elsevier.

Kronenberg, F., Pollard, N., & Sakellariou, D. (Eds.). (2011). *Occupational therapy without borders (Volume 2): Towards an ecology of occupation based practices*. London: Elsevier.

Lane, S. J., Lynn, J. Z., & Reynolds, S. (2010). Sensory modulation: A neuroscience and behavioral overview. *OT Practice, 15*(21), CE1–CE8.

Larson, E., Wood, W., & Clark, F. (2003). Occupational science: Building the science and practice of occupation through an academic discipline. In W. Blesedell Crepeau, E. Cohn, & B. Schell (Eds.), *Willard and Spackman's occupational therapy* (10th ed.). Philadelphia: Lippincott Williams & Wilkins.

Law, M. (Ed.). (1998). *Client centered occupational therapy*. Thorofare, NJ: Slack.

Le Boutillier, C., & Croucher, A. (2010). Social inclusion and mental health. *British Journal of Occupational Therapy, 73*(3), 136–139.

Lim, S., Kattapuram, A., & Lian, W. (2007). Evaluation of a pilot clinic-based social skills group. *British Journal of Occupational Therapy, 70*(1), 35–39.

Lin, K., Smith, M., & Ortiz, V. (2001). Culture and psychopharmacology. *Psychiatric Clinics of North America, 24*(3), 523–538.

Linehan, M. M., Dimeff, L. A., Reynolds, F. K., Comtois, K. A., Welch, S. S., et al. (2002). Dialectical behavior therapy versus comprehensive validation therapy plus 12-step for the treatment of opioid dependent women meeting criteria for borderline personality disorder. *Drug and Alcohol Dependence, 67*(1), 13–26.

Luiselli, J., Bass, J., & Whitcomb, S. (2010). Teaching applied behavior analysis knowledge competencies to direct-care service providers: Outcome assessment and social validation of a training program. *Behavior Modification, 34*(5) 403–414.

Mackenzie, A., & Beecraft, S. (2004). The use of psychodynamic observation as a tool for learning and reflective practice when working with older adults. *British Journal of Occupational Therapy, 67*(12), 533–539.

Maslow, A. H. (1968). *Toward a psychology of being*. New York: Van Nostrand-Reinhold.

Max-Neef, M. (1991). *Human scale development: Conception, application and further reflections*. New York: Apex Press.

Miller, R., Seig, K., Ludwig, F., Shortridge, S., & Van Deusen, J. (1988). *Six perspectives on theory for the practice of occupational therapy*. Rockville, MD: Aspen.

Molinari, V., & Edelstein, B. (2011). Commentary on the current status and the future of behavior therapy in long-term care settings. *Behavior Therapy, 42,* 59–65.

Moore, J. (2010). Philosophy of science, with special consideration given to behaviorism as the philosophy of the science of behavior. *The Psychological Record, 60,* 137–150.

Moro, C. (2007). A comprehensive literature review defining self-mutilation and occupational therapy intervention approaches: Dialectical behavior therapy and sensory integration. *Occupational Therapy in Mental Health, 23*(1), 55–67.

Mosey, A. C. (1980). A model for occupational therapy. *Occupational Therapy in Mental Health, 1,* 11–31.

Neisser, U. (1976). *Cognition and reality.* San Francisco: Freeman.

O'Leary, K. D., & Wilson, G. T. (1987). *Behavior therapy: Application and outcome.* Englewood Cliffs, NJ: Prentice-Hall.

Ovsiew, F. (2009). Neuropsychiatry and behavioral neurology. In B. J. Sadock, V. A. Sadock, & P. Ruiz (Eds.), *Kaplan and Sadock's comprehensive textbook of psychiatry* (9th ed.). Philadelphia: Lippincott Williams & Wilkins.

Patterson, C. H. (1989). Eclecticism in psychotherapy: Is integration possible? *Psychotherapy, 26,* 157–161.

Pistrang, N., Barker, C., & Humphreys, K. (2010). The contributions of mutual help groups for mental health problems to psychological well-being: A systematic review. In L. D. Brown & S. Wituk, (Eds.), *Mental health self-help: Consumer and family initiatives* (pp. 61–85). New York: Springer Science + Business Media. doi:10.1007/978-1-4419-6253-9_4

Reilly, M. (1962). Occupational therapy can be one of the greatest ideas of twentieth century medicine. *American Journal of Occupational Therapy, 16,* 1–16.

Richard, L., & Knis-Matthews, L. (2010). Are we really client centered? Using the Canadian Occupational Performance Measure to see how the client's goals connect with the goals of the occupational therapist. *Occupational Therapy in Mental Health, 26*(1), 51–66.

Rogers, C. R. (1942). *Counseling and psychotherapy: Newer concepts in practice.* Boston: Houghton Mifflin.

Rogers, C. R. (1951). *Client-centered therapy: Its current practice, implications, and theory.* Boston: Houghton Mifflin.

Rogers, C. R. (1961). *On becoming a person: A therapist's view of psychotherapy.* Boston: Houghton Mifflin.

Rosenzweig, M. R., Leiman, A. L., & Breedlove, S. M. (2001). *Biological psychology: An introduction to behavioral, cognitive, & clinical neuroscience* (3rd ed.). Sunderland, MA: Sinauer.

Rotter, J. B. (1966). Generalized expectancies for internal versus external control of reinforcement. *Psychological Monographs, 80*(1).

Rowan, J. (1999). Ascent and descent in Maslow's theory. *Journal of Humanistic Psychology, 39,* 125–133.

Rowan, J. (2004). *A guide to humanistic psychology.* Alameda, CA: Association for Humanistic Psychology.

Russell, A., & Lloyd, C. (2004). Partnerships in mental health: Addressing barriers to social inclusion. *International Journal of Therapy and Rehabilitation, 11*(6), 267–274.

Sadock, B., & Sadock, V. (2003). *Kaplan and Sadock's synopsis of psychiatry* (9th ed.). Philadelphia: Lippincott Williams & Wilkins.

Schneider, F., Backes, V., & Mathiak, K. (2009). Brain imaging: On the way toward a therapeutic discipline. *European Archives of Psychiatry and Clinical Neuroscience, 259*(Suppl 2), S143–S147.

Schreibman, L. (1985). Backward chaining. In A. S. Bellack & M. Hersen (Eds.), *Dictionary of behavior therapy techniques* (p. 22). New York: Pergamon.

Schultz, S. (2009). Theory of occupational adaptation. In E. Blesedell Crepeau, E. Cohn, & B. Boyt Schell (Eds.), *Willard and Spackman's occupational therapy* (11th ed.). Philadelphia: Lippincott Williams & Wilkins.

Seligman, S. (1994). Applying psychoanalysis in an unconventional context. *Psychoanalytic Study of the Child, 49,* 481–500.

Shane, S., Nicolaou, N., Cherkas, L., & Spector, T. D. (2010). Genetics, the Big Five, and the tendency to be self-employed. *Journal of Applied Psychology, 95*(6), 1154–1162.

Sheffer, M., & Harlock, S. (1980). Tell us what your drawings say. *Occupational Therapy in Mental Health, 1*, 21–38.

Skinner, B. F. (1938). *The behavior of organisms: An experimental analysis.* New York: Appleton-Century-Crofts.

Skinner, B. F. (1953). *Science and human behavior.* New York: Macmillan.

Skinner, B. F. (1971). *Beyond freedom and dignity.* New York: Knopf.

Sroufe, L. A. (1998). The role of infant-caregiver attachment in development. In T. Nezworski (Ed.), *Clinical implications of attachment* (pp. 18–38). New York: Erlbaum.

Sroufe, L. A., & Waters, E. (1977). Attachment as an organizational construct. *Child Development, 48*, 1184–1199.

Stan, A. D., Lesselyong, A., & Ghose, S. (2009). Cellular and molecular neuropathology of schizophrenia. In B. J. Sadock, V. A. Sadock, & P. Ruiz (Eds.), *Kaplan and Sadock's comprehensive textbook of psychiatry* (9th ed.). Philadelphia: Lippincott Williams & Wilkins.

Stern, D. (1985). *The interpersonal world of the infant.* New York: Basic.

Stern, D. N. (2003). *Attachment and intersubjectivity.* Paper presented at the New Developments in Attachment Theory: Applications to Clinical Practice, Los Angeles, CA.

Stern, D. N., Sander, L. W., Nahum, J. P., Harrison, A. M., Lyons-Ruth, K., Morgan, A. C., et al. (1998). Non-interpretive mechanisms in psychoanalytic therapy: The "something more" than interpretation. *International Journal of Psycho-Analysis, 79*, 903–921.

Stoffel, V. C., & Moyers, P. A. (2004). An evidence-based and occupational perspective of interventions for persons with substance-use disorders. *American Journal of Occupational Therapy, 58*(5), 570–586.

Stolorow, R. (1994). The intersubjective context of intrapsychic experience. In R. Stolorow, G. Atwood, & B. Brandchaft (Eds.), *The intersubjective perspective.* Northvale, NJ: Jason Aronson.

Stolorow, R., Atwood, G., & Brandchaft, B. (Eds.). (1994). *The intersubjective perspective.* Northvale, NJ: Jason Aronson.

Strong, J. (1998). Incorporating cognitive-behavioral therapy with occupational therapy: A comparative study with patients with low back pain. *Journal of Occupational Rehabilitation, 8*(1), 61–71.

Sumsion, T., & Lencucha, R. (2007). Balancing challenges and facilitating factors when implementing client-centered collaboration in a mental health setting. *British Journal of Occupational Therapy, 70*(12), 513–520.

Tang, M. (2001). Clinical outcome and client satisfaction of an anger management group program. *Canadian Journal of Occupational Therapy, 68*(4), 228–236.

Thorndike, E. L. (1898). Animal intelligence: An experimental study of the associative processes in animals. *Psychological Review Monograph Supplement, 2*(8).

Townsend, E. (2003). Occupational justice: Ethical, moral and civic principles for an inclusive world. Keynote presentation at the Annual Conference of the European Network of Occupational Therapy Educators, Czech Republic, Prague.

Townsend, E., & Wilcock, A. (2004). Occupational justice and client-centered practice: A dialogue in progress *Canadian Journal of Occupational Therapy 71*(2),75–87.

Tutu, D. (2011). Forward 1. In F. Kronenberg, N. Pollard, & D. Sakellariou (Eds.), *Occupational therapy without borders (Volume 2): Towards an ecology of occupation based practices* (p. ix). London: Elsevier.

Tyrka, A., Wier, L. M., Price, L. H., Rikhye, K., Ross, N. S., Anderson, G. M., et al. (2008). Cortisol and ACTH responses to the Dex/CRH Test: Influence of temperament. *Hormones & Behavior, 53*(4), 518–525.

Van Vliet, K. (2009). The role of attributions in the process of overcoming shame: A qualitative analysis. *Psychology & Psychotherapy: Theory, Research & Practice, 82*(Part 2), 137–152.

Weiss, J. (1993). *How psychotherapy works.* New York: Guilford.

Wingenfeld, K., Spitzer, C., Rullkötter, N., & Löwe, B. (2009). Borderline personality disorder: Hypothalamus pituitary adrenal axis and findings from neuroimaging studies. *Psychoneuroendocrinology, 35*, 154–170.

Yancosek, K., & Howell, D. (2010). Integrating the dynamical systems theory, the task-oriented approach, and the practice framework for clinical reasoning. *Occupational Therapy in Health Care, 24*(3), 223–238.

Yerxa, E. J. (1967). Authentic occupational therapy. *American Journal of Occupational Therapy, 21*, 1–9.

Zeanah, C. H., & Anders, T. F. (1987). Subjectivity in parent-infant relationships: A discussion of internal working models. *Infant Mental Health Journal, 8*(3), 237–249.

SUGGESTED RESOURCES

Bruce, M., & Borg, B. (2001). *Psychosocial frames of reference: Core for occupation-based practice* (3rd ed.). Thorofare, NJ: Slack.

Canadian Association of Occupational Therapists. (1993). *Occupational therapy guidelines for client-centered mental health practice.* Toronto: Minister of Supply and Services.

Cole, M. B. (2005). *Group dynamics in occupational therapy, the theoretical basis and practice application of group intervention* (3rd ed.). Thorofare, NJ: Slack.

Creek, J., & Lougher, L. (Ed.). (2008). *Occupational therapy and mental health* (4th ed.). New York: Churchill Livingstone.

Fearing, V., & Clark, J. (2000). *Individuals in context: A practical guide to client centered practice.* Thorofare, NJ: Slack.

Hagedorn, R. (2001). *Foundations for practice in occupational therapy* (3rd ed.). New York: Churchill Livingstone.

Korb-Khalsa, K., Leutenberg, E., & Leutenberg Brodsky, A. (2001). *Life management skills V: Reproducible activity handouts created for facilitators.* Beachwood, OH: Wellness Reproductions.

Morihisa, J. M. (Ed.). (2001). *Advances in brain imaging.* Washington, DC: American Psychiatric Publishing.

Mosey, A. C. (1986). *Psychosocial components of occupational therapy.* New York: Raven.

Rogers, C. (1965). *Client-centered therapy: Its current practice, implications and theory.* Boston: Houghton Mifflin.

Schwartzberg, S. (2002). *Interactive reasoning in the practice of occupational therapy.* Upper Saddle River, NJ: Prentice-Hall.

Shannon, P. (1977). The derailment of occupational therapy. *American Journal of Occupational Therapy, 31*(4), 229–234.

Websites

Center for Psychiatric Rehabilitation (affiliated with Sargent College of Health and Rehabilitation Sciences at Boston University): http://www.bu.edu/cpr/

Association for Humanistic Psychology: http://www.ahpweb.org/aboutahp/whatis.html

Official Abraham Maslow Publication site: http://www.maslow.com/

Beck Institute for Cognitive Behavior Therapy: http://www.beckinstitute.org/

The Albert Ellis Institute: http://www.rebt.org/

International Association for Contemporary Psychoanalysis and Psychotherapy: http://www.iarpp.net/about/index.html

Self- Psychology: http://www.selfpsychology.com/bibliogr.htm

International Association for Psychoanalytic Self Psychology: http://www.selfpsychology.com/bibliogr.htm

P A R T   III

Diagnosis and Dysfunction

The first chapter in Part III on diagnosis and psychopathology (Chapter 6) discusses the significant changes occurring, and that are expected to occur, with the diagnostic process used in mental health practice and reviews the major symptoms seen with mental illness. The procedures of diagnosis are being influenced first by a recovery perspective and also by the desire to align more closely with an international perspective on the process. It remains to be seen how proposed changes will unfold in service delivery but there are many opportunities for occupational therapists who are knowledgeable and well prepared for these changes. Despite the many controversies surrounding the diagnostic process and the identification of psychopathology, it is the authors' beliefs that a thorough understanding of both psychopathology and diagnosis is critical in providing competent mental health care. However, this background alone is not sufficient. Therefore, each chapter in this section addresses symptoms and diagnosis and places this information in context while discussing environments, assessment, and interventions in a client-centered, occupation-based approach.

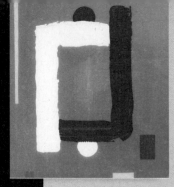

Chapter 6

Diagnosis and Psychopathology

Anne MacRae, PhD, OTR/L, BCMH, FAOTA

◼ KEY TERMS

comorbidity

compliance

diagnosis

dysfunction

executive function

hoarding

psychopathology

psychotropic

shared decision making

symptom

telepsychiatry

CHAPTER OUTLINE

Introduction

Clinical Terminology

Diagnosis

    Diagnostic Controversy

    Diagnostic Classification

    The *Diagnostic and Statistical Manual (DSM)*

    The Evolution of the Diagnostic Process

Psychopathology

    Thought

    Language

    Perception and Sensation

    Affect

    Orientation

    Memory

    Energy and Motoric Response

Psychiatric Intervention in the Era of Recovery
    Psychotropic Medication
    Access and Technology
Summary

INTRODUCTION

The purpose of this chapter is to provide a brief overview of the clinical perspective of diagnoses and symptoms of mental illness. The evolution of this clinical perspective has been influenced by and can be viewed as part of the recovery perspective. Delivery of clinical services is also going through dramatic changes based on research, an orientation toward recovery, and technology.

CLINICAL TERMINOLOGY

The terminology used in mental health settings can often be confusing, especially since the general public often misuses the terms. It is important to be as specific as possible and to be clear as to whether a phenomenon is a **symptom**, **dysfunction**, or **diagnosis**, even though there is often much overlap. In other words, an individual may experience a particular symptom that is typical of a specific disorder but still not meet the criteria for that diagnosis. Moreover, neither the symptom nor the diagnosis will give the clinician a true indication about the level or type of dysfunction. It is a common error to assume that some diagnoses automatically imply a greater level of dysfunction. However, it is not possible to determine occupational or functional performance based on diagnosis or symptoms alone. An individual's strengths, prior level of functioning, and support systems, must also be considered. The following case illustrations compare brief psychiatric histories of three people in order to show the differences between symptoms, diagnosis, and dysfunction.

CASE ILLUSTRATION

Symptoms, Diagnosis, and Dysfunction

Ms. Jones complains of feeling bored and depressed (symptoms). She has alienated all of her friends and is now isolated from social contact (dysfunction). Ms. Jones also meets the criteria for borderline personality disorder (diagnosis).

Mr. Nguyen has recently been fired from his job for reportedly "slipshod" work (dysfunction). His doctor has been treating him for dysthymic disorder (diagnosis) for several years, but lately Mr. Nguyen has been feeling more lethargic and melancholic (symptoms).

Mrs. Garcia is hospitalized for an episode of major depression (diagnosis). She expresses feelings of hopelessness and suicidal ideation (symptoms) and is disinterested in performing basic self-care tasks such as caring for personal hygiene (dysfunction).

DIAGNOSIS

Although occupational therapists are not responsible for determining diagnosis, knowledge of diagnostic terminology and criteria is essential for effective communication with the clinical team and occupational therapists often contribute to the diagnostic process by providing the team with specific information from evaluations. This includes an analysis of the sociocultural and environmental contexts affecting the individual's life as well as the impact an individual's symptoms may have on his or her ability to perform life tasks.

The determination of a clinical diagnosis in psychiatry is, at best, an inexact process based on both deductive and inductive reasoning. One view of this process is that it is a constructive way of ordering knowledge about a person's dysfunction in order to better understand the mental illness. However, diagnoses are also viewed by some as a destructive force that serves only to inappropriately label and dehumanize individuals (Glackin, 2010; McGruder, 2001).

Diagnostic Controversy

There are inherent dangers in labeling, and it is the clinician's responsibility not to make assumptions about an individual's behavior or abilities based on diagnosis alone. On the other hand, a structured diagnostic process attempts to make psychiatric terminology more uniform, which is important because of the stigma attached to mental illness. The implications of these disorders at a societal level are great, which means that the careless use of volatile terms must be avoided, regardless of the purpose of diagnosis. Indeed, the occupational therapist can play an important role in educating the public about the myths of mental illness and the misuse of clinical terminology. For example, calling someone "a schizophrenic" implies that the individual's main identifying feature is an illness, which is simplistic and dehumanizing. It is both more appropriate and more accurate to identify the individual as a "person with schizophrenia." Figure 6-1 suggests other ways to use labels intelligently and sensitively. Figure 6-2 contains quotes from mental health clients who participated in a focus group that describe the ambivalence felt regarding psychiatric diagnosis.

LANGUAGE

Mental illnesses are frequently the subject of news stories, or of dramatic films or television programs. NAMI, the Nation's Voice on Mental Illness, offers the following guidelines for use of medical and slang terms about mental illnesses:

- words like "crazy," "nuts," "wacko," "sicko," "psycho," "lunatic," "demented," and "loony" are offensive

- terms like "insane" are inappropriate except when used in a specific medical or legal context (e.g., the term "criminally insane" in a courtroom scene)

- referring to a "person with a severe mental illness" is preferable to "the mentally ill," which depersonalizes—highlighting the illness, not the person

- terms like "schizophrenia" and "manic depressive illness" have very specific meanings and apply only to certain groups of people; such scientific labels should be checked carefully for accuracy; they should not be used to refer to "schizophrenic weather" or other uses unrelated to the illnesses themselves

■ ■ ■ ■ ■ ■ ■

For more information, contact the NAMI, a self-help organization providing mutual support, public education, research, and advocacy for people with serious mental illnesses:

Public Relations Director
National Alliance for the Mentally Ill
2107 Wilson Boulevard,
Suite Colonial Place Three
Arlington, VA 22201
www/nami.org

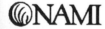

ABOUT MENTAL ILLNESS

FIGURE 6-1. Language About Mental Illness
Reprinted with permission from NAMI

Another criticism of the diagnostic process is the lack of precise data on psychiatric illness. Although knowledge of the structure and chemistry of the brain is growing, it is rare that measurable or visible objective data such as X-rays and blood tests, as are used in physical diagnosis, can be used in psychiatry. The following case illustration demonstrates the subjective nature of psychiatric diagnosis.

Still another significant concern about diagnosis is cultural bias, specifically, a white, male, Judeo-Christian orientation. This issue is beginning to be addressed, but

- It's sort of weird, like a label stuck on my forehead.
- My diagnosis of bipolar disorder seems to make me think that's all of me. It isn't though. There is so much more to me than my diagnosis of a mental illness.
- I guess there has to be different diagnoses. It gives the doctors something to work on and hopefully prescribe the right medication.
- The diagnosis of a mental illness is not so different than a medical diagnosis. It helps everyone understand his or her disease or problem.
- If only the "normies" could understand that the diagnosis of a mental illness is only a way to figure out how to help the client, just like with a medical diagnosis, then it wouldn't be such a bad thing.
- My diagnosis of schizophrenia has followed me around my entire adult life. It is like a plague. I hate it. It's like being called a wart, and having a wart sitting right in the middle of my forehead!
- There are so many different diagnoses. I always wonder how the doctors come up with the right one, or if maybe they just guess

FIGURE 6-2. Client Attitudes About Diagnosis

© Cengage Learning 2013

CASE ILLUSTRATION

—Brian's Many Diagnoses

Brian is a 58-year-old man who was first diagnosed with depression in his senior year of high school after fracturing his neck. With the physical pain, he remembers that the emotional pain that had been hidden suddenly rushed to the surface and he could no longer control it. His diagnosis of depression was only the first of many more diagnoses to come. Over the years, he recalls being diagnosed with bipolar disorder, borderline personality disorder, schizophrenia, schizoaffective disorder, post-traumatic stress disorder, and others. He isn't sure if any of those diagnoses were correct. Brian had symptoms that fit into just about all of those diagnoses at one time or another, but the diagnoses seemed to change with new psychiatrists and therapists. He now wonders if the different medications prescribed for his various diagnoses were possibly the wrong ones. He'll never know, but still thinks about what would have happened if he had one psychiatrist, one therapist, and one [correct] diagnosis.

Discussion

There are many reasons why a diagnosis may change, including the differing theoretical perspectives of the primary clinician. However, diagnoses may also change because of the adopting of new criteria and diagnostic procedures by the psychiatric establishment, changing environmental stressors of the client, the development of new symptoms, or even new information coming to light within the therapeutic relationship. Regardless of the reasons for changing a client's diagnosis, this story demonstrates the need for caution again over reliance or interpretation based on diagnosis alone.

it remains essential that clinicians be aware of the inherent ethnocentrism found in the current diagnostic system. "Careful attention to the sociocultural dimensions of mental illness serves both a scientific and social justice agenda. For example, when assessment fails to attend to sociocultural factors, it risks misdiagnosis and the perpetuation of clinical stereotypes based on race, ethnicity, gender, religion, or sexual orientation, among other factors, which can lead to mental healthcare disparities" (Alarcon et al., 2009, p. 559). It has also been suggested that not taking into account all contextual factors has caused an increase in false positive diagnoses in community-based treatment (Wakefield, 2010). As psychiatric care continues to shift away from an institutional model, it is critical that the complex and interrelated stress of life events be taken into consideration before determining a diagnosis. Given these limitations, why are diagnoses used at all? Despite legitimate controversy, the diagnostic process helps facilitate interdisciplinary communication and fosters research, both of which are essential for high-quality mental health care. It is hoped that as research continues, the process of diagnosing will become increasingly objective, culturally sensitive, and accurate.

Diagnostic Classification

The most commonly used instrument to record diagnoses, disorders, and symptoms is the World Health Organization's (WHO) *International Classification of Diseases,* currently in its 10th edition (*ICD-10*) with the 11th edition in development.

WHO also publishes a companion document known as the *International Classification of Function* (*ICF*), which not only covers the diagnostic concerns of body structure and functions but also includes ratings of activities and participation and contextual factors such as the influence of personal causation and environment (WHO, 2001). The *ICF* is very consistent with an occupational therapy approach and indeed was used to develop the language of the first edition of the Occupational Therapy Practice Framework (American Occupational Therapy Association [AOTA], 2002). Table 6-1 is an overview of the *ICF* and its structures.

The *Diagnostic and Statistical Manual (DSM)*

The *ICD* and the *ICF* are not limited to mental illness and do not contain the diagnostic specificity found in the American Psychiatric Association's (APA) *Diagnostic and Statistical Manual* (*DSM*). This manual is a significant part of the academic curricula of mental health professionals, especially in the United States. Furthermore, the "DSM not only influences how mental health specialists diagnose and treat their patients but also sways how US insurance companies decide which disorders to cover, how pharmaceutical companies design clinical trials and how funding agencies decide which research to fund" (Hebebrand & Buitelaar, 2011, p. 57). With such widespread influence, it is sometimes difficult

TABLE 6-1. An Overview of *ICF*

	Part 1: Functioning and Disability		Part 2: Contextual Factors	
Components	Body Functions and Structures	Activities and Participation	Environmental Factors	Personal Factors
Domains	Body functions Body structures	Life areas (tasks, actions)	External influences on functioning and disability	Internal influences on functioning and disability
Constructs	Change in body functions (physiological) Change in body structures (anatomical)	Capacity Executing tasks in a standard environment Performance Executing tasks in the current environment	Facilitating or hindering impact of features of the physical, social, and attitudinal world	Impact of attributes of the person
Positive aspect (Functioning)	Functional and structural integrity	Activities participation	Facilitators	Not applicable
Negative aspect (Disability)	Impairment	Activity limitation Participation restriction	Barriers/hindrances	Not applicable

Source: From *International Classification of Functioning, Disability and Health (ICF)* (WHO, 2001). Reprinted with permission of the World Health Organization (WHO), and all rights are reserved by the organization.

to keep in mind that the information being presented is not clear-cut, concrete, or complete. It is important to analyze the data critically and be aware of its limitations. Furthermore, the process of evaluation and treatment planning is far more comprehensive than can be covered in a manual such as the *DSM*, and each particular discipline has something unique and specific to offer. It is important to be familiar with the information in the *DSM*; however, it should not be assumed that this knowledge is all that is required for practice, as it barely constitutes a beginning.

Although the APA states that the *DSM* is atheoretical, theories pervade both our conscious and unconscious thought, so it may not be possible to eliminate theoretical bias. However, the association did make a serious attempt to avoid defining disorders based on the beliefs of a particular school of thought. This is a valuable unifying concept for all the professions involved in mental health because of the diversity of beliefs that are found in practice, particularly regarding the etiology of mental illness. Rather than defining disorders based on an individual theory, such as behaviorism or psychoanalytic thought, a biopsychosocial approach to assessment is used. This model is an attempt to be holistic by providing a wide range of information without necessarily referring to the etiology of the disorder or defining it according to one theoretical belief. Figure 6-3 illustrates the communication difficulties encountered when theoretic beliefs are the sole basis of diagnosis. While various theories have significance for treatment, diagnosis becomes problematic when clinicians base their diagnosis solely on theoretical premises.

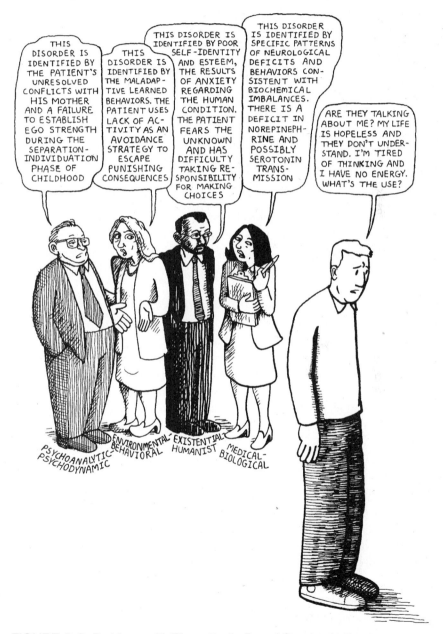

FIGURE 6-3. Problems with Theoretically-Based Communication

The Evolution of the Diagnostic Process

In an effort to capture a biopsychosocial view of diagnosis, the *DSM-III* (APA, 1980) through the *DSM-IV-TR* (APA, 2000) used a multi-axial system, with each axis addressing a different domain. The intent was to minimize the likelihood that pertinent information would be overlooked in interdisciplinary treatment planning.

However, criticism mounted regarding the accuracy and practicality of the multi-axial system and various DSM-5 task forces and study groups, as well as other researchers, have recommended significant changes. According to the DSM-5 development website (APA, n.d.), the current recommendation is to "collapse Axes I, II, and III into one axis that contains all psychiatric and general medical diagnoses. This change would bring DSM-5 into greater harmony with the single-axis approach used by the international community." This proposed change also reflects the growing awareness of the **comorbidity** of physical and mental disorders because well over half of all people with mental illness have at least one co-occurring physical illness. It remains to be seen how service delivery models will evolve to reflect this understanding. However, new organizational and financial models are being explored that can more efficiently and effectively address comorbidity (Druss & Reisinger Walker, 2011).

Also under consideration is using *ICD* codes in place of Axis IV ratings to document psychosocial and environmental problems. Axis V of the *DSM IV-TR* (APA, 2000) is the Global Assessment of Functioning (GAF). Although this scale has been widely used in research, its use in the clinical diagnostic process is minimal. According to Soderberg, Tungstrom, and Armelius (2005), "clinical raters can use the GAF in a sufficiently reliable way to enable use of the ratings at an aggregated level. To use the scale for an individual patient, special procedures are required" (p. 438). The DSM-5 Impairment and Disability Study Group has recommended that the DSM-5 adopt the strategies used in the *ICD* and *ICF* that assess associated disability and dysfunction separately from diagnosis. In addition, an effort is under way to identify and develop more, well-designed tools for functional assessment (APA, n.d.). This is obviously an area where the specific expertise of occupational therapy could be of great benefit and occupational therapists are encouraged to continue developing, researching, and publishing such assessments.

There is also a profound shift away from using the current categorical approach because the "*DSM–IV* routinely fails in the goal of guiding the clinician to the presence of one specific disorder, despite the best efforts of the leading clinicians and researchers who have authored the manual" (Widiger & Samuel, 2005). A categorical approach requires the presence of a specific number of symptoms, within a set time frame, to warrant a diagnosis and therefore be eligible for treatment. This is simply not consistent with the reality of people's experiences with mental illness or the observations of countless clinicians. More often than not, a client will present with a constellation of symptoms across a spectrum of disorders but not necessarily meeting the number of criteria required for any or all of the potential diagnoses (Regier, Narrow, Kuhl, & Kupfer, 2009). This leads to the dilemma of potentially underdiagnosing or overdiagnosing, because the complexity, severity, and variability of individual experiences cannot be captured with rigid predetermined criteria. The approach that is suggested for the DSM-5 and appears to have strong support in the clinical and scholarly community is the use of dimensional assessment, "intended to make diagnoses of mental disorders a matter of degree, rather than just a yes or no assessment" (CMAJ, 2010, p. 16).

One potential benefit of using a dimensional rather than categorical assessment is the possible reduction of stigma associated with diagnostic labels (Ben-Zeev, Young, & Corrigan, 2010). Dimensional assessment might also better capture "the first-person experience of mental illness. This basis would ensure that the *DSM* truly represents the experience of mental illness and not how mental illness appears to an outside observer (i.e., clinician)" (Flanagan & Blashfield, 2010, p. 474). It remains to be seen how dimensional assessment is incorporated into the DSM-5 and how it will be operationalized in practice.

One difficulty with all diagnostic models is the focus on mental illness rather than mental wellness. Slade (2009) suggests that the conceptual framework, *The Complete State Model of Mental Health,* originally presented by Corey Keyes, "provides a better match with the values of recovery" (p. 126). This model, presented in Chapter 3, presents both the subjective experiences of wellness with the presence of (illness) symptoms. This holistic, person-centered view of the experience of mental illness is not only consistent with a recovery perspective, but also aligns with the occupational therapy perspective of understanding context, meaning, and inclusion, as well as capitalizing on an individual's strengths to improve overall function.

Attitudes and procedures regarding the diagnostic process are undergoing dramatic shifts with the trend toward a wellness and recovery perspective. Since part of this perspective is a focus on context and function, occupational therapists have a valuable opportunity to increase their visibility and influence in mental health practice by sharing their specific expertise in these areas.

PSYCHOPATHOLOGY

Inherent in the diagnostic process is the recognition of specific symptoms of mental illness. While the trend in mental health practice is toward minimizing the focus on symptoms alone and avoiding overpathologizing behavior, appropriate and effective treatment planning is dependent on identifying and understanding the symptoms of mental illness and the various ways they can interfere with a person's recovery. Symptoms of mental illness may present in a wide variety of combinations, and there are various schemas for organizing the information. The following is one example of a categorical organization of **psychopathology** and descriptions of common symptoms within each category.

Thought

Thought includes what are considered to be the higher intellectual functions of abstraction, reasoning, judgment, and analysis. Common deficits seen in this area are concrete thinking and an inability to recognize or correct errors (which may be due to increased impulsivity). Concrete thinking includes thought processes focused on immediate experiences and specific objects or events as well as an inability to think metaphorically or abstractly. Occupational therapists also pay particular attention to one's **executive function**, which is the ability to connect these mental processes with current actions. People with deficits in executive function have difficulty in planning, organizing, and strategizing.

A specific form of psychopathology involving the content of thought is delusions, which are deep-seated beliefs not based in reality. The presentation of factual proof will not typically change such beliefs. There are many types of delusions, including delusions of grandeur as well as self-deprecating and paranoid delusions. These are typically not an exaggeration of real experiences, but rather an essentially inaccurate, though powerful, belief. For example, an individual with a delusion of grandeur may believe he or she has supernatural powers, is a famous historical figure, or has an important secret mission to accomplish. Some delusions are relatively harmless with little associated dysfunction, while others leave an individual extremely incapacitated in daily living activities or, as sometimes is the case with paranoid delusions, make him or her a danger to self or others.

Another form of disordered thought is obsession, which is a specific and repetitive thought that is typically unwanted and cannot be eliminated by reason. Obsessions are often found in conjunction with compulsions, whereby a person attempts to extinguish the obsession by acting upon it. Although obsessive-compulsive disorder (OCD) is a diagnosis, it is possible to have either or both symptoms without meeting the criteria for OCD or any other diagnosis. Again, the level of associated dysfunction is quite variable. The practice of **hoarding** has received much attention in the popular as well as scholarly literature. This behavior is not limited to OCD and may be found in people with no diagnosis or with any of the anxiety disorders, depression, or dementia. There is an ongoing debate as to whether or not hoarding should be considered its own diagnostic category. Dr. Sanjaya Saxena concluded that "On the basis of phenomenology, comorbidity patterns, family and genetic studies, and neuroimaging data, compulsive hoarding syndrome appears to be a discrete entity with a unique and characteristic pattern of core symptoms, associated features, and neurobiological abnormalities that differ from OCD" (First, 2006). One of these features is that there appears to be a relationship between the severity of hoarding behavior and a history of stressful or traumatic life events (Tolin, Meunier, Frost, & Steketee, 2010).

Language

Speech disturbances are often considered to be part of thought disorder, but they are so common in severe mental illness that it is easier to study them as a separate category. Some people who experience these symptoms seem oblivious to the oddity of their speech, but other people find it exhausting to engage in casual conversation and may avoid it whenever possible. Occupational therapists must be knowledgeable of these symptoms in order to appreciate the effort clients may be expending in conversation and also to understand the meaning of their communication. Table 6-2 provides examples of some of the abnormal speech patterns that can occur with severe mental illness.

TABLE 6-2. Abnormal Speech Patterns Associated with Mental Illness

Term	Description	Example
Concreteness	Extremely literal verbal responses due to concrete thinking patterns. The speaker does not recognize the nuances of language, including abstractions or metaphors.	"Reading can open a whole new world." *Response:* "And then the lava flows out of the cracks."
Loosening of Associations	Ideas shift from one subject to another that is completely unrelated. The speaker does not show any awareness that the topics are unconnected.	"What is your name?" *Response:* "A rose by any other name . . . I wish I could get out of here . . . Jigsaw puzzles are fun."
Perseveration	Repetition of the same word, phrase, or idea. Also, an inability to shift from one task to another.	"What do you want to do today?" *Response:* "Today is Tuesday, I always do wash on Tuesday, always on Tuesday it's wash."
Circumstantiality and Tangentiality	The person digresses, giving unnecessary, irrelevant information. When speech is circumstantial there is difficulty getting to the point of the conversation, yet in the person's mind, the answers are related. In tangential speech the person starts answering a question but then rapidly digresses.	"When were you in the hospital?" *Circumstantial response:* "I went to this great concert last summer after I visited my aunt." *Tangential response:* "In the fall . . . the leaves were so beautiful . . . They were like my paintings . . . My art is my soul."
Echolalia	Repetition (echo) of the words and phrases of others. This speech is repetitive and persistent.	"What is your name?" *Response:* "What is your name? Your name, your name."
Clanging	The sound or rhyme of the words takes precedence over the meaning or content of the replies.	"What is your occupation?" *Response:* "I used to be a lawyer, now a liar, lollipops, licenses, and licorice."
Neologism	An invented word that may closely resemble an existing word or may be known only to the individual.	"Why were you admitted to the hospital?" *Response:* "It come from too much normiation, a sort of infesteration of some sort. I was being institized."

Although language is usually considered a cognitive ability, speech or language production is motoric in nature. A decreased intelligibility of speech (dysarthria) may be due to long- and short-term side effects of psychotropic medication. Also, in general, illnesses that affect the nervous system have the potential for causing a variety of problems that can interfere with the production of speech and language.

Perception and Sensation

Perception is the ability to attain information via the senses and then process and interpret the stimuli. Another closely related term is *sensory processing*. Although problems in both areas can exist independently, they often overlap and it is sometimes difficult to clearly identify the resulting dysfunction as attributable to one or the other. Perception is usually considered a cognitive process with the emphasis on interpretation, whereas the term *sensory-processing deficits* implies that the dysfunction is in the delivery or integration of the sensory message. It is well documented that people with persistent mental illness (particularly schizophrenia) commonly experience hallucinations, but it is also true that there is a higher than average incidence of other perceptual disturbances, as well as problems with sensory processing and integration, which are found in this population (Javitt, 2009; Leitman et al., 2010). These deficits include distorted time sense and spatial awareness, poor visual perception, poor body scheme, hyper- or hyposensitivity to stimuli, and astereognosis, which is the inability to identify common objects by touch. Also, people with serious mental illness may display a variety of sensorimotor symptoms either as a direct result of the illness or as side effects of psychotropic medication. These include abnormal muscle tone, abnormal gait, and apraxia, which is an inability to plan and coordinate complex motor actions. In addition, a decreased pain and temperature response as well as an increased sensitivity to sunlight may also be found in people with severe mental illness. These deficits are often subtle and may go unrecognized. However, a careful evaluation of these possible conditions is essential, as they pose potential safety threats to the individual.

Hallucinations

Hallucinations are perceptual images experienced as sensations but not based on actual stimulation from the external environment. Hallucinations can involve any of the senses: visual (seeing images), auditory (hearing voices or sounds), tactile (feeling sensations on the skin surface), gustatory (taste), olfactory (smell), and somatic (feeling sensations within the body). There have been many attempts to correlate kinds of hallucination with an actual diagnosis, but care must be taken not to oversimplify the relationship between symptom and diagnosis. For example, there are many theories regarding damage to the brain and the presence of visual and tactile hallucinations, yet there are also many exceptions. Nevertheless, there are some significant patterns regarding kinds of hallucinations and diagnosis. For example, visual or olfactory hallucinations may precede grand mal seizures. Tactile hallucinations are often experienced during alcohol or drug withdrawal, and gustatory hallucinations may indicate brain trauma.

Hallucinations seem very real to the person experiencing them and can cause dysfunction in several ways. The relationship between the manifestation of hallucinations and specific dysfunctions is described in the model of functional deficits (MacRae, 1997) and shown in Table 6-3.

The model of functional deficits is a framework for examining the phenomenon of hallucinations from an occupational therapy perspective. In this model, various types of dysfunction are correlated to specific manifestations of hallucinations.

For example, when the dominant feature of the hallucinations is the *content* (such as what the voices are saying), typically there is evidence of poor self-esteem and observations may include frequent self-deprecating remarks, poor posture, lack of social interaction, and poor motivation. However, when the dominant feature of the hallucinations is the *intrusiveness* of the phenomenon, dysfunctions will more

TABLE 6-3. Model of Functional Deficits Associated with Hallucinations

Classification		Observable Behavior
Class 0	Insufficient information	None identifiable.
Class I	No hallucinations	None.
Class II	Intermittent hallucinations with minimal or no functional deficits	Phenomena reported upon questioning or in appropriate settings. Individual may appear withdrawn.
Class III	Intermittent or persistent hallucinations with functional deficits related to the content of the phenomena	Evidence of poor self-esteem, such as frequent self-deprecating remarks, poor posture, lack of social interaction, and poor motivation.
Class IV	Intermittent or persistent hallucinations with functional deficits directly related to the intrusiveness of the phenomena	Inappropriate behavior while apparently responding to internal stimuli. Inappropriate affect such as giggling not related to the outside environment. Conversations with the self. Poor attention to the task on hand but can be redirected to task and surroundings.
Class V	Intermittent or persistent hallucinations with functional deficits related to *both* content and intrusiveness of the phenomena	See Classes III and IV.
Class VI	Persistent hallucinations with profound functional deficits. Generally acute	Inability to appropriately respond to the external environment.

Adapted from MacRae (1997)

likely include inappropriate behavior while apparently responding to internal stimuli. Observations might include behaviors such as giggling for no apparent reason, conversations with the self, and poor attention to tasks.

Illusions

A milder form of perceptual distortion is an illusion, in which the outside object causing the stimuli is real but the person misinterprets the object (for example, a lamppost may be mistaken for a robot). Like hallucinations, illusions may involve any of the senses, but auditory and visual illusions are most common.

Affect

Affect refers to the observable behavior representing one's emotions, but (as shown in Figure 6-4, which depicts classical drama masks) it is not always possible to know what someone is feeling. It is also sometimes difficult to determine a pathological affect because there are normal fluctuations in everyone's emotional state. The demonstration of emotions is partially dictated by culture, so awareness of and sensitivity to a person's background are essential. Disturbances of affect can be a direct result of a mental illness or a neurological disorder such as cerebrovascular accident (CVA). Changes in affect can also be drug induced. *Flat affect* refers to a lack of observable emotion. Other emotional states, such as anxiety or hostility, may be considered pathologic if the emotional state is either inappropriate or out of proportion to the environmental stimuli.

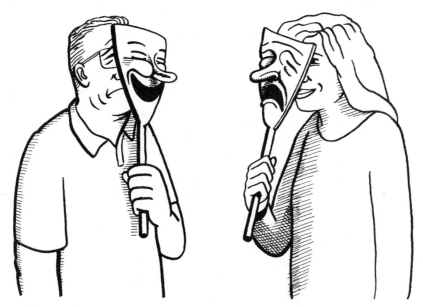

FIGURE 6-4. Affect is an Observable Behavior Representing Emotion

Slade, M. Personal Recovery and Mental Illness: A Guide for Mental Health Professionals. Figure 14-1, p. 127. Copyright ©2009 Mike Slade. Reprinted with the permission of Cambridge University Press.

Depression

Depression is one of the most common affective symptoms. It may be seen with many psychiatric diagnoses, including not only major depression and dysthymic disorder but also schizophrenia, the dementias, and personality disorders. Mania is a condition in which the individual responds in an eager, exuberant, and even joyful manner, regardless of the environmental reality. Although mania is considered a disordered affect, the dysfunction resulting from the manic state is usually caused by the associated features of poor judgment and impulsivity. Therefore, mania might best be described as a syndrome consisting of affect, thought, and motor dysfunctions.

Lability

Lability is a state of unstable emotions, which may present in many different ways. For example, one individual may swing rapidly between laughter and tears, while another person may cry uncontrollably yet be unable to identify a reason for the tears. Paying particular attention to the individual's previous level of emotional display and cultural background is necessary to identify a true lability accurately.

Because *affect* refers only to the observable behavior associated with feelings, it is difficult to categorize or even identify some altered or impaired feelings. For example, a person with a mental illness may experience intense feelings of rage and yet have no visible signs of such intense feelings. Another altered emotional state common in mental illness is anhedonia, which is an inability to experience pleasure. Some individuals experience a milder form of this symptom known as hypohedonia, which is defined as a decreased ability to experience pleasure.

Orientation

Orientation refers to a person's awareness of time, place, and person. Typically, the first orientation to be lost is time. The individual may know where and who he or she is, yet not know the date, month, or even year. The second orientation to be lost is orientation to place, and the last is orientation to person, which includes the recognition of both the self and significant others. This pattern is so predictable that a standard method of charting has been developed to represent orientation: O (orientation) $\times$ 3 means that the individual is oriented to time, place, and person; O $\times$ 2 means orientation is to place and person only; and O $\times$ 1 means that the person is oriented only to person. If orientation was lost in a different order than that of time, place, and person, this must be explicitly stated. Table 6-4 provides examples of this form of documentation.

Memory

The most common categorization of memory is the simple division into short term and long term. However, memory is quite complex and further categorization is helpful to determine specific functional deficits associated with its loss. Table 6-5 describes one classification system of types of memory and their clinical significance.

TABLE 6-4. Orientation of Time, Place, and Person

Description	Clinical Interpretation	Charting
Mrs. Wong states that she is in Hong Kong in 1948 when she is actually in present-day San Francisco. She recognizes her children and can report her own name.	Mrs. Wong is not oriented to place or time; she is oriented to person.	0 × 1
Mr. Geary recognizes all of his family members, as well as his doctor. He is aware that he is presently hospitalized in his hometown but frequently is unclear about the day and month and occasionally does not know the year.	Mr. Geary is clearly oriented to person and place; however, his time disorientation fluctuates in severity.	0 × 2
Ms. Tenaka was administered a mental status exam during which she was able to accurately report her name, her presence in the psychiatric emergency room, and the correct date.	Ms. Tenaka is fully oriented to time, place, and person.	0 × 3

© Cengage Learning 2013

TABLE 6-5. Types of Memory

Type	Description	Example
Procedural memory	An automatic sequence of behavior such as conditioned responses	Despite significant deterioration of her mental status, Mrs. Makiba remembers to retrieve the newspaper from the porch and make a pot of coffee by 8 A.M as she has done every day for years.
Declarative memory	Memory specific to consciously learned facts such as school subjects	Mr. Alvarado is diagnosed with schizophrenia. He has a history of failure in jobs and has been unable to pass classes at the community college due to poor attendance. Nevertheless, he is able to recall much of the material from the lectures he was able to attend and he is quite knowledgeable about current events.
Semantic memory	The knowledge of the meaning of words and the ability to classify information or ideas	Mr. Hackett lives in a supervised residential care home, where he is considered to be quite proficient at solitary crossword puzzles.
Episodic memory	The knowledge of personal experiences	Mrs. Yen spends three mornings a week meeting at the cultural center, where she enjoys sharing stories and reminiscing with her friends.
Prospective memory	The capacity to remember to carry out actions in the future. In essence, "to remember to remember"	After a home evaluation, the occupational therapist concluded that Ms. Cohen can live independently. She has been able to keep all her appointments and safely operates a stove in the kitchen.

© Cengage Learning 2013

A knowledge of these specific types of memory will help the clinician identify an individual's assets as well as deficits and plan treatment accordingly. For example, procedural memory is often retained when declarative memory is not. By designing a treatment plan that allows desired responses to become automatic, the therapist can help clients become more functional.

Another example of clinical significance is the identification of prospective memory, which is important for independent living. Examples of prospective memory include remembering to pay bills, go to the doctor, and turn off the stove.

People who have severe memory deficits, as is found with many neurocognitive disorders or a substance-induced persisting amnestic disorder, often engage in confabulation. Confabulation is the unknowing fabrication of events to fill in the gaps of true memory. It is not intentional lying, as the person is not aware that he or she is doing so. It is also not delusional, as the person will not be particularly invested in, or attached to, the confabulated statements.

Energy and Motoric Response

Observable changes in the energy or activity level of a person with a mental illness are sometimes assumed to be a consequence of **psychotropic** medications. While drugs can have such effects, it is also common to experience increased or decreased energy levels due directly to a mental illness. It is not always possible to predict when, or if, this fluctuation will accompany a mental illness or what form it will take. For example, one person with depression may appear lethargic while another person is quite agitated and yet a third person with depression shows little or no change in energy level.

Many people with serious mental illness experience disruption of the sleep–wake cycle. For example, either excessive or insufficient sleep patterns are often found in people experiencing major depression. Too little or too much sleep can contribute to poor overall functioning and to worsening of other symptoms. "Rest and sleep" is an area of occupation that "includes activities related to obtaining restorative rest and sleep that supports healthy active engagement in other areas of occupation" (AOTA, 2008, p. 632).

Changes in sleep patterns can also be the result of psychotropic medication. Medication-induced sleep problems may be resolved by changes in dose, frequency, or time of administration of medication.

Specific motor symptoms may be related to the severity of the mental disorder. For example, catatonia, which is rigidity or immobility, would most likely be observed during an acute and severe psychotic episode rather than as a persistent state. Other possible symptoms involving motor function are stereotypy, the repetition of apparently senseless actions; tics, involving muscular spasms or twitching; and compulsions, which are repetitive, irrational behaviors acted out in response to an overwhelming urge.

PSYCHIATRIC INTERVENTION IN THE ERA OF RECOVERY

Diagnoses and symptoms are the traditional focus of a medical or clinical orientation to the treatment of mental illness. However, as discussed in Chapter 1, the specific expertise that is part of this orientation can be a critical part of an individual's road to recovery. "The change in a recovery-focused service is that this expertise is meshed with the consumer's expertise about their own values, beliefs, goals, and preferred approaches to meeting challenges. In a partnership relationship, the job of the clinician is to help the person come to the best choice *for them*" (Slade, 2009, p. 173).

One approach that is gaining acceptance is establishing formalized **shared decision making**. According to Torrey and Drake (2010), "the mental health studies demonstrate that shared decision making interventions improve decision making (more knowledge, participation, and congruence with values), and some studies have shown improved adherence with treatment and satisfaction with care" (p. 434). However, Mahone (2008) reports that although shared decision making and self-management techniques appear to be accepted in mental health treatment, an attitude of acceptance is often not found regarding self-management of medication.

Psychotropic Medication

Psychotropic medication is now the most common form of treatment for many mental illnesses. However, psychopharmacology is not without controversy and pharmaceuticals rarely work in isolation to control all of the symptoms and deficits found in persons with mental illness; drug therapy should be viewed as one possible facet of comprehensive, interdisciplinary treatment. **Compliance** with prescribed medication regimes is often the primary goal and focus of clinically oriented intervention. But, "compliance is rooted in medical paternalism and is at odds with principles of person centered care and evidence based medicine" (Deegan & Drake, 2006, p. 1636). Prescribing clinicians walk a fine line between respecting the rights of the client to choose a course of treatment and ensuring that the client has access to information and understands all of the positive and negative consequences of taking or not taking prescribed medication. In an effort to improve communication regarding medication choices, several tools are now being utilized. One such tool, called CommonGround, was created by Dr. Patricia E. Deegan based on a pilot study conducted by Deegan, Rapp, Holter, and Riefer (2008). CommonGround is a computer-based program designed to help the client prepare for the visit with the psychiatrist by guiding him or her in developing a one-page health report listing concerns and personal goals as well as summarizing progress. The goal of this process is to arrive at a shared decision, which is then printed so the client will have a reminder of the agreed-upon course of treatment and steps for recovery.

Additional tools include the Wellness Recovery Action Plan (WRAP) (discussed in Chapter 1), as well as other psychiatric advance directives. These directives are developed when the individual is stable, in order to retain some control over treatment when in crisis. While many people complete such plans without professional help, a shared decision-making process with a member or members of the professional team does have some benefits. "Many consumers engage a provider in creation of directives to facilitate decisions about treatment, confirm details of previous treatment, ensure timely access to the document, or provide clarification" (Henderson, Lee, Herman, & Dragatsi, 2009, p. 1390).

Although occupational therapists do not prescribe medication, the occupational therapy focus on function (doing) provides an ideal perspective from which to observe the effectiveness of the medication regimen and work with both the team and the client to establish an individualized and optimum plan of treatment. Table 6-6 lists

TABLE 6-6. Interventions for Medication Management

Reason	Description	Interventions
Delusions or beliefs of potential harm	Paranoid delusions may include fears of poisoning or other physical damage. However, clients also may refuse medication based on nonpathological belief systems grounded in their sociocultural and religious upbringing.	Trust building—Clients who have a solid therapeutic relationship with someone in the system are less likely to think they will come to harm. Correcting misinformation— erroneous beliefs such as an individual's fear of becoming a "drug addict"—can be addressed through education.
Admission of illness	Denial is a common reaction to the onset of severe, especially chronic, illness. With psychiatric disorders, there are the added problems of dealing with social stigma and the possible presence of thought disorder.	Create an accepting environment—Rather than attempting to "convince" someone of his or her illness, it is important to convey that individuals are accepted for who they are. Peer counseling—Often clients can benefit from hearing about the personal experience of others. Education—The realities of the illness may not be as frightening as the assumptions. It is important for clients to know that many people are able to live satisfying and productive lives with the presence of a mental illness.
Side effects	Individual reaction to psychotropic medication is extremely variable. Many side effects disappear or decrease with time. However, others may be ongoing and difficult to tolerate or manage.	Medical interventions—May include switching medications or reducing dosages as well as adding additional medications. Educational techniques (individual or group) for medication management— May include instruction in nutrition (increasing fluid and fiber, decreasing caffeine); avoidance of direct sunlight (sunscreen, outing schedule, hats, etc.); regulation of sleep and exercise as well as relaxation techniques.
Cognitive deficits	Deficits may include poor memory, confusion, poor time orientation, concrete thinking, poor organizational skills	Medical intervention—Simplify regime by decreasing dosages per day and using long-acting agents. Supervision—Health care staff or appropriately instructed caregivers. Memory and orientation strategies—Reminder notes, pill organizers, schedules.
Perceived loss of freedom	Complaints of restrictive monitoring and dislike of precautions, including recommendations to avoid caffeine or alcohol as well as the necessity for remaining on a schedule and reporting to the clinic for follow-up lab work.	Education—Clients are more likely to adhere to recommendations if they understand the consequences of avoiding advice. Change of medication—Choice may be for a medication with limited side effects or precautions even if it is considered less effective than alternatives. Adaptation of daily living—Helping client switch to decaffeinated nonalcoholic beverages, use of calendar, day planner, and/or clock and visual reminders.

commonly cited reasons for refusal or inability to take medication and some techniques that the occupational therapist or other team members may use to help the individual adhere to prescribed treatment. However, the ultimate choice remains the client's and that must be respected.

Access and Technology

Technology has dramatically facilitated the ability of people with mental illness to be informed and involved in their choice of treatments. The Internet is not only a source of information about conditions; it also provides access to support and advocacy groups, legal advice, and networking sites. (See Suggested Resources in this chapter and also in Chapter 1.) In addition, there are computer programs that also facilitate recovery-oriented interventions. For example, the previously mentioned Common-Ground program provides many informational links that can be used along with the generated shared decision plan.

Research conducted by Borzekowski et al. (2009) found that one third of the study participants used the Internet and over one half of the younger participants specifically used the Internet for health information. But even among "Internet non-users there was still interest in finding health information online; however, expense, lack of computer skills or knowledge, and difficulties with typing and reading prevented doing so" (p. 1265). Wellness Centers and other community-based services for people with mental illness often have Internet-capable computers for client use and are now routinely offering computer classes. An occupational therapist can evaluate for universal accessibility, such as ergonomically correct workstations and keyboards, as well as speech and vision adaptations.

Technology not only provides access to information but also to direct treatment. It is well documented that there is great shortage of psychiatric services especially in rural areas (Rural Healthy People, 2010; WHO, 2009). **Telepsychiatry** is one innovative technology developed to reduce this disparity. It is used to provide an array of services including diagnosis and assessment, as well as individual and group therapy. However, it is most widely used for medication management. Although primarily found in rural areas, it has also been introduced in areas with other underserved populations (Anthony, 1996; Hilty, Nesbitt, Kuenneth, Cruz, & Hales, 2007; Morgan, Patrick, & Magaletta, 2008; Savin, Garry, Zuccaro, & Novins, 2006). Telepsychiatry may also be useful situationally. "For example, certain psychological stressors—such as social anxiety, agoraphobia, or even physical challenges such as chronic pain or limited mobility—may make accessing services in the traditional face-to-face environment nearly impossible" (Simms, Gibson, & O'Donnell, 2011, p. 41). A systematic review conducted by García-Lizana and Muñoz-Mayorga (2010) suggests that there is "a strong hypothesis that videoconference-based treatment obtains the same results as face-to-face therapy" (p. 1).

An interesting and somewhat unexpected outcome of telepsychiatry is improved collaboration, communication, and effective teamwork among professionals (APA, 2011). This is, however, contingent on having a coordinator, who uses the available technology to disseminate information in a timely manner to all stakeholders. This is especially important when services are provided by different entities in different geographical locations such as occurs when a client is hospitalized.

In general, there is a high level of client satisfaction with telepsychiatry (APA, 2011) after an initial period of adjustment to the technology. The older population, with less experience with technology, as well as people who may be quite symptomatic, tend to require greater time to adjust to telepsychiatry but do eventually appear to gain equal benefit. Figure 6-5 describes a typical arrangement for a telepsychiatry appointment with a photograph of a client and her "on screen" psychiatrist.

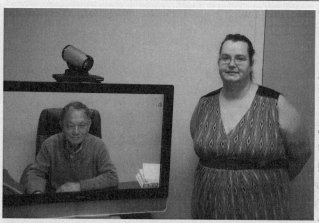

The interval between "telepsych" appointments varies depending on client concerns, new symptoms, side effects of medication, or any changes in medications, but the average length of time between appointments ranges between 2 and 12 weeks. Children are usually seen at more frequent intervals. The length of each session is also dictated by the individual needs of the client but routine appointments are generally between 15 and 30 minutes. The initial telepsych appointment, or an appointment after a major change in status such as discharge from the hospital, is typically at least 90 minutes. This allows for a thorough review of all medications, including those prescribed by primary care physicians, as well as the ordering of new prescriptions and necessary lab work. This investment of time is also crucial for relationship building between the psychiatrist and client.

The client is encouraged to prepare a list of questions prior to the session and a brief report on his or her health. This may be done informally or with the use of a specifically designed tool. The technology includes a video screen with camera and

(Continues)

FIGURE 6-5. A Telepsychiatry Session

audio capability for both the client and the psychiatrist. The environment is arranged for adequate light, minimal noise interference, and privacy. Although the client has the right to a private session with the psychiatrist, it is strongly recommended that another care provider, such as the psychiatric nurse or case manager, be present to later clarify communication from the psychiatrist and provide additional information to the psychiatrist as needed. Some sessions may also include family members or other support persons for the client.

FIGURE 6-5. A Telepsychiatry Session (*continued*)

SUMMARY

The delivery of mental health services is going through a period of rapid transformation in which occupational therapists, as all mental health clinicians, must align their practice with new trends. Many of the diagnostic controversies discussed in this chapter are being addressed through the revision of the *DSM* and *ICD*, as well as through the development of additional models to explain mental illness. However, it remains to be seen how these revisions will transform practice. Especially in this time of great change, clinicians practicing in the field need to be as specific and clear as possible in professional discussions and documentation, and further develop collaborative models of service, together with people with the lived experience of mental illness, as well as their support networks and communities. Furthermore, clinicians can be role models for the sensitive use of terminology and advocates for educating the public about mental health.

The changes in perspective seen in the revision of the diagnostic process are very much in line with the philosophy and practice of occupational therapy. Therefore, the profession has an opportunity to not only be responsive to changes but also be proactive leaders in this new paradigm.

Occupational therapists primarily focus their practice on the alleviation of dysfunction for engagement in occupation, but a thorough understanding of symptoms and diagnoses is essential for all clinicians working in mental health. People with mental illness present with a range of symptoms and dysfunctions of varying frequency and severity, and it is not possible in this chapter to do justice to all presentations. However, forthcoming chapters on specific disorders provide more in-depth discussions of commonly seen diagnoses, dysfunctions, and symptoms.

Acknowledgment: Material for the diagnostic case illustration and client quotes regarding diagnosis was gathered in focus groups conducted by Carol Underwood. Invaluable assistance on the telepsychiatry discussion was provided by Sally Mann, RN.

REVIEW QUESTIONS

1. How does the use of clinical terminology help or hinder the recovery process?
2. What is the role of the occupational therapist in the diagnostic process?
3. How would you justify the use of the *DSM* for diagnosis? What argument would you offer against use of the *DSM*?
4. How can technology promote recovery?

REFERENCES

Alarcon, R., Becker, A., Lewis-Fernandez, R., Like, R., Desai, P., Foulks, E., et al. (2009). Issues for DSM-V: The role of culture in psychiatric diagnosis. *The Journal of Nervous and Mental Disease, 197,* 559–560.

American Occupational Therapy Association (AOTA). (2002). Occupational therapy practice framework: Domain and process. *American Journal of Occupational Therapy, 56*(6), 614–639.

American Occupational Therapy Association (AOTA). (2008). Occupational therapy practice framework: Domain and process (2nd ed.). *American Journal of Occupational Therapy, 62,* 625–683.

American Psychiatric Association (APA). (1980). *Diagnostic and statistical manual of mental disorders* (3rd ed.). Washington, DC: Author.

American Psychiatric Association (APA). (2000). *Diagnostic and statistical manual of mental disorders* (4th ed., text revision). Washington, DC: Author.

American Psychiatric Association (2011). *Telepsychiatry.* Underserved Clearinghouse. Linked Document. Retrieved from http://www.psych.org

American Psychiatric Association. (n.d.). DSM-5 Development. Retrieved from http://www.dsm5.org

Anthony, G. (1996). Telepsychiatry in Appalachia. *The American Behavioral Scientist, 39*(5), 602–615.

Ben-Zeev, D., Young, M., & Corrigan, P. (2010). DSM-V and the stigma of mental illness. *Journal of Mental Health, 19*(4), 318–327.

Borzekowski, D., Leith, J., Medoff, D., Potts, W., Dixon, L., Balis, T., et al. (2009). Use of the Internet and other media for health information among clinic outpatients with serious mental illness. *Psychiatric Services, 60*(9), 1265–1268.

CMAJ. (2010). Changes to mental illness handbook not taken lightly. *Canadian Medical Association Journal,* 15–16.

Deegan, P., Rapp, C., Holter, M., & Riefer, M. (2008). A program to support shared decision making in an outpatient psychiatric medication clinic. *Psychiatric Services, 59,* 603–605.

Deegan, P., & Drake, R. (2006). Shared decision making and medication management in the recovery process. *Psychiatric Services,* 57. 1636–1639.

Druss, B., & Reisinger Walker, E. (2011). *The Synthesis Project: Mental Disorders and Medical Comorbidity.* Robert Wood Johnson Foundation.

First, M. (Ed.). (2006). *Obsessive compulsive spectrum disorders conference proceedings.* Washington, DC: American Psychiatric Association.

Flanagan, E., & Blashfield, R. (2010). Increasing clinical utility by aligning the *DSM* and ICD with clinicians' conceptualizations. *Professional Psychology: Research and Practice, 41*(6), 474–481.

García-Lizana, F., & Muñoz-Mayorga, I. (2010). What about telepsychiatry? A systematic review. *The Primary Care Companion to the Journal of Clinical Psychiatry, 12*(2), 19.

Glackin, S. (2010). Tolerance and illness: The politics of medical and psychiatric classification. *Journal of Medicine and Philosophy, 35,* 449–465.

Hebebrand, J., & Buitelaar, J. (2011). On the way to DSM-V. *European Child & Adolescent Psychiatry, 20*, 57–60.

Henderson, C., Lee, R., Herman, D., & Dragatsi, D. (2009). From psychiatric advance directives to the joint crisis plan. *Psychiatric Services, 60*(10), 1390.

Hilty, D., Nesbitt, T., Kuenneth, C., Cruz, G., & Hales, R. (2007). Rural versus suburban primary care needs, utilization, and satisfaction with telepsychiatric consultation. *The Journal of Rural Health, 23*(2), 163–165.

Javitt, D. (2009). Sensory processing in schizophrenia: Neither simple nor intact. *Schizophrenia Bulletin, 35*(6) 1059–1064.

Leitman, D., Sehatpour, P., Higgins, B., Foxe, J., Silipo, G., & Javitt, D. (2010). Sensory deficits and distributed hierarchical dysfunction in schizophrenia. *American Journal of Psychiatry, 167*, 818–827.

MacRae, A. (1997). The model of functional deficits associated with hallucinations. *American Journal of Occupational Therapy, 51*, 57–63.

Mahone, I. (2008). Shared decision making and serious mental illness. *Archives of Psychiatric Nursing, 22*(6), 334–343.

McGruder, J. (2001). Life experience is not a disease or why medicalizing madness is counterproductive to recovery. *Occupational Therapy in Mental Health, 17*, 59–80.

Morgan, R., Patrick, A., & Magaletta, P. (2008). Does the use of telemental health alter the treatment experience? Inmates' perceptions of telemental health versus face-to-face treatment modalities. *Journal of Consulting and Clinical Psychology, 76*(1), 158–162.

Regier, D., Narrow, W., Kuhl, E., & Kupfer, D. (2009). The conceptual development of DSM-V. *American Journal of Psychiatry, 166(6)*, 645–650.

Rural Healthy People 2010—*Healthy People 2010: A Companion Document for Rural Areas.* Retrieved from http://www.srph.tamhsc.edu/centers/rhp2010/

Savin, D., Garry, M., Zuccaro, P., & Novins, D. (2006). Telepsychiatry for treating rural American Indian youth. *Journal of the American Academy of Child and Adolescent Psychiatry, 45*(4), 484–488.

Simms, D., Gibson, K., & O'Donnell, S. (2011). To use or not to use: Clinicians' perceptions of telemental health. *Canadian Psychology, 52*(1), 41–51.

Slade, M. (2009). *Personal recovery and mental illness: a guide for mental health professionals.* New York: Cambridge University Press.

Soderberg, P., Tungstrom, S., & Armelius, B. (2005). Reliability of Global Assessment of Functioning ratings made by clinical psychiatric staff. *Psychiatric Services, 56*(4), 434–438.

Tolin, D., Meunier, S., Frost, R., & Steketee, G. (2010). Course of compulsive hoarding and its relationship to life events. *Depression and Anxiety, 27*(9), 829–838.

Torrey, W., & Drake, R. (2010). Practicing shared decision making in the outpatient psychiatric care of adults with severe mental illnesses: Redesigning care for the future. *Community Mental Health, 46*, 433–440.

Wakefield, J. (2010). Misdiagnosing normality: Psychiatry's failure to address the problem of false positive diagnosis of mental disorder in a changing professional environment. *Journal of Mental Health, 19*(4), 337–351.

Widiger, T., & Samuel, D. (2005). Diagnostic categories or dimensions? A question for the Diagnostic and Statistical Manual of Mental Disorders—Fifth Edition. *Journal of Abnormal Psychology, 114*(4), 494–504.

World Health Organization (WHO). (2001). *International classification of functioning, disability and health (ICF).* Geneva: WHO.

World Health Organization (WHO). (2009). *Increasing access to health workers in remote and rural areas through improved retention.* Retrieved from http://www.who.int/hrh/migration/background_paper.pdf

SUGGESTED RESOURCES

Medical Terminology

Many new terms have been introduced in this chapter that will also be used in other chapters. Therefore, it is strongly recommended that students have at least one medical dictionary to study clinical terminology. Suggested sources include the most recent editions of the following:

Dorland's medical dictionary. Philadelphia: Saunders.

Miller, B., & Keane, C. *Encyclopedia and dictionary of medicine, nursing, and allied health.* Philadelphia: Saunders.

Taber's cyclopedic medical dictionary. Philadelphia: F.A. Davis.

Websites

American Psychiatric Association: http://www.psych.org

Common Ground: http://www.patdeegan.com/commonground

DSM-5 Development: http://www.dsm5.org

MedlinePlus-National Library of Medicine: http://www.nlm.nih.gov/medlineplus/

Physicians' Desk Reference (PDRhealth): http://www.pdrhealth.com/

World Health Organization (WHO)–ICD: http://www.who.int/classifications/icd/en/

World Health Organization (WHO)–ICF: http://www.who.int/classifications/icf/en/

In addition, please see the list of related resources in Chapter 1.

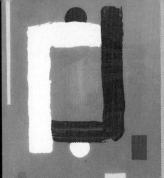

Chapter 7

Schizophrenia

Anne MacRae, PhD, OTR/L, BCMH, FAOTA
Lynne Andonian, PhD, OTR/L

KEY TERMS

cognitive deficits

extrapyramidal symptoms (EPS)

negative symptoms

positive symptoms

psychosis

CHAPTER OUTLINE

Introduction
Myths and Misconceptions
     Eight Common Myths
Etiology of Schizophrenia
Diagnosis of Schizophrenia
Positive Symptoms
     Delusions
     Sensory Deficits and Perceptual Distortion
Negative Symptoms
Prognosis
Collaborative Treatment
     Goal Attainment
     Psychotropic Medication
Occupational Therapy Intervention
     Evaluation
     Treatment
Summary

INTRODUCTION

Schizophrenia is a common disorder affecting approximately one in every 100 people. According to the National Institute of Mental Health (NIMH), approximately two million people will develop schizophrenia in their lifetime.

The disorder of schizophrenia has probably existed as long as humankind, but it has been interpreted in various physical, emotional, and spiritual ways by different generations and cultures. Even after the condition was recognized as a specific disease entity, diagnostic criteria have varied historically as well as geographically. In other words, depending on when and where diagnosticians were trained, they may or may not agree on the diagnosis of schizophrenia. Kraepelin (1919/1971) was one of the first European clinicians to recognize schizophrenia as a specific disease process. He called the condition dementia praecox because of its relatively early onset (usually in young adulthood) and its tendency to produce cognitive and behavioral changes in the individual. Bleuler (1911/1950) concluded that the term *dementia praecox* was essentially inadequate because there was not always cognitive deterioration and the disorder was not necessarily degenerative, as had been thought by Kraeplin. It was Bleuler who first suggested that schizophrenia was really one of several possible diseases that present in similar fashion. Therefore, he suggested that the term *dementia praecox* be replaced with *the group of schizophrenias*. Current diagnostic criteria have been strongly influenced by Kurt Schneider's (1959) identification of "first rank" symptoms of schizophrenia. These symptoms primarily consist of hallucinations (auditory especially), delusions, and bizarre behavior. This emphasis on the psychotic or **positive symptoms** of the disorder may not give an accurate representation of the functional level of people with schizophrenia.

Schizophrenia is referred to as a thought disorder, but not all forms of the disorder include long-term **cognitive deficits**. It is also referred to as a psychotic disorder, yet **psychosis** may be present only for some period during the course of the disease, not as a chronic condition. Both the terms *psychotic* and *thought disorder* could be applied to other conditions and lack the specificity needed to identify schizophrenia accurately.

MYTHS AND MISCONCEPTIONS

To this day, the term *schizophrenia* is often misused and the concept is frequently misunderstood. The misconceptions regarding this condition are rampant and must be dispelled before any meaningful understanding can be reached.

Eight Common Myths

Myth #1: "Split personality"

A person suffering from schizophrenia does not have a split personality. This is an unfortunate, and essentially inaccurate, description. Schizophrenia is not a personality disorder. The concept of split personality more accurately describes multiple personality disorder, which is now referred to as dissociative identity disorder.

Myth #2: Bad parenting

People with schizophrenia are not a product of bad parenting. No one can cause another person to have schizophrenia. It is caused by a combination of factors, including hereditary predisposition. If someone who inherits the predisposition to schizophrenia is in a particularly stressful environment, the illness may manifest itself earlier, have greater severity and frequency, and lead to a poorer outcome, but environment alone is not believed to cause the disorder. The vast majority of people who experience even catastrophic levels of stress do not develop schizophrenia. Although the popularity of this myth is waning, it still persists and is particularly damaging and painful to families—the very people who might best support people with schizophrenia.

Myth #3: Drug experimentation

Schizophrenia is not caused by taking drugs, yet recent studies show that those who use cannabis may have a more acute mode of onset for their first psychotic episode and those who had a first psychotic episode used substances three to five times more than the general population (Mazzoncini et al., 2010). Drug experimentation does not cause schizophrenia, yet it may be a risk factor, in combination with other gene and environmental interactions, for those who are genetically predisposed to the disorder (Kuepper et al., 2010). It is not uncommon for people with schizophrenia to have a coexisting diagnosis of substance abuse. In many cases, people with schizophrenia use drugs and alcohol in a maladaptive attempt to control their symptoms and the related distress.

Myth #4: Lack of motivation

People with schizophrenia do indeed try to get better. No one wants to have a disorder such as schizophrenia. People who take their prescribed medication and maintain psychosocial support usually fare better, but dysfunction may persist regardless of the level of treatment or consistency in taking medication. Psychotropic medication typically dampens or reduces the severity of the more obvious symptoms, but they often fail to eliminate them. There are a variety of reasons why someone may not be consistent with treatment. In some cases, appropriate treatment is simply unavailable. People with schizophrenia benefit the most from consistent and maintained intervention, yet community and outreach programs are scarce. Side effects of medications are problematic and may also affect the consistency of treatment—up to 54% of people taking atypical antipsychotics reported side effects such as "weight gain/hunger, tiredness/lethargy, and lack of coordination/muscle problems, such as tenderness, twitches, and tremors. Of those experiencing a side effect, less than 25 percent reported this side effect to their physician" (Cascade, Kalali, Mehra, & Meyer, 2010, p. 9).

Myth #5: Rising incidence

The incidence of schizophrenia is not on the rise, and there is no evidence to support the myth that it is increasing. However, modern Western society is stressful, particularly in the urban areas, so there may be a trend for people with schizophrenia to be more seriously disabled by the condition. Moreover, the deinstitutionalization movement created a situation in which people with schizophrenia are more visible in the community. This has had some positive effects but also many negative ones. Official estimates of the numbers of people who are homeless and have schizophrenia range from 15% to 35%, yet it may be much higher as it is difficult to measure (Folsom et al., 2005).

Myth #6: Institutionalization and disability

People with schizophrenia do not always live in institutions and are not always profoundly disabled. While it is true that in the past there were greater numbers of people who were institutionalized, they never constituted the majority of people who have schizophrenia. Most people with the disorder live with families, in residential care facilities in the community, or independently. The disorder has the potential for being gravely disabling, and it is a serious mental illness. However, the actual functional deficits are highly variable, and it is possible for some people to work, go to school, and raise a family.

Myth #7: Low intelligence

People with schizophrenia do not have below-average intelligence. Instead, the actual range of IQs of people with schizophrenia is highly variable. It is possible to have schizophrenia and be quite brilliant; it is also possible to have a coexisting developmental disability. Many, but not all, people with schizophrenia have a variety of cognitive deficits, but these do not necessarily include decreased intelligence. Rather, the executive function required to coordinate abstraction, judgment, and processing time with purposeful action may be impaired, which can be misinterpreted as low intelligence. "Executive impairment is one of the most robust and central deficits to be associated with schizophrenia and is seen across stages of the illness" (Liu et al., 2011, p. 87).

Myth #8: Danger and violence

People with schizophrenia are generally not dangerous and violent. This is a persistent and highly damaging myth largely fostered by the media. Although a statistical relationship does exist between schizophrenia and violence, only a small proportion of societal violence (less than 10%) can be attributed to people with schizophrenia (Walsh, 2002). People who are actively psychotic, particularly if they are paranoid, sometimes do become very violent, and this can be understandably frightening.

However, the typical profile of a violent offender is a young man with a history of violence and substance abuse, who may or may not have an untreated mental illness. Statistically, people who have schizophrenia, who live in the community, are no more likely to commit a serious crime than are people in the general population.

People with psychotic symptoms are more likely to hurt themselves than someone else (MacRae, 1993). Self-inflicted violence includes a wide variety of injuries, including mutilation and starvation. It also unfortunately includes successful suicide attempts. Current estimates of suicide by people with schizophrenia range from 5% to 10% with the greatest prevalence of suicide at illness onset (Palmer, Pankratz, & Bostwick, 2005). As many as 10% to 25% of people with schizophrenia attempt suicide (Robinson et al., 2009). It is also true that family members or significant others may sometimes be the target of violent outbursts.

Several recent reports have indicated that violent crimes committed by people with serious mental illness are on the rise. One explanation for this is the increased number of people with dual diagnoses. Clearly, violence related to drug and alcohol use is a significant problem, regardless of whether there is concurrent schizophrenia (see also Chapters 21 and 24).

Another explanation for this increase in violence is the shortage of appropriate treatment. As cutbacks in mental health and social services continue, people are forced to do without necessary treatment, become more disenfranchised, and experience both acute exacerbations and gradual decompensations of their illness. It could well be true that if the present trends continue, what started out as a myth about violence may become a self-fulfilling prophecy.

ETIOLOGY OF SCHIZOPHRENIA

Ideas regarding the cause of schizophrenia are constantly changing, but it is now generally accepted that there is some level of organic involvement, and many believe that at least a predisposition to the disease is hereditary. Stress may play a role in the onset of episodes and the severity of the disorder, but it is not the single causative factor.

Much of the neurological information about people with schizophrenia is due to the development of technology, including computerized tomography (CT), magnetic resonance imaging (MRI), magnetoencephalography (MEG), and positron emission tomography (PET) (Schneider, Backes, & Mathiak, 2009). Unfortunately, however, understanding of the findings lags behind the information explosion created by these new technologies. The list of hypothesized causes of schizophrenia is somewhat daunting and may, on the surface, seem contradictory, but it highlights the need for much further research. Currently in the United States, research dollars available to study schizophrenia are only a small fraction of the money spent to research other diseases. Also complicating the research efforts is the awareness that schizophrenia, like many other diseases, is probably caused by a combination of many factors. One of the criticisms of neurologic, and particularly structural, theories of etiology is that they cannot account for the episodic nature of the disease in some people or for its highly variable clinical outcome. Research is currently focusing on the interaction of many variables such as environment, genes, and neurotransmitters rather than a single entity (Kuepper et al., 2010; Watanabe, Someya, & Nawa, 2010).

Many different structural anomalies have been discovered in the brains of people with schizophrenia. These include lesions in the brain stem, enlargement of the ventricles, brain atrophy, and abnormalities in the limbic structures, cerebellum, and corpus callosum. There is a growing body of evidence that frontal lobe dysfunction, possibly related to the basal ganglia, plays a role in the development of **negative symptoms**. Structural abnormalities in the brain are clearly more common in people with schizophrenia than in the general population. However, the clinical significance of these findings is far from understood. The NIMH is currently conducting research exploring the human genome and the possibility that schizophrenia is a developmental disability that manifests itself after puberty. Possessing a given gene explains less than 50% of the causality of mental illnesses, supporting the assumption that multiple factors influence the development of schizophrenia (Andreasen, 2001). Genetic variants in catechol-O-methyltransferase (COMT) might be involved in the modulation of neurocognitive functions and increase the risk of schizophrenia (Liao et al., 2009).

One of the most prevalent theories of etiology concerns the role of the neurotransmitter dopamine. It is hypothesized that people with schizophrenia have either an excess of dopamine or an excessive quantity of dopamine receptors, making the neurotransmitter more effective. No reliable measure presently exists to determine specific amounts of neurotransmitters in the brain, but it is known that antipsychotic medication, which often decreases overtly psychotic symptoms, affects dopamine levels. Therefore, it might be assumed that excessive dopamine is particularly related to positive symptoms. Although there has been a tremendous amount of emphasis placed on the role of dopamine, other neurotransmitters, specifically norepinephrine, serotonin, and glutamate, as well as certain neuropeptides, are also being studied (Tibbo, Hanstock, Valiakalayil, & Allen, 2004). A new atypical antipsychotic acting on both dopamine and serotonin receptors is asenapine, which has been found to be efficacious on positive symptoms with less weight gain, which is a notable difference compared with the other atypical agents (Minassian & Young, 2010). Newer research by researchers is focusing on the receptors that normalize glutamate neurotransmission (Hui, Wardwell, & Tsai, 2009).

Another promising area of research is the role of a virus or viruses in the development of schizophrenia. There are viruses that stay inactive for many years and then start to grow slowly. Thus, it is hypothesized that a possible cause of schizophrenia is exposure to certain viruses prenatally while involved areas of the brain are being developed (Buka, Cannon, Torrey, & Yolken, 2007; Boksa, 2008). The person's subsequent deterioration in adolescence or young adulthood may be the direct result of a virus or an autoimmune reaction triggered by a virus. Evidence to support this theory is growing. For example, there is a higher than average incidence of people with schizophrenia who are born in the winter or spring months, which coincides with the epidemiological patterns of many viruses. Moreover, low birth weight is more common than average in people with schizophrenia, possibly suggesting a viral infection *in utero*. Research suggests that advanced paternal age at the time of birth of the offspring may also be a risk factor for adult schizophrenia (Brown et al., 2002).

There are many theories about the role of food substances in both the cause and treatment of schizophrenia. One promising area of research is in the use of fish oil or other fatty acids that have been found to reduce inflammation in the body. A research literature review conducted by the Cochrane Collaboration Project concluded that polyunsaturated fatty acid supplementation to standard treatment or as primary intervention for schizophrenia may be acceptable to people with schizophrenia and have a moderately positive effect (Joy, Mumby-Croft, & Joy, 2002; Peet, 2002). Inflammatory immune processes have been implicated in the etiology of schizophrenia. Abnormal levels of specific cytokines, regulators of immune/inflammatory reactions and brain development, are found in both the brain and peripheral blood of patients with schizophrenia (Watanabe et al., 2010), thus reducing inflammation may be relevant for people with schizophrenia.

Other deficiencies in diet and vitamins have also been examined as possible causes of schizophrenia, but so far the results have been largely discounted or considered to be anecdotal. Nevertheless, considering what is still unknown about neurochemistry, these avenues of study may still hold promise.

DIAGNOSIS OF SCHIZOPHRENIA

There is criticism that schizophrenia tends to be overdiagnosed, particularly with people demonstrating bizarre or flagrant behaviors. Some societies more than others appear to tolerate "eccentric" behavior without necessarily considering it pathological. For a person to act "odd" or "different" does not necessarily mean that he or she has a disease. Even with the presence of obvious psychosis, it cannot be assumed that a pathological condition exists. For example, it has been well documented that hallucinations can occur as part of specific religious and cultural rituals, drug-induced behavior, or even within the realm of "normal" experience (MacRae, 1991).

One way of classifying schizophrenia is to differentiate the predominance of either positive symptoms or negative symptoms. In some cases there may be interplay between positive and negative symptoms. For example, deficits in perception (usually considered a positive symptom) "may contribute to the muted world experience of patients with persistent negative symptoms of schizophrenia" (Doniger, Silipo, Rabinowicz, Snodgrass, & Javitt, 2001, p. 1818). People with schizophrenia may have a combination of both positive and negative symptoms and the prominence of positive symptoms or negative symptoms may also change in the individual over the course of the illness (Mancevski et al, 2007).

Recently researchers have developed a conceptualization of *deficit* and *nondeficit schizophrenia* to describe the heterogeneity of the disorder and to categorize the predominance of positive and negative symptoms, the level of disorganization, and the presence of mood symptoms (Cohen, Brown, & Minor, 2010). Deficit schizophrenia is a conceptualization of the disorder focused on the predominant negative symptoms that are enduring (i.e., last longer than one year) and not attributable to other sources such as "depression, co-occurring substance abuse, intellectual disability, social isolation, paranoia, disorganization etc." (Cohen et al., 2010, p. 122). The diagnosis is based upon a well-validated semi-structured interview, the Schedule for Deficit Syndrome (Kirkpatrick, Buchanan, McKenney, Alphs, & Carpenter, 1989). Nondeficit schizophrenia is characterized by the prominence of positive symptoms and has been found to have slightly more severe mood symptoms. The differences in deficit and nondeficit schizophrenia in regard to level of disorganization have been inconsistent. Some studies have found more severe disorganization symptoms in deficit schizophrenia while other studies have found negligible differences between the two groups (Cohen et al., 2010).

POSITIVE SYMPTOMS

The most common positive symptoms associated with schizophrenia are delusions and perceptual distortions, especially hallucinations. However, various other perceptual and behavioral disturbances, such as uncontrolled laughing or silliness, may also present as positive symptoms. Language disturbances may include bizarre speech, echolalia, and, more frequently, circumstantiality, tangentiality, loosening of associations, incoherency, and pressured speech. Changes are possible in motoric responses, including pacing, rocking, restlessness, and lethargy, as well as disturbances of sleep patterns. It is important to recognize that the range and severity of symptoms vary with the individual. It has been thought that those with more positive symptoms may have less cognitive deficits than those with more negative symptoms. Generally those with positive symptoms may have a fluctuating course of exacerbations and remissions, compared with those with more prominent negative symptoms who tend to have a more chronic course of the illness without remissions (Strauss, Harrow, Grossman, & Rosen, 2010). Those with positive symptoms may respond well to antipsychotic medication; thus the major symptoms of hearing voices may be controlled or dampened through the use of medications.

Delusions

Delusions vary in content. Typical delusions found with schizophrenia are considered bizarre in that they are implausible within the context of the individual's environment and culture. William Bowden, a man diagnosed with schizophrenia, paranoid type, described the intractable nature of delusional thinking in this first-person account: "My belief has withstood attack from anyone I've shared it with. It is also something that I truly wish would stop. I also wish, even if this phenomenon is true, that I did not believe it" (Bowden, 1993, p. 165).

Paranoid delusions are certainly not limited to schizophrenia, but they do partially account for the suspicious and guarded behavior sometimes seen with the disorder. The delusions of schizophrenia also take various forms of presentation. For example, a delusion may be in the form of thought broadcasting, which occurs when the individual believes that his or her thoughts can be transmitted and that others can hear the thoughts. Thought insertion and thought withdrawal are the beliefs that someone or something is responsible for either putting thoughts into one's brain or removing one's thoughts (and ability to think). Thought control is also attributed to someone other than the person having the delusion and usually also implies action control (for example, someone who commits a crime and attributes the action to the force of a spirit or devil).

Presentations of thought broadcasting, insertion, withdrawal, and control are relatively consistent throughout different cultures and in historical reports of suspected delusions. What does change is the individual's rationale for what is happening. Thus, descriptions of these phenomena are remarkably similar throughout the world except for the individual's explanation for the phenomena. For example, a person who experienced a delusion of thought control in the European Middle Ages would have typically explained the control as coming from a demonic force, while in the decade of the 1950s in the United States, when the Cold War was raging, it was common for "the communists" to be blamed for thought control delusions. It is understandable that people would attempt to explain something happening to them that is out of the realm of the ordinary; therefore, these rationales are usually common themes found in the culture. The forms of the rationale may be political, religious, supernatural, scientific, or pseudo-scientific.

Sensory Deficits and Perceptual Distortion

Hallucinations are probably the most common perceptual disturbance found in schizophrenia, particularly in acute phases of the disorder. However, illusions are also possible, as well as poor body schema and personal boundaries, tactile defensiveness, and distorted figure-ground spatial and time relations (Olson, 2010; Tanaka et al., 2007).

Sensory deficits were not originally considered among the "first rank" symptoms of schizophrenia because it was originally thought that sensory function was not affected by the disorder and the patient's sensory descriptions were attributed to emotional or cognitive interpretations (Javitt, 2009). The relationship between sensory processing, perceptual distortion, and cognitive functions remains unclear. However, the renewed interest in sensory deficits in schizophrenia has opened the way for new research and potential treatments including sensory modulation as indicated in Table 7-1 (Brown, Cromwell, Filion, Dunn, & Tollefson, 2002; Dunn, 2001).

Distemporality does not fit neatly into a description of positive or negative symptoms, as it includes perceptual distortion and disorientation but also behaviorally presents as avolition. People with schizophrenia often report a sense of being stuck in present time, living only in the moment and unable to process the events of the past or determine a future course. Fuchs (2007) stated that the integration of past,

TABLE 7-1. Occupational Therapy Treatment Formats for People with Schizophrenia

Types	Comments
Structured tasks	Provide habit training, diversion, coping skills, and time management training. Potential for leisure skill development. May also build self-esteem through successful completion.
Expressive activities	Nonverbal communication, emotional and creative outlets. Potential for leisure skill development. May also build self-esteem through successful completion (Crawford et al., 2010; Griffiths & Corr, 2007).
Functional living skills	May include basic self-care (Mairs & Bradshaw, 2004), including hygiene, grooming, and dressing. Also includes independent living skills such as meal preparation (Grimm et al., 2009; Duncombe, 2004), computer skills, grocery shopping (Brown, Rempfer, & Hamera, 2002), and money management.
Sensory modulation	May include identifying sensory needs (may be alerting or calming) and how to address these needs through a sensory diet that may involve simple specific activities (e.g., rocking in a chair or chewing peppermint gum) as self-directed strategies to manage mood and energy levels (Champagne, Koomar, & Olson, 2010).
Psychoeducation	Can be used to teach living skills but is also used for teaching symptom management (Chan, Lee, & Chan, 2007), wellness recovery action plans (Copeland, 2001), health and safety awareness (may be related to nutrition, exercise, smoking, healthy choices) (Luboshitzky, & Gaber, 2000), self and group advocacy, and assertiveness training.
Social participation	May include developing links with community groups and facilitating social inclusion, sense of belonging, and friendships, relationships, and memberships (i.e., church, family, peer-based groups, advocacy groups, groups based on shared interests within the physical community, and virtual/web-based groups) (Roy et al., 2009).
Social skills training	Especially effective in groups; includes verbal and nonverbal communication. Role playing is one technique used (Lloyd, Waghorn, Williams, Harris, & Capra, 2008).
Vocational/educational training	Includes basic skill preparation, supported employment (Waghorn, Lloyd, & Clune, 2009) as well as time management and social skills. Vocational pursuits must be carefully graded and may require ongoing support. May also address educational goals related to completing GED or continuing education, or college (Robson, Waghorn, Sherring, & Morris, 2010; Gutman, Kerner, Zombek, Dulek, & Ramsey, 2009).

present, and future enables people to direct themselves toward objects and goals in a meaningful way. In contrast, symptoms of schizophrenia may prevent the "continuous intertwining of succeeding moments, . . . [which] leads to a loss of the tacit or operative intentionality that carries the acts of perceiving, thinking and acting" (p. 229). This area of temporality continues to be overlooked in evaluation and intervention, yet anecdotal evidence shows this continues to dramatically affect people's occupational performance.

Hallucinations are considered one of the hallmark symptoms of schizophrenia, but it has often been inaccurately considered that only auditory hallucinations are found in this disorder. Auditory hallucinations are probably the most common presentation, and they may lead to the greatest personal distress, possibly causing them to be reported with greater frequency. However, it is the phenomenon of multiple presentations of hallucinations that probably causes the greatest level of dysfunction. In other words, the more senses are involved with hallucinatory experiences, the more difficult it is for an individual to stay oriented to reality (MacRae, 1993).

Interestingly, the vividness or frequency of the hallucinations is not necessarily indicative of the severity of the disorder. Some people with quite pronounced perceptual distortion manage to develop adequate coping skills, while others with only a minimal disturbance remain severely impaired. In schizophrenia, the presence of negative symptoms, cognitive deficits, and a poor ability to manage environmental stimuli decreases the ability to cope with hallucinations, therefore creating a greater level of dysfunction.

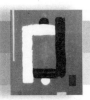

CASE ILLUSTRATION

Maureen—Positive Symptoms

Maureen is a 23-year-old college student who was accompanied by her roommate to the Emergency Psychiatric Services at the county hospital. She arrived in a wildly agitated state, claiming, "They are all trying to kill me." During an initial interview, Maureen admitted that she had been hearing voices commanding her to kill herself. The voices had apparently worsened over the last several days to the point where she was unable to sleep or concentrate on any activities. It was decided that Maureen was a danger to herself, and she was admitted to the acute inpatient locked unit. Further interviews revealed that Maureen had a history of repeated psychotic episodes starting in high school. Six years ago she had been diagnosed with schizophrenia, paranoid type. When she took her medication, her symptoms remained under control and she was able to function relatively well. However, her attempts to finish college had been hampered by acute exacerbations of her illness at times when she stopped taking her medication.

Discussion

Maureen's behavior is characteristic of someone with predominantly positive symptoms, minimal cognitive deficits, a fluctuating course of exacerbations and remissions, and good response to antipsychotic medication, which aids her functioning.

NEGATIVE SYMPTOMS

Many researchers and theorists are concentrating on negative symptoms in schizophrenia to better understand the disorder and how to best intervene. Those with more prominent negative symptoms generally respond poorly to typical antipsychotic medication but may experience a reduction of negative symptoms with an atypical agent. Nonmedical interventions are also being explored to manage the negative symptoms, which have been described through the work of Nancy Andreasen, who developed the Scale for the Assessment of Negative Symptoms (Andreasen, 1984). The scale includes the following broad categories:

- Affective flattening or blunting—a limited ability to express emotions and feelings
- Alogia—impoverished thought process that is manifested in speech patterns
- Avolition—a lack of interest or energy unaccompanied by depressed affect
- Anhedonia—an inability to experience pleasure or sustain interest in activities
- Inattention—an inability, of which the person may be unaware, to sustain concentration or attention

From an occupational therapy perspective, the term *hypohedonia* (decreased enjoyment) rather than *anhedonia* probably more accurately reflects the emotions, affect, and potential of the person with prominent negative symptoms of schizophrenia (Krupa & Thornton, 1986). A study conducted by Bejerholm (2010) examining occupational balance in people with schizophrenia suggests that people with schizophrenia, even with negative symptoms, are engaged in occupations that give pleasure and structure to daily life. However, not surprisingly, negative symptoms were significantly correlated with greater likelihood of being under-occupied (Bejerholm, 2010). Because negative symptoms are most often observed during sustained and social activity, the occupational therapist has a critical role in the accurate assessment of function. Given that many with prominent negative symptoms experience deficits in their teenage years or young adulthood, skills generally developed at that time of life related to home management and community mobility may not be developed. Moreover, the occupational therapy emphasis on activities of self-care, work, and leisure makes it essential that the therapist understand the nature of negative symptoms. A meaningful treatment plan reflects an awareness of these symptoms and efforts to be made to help the individual cope with, and compensate for, existing deficits.

CASE ILLUSTRATION

James—Negative Symptoms

James has lived in a residential care facility for the past seven years. He has not been hospitalized since living in this home but had several hospitalizations in the five years prior to this move. James takes antipsychotic medication, which seems to completely control the hallucinations he experienced in the past. Nevertheless, even in the absence of psychosis, James remains unable to function independently. He reports that he does nothing all day but has no plans for changing his lifestyle. He has been enrolled in several rehabilitative programs, including sheltered workshops, but was unable to follow through with their recommendations.

James also attempted to complete an associate's degree at the local community college but dropped out during his first semester. Poor attendance and difficulty attending to tasks were the primary reasons for this cycle of failure. James also has great difficulty in social situations. He tends to be passive, avoiding conversation and relationships even though he states he is lonely.

Discussion

James's functioning is severely influenced by his negative symptoms of avolition, anhedonia, and inattention.

PROGNOSIS

Schizophrenia is a serious and persistent mental illness, but data on its prognosis are unreliable, due to "the wide heterogeneity of its long-term course and outcome, as well as the variable effects of different treatments on schizophrenia symptoms" (Andreasen et al., 2005, p. 441). A 20-year longitudinal study showed very different rates of recovery for those with deficit compared with nondeficit schizophrenia. Strauss, Harrow, Grossman, and Rosen (2010) found, "the deficit syndrome represents a persistently impaired subsample of schizophrenia patients, with continuous social, occupational, and symptom impairment. In contrast, nondeficit syndrome schizophrenia patients showed at least some periods of remission or recovery" (p. 788) and marked improvement in vocational functioning later in the course of the illness.

The severity and prognosis of schizophrenia may be affected by cultural and environmental influences. For example, the World Health Organization (WHO, 2010) concluded that schizophrenia has a more benign course in the Third World. This may be explained by different family structures and types of treatment, a less urban environment, or the possibility that the disorder found in the Third World may have a different biological basis. Severity and clinical presentation are also partially determined by gender. The prevalence is greater in men than in women and women generally have a later onset of the disorder than men with the potential for a more benign course (Abel, Drake, & Goldstein, 2010). It is unclear if the differences are related to socio-cultural factors or biological differences, yet there is recent evidence that implicates biological factors. Abel et al. (2010) found, "Findings of sex differences in brain morphology are inconsistent but occur in areas that normally show sexual dimorphism, implying that the same factors are important drivers of sex differences in both normal neurodevelopmental processes and those associated with schizophrenia" (p. 417). Women also experience a greater side effect burden than men when taking antipsychotic medications (Seeman, 2010).

The long-held belief that schizophrenia is always a chronic and possibly deteriorating condition is currently being challenged. It has been suggested that some people with schizophrenia may have a natural remission after two to three decades. In other words, recovery rates may actually be much higher than previously estimated, but only after a prolonged course of illness (possibly 20 to 30 years). Factors that are associated with recovering from schizophrenia are shorter durations of untreated psychosis, coping and problem solving skills, and continuity of treatment (Liberman & Kopelowicz, 2005). A recent European study found that prognosis was better for younger patients with lower baseline clinical severity (Treuer, Martenyi, Saylan, & Dyachkova, 2010) and researchers are beginning to conceptualize remission and recovery models for schizophrenia (Andreasen et al., 2005; Ford, 2010). According to Liberman and Koelowicz:

> Long-term follow-up studies of persons who had experienced severe forms of schizophrenia earlier in their lives have discovered that over 50 percent of these individuals are living what may be considered "normal" lives—working, socializing, playing, living without close supervision and with little or no psychotic symptoms—20 to 30 years after their illness began. These "recoveries" have been documented in Japan, Germany, Switzerland, Scotland, France, and the USA. (1994, p. 67)

Research continues to support the concept of recovery from even the most serious of mental illnesses (see Chapter 1 for further discussion) and these studies have many ramifications for treatment. Hypothetically, if a young man developed schizophrenia at the age of 17, by the time he was 40 years old the disease might have run its course, but by that time his identity will also be firmly entrenched as a "disabled person." Many functional deficits would continue because of lifestyle, habits, and societal expectations and, most important, because of the missed developmental milestones of adolescence and young adulthood such as moving away from parents' home for independent living or getting a driver's license. Role dysfunction, which is considered an integral part of schizophrenia, may be minimized if aggressive rehabilitation is provided early in the course of illness. Occupational therapy interventions for people with first episode psychosis may address issues such as occupational and social roles and "the management of energy level, communication and social skills training, residential stability, academic and work rehabilitation and attention to physical features of the home, school and work environments" (Roy, Rousseau, Fortier, & Mottard, 2009, p. 424).

It also must be acknowledged that poor prognosis may be linked to inadequate treatment. It has been repeatedly documented that outcome is improved when people with schizophrenia are given comprehensive and consistent long-term treatment. It is possible that if such treatment were universally available, there would be a higher incidence of full recovery. It is certain that, given comprehensive and consistent treatment, functional outcome and quality of life would be improved even if the course of the disease remains chronic.

COLLABORATIVE TREATMENT

Collaborative treatment refers to the interdisciplinary members of a given treatment team, as well as the consumers of mental health services and their significant others or family members. In the acute phase of illness, hospital treatment may be necessary and beneficial, but typical hospitalization stays have shortened considerably over the last decade, and in the United States they are often only three to seven days in length. The hospitalization of people with schizophrenia usually only occurs when the individual has a severe psychotic episode, has grossly decompensated in function, and is considered either a danger to the self, a danger to others, or gravely disabled. The primary goal of acute hospitalization is to provide a thorough evaluation and stabilize the person on medication. Acute care hospitalizations also help stabilize clients by providing a safe environment with adequate rest and nutrition. This is becoming especially pertinent due to the incidence of homelessness among people with schizophrenia. Depending on the length of stay, the beginnings of a rehabilitation program may be commenced, but it is unrealistic to assume that brief hospitalizations will serve as sufficient intervention. People with schizophrenia require consistent treatment, typically of long duration, with a combined interdisciplinary approach. "Compared with those receiving medication only, patients with early-stage schizophrenia receiving medication and psychosocial intervention have a lower rate of treatment discontinuation or change, a lower risk of relapse, and improved insight, quality of life, and social functioning" as well as higher rates of obtaining employment or accessing education (Guo et al., 2010, p. 895). Treatment should include psychotropic medication, supportive services, and rehabilitation that includes both verbal and activity-based therapies.

Goal Attainment

A key component of an interdisciplinary treatment plan is setting the goals of treatment and developing a plan for attaining the goals. Ideally, these goals are determined by the individual in conjunction with the team. This cornerstone of client-centered practice "does not negate the importance of professional expertise, but is guided by a commitment to listen and respond to each client. The clients' personal knowledge and experience of living with a mental illness enable them to explain their lives, goals, and plans and allows them to seek personal meaning in their lives" (Dressler & MacRae, 1998, p. 37). It is highly desirable to also include the family and significant others, provided the person in treatment consents. Unfortunately, there are many constraints to this ideal situation. The trend toward managed care has placed great limits on the amount of services that can be provided, and too often, services are predetermined by agency mandate. Moreover, Western society has a long history of an authoritarian approach to health care, whereby professionals are viewed as "experts" who know what is best for the client. Although the "expert" model is changing to a more collaborative one, vestiges of the authoritarian health care system remain in practice. (See Chapter 1 for further discussion.)

Cooperative goal setting can also be hampered by the individual's pathology. People with delusions, poor insight, concrete thinking, or avolition may be incapable of healthy and realistic goal setting. Nevertheless, within the person's capabilities, every effort should be made to seek out and honor his or her expressed interests and desires, even if they sometimes conflict with the team's opinion.

CASE ILLUSTRATION

Diamond—Goal-Setting Conflict

Diamond, 38, has been diagnosed with schizophrenia, undifferentiated type. She has a long history of repetitive decompensations while living in the community. During her most recent hospitalization, the team recommended that she be placed in a residential care facility to help monitor her symptoms and medication. Diamond strongly objected, stating that she likes living alone in an apartment and that her goal is to return to independent living. After repeated discussions with the team, Diamond reluctantly agreed to the placement. Two weeks later, Diamond walked out of the facility and has not gotten in touch with her therapist in the ensuing month.

Discussion

This scenario might have been avoided if more effort had been made to comprehend Diamond's goals. While a residential care facility may be a safer alternative than independent living, it cannot be a feasible alternative without the individual's cooperation. Negotiation about follow-up care in the community, including day treatment and case management options, might have addressed the team's legitimate concerns while allowing Diamond to remain in an independent living situation.

Agreement as to what are "realistic" goals is not an easy task. The goals of the treatment team members may be quite different from those of the person with schizophrenia, whose ideas may also differ from the goals and expectations of the family. Professionals have been accused of contributing to chronicity by fostering dependency on the system and discouraging individuals from pursuing goals of independence in housing, employment, or school. On the other hand, for some people the demands of independent living exacerbate their symptoms, leading to a cycle of failure. Either overestimating or underestimating a person's potential can have adverse effects, so it is essential that goal setting not be based on diagnosis or preconceived ideas of outcome but rather be founded on an assessment of the particular individual's strengths, deficits, interests, needs, and level of support. In client-centered occupational therapy, "the targeted outcome is a vision of the future shared by the client and therapist and driven by the dream and desire of the individual. Dreams are unique to each individual, thus, targeted outcomes will also be" (Clark & Bell, 2000, p. 80).

Setting goals is only the first step. Working with a recovery orientation, it is very important to have an agreed-upon plan for reaching these goals within a realistic, but flexible, timeframe. Special attention must be given to understanding the entire social context, including support systems and external constraints. Goal attainment is a process that invariably has setbacks as well as unexpected accomplishments, Therefore, periodic review and possibly modification of goals are essential.

Psychotropic Medication

A significant part of the treatment of schizophrenia involves antipsychotic medication prescribed by a physician. However, the role of drug therapy has often been misunderstood. Antipsychotic medication does not cure schizophrenia. It typically decreases symptoms, but treatment that involves only drug therapy is inadequate. The primary benefit of psychotropic medication is to stabilize the individual sufficiently that he or she may benefit from other treatment. Medication ideally is viewed not as a panacea, but as part of a multipronged treatment approach that also includes peer support groups, skill development groups, opportunities for work and contributing to the community, and memberships (within home environments, community groups, or support services) that generate a sense of belonging.

In the 1990s the atypical antipsychotic agents, such as clozapine, risperidone, and olanzapine, were introduced and hailed as a major breakthrough in the treatment of schizophrenia in terms of offering greater choices of medications with less side effects (Gray & Roth, 2007). More recently asenapine was introduced (Minassian & Young, 2010). Some people switching from one of the earlier medications, such as haloperidol, experienced a significant reduction in both symptoms and side effects (Csernansky, Mahmoud, & Brenner, 2002), yet the hope that atypical antipsychotics would better address the negative and cognitive symptoms of schizophrenia has not been consistently supported across studies (Gray & Roth, 2007). While atypicals have less side effects, and no **extrapyramidal symptoms (EPS)**, they do have significant side effects of their own including weight gain and risk of diabetes. Some researchers are proposing that no single medication will succeed in addressing positive symptoms, negative symptoms, and cognitive deficits and rather that specific medications will need to be developed to target each aspect separately (Gray & Roth, 2007).

Current research on medication for schizophrenia continues to focus on medications targeting dopamine receptors, serotonin receptors, adrenergic receptors (which are thought to hold promise in improving cognitive performance), acetylcholine receptors, and glutamate receptors. Another avenue for medication development is targeting the genes or their associated pathways associated with schizophrenia, such as COMT, which appears related to the control of glutamate transmission, to develop novel treatments (Gray & Roth, 2007).

Side effects do occur with antipsychotic medication, including EPS, autonomic nervous system signs, endocrine side effects, weight gain, and skin changes. Therefore, it is important that drug trials be closely monitored to determine the best choice of drug and optimum dosage to prevent overmedication. In the medical model, there is often an overemphasis on decreasing symptoms, even at the expense of overall function. For example, a person on relatively high dosages of medication may experience a complete elimination of hallucinations but be too sedated to engage in meaningful activity, while a lower dose may cause some of the positive symptoms to persist but allow the individual to continue functioning while coping with the symptoms.

As mentioned previously, medication for schizophrenia continues to focus on targeting dopamine receptors, serotonin receptors, adrenergic receptors (which are thought to hold promise in improving cognitive performance), acetylcholine receptors, and glutamate receptors. Many of the drugs in development are related to dopamine in the brain. For example, Tuominen, Tiihonen, and Wahlbeck (2005) found that "Brain glutamate is thought to mediate symptoms in schizophrenia due to the influence of glutamate neurons on the dopaminergic transmission in the brain. It might be possible to decrease negative symptoms and the cognitive impairment of people with schizophrenia by treatment with glutamatergic drugs" (p. 225). It is theorized that the typical antipsychotic agents primarily act as antagonists of typical dopamine. Their therapeutic effect is believed to come from blockage of dopamine in the frontal cortex and limbic system, which is responsible for behavior and affect. Moreover, medications, such as clozapine, may influence serotonergic responses directly, which then affects dopamine systems. Kohlrausch et al. (2010) found, "Clozapine's action results from interactions between dopaminergic and serotonergic neurotransmitter systems and since clozapine appears to exert its effect strongly through the serotonergic systems, alterations in serotonin synaptic levels may influence antipsychotic response" (p. 1158).

A major concern in drug therapy for people with schizophrenia is a relatively high incidence of noncompliance. Given the extent of side effects experienced with these medications, it should not be a surprise that people may not want to take their medication, but there are many additional reasons for noncompliance. People with schizophrenia find themselves in a paradoxical situation in that the very symptoms that need treatment may prevent them from taking their medication. These symptoms may include delusional thinking regarding the harm of the drugs or lack of insight regarding their illness. Moreover, people with schizophrenia often have cognitive deficits such as forgetfulness, confusion, and poor time orientation, making it difficult for them to manage medication independently.

Noncompliance can be minimized by providing education and supportive interventions to help the individual manage both symptoms and side effects. Moreover, people with cognitive deficits can benefit from simplified drug regimens and time and memory management techniques. However, the most important predictor of compliance is the therapeutic relationship and level of trust the individual feels with the prescribing physician and treatment team as a whole. Listening to the concerns of the client and acknowledging their experiences with medication are essential for both the prescribing physician and the treatment team. Unfortunately, the current state of mental health care makes it difficult for a consistent treatment team to follow people, who frequently become "lost in the system."

OCCUPATIONAL THERAPY INTERVENTION

Team treatment of people with schizophrenia is common and, depending on the model of treatment used, various disciplines may be involved. For the purposes of this chapter, discussion is limited to the role of the occupational therapist. It must be acknowledged, however, that in some team approaches, several disciplines may overlap with occupational therapy or conduct evaluation and treatments typically viewed as occupational therapy. In some cases, occupational therapists may also take on roles outside their traditional domain. Regardless of the model of intervention, the needs of the client should drive the services provided.

Evaluation

The choice of assessment tools is influenced by the therapist's theoretical frame of reference, familiarity, and the purpose of the assessment. In working with people with serious mental illness, it is important to do top-down practical assessments of daily functioning—that is, focusing on the daily life skills such as doing one's laundry rather than the component skills such as sequencing the steps of an activity. Having the opportunity to observe occupational performance within the home environment is a rich resource for gaining practical knowledge of the "real life" of the clients with whom one works.

There is a dearth of updated, current, and standardized community living skill assessments for people with schizophrenia. The Kohlman Evaluation of Living Skills (KELS) (Kohlman Thomson, 1992) and the Executive Function Performance Test (EFPT) (Baum et al., 2008) are easily administered and provide information on an individual's ability to perform a variety of tasks necessary for independent living. Unfortunately, the money management and phone use portion of these assessments do not reflect the updated skill set related to online banking, ATM cards, and mobile phones. The Independent Living Skills Assessment (ILS) (Johnson, Vinnicombe, & Merrill, 1980) may also be used with this population. The Milwaukee Evaluation of Daily Living Skills (MEDLS) (Haertlein, 1995) offers the opportunity to tailor the assessment by administering the evaluation of only the specific skills in question (e.g., eyeglass care) rather than the entire evaluation. The Test of Grocery Shopping Skills (Hamera, & Brown, 2000) occurs in a grocery store (*in vivo*) and reflects a top-down approach. Community living skills evaluations are not diagnostic tools; they do not give specific information on the causes of dysfunction. For this reason, they are not sufficiently sensitive tools for treatment planning. However, they may be valuable for determining needed skills and supports for community living. Given the changes in technology, the individuality of people's skills, and the variability of living situations, it may not be possible to administer the living skills assessments in a standardized manner; the client's environment and context must primarily drive the assessment process.

Another functional evaluation is the Assessment of Motor and Process Skills (AMPS) developed by Anne Fisher. "The AMPS is an observational assessment that permits the simultaneous evaluation of motor and process skills as a person performs two or three complex or instrumental activity of daily living (IADL) tasks (e.g., meal preparation, home maintenance, laundry) of his or her choice" (Fisher, Liu, Velozo, & Pan, 1992, p. 878). The AMPS is not specific to any diagnosis, but considering that people with schizophrenia often have both cognitive and sensorimotor deficits that result in dysfunction, it is very useful for this population. One limitation of the AMPS is the lengthy training process required to become a calibrated administrator of the assessment, which, while necessary, prevents its widespread use currently.

The Adult Sensory Profile (Brown, Tollefson, Dunn, Cromwell, & Filion, 2001) is being used across mental health settings and diagnoses. Considering the sensory-processing deficits and perceptual distortions found in schizophrenia, this assessment may be valuable in developing successful interventions, especially in the areas of coping strategies, sensory modulation, and environmental modifications.

Occupational therapists also use an interview to build a therapeutic relationship, determine interests and skills, and develop goals. A particularly useful interview format is the Canadian Occupational Performance Measure (COPM) (Law et al., 2005), which measures the client's self-perception of occupational performance by using a semi-structured interview. The structure of the COPM helps the client and therapist develop goals that are both realistic and applicable for occupational therapy intervention. It can also be used as an outcome measure of the client's perception of performance and satisfaction, if it is administered at the beginning of treatment and then readministered at the time of discharge (Schindler, 2010; Law et al., 2005). The Occupational Performance History Interview (OPHI-II) offers a structured interview format using scales to rate occupational identity, occupational competency, and occupational behavior settings; the scales have been found to be valid across age, diagnosis, and six languages (Kielhofner, Mallinson, Forsyth, & Lai, 2001). Self-report assessments may also be used, such as the Occupational Self Assessment (OSA) (Kielhofner & Forsyth, 2001), the Role Checklist (Dickerson & Oakley, 1995), and the Kawa Model (Iwama, Thomson, & Macdonald, 2009; Richardson, Jobson, & Miles, 2010); these measures are most useful when given in conjunction with an interview. An interview also discloses much information regarding symptoms related to thought processes, but it is not the most effective method of determining function. A more useful tool for evaluating the functional skills of people with schizophrenia is task analysis. The observation of an individual engaged in routine activities provides a wealth of information about functioning that could not be uncovered through an interview. One such observation-based assessment is the Assessments and Communication of Interaction Skills (ACIS) (Forsyth, Lai, & Kielhofner, 1999), which is based upon the Model of Human Occupation and describes the social interaction skills of adults.

Treatment

Group work is the most common approach used by occupational therapists in mental health. (For discussion of groups, see Chapter 20.) Groups are especially effective for building social skills, but the importance of one-to-one personal contact should not be underestimated, especially in the early stages of treatment, when it aids in developing a relationship and performing evaluation. Unfortunately, occupational therapists working with budget and time constraints often must limit individual treatments. One-to-one contact is vital for individuals who are withdrawn or are too psychotic to benefit from a group approach. The stimulation of an activity group may place undue demands on some people and exacerbate their symptoms.

In addition, individual contact is often a prelude to group involvement. It is helpful if the occupational therapist in a one-to-one interaction explains the purpose of the available groups, and personally invites the individual to join. Attendance and participation in group activities is much more likely if the person already has a relationship with the group leader and knows what to expect. Research indicates that clients on inpatient units value group approaches and content that provide a supportive milieu, respect clients' comfort levels in self-disclosure and readiness to attend groups, and link occupational therapy activities with psychoeducational topics to integrate learning (Cowls & Hale, 2005)

Individual intervention is often thought to be too expensive, but in fact it is possible to meet specific objectives in a time- and cost-effective manner. For example, an occupational therapist may visit individual rooms on an inpatient unit with a cart stocked with grooming supplies. In this way, the therapist engages in one-to-one contact with clients while providing evaluation and treatment. This activity gives the therapist an opportunity to check in with clients at the beginning of the day. Introductions and orientation to occupational therapy occur simultaneously with activity of daily living (ADL) evaluation and treatment. The actual contact may be quite brief, yet this form of individual treatment paves the way for more sustained one-to-one and group activities. Individual occupational therapy intervention for community dwelling people with schizophrenia has been found to be effective in promoting social functioning in areas such as relationships and recreation (Cook, Chambers, & Coleman, 2009). People with schizophrenia also found occupational therapy helpful with trying new activities, stabilizing one's sleep pattern, routinely accomplishing self-care activities, and the pursuit of leisure, education, and work activities (Cook & Chambers, 2009). Interestingly, it was found that "people did not separate different aspects of their lives. What helped them with their mental health also helped them to choose and do the things that they wanted to do in their daily lives and vice versa" (Cook & Chambers, 2009, p. 243). Although occupational therapists structure their interventions on the individual's strengths, understanding the pathology of the illness is also essential. People who display positive symptoms, especially hallucinations, benefit from activities that divert attention from their symptoms. In the process, the individual can learn self-help coping strategies to minimize the intrusiveness of positive symptoms. However, it is only when people can clearly identify activities with *personal meaning or purpose* that they are able to see them as a viable method of symptom management. While random applications of activities sometimes provides a temporary distraction from hallucinations, it is the use of activities that bolsters the sense of personal achievement and mastery that are consistently deemed as most successful in coping with hallucinations and other positive symptoms (MacRae, 1993; Ivarsson, Soderback, & Ternestedt, 2002). Occupational therapists may reinforce this realization of achievement and its effect on symptoms by facilitating a feedback loop with individuals. For example, therapists may ask individuals to rate their mood or severity of symptoms before engaging in an activity and then after the activity to compare and discuss any changes that may have occurred. The occupational therapist may help the individual make the link between the experience of doing an activity and how they feel quite directly and overtly, which may help individuals to implement activities as coping strategies in their own lives. Negative symptoms have a more profound effect than positive symptoms on an individual's overall ability to function. Understanding that negative symptoms are part of the disease process and not necessarily a learned maladaptive behavior can help the clinician structure interventions to compensate for these deficits. Individuals who display negative symptoms often need highly structured activities with concrete expectations and goals. Specific skill training and psychoeducation are very beneficial to people with negative symptoms, but many individuals need ongoing support to utilize their skills.

Improving overall quality of life for people with schizophrenia is one of the main objectives of treatment. In research conducted by Laliberte-Rodman, Yu, Scott, and Pajouhandeh (2000), three major themes regarding quality of life were identified through the use of focus groups consisting of subjects with schizophrenia, a consumer facilitator, and a nonconsumer facilitator. These themes are managing time, connecting and belonging, and making choices and maintaining control. Occupational therapy techniques and interventions are ideal for mastering and fulfilling these quality-of life-concerns.

Considering the global dysfunction associated with schizophrenia, there is a wide range of possible interventions, which address the occupational performance areas of self-care, work, and leisure as well as the performance components of motor, sensory-integrative, cognitive, psychological, and social functioning. Most activities can address more than one component or area, and the therapist must adapt and grade the activities to best meet the needs of the individual patient or group. Treatment goals may be accomplished in many different ways using a variety of individual and group techniques. Table 7-1 describes some of the specific treatment formats used with this population by occupational therapists.

SUMMARY

Schizophrenia is a complicated disorder affecting over 24 million people throughout the world (WHO, 2010). Its effects can be devastating on a person's ability to function but individuals with schizophrenia additionally experience dysfunction from society's reaction to them for being ill. Schizophrenia is largely misunderstood by the general public, and clinicians have a responsibility to combat the myths and misconceptions about this disorder. The diagnostic trend toward dimensional assessment rather that categorization will likely have the biggest impact on people with serious mental illnesses such as schizophrenia, by reducing stigma and inappropriate labeling. (See Chapter 6 for further discussion.) Knowledge of the underlying pathology of the illness, an ability to work with a team approach, and a willingness to relate to the person with schizophrenia are essential for successful intervention and support for recovery.

REVIEW QUESTIONS

1. Why is schizophrenia commonly misunderstood?
2. What is believed to be the cause of schizophrenia?
3. How does the presence of positive symptoms affect occupational therapy intervention?
4. How does the presence of negative symptoms affect occupational therapy intervention?
5. How does occupational therapy intervention for people with schizophrenia differ from other mental health professions?

REFERENCES

Abel, K. M., Drake, R., & Goldstein, J. M. (2010). Sex differences in schizophrenia. *International Review of Psychiatry, 22*(5), 417–428.

Andreasen, N. (1984). *Scale for the Assessment of Negative Symptoms (SANS).* Iowa City: University of Iowa Press.

Andreasen, N. (2001). *Brave new brain: Conquering mental illness in the era of the genome.* Oxford, UK: Oxford University Press.

Andreasen, N. C., Carpenter, W. T., Jr., Kane, J. M., Lasser, R. A., Marder, S. R., & Weinberger, D. R. (2005). Remission in schizophrenia: Proposed criteria and rationale for consensus. *American Journal of Psychiatry, 162*(3), 441–449. Retrieved from EBSCO*host* database.

Baum, C., Connor, L., Morrison, T., Hahn, M., Dromerick, A., & Edwards, D. (2008). Reliability, validity, and clinical utility of the Executive Function Performance Test: A measure of executive function in a sample of people with stroke. *American Journal of Occupational Therapy, 62*(4), 446–455.

Bejerholm, U. (2010). Occupational balance in people with schizophrenia. *Occupational Therapy in Mental Health, 26*(1), 1–17.

Bleuler, E. (1950). *Dementia praecox, or the group of schizophrenias* (J. Zinkin, Trans.). New York: International Universities Press. (Original work published in 1911)

Boksa, P. (2008). Maternal infection during pregnancy and schizophrenia. *Journal of Psychiatry & Neuroscience, 33*(3), 183–185.

Bowden, W. (1993). First person account: The onset of paranoia. *Schizophrenia Bulletin, 19*(1), 165–167.

Brown, A., Schaefer, C., Wyatt, R., Begg, M., Goetz, R., Bresnahan, M., et al. (2002). Paternal age and the risk of schizophrenia in adult offspring. *American Journal of Psychiatry, 159,* 1528–1533.

Brown, C., Cromwell, R. L., Filion, D., Dunn, W., & Tollefson, N. (2002). Sensory processing in schizophrenia: Missing and avoiding information. *Schizophrenia Research, 55*(1/2), 187. Retrieved from EBSCO*host* database.

Brown, C., Rempfer, M., & Hamera, E. (2002). Teaching grocery shopping skills to people with schizophrenia. *OTJR: Occupation, Participation, and Health, 22*(suppl. 1), 90S–91S.

Brown, C., Tollefson, N., Dunn, W., Cromwell, R., & Filion, D. (2001). The Adult Sensory Profile: Measuring patterns of sensory processing. *American Journal of Occupational Therapy, 55*(1), 75–82.

Buka, S. L., Cannon, T. D., Torrey, E. F., & Yolken, R. H. (2007). Maternal exposure to herpes simplex virus and risk of psychosis among adult offspring. *Biological Psychiatry, 63*(8), 809–815.

Cascade, E., Kalali, A. H., Mehra, S., & Meyer, J. M. (2010). Real-world data on atypical antipsychotic medication side effects. *Psychiatry* (Edgemont), *7*(7), 9–12.

Champagne, T., Koomar, J., & Olson, L. (2010). Sensory processing evaluation and intervention in mental health. *OT Practice, 15*(5), CE-1–8.

Chan, S., Lee, S., & Chan, I. (2007). TRIP: A psycho-educational programme in Hong Kong for people with schizophrenia. *Occupational Therapy International, 14*(2), 86–98. Retrieved from EBSCO-*host* database.

Clark, J., & Bell, B. (2000). Collaborating on targeted outcomes and making action plans. In V. Fearing & J. Clark (Eds.), *Individuals in context: A practical guide to client-centered practice.* Thorofare, NJ: Slack.

Cohen, A. S., Brown, L. A., & Minor, K. S. (2010). The psychiatric symptomatology of deficit schizophrenia: A meta-analysis. *Schizophrenia Research, 118*(1-3), 122–127.

Cook, S., & Chambers, E. (2009). What helps and hinders people with psychotic conditions doing what they want in their daily lives. *British Journal of Occupational Therapy, 72*(6), 238–248.

Cook, S., Chambers, E., & Coleman, J. (2009). Occupational therapy for people with psychotic conditions in community settings: A pilot randomized controlled trial. *Clinical Rehabilitation, 23*(1), 40–52. Retrieved from EBSCO*host* database.

Copeland, M. (2001). Wellness Recovery Action Plan: A system for monitoring, reducing and eliminating uncomfortable or dangerous physical symptoms and emotional feelings. *Occupational Therapy in Mental Health, 17*(3/4), 127–150. Retrieved from EBSCO*host* database.

Cowls, J., & Hale, S. (2005). It's the activity that counts: What clients value in psycho-educational groups. *Canadian Journal of Occupational Therapy, 72*(3), 176–182.

Crawford, M. J., Killaspy, H., Kalaitzaki, E., Barrett, B., Byford, S., Patterson, S., et al. (2010). The MATISSE study: A randomised trial of group art therapy for people with schizophrenia. *BMC Psychiatry*, 1065–1073. Retrieved from doi:10.1186/1471-244X-10-65

Csernansky, J., Mahmoud, R., & Brenner, R. (2002). A comparison of risperidone and haloperidol for the prevention of relapse in patients with schizophrenia. *New England Journal of Medicine, 346*(1), 16–22.

Dickerson, A. E., & Oakley, F. (1995). Comparing the roles of community-living persons and patient populations. *American Journal of Occupational Therapy, 49*(3), 221–228.

Doniger, G., Silipo, G., Rabinowicz, E., Snodgrass, J., & Javitt, D. (2001). Impaired sensory processing as a basis for object-recognition deficits in schizophrenia. *American Journal of Psychiatry, 158*(11), 1818–1826.

Dressler, J., & MacRae, A. (1998). Advocacy, partnerships, and client centered practice. *Occupational Therapy in Mental Health, 14*(1/2), 35–43.

Duncombe, L. (2004). Comparing learning cooking in home and clinic for people with schizophrenia. *The American Journal of Occupational Therapy, 58*(3), 272–278.

Dunn, W. (2001). The 2001 Eleanor Clarke Slagle Lecture. The sensations of everyday life: empirical, theoretical, and pragmatic considerations. *American Journal of Occupational Therapy, 55*(6), 608–620. Retrieved from EBSCO*host* database.

Fisher, A., Liu, Y., Velozo, C., & Pan, A. W. (1992). Cross-cultural assessment of process skills. *American Journal of Occupational Therapy, 46*(10), 876–885.

Folsom, D. P., Hawthorne, W., Lindamer, L. Gilmer, T., Bailey, A., Golshan, S., et al. (2005). Prevalence and risk factors for homelessness and utilization of mental health services among 10,340 patients with serious mental illness in a large public mental health system. *American Journal of Psychiatry, 162*, 370–376.

Ford, K. (2010). The concept of remission for people with schizophrenia. *Mental Health Practice, 13*(5), 22–25.

Forsyth, K., Lai, J., & Kielhofner, G. (1999). The assessment of communication and interaction skills (ACIS): Measurement properties. *British Journal of Occupational Therapy 62*(2), 69–74.

Fuchs, T. (2007). The temporal structure of intentionality and its disturbance in schizophrenia. *Psychopathology, 40*(4), 229–235. Retrieved from doi:10.1159/000101365

Gray, J. A., & Roth, B. L. (2007). The pipeline and future of drug development in schizophrenia. *Molecular Psychiatry, 12*(10), 904–922.

Griffiths, S., & Corr, S. (2007). The use of creative activities with people with mental health problems: A survey of occupational therapists. *British Journal of Occupational Therapy, 70*(3), 107–114.

Grimm, E., Meus, J., Brown, C., Exley, S., Hartman, S., Hays, C., et al. (2009). Meal preparation: comparing treatment approaches to increase acquisition of skills for adults with schizophrenic disorders. *OTJR: Occupation, Participation & Health, 29*(4), 148–153. Retrieved from EBSCO*host* database.

Guo, X., Zhai, J., Liu, Z., Fang, M., Wang, B., Wang, C., et al. (2010). Effect of antipsychotic medication alone vs combined with psychosocial intervention on outcomes of early-stage schizophrenia: A randomized, 1-year study. *Archives of General Psychiatry, 67*(9), 895–904. Retrieved from doi:10.1001/archgenpsychiatry.2010.105

Gutman, S. A., Kerner, R., Zombek, I., Dulek, J., & Ramsey, C.A. (2009). Supported education for adults with psychiatric disabilities: Effectiveness of an occupational therapy program. *American Journal of Occupational Therapy, 63*, 245–254. Retrieved from doi: 10.5014/ajot.63.3.245

Haertlein, C. (1995). Validity and reliability of the Milwaukee Evaluation of Daily Living Skills (MEDLS). In *Conference abstracts and resources 1995: The American Occupational Therapy Association's 1995 annual conference and exposition, Saturday, April 8–Wednesday, April 12, 1995, Colorado Convention Center, Denver, Colorado* (pp. 159–160). Bethesda, MD: American Occupational Therapy Association.

Hamera, E., & Brown, C. (2000). Developing a context-based performance measure for persons with schizophrenia: the Test of Grocery Shopping Skills. *American Journal of Occupational Therapy, 54*(1), 20–25. Retrieved from EBSCO*host* database.

Hui, C., Wardwell, B., & Tsai, G. E. (2009). Novel therapies for schizophrenia: understanding the glutamatergic synapse and potential targets for altering N-methyl-D-aspartate neurotransmission. *Recent patents on CNS drug discovery. 4*(3), 220–238.

Ivarsson, A., Soderback, I., & Ternestedt, B. (2002). The meaning and form of occupational therapy as experienced by women with psychosis. *Scandinavian Journal of Caring Science, 16*, 103–110.

Iwama, M., Thomson N. A., & Macdonald R. A. (2009). The Kawa Model; the power of culturally responsive occupational therapy. *Disability and Rehabilitation, 31*(14), 1125–1135.

Javitt, D. (2009). Sensory processing in schizophrenia: Neither simple nor intact. *Schizophrenia Bulletin, 35*(6), 1059–1064.

Johnson, T., Vinnicombe, B., & Merrill, G. (1980). The independent living skills evaluation. *Occupational Therapy in Mental Health, 1*, 5–18.

Joy, C. B., Mumby-Croft, R., & Joy, L. A. (2002). Polyunsaturated fatty acid (fish or evening primrose oil) for schizophrenia (Cochrane Review). *The Cochrane Library*, Issue 3. Oxford: Update Software.

Kielhofner, G., & Forsyth, K. (2001). Measurement properties of a client self-report for treatment planning and documenting therapy outcomes. *Scandinavian Journal of Occupational Therapy 8*(3), 131–139.

Kielhofner, G., Mallinson, T., Forsyth, K., & Lai, J. (2001). Psychometric properties of the second version of the Occupational Performance History Interview (OPHI-II). *American Journal of Occupational Therapy, 55*(3), 260–267.

Kirkpatrick, B., Buchanan, R. W., McKenney, P. D., Alphs, L. D., & Carpenter, W. T. (1989). The Schedule for the Deficit Syndrome: An instrument for research in schizophrenia. *Psychiatry Research, 30*(2), 119–123.

Kohlman Thomson, L. (1992). *The Kohlman Evaluation of Living Skills* (3rd ed.). Bethesda, MD: American Occupational Therapy Association.

Kohlrausch, F. B., Salatino-Oliveira, A., Gama, C. S., Lobato, M., Belmonte-de-Abreu, P., & Hutz, M. H. (2010). Influence of serotonin transporter gene polymorphisms on clozapine response in Brazilian schizophrenics. *Journal of Psychiatric Research, 44*(16), 1158–1162.

Kraepelin, E. (1971). *Dementia praecox and paraphrenia* (R. M. Barclay & G. M. Robertson, Trans. & Eds.). Edinburgh: E. & S. Livingstone. (Original work published in 1919)

Krupa, T., & Thornton, J. (1986). The pleasure deficit in schizophrenia. *Occupational Therapy in Mental Health, 6*(2), 65–78.

Kuepper, R., Morrison, P., van Os, J., Murray, R., Kenis, G., & Henquet, C. (2010). Does dopamine mediate the psychosis-inducing effects of cannabis? A review and integration of findings across disciplines. *Schizophrenia Research, 121*(1-3), 107–117.

Laliberte-Radman, D., Yu, B., Scott, D., & Pajouhandeh, P. (2000). Exploring the perspective of persons with schizophrenia regarding quality of life. *American Journal of Occupational Therapy, 54*(2), 137–147.

Law, M., Baptiste, S., Carswell, A., McColl, M., Polatajko, H., & Pollock, N. (2005). *Canadian Occupational Performance Measure Manual (COPM)* (4th ed.). Thorofare, NJ: Slack.

Liao, S. Y., Lin, S. H., Liu, C. M., Hsieh, M. H., Hwang, T. J., Liu, et al. (2009). Genetic variants in COMT and neurocognitive impairment in families of patients with schizophrenia. *Genes, Brain & Behavior, 8*(2), 228–237.

Liberman, R. P., & Kopelowicz, A. (1994). Recovery from schizophrenia: Is the time right? *Journal of the California Alliance for the Mentally Ill, 5*(3), 67–69.

Liberman, R. P., & Kopelowicz, A. (2005). Recovery from Schizophrenia: A Concept in Search of Research. *Psychiatric Services 56*(6), 735–742.

Liu, K., Chan, R., Chan, K., Tang, J., Chiu, C., Lam, M., et al. (2011). Executive function in first-episode schizophrenia: A three-year longitudinal study of an ecologically valid test. *Schizophrenia Research 126*, 87–92.

Lloyd, C., Waghorn, G., Williams, P., Harris, M., & Capra, C. (2008). Early psychosis: treatment issues and the role of occupational therapy. *British Journal of Occupational Therapy, 71*(7), 297–304. Retrieved from EBSCO*host* database.

Luboshitzky, D., & Gaber, L. (2000). Collaborative therapeutic homework model in occupational therapy. *Occupational Therapy in Mental Health, 15*(1), 43–60. Retrieved from EBSCO*host* database.

MacRae, A. (1991). An overview of theory and research on hallucinations: Implications for occupational therapy intervention. *Occupational Therapy in Mental Health, 11*(4), 41–60.

MacRae, A. (1993). *Coping with hallucinations: A phenomenological study of the everyday lived experience of people with hallucinatory psychosis.* Ann Arbor, MI: University Microfilms.

Mairs, H., & Bradshaw, T. (2004). Life skills training in schizophrenia. *British Journal of Occupational Therapy, 67*(5), 217–224. Retrieved from EBSCO*host* database.

Mancevski, B., Keilp, J., Kurzon, M., Berman, R. M., Ortakov, V., Harkavy-Friedman, et al. (2007). Lifelong course of positive and negative symptoms in chronically institutionalized patients with schizophrenia. *Psychopathology, 40*(2), 83–92.

Mazzoncini, R., Donoghue, K., Hart, J., Morgan, C., Doody, G. A., Dazzan, P., et al. (2010). Illicit substance use and its correlates in first episode psychosis. *Acta Psychiatrica Scandinavica, 121*(5), 351–358.

Minassian, A., & Young, J. W. (2010). Evaluation of the clinical efficacy of asenapine in schizophrenia. *Expert Opinion on Pharmacotherapy, 11*(12), 2107–2015.

Olson, L. (2010). Examining schizophrenia and sensory modulation disorder: a review of the literature. *Sensory Integration Special Interest Section Quarterly, 33*(1), 1–3. Retrieved from EBSCO*host* database.

Palmer, B. A., Pankratz, V. S., & Bostwick, J. M. (2005). The lifetime risk of suicide in schizophrenia: A reexamination. *Archives of General Psychiatry, 62,* 247–253.

Peet, M. (2002). Essential fatty acids: theoretical aspects and treatment implications for schizophrenia and depression. *Advances in Psychiatric Treatment, 8*(3), 223–229.

Richardson, P., Jobson, B., & Miles, S. (2010). Using the Kawa model: a practice report. *Mental Health Occupational Therapy, 15*(3), 82–85.

Robinson, J., Cotton, S., Conus, P., Schimmelmann, B. G., McGorry, P., & Lambert, M. (2009). Prevalence and predictors of suicide attempt in an incidence cohort of 661 young people with first-episode psychosis. *Australian and New Zealand Journal of Psychiatry, 43*(2), 149–157.

Robson, E., Waghorn, G., Sherring, J., & Morris, A. (2010). Preliminary outcomes from an individualised supported education programme delivered by a community mental health service. *British Journal of Occupational Therapy, 73*(10), 481–486. Retrieved from EBSCO*host* database.

Roy, L., Rousseau, J., Fortier, P., & Mottard, J. (2009). Perception of community functioning in young adults with recent-onset psychosis: Implications for practice. *British Journal of Occupational Therapy, 72*(10), 424–433. Retrieved from EBSCO*host* database.

Schindler, V. (2010). A client-centered, occupation-based occupational therapy programme for adults with psychiatric diagnoses. *Occupational Therapy International, 17*(3), 105–112.

Schneider, K. (1959). *Clinical psychopathology* (M. W. Hamilton, Trans.). London & New York: Grune & Stratton.

Schneider, F., Backes, V., & Mathiak, K. (2009). Brain imaging: on the way toward a therapeutic discipline. *European Archives of Psychiatry and Clinical Neuroscience, 259*(Suppl 2), S143–S147.

Seeman, M. V. (2010). Schizophrenia: Women bear a disproportionate toll of antipsychotic side effects. *Journal of the American Psychiatric Nurses Association, 16*(1), 21–29.

Strauss, G. P., Harrow, L., Grossman, L. S., & Rosen, C. (2010). Periods of recovery in deficit syndrome schizophrenia: A 20-year multi–follow-up longitudinal study. *Schizophrenia Bulletin, 36*(4), 788–799.

Tanaka, G., Mori, S., Inadomi, H., Hamada, Y., Ohta, Y., & Ozawa, H. (2007). Clear distinction between preattentive and attentive process in schizophrenia by visual search performance. *Psychiatry Research, 149*(1-3), 25–31. Retrieved from doi:10.1016/j.psychres.2006.01.014

Tibbo, P., Hanstock, C., Valiakalayil, A., & Allen, P. (2004). 3-T proton MRS investigation of glutamate and glutamine in adolescents at high genetic risk for schizophrenia. *American Journal of Psychiatry, 161,* 1116–1118.

Treuer, T., Martenyi, F., Saylan, M., & Dyachkova, Y. (2010). Factors associated with achieving minimally symptomatic status by patients with schizophrenia: results from the 3-year intercontinental schizophrenia outpatients health outcomes study. *International Journal of Clinical Practice, 64*(6), 697–706.

Tuominen, H. J., Tiihonen, J., & Wahlbeck, K. (2005). Glutamatergic drugs for schizophrenia: a systematic review and meta-analysis. *Schizophrenia Research, 72*(2/3), 225–234.

Waghorn, G., Lloyd, C., & Clune, A. (2009). Reviewing the theory and practice of occupational therapy in mental health rehabilitation. *British Journal of Occupational Therapy, 72*(7), 314–323. Retrieved from EBSCO*host* database.

Walsh, E. (2002). Violence and schizophrenia: examining the evidence. *The British Journal of Psychiatry, 180*(6), 490–495.

Watanabe, Y., Someya, T., & Nawa, H. (2010). Cytokine hypothesis of schizophrenia pathogenesis: Evidence from human studies and animal models. *Psychiatry & Clinical Neurosciences, 64*(3), 217–230.

World Health Organization. (WHO) (2010). Schizophrenia: What is schizophrenia? Retrieved from http://www.who.int/mental_health/management/schizophrenia/en/

SUGGESTED RESOURCES

The reader is encouraged to also explore the extensive website resources list in Chapter 1.

Cook, S., Chambers, E., & Coleman, J. (2009). Occupational therapy for people with psychotic conditions in community settings: A pilot randomized controlled trial. *Clinical Rehabilitation, 23*(1), 40–52.

Copeland, M. (2001). Wellness Recovery Action Plan: A system for monitoring, reducing and eliminating uncomfortable or dangerous physical symptoms and emotional feelings. *Occupational Therapy in Mental Health, 17*(3/4), 127–150.

Krupa, T., Edgelow, D., Radloff-Gabriel, D., Mieras, C., Almas, A., Perry, A., et al. (2010). *Action over inertia: Addressing the activity-health needs of individuals with serious mental illness.* Ottawa: CAOT publications.

Olson, L. (2010). Examining schizophrenia and sensory modulation disorder: A review of the literature. *Sensory Integration Special Interest Section Quarterly, 33*(1), 1–3. Retrieved from EBSCO*host* database.

Chapter 8

Mood Disorders

Elizabeth Cara, PhD, OTR, MFT

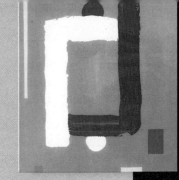

KEY TERMS

affect

cyclothymia

depression

dysthymia

mania

melancholia

mood

referential thinking

CHAPTER OUTLINE

Introduction

Diagnostic Criteria

    Episodes

    Disorders

    Specifiers

Causes, Occurrence, and Theories of Mood Disorders

    Causes and Occurrence

    Other Theories

Clinical Picture

Common Evaluation and Management

    Evaluation

    Management

Occupational Therapy Treatment and Intervention

    Interpersonal Approach

    Person-to-Person Interventions

    System Interventions

Summary

INTRODUCTION

Mood disorders have been described throughout history. Descriptions of depressive episodes are found in the Old Testament and in classical Greek literature. Originally, in ancient times, they were thought to be a curse of the gods, and therefore, sufferers were treated by priests. In the sixth century BC, Hippocrates, "the father of physicians," introduced the terms **melancholia** and **mania** in clinical descriptions that are still accurate today. He also placed mental functioning, or malfunctioning, in the brain rather than in the spirit. Therefore, mania and melancholia became the domain of the medical doctor rather than the priest. The first text devoted to "affective illness" was published in England in 1621 and cited causes that continue to be considered today, such as diet, biological rhythms, alcohol, and love and grief. The first modern psychiatrist suggested that a disturbance in **mood** most likely was underlying most forms of depression and some psychoses. Although the disorders continued to be recognized throughout different periods of history, it was not until recently, in the nineteenth century, that the current diagnostic properties of manic and depressive illness were formally categorized (Sadock, Sadock, & Ruiz, 2009). Initially, the disorders were considered "affective disorders" and *affect* and *mood* are often used interchangeably, but are different. **Affect** is described as " . . . the subjective experience or expression of a feeling state (emotion) . . . in contrast to mood, which refers to a more pervasive and sustained emotional 'climate', affect refers to more fluctuating changes in emotional 'weather'" (First, Frances, & Pincus, 2004, p. 185). The current accepted term used in *DSM-IV-TR* is *mood disorders*.

Many people living in the twenty-first century can identify with the term **depression** because they have some idea of what it feels like to be sad, blue, "under the weather," or to temporarily lose a sense of meaning in their lives. Many people can also identify with the term *mania*, because, due to today's fast-moving society, they have some idea of what it is like to feel "pressured," "pressed," "speedy," or "hyper." Perhaps because of our general ability to experience a range of emotions, depression and mania (to a lesser extent) have become household words.

Perhaps because these terms have become familiar and because, generally, people can identify the emotions associated with each term, beginning clinicians are often not prepared for the depth of the symptoms or for how extremely and strongly mood and behavior are affected. Although recognizing that there is a range of severity of symptoms accompanying depression and mania, this chapter will refer mostly to the extreme syndromes or symptoms of mania and major depression.

DIAGNOSTIC CRITERIA

The *DSM-IV-TR* (APA, 2000) describes a group of disorders with the essential feature of a disturbance in mood that is not due to any other mental or physical disorder, medication, substance use, or other psychiatric condition. These disorders are classified as *mood disorders*. Former classifications described the same disorders as *affective disorders*, so this term may be used interchangeably (Sadock et al., 2009) but as noted above the correct term is mood disorders.

The *DSM-IV-TR* uses three groups of criteria to diagnose problems regarding mood: episodes, disorders, and specifiers that describe a most recent episode and a recurrent course (Morrison, 2007). *DSM-IV-TR* divides mood disorders into bipolar disorders and depressive disorders. The essential feature of a bipolar disorder is the presence of one or more manic episodes (often with a history of at least one major depressive episode). The essential feature of depressive disorders is one or more periods of depression, but not necessarily with a manic episodic history. **Dysthymia** is a milder form of major depressive episode, but it lasts for a longer period of time. **Cyclothymia** is a milder form of bipolar disorder, and it also has a longer duration. Bipolar and depressive disorders range from mild to severe and may include psychotic features. They usually cause considerable distress and/or impairment in all occupational areas of functioning.

Episodes

A mood episode refers to any time at which a client feels abnormally happy or sad. The mood disorders are constructed from these episodes; that is, the episodes are the foundation from which the disorders are arranged (Morrison, 2007).

Major Depressive

At least five of the following symptoms must be present for two weeks and represent a change from previous level of functioning. At least one of the symptoms is either depressed mood or loss of interest and pleasure.

1. Daily depressed mood, indicated by subjective report or the observation of others. In children or adolescents, the mood can be irritable.
2. Very marked decrease of interest or pleasure in most daily activities.
3. Significant weight loss (when not dieting) or weight gain or significant increase or decrease in appetite. For children this could be represented by failure to gain expected weight through normal growth.
4. Inability to sleep or sleeping most of the day.
5. Psychomotor agitation or its opposite, psychomotor retardation.
6. Extreme fatigue or loss of energy.
7. Feelings of extreme worthlessness or inappropriate guilt nearly every day.
8. Indecisiveness or lack of concentration.
9. Recurring thoughts of death, suicidal ideas, or a suicidal plan or attempt.

Manic

There is a distinct period of abnormal, elevated, expansive, or irritable mood lasting at least one week. During this period at least three or more of the following symptoms are significantly present. There may be psychotic features or hospitalization may be necessary to prevent harm to the self or others.

1. Grandiosity or overinflated self-esteem
2. Decreased need for sleep
3. Talking more than usual or pressured talking
4. The experience that thoughts are racing
5. Extreme distractibility
6. Increase in goal-directed activity (this can take form in different areas, e.g., socially, at work or school, or sexually) or psychomotor agitation
7. Excessive involvement in pleasurable activities that have the potential for later painful consequences (such as buying sprees, imprudent investments, or indiscreet sexual activity)

Hypomanic

The elevated mood must last at least four days, be observably different from the usual nondepressed mood, and include three of the symptoms of mania. The episode does not cause marked impairment in occupational or social functioning, call for hospitalization, or include psychotic features.

Mixed

The criteria for both manic and major depressive episodes are met nearly every day for at least one week. The impairment in functioning is identical to that of the manic and major depressive episodes.

Disorders

A disorder is a pattern of illness due to an abnormal mood. Most people who have a mood disorder experience depression at some times, and some also have high moods. Most mood disorders are diagnosed on the basis of a mood episode (Morrison, 2007).

Major Depressive Disorder

A major depressive disorder, single episode, is diagnosed if there is a single major depressive episode and there has never been a manic, mixed, or hypomanic episode. A major depressive disorder, recurrent episode, is diagnosed if there have been two or more major depressive episodes at least two months apart and there has never been a manic, mixed, or hypomanic episode. A dysthymic disorder is a depressed mood that lasts most of the day for a majority of days over at least two years. In children and adolescents the mood can be irritable, and symptoms must be present for at least one year. To qualify for diagnosis, during the period of symptoms, the person should not have been symptom free for more than two months at a time and he or she should have experienced no major depressive, manic, mixed, or hypomanic episode or cyclothymic disorder. There also must be at least two of the following symptoms:

1. Poor appetite or overeating
2. Insomnia or too much sleeping
3. Fatigue
4. Low self-esteem
5. Poor concentration or difficulty with decisions
6. Hopelessness

Bipolar Disorders

The various bipolar disorders are distinguished by the presence of either a manic episode or a major depressive episode. They are classified as either bipolar I or bipolar II, depending on which is the dominant mood. Bipolar I features a dominant manic mood, and bipolar II features a dominant depressed mood. As with the other disorders, the symptoms cause significant distress or impairment in important daily areas of functioning; they are not the result of use of a substance, medication, or medical condition; and they cannot be better accounted for by positing the existence of other disorders.

In bipolar I, single manic episode, there is the presence of a manic episode and there have been no major depressive episodes in the past. In bipolar I, most recent episode hypomanic, there is currently a hypomanic episode and there has been at least one manic or mixed episode in the past. In bipolar I, most recent episode manic, there is a manic episode and there has been at least one major depressive, manic, or mixed episode in the past. In bipolar I, most recent episode mixed, there is a mixed episode and there has been at least one major depressive, manic, or mixed episode in the past. Finally, in bipolar I, most recent episode depressed, there is currently a major depressive episode and there has been in the past at least one manic or mixed episode.

In bipolar II, there is one or more major depressive episodes and at least one hypomanic episode in the past, but there has never been a manic or mixed episode. In cyclothymic disorder there have been periods of hypomanic symptoms with periods of depressive symptoms for at least two years and the person has not been symptom free for more than two months. Moreover, there has been no major depressive, manic, or mixed episode during that time (APA, 2000)

Specifiers

Specifiers are descriptors that help qualify disorders or episodes. One set describes the most recent major depressive episode and manic episode. "Atypical features" describes individuals who eat and sleep a lot, feel weighted down and almost immobile, and are extremely sensitive to rejection. "Melancholic features" describes what can be considered the classic features of depression: early morning awakening with a mood that improves later in the day, loss of appetite, guilt, and feeling slowed down or agitated, with loss of interest and pleasure in those events and experiences that usually bring pleasure. "Catatonia" describes features of either extreme motor hyperactivity or extreme inactivity. "Postpartum onset" describes either a manic or a depressed episode experienced by a woman within a month of giving birth.

The other set of descriptors describes the overall course of a disorder. "With or without full interepisode recovery" describes the presence or absence of symptoms between episodes. "Rapid cycling" describes a person who has had at least four episodes within a year. "Seasonal pattern" describes those who become ill with regularity at the same time each year.

CAUSES, OCCURRENCE, AND THEORIES OF MOOD DISORDERS

In all industrialized countries, major depression is twice as common in females as in males (NIMH, 2011; Sadock et al., 2009); depressive disorders affect 1 in 5 women and 1 in 10 men. Reasons for this difference include hormonal and endocrine system involvement and other gender-related stresses, such as childbirth and social conditions related to women's sex roles (NIMH, 2011; see also Bracegirdle, 1991; Feder, 1990, 1991) and other typical stressors (Harkness et al., 2010). Bipolar disorder is reported to be almost equally common among males and females. Major depression is 1.5 to 3 times more common among relatives of people with the disorder than in the general population. Bipolar disorder clearly occurs at a much higher rate in first-degree relatives. The conventional estimate was up 1.2% of the adult population with bipolar disorder. However, data now indicate that it may be prevalent in up to 5% of the population. The average age of onset of bipolar disorder in the United States is 20 years for men and 25 for women though in more than half of the cases onset is in adolescence. However, the incidence of mood disorders may be increasing in younger age groups: Mood disorders are being diagnosed more often in children and adolescents and there may be a continuum between juvenile and adult mood disorders (Sadock et. al., 2009). The lifetime prevalence of major depressive disorder ranges from 4.4% to 5.8% for those 18 and older though a 12-month prevalence rate was as high as 9.5% (NIMH, 2011), although some (APA, 2000) estimate the prevalence of major depression as high as 26% for women and 12% for men. The age of onset for major depression varies from children to adults but the average age is between 30 and 35 (NIMH, 2011; Sadock et al., 2009). An interesting statistic is that the incidence of depression has increased among individuals who matured after World War II, and the age of onset for a major depressive episode has decreased (Blazer & Hybels, 2008; NIMH, 2011; Pelissolo & Lepine, 2001).

Causes and Occurrence

The causes of mood disorders are unknown; however, most agree that there are multiple factors involved in mood disorders, such as genetic/biochemical, psychosocial, and socio-environmental, which interact in very complex ways (Sadock et al., 2009). Table 8-1 discusses the factors implicated in both mood disorders.

Physical diseases such as Addison's and Cushing's disease, thyroid disorders, diabetes, syphilis, multiple sclerosis, and chronic brain syndromes related to arteriosclerosis may induce depression. Thyroid disorders may also be implicated in bipolar illness, although thyroid disorders are generally ruled out prior to making the bipolar diagnosis. Other physical disorders are associated with depression, including mononucleosis, anemia, malignancies, hypoglycemia, colitis, congestive heart failure, rheumatoid arthritis, and asthma. Some medications are also associated with depression, including antiparkinsonian agents, hormones, steroids, and antihypertensives (Sadock et al., 2009).

Other Theories

Various authors present interesting theoretical ideas regarding major depressive and bipolar illnesses. There was an explosion of information in the 1990s, particularly regarding bipolar illness. When discussing the centrality of cycling to the bipolar disorder, Koukopoulos, Sani, Koukopoulos, and Girardi (2000) believe that there is not a unipolar disorder but more likely recurrent depressions preceded or followed by mild hypomanias, and that cyclothymic or hyperthymic clients belong to the bipolar group. They think of bipolar disorder in terms of energy. There is an increased level of energy in mania and a decreased need for sleep. Periods of excitement, like a fire, consume much energy and may exhaust the biological processes that create it. As a result of this exhaustion, depression occurs and a genetic flaw may then prevent recovery of the energy, leading to long-lasting depression.

Temperament is also related to both major depression and bipolar illness and "affective disorders predominantly arise in persons with great emotional reactivity" (Bylsma, Morris, & Rottenberg, 2008; Koukopoulos et al., 2000, p. 330). Temperaments may be dysthymic (depressive), hyperthymic (manic), irritable, or cyclothymic (cycling) (Akiskal, as cited in Koukopoulos et al., 2000). Although the concept of bipolar I and bipolar II was used in the *DSM-IV-TR*, there is much support (Marneros & Angst, 2010; Marneros, 2000) for a spectrum of disorders on a continuum of affectivity (see Table 8-1) that distinguishes between hypomania, cyclothymia, mania, mania and mild depression, mania and major depression, and major depression and hypomania. Usually there is a normal level of human behavior and activity that moves

TABLE 8-1. Major Etiologic Theories of Depression and Bipolar Illnesses

	Depression	Bipolar
Biochemical	The neuronal response may be influenced by multiple signals from serotonin and other neurotransmitters such as acetylcholine, melatonin, norepinephrine, hormones, or neuropeptides that modulate mood (Loosen et al., 2000). The hypothalamic-pituitary-adrenal (HPA) and hypothalamic-pituitary-thyroid (HPT) systems are believed to be involved in major depression (Sadock et al., 2009).	As in depression, the neuronal response may be influenced by multiple signals from serotonin and other neurotransmitters such as acetylcholine, melatonin, norepinephrine, hormones, or neuropeptides that modulate mood (Loosen et al., 2000).
Neuroendocrine	Almost half of those with major depression show a higher secretion of cortisol than those who are not depressed. The level returns to normal when depression abates. A small dose of thyroid hormone accelerates the effects of antidepressants in women and for both sexes the hormone is responsible for making those who do not respond to antidepressants more responsive than usual (Loosen et al., 2000).	Stress affects the hypothalamic-pituitary-adrenal (HPA) axis; the HPA then disrupts social and circadian rhythms, leading to mood instability (Hlastala & Frank, 2000).
Genetic	Family studies, twin studies, and adoption studies support the role of genes in transmission of major depressive disorder (Tsuang & Faraone, 2000; Sadock et al., 2009).	Family studies, twin studies, and adoption studies support the role of genes in transmission of bipolar disorder (Tsuang & Faraone, 2000).
Socio-environmental	Life events, particularly the death or loss of a loved one. Support for other predisposing factors in combination with life events is the fact that fewer than 20% of those who report a loss become depressed. Problems with attachment or affectional bonds in early childhood predispose the individual to depressive episodes with later loss and trauma (Bowlby, 1988; Cassidy & Shaver, 2008).	Life events, such as a change in social roles (becoming a parent or getting a divorce), changes in routines (travel across time zones), loss (death of a loved one), or birth of a child (Hlastala & Frank, 2000) precipitate manic episodes.
Psychosocial	Behavioral theories concerning control and reinforcement predominated in the late twentieth century; currently, however, a popular behavioral theory is that depression develops when a person cognitively misinterprets life events and develops a cognitive triad of a negative view of self, of the experience, and of the future. The views one keeps in the mind are called schemas or schemata and all events become interpreted through the negative schemata (Beck, 1973, 1976; Loosen et al., 2000). Seligman (cited in Sadock et. al., 2009) proposed that depression results from learned helplessness—a belief that it is futile to initiate action because the action will not prevent adversity.	People with bipolar illness may be affected by family members and relatives who often explicitly express (often critical) emotions. These high emotion expression (HEE) families may promote relapses in the early stages of the illness, depending on the bipolar person's style, self-concept, age, psychological status, rehabilitation planning, and social environment (Mundt, Kronmuller, & Backenstraf, 2000; Myin-Germeys et al., 2003).

TABLE 8-1. Continued

	Depression	Bipolar
Psychophysiological	Affective disturbance is associated with lack of daylight (called seasonal affective disorder, or SAD). People tend to be depressed in fall and winter, but not so in spring and summer (Lewy et al, 2009).	Physiological cycles are influenced by the seasons and the environment, so in bipolar illness the individual is not able to mediate adaptation to changes in the physical environment (Koch, 2010; Koukopoulos et al., 2000; Rosenthal, 2009).

© Cengage Learning 2013

between the two poles of depression and mania. However, with some people there is a disruption of the normal homeostasis, with resulting restriction as in depressive disorders or expansion as in bipolar disorders. The spectrum has expanded to encompass diagnostic subgroups called *soft bipolar spectrum* (described by Akiskal, as cited in Marneros & Angst, 2000b, p. 26). Likewise, the DSM-V mood disorder work group proposes that severity dimensions of factors that determine treatment outcome be included with the categorical mood diagnosis. They propose an anxiety and suicide assessment dimension across all mood disorder categories (updated June 3, 2010). They also are considering a substance abuse severity dimension. There is also consideration that Premenstrual Dysphoric Disorder (PMDD) could be a separate and distinct disorder from mood disorders or a specifier for mood disorders.

This soft spectrum of affectivity (Marneros, 2000; Marneros & Angst, 2000b) would include a bipolar III classification of recurrent depression that changes to hypomania with antidepressant treatment and the speculation that people with hyperthymic temperaments belong to the bipolar spectrum and that certain personality disorders, such as histrionic-sociopathic or borderline-narcissistic, may belong to cyclothymic temperaments. Support for this soft spectrum could be found in the fact that 84% of those who have a bipolar disorder also have another disorder. Of those who have a comorbid condition, over 50% have an Axis I or Axis III disorder and up to 30% have a coexisting Axis II personality disorder. However, these subgroups need to be researched further to move beyond speculation.

The kindling and sensitization model of recurrent affective disorders (Bender & Alloy, 2011; Hlastala & Frank, 2000) proposes that people with bipolar illness become so sensitized to stress because of so many episodes that they eventually only require the slightest stimulus to precipitate an episode. Also, the episodes will be increasingly severe and time between episodes will shorten. So far, research has been equivocal, with about an equal number of studies supporting or not supporting the hypothesis. Age, symptom severity, type of bipolar illness, and other factors, such as self-esteem, relationships, social support, and personality, may be important mediating factors in the role of sensitization as well as a newer theory of a behavioral activation system, responsible for motivation, action, and goal striving that is overreactive (Bender & Alloy).

Another interesting speculation (Crow, 2000) is an evolutionary theory connecting the division of the spheres of the brain and language acquisition with bipolar disorders as well as psychotic disorders. This theory proposes that the same gene responsible for the evolution of language in humans was also responsible for the psychoses. Furthermore, the psychoses and affective disorders can be viewed on a continuum, with the schizophrenic disorders developing first in a person followed later by the affective disorders. Crow puts forth evidence for his hypothesis by correlating the psychotic symptoms of thought insertion, withdrawal, and broadcast and auditory hallucinations with a language disorder (indeed, they are classified as disorders of language in *DSM-IV-TR*). Additionally, some affective symptoms, such as pressured speech or mutism, are also disorders of speech production. Further evidence that the disorders relate to brain lateralization are that affective disorders are often associated with spatial orientation and face recognition difficulty generally attributed to the nondominant hemisphere. Also, many who have psychotic or affective disorders are ambidextrous, and thus lateralization is not specialized.

Another evolutionary theory (Gilbert, 2000) focuses on depression. The author proposes that an evolutionary-biological model, the social competition model, is involved in mood disorders, primarily depression. According to this model, humans, like nonhuman primates, developed strategies for dominance and control or submission in conflicts that are related ultimately to survival. In every conflict a person has to decide if she or he can be victorious (dominate and control) or not. Just as in other evolutionary mechanisms like attachment, if one assesses a situation to be such that she or he cannot win, then she or he will involuntarily trigger submission strategies. These dominant or submission strategies involve actual behavior to fight or flee and internal mechanisms to read the situation and activate or deactivate physiological mechanisms, such as arousal or inhibition of the HPT axis.

Sloman and Gilbert (2000) propose that depressed people find themselves in situations or instances that can be actual or imagined that they believe they cannot control. Therefore, "involuntary defeat strategies" (IDS) are activated. Thus the individual avoids defeat and accommodates to control. However, the depression results when the IDS are not deactivated and areas for fight are suppressed and flight are blocked. The IDS continue and result in physiological and intrapsychic signals that both lead to depression and continue the maladaptive strategies. Some situations typical of arrested fight and resulting anger of suppression are dependence on the object of one's own anger as in a boss who could fire an employee, or a spouse who could leave the partner, or fear of making a fool of oneself, or shame for one's anger. Some typical situations of arrested flight leading to feelings of entrapment are external, such as loss of resources or lack of alternatives, or internal, such as fear of asking for help due to worry about what the other may think, fear that one cannot cope alone, or moral concerns about hurting others and resulting guilt. Ironically, the same cortical advantages that humans evolved that enable self-awareness, self-evaluation, anticipation, and planning are also responsible for the maladaptive internalization of signals that activate the subordinate psychobiological response patterns.

CLINICAL PICTURE

Most people experience varying moods at different times in their lives. Generally, moods can be described as ranging from happiness, elation, and joy to sadness, despair, and hopelessness. The usual feelings that one experiences in daily life should not be confused with the syndromes of mania and depression. Most happy, energetic people do not have a manic disorder, and unhappiness or sadness does not signal a depressive disorder. Both the manic and depressive disorders can be viewed according to the degree and duration of symptoms. Like other disorders they have to be viewed in the context of how an individual usually functions and to what degree and how long a change in function occurs.

Individuals experiencing a manic episode present themselves with a very elevated mood and their behavior is generally very expansive and irritable. There is heightened psychomotor activity, and they speak, think, and move very rapidly. Usually they have seemingly boundless energy. Often they feel very creative, and indeed, they are usually flooded with some ideas that are imaginative. Popular lore would have us envy those who are manic for their creative qualities. However, although there may be heightened motor activity, there is usually little productivity. An individual who is manic rarely completes projects; attention is fragmented and activity has a purposeless quality to it. Increased activity often takes the form of sexual provocativeness and promiscuity, exaggerated political and religious concern, or purchasing many expensive items regardless of their affordability. Essentially, all activities are carried out with a gross lack of judgment.

An individual who is manic may be euphoric and have an infectious quality, but there is also an accompanying quality of being "driven." He or she may be humorous but, due to a low frustration tolerance, may also easily become irritable and angry. The grandiose behavior and sense of importance may give way to psychotic delusions. It is not unusual to think that one is God, and an individual may show considerable contempt for other people. Due to this grandiosity; frequent, loud speech; and an interruptive manner accompanied by poor social judgment, those with manic behavior are often socially rejected (Kaplan & Sadock, 1989, 1991). Often, beginning professionals find it difficult to simply "be with" someone who is manic, and therefore should seek out clinical supervision for assistance in tolerating this behavior and working effectively.

In my clinical experience, in the realm of occupational therapy, their heightened activity, difficulty concentrating and attending to tasks, distractibility, and intrusiveness often make individuals experiencing a manic episode candidates for individual treatment with engagement in simple concrete tasks or movement. Working with those who are manic often calls on one's best idea of the therapeutic use of self and the use of a full repertoire of interpersonal skills. At the same time, it also calls for the use of concrete and simple tasks or activities. The seeming contradiction involving requirements of simplicity, on one hand, and the use of complex interpersonal skills, on the other, is often confusing and difficult for new clinicians. Again, this is a time to seek out clinical supervision. Table 8-2 lists major symptoms of mania and depression.

Individuals with major depression present themselves as hopeless with a very despairing mood and their behavior is usually passive and withdrawn. There is usually a marked lack of energy, and they speak, think, and move very slowly. However, this psychomotor retardation (slow movements) can also be accompanied by anxiety and agitation, called *psychomotor agitation*. Often, the person complains of not experiencing pleasure, and indeed, is often unable to accept or experience humor in naturally humorous situations. The person with major depression will experience most activity as overwhelming and burdensome. Often, the person will be unable to initiate activity or may vacillate and be unable to make a decision, even the simplest of ones.

Often individuals have trouble concentrating or organizing thinking, usually feel worthless, and make many negative statements about themselves. Often they feel an overwhelming sense of guilt for some imaginary crimes and they often imagine that they are the cause of someone else's misfortune (called **referential thinking**).

TABLE 8-2. Clinical Picture: Major Symptoms of Depression and Mania

Symptoms	Depression	Mania
Emotional	Depleted mood	Euphoric mood
	Hopelessness	Grandiosity
	Decreased sense of humor	
	Lack of pleasure	
Cognitive	Negative thinking	Grandiose, expansive thinking
	Decreased concentration and attention	Decreased concentration and attention
	Indecision	
Motivational	Decreased energy	Increased energy
	Paralysis of will and initiation	Agitation
	Avoidance or escapist wishes	Distraction
		Low frustration tolerance
Self-concept	Worthlessness	Inflated sense of worth and power
	Guilt	
Vegetative	Loss of appetite	Loss of appetite
	Sleep disturbance	Sleep disturbance
	Loss of sexual desire	Increased sexual preoccupation

Because of their negativity, hopelessness, ambivalence, and lack of humor, they may repel people. The palpable depressed mood or agitated behavior can be difficult to be around. Also, their indecision and ambivalence may make them appear overly dependent. Just as with a person who is manic, it may be difficult for new clinicians to empathize with a person who is depressed, or to tolerate dependency. There may be a tendency to push persons with depression to do things that they are unable to do, or to reject their dependent behavior. If this is the case, then seeking clinical supervision for assistance is indicated just as it is in working with people who are manic.

Suicidal thoughts are experienced by some people who suffer from depression (Beck, 1973; see also Hemphill, 1992). The most dangerous periods often are in the beginning, usually when the person is most anxious and help is not present, and in the later remission period, when the person begins to feel better and then may become frightened of a relapse. At this time, he or she will have regained energy and be able to think clearly enough to commit suicide. It is important to take suicidal statements seriously and inquire if an individual has the means (usually a gun or pills) and a formulated plan. All statements and other information should be immediately reported to the primary therapist and the treatment team.

In the occupational therapy clinic, people who are depressed may have difficulty initiating any task or may protest often that they can do nothing. They may require much prompting and activities that are concrete and simple. They may take a very long time to complete a task or obsess over a perceived error. An individual who is manic may display the opposite behavior, initiating too many tasks, stating that he or she can do everything and anything, flitting from task to task, denying any errors, and requiring much attention and prompting to contain or stop behavior.

In community settings people who are depressed will be unobtrusive and quiet and may seem shy or asocial. They may not be noticed because they typically will not initiate conversation or actions and will not be participative. They may display ambivalence and take time to choose or make a decision. While those who have depression may be unnoticed, those who are on the manic spectrum may present the opposite picture. They may seem obtrusive and interfering and somewhat obnoxious. They may initiate conversation or act impulsively or they may "take over" in a conversation or group. Indeed, they may interrupt any occupation; for example, when I have been sitting in a café reading quietly, an individual who is hypermanic has interfered and initiated conversation more than once, and the interaction stops only when I have ended it.

COMMON EVALUATION AND MANAGEMENT

There are some common strategies of evaluation and management for depressive and manic disorders that are recognized by most disciplines working in psychiatric settings.

Evaluation

The intensity, severity, and duration of symptoms are obtained by observation, interview, and history taking. Since life events such as loss or psychosocial stressors (e.g., divorce or abusive relationships) are implicated in the timing of both depressive and manic episodes (APA, 2002, 2010; Hlastala & Frank, 2000; Hundt, Nelson-Gray, Kimbrel, Mitchell, & Kwapil, 2007), a life events inventory may be used to supplement a careful history. Some scales are used by other professionals, most notably, the Hamilton Rating Scale for Depression (HRSD) and the Beck Depression Inventory (BDI) (Beck, 1978), and later, similar versions (Burns, 1989), which are easily answered questions referring to symptoms. Due to biological research there are also tests that measure the disorders by various biological means (Sadock et al., 2009). However, they are expensive and their use and diagnostic efficiency are still questionable.

Usually, symptoms of mania, such as pressured speech, psychomotor agitation, and grandiosity, are easily observable. An interview and a recent history usually supplement the evaluation. Often, family members may aid in the history. The task is to differentiate the types of bipolar illness from major depressive disorder and other psychotic disorders.

People with major depression and bipolar illness will often have other disorders concurrently with the manic or depressive ones. Having more than one condition at the same time is called comorbidity. Alcohol abuse is frequently comorbid with major depression and bipolar disorders (APA, 2002, 2010; Kassel & Veilleux, 2010). There is a relationship between substance abuse and emotional disorders but the nature of it is not well understood. Because it changes over time and the relationship is stronger for dependence than abuse. The prevalence of anxiety and depression is significantly higher among substance abusers relative to those who use but do not abuse. Those who have higher levels of emotional distress are more likely to use and abuse drugs and people who abuse drugs are more likely to experience disorders of mood. The relationship between emotional disorders and substance use problems is stronger for women than for men, and comorbidity rates differ by country and ethnicity.

Panic and obsessive-compulsive disorders are common with depression (APA, 2010) and over 50% of those with bipolar disorder are said to have a comorbid major disorder or physical condition, while over 30% have a comorbid personality disorder (Marneros, 2000). In one interesting study (Kotov, Gamez, Schmidt, & Watson, 2010) of the correlation between major higher order personality traits (called the Big Five or Big Three Factors) in which most people are considered to have a combination or different degrees of neuroticism, disinhibition, extaversion, openness, agreeableness, and conscientiousness, the mental disorders of depression, anxiety, and substance abuse have similar factors or are linked by their traits. These disorders were linked most strongly by the factors of high neuroticism and low conscientiousness followed by low extraversion.

Management

Psychotherapy and medications are common methods of managing depression and bipolar disorders (APA, 2002, 2010; Belmaker & Yaroslavsky, 2000; Gabbard, 2009; Leahy, 2004; Maj, Totorella, & Bartoli, 2000; Moller & Grunze, 2000; Sadock et al., 2009; Thase, 2000). The kindling and desensitization hypothesis has resulted in more aggressive treatment for the first episodes, primarily for bipolar disorders, less so for major depression, with the belief that later episodes will be prevented or that they will be less severe and shorter in duration. Indeed there is now evidence that each manic or depressive episode is associated with decrements in the neuroprotective brain-derived neurotropic factor (BDNF); that is, each episode can facilitate changes in the brain neurons or systems and make the brain more vulnerable to the illness. Therefore, early and sustained treatment is advocated (Sadock et al., 2009).

Medicines that are mood stabilizers for bipolar disorder are lithium and anti-convulsants such as carbamazepine and valproate (Nasrallah, Ketter, & Kalali, 2006). Sometimes antipsychotic medicines, including the newer ones, such as clozapine, are used for acute manic episodes (Sadock et al., 2009). Some (Belmaker & Yaroslavsky, 2000) advocate "rational polypharmacy," a combination of anticonvulsants, lithium, and neuroleptics, and believe that since mania is a symptom of both bipolar I and II that it should be the target of treatment (Koukopoulos et al., 2000).

Optimal medicines for major depression are selective serotonin reuptake inhibitors (SSRIs) and tricyclic medicines; common brand names are Norpramin, Vivactil, Aventyl, Ludiomil, Celexa, Lexapro, Prozac, Luvox, Paxil, Zoloft, Elavil, Tofranil, Effexor, Cymbalta, Wellbutrin, and Anafranil, and so on. The medicines are grouped according to the serotonin site that they influence and their mechanism of action, that is, presynaptic, postsynaptic, or both (Sadock et al., 2009). Monoamine oxidase inhibitors (MAOIs) are recommended for those who do not respond to other medicine, and electroconvulsive therapy (ECT) is still an option for those who are unresponsive to treatment (Sadock et al., 2009). A combination of medicine and psychotherapy is more effective than medicine alone for those with dysthymia. Those who have comorbid obsessive-compulsive, avoidant, dependent, borderline, or narcissistic personality disorders respond to SSRIs and MAOIs rather than tricyclics (APA, 2001).

Evidence-based practice indicates that cognitive-behavioral therapy (CBT) and interpersonal therapy (IPT) are the most effective psychotherapy treatments for depression (Hollon & DeRubeis, 2004; Markowitz, 1998; Markowitz & Weissman, 2009; Scott, 2004), particularly for acute episodes (Roth & Fonagy, 2005; Sadock et al., 2009). These therapies work for short-term episodes and when given from 4 to 20 sessions. However, their efficacy becomes weaker after 20 sessions. Also, the two therapies have not proved to be as effective for severe depression, though IPT was more effective than CBT for more severe depression and more recent studies indicated that cognitive therapy and medicine were equally effective (Hollon & DeRubeis, 2004). Behavior therapy may be as effective as CBT and IPT, but there have not been enough randomly controlled studies to verify its efficacy (APA, 2010). Marriage and family therapy may be effective for decreasing major depressive symptoms and prevent relapse but if there is marital distress it may delay recovery and increase vulnerability to major depression (APA, 2010). Short-term psychodynamic therapy has not proved to be as effective as CBT and IPT and it is unclear how effective long-term psychoanalytic therapy is for depression. IPT (Frank et al., 2008; Markowitz, 1998; Markowitz & Weissman, 2009) focuses on social and interpersonal relationship functioning. It deals with disturbances between the depressed person and others in the environment. In a very structured way the therapist together with the client determines interpersonal problems in the here and now and then the therapist links the problems to the interpersonal problem area. Usually problem areas are classified as ones of grief (complicated bereavement), role disputes (conflicts with significant others), role transitions (moving, changing jobs), or interpersonal deficits (lack of social skills). The therapist very directively works with the client on two problems that the client determines are most emotionally charged using various techniques such as psychoeducation, prescribing activity and socialization, using contracts, and capitalizing on a therapeutic alliance. Family therapy aids in maintaining support for the individual in the environment. Behavioral therapy for depressive disorders is designed to alter behaviors that may be keeping a person isolated or feeling defeated. It also deals with changing life patterns or situations in the environment that may be negative reinforcers. It may involve skills training, such as assertiveness, self-monitoring, and activity scheduling (APA, 2010). Cognitive therapy (Persons, Davidson, & Tompkins, 2001) is designed to change negative thinking processes that contribute to depression. Distorted thinking is targeted, and the here-and-now therapy interactions and current life situations are the focus for changing thinking.

Research indicates that peer-support interventions are effective for depression (Pfeiffer, Heisler, Piette, Rogers, & Valenstein, 2010). Although a meta-analysis indicated that populations studied were very diverse, peer support was rated as effective as CBT groups. Peer support interventions follow a recovery-based model and have the potential to be cost-effective as well as the ability to reach a broad range of individuals.

More recent therapies for bipolar disorder are Family Focused Therapy (FFT) (David Miklowitz), Interpersonal Social Rhythm Therapy (IPSRT) (Ellen Frank), and a biological approach to depression that integrates other models such as education, coping skills, and family involvement (Stephen Shuchter and Sidney Zisook) (cited in Sadock et al., 2009). These therapies are very much like occupational therapy in different aspects.

Psychoanalytic theories attempt to change personality structure. This means targeting for change an individual's experience of trust, intimacy, dealing with loss, coping mechanisms, and recognition of a range of emotions. Usually problems are thought to stem from relationships in early childhood. The therapy process utilizes *transference*; that is, the client transfers perceptions and feelings about important childhood figures and events to the therapist and the therapy situation. Typically these are then interpreted by the therapist and discussed and explored together. In the short-term versions, the therapist quickly points out transference reactions and immediately uses the present session to explore and correct behavior carried over from the past.

Psychotherapy has been emphasized for bipolar disorder (Gabbard, 2009; Leahy, 2004). Studies (Marneros & Angst, 2000a; Roth & Fonagy, 2005) show that psychosocial events contribute to the first manic episode and to the timing of subsequent episodes, there are role disturbances between episodes, and medicines such as lithium may be effective for only half of those who take it. Also, psychotherapy is indicated because those with most severe symptoms may experience low self-esteem and fear of recurrence and have social consequences to repair. They also may have interpersonal, family, and vocational problems (Hackman, Ram, & Dixon, 1999).

The use of ECT has stirred controversy for many years (Sadock, Sadock, & Ruiz, 2009) although 80% to 90% respond to ECT (APA, 2010). Some claim it caused a permanent loss of memory, while others claim that ECT was the only intervention that aided their recovery. Some people claim that the practice should be outlawed, and it is illegal in several states. Others point to recent advances in administration of the treatment that make it less harmful. Typically 6 to 12 and not more than 20 treatments are administered (APA, 2010). The method of delivery includes giving a general anesthetic along with a muscle relaxant and then placing electrodes usually bilaterally, which causes a seizure consisting of muscular contractions in face, jaw, and plantar extensions for about 30 to 60 seconds. ECT can be extremely effective when there are very severe symptoms, such as psychomotor retardation, early morning awakening, agitation, decreased appetite and weight, psychotic symptoms, or little response to other antidepressant medications (Pagnin, 2004). It is indicated when there is a high risk of suicide or danger to physical health. The mode of action of ECT is thought to be brought about through physiological and biochemical changes in the brain, caused by the seizure. Neurochemical changes are thought to produce changes in neurotransmitter function. Physiological changes are thought to be affected by the reduction of activity in the brain following the seizure.

Studies show an immediate loss of memory shortly after treatment, though clients are back to their baseline memory six months later. Unwanted effects of ECT include anxiety and headache immediately afterward; confusion, nausea, and vertigo a few hours afterward; and some muscle pain. The contraindications include respiratory infections, heart disease, aneurysms, and certain other drugs, such as reserpine. Obviously, the procedure's benefits and risks should be adequately and clearly explained, and the client must sign a standard consent form. Other forms of medicine, such as the newer neurotransmitter drugs, are less controversial (Sadock et al., 2009) but nevertheless, ECT remains a topic of popular discussion.

OCCUPATIONAL THERAPY TREATMENT AND INTERVENTION

Various occupational therapy evaluations may be used depending on which context or performance area and components are being assessed or which occupational therapy model is followed (see Devereaux & Carlson, 1992). There is not yet an occupational therapy assessment specific to depression or bipolar disorders. Notwithstanding that fact, the therapist should always evaluate a client according to the severity of the mood disorder. A person's behavior and statements will indicate the stage of functioning on a *mood continuum*. Where a person's behavior falls on this continuum will indicate a different treatment and interpersonal approach (see Figure 8-1). The following Case Illustrations demonstrate the difference in people's symptoms, whether severely depressed or severely manic. However, despite different symptoms, their behavior fits on the far ends of the mood continuum and therefore necessitates a similar approach and treatment.

Occupational therapists' training in analyzing and grading activities means that interventions can, and should, be tailored for anyone at any stage of the mood continuum. Moreover, an occupational therapist's interpersonal approach should also be tailored to stages of the mood continuum (see Figure 8-1).

At the extreme ends of the continuum, represented by severe depression and hypermania, the therapist's focus is on providing structure and meeting demands. Interventions should be concrete and tangible, and activities should be short term, simple, and success enhancing. The surrounding environment should be carefully

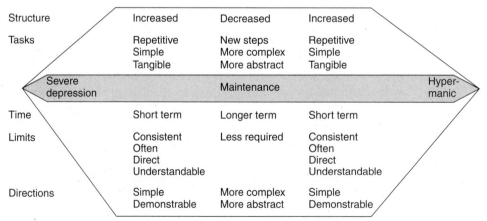

Structure	Increased	Decreased	Increased	
Tasks	Repetitive Simple Tangible	New steps More complex More abstract	Repetitive Simple Tangible	
Severe depression		Maintenance		Hyper-manic
Time	Short term	Longer term	Short term	
Limits	Consistent Often Direct Understandable	Less required	Consistent Often Direct Understandable	
Directions	Simple Demonstrable	More complex More abstract	Simple Demonstrable	

FIGURE 8-1. The Mood Continuum
© Cengage Learning 2013

CASE ILLUSTRATION

Tae—Severely Depressed

On Tuesday, Tae did not show up for the partial hospitalization occupational therapy group, "About Depression." When he was called by his therapist, he reported that he was still in bed, he had been there since Friday, and this was the first time he had answered the phone in three days. He reported that he had been ruminating about his life and obsessively thinking that he had hurt another client because of his remarks in a community meeting at the program. He felt as if he could hardly move from his house. However, after reassurance that he was missed and was expected at the program, he said he would try to make it. With prompting from the therapist that she was counting on him, he agreed to come in the next day. Tae did not come the next day and continued to be homebound and noncommunicative. Because the occupational therapist was able to provide home visits, she went to his home. He answered the door and was cordial and agreed that he needed motivation to leave the house. The therapist and he designed a concrete, step-by-step list of the exact tasks and times that he would accomplish getting out of bed, dressing, leaving the house, and taking the bus to his group. They included incentives, such as the therapist phoning him the next morning, an agreement to call her on his cell phone from the bus-stop, and rewards, such as a café-latte from the hospital café.

Discussion

Tae had difficulty initiating any task and required much prompting to follow through. He obsessed over self-referential remarks that he perceived as wrong and harmful. He responded to concrete and structured behaviors by the OTR including the therapist going to his house, working on written lists with him, phone contacts, and rewards that were usually pleasurable.

CASE ILLUSTRATION

Maria—Hypermanic

Maria entered the occupational therapy group early, bringing five other clients with her. She proceeded to walk around the room, taking something from every cabinet and announcing how she would lead the group. Before the therapist caught up with her, she commented coquettishly on how sexy the occupational therapist looked and suggested that maybe they could get together since she was available. While thanking her for her willingness to assist and her flattering comments, the OTR assured her that he could aptly lead the group and asked her to take a seat.

Discussion

Maria initiated too many tasks, and did so in a grandiose and expansive manner, in addition to making inappropriate remarks to the therapist. Even though her symptoms were quite the opposite of Tae's, she, too, responded to a direct approach by the OTR.

arranged so as not to be too distracting. The therapist also should make decisions, provide clear expectations and parameters for activities, and provide limits on expansive behavior and validation for depressed behavior. The therapist's focus is on creating an external structure for the clients. Craft and exercise activities in short segments of 30 to 45 minutes can be most useful at this stage.

As a person improves and moves toward the middle, maintenance stage of the continuum, more abstract activities with more complex steps that require more time can be incorporated. Activities can include more client decision making and fewer limits. Clients can be expected to take more responsibility for functioning and for reflection on their behavior and thoughts. The therapist's focus is to assist the client to realize his or her internal abilities and resources. Useful groups are daily living and vocational, problem solving, and expressive activities; these can be an hour or longer.

The occupational therapy emphasis on independent functioning often leads beginners to insist on independent functioning and decision making from all people at all times. However, occupational therapy also advocates meeting a person at his or her particular level. If an individual clearly is unable to make independent decisions or to engage in daily activities, the occupational therapist should adjust to meet the demands of the person and the environment. Following the concept of the mood continuum helps a therapist know when to focus on the external or internal environments. It allows the OTR to flexibly provide treatment according to whatever the person (internal environment) and stage of the disorder (external environment) require.

Interpersonal Approach

Many occupational therapists may find themselves charmed by an individual who is manic and drawn to take inordinate responsibility for the individual who is depressed. They may be overwhelmed by overactive, expansive behavior or extreme depression. They may become impatient and frustrated. Beginners often make the mistake of expecting too much and therefore frustrating their clients.

When working with someone who is depressed, it is essential to relate with understanding and empathy. The client will not benefit from a "snap out of it" attitude. The depressed individual already feels sad, worthless, humorless, and, often, guilty. Depressed individuals may subject themselves to mental punishment because they are depressed and have been unable to change their condition. They may be stuck in a cycle of negative ruminations. If depressed people could benefit from badgering, they would not be depressed and would certainly help themselves. Often, the tendency is to treat them in an authoritarian manner, and sometimes staff members are unable to tolerate ruminating or negativistic behavior. Some find it difficult to work with people who may not respond immediately or may not be expressive. Although the tendency may be to "encourage independence" and setting limits or to help people see the brighter, often reality-based, alternative, one should provide the opposite: understanding and empathic responses and a validation of the client's feelings or thoughts. Particularly in the early stages of the disorder, one should permit dependence in the form of information about the depressive process and assurance that the person will get better although he or she may not know or feel it now.

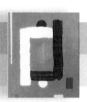

CASE ILLUSTRATION

Lizzie—Handling Depressed Behavior

Initially, when Lizzie came to the occupational therapy group she would often sit alone and refuse to work on anything. She felt as if she could hardly move—as if she had a 100-pound pack on her back. To think about making a decision precipitated panic. She worried that she would never get better and would continue to fall into what she described as a "black hole." When approached, she would only ruminate about the "black hole," and most interactions were negative statements about herself and her past, present, and future life. People on the unit stayed away from her, and the staff avoided her or attempted to provide reality testing by reviewing how her life "really" was. She became more depressed

and hopeless, certain that others hated her, did not understand her, and maybe were unable to help her.

The OTR provided a different approach. She validated Lizzie's statements of how she felt, acknowledged that her state was indeed painful and difficult, and stated that although it seemed there was no light at the end of the tunnel, Lizzie would indeed get better. The therapist shared the information that she had worked with many people who had been severely depressed and had felt similarly hopeless, and that through treatment they did return to former functioning. The OTR was not put off by negative statements and continued to initiate contact. She continued to provide empathic responses and to invite Lizzie to participate in structured groups that included movement and working on very short-term activities. Lizzie's ruminations did not completely stop; however, they decreased. She felt that someone seemed to understand her, did not reject her, and was competent to help. She attempted to participate in groups and began to sense some hope.

Discussion

Lizzie demonstrated symptoms and behaviors of depression, negative ruminations, immobility, and hopelessness. These often are responded to with a positive manner that is not perceived as genuine. However, when the therapist responded in an understanding and validating manner and with structure in activities, Lizzie's behavior changed for the better.

When working with an individual who is experiencing a manic episode, it is also essential to relate with understanding and empathy. Empathy means being present and able to tolerate manic behavior that may be grandiose, obnoxious, intrusive, and egocentric. Just as with someone who is severely depressed, the person who is severely manic does not deliberately desire to be this way. This client will also not benefit from a heavily authoritarian approach, but he or she will benefit when a therapist consistently demonstrates the ability to be with the client and is not "turned off" by the individual's often overwhelming behavior. In addition, the client will benefit from direction providing parameters of acceptable behavior, and an honest appraisal of behavior presented in a gentle yet firm, matter-of-fact way. It is not unusual for clients to recognize, acknowledge, and apologize for their behavior when they are less symptomatic.

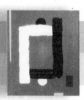

CASE ILLUSTRATION

Jeremy—Handling Manic Behavior

Jeremy entered the occupational therapy evaluation group with expansive, grandiose behavior, talking about why he did not need the group. He spoke in a nonstop, stream-of-consciousness manner, with pressured speech. He was unable to remain in one place and was distracted by almost everybody and everything in the room.

When approached by the OTR, he proceeded to tell her how attractive she was, asked if she was married, and told her how "good" he could be with women. The OTR asked him to begin the assessment. He did not think that he needed to be assessed and stated that, in fact, he could probably "assess" and help her. She stated that she understood that he felt wonderful and probably wanted to make a connection with her, but his behavior was out of line, and, indeed, would distance her, which was probably opposite of what he wanted. Jeremy did begin the assessment but after two minutes, he became distracted in an agitated way and declared to all that this was childish and the OTR "did not have a clue." The OTR gently asked him to return to the activity and continued. Occasionally she validated how agitated and disconnected his behavior made him feel.

When Jeremy's manic behavior subsided, following two weeks of hospitalization and lithium treatment, he thanked the OTR for giving him directions and reminders to return to his activity at a time when he became distracted every few minutes. He also apologized for any behavior that was offensive or insulting, adding that he actually liked the therapist because she was able to tolerate and withstand sexual innuendoes by pointing out what was not acceptable and did so without becoming angry or withdrawing from him.

Discussion

The OTR's approach to Jeremy's manic behavior was also empathic, direct, and consistent, demonstrating her ability to tolerate his behavior and, therefore, conveying that she valued him.

Person-to-Person Interventions

Evidence-based practice supports cognitive-behavioral and interpersonal therapies in psychotherapy, primarily for clients with depression and less so for those with bipolar illnesses. As yet there are few research studies that support occupational therapy in general. However, in practice occupational therapists may use techniques or strategies specified by CBT or IPT. In fact, occupational therapists implicitly may have used some of the interventions from both schools, such as focusing on thoughts, activity schedules, and social skills training, for many decades. Occupational therapy also focuses on some of the same areas specified in CBT or IPT manuals, such as role disputes and transitions, explicit rehabilitation planning, or job coaching for employment. Although research should validate the efficacy of occupational therapy's unique contributions (for interesting avenues of research, see Gutman & Biel, 2001), specifying the use of CBT and IPT strategies in practice would provide common ground for dialogues with other professions and eventually might differentiate the uniqueness of occupational therapy strategies and dimensions from these other domains.

Following are practical occupational therapy interventions that can be delivered in a way that makes use of techniques or strategies specified by other schools of therapy. Treatment addresses all symptoms—emotional, cognitive, motivational, self-concept, and vegetative. See Table 8-2 for symptoms of depression and mania.

Particularly when addressing motivational symptoms, occupational therapy provides interventions that directly relate to changing behavior. For an individual who is depressed, it provides evidence of the ability to continue with occupations of everyday life and provides concrete proof, often through working with and mastering crafts, of a continued ability to function. For an individual who is manic, it provides concrete structure through which to focus attention. Concrete evidence of a remaining ability to function combats helplessness and distractibility with hope and defense, which are key motivational symptoms.

Occupational therapy can experientially contract or disprove negative thoughts through its focus on functioning in the everyday occupations and activities of daily life. Occupational therapy can intervene in the depressed person's negative cycle of misconstruing experiences as defeating, regarding oneself as deficient or morally defective, and viewing the future in a negative way. Through its focus on the activities of daily life, occupational therapy can intervene in the manic person's expansive and grandiose cycle by providing a structured environment and activities through which to organize and monitor behavior. Tables 8-3 and 8-4 outline the symptoms, problems, and interventions involved in depression and mania (see also Boswell, 1989; Centoni & Tallant, 1986; Devereaux & Carlson, 1992; Feder, 1991; Hutcheson, Ferguson, Nish, & Gill, 2010; Meyers, 1991; Stein & Smith, 1989).

Table 8-3 focuses on interventions for depression. Pervasive symptoms of depression lead to problems in all areas of performance, patterns, and skills (AOTA, 2008) particularly cognitive and social. Treatment focuses on changing behavior, changing the environment, or changing internal appraisals. The most prevalent emotional symptoms of depression will manifest in a loss of volition (Cole, 2010) and loss of interest in formerly valued activities or the pursuit of only one interest in an exclusive and/or compulsive manner. The individual will tend to withdraw from others and become isolated. Sleep will be disordered. Some common interventions are to engage the individual in activities that he or she values or has valued in the past and to provide opportunities to engage in different activities or in activities within a group setting. Sometimes an individual will be reluctant to engage in any activities or group; however, the therapist should maintain an approach that is inviting and confident without being authoritarian and overly demanding. Providing activities that do not require too many choices or steps to complete, and perhaps allowing a person to work while in the presence of others but not necessarily interact, will enhance engagement. A more behavioral intervention is to ask the client to monitor the pleasure or value received from working on, and completing, an activity. This can be a self-report, and it often is more effective if a simple, concrete scale is constructed. When a person is less severely depressed (on the mid-stage of the mood continuum), values clarification activities may be introduced.

Cognitive and motivational symptoms will manifest in indecision and ambivalence, difficulty concentrating and attending, difficulty initiating or sustaining activities, and the expression of negative thoughts predominantly rather than positive ones. Activities or occupations that do not require too many choices, can

TABLE 8-3. Interventions for Depression

Symptoms	Problems	Interventions
Emotional	Loss of interest in formerly valued activities or pursuit of narrow or single interests exclusively and in a compulsive manner. Tendency to isolate oneself and withdraw from others.	Engage in valued activities. Expand opportunities to engage in other than one activity. Monitor value and pleasure while doing or completing activities and engage in values clarification activities.
Cognitive and motivational	Indecision and ambivalence. Inability to concentrate and attend to usual daily activities. Negative attitudes that predominate in all usual activities. Inability to initiate or sustain activity. Tendency to isolate.	Engage in group activities, Initially provide occupations and do not require too many choices. Provide opportunities to successfully accomplish short-term, simple, concrete activities. Engage in movement activities and mindfulness-based activities. Set realistic, step-by-step goals and behavioral "to do" lists, grading activities and environment for successful completion. Reestablish normal routines: structured planning of daily occupations, simple behavioral lists. Engage in cognitive therapy (i.e., recognizing, monitoring, and changing thoughts). Perform reality testing and question unrealistic beliefs. Engage in psychoeducational groups concerning symptoms and behavior, such as recognizing precursors to mood changes and managing medicines.
Self-concept	Worthlessness and guilt.	Provide opportunities to successfully accomplish short-term, simple, concrete activities. Set realistic, step-by-step goals and behavioral "to do" lists; grading activities and environment for successful completion. Perform cognitive therapy; challenge distorted ideas. Engage in activities that focus on self-exploration, such as recognizing and dealing with emotions, self-expression, and self-exploration through creative media and expanding coping styles.
Vegetative	Failure to sustain basic needs for food, rest, etc.	Provide external structure.

TABLE 8-4. Interventions for Mania

Symptoms	Problems	Interventions
Emotional	Overinflated or exaggerated interest and meaning attributed to all areas of life.	Offer an honest, realistic appraisal of behavior and end products while engaging in activities or occupations. Elicit clients' appraisals and reflection regarding their behavior and end products after engaging in activities.
Cognitive and motivational	Increased energy resulting in distractibility, initiation of too many activities, and inability to sustain activity. Inability to concentrate and attend to usual daily activities. Inability to follow through on decisions. Unrealistically positive attitudes that predominate in all usual daily activities.	Provide opportunities to engage in concrete, short-term activities that include more than two steps. Use mindfulness-based therapies. Provide clear expectations for behavior and end products. Arrange a distraction-free environment. Assist client to return to goal-directed action whenever distracted. Eventually assist in goal setting and planning and in anticipating the consequences of actions by monitoring behavior during activities.
Self-concept	Inflated, unrealistic sense of worth and efficacy. Failure to take responsibility for consequences of behavior.	Display an accepting, tolerant attitude. Offer an honest, realistic appraisal of behavior and end products while engaging in occupations. Engage in activities that focus on self-exploration, such as recognizing and dealing with emotions, self-expression, and self-exploration through creative media and expanding coping styles.
Vegetative	Failure to sustain basic needs.	Provide external structure.

© Cengage Learning 2013

be accomplished successfully in a short time, and are tangible may enhance a person's motivation and self-concept. More behavioral interventions of setting and listing step-by-step, easily achieved goals and crossing them off when accomplished will enhance motivation. Cognitive interventions, such as recognizing and monitoring negative thoughts, changing the internal "tapes" one plays over and over, and questioning unrealistic beliefs can be directed toward cognitive symptoms. Psychoeducational groups concerning symptoms, behavior, recognizing precursors to mood changes, managing medicines, and expanding coping strategies can also address cognitive problems.

Symptoms that relate to one's self-concept are expressed as feelings or thoughts of worthlessness or guilt. Again, short-term, concrete activities that can be quickly mastered and completed will add to a person's sense of self. In addition, behavioral interventions that show that goals have been achieved usually also enhance self-esteem. Cognitive interventions that directly challenge self-distortions and expressive interventions that focus on self-awareness, self-expression, and self-exploration will model the power of self-reflection and self-expression. Self-exploration can also include exploring and changing styles of coping. Again, it is important to be aware of where a person is located on the mood continuum when introducing interventions that require energy, initiation, imagination, and problem solving.

Table 8-4 focuses on interventions for mania. Emotional symptoms of mania will usually manifest in a person having an overinflated or exaggerated interest in various activities and perhaps attributing excessive meaning to all objects and people in life. Interventions can center around engagement in activities or occupations. The occupational therapist can offer honest, realistic appraisals of an individual's behavior while engaged in activities or can make honest, realistic appraisals of end products. The therapist may elicit the client's appraisal and reflection concerning his or her own behavior and products. Sometimes reality testing (e.g., Socratic questioning) utilizing an appropriate tone may be productively employed, even though this may not bring about an immediate change in behavior. Again, the approach depends on where the behavior is located on the mood continuum.

Cognitive and motivational symptoms may result in distractibility, inability to concentrate and attend, and a desire to initiate too many activities, usually all at once. Once activities have been initiated there may be difficulty following through, and in spite of this inability, there may also be an unrealistic appraisal of the person's abilities. Just as with an individual who is depressed, it is important to provide opportunities to engage in concrete, short-term activities that do not contain many steps. It is also important to provide an environment with few distractions, including noises and visual stimulation. In addition, whenever possible the OTR should provide clear expectations for behavior and assist the client to return to the goal whenever he or she becomes distracted.

Symptoms involving one's concept of self will usually result in the expression of inflated, unrealistic ideas about oneself and one's effectiveness, often accompanied by a failure to assume responsibility for any consequences related to one's behavior. An approach that is genuine, authentic, and accepting, even while offering clear limits, is suggested, along with an honest, realistic appraisal of the person's behavior and the end products. It is particularly important to assess where a person with mania is located on the mood continuum. Those on the farther ends may have difficulty being in, and may indeed disrupt, a group setting. Engaging in self-exploration and self-expression can be helpful for symptoms relating to self-concept and for expanding coping styles, but these interventions are usually most helpful when a person has moved to the middle of the mood continuum.

System Interventions

Intervention strategies in different programs (Hackman, Ram, & Dixon, 1999; Linroth, Zander, Forde, Hanley, & Lins, 1996) address both depression and bipolar illness. Often the community or outpatient (Yakobina, Yakobina, & Tallant, 1997) programs use CBT and IPT strategies.

People with severe depression and bipolar illness may require continuing care after hospitalization. Typically, they may be referred for maintenance for a period of time in a partial hospitalization or day treatment program. Often the day program consists of various levels of treatment directed to people with illnesses varying from severe to mild. Sometimes treatment will take place in the clients' homes or other places in the community (Hackman, Ram, & Dixon, 1999). Usually, there is an intake period where the clients and staff can observe each other and make decisions about which treatment groups would be most beneficial. Then there is a period of time in which the clients work in groups to achieve goals that they have established themselves. Prior to discharge, clients often will anticipate how to prevent relapses after they have left the program. Sometimes there are visits within a few months or a year for "tuneups" (Linroth et al., 1996). Self-help centers (Swarbrick & Ellis, 2009) and peer-support self-help groups, mentioned earlier (Pfeiffer et al., 2010), are also recovery-based programs that provide empowerment, advocacy, socialization, recreation, coping skills, and prevention of relapses.

Groups often address skill development, problem solving, managing symptoms, coping with daily life stressors, simply recognizing pleasure and humor, and self-awareness (including not being so intense) (Linroth et al., 1996). Groups also address employment and vocational issues (Helfrich & Rivera, 2006; see also Hees, Koeter, deVries, Ooterman, & Schene, 2010, for a randomized controlled pilot study in the workplace), managing and coping with stigmatizing behaviors from others, medicine compliance, and family psychoeducation (Hackman, Ram, & Dixon, 1999). These latter groups are particularly important for people with bipolar illness who have more of a community than previously was thought (Hackman, Ram, & Dixon, 1999; Kusznir Scott, Cooke, & Young,1996; Tse & Walsh, 2001).

Following are the treatment processes for Lizzie and Jeremy, which illustrate occupational therapy interventions.

CASE ILLUSTRATION

Lizzie—Treatment Process

Observation while performing crafts from the Allen Diagnostic Module (Earhart, Allen, & Blue, 1993) indicated that Lizzie was slow to engage, and many comments indicated a lack of interest in what she was doing. A self-report checklist adapted from the Burns Depression

Checklist (Burns, 1989) indicated a high score of 40, indicating particularly that Lizzie felt very sad, discouraged, worthless, inferior, guilty, and unattractive. She was indecisive and irritable, had lost interest in life, and was generally unmotivated. An Occupational Performance History interview (OPHI-II) indicated a history of being newly divorced. She worried about losing her job due to downsizing and feared she would not be able to support her two children. She had become isolated, stopped going to work, and attempted suicide. She felt guilty that she was now hospitalized.

The Occupational Self Assessment (Baron, Kielhofner, Iyenger, Goldhammer, & Wolenski, 2002) indicated that Lizzie liked to cook and bake; she had formerly enjoyed tennis and running and had belonged to a book club. Since her marital separation she had not pursued any of these activities. She reported that she had a few close friends but had withdrawn from them because she felt she was a burden and was generally not presentable to people. She did not see the point in participating in occupational therapy groups since she was feeling hopeless and negative about the present and future. However, she agreed to attend some groups.

Initially she attended a movement/exercise group after being sought out by the leader every day. It was difficult for her to follow the simple exercises, though she eventually did look forward to the group and expressed relief that she could just follow directions and did not have to initiate interactions. At the same time she attended a parallel group where people worked on individual craft projects, and after a few days she finally agreed to start a project after admiring another member's finished work. She found that, although she generally had negative things to say about the project, she actually felt some sense of accomplishment. She also was relieved that she did not have to make decisions or "process her feelings." Within a week she had become an active member and finished projects for both herself and her children.

After a few days, she attended a "Learning about Depression" workshop. She enjoyed receiving a handout about depression, and she was surprised at what she learned from the different theories. She gave the handout to her family and they were able to discuss their concerns about her.

Lizzie was discharged to a partial hospitalization program. She attended a medication management group, a "Learning about Feelings" group, and a group titled, "Preventing Depression/Coping Differently" three times a week in the occupational therapy program. In addition, she participated in a sports group and a community resource group, in which she identified resources in the community, such as Parents without Partners and a 12-step group addressing self-confidence. The OTR worked individually with her to help her learn vocational skills and interests. She completed a vocational assessment (APTICOM®), consisting of aptitude, interest, and skills tests (Vocational Research Institute, cited in Asher, 1996). She began to focus on obtaining a job and to explore alternative careers. She eventually attended the partial program one day a week while she began to work at a new job three days a week. Eventually she began to work full-time and was discharged from the day program. She enjoyed a continuing education group sponsored by the partial program, which focused on self-exploration through creative media.

Discussion

Initially, Lizzie was severely depressed but without cognitive impairment, as indicated on the assessments. Her occupational profile yielded her former interests and present concerns. An analysis of occupational performance identified client factors such as guilt, isolation, and fear that were barriers to engagement in occupation and strengths such as her intellect and intact communication skills. The analysis also identified the contexts, such as work, sports, and community self-help programs in which she desired participation. She responded initially to structured interventions that did not require too much independent decision making and would demonstrate her ability to continue to function. She was able to utilize information regarding her disease, and later, as she improved, to utilize interventions that required more thought and independent decision making. She also responded to a reasoned approach of empathy and validation of her experience.

CASE ILLUSTRATION

Jeremy—The Treatment Process

During his hospitalization, Jeremy was able to attend a directive group (Kaplan, 1986). With structured treatment directed toward his behavior that initially was represented on the extreme ends of the mood continuum (see Figure 8-1), his mood stabilized and he prepared for discharge by attending a "Recovery in the Community" predischarge group. This group essentially engaged members in anticipating problem areas that they might experience after leaving the hospital. After anticipating future difficulties, they worked together to set up ways to handle the potential problems, but they also focused on ways in which they could have a balance to the more intense focus on problems. Initially, Jeremy had a hard time anticipating problems and blithely stated that he could handle anything that came up. With the occupational therapist's Socratic questioning and peer support from the group members, he came to think that maybe he could benefit from continuing treatment, at least two days per week; he was particularly apprehensive about returning to work.

After discharge he attended a partial hospitalization program for two days a week for four weeks. In the program with the facilitation of his occupational therapist and the other members he established goals for repairing family and work relationships and for putting in place ways in which he could deal with distressing situations in his home and work life. He attended a family psychoeducation group offered by social workers and an occupational therapy group that discussed interpersonal skills, particularly how to get along with co-workers. His occupational therapist also worked individually with him to assess his workplace using the Work Environment Impact Scale (Moore-Corner, Kielhofner, & Olson, 1998) to analyze his work situations and develop necessary social and physical accommodations. He was able to recognize which work situations were a hindrance to him, such as having more than one project boss and taking on too many projects at the same time. He was able to recognize how some of his behaviors,

particularly when he was manic, caused people at work to stay away from him, thus causing him to feel isolated and unsupported. He successfully graduated from the partial program after three weeks, but returned each quarter or when needed for maintenance therapy.

Discussion

Initially Jeremy's behavior was very manic and he had difficulty being in a group setting. With structured treatment in addition to valproate, his behavior moved more to the middle of the mood continuum (see Figure 8-1). At first he did not acknowledge that he needed to plan a rehabilitation program that would maintain stability, but his occupational therapist and occupational therapy group facilitated self-awareness. He used a postdischarge partial hospitalization program to tackle work and family issues.

SUMMARY

Mood disorders have been described throughout history. Initially, melancholia and mania were thought to be curses of the gods. Over the centuries, environmental and biological theories have emerged and mood disorders were classified as depressive and bipolar disorders. Research on, and treatment of, mood disorders addresses biology, personality, behavior, cognition, and life events.

Mania and depression represent opposite ends of what can be considered more than a mood disorder because both include multiple symptoms, which may be emotional, cognitive, motivational, or vegetative. Occupational therapy treatment consists of changing behavior, arranging the environment, and changing internal appraisals. One should tailor the therapy to the severity of the mood disorder. Occupational therapy is particularly important for mood disorders because of its use of tangible, concrete activities and its focus on everyday occupations and motivation.

REVIEW QUESTIONS

1. What are some reasons for the prevalence of depression in females?
2. Which theories of mood disorders are addressed in occupational therapy treatment?
3. Explain the mood continuum. Why is it important?
4. Name one intervention for cognitive and motivational problems for an individual who is manic.
5. Name one intervention for emotional problems of depression.

REFERENCES

American Occupational Therapy Association (AOTA). (2008). The occupational therapy practice framework: Domain and process. *American Journal of Occupational Therapy, 62*(6), 625–683.

American Psychiatric Association (APA). (2000). *Diagnostic and statistical manual of mental disorders* (4th ed., text rev.). Washington, DC: Author.

American Psychiatric Association (APA). (2002). *Practice guidelines for the treatment of patients with bipolar disorder.* Retrieved from www.psychiatryonline.com/com/comcontent .aspx?aID=50226

American Psychiatric Association (APA). (2010). *Practice guidelines for the treatment of patients with major depressive disorder.* Retrieved from www.psychiatryonline.com/pracGuide/ pracGuideTopic_7.aspx

Asher, I. E. (1996). *Occupational therapy assessment tools: An annotated index* (2nd ed.). Bethesda, MD: American Occupational Therapy Association.

Baron, K., Kielhofner, G., Iyenger, A., Goldhammer, V., & Wolenski, J. (2002). *The Occupational Self Assessment (OSA) (Version 2.0).* Chicago: Model of Human Occupation Clearinghouse, Department of Occupational Therapy, College of Applied Health Sciences, University of Illinois at Chicago.

Beck, A. (1973). *Depression: Causes and treatment: The diagnosis and management of depression.* Philadelphia: University of Pennsylvania Press.

Beck, A. (1976). *Cognitive therapy and the emotional disorders.* New York: International Universities Press.

Beck, A. (1978). *Beck Depression Inventory.* San Antonio: Psychological Corporation.

Belmaker, R. H., & Yaroslavsky, Y. (2000). Perspectives for new pharmacological interventions. In J. Soares & S. Gershon (Eds.), *Bipolar disorders: Basic mechanisms and therapeutic implications* (pp. 507–528). New York: Marcel Dekker.

Bender, R., & Alloy, L. (2011). Life stress and kindling in bipolar disorder: Review of the evidence and integration with emerging biopsychosocial theories. *Clinical Psychology Review, 31*(3), 383–396. Retrieved from doi: 10.1016/j.cpr2011.01.004

Blazer, D., & Hybels, C. (2008). Epidemiology of psychiatric illness. In S. H. Fatemi & P. Clayton (Eds.), *The medical basis of psychiatry, Part IV* (3rd ed., pp. 547–559). Retrieved from doi: 10.1007/978-1-59745-252-6_32

Boswell, S. (1989). A social support group for depressed people. *Australian Occupational Therapy Journal, 36*(1), 34–41.

Bowlby, J. (1988). *A secure base: Parent-child attachment and healthy human development* (Chap 2, pp. 20–38). New York: Basic Books.

Bracegirdle, H. (1991). The female stereotype and occupational therapy for women with depression. *British Journal of Occupational Therapy, 54*(5), 193–194.

Burns, D. (1989). *The feeling good handbook: The new mood therapy*. New York: Plume/Penguin.

Bylsma, L., Morris, B., & Rottenberg, J. (2008). A meta-analysis of emotional reactivity in major depressive disorder. *Clinical Psychology Review, 28*(4), 676–691. Retrieved from doi: 6/j .cpr.2007.10.001

Cassidy, J., & Shaver, P. (Eds.). (2008). *Handbook of attachment: Theory, research, and clinical applications*. New York: Guilford.

Centoni, M., & Tallant, B. (1986). The projective use of drawings as a treatment technique with the depressed unemployed male. *Canadian Journal of Occupational Therapy, 53*(2), 81–87.

Cole, F. (2010). Physical activity for its mental health benefits: conceptualizing participation within the model of human occupation. *British Journal of Occupational Therapy, 73*(12), 607–615. Retrieved from doi: 10.4276/030802210X12918167234280

Crow, T. J. (2000). Bipolar shifts as disorders of the bi-hemispheric integration of language: Implications for the genetic origins of the psychotic continuum. In A. Marneros & J. Angst (Eds.), *Bipolar disorders: 100 years after manic-depressive insanity* (pp. 335–348). Boston: Kluwer Academic.

Devereaux, E., & Carlson, M. (1992). Health policy: The role of occupational therapy in the management of depression. *American Occupational Therapy Association, 465*(2), 175–180.

Earhart, C. A., Allen, C. K., & Blue, T. (1993). *Allen Diagnostic Module: The manual*. Colchester, CT: S & S Worldwide.

Feder, J. (1990). Occupational stress and the depressed female client. *Work: A Journal of Prevention, Assessment and Rehabilitation, 1*(2), 55–62.

Feder, J. (1991). Women, depression and work: Treatment strategies for the depressed patient. *Occupational Therapy Practice, 2*(4), 58–67.

First, M. B., Frances, A., & Pincus, H. A. (2004). *DSM-IV-TR Guidebook: The essential companion to the Diagnostic and Statistical Manual of Mental Disorders, Fourth Edition, Text Revision*. Washington, DC: American Psychiatric Publishing.

Frank, E. Soreca, I., Schwartz, H., Fagiolini, A., Mallinger, A., Thase, M., et al. (2008). The role of interpersonal and social rhythm therapy in improving occupational functioning in patients with bipolar disorder. *American Journal of Psychiatry, 165*, 1559–1565. Retrieved from http://www .ajp.psychiatryonline.org

Gabbard, G. (2009). *Textbook of psychotherapeutic treatments*. PsychiatryOnline.com: American Psychiatric Publishing. Retrieved from doi: 10.1176/appi.books.9781585623648

Gilbert, P. (2000). Varieties of submissive behavior as forms of social defense: Their evolution and role in depression. In L. Sloman & P. Gilbert (Eds.), *Subordination and defeat: An evolutionary approach to mood disorders and their therapy* (pp. 3–45). London: Erlbaum.

Gutman, S. A., & Biel, L. (2001). Abstract: Promoting the neurologic substrates of well-being through occupation. *Occupational Therapy in Mental Health, 17*(1), 1–22.

Hackman, A. L., Ram, R. N., & Dixon, L. B. (1999). Psychosocial treatment of bipolar disorder in the public sector: Program for assertive community treatment. In J. Goldberg & M. Harrow (Eds.), *Bipolar disorders: Clinical course and outcome* (pp. 259–274). Washington, DC: American Psychiatric Press.

Harkness, K., Alavi, N., Monroe, S., Slavich, G., Gotlib, I., & Bagby, R.M. (2010). Gender differences in life events prior to onset of major depressive disorder: The moderating effect of age. *Journal of Abnormal Psychology, 119*, 4, 791–803.

Hees, L, Koeter, M., deVries, G. Ooteman, W., & Schene, A. (2010). Effectiveness of adjuvant occupational therapy in employees with depression: Design of a randomized controlled trial. *BMC Public Health, 10*(558), 2–9. Retrieved from doi: 10.1186/1471-2458/10/558/prepub

Helfrich, C., & Rivera, Y. (2006). Employment skills and domestic violence survivors: A shelter-based intervention. *Occupational Therapy in Mental Health, 22*(1), 33–48.

Hemphill, B. (1992). Depression among suicidal elderly: A life-threatening illness. *Occupational Therapy Practice, 4*(1), 61–66.

Hlastala, S. A., & Frank, E. (2000). Biology versus environment: Stressors in the pathophysiology of bipolar disorder. In J. C. Soares & S. Gershon (Eds.), *Bipolar disorders: Basic mechanisms and therapeutic implications* (pp. 353–372). New York: Marcel Dekker.

Hollon, S., & DeRubeis, R. (2004). Effectiveness of treatment for depression. In R. Leahy (Ed.). *Contemporary cognitive therapy: Theory, research and practice* (pp. 45–61). New York: Guilford.

Hundt, N., Nelson-Gray, R., Kimbrel, M., Mitchell, J., & Kwapil, T. (2007). The interaction of reinforcement sensitivity and life events in the prediction of anhedonic depression and mixed-anxiety depression symptoms. *Personality and Individual Differences, 43*(5), 1001–1012. Retrieved from http://www.sciencedirect.com

Hutcheson, C., Ferguson, H., Nish, G., & Gill, L. (2010). Promoting mental wellbeing through activity in a mental health hospital. *British Journal of Occupational Therapy, 73*(3), 121–128. Retrieved from doi:104276/0308022 10X12682330090497

Kaplan, H., & Sadock, B. (1989). *Comprehensive textbook of psychiatry* (5th ed.). Baltimore: Williams & Wilkins.

Kaplan, H., & Sadock, B. (1991). *Synopsis of psychiatry: Behavioral sciences: Clinical psychology* (6th ed.). Baltimore: Williams & Wilkins.

Kaplan, K. L. (1986). The directive group: Short term treatment for psychiatric patients with a minimal level of functioning. *American Journal of Occupational Therapy, 40*, 474–481.

Kassel, J. D., & Veilleux, J. C. (2010) Introduction: The complex interplay between substance abuse and emotion. In J. D. Kassel (Ed.), *Substance abuse and emotion* (pp. 3–11). Washington, DC: American Psychological Association.

Koch, H. (2010). Seasonality of psychiatric disease exacerbation assessed by evaluation of a consultancy service: A retrospective pilot study. *Biological Rhythm Research, 41*(2), 159–163. Retrieved from doi: 10.1080/0929101090324821

Kotov, R., Gamez, W., Schmidt, F., & Watson, D. (2010). Linking "big" personality traits to anxiety, depressive, and substance use disorders: A meta-analysis. *Psychological Bulletin, 136*(5), 768–821.

Koukopoulos, A., Sani, G., Koukopoulos, A. E., & Girardi, P. (2000). In A. Marneros & J. Angst (Eds.), *Bipolar disorders: 100 years after manic-depressive insanity* (pp. 315–334). Boston: Kluwer Academic.

Kusznir, A., Scott, E., Cooke, R. G., & Young, L. T. (1996). Functional consequences of bipolar affective disorder: An occupational therapy perspective [Abstract]. *Canadian Journal of Occupational Therapy, 63*(5), 313–332.

Leahy, R. (Ed.) (2004). *Contemporary cognitive therapy: Theory, research, and practice*. New York: Guilford.

Lewy, A., Emens, J., Songer, J., Sims, N., Laurie, A., Fiala, S., et al. (2009). Winter depression: Integrating mood, circadian rhythms, and the sleep/wake and light/dark cycles into a bio-psycho-social-environmental model. *Sleep Medicine Clinics, 4*(2), 285–299. Retrieved from doi: 10.1016/j.jsmc.2009.02.003

Linroth, R., Zander, S., Forde, S., Hanley, M., & Lins, J. (1996). Ramsey county day treatment services: Day treatment to extended day treatment centers to focus groups. *Occupational Therapy in Health Care, 10*(2), 89–103.

Loosen, P. T., Beyer, J. L., Sells, S. R., Gurtsman, H. E., Shelton, R. C., Baird, R. P., et al. (2000). Mood disorders. In M. H. Evbert, P. T. Loosen, & B. Nurcombe (Eds.), *Current diagnosis and treatment in psychiatry* (pp. 290–327). New York: Lange Medical Books/McGraw Hill.

Maj. M., Tortorella, A., & Bartoli, L. (2000). Mood stabilizers in bipolar disorder. In A. Marneros & J. Angst (Eds.), *Bipolar disorders: 100 years after manic-depressive insanity* (pp. 461–464). Boston: Kluwer Academic.

Markowitz, J. C. (1998). *Interpersonal psychotherapy for dysthymic disorder.* Washington, DC: American Psychiatric Press.

Markowitz, J. C., & Weissman, M. M. (2009). In G. Gabbard (Ed.), *Textbook of psychotherapeutic treatments*, pp. 339–364. Arlington, VA: American Psychiatric Publishing, Inc.

Marneros, A. (2000). On entities and continuities of bipolar disorders. In A. Marneros & J. Angst (Eds.), *Bipolar disorders: 100 years after manic-depressive insanity* (pp. 461–464). Boston: Kluwer Academic.

Marneros, A., & Angst, J. (2000a). The prognosis of bipolar disorders: Course and outcome. In A. Marneros & J. Angst (Eds.), *Bipolar disorders: 100 years after manic-depressive insanity* (pp. 406–436). Boston: Kluwer Academic.

Marneros, A., & Angst, J. (2000b). Bipolar disorders: Roots and evaluation. In A. Marneros & J. Angst (Eds.), *Bipolar disorders: 100 years after manic-depressive insanity* (pp. 1–35). Boston: Kluwer Academic.

Marneros, A., & Angst, J. (Eds.). (2010). *Bipolar disorders: 100 years after manic-depressive insanity.* Boston: Kluwer Academic.

Meyers, J. (1991). Clinical differentiation between dementia and depression. *Gerontology Special Interest Section Newsletter (American Occupational Therapy Association), 14*(1), 5–6.

Moller, H. J., & Grunze, H. (2000). Antidepressant treatment of bipolar depression. In A. Marneros & J. Angst (Eds.), *Bipolar disorders: 100 years after manic-depressive insanity* (pp. 387–403). Boston: Kluwer Academic.

Morrison, J. (2007). *DSM-IV made easier: Principles and techniques for mental health clinicians.* New York: Guilford.

Mundt, C., Kronmuller, K., & Backenstraf, S. (2000). Interactional styles in bipolar disorder. In A. Marneros & J. Angst (Eds.), *Bipolar disorders: 100 years after manic-depressive insanity* (pp. 201–213). Boston: Kluwer Academic.

Myin-Germeys, I., Peeters, F., Havermans, R., Nicolson, N., deVries, M., Delespaul, P., et al. (2003). Emotional reactivity to daily life stress in psychosis, and affective disorder: an experience sampling study. *Acta Psychiatrica Scandinavica, 107*, 24–131. Retrieved from doi: 10.1034/j.1600-0447.2003.02025.x

Nasrallah, H., Ketter, T., & Kalali, A. (2006). Carbamazepine and valproate for the treatment of bipolar disorder: A review of the literature. *Journal of Affective Disorders, 95*, 69–78. Retrieved from doi: 10.1016/j.jad.2006.04.030

National Institute of Mental Health (NIMH). (2011). Retrieved from http://www.nimh.nih.gov/healthtopics

Pagnin, P. (2004). Efficacy of ECT in Depression: A meta-analytic review. *The Journal of ECT, 20*(1), 13–20.

Pelissolo, A., & Lepine, P. (2001). Epidemiology of depression and anxiety disorders. In S. A. Montgomery & J. A. den Doer (Eds.), *SSRIs in depression and anxiety* (pp. 1–23). New York: Wiley.

Persons, J. B., Davidson, J., & Tompkins, M. A. (2001). *Essential components of cognitive-behavior therapy for depression.* Washington, DC: American Psychological Association.

Pfeiffer, P., Heisler, M., Piette, J., Rogers, M., & Valenstein, M. (2010). Efficacy of peer support interventions for depression: a meta-analysis. *General Hospital Psychiatry, 33*, 1, 29–36. Retrieved from doi: 10.1016/j.genhosppsych.2010.10.002

Rosenthal, N. (2009). Issues for DSM-V: Seasonal affective disorder and seasonality. *American Journal of Psychiatry, 162*(8), 852–853. Retrieved from doi: 10.1176/appi.ajp.2009.09020188

Roth, A., & Fonagy, P. (2005). *What works for whom?* New York: Guilford.

Sadock, B., Sadock, V., & Ruiz, P. (Eds.). (2009). *Kaplan and Sadock's comprehensive textbook of psychiatry* (9th ed.), Philadelphia: Lippincott, Williams and Wilkins.

Scott, J. (2004). Cognitive therapy of bipolar disorders. In R. Leahy (Ed.), *Contemporary cognitive therapy: Theory, research and practice* (pp. 228–243). New York: Guilford.

Sloman, L., & Gilbert, P. (Eds.). (2000). *Subordination and defeat: An evolutionary approach to mood disorders and their therapy.* London: Erlbaum.

Stein, F., & Smith, J. (1989). Short-term stress management programme with acutely depressed in-patients. *Canadian Journal of Occupational Therapy, 56*(4), 185–191.

Swarbrick, M., & Ellis, J. (2009). Peer-operated self-help centers. *Occupational Therapy in Mental Health, 25,* 239–251.

Thase, M. E. (2000). Modulation of biological factors by psychotherapeutic interventions. In J. Soares & S. Gershon (Eds.), *Bipolar disorders: Basic mechanisms and therapeutic implications* (pp. 373–385). New York: Marcel Dekker.

Tse, S. S., & Walsh, A. E. S. (2001). How does work work for people with bipolar affective disorder? [Abstract]. *Occupational Therapy International, 8*(3), 210–225.

Tsuang, M. T., & Faraone, S. (2000). The genetic epidemiology of bipolar disorder. In A. Marneros & J. Angst (Eds.), *Bipolar disorders: 100 years after manic-depressive insanity* (pp. 231–241). Boston: Kluwer Academic.

Yakobina, Y., Yakobina, S., & Tallant, B. K. (1997). I came, I thought, I conquered: Cognitive behavior approach applied in occupational therapy for the treatment of depressed (dysthymic) females [Abstract]. *Occupational Therapy in Mental Health, 13*(4), 59–73.

SUGGESTED RESOURCES

Popular Books About Depression and Mania

Berger, D., & Berger, L. (1991). *We heard the angels of madness: A family guide to coping with manic depression.* New York: William Morrow.

Gold, M. (1995). *The good news about depression: Cures and treatments in the new age of psychiatry.* New York: Bantam.

Ingersoll, B. D. (1995). *Lonely, sad and angry: A parent's guide to depression in children and adolescents.* New York: Doubleday.

Jamison, K. R. (1995). *An unquiet mind: A memoir of moods and madness.* New York: Vintage.

Rosen, L. (1996). *When someone you love is depressed: How to help your loved one without losing yourself.* New York: Free Press.

Salmans, S. (1995). *Depression: Questions you have—Answers you need.* Allentown, PA: People's Medical Society.

Styron, W. (1990). *Darkness visible: A memoir of madness.* New York: Vintage.

Popular Self-Help Books

Colgrove, M., Bloomfield, H., & McWilliams, P. (Eds.). (1991). *How to survive the loss of a love.* Los Angeles: Prelude.

Copeland, M. E. (1994). *Living without depression and manic depression: A workbook for maintaining mood stability.* Oakland, CA: New Harbinger.

Emery, G. (1988). *Getting un-depressed: How a woman can change her life through cognitive therapy* (rev. ed.). New York: Touchstone.

Greenberger, D., & Padesky, C. A. (1995). *Mind over mood: Change how you feel by changing the way you think.* New York: Guilford.

Lange, A., & Jakubowski, P. (1976). *Cognitive behavioral procedures for trainers.* New York: Research Press.

Young, J. E., & Klosko, J. S. (1993). *Reinventing your life: How to break free from negative life patterns and feel good again.* New York: Plume/Penguin.

Websites

Mood Disorders:

    http://www.surgeongeneral.gov/library/mentalhealth/chapter4/sec3.html

Depression Video:

    http://www.youtube.com/watch?v=xCeOAZSFbME

    http://www.youtube.com/watch?v=NWY_NPJ39iQ

Bipolar video:

    http://www.youtube.com/watch?v=KtHXzDqXy3w

Depression:

    http://www.ncbi.nlm.nih.gov/pubmedhealth/PMH0001941/

    http://www.webmd.com/depression/default.htm

    http://www.mayoclinic.com/health/depression/DS00175

    http://www.nimh.nih.gov/health/publications/depression/complete-index.shtml

    http://helpguide.org/mental/depression_signs_types_diagnosis_treatment.htm

Mania:

    http://www.webmd.com/bipolar-disorder/guide/hypomania-mania-symptoms

    http://psychcentral.com/disorders/sx9.htm

    http://www.webmd.com/bipolar-disorder/managing-a-manic-episode

Bipolar:

    http://www.healthline.com/health/bipolar-disorder

    http://www.dbsalliance.org/site/PageServer?pagename=about_maniascreener

    http://helpguide.org/mental/bipolar_disorder_symptoms_treatment.htm

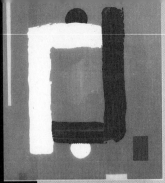

Chapter 9

Anxiety Disorders

Elizabeth Cara, PhD, OTR/L, MFC

KEY TERMS

autogenic training

benzodiazapines

compulsions

depersonalization

derealization

mindfulness

obsessions

psychogenic

sensory overresponsive type (SOR)

vasodilatation

CHAPTER OUTLINE

Introduction

Encountering People with Anxiety Disorders: Settings

    Acute Inpatient

    Outpatient

    Home Care

Description of Anxiety Disorders

Impact on Daily Functioning

DSM-IV-TR Descriptions of Anxiety

    Panic Attack

    Agoraphobia

    Panic Disorder Without and with Agoraphobia

    Specific Phobia

    Social Phobia

    Obsessive-Compulsive Disorder (OCD)

    Post-Traumatic Stress Disorder (PTSD)

    Acute Stress Disorder

    Generalized Anxiety Disorder (GAD)

Anxiety Disorder Due to a General Medical Condition
Substance-Induced Anxiety Disorder
General Treatment Strategies
Psychopharmacology
Counseling
Cognitive-Behavioral Treatment
Mindfulness
Behavioral Approaches
Biofeedback
Meditation
Eye Movement Desensitization and Reprocessing (EMDR)
Interpersonal Skills Training
Occupational Therapy and Self-Management Techniques
Assessment
Treatment Interventions
Relaxation Training
Assertiveness and General Social Skills Training
Sensory Modulation Interventions
Goals
Treatment
Summary

INTRODUCTION

The occupational therapist invites a client on the psychiatric unit, a 35-year-old man who was found pacing the floors, to attend a stress management group. Wringing his hands, trembling as he talks, and speaking quickly, the client refuses to attend the group and states he is too anxious to concentrate. This man has been diagnosed with generalized anxiety disorder (GAD) and depression; he is a challenge to the occupational therapist, who wonders how to best intervene and make a therapeutic connection. People experience many kinds and degrees of anxiety, but only when anxiety markedly interferes with daily function and the fear is inappropriate to the persons' life circumstances is it called clinical anxiety (McClure-Tone & Pine, 2009).

The origin of the word *anxiety* lies in the Greek root *angh,* meaning both "to press tight" and "to be heavy with grief" (Taylor & Arnow, 1988), and more recently, in the Latin word *anxietas,* meaning "troubled mind" (Sims & Snaith, 1988). Anxiety disorders are often the most common psychiatric disorders and yet the least treated ones.

Approximately 29% of adults and 20% to 25% of adolescents in the United States (Merikangas & Kalaydjian, 2009; NIMH, 2011), can expect to have an anxiety disorder in his or her lifetime; women outnumber men two to one in this population. The number of words in the English vocabulary that describe anxiety highlights its pervasiveness—witness the words *worry, edginess, panic, fright, alarm, terror, jitters, jumpiness,* and *uneasiness*. Anxiety is linked to our primitive fight-or-flight response that, when activated, prepares the body biochemically for meeting possible danger. The heart rate and blood pressure rise, blood goes to the large muscles, adrenaline is secreted, and sensory functions such as sight and hearing become keener.

ENCOUNTERING PEOPLE WITH ANXIETY DISORDERS: SETTINGS

Anxiety is a concern that needs to be addressed in all practice areas, including home and physical rehabilitation settings, due to the related loss of function, uncertainty of prognosis, chronicity of symptoms, and other serious related issues. One study of patients in primary care settings revealed that at least 19% had at least one anxiety disorder and many were untreated (Kroenke, Spitzer, Williams, Monahan, & Lowe, 2007). It is a disorder that is not limited to any age group and is diagnosed in young children as well as older adults. In this chapter, anxiety disorders will be discussed in adult psychiatric populations in psychiatric settings; however, the interventions can be used with almost all ages and in any setting.

Acute Inpatient

The occupational therapist is likely to encounter clients with anxiety disorders on inpatient psychiatric units. Their symptoms are usually so severe that they are unable to function in their daily lives. This incapacitation may sometimes include suicidal thoughts or actual suicide attempts. In both instances, the safe and, perhaps, locked environment of a hospital meets the immediate need for structure and external control.

Outpatient

Clients are often referred to outpatient programs, usually called partial hospitalization programs, if (1) they require further intervention following hospitalization and are unable to immediately return to their former occupations or (2) they need considerable support and structure but are able to manage outside the hospital. In either case, people may be living at home, in halfway houses, or in other special living arrangements. Clients with anxiety disorders as a primary diagnosis are usually able to function outside the hospital despite their distressing symptoms.

Home Care

Occupational therapists work in home care programs for clients with psychiatric as well as physical dysfunction. Isolated at home and too impaired to participate in a structured day program, people with anxiety disorders such as agoraphobia (fear of leaving the house) or obsessive-compulsive behavior (OCD) (involving intrusive thoughts and ritualized behavior) may benefit from one-on-one programs in time management, activities of daily living, and community reentry.

Those who have physical illnesses that require home or rehabilitation treatment may also experience anxiety subsequent to their disease or condition. Occupational therapist practitioners will also encounter people with GAD in any settings that will treat those with physical conditions. In addition, school settings for children and adults will also include people with heightened anxiety due to the stresses of these occupations. Lastly, occupational therapists will most likely encounter employees who have anxiety disorders that may prevent them from working or increase absenteeism rates.

Changes in health care have dramatically shortened lengths of stay in acute hospital settings. As a consequence of the reduction in client care days, occupational therapists must now focus more on evaluation than on treatment and be ready to make recommendations for discharge early in the hospitalization. Anxiety, especially if it takes a chronic course, will usually not be fully resolved during an inpatient stay. Occupational therapists in these settings must be prepared to help identify problem areas in functioning, begin intervention, and solve problems related to the discharge environment with the client and, often, with family members. The consideration of the entire continuity of client care becomes a crucial piece in treatment so that gains made in one environment may be carried over to the next. Communication with professionals working with the client in a prehospital or posthospital setting helps to both accelerate and consolidate treatment plans and recommendations.

The Occupational Therapy Practice Framework (OTPF) (AOTA, 2008) also designates communities and populations as clients. Anxiety disorders will also generally be encountered in communities and populations as well as organizations. Therefore, evaluation and consultation approaches should be an occupational therapy approach.

DESCRIPTION OF ANXIETY DISORDERS

The *Diagnostic and Statistical Manual of Mental Disorders,* Fourth Edition (*DSM-IV-TR*) (APA, 2000), describes a number of anxiety disorders that may occur alone or concomitantly with other *DSM-IV-TR* diagnoses. Although the next edition currently in development (DSM-5) may be different and add disorders, such as hoarding, to this classification, the *DSM-IV-TR* conditions are described here (see Chapter 6, Diagnosis and Psychopathology for more information regarding the DSM-5 format). For example, OCD may overlay another Axis I disorder, major depressive disorder. In this case, an individual may have an agitated depression manifested by sleeplessness, excessive motor activity, and extreme feelings of worthlessness (major depressive disorder) compounded by a compelling need to follow rigid behaviors, such as pacing a certain number of times around the halls of the hospital (OCD). However, anxiety is also frequently a component of other psychiatric illnesses without necessarily meeting the definition of a true *DSM-IV* diagnosis of anxiety disorder. The *International Classification of Diseases (ICD-10)* (WHO, 2011) also describes similar anxiety disorders and its dimensions in addition to one not in the *DSM-IV-TR*, mixed anxiety and depression.

Several different kinds of anxiety are defined in Figure 9-1. For example, people with diagnoses such as eating disorders, personality disorders, and schizophrenia are often highly anxious. Many have trait anxiety or enduring personality patterns of anxiety. In addition, people without any history of mental disorders commonly experience acute anxiety—time-limited periods of anxiety—when, for example, undergoing uncomfortable, and perhaps, life-threatening medical procedures. The mere prospect of dealing with an aversive event such as diagnostic testing, chemotherapy, radiation, or surgery may produce intense levels of anxiety (often called *anticipatory anxiety*). In these examples, the anxiety often diminishes with emotional support and the termination of the stressor. However, there are times when anxiety repeatedly arises around new stressors even after the resolution of the initial ones. In these circumstances the anxiety is labeled *chronic anxiety*. There are also circumstances when anxiety continues but is generalized and vague without an identifiable stressor. In this case, it is called *free-floating anxiety*.

There are certain medical diseases and conditions that are also likely to produce states or acute experiences of anxiety. However, these symptoms of worry, or even panic, often subside when the medical reason is resolved. Examples include hyperthyroidism, estrogen loss occurring in menopause, congestive heart failure, asthma, hypoglycemia, and temporal lobe epilepsy (Taylor & Arnow, 1988). A number of medications and nonprescription drugs may either cause or worsen acute anxiety symptoms. These include anticholinergic drugs, steroids, aspirin, cocaine, amphetamines, and hallucinogens (Taylor & Arnow, 1988). Caffeine and nicotine, two commonly ingested substances, may also produce symptoms of anxiety. Moreover, withdrawal from alcohol or other addictive substances presents a high risk for acute anxiety states.

The difference between normal anxiety (worry that propels one to act), and clinical anxiety (worry that disrupts function) is not always easily or clearly defined. Anxiety in a limited dose is universal, normal, appropriate, and adaptive as a

---

Anxiety: unpleasant emotional, cognitive, behavioral, or physical experiences of stress.

Trait Anxiety: enduring personality style that manifests persistent anxiety.

Acute Anxiety: time-limited anxiety that diminishes with resolution of the problem.

Anticipatory Anxiety: predictive anxiety in response to future actual or imagined situations.

Chronic Anxiety: anxiety that persists, developing around new stressors after immediate problems are resolved.

Free-Floating Anxiety: generalized anxiety, which may be vague in origin.

Clinical Anxiety: disruption in function due to anxiety.

FIGURE 9-1. Definitions of Different Kinds of Anxiety
© Cengage Learning 2013

protection from potential threat. It is almost always associated with the anticipation of future events accompanied by expected loss or pain (Sims & Snaith, 1988; Stein, Hollander, & Rothbaum, 2010). It can be the force that propels people to act, cope, and even perform more efficiently. For example, most college students experience a normal level of anxiety as they prepare for final exams, which usually helps induce studying.

On the other hand, anxiety is often defined as abnormal when it hinders rather than helps the individual. If the person's response to a stimulus is greater than one would expect, if his or her feelings of anxiety persist after the stimulus is removed, or if anxiety is ineffective in dealing with the threat of the stimulus, the anxiety may be called abnormal (Sims & Snaith, 1988; Stein et al., 2010). Anxiety of this proportion has been likened to having a faulty burglar alarm that signals nonexistent danger (Agras, 1985). For example, if the college students' anxiety prevents them from taking other exams, then it becomes abnormal.

Clinical anxiety is the name given to abnormal anxiety when it clearly affects and hinders daily function and is no longer serviceable. Anxiety becomes disabling when it persists without stimulating positive action to resolve the stressor or ward off distress. For instance, a woman with intense anxiety was so incapacitated by the feelings of terror associated with an upcoming job layoff that she was unable to develop an alternative survival plan for herself. Such clinical anxiety is seen in many people hospitalized on psychiatric units.

When action is taken to diminish the anticipated threat, there is a great possibility that the anxiety will be reduced. For example, clients who are preparing for discharge from the psychiatric hospital are often very anxious about responding to future inquiries about their hospitalization. They feel vulnerable to the feared onslaught of questions by friends and family and are effectively addressed in an assertiveness group led by an occupational therapist; anxiety related to this issue will likely decrease. Clients report feeling more prepared to encounter others after discharge when they have learned and practiced direct forms of communication.

Anxiety can affect a person physiologically, emotionally, behaviorally, and cognitively. Several parts of the brain are implicated in the production of fear and anxiety. Using brain imaging technology and neurochemical techniques, the amygdala and the hippocampus play significant roles in most anxiety disorders (National Institute of Mental Health [NIMH], n.d.). See Table 9-1 for a list of symptoms of anxiety in each area.

IMPACT ON DAILY FUNCTIONING

The impact of anxiety on a person's life may be dramatic and may affect all aspects of functioning, including work, social life, self-care, parenting, and leisure activities. Performance in all roles may dramatically decline as anxiety symptoms persist.

TABLE 9-1. Symptoms of Anxiety

Emotional	Physiological	Cognitive	Behavioral
Feeling uneasy, off-balance.	*Cardiovascular:* increased heart rate (tachycardia), chest pain and pressure.	Confusion.	Preoccupied with internal thoughts.
Feeling overwhelmed.		Poor memory.	Immobile, withdrawn.
Feeling a sense of impending doom.	*Gastrointestinal:* diarrhea, constipation, nausea, vomiting, gas, cramps, and loss of appetite.	Distractibility, poor concentration.	Overactive, restless, agitated.
Feeling helpless and out of control.		Thought blocking.	Excess or decreased consumption of substances and/or food.
Feeling one is going insane.	*Respiratory:* dyspnea (shortness of breath) and choking sensations.	Loss of perspective, cognitive distortion including catastrophic thinking and negative self-evaluation.	Rituals to alleviate anxiety.
Depersonalization (having feelings of unreality, as if in a dream).	*Urinary:* frequency and urgency of urination.	Obsessive thoughts.	
Derealization (feeling detached from one's surroundings).	*Genital:* loss of libido, premature ejaculation, and amenorrhea.	Fears of loss of control, going crazy, injury, death, and not coping.	
	Autonomic: sweating, flushing, dry mouth, dizziness, and fainting.	Poor problem solving.	
	Muscular: twitching, tremors, spasms, tension, cramping, hypervigilance.		

NOTE: Some of the self-help behavioral methods sought to reduce discomfort may be unintentionally self-destructive and therefore not adaptive. For example, addiction to prescription medications and alcohol, extreme isolation, and regression are common secondary problems that develop from immediate, or nonadaptive, behavioral solutions.

© Cengage Learning 2013

Employment may suffer because of cognitive impairment. Concentration, problem solving, and memory may all be markedly affected by episodes of acute anxiety, primarily because the individual's primary focus is directed toward combating unpleasant symptoms and not to the task at hand. Tardiness, inaccuracy in completing work, and distractibility are some of the problem behaviors that develop in people who experience persistent anxiety. For example, one client with OCD spent so many hours performing ritualistic hand and clothes washing that he was unable to maintain his required work schedule. Social relationships may decline as the person restricts activities and therefore becomes unavailable to others.

There is also the likelihood that others will be alienated by the rigidity and withdrawal of the anxious person. For example, a woman with panic attacks stopped attending her church and volunteer activities and became reclusive in her small apartment. After some period of time, friends and acquaintances associated with these activities no longer called her because of her continued self-imposed isolation and their experience of personal rejection.

Many persons experience stress with their partners as they curtail previously shared activities or become overreliant on them for assistance. For example, the husband of a client with agoraphobia became resentful of his wife's dependency when she would not leave the house without him, even to complete the smallest task. The decrease in function may affect homemaking, grooming, and parenting activities, as well as leisure occupations. The woman described here sought help from friends to transport her children to school and to her medical appointments when her husband was not available. Another client, an elderly man who was coping poorly with a GAD, abandoned his avid avocational interest in the stock market because of difficulty in concentrating on the newspaper figures.

Depression commonly develops secondarily to anxiety symptoms. People often feel a sense of desperation as various forms of anxiety immobilize them or cause severe discomfort; therefore, the potential for suicide can be high. From a medical standpoint, clients are prone to certain physical diseases, such as heart problems and gastrointestinal disorders like ulcerative colitis and stomach ulcers. Figure 9-2 highlights the impact of anxiety disorders on daily functioning.

DSM-IV-TR DESCRIPTIONS OF ANXIETY

There are 10 major diagnostic groups related to anxiety in the *DSM-IV-TR* (APA, 2000). The *ICD-10* lists similar diagnostic groups (WHO, 2011) with one exception; the *ICD-10* has a category (41.2) for mixed anxiety and depression, which seems to be an apt

---

Work: poor habits due to problems in concentration and time management.

Social Relationships: diminished due to restriction of activity and isolation.

Marital Relationships: decrease in shared activities, dependency on spouse.

Activities of Daily Living: homemaking, grooming, and parenting may be inadequate secondary to poor concentration, depression, and physical symptoms.

Leisure Activities: pleasurable activities may be neglected, primarily because of an inability to sustain sufficient attention.

Depression: feelings of low self-esteem and despair may result, hindering involvement in customary activities.

Medical Status: susceptibility to numerous diseases such as colitis, ulcers, heart disease, stroke, and respiratory disorders, which may decrease the ability to work, care for the self, and engage in pleasurable activities alone or with family and friends.

FIGURE 9-2. Impact of Anxiety Disorders on Daily Functioning
© Cengage Learning 2013

description recognizing the high comorbidity of anxiety and depression. A description of each group, with typical symptoms, follows.

Panic Attack

The term *panic attack* defines a limited period of intense fear or distress in which four or more of the following symptoms progress rapidly and peak within 10 minutes: cardiac symptoms (palpitations, pounding, rapid heartbeat), trembling, shortness of breath, feelings of suffocation, chest pain, sensations of choking, nausea or abdominal distress, dizziness or lightheadedness, **derealization**, fear of losing control or going crazy, fear of dying, paresthesias (numbness or tingling), and chills or hot flashes. Panic attacks are most often associated with panic disorder but may also develop in those who have social phobias as well as other anxiety disorders.

Agoraphobia

Usually thought of as a reaction to repeated panic attacks, agoraphobia is often an avoidance of, or suffering through, situations where it might be difficult or embarrassing to leave in the event of a panic attack. Feelings of terror that assistance might not be available in the event of a panic attack is a major feature of this condition and leads to restriction of activity in respect to destination and conditions of travel. People with agoraphobia frequently will not travel without a companion. Although it is in itself not a disorder, this term is included in the description of three of the anxiety disorders.

Panic Disorder Without and With Agoraphobia

These distressing conditions usually first appear in teenage or early adult years and may be related to life transitions. Twice as many women as men suffer from panic disorder. An individual has repeated and unexpected panic attacks with at least one attack followed by persistent worry of having additional attacks or dealing with the consequences of an attack. Attacks may occur in clusters or more randomly over longer timeframes. Losing control of one's feelings is a major concern of people with this disorder. To accommodate their anxieties, many people will go to great lengths to avoid those circumstances where fear of panic attacks is strong, such as standing in long lines or crossing bridges. This is called *situational avoidance*. Panic disorder often is accompanied by depression, alcohol abuse, and/or multiple phobias.

Specific Phobia

This disorder, frequently beginning in childhood or the mid-20s, is characterized by recurrent illogical and excessive fear and anxiety, evoked during either the expectation of, or an actual encounter with, a particular stimulus, object, or situation. The stimulus can exist in real life or be imagined, such as what might be seen in a video, book, or dream. The object or situation is fiercely avoided though there is usually insight that the reaction is exaggerated and irrational. The anxiety responses dissipate if the stimulus is weakened or removed. A phobia in one subtype often leads to other phobias in the same subgroup. The degree to which a phobia impairs functioning appears to relate to the ease and success of avoiding the stressor. One is impaired if behaviors interfere considerably with daily life, such as missing work or giving up a social life. Animals are the most common phobias, followed by spiders, bats, and rats.

Social Phobia

This disorder, also called social anxiety disorder, refers to excessive fears of potentially humiliating social or performance situations in which there is the anticipation of examination or judgment by others. Extreme self-consciousness and worry about ridicule are key factors in limiting social contacts. Concerns about one's mind going blank, having a panic attack, or losing bladder control are some of the fears that may plague a person well in advance of an event. In most cases the disruption in the person's life is not debilitating and may be focused on discreet situations, such as avoiding eating in front of others. In other circumstances, however, there may be a more pronounced interference with work and social activities, such as compromising possible achievement by quitting a job when duties expand to public speaking or refusing dates with potential lifetime mates.

Obsessive-Compulsive Disorder (OCD)

This serious and somewhat rare disorder, usually beginning in adolescence or young adulthood, is characterized by recurrent **obsessions** and **compulsions** that cause anxiety or great distress to the individual. Obsessions are persistent thoughts and images that are experienced as intrusive and unwanted. The content often concerns an exaggeration of usual fears. Examples of obsessions are aggressive thoughts, fear of acting improperly, and repeated questioning whether appliances were turned off. Compulsions are the behaviors devised to neutralize or reduce unwanted thoughts and may not be related directly to the obsession. Counting the number of items in a room, hoarding, hair pulling, and persistent hand washing are some of the behaviors devised to reduce obsessions. When attempts are made to curb these disturbing behaviors, the individual experiences surges of anxiety. Although the individual realizes that the compulsive behaviors, which are attempts to reduce tension, are ultimately fruitless and time-consuming, he or she feels unable to stop them and experiences surges of anxiety when attempts are made to do so. These odd behaviors often may lead to the alienation of others. Because they can be extremely time-consuming (more than one hour daily), they often interfere with occupational functioning and work, school, social, self-care, and homemaking routines. Other Axis I diagnoses commonly coexist with OCD, especially depression and eating disorders. Believing affected individuals share traits with people with phobias, Liebgold (2000) has labeled this group "phobocs." He offers educational information as well as exercises in a handbook (Liebgold, 2000) designed for both professionals and clients.

Post-Traumatic Stress Disorder (PTSD)

This disorder, more common in women than men, occurs in people who have been exposed to an overwhelming traumatic event that continues to impact their current daily functioning and causes them severe distress. It occurs in adults but can occur in childhood. There is some evidence that the disorder does run in families (NIMH, n.d.). Exposure to the trauma can be either in the form of witnessing it, such as seeing a murder, or by personally experiencing it, such as living through childhood sexual abuse. The occurrence in most cases is either a perceived or actual life-threatening situation in which terror and helplessness are responses. Natural disasters, combat, mass causalities, serious medical conditions, rape, domestic violence, accidents, and observing the death of a loved one are all calamities that might lead to post-traumatic stress disorder (PTSD) (NIMH, n.d.).

People reexperience the trauma in different ways but the overwhelming symptoms are anxiety and hypersensitivity and a cluster of symptoms of intrusion, arousal, and avoidance (Lazar & Offenkranz, 2010). Reoccurring dreams or nightmares, intrusive images, or thoughts, called flashbacks, are key to keeping the trauma alive. "Triggers" that evoke the memories can be in the form of smells, sounds, or images. Avoidance of situations where symptoms might occur is a common strategy used by those with this disorder. People also may feel emotionally numb and disconnected to others and at the same time hypervigilant to their surroundings.

The symptoms continue for more than one month and most often occur in close proximity to the traumatic event. Following the 9/11 World Trade Center catastrophe, many cases of PTSD were reported and emergency health care workers streamed in to help victims cope. One study cited 67,000 residents living below 110th Street in Manhattan suffering from the condition. The disorder may also develop months or years following the trauma. For example, a Bosnian refugee, hospitalized for PTSD, had suddenly developed the symptoms of this disorder many years after fleeing his homeland while watching a TV documentary about his country.

Sometimes the disorder is resolved fairly quickly, but other times, it may turn into a chronic, debilitating condition with varying ranges of impairment. Substance abuse and violence, especially related to combat stress, may lead to confrontation with the law. Chronic depression may result in suicide attempts and difficulty with interpersonal relationships.

Acute Stress Disorder

Acute stress disorder is similar to PTSD in respect to the exposure to a traumatic event and the response of horror, terror, and powerlessness. However, the symptoms of this disorder develop within one month of the event and last only from two days to one month following the exposure. In addition to experiencing at least one symptom of each

PTSD cluster (e.g., flashbacks, dreams, and avoidance of the stimuli), an individual feels a sense of detachment. She or he must also exhibit several dissociative symptoms such as numbing, derealization, **depersonalization**, and amnesia. The world seems dream-like and the individual may feel her or his feelings and body are disconnected. During a major California earthquake a woman could not recall how she had sustained cuts and bruises while trying to evacuate a store. After the earthquake others confessed to waking up frequently during the night with cold sweats and a rapid heartbeat. Although it was very helpful at times for them to talk about the trauma, this was balanced by their need to stay distanced from the event and avoid discussing it or viewing the damage.

Generalized Anxiety Disorder (GAD)

This common disorder describes persistent, uncontrollable, and excessive anxiety or worry. It appears twice as often in women than men and develops gradually from childhood to middle age. People often present a pessimistic outlook because they are continually anticipating problems in everyday life. The focus of the worry can change, from work, school, friends, and family to finances. There may be little variation in the intensity of the anxiety experienced, whether it is related to the outcome of a school exam or to the deteriorating health of a family member. People with GAD may be aware of the exaggeration of their worry but feel unable to control it.

Symptoms range from sleep disturbances to fatigue and muscle tension. Abundant sweating, gastrointestinal distress, headaches, lightheadedness, and irritability are common as well as an inability to relax. In addition to not being able to manage excessive anxiety, to have the diagnosis of GAD someone must have experienced the anxiety for at least six months. Generalized anxiety disorder rarely occurs as a primary diagnosis but major depressive disorder and other anxiety orders frequently occur simultaneously.

Anxiety Disorder Due to a General Medical Condition

Anxiety in this group is due to the physiological causes of a medical problem. Any of the previously mentioned anxiety symptoms may be present. For example, rapid pulse caused by cardiac disease may lead to clinical symptoms of anxiety.

Substance-Induced Anxiety Disorder

The physiological effect of a drug medication or toxin causes substance-induced anxiety. The anxiety may be manifested in a variety of ways, as described thus far.

GENERAL TREATMENT STRATEGIES

A variety of treatments are used to diminish the symptoms of anxiety and promote more adaptive functioning. Treatments range from medications to self-management techniques. Figure 9-3 lists types of general treatment strategies.

Psychopharmacology
Counseling
Cognitive-Behavioral Approaches
Mindfulness
Behavioral Approaches (exposure, desensitization)
Biofeedback and Meditation
EMDR
Interpersonal Skills Training
Occupational Therapy and Self-Management Techniques

NOTE: These common strategies for treatment of anxiety disorders require expertise and training, and some are more likely to be utilized by certain professionals. For example, psychiatrists prescribe medication, psychologists may provide psychotherapy and exposure therapy, and social workers or marriage and family counselors often provide couples therapy.

FIGURE 9-3. Treatment Strategies for Anxiety Disorders
© Cengage Learning 2013

Psychopharmacology

Medications addressing the physiological component of anxiety are prescribed most often for the relief of both acute attacks of anxiety and for chronic conditions (see Figure 9-4). They are used in conjunction with other types of therapy, such as cognitive-behavioral therapy (Dozois & Dobson, 2004; Lazar & Offenkranz, 2010; NIMH, n.d.; Ravindran & Stein, 2009; Rosenblatt, 2010). Their aim is to reduce the level of arousal through regulation of neurotransmitters and activating hormones in the brain. There are several groups of medications that work in this way. Antianxiety drugs, such as **benzodiazapines**, are effective for acute anxiety such as those present in panic attacks, generalized anxiety, social anxiety, and phobias, and they quickly reduce distressing symptoms of trembling and rapid heart beat. They are used as short-term therapy or as needed secondary to tolerance. They may be beneficial in the short term (2 to 12 months); however, they may lead to drug dependence and drug tolerance and are therefore not suited to long-term use. Examples of benzodiazapines are Ativan (lorazepam) and Klonopin (clonazepam). See Figure 9-4 for a list of common medications.

Antidepressant medications are the best long-term treatment and are also commonly prescribed for anxiety disorders, especially when an affective disorder coexists. However, the side effects of these drugs, such as lethargy, gastrointestinal symptoms, and sexual dysfunction, may not be tolerated well and therefore may be discontinued prematurely. The newest classification of antidepressants, selective serotonin reuptake inhibitors (SSRIs), have fewer unpleasant consequences than the earlier drugs. Prozac (fluoxetine) and Zoloft (sertraline) are examples of SSRIs, and may be useful for people with symptoms of OCD, PTSD, panic disorder, and social phobia. The older, tricyclic antidepressants, such as Tofranil (imipramine), may be especially helpful for individuals with panic disorder. Monoamine oxidase inhibitors (MAOIs) are the third and oldest class of antidepressants, which work by blocking enzymes that break up important neurotransmitters. Because of potentially serious side effects if used

CLASS OF DRUGS Brand and (Generic)	Panic Disorder	GAD	Specific Phobia	Social Phobia	OCD	PTSD
BENZODIAZEPINES Ativan (lorazepam), Klonopin (clonazepam), Librium (chlordiazepoxide), Centrax (prazepam), Restoril (temazepam), Serax (oxazepam), Valium (diazepam), Xanax (alprazolam)	X	X	X	X		
ANTIDEPRESSANTS						
Selective Serotonin Reuptake Inhibitors (SSRIs): Prozac (fluoxetine), Luvox (fluvoxamine), Zoloft (setraline), Paxil (paroxetine), Celexa (citalopram)	X			X	X	X
Tricyclics (TCAs): Tofranil (imipramine), Anafranil (clomipramine), Aventyl (nortriptyline), Ludiomil (maprotiline), Norpramin (desipramine), Sinequan (doxepin), Elavil (amitriptyline)	X				X (Anafranil)	X
Monoamine Oxidase Inhibitors (MAOIs): Nardil (phenelzine), Parnate (tranylcypromine), Marplan (isocarboxazid), Eldepryl (selegilene)	X					X
OTHER ANTIDEPRESSANTS Effexor (venlafaxine), Serzone (nefaxadone)	X	X		X	X	
BETA-BLOCKERS Inderal (propranolol), Tenormin (atenolol)				X		
ANTICONVULSANTS Neurontin (gabapentin)				X		
AZASIPIRONES BuSpar (buspirone)		X				

FIGURE 9-4. Medications Frequently Used with Anxiety Disorders.

Adapted from Anxiety Disorders Association of America website: http://www.adaa.org/AnxietyDisorderInfor/Medications.cfm 6/03

in conjunction with prohibited foods and medications, MAOIs are commonly prescribed only after other antidepressants have failed. Nardil (phenelzine) is an MAOI that is an effective treatment for panic attacks as well as PTSD.

Heart medications such as beta-blockers like propranolol (Inderal) are sometimes used for social phobias. Also, antipsychotic drugs have proven successful in treating anxiety disorders in which symptoms are so debilitating as to prevent functioning or where delusions are present.

Counseling

There are many verbal approaches designed to help decrease anxiety in its maladaptive form. They range from intense, long-term treatment, such as psychoanalysis, to short-term, supportive treatment, such as cognitive therapy. Psychotherapy addresses the immediate relief of symptoms and has a direct focus on immediate, pressing issues; supportive psychotherapy enhances the ability to cope through education, reassurance, and empathy. Cognitive interventions help clients to identify faulty, irrational thinking regarding perceived dangers and to substitute more realistic thoughts.

Cognitive-Behavioral Treatment

Cognitive-behavioral treatment (CBT) is the first-treatment for anxiety disorders (Huppert, Cahill & Foa, 2009). Research has shown its efficacy and also cost-effectiveness (Craske, 2009; Lazar & Offenkranz, 2010; Mueser, Rosenberg, & Rosenberg, 2009). Cognitive-behavioral treatment rests on a psychological model of anxiety disorders, Emotional Processing Theory. In this theory, a cognitive fear structure contains a meaning (usually largely irrational) of a dangerous stimulus and a response that helps one avoid the dangerous stimulus. The fear structure typically contains associations or prior memories that set off physiological or behavioral responses, or a fight or flight reaction. Usually in anxiety disorders the associations do not reflect reality and the avoidance becomes habitual. In the treatment, or emotional processing, the person confronts the feared stimulus that is activated, either confronted or symbolically confronted, and then new information not compatible with the irrationality of the fear structure is available for processing. So, helping clients to actually or symbolically confront fears in a safe situation where they can change their response or recognize that they have survived despite the physiological or cognitive emotions can reduce their fear and decrease avoidance. In this theory, two conditions are necessary: activation of the fear and reduction of the fear in the session or between sessions.

For example, a cognitive treatment may be accomplished through various strategies, including challenging negative thinking and global generalizations. Someone who is convinced that the decrease in the number of e-mails received from her best friend signifies rejection, for example, may be helped to see other possible causes for the change in the friend's behavior. Alternative explanations for her friend's decreased communication could be increased workload on the job, illness, more involvement in her outside pursuits, or marital pressure to spend more time with her spouse and less time on the Internet. Furthermore, the client may have made startling negative generalizations about herself from her perhaps erroneous interpretation of this one specific event. Sweeping statements may take this form: I upset my friend, I'm insensitive, I'm unable to sustain friendships, I'm unlikable, I'm a loser. In this case, the psychotherapist would help the client focus on the specific situation in question and challenge notions that possible rejection by one friend does not signify general unworthiness. This method may be accomplished through seeking "proof" to support these notions. Educational sessions and homework assignments may help to support cognitive interventions.

Another example of cognitive treatment may address constant worrying and ruminations. A client could not stop thinking that she had made a huge mistake that might cause her to lose her job. These thoughts intruded on her daily activities. She was instructed to make a list of the worst thoughts and to read them out loud to herself twice a day, for at least 15 minutes per session. If she was unable to do this then the therapist made a list with her and recorded the list for her to listen to. After about five days of this activity, called "flooding," her ruminations decreased and did not seem so important.

Mindfulness

Mindfulness-based therapy (MBT) is a current approach to treatment for anxiety (and depression) (Evans et al., 2008; Hofmann, Sawyer, Witt, & Oh, 2010). Such approaches are based on ancient Buddhist and Yoga practices and may be used in a form of mindfulness-based cognitive therapy and mindfulness-based stress reduction. **Mindfulness** is a mental state of being aware of one's sensations, thoughts, bodily states, consciousness, and the environment, while also being accepting, open, and curious (Hofmann et al., 2010). Thus it is achieving a state of focus in the present moment without making judgments. In mindfulness an individual regulates his or her attention and orients himself or herself to the present. The basic idea of mindfulness is that by staying present in and not judging the present moment relieves stress. This strategy works because it counteracts the tendency to think of the past or the future, thoughts believed to contribute to feelings of depression and anxiety. Also, by educating people to respond to stressful situations more reflectively rather than reflexively, MBT can counter avoidance strategies, which may be attempts to alter frequency of unwanted internal experiences. Thus MBT can eliminate the maladaptive strategies that are believed to contribute to the maintenance of many, if not all, emotional disorders. In addition, there is an emphasis on slow and deep breathing involved in mindfulness meditation that may decrease bodily symptoms of distress by balancing the sympathetic and parasympathetic systems.

There were relatively few quantitative studies of MBT until recently. Hofmann et al. (2010) conducted a thorough meta-analysis of 720 qualitative and quantitative studies, including analysis of 39 random-controlled studies. They found that overall MBT did reduce anxiety (and depression) in those individuals with anxiety and depression, more so in those with anxiety and depression disorders. So, MBT approaches would be good additions to an occupational therapy practitioner's toolbox, particularly with MBT's behavioral or "doing" component. In addition, MBT's encouragement of emotional regulation skills is also part of occupational therapy's domain of practice (AOTA, 2008) and outcomes of health and wellness.

Behavioral Approaches

Once irrational ideas are identified, behavioral strategies may be applied to practice new behaviors. There is a broad range of behavioral interventions and many are combined to be the most effective.

In Vivo Exposure Therapy

Exposure therapy, also called "programmed practice" (Agras & Berkowitz, 1994), focuses entirely on real encounters with the objects of the individual's anxiety, while helping him or her to use a variety of techniques (i.e., deep breathing and positive self-talk) to master the situation. Because of its *in vivo* (real-life) component, exposure therapy appears to be a highly effective and powerful treatment, which helps to weaken fear and the subsequent avoidant responses, especially with persons with phobic, panic, and obsessive-compulsive disorders.

Imaginal Exposure

Similar to *in vivo* exposure, imaginal exposure has the client close his eyes and then imagine the feared stimuli instead of actually confronting it. This exposure helps habituate clients to the memory of the feared stimulus and to distinguish between an actual traumatic stimulus and the non-harmful memory of it. Imaginal exposure is used also when *in vivo* exposure is not safe or feasible (Huppert et al., 2009).

Virtual Exposure

A variant of exposure therapy, virtual reality-enhanced exposure significantly decreased those affected with PTSD after the World Trade Center attacks of 9/11/2001 (Lazar & Offenkranz, 2010). Clients viewed computer-generated 3-D sequences in increasingly intense increments. The virtual exposure significantly decreased all symptoms. Virtual exposure has also been tested with children experiencing anxiety in the classroom and combat veterans (Lisetti et al., 2009) using avatars in a 3-D environment.

Systematic Desensitization

Although one of the first exposure techniques, systematic desensitization has fallen out of favor with therapists and researchers (Huppert et al., 2009). Systematic desensitization is a type of incremental exposure that attempts to systematically diminish anxiety related to specific fears primarily through the use of imagery and relaxation and then real contact with the image of or actual object. Used most often with phobic disorders, a trained therapist helps the client devise a hierarchical list of, usually, 10 items to break down the fear into steps according to the subjective rating of their intensity (Wolpe, 1973). For example, someone who fears rats would likely rank touching a rat as very challenging, while looking at a picture of a rat might be the least threatening. Starting with the least troubling item on the list and coupling progressive relaxation with visualization, the person advances up the hierarchy once each level is mastered as evidenced by the absence of an anxiety response. A variation of this intervention is participant modeling (Bandura, 1977), whereby the therapist interacts with the feared object or situation and then encourages the client to interact jointly before performing alone.

Interoceptive Desensitization

Interoceptive desensitization refers to evoking fear in a controlled setting to help manage the symptoms before they mushroom into unmanageable anxiety, as in the case with someone with panic attacks (Bourne, 2011; Huppert et al., 2009). Essentially, panic-like sensations are induced with the goal of finding activities that produce similar sensations to the avoided situation. The client then is assisted to distinguish normal responses from the pathological ones, learn that the sensations do not cause harm, and experience a sense of control over them. For instance, someone who fears heights could practice spinning on a desk chair, look at videos of people on roller coasters, and then participate in virtual video games where dizziness might be evoked. Eventually, the real situation is tackled.

Exposure and Response Prevention (ERP)

Exposure and response prevention (ERP) (Bourne, 2011; Huppert et al., 2009) is a treatment applied to people with OCD whereby usual behaviors devised by the client to ward off anxiety caused by obsessional thinking are gradually prevented. For example, a client with OCD was perceptually fearful of germs and scrubbed his hands at least 50 times a day for about six minutes each time. The ERP program slowly and systematically first exposed him to the feared stimulus, in this case, touching doorknobs, and prevented him from the ritual hand washing by incremental restrictions of the behavior. This was accomplished both by curtailing the number of hand washing episodes per day and by the length of time of each hand washing occurrence. Exposure and response prevention has also been proposed for treatment of eating disorders where the rituals associated with anorexia nervosa are obsessional. Clients are exposed to feared foods and systematically prevented from using their rituals to avoid the feared food (Steinglass et al., 2011).

Biofeedback

Biofeedback has evolved with the use of portable devices (Reiner, 2008), which are inexpensive for most clinics, and can be used at home (Ratanasiripong, Sverduk, Hayashino, & Prince, 2010) or other environments (McLay & Spira, 2009). The goal of biofeedback is to decrease arousal by providing the client with objective data about, and then helping him or her gain control over, biological states that are normally involuntary. Biofeedback techniques target and attempt to alter changes in heart rate, blood pressure, sweating, and skin temperature by providing feedback through instrumentation. (Electrodes, blood pressure indicators, and finger sensors in contact with the body are examples of devices used to provide data that tracks how the treatments are impacting physical condition.) Once information is received, the client learns methods of altering the body functions to reduce anxiety. Biofeedback may be seen as a type of behavioral therapy in that objective, observable data are the focus.

Meditation

Meditation has been used for those with anxiety disorders and includes styles that draw from both Western and Eastern practices, although research regarding the efficacy of meditation is lacking (Krisanaprakornkit, Piyavhatkul, & Laopaiboon, 2009). Calm breathing, thought focusing, repetition of sounds, and posture are aspects that are stressed in varying ways. Mindful meditation has been used for chronic conditions, both physiological and psychological, especially PTSD. What makes this practice unique is that the participant is instructed to observe thoughts without judging, instead of ridding himself or herself of them (Freeman & Lawlis, 2001). Studies have shown that during meditation, heart rate, respiration, anxiety level, and oxygen consumption are lowered and positive mood states are raised (Freeman & Lawlis, 2001). Other relaxation exercises are discussed in more detail in the Occupational Therapy and Self-Management Techniques section in this chapter.

Eye Movement Desensitization and Reprocessing (EMDR)

This approach, developed by Shapiro and Maxfield (2002) is used to treat a range of psychological disorders from PTSD to phobias (Spector, 2007). This multifaceted and short-term form of psychotherapy draws from cognitive-behavioral approaches, combining eye movements with evocation of feelings, sensations, thoughts, and memories in order to reprocess them in the brain. Negative feelings such as anxiety associated with memories of traumatic events are induced during directed experiences by a trained therapist, who combines eye exercises with verbal instructions. Clients are instructed to track a light or the therapist's finger as it moves back and forth horizontally. This intervention stimulates both sides of the brain. The expected result is that the client gains insight and assumes more adaptive and integrated behavior.

Research in the field of anxiety disorders has investigated the effectiveness of different types of therapeutic interventions. These results as described by Roth and Fonagy (1996), by Lazar (2010), and by the NIMH (2011) are summarized as follows. For panic disorder, cognitive and exposure therapy in combination with applied relaxation are most helpful. Systematic desensitization is the treatment of choice for someone with a specific phobia. A combination of social skills training and exposure therapy is most useful for an individual treated for social phobia. In addition to tricyclic medications, someone with OCD would be most helped by mass exposure and response prevention for behavioral aspects of the condition and cognitive therapy for ruminations. Those managing symptoms of PTSD would benefit from anxiety management strategies, especially CBT and psychoeducation, in some cases (Lazar & Offenkranz, 2010). Cognitive-behavioral treatment has also been most effective with individuals with GAD in conjunction with short-term use of benzodiazapines.

Interpersonal Skills Training

Those who have a social anxiety disorder may have deficits in their interpersonal interaction skills. Therefore, they may avoid all social contact, which then further limits their social support (Huppert et al., 2009). Therefore, interpersonal skills training, such as assertiveness training, or basic training on how to initiate, maintain, and end conversations, is suggested.

OCCUPATIONAL THERAPY AND SELF-MANAGEMENT TECHNIQUES

Most of the anxiety disorders have a chronic course with periods of remission. Therefore, the foremost task is learning how to manage anxiety in order to continue functioning and to face, rather than avoid, situations that irrationally generate fear. The avoidance of fear-producing stimuli is an attempt at self-protection, but it is maladaptive if it interferes with the fulfillment of environmental and internal needs (Depoy & Kolodner, 1991). Avoidant behavior also reinforces a sense of helplessness. Occupational therapists can help people develop a range of self-efficacy techniques that help to increase the feeling of influence or mastery over one's circumstances (Bandura, 1995, 1997). A problem-focused approach is especially useful with this population, for it helps people to respond rationally, rather than emotionally, to potentially fear-producing situations. Self-efficacy has been said to be a major factor in fear reduction (Taylor & Arnow, 1988). In fact, self-efficacy as a goal is a major tenet of the Model of Human Occupation and so addressing self-efficacy fits seamlessly with an occupational therapy approach (Kielhofner, 2007). As well, the OTPF (AOTA, 2008) suggests that interventions can be made in performance areas of social, leisure, self-care, rest, and sleep and in emotional regulation and coping skills.

ASSESSMENT

Many tools exist for measuring the degree and type of anxiety. Occupational therapists, provided they have the required education, qualifications, and experience in using these general anxiety measurement tools, sometimes administer them in research settings. The Hospital Anxiety and Depression Scale (HAD) (Zigmond & Snaith, 1983) is composed of 14 questions that identify levels of both factors in hospitalized clients. Differentiating between state and trait anxiety, the State/Trait Anxiety Inventory (STAI) (Spielberger, 1983) looks at whether anxiety is either a temporary or more permanent condition. A third general anxiety assessment is the Institute for Personality and Ability Testing (IPAT) anxiety scale (Krug, Scheier, & Cattell, 1976). (Raymond Cattel, 1905–1998, was a prolific and productive psychologist who founded the institute and studied psychological assessments throughout his life.) This self-assessment of 40 questions investigates factors such as tension and guilt-proneness and measures clinical anxiety. This measure is typically used with a clinical population. Physiological measures of heart rate and body temperature are also used as indicators of changes in heart rate. By using these immediately in conjunction with interventions, clinicians can help clients monitor probable decrease in levels of anxiety. Typically occupational therapists are interested in how anxiety impacts daily functioning. Their target, therefore, is assessing impairment caused by anxiety.

In order to develop strategies for improved functioning, the level of impairment of the person with anxiety must be assessed. The assessments serve to highlight the extent of the disorder's interference in daily life activities.

Interviews, surveys, observation of performance, role checklists, function questionnaires, self-assessment of activities, and activity configurations listed in Figures 9-5 through 9-8 elicit information about how anxiety impacts a person's life. For example, accounting for daily activities by filling out typical schedules (Figure 9-5) reveals significant information in respect to role functioning as well as productive activities (Figures 9-6 and 9-7). Someone with agoraphobia may stay indoors the majority of each day, during which time expected activities are not performed, with the roles of hobbyist, homemaker, or worker being lost. Also, although self-assessment (Figure 9-7) is used most often to target interventions (discussed in the next section) and develop an occupational therapy program, the assessment also indicates the impact of anxiety on daily activities.

ROLE CHECKLIST

NAME _____ AGE_____ DATE_____

SEX: ☐ MALE ☐ FEMALE   ARE YOU RETIRED: ☐ YES ☐ NO

MARITAL STATUS: ☐ SINGLE ☐ MARRIED ☐ SEPARATED ☐ DIVORCED ☐ WIDOWED

The purpose of this checklist is to identify the major roles in your life. The checklist, which is divided into two parts, presents 10 roles and defines each one.

PART I

Beside each role, indicate, by checking the appropriate column, if you performed the role in the past, if you presently perform the role, and if you plan to perform the role in the future. You may check more than one column for each role. For example, if you volunteered in the past, do not volunteer at present, but plan to in the future, you would check the past and future columns.

ROLE	PAST	PRESENT	FUTURE
STUDENT: Attending school on a part-time or full-time basis.			
WORKER: Part-time or full-time paid employment.			
VOLUNTEER: Donating services, *at least once a week,* to a hospital, school, community, political campaign, and so forth.			
CARE GIVER: Responsibility, *at least once a week,* for the care of someone such as a child, spouse, relative, or friend.			
HOME MAINTAINER: Responsibility, *at least once a week,* for the upkeep of the home such as housecleaning or yardwork.			
FRIEND: Spending time or doing something, *at least once a week,* with a friend.			
FAMILY MEMBER: Spending time or doing something, *at least once a week,* with a family member such as a child, spouse, parent, or other relative.			
RELIGIOUS PARTICIPANT: Involvement, *at least once a week,* in groups or activities affiliated with one's religion (excluding worship).			
HOBBYIST/AMATEUR: Involvement, *at least once a week,* in a hobby or amateur activity such as sewing, playing a musical instrument, woodworking, sports, the theater, or participation in a club or team.			
PARTICIPANT IN ORGANIZATIONS: Involvement, *at least once a week,* in organizations such as the American Legion, National Organization for Women, Parents Without Partners, Weight Watchers, and so forth.			
OTHER:_____ A role not listed which you have performed, are presently performing, and/or plan to perform. Write the role on the line above and check the appropriate column(s).			

FIGURE 9-5. Role Checklist

Reprinted with permission from Frances Oakley, MS, OTR, FAOTA

(Continues)

PART II

The same roles are listed below. Next to *each* role check the column which best indicates how valuable or important the role is to you. Answer for *each role,* even if you have never performed or do not plan to perform the role.

ROLE	NOT AT ALL VALUABLE	SOMEWHAT VALUABLE	VERY VALUABLE
STUDENT: Attending school on a part-time or full-time basis.			
WORKER: Part-time or full-time paid employment.			
VOLUNTEER: Donating services, *at least once a week,* to a hospital, school, community, political campaign, and so forth.			
CARE GIVER: Responsibility, *at least once a week,* for the care of someone such as a child, spouse, relative, or friend.			
HOME MAINTAINER: Responsibility, *at least once a week,* for the upkeep of the home such as housecleaning or yardwork.			
FRIEND: Spending time or doing something, *at least once a week,* with a friend.			
FAMILY MEMBER: Spending time or doing something, *at least once a week,* with a family member such as a child, spouse, parent, or other relative.			
RELIGIOUS PARTICIPANT: Involvement, *at least once a week,* in groups or activities affiliated with one's religion (excluding worship).			
HOBBYIST/AMATEUR: Involvement, *at least once a week,* in a hobby or amateur activity such as sewing, playing a musical instrument, woodworking, sports, the theater, or participation in a club or team.			
PARTICIPANT IN ORGANIZATIONS: Involvement, *at least once a week,* in organizations such as the American Legion, National Organization for Women, Parents Without Partners, Weight Watchers, and so forth.			
OTHER:_____ A role not listed which you have performed, are presently performing, and/or plan to perform. Write the role on the line above and check the appropriate column(s).			

FIGURE 9-5. Role Checklist (*continued*)

Reprinted with permission from Frances Oakley, MS, OTR, FAOTA

TREATMENT INTERVENTIONS

The primary occupational therapy interventions utilized with anxiety disorders are listed in Table 9-2. The selection of strategies will depend on the nature of the disorder, the setting in which the client is being treated, and the environment to which the person will return. There is a broad application of principles, including approaches

WORK

The extent to which my work is impaired because of anxiety

0	1	2	3	4	5	6	7	8	9	10
Never		Slightly			Moderately		Markedly		Very Severely	

SOCIAL ACTIVITIES

The extent to which my social life is impaired because of anxiety
(going out with friends, dating, outings, entertaining)

0	1	2	3	4	5	6	7	8	9	10
Never		Slightly			Moderately		Markedly		Very Severely	

LEISURE ACTIVITIES

The extent to which engagement in leisure activities is impaired because of anxiety
(hobbies, use of free time)

0	1	2	3	4	5	6	7	8	9	10
Never		Slightly			Moderately		Markedly		Very Severely	

HOME, SELF-MAINTENANCE, AND FAMILY RESPONSIBILITIES

The extent to which my ability to care for myself and others is impaired by my anxiety
(cleaning house, meal preparation, carpooling, doing laundry, paying bills, grooming)

0	1	2	3	4	5	6	7	8	9	10
Never		Slightly			Moderately		Markedly		Very Severely	

FIGURE 9-6. Function Questionnaire

Adapted from the Fear Questionnaire in Taylor & Arnow, 1988

for people suffering more severe impairment (Stein & Nikolic, 1989). Most of the approaches listed in the table have emerged from other disciplines, most notably from psychology and from health and wellness. However, they have become widely used by professionals of all disciplines who practice in mental health. Occupational therapists use the techniques to enhance occupational therapy goals and for engagement in occupation to support participation in context. Naturally, it is assumed that, when employing any strategy, the therapist will become competent through education and training.

There is some evidence that occupational therapists use the assessments and the following methods in different combinations in different groups (Prior, 1998; Rosier, Williams, & Ryrie, 1998). For example, Prior (1998) reported the success of

TABLE 9-2. Occupational Therapy and Self-Management Techniques

- *Relaxation Training*
  Breathing Exercises
  Progressive Muscle Relaxation
  Visualization
  Autogenic Training
- *Assertiveness Training*
- *Community Mobility/Reentry*
- *Expressive Activities*
  Journal Writing
  Craft and Art Activities
- *Functional Behavioral Training*
- *Education/Lifestyle Alterations*
- *Rational/Cognitive Approaches*
- *Time Management*

© Cengage Learning 2013

a six-week anxiety management course at a day hospital that used the HAD scale and the STAI as dependent measures. In addition, clients valued the course as determined by a client satisfaction questionnaire. Strategies used in the six sessions were education and use of homework, breathing, relaxation, cognitive-behavioral methods, and assertiveness. Rosier et al. (1998) discussed an anxiety management group in a community mental health setting where anxiety management was identified by occupational therapists as the second most frequent intervention after activities of daily living (ADLs). In their seven-week group they used psychoeducation, progressive muscle relaxation, lifestyle assessment, cognitive-behavioral techniques, guided imagery, musical relaxation, and homework. The efficacy of the group was assessed by a client satisfaction questionnaire six weeks after the group's conclusion.

Relaxation Training

Relaxation training can be an effective intervention to help people with anxiety disorders diminish arousal states and ultimately cope with stress; the relaxation response and a feeling of well-being are incompatible with anxiety. Initially, clients usually require external direction, but the overall goal is to teach them to recognize and manage their own anxiety while it is "young" (still of short duration) to prevent major anxiety attacks, as well as to avert attacks if they occur. It is important to help people generalize from treatment sessions to the variety of life situations where anxiety is likely to occur. The Function Questionnaire (see Figure 9-6) targets these areas effectively. The client rates the extent to which anxiety interferes with daily activities from a quantitative and qualitative standpoint. The next step is to focus on these areas one at a time and strategize how

Self-Assessment of Activities

Name:_____

Date:_____

This checklist will be used to help develop an Occupational Therapy program for you. Mark the appropriate column for each item and add any comments you feel would be helpful.

Activity	Never a problem	Sometimes a problem	Always a problem	N.A.	Comments
Grooming					
Bathing or showering					
Preparing meals					
Food shopping					
Doing errands					
House cleaning					
Doing yardwork					
Caring for others					
Managing money					
Transportation					
Socializing					
Attending school					
Working					
Volunteering					
Exercising					
Concentrating					
Problem solving					
Communicating					
Coping with stress					
Managing time					
Managing impulses					
Doing leisure activities					

FIGURE 9-7. Self-Assessment of Activities

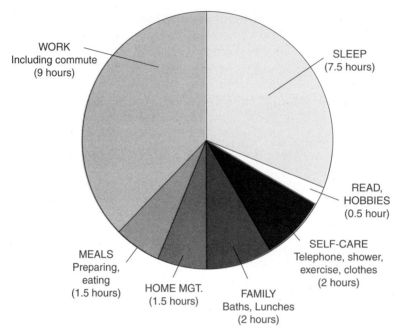

FIGURE 9-8. Activity Configuration
© Cengage Learning 2013

relaxation techniques could be incorporated into the activities. For example, this method was successful with a construction worker who often became panicky when working on roofs. Utilizing abdominal breathing just before she went on the roof or while she was working on it greatly helped to reduce her symptoms of rapid pulse and queasiness.

Typically, occupational therapists teach a variety of relaxation skills (after they themselves have been sufficiently trained). These skills include deep breathing, progressive muscle relaxation, visualization, and **autogenic training** among others. As described by Benson (1976), who is a pioneer of relaxation training, all relaxation interventions involve the following: (1) the person has a passive attitude, (2) there is a decrease in muscle tone, (3) the environment is quiet, and (4) a mental device is used, such as an image or sound. Anxious people often lack the ability to engage in all steps of the relaxation activity; therefore, it is helpful to teach specific relaxation exercises that have an action component in addition to the distraction of a mental device. Progressive muscle relaxation (discussed in a subsequent section) has this feature. Sessions usually last up to about 30 minutes. Because of the quiet atmosphere generated by the relaxation training, it is wise to include people with the same attention span and to exclude those who are extremely restless or distractible. People should be given the option of keeping their eyes open or closed and the choice of sitting in a chair or sitting or lying on the floor. A protective covering such as a sheet should be available for hygienic reasons. If an individual chooses to use a chair, the therapist should make certain that there is back support by putting the chair against the wall. This will protect the person's neck from possible injury should he or she fall asleep.

Each person will have a preferred technique. Therefore, it is helpful to briefly introduce a variety of methods so as to gain feedback from the client as to which is the most useful. This can be accomplished by having people rate their subjective levels of anxiety on a scale from 1 to 10 before and after the exercises, by taking respiratory and heart rates before and after tasks, by asking which exercise was the most effective, or by observing the person's apparent level of concentration during the exercises. Sampling a variety of relaxation techniques within one session has the advantage of addressing problems of limited attention span and restricted opportunities for treatment due to the increasingly short lengths of stay on inpatient units or treatment in a home setting.

Making personalized audiotapes for relaxation can be extremely helpful, but commercial tapes are also readily available in a variety of forms, from soothing music or nature sounds to directed sessions. When making or selecting tapes, it is essential to consider the concentration level as well as the particular needs of each person. If given a choice, most people will state a preference for either a male or female narrator; therefore, having both available is useful. Some clinicians are finding that having clients make their own tapes facilitates a deeper sense of personal control (H. Stein, personal communication, June 2, 2003, Grand Rounds, Stanford Hospital and Clinics). Once the individual learns and masters the selected techniques, he or she should be helped to apply the skill to everyday barriers. For example, a person with social phobia may learn to practice a few minutes of deep breathing before meeting coworkers for lunch, an individual with agoraphobia may visualize a pleasant spot before leaving the house, and a person with PTSD may engage in relaxation exercises to counteract insomnia.

People should also be encouraged to differentiate, and then apply, other resources they have previously used to enhance the relaxation process, such as music, meditation, lighting, warm baths, and humor.

Breathing Exercises

Abdominal breathing can effectively address relaxation, especially when people learn to self-monitor the technique by placing their hands on the abdomen and witnessing their hands rise on inhalation. This is a logical first task for an individual with an anxiety disorder for it can be short in duration and requires limited direction. However, clients should be introduced to this technique slowly to avoid lightheadedness from the increased oxygen consumption. Breathing exercises have been found to be a useful strategy to use during panic attacks (Clark, Salkovskis & Chalkley, 1985), with the addition of the client counting to five between breaths. Under stress, many anxious people hyperventilate, causing blood chemistry changes that lead to unpleasant sensations, such as dizziness. It is this reaction that may actually precipitate the panic and fear. Respiratory control by means of slow, paced breathing counteracts the patterns of hyperventilation thought to contribute to acute anxiety attacks. Sometimes other types of breathing exercises are more effective or can be used in conjunction with abdominal breathing. Imagining the words, "I am," as one inhales, and, "relaxed," as one exhales helps to slow the breath and focus on breathing patterns. Synchronizing breathing with counting slowly or the visualization of color is also effective. Clients seem to respond favorably to imagining the inhalation of clear colors, such as yellow or blue, and the exhalation of gray.

Progressive Muscle Relaxation

Progressive muscle relaxation, which was first described by Jacobson (1938), teaches clients to tighten and release voluntary muscle groups slowly and methodically in a progressive fashion, thereby contrasting the states of tension and relaxation. This technique offers a discharge of tension as a means to achieve a state of deep relaxation, with the underlying hypothesis that relaxation of the body leads to relaxation of the mind. For clients with limited concentration, the active involvement of tensing and relaxing can be more engaging and therefore more successful than pure mental activity. Daily sessions are recommended for practicing and mastering the technique.

Visualization

Picturing a pleasant scene is another method used to enhance the relaxation response. It is easiest for people to activate images after anxiety has partially subsided; therefore, it is recommended to precede visualization with breathing exercises. Soothing music may also help to evoke images, but some people will still need guidance. If the therapist provides mental pictures for the client such as floating or diving into water, it is important to know beforehand that the images selected are pleasant. Directions can include visualizing a leaf floating in a stream, walking in a meadow or strolling by a pond, returning to a happy childhood place, imagining a fantasy place, or picturing a comfortable place in one's home. By presenting only a general direction and structure, such as saying, "Imagine a beautiful place you've seen," the therapist encourages the client to fill in more of his or her personal experience. The exercise then becomes more interactive and the client may feel a stronger sense of participation and control. If the client is unable to evoke images easily, simply picturing colors may provide a sufficient degree of pleasant sensation. Visualization exercises are contraindicated for patients experiencing perceptual distortions (hallucinations) or thought disorders (delusions) because these exercises can intensify the psychotic experience and become frightening. If visualization exercises stimulate flashbacks of distressing events in people who have PTSD, another form of relaxation should be introduced. Before beginning the task, the occupational therapist should always inform clients to open their eyes if the exercise evokes unpleasant feelings. The therapist should assume this may be happening if he or she observes crying, restlessness, or the eyes suddenly opening. Visualization methods can also be adapted for use with children.

Autogenic Training

Autogenic training, which was developed by German neurologist H. H. Shultz, teaches the body and mind to relax through the person's own verbal commands. The intent is to relax the voluntary and involuntary muscles to provide **vasodilatation** and help regulate the circulatory and respiratory systems (Davis, Eshelman, & McKay, 2008; Levy, 2008).

The occupational therapist can introduce several of the exercises, which are learned methodically over several weeks. They consist of imagining the limbs as heavy and warm, the heart as beating regularly and calmly, the lungs as operating regularly, the solar plexus as feeling warm, and the forehead as feeling cool. Since this method of relaxation has a strong effect on body physiology, it is not recommended for people with serious medical problems. In addition, it is contraindicated for children and for people with severe psychiatric disorders.

Assertiveness and General Social Skills Training

Clients with anxiety disorders often manifest passive behavior. This may be due in part to fears related to anticipated embarrassment in social situations in which they may feel they will have no control. This is particularly true of clients with social phobias and GAD. For example, a young man with generalized anxiety and depression was exceedingly lonely. Terrified to attend social functions, where he could possibly meet a potential mate, he ruminated about rejection and humiliation. He was unsure of how to approach strangers, initiate conversation, or sustain friendships. The cycle continued as he further isolated himself despite craving social contact, which he did in part to manage his anxiety. This client attended assertiveness groups while on a psychiatric unit and was referred to a community class at discharge. The OT group included the following stages: (1) understanding the components of assertive behavior, including differentiation between styles; (2) identifying personal styles and blocks to behaving assertively, including irrational beliefs and fears; and (3) practicing assertive communication and the principles and applications of good communication practices through role-play situations. Assertiveness training was popular in the 1970s but is no less useful for those with disorders (as well as for therapists [Mays, 1987]). Assertiveness training (Alberti & Emmons, 1990; Gaddis, 2010; Smith, 1975) helped him to reduce anxiety and taught him to confront intimidating social situations in a way that offered more personal control. Assertiveness training can be an effective means of helping people reduce anxiety because it can help people confront intimidating situations in a way that offers more personal control.

Social skills group can be helpful by teaching other appropriate ways of interacting with others. Topics such as eye contact and other nonverbal communication and problem-solving uncomfortable situations are usually explored through discussion, educational materials, and role playing.

Community Mobility and Reentry

Isolation is a serious problem for people with anxiety disorders, who may completely withdraw from friends, family, leisure activities, and work in order to curb their anxiety. Not only does such constraint lead to loneliness and depression, but the absence of physical and emotional outlets can also contribute to maintaining the anxiety cycle. With restricted activity, people may become even more focused on their thoughts, sensations, and other internal experiences. Clients with anxiety may benefit from locating community resources that draw on former or current interests and simultaneously provide contact with other people. Some feel most supported in activities provided by mental health agencies, such as support groups or social events, because here they can receive direct help with their anxiety while also engaging in the activity at hand. Other clients feel more comfortable in small classes such as private art, music, or bridge classes, which are offered in many communities. Many prefer noncompetitive enrichment classes over junior college courses such as those offered by adult education programs. The occupational therapist can help locate appropriate programs during an individual or group treatment session.

Expressive Activities

Clients experiencing anxiety disorders may benefit from engaging in expressive activities, which provide an outlet and release for the physical and emotional turbulence associated with anxiety. Family members and friends may have limited tolerance for discussing the client's repetitive concerns, so self-reliance techniques can help to preserve social relationships as well as promote independence.

Journal and Diary Writing. A journal can become a focus and receptacle for distressing thoughts. The symbolic act of writing down concerns and feelings may help the individual become better able to dismiss the troublesome emotions once the book is closed. It is been demonstrated that writing about stressful events can reduce physiological symptoms present in some illnesses (Booth & Petrie, 2002; Pennebaker, 2004, 2007; Smyth, Stone, Hurewitz, & Kaell, 1999). When using a diary, a person has control over the expression of content and amount of time devoted to addressing symptoms. For example, a woman in her early 30s with OCD annoyed her mother, who lived next door, by her persistent criticism of her mother's perceived lack of attention to home maintenance and safety. To improve their relationship, the daughter began to write these worries in a notebook rather than discuss them with her mother, who did not perceive that there was a problem.

Sometimes keeping a journal or diary is suggested by a psychologist or psychiatrist as a means for recording specific anxiety disorder symptoms such as those of panic attacks or phobias. The information included may concern the times during the day when the symptoms emerge, the nature and intensity of the symptoms, and events occurring prior to or after the attack. These data help the person with anxiety achieve some control over the symptoms by recognizing their patterns, precipitants, and consequences.

Craft and Art Activities. Structured craft and expressive art activities both have a place in the treatment of anxiety disorders. In structured crafts, the limits of a repetitive and predictive project can offer reassurance to the fearful person and help to contain anxiety. Clients with anxiety disorders often prefer projects with true boundaries, such as plastic "stained glass," sophisticated coloring sheets, and mosaics. Simple greeting cards may have the same effect. Completing these tasks successfully also provides a sense of mastery through accomplishment and increases clients' perceived sense of effectiveness.

The more expressive art activities may offer a release of tension through physical activity, such as ripping paper or using a stippling brush for painting designs on paper or cloth, and thus provide an acceptable substitute for an otherwise inappropriate expression of anxiety. For example, a client with multiple diagnoses including borderline personality disorder repeatedly burned herself with lit cigarettes in order to find relief from intolerable levels of anxiety. The occupational therapist provided her with a large body outline on which she was able to draw cigarette burns when she felt overcome by these impulses. Another client, a middle-aged man with schizophrenia and OCD, was encouraged to draw with large felt pens whenever he began to frantically pace, wring his hands, or shake. His subsequent drawings were usually highly controlled, for example, portraying multi-tiled houses and paved roads, but his obsessive behavior decreased (see Figure 9-9).

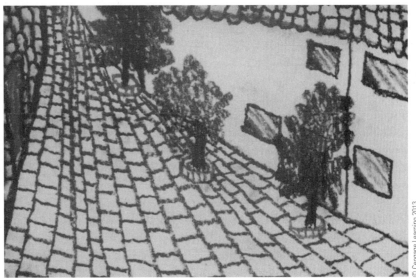

© Cengage Learning 2013

FIGURE 9-9. Client Drawing in Which Anxiety Is Expressed and Channeled

Expressive art activities may also stimulate self-understanding through the content that emerges. For example, in a group activity, a young mother with tenacious abdominal **psychogenic** pain and anxiety inadvertently drew a representation of her pain similar to the symbol she drew for her husband. When she discussed these similarities with her psychotherapist, she was able to connect the pain in her stomach to anger at her husband for not participating in any of the parenting responsibilities. All the expressive techniques discussed in this section are personally gratifying and increase the internal sense of control and self-mastery.

Functional Behavioral Training

A psychologist or psychiatrist may ask the occupational therapist to assist in carrying out behavioral programs that directly deal with improving functioning by decreasing symptoms as they relate to daily activities. For example, the plan may take the form of accompanying an agoraphobic client on a community outing to combat anxiety symptoms while riding a bus or going to a store. This intervention (previously referred to as exposure therapy) addresses avoidant behavior and can be an effective approach in treating some of the anxiety disorders, particularly phobias.

The occupational therapist may help the client negotiate difficult tasks through instruction in breathing exercises, refuting irrational thoughts, or suggesting that he or she confront unpleasant sensations as if "riding the wave." More experienced occupational therapists may actually take part in devising the behavioral plan for decreasing symptoms. This might include helping the person identify target behaviors and then breaking them down into smaller, manageable steps. This is traditionally called *grading the activity* by occupational therapists. For example, one client with agoraphobia wanted to be able to go back to his favorite coffeehouse a few times a week. The occupational therapist guided him in making a plan—walking first one block from home with her, walking alone on the same route, buying a newspaper in front of the coffeehouse, and so forth. Another occupational therapist assisted a young woman with OCD who had a fixation on soiled clothes and contamination of the washing machine, which prevented her from performing adequate hygiene routines as she felt impelled to wear the same, unwashed, clothes day after day. The occupational therapist helped her counteract these fears through relaxation training and visualization prior to, and during, the actual laundry activity, resulting in the client being able to carry out the task and thus achieve adequate hygiene.

Education and Lifestyle Alterations

The relationship between internal (inherent to an individual) and external (outside) factors and anxiety is often not understood by those experiencing anxiety disorders. In particular, reducing caffeine intake, eliminating non–medically prescribed drugs, exercising regularly, eating a balanced diet, maintaining appropriate weight, sleeping sufficiently, lowering blood pressure, increasing leisure involvement, and managing time effectively are all elements that can positively affect one's ability to cope with anxiety. Sufferers of panic attacks tend to experience fewer attacks when their overall state of arousal is diminished by attending to some of these basic suggestions (Stein et al., 2010; Taylor & Arnow, 1988).

Rational-Cognitive Approaches

The occupational therapist may assist people in coping more effectively by utilizing cognitive interventions (Dryden, 2003; Ellis, 1976) (provided he or she is properly trained in the techniques). Anxious clients are often highly perfectionistic and consequently self-critical of their current or anticipated behavior. They worry in the form of engaging in negative self-talk about their finances, health, job performance, and relationships, expecting failure in every area (Wright & Beck, 1994). The worry becomes even more magnified in OCD. This negative thinking is both time-consuming and self-defeating and usually distorts reality. Cognitive strategies attempt to help replace negative self-talk statements with more favorable ones. One technique is to teach clients to make positive self-statements. For example, when asked to participate in a drawing activity, a good number of clients will disqualify themselves by saying: "I am a terrible artist. I can't do this." The occupational therapist can suggest a reframe of the statement such as, "It makes me nervous to draw but at least I'll give it a try." Another strategy is to help clients relabel internally directed, destructive emotions as more neutral and appropriate ones. For instance, anxiety at failing to meet work deadlines can be changed to "concern," feelings of worthlessness at being criticized can be changed to "annoyance," and guilt at criticizing a child can be changed to "regret" (Davis et al., 2008). These interventions seem to be most effective when they are presented as paper-and-pencil exercises, perhaps because problem solving through writing causes a delay in emotional response. The task can also be applied as a self-management strategy whereby the individual tracks responses over time.

Time Management

Anxiety is often manifested by paralysis in goal-directed activity, which arises as a by-product of fears of failure, decreased concentration, or preoccupation with the stressor. Inactivity is further perpetuated by a lack of task mastery, which would likely enhance feelings of self-control and self-esteem. Instead, anxiety is often intensified by the failure to adequately meet personal and environmental demands. Clients may be surprised at the amount of nonproductive time they encounter in a 24-hour day. This is effectively illustrated by an assessment of daily activities whereby clients account for their time hour by hour in either a graphic or a written format. Learning effective time management techniques is a useful strategy for people with anxiety disorders. For example, the occupational therapist can teach how to prioritize tasks and break them down into manageable and attainable steps. People usually respond favorably to schedules and "to do" lists. Sometimes actually incorporating "worry time" into the daily routine helps to decrease the behavior. For example, one person was horrified that she had written down "worry" as a daily activity that consumed six hours a day. She was helped to plan more productive substitute activities during the vulnerable times of the day. This plan also provided her with access to her former hobbies; for example, she elected to write letters, knit, and practice computer graphics during those times.

Sensory Modulation Interventions

There is growing research connecting sensory defensiveness in adults with increased levels of anxiety, depression, and maladjustment (Kinnealey & Fuiek, 1999; Kinnealey, Koenig, & Smith, 2011). Hypersensitivity as well as hyposensitivity to sensory stimuli and difficulty modulating and integrating input are characteristics of sensory defensive individuals. A newer term is described by Kinnealey et al. (2011) as **sensory overresponsive type (SOR)** and refers to hypersensitivity and sensory defensiveness. As with clinical anxiety disorders, to outsiders these sources of anxiety, of difficulty in sensory processing, may look harmless when in fact they cause great distress, even leading to panic attacks in the sufferers. Exposure to many sources of sensory input, including certain noises, unexpected movement, tastes, smells, and physical touch, may be interpreted as aversive and anxiety-producing, and therefore are either avoided or approached with great caution (Kinnealey et al., 2011; Kinnealey, Oliver, & Wilbarger, 1995). This vulnerability to the environment and decreased coping strategies may lead to significant restrictions in daily activities in order to avoid anxiety and distress, and greatly influences all aspects of life.

It is postulated that since many symptoms of sensory defensiveness may be interchangeable with those of mental disorders, especially GAD, panic disorder, and phobias, poor sensory regulation may actually contribute to the development of anxiety disorders. For instance, someone with tactile defensiveness who avoided going on subways because of the aversive nature of being in physical contact with crowds could also be labeled as having a phobia of subways. On the other hand, because of the pervasive impact on all aspects of one's life, it has been suggested that sensory defensiveness should be viewed as a stand-alone diagnosis, "sensory affective disorder," which encompasses both the physical and emotional aspects of the condition (Wilberger, cited in Heller, 2002) or as a type of sensory modulation disorder (Kinnealey et al., 2011).

Research is exploring sensory integration interventions for decreasing levels of anxiety such as deep pressure, tactile, and proprioceptive activities in both adults and children. Providing a "sensory diet" in order to maintain a balance of arousal and tolerance while incorporating a person's interests and needs is described in the literature (Kinnealey et al., 1995). A personal account by a psychologist, survivor, and client advocate, Dr. Pat Deegan, praises the work of an occupational therapist, specializing in treating sensory defensiveness in adults, for her assistance in helping Deegan, as an adult, resolve childhood abuse issues through sensory interventions: joint compression, tactile brushing, and sand blankets (Deegan, 2001). Numerous practical, everyday strategies for managing sensory defensiveness in adults are described in Heller's book *Too Loud, Too Bright, Too Fast, Too Tight* (2002). Recommendations cover a range of topics from doing physical exercises to making the environment more pleasing.

Champagne with other professionals (Champagne, 2011; Champagne & Stromberg, 2004; LeBel & Champagne, 2010; LeBel, Champagne, Stromberg, & Coyle, 2010a) has pioneered the use of sensory approaches in mental health settings. She advocates for sensory processing programs in acute psychiatric settings and large psychiatric systems to ameliorate anxiety and the effects of trauma. (See also Chapter 10, Personality Disorders.)

CASE ILLUSTRATION

Sharman—Occupational Therapy Assessment and Treatment

A young, single woman reported problems in job performance following the development of a phobia and subsequent depression. Her usual route to work included driving on a particularly busy street where she had witnessed a catastrophic car accident. Shortly after the accident she developed acute anxiety when driving on this street, so she began to take a more circuitous route to avoid the scene of the accident, which invariably made her late for work. She also became highly distractible, especially during the last hour of the workday as she mentally prepared to go home. In addition, she had difficulty organizing her various work tasks and had been counseled by her employer on several occasions. As her anxiety mounted about losing her job and her performance declined, she took a leave from work in order to attend a partial hospitalization program.

Assessment

Sharman's Role Checklist (see Figure 9-10) indicated difficulty in performing the worker role and the high value Sharman placed on it. The Function Questionnaire (see Figure 9-11) indicated moderate to severe impairment in work because of anxiety. Sharman's Self-Assessment of Activities (see Figure 9-12) reported problems in concentration, job insecurity, excessive worry, poor coping strategies, and problem solving, and Sharman's Activity Configuration (see Figure 9-13) indicated that not enough time was allotted for commuting.

In reviewing the results with Sharman, the occupational therapist confirmed her strong motivation to be able to resume her usual roles, particularly that of employee. Research was shared with Sharman (Prior, 1998) demonstrating that a short-term anxiety management course at a mental health day hospital significantly decreased anxiety in its attendees, as measured by the Hospital Anxiety and Depression Scale (Zigmond & Snaith, 1983). The groups were also rated highly in respect to helpfulness. The content of the course covered the

ROLE CHECKLIST

NAME ___S.T._____ AGE __26____ DATE _2-24-95___

SEX: ☐ MALE ☑ FEMALE ARE YOU RETIRED: ☐ YES ☑ NO

MARITAL STATUS: ☑ SINGLE ☐ MARRIED ☐ SEPARATED ☐ DIVORCED ☐ WIDOWED

The purpose of this checklist is to identify the major roles in your life. The checklist, which is divided into two parts, presents 10 roles and defines each one.

PART I

Beside each role, indicate, by checking the appropriate column, if you performed the role in the past, if you presently perform the role, and if you plan to perform the role in the future. You may check more than one column for each role. For example, if you volunteered in the past, do not volunteer at present, but plan to in the future, you would check the past and future columns.

ROLE	PAST	PRESENT	FUTURE
STUDENT: Attending school on a part-time or full-time basis.	✓		
WORKER: Part-time or full-time paid employment.	✓	✓	✓
VOLUNTEER: Donating services, **at least once a week,** to a hospital, school, community, political campaign, and so forth.	✓		
CARE GIVER: Responsibility, **at least once a week,** for the care of someone such as a child, spouse, relative, or friend.			✓
HOME MAINTAINER: Responsibility, **at least once a week,** for the upkeep of the home such as housecleaning or yardwork.	✓	✓	✓
FRIEND: Spending time or doing something, **at least once a week,** with a friend.	✓	✓	✓
FAMILY MEMBER: Spending time or doing something, **at least once a week,** with a family member such as a child, spouse, parent, or other relative.	✓		✓
RELIGIOUS PARTICIPANT: Involvement, **at least once a week,** in groups or activities affiliated with one's religion (excluding worship).	✓		
HOBBYIST/AMATEUR: Involvement, **at least once a week,** in a hobby or amateur activity such as sewing, playing a musical instrument, woodworking, sports, the theater, or participation in a club or team.	✓		✓
PARTICIPANT IN ORGANIZATIONS: Involvement, **at least once a week,** in organizations such as the American Legion, National Organization for Women, Parents Without Partners, Weight Watchers, and so forth.			
OTHER:_____ A role not listed which you have performed, are presently performing, and/or plan to perform. Write the role on the line above and check the appropriate column(s).			

FIGURE 9-10. Sharman's Role Checklist

(Continues)

Reprinted with permission from Frances Oakley, MS, OTR, FAOTA

PART II

The same roles are listed below. Next to *each* role check the column which best indicates how valuable or important the role is to you. Answer for *each role,* even if you have never performed or do not plan to perform the role.

ROLE	NOT AT ALL VALUABLE	SOMEWHAT VALUABLE	VERY VALUABLE
STUDENT: Attending school on a part-time or full-time basis.		✓	
WORKER: Part-time or full-time paid employment.			✓
VOLUNTEER: Donating services, *at least once a week,* to a hospital, school, community, political campaign, and so forth.		✓	
CARE GIVER: Responsibility, *at least once a week,* for the care of someone such as a child, spouse, relative, or friend.		✓	
HOME MAINTAINER: Responsibility, *at least once a week,* for the upkeep of the home such as housecleaning or yardwork.		✓	
FRIEND: Spending time or doing something, *at least once a week,* with a friend.			✓
FAMILY MEMBER: Spending time or doing something, *at least once a week,* with a family member such as a child, spouse, parent, or other relative.		✓	
RELIGIOUS PARTICIPANT: Involvement, *at least once a week,* in groups or activities affiliated with one's religion (excluding worship).		✓	
HOBBYIST/AMATEUR: Involvement, *at least once a week,* in a hobby or amateur activity such as sewing, playing a musical instrument, woodworking, sports, the theater, or participation in a club or team.			✓
PARTICIPANT IN ORGANIZATIONS: Involvement, *at least once a week,* in organizations such as the American Legion, National Organization for Women, Parents Without Partners, Weight Watchers, and so forth.	✓		
OTHER:_____ A role not listed which you have performed, are presently performing, and/or plan to perform. Write the role on the line above and check the appropriate column(s).			

FIGURE 9-10. Sharman's Role Checklist (*continued*)

FUNCTION QUESTIONNAIRE WORK

The extent to which my work is impaired because of anxiety

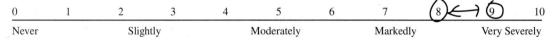

0	1	2	3	4	5	6	7	8	9	10
Never		Slightly			Moderately			Markedly		Very Severely

SOCIAL ACTIVITIES

The extent to which my social life is impaired because of anxiety
(going out with friends, dating, outings, entertaining)

0	1	2	3	4	5	6	7	8	9	10
Never		Slightly			Moderately			Markedly		Very Severely

LEISURE ACTIVITIES

The extent to which engagement in leisure activities is impaired because of anxiety
(hobbies, use of free time)

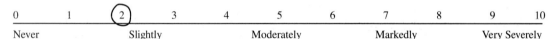

0	1	2	3	4	5	6	7	8	9	10
Never		Slightly			Moderately			Markedly		Very Severely

HOME, SELF-MAINTENANCE, AND FAMILY RESPONSIBILITIES

The extent to which my ability to care for myself and others is impaired by my anxiety
(cleaning house, meal preparation, carpooling, doing laundry, paying bills, grooming)

0	1	2	3	4	5	6	7	8	9	10
Never		Slightly			Moderately			Markedly		Very Severely

FIGURE 9-11. Sharman's Function Questionnaire
© Cengage Learning 2013

nature of the anxiety and learning techniques for managing it. Homework was included in addition to the class exercises in cognitive and behavioral aspects, breathing and relaxation, and assertiveness. A second study giving credence to a short-term stress management group for inpatients using a cognitive-behavioral and psychoeducational approach was also described to Sharman (Stein & Smith, 1989). The primary diagnosis of these hospitalized clients was depression, but they too showed significant decrease on the State-Trait Anxiety Inventory (Spielberger, 1983) following attendance in the six-session course. As with the other program, they were taught a variety of relaxation techniques and communication skills, but also learned biofeedback and pleasant visualization to reduce anxiety.

Self-Assessment of Activities

Name: S T

Date: 2-24-95

This checklist will be used to help develop an Occupational Therapy program for you. Mark the appropriate column for each item and add any comments you feel would be helpful.

Activity	Never a problem	Sometimes a problem	Always a problem	N.A.	Comments
Grooming	✓				
Bathing or showering		✓			I tend to stay in too long-- 20 minutes
Preparing meals	✓				
Food shopping		✓			I don't like to drive to supermarket
Doing errands		✓			If I have to go down a particular street
House cleaning	✓				
Doing yardwork	✓				
Caring for others				✓	
Managing money	✓				
Transportation			✓		I am having difficulty driving-- very anxious
Socializing					
Attending school				✓	
Working			✓		Not as focused or organized as I used to be
Volunteering				✓	
Exercising	✓				
Concentrating			✓		I worry all the time about work, driving.
Problem solving		✓			I can't seem to figure out my problems
Communicating		✓			Most people O.K. but I avoid my boss
Coping with stress			✓		I get overwhelmed by anxiety
Managing time			✓		Always a problem regarding getting to work
Managing impulses		✓			
Doing leisure activities		✓			Not as motivated as in past

FIGURE 9-12. Sharman's Self-Assessment of Activities

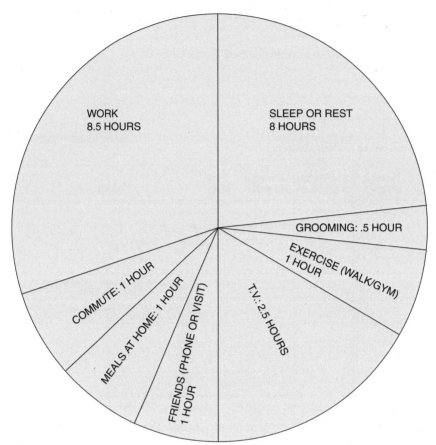

FIGURE 9-13. Sharman's Activity Configuration Prior to Treatment
© Cengage Learning 2013

GOALS

The overall goal of the occupational therapy program was to assist the client in functioning more effectively in her role as worker, particularly through improved coping strategies. After hearing the evidence about the success of stress management groups in decreasing anxiety, she agreed to attend a similar group three times a week for an hour as well as to work individually with the OTR three times a week for half-hour sessions. In addition, she joined the leisure exploration simulation groups, which each met for one hour weekly. The objectives and interventions to reach this goal were as follows:

Objective	Intervention	Method
1. Client will have knowledge of alternative forms of transportation	Community mobility through exploration of resources— bus routes, carpool accessibility, and alternative routes for driving	Individual OT Session
2. Client will plan daily schedule to ensure arriving at work on time	Training in time management—prioritization of activities and strategies to follow schedule	Individual OT Session
3. Client will learn and apply one method of relaxation to decrease general anxiety and to facilitate getting to work	Relaxation training—breathing and visualization exercises	Stress Management Group
4. Client will concentrate for 60 minutes on one task while at the program and for 60 minutes on one task at home	Leisure and job simulation activities	Leisure Group and Homework
5. Client will apply one strategy to neutralize fears that impede performance	Cognitive techniques focused on rational thinking	Stress Management Group

© Cengage Learning 2013

TREATMENT

The occupational therapy program proceeded as follows:

Learning and applying relaxation techniques: Sharman's anxiety was focused primarily on the witnessed accident as she thought about or actually commuted to and from work. However, merely thinking about the accident or about her work problems throughout the day caused rapid heartbeat, nausea, and poor concentration. The occupational therapist initially instructed Sharman in abdominal breathing during a group session. This method taught her to use her lungs more fully through deep breathing, since anxiety symptoms may be exacerbated with shallow breathing. She was trained to be aware of her abdomen rising as she took slow and deep breaths. Her position was supine on the floor on a blanket with her legs bent.

Sharman was told to practice this exercise once a day supine and one or two times a day in a sitting position. Each session was to last two minutes in the beginning and later to be expanded to about five minutes. In addition, she was coached to make use of this technique immediately while sitting in her chair whenever she experienced an initial sign of anxiety. She was also cautioned to return to her normal breathing patterns if she experienced any lightheadedness from increased oxygen flow. Sharman developed skill in using this breathing technique to combat her anxiety symptoms, such as nausea and poor concentration, and subsequently felt less helpless when symptoms appeared during the day.

Visualization and breathing were combined for the second phase. First, the occupational therapist, in an individual session, helped Sharman identify and visualize in her imagination a comfortable, safe place. To help guide the exercise, the OT instructed her to describe places she had been that inspired a sense of well-being. Since Sharman particularly enjoyed the ocean, this was incorporated in the visualization. After first directing her in abdominal breathing, the OT instructed her to imagine being at the beach, while combining sounds, noises, and smells into the picture to strengthen the image. Two 10- to 15-minute sessions a day, to be done at home independently, were prescribed once Sharman had learned to concentrate and attain a state of relaxation with the therapist's assistance. After two weeks, she was able to perform this exercise independently and practiced it before going to the program, work, and bed.

The final phase of training focused on the client visualizing, after completing the two previous steps, driving down the dreaded street in her car. When anxiety surfaced during this exercise, she was told to return to the calming image she had learned to picture. She reported difficulty mastering this aspect of treatment although she continued to practice regularly at home as well as deal with the phobia directly with a psychologist using desensitization techniques, by alleviating anxiety through controlled exposure to the scene of the accident.

Overcoming irrational fears: Sharman reported worrying excessively about projected failures; that is, being shunned by her coworkers, being fired by her boss, having an anxiety attack while driving, and a host of other events. This response led to a heightened state of arousal and caused her either to avoid important activities or feel distressed while doing them. This negative thinking contributed to her depressive symptoms as well. Sharman responded well to the stress management group session in which cognitive strategies were discussed. The occupational therapist helped her develop more realistic ways to perceive current and future events through changing her self-talk about the expected outcome. This was accomplished by first assisting Sharman in completing worksheets that helped to challenge her irrational thinking and then substitute more realistic thinking. The "Daily Mood Log" (Burns, 1993) was one effective tool for this. Here, using a three-column form, she first documented her negative thoughts, then her distorted thoughts (taken from a preprinted list), and finally positive thoughts she could substitute. Her challenge to her worry that she would be rejected by her coworkers was this was "jumping to conclusions." There was no evidence that others viewed her as defective or weak since she had to take a leave from work. In fact, she had received a few phone calls inquiring about her well-being from people with whom she worked. Her positive thoughts included: (1) people will likely be supportive of my actions to get help; (2) others could feel closer to me since I have exposed my vulnerabilities; and (3) even if the people at work reject me, there are many others who like me and it does not mean I am a bad person. Other cognitive strategies included telling herself that her life would not come to an end if she were fired and that searching for a new job would be an inconvenience rather than a failure. She further reminded herself that many others had lived through this experience and had even found the subsequent change rewarding. *Improving concentration:* Sharman had reported difficulty attending to work tasks. Simulated leisure and work activities were introduced into the treatment program with the goal to work for 60 minutes uninterrupted in occupational therapy and then 60 minutes at home on predefined tasks. If she did work tasks in the program, she did a leisure activity at home, and vice versa.

In the past Sharman had enjoyed ceramics, and in particular, making necklaces. She readily accepted the idea of making jewelry using commercial beads and other materials. Sessions were initially 15 to 30 minutes long and involved uncomplicated techniques such as stringing beads for simple necklaces, but as her concentration improved, they were lengthened to 60 minutes and made to incorporate more complex tasks such as making fashion earrings and constructing beads from a quick-drying substitute clay material. She became so enthusiastic about this activity that she started going to yard sales to buy old, inexpensive jewelry to rework for her new hobby. She also found that engaging in this task helped to dissipate her anxiety at times when it surfaced at home. Sharman's employment was as office assistant, and her workload consisted of a variety of clerical tasks. The occupational therapist was able to simulate some of these activities by requesting participation in a volunteer project the program had undertaken (assisting with a blood drive). Making up a flyer on the computer, writing letters to local businesses and organizations for support, and compiling blood donation packets were some of the tasks involved. Sharman also made a list of related jobs she needed to accomplish at home; specifically, reorganizing her financial files, working on her tax return, and updating her computer records. She made agreements with the occupational therapist as to the specific tasks and deadlines for jobs to be done at home.

Arriving at work on time: Sharman's late arrival at work was generally the result of not allowing enough time for the task. She was used to her usual half-hour commute prior to the development of the phobia. The OT helped her to adjust other activities by reprioritizing them in order to accommodate the extra one to two hours (round trip) now needed when she drove herself by the longer alternate route. By categorizing her activities away from work from most valued to least valued (Lakein, 1973), she decided to decrease her evening time watching television ("least valued") and to wake up one hour earlier. To make the transition to the earlier wake-up time, she decided to prepare and lay out her clothes the night before, reduce her lengthy shower time, and read only half the newspaper over breakfast. As Sharman advanced in her partial hospitalization treatment program, she discarded television altogether and replaced it with a new hobby and therapy "homework."

In all these activities, the occupational therapist strategized with the client on ways to stay focused on the task at hand. Creating an uncluttered work environment and removing distracting stimuli proved helpful. At home, Sharman turned off her telephone for one hour while she worked, and she agreed to get up from her desk only once during that time. If distracted, she was able to cue herself by saying, "I am able to focus on this task," and doing one minute of deep breathing. Sharman reported increased concentration and was able to meet her goals.

Sharman stayed in the partial hospitalization program for four weeks and then returned to work, commuting by bus. She planned to join a carpool the following month, paying a small fee to members so that she would not be required to drive until her phobia was more resolved through continued work on this issue with her psychologist. She employed relaxation techniques and cognitive strategies to cope with anxiety throughout the day and reported a notable reduction in anxiety and improved concentration. Leisure activities also served as an outlet for her tension as well as a focus through which to override her irrational thoughts. Sharman made the transition into a new daily schedule in order to wake up earlier starting before her actual return to work and consequently was no longer late to her job. She became more self-confident as she showed improved performance in her worker role as well as a newly developed role as a hobbyist.

SUMMARY

Occupational therapists work with people with anxiety disorders in a variety of treatment settings from acute psychiatric hospitals to home care programs. As changes in health care policies reduce the length of hospital stays, treatment is occurring more often in community settings.

Anxiety may be a mental disorder, as outlined in *DSM-IV-TR,* or it may be a component of a physical or other psychiatric illness. The major disorders described in *DSM-IV-TR* include panic disorder without and with agoraphobia, agoraphobia without history of panic attacks, specific phobia, social phobia, obsessive-compulsive disorder (OCD), post-traumatic stress disorder (PTSD), acute stress disorder, and generalized anxiety disorder (GAD). When anxiety accompanies a physical illness, it may actually have been induced by a hormonal imbalance or other medical condition. On the other hand, anxiety may be the outcome of coping with a life-threatening illness and thus be likely to dissipate when the medical problem is resolved.

Differentiating between a true anxiety syndrome and normal anxiety is sometimes difficult. Anxiety is universal and often helpful, being related to the fight-or-flight response. However, when anxiety impairs rather than enhances functional performance, it becomes pathological. Anxiety symptoms fall into several categories: emotional, physiological, cognitive, and behavioral. Usually people experience some symptoms in each of these areas.

Treatment strategies aim to reduce symptoms, prevent relapse, and improve functioning. Approaches used by other health professionals include medications, psychotherapy, biofeedback, cognitive interventions, systematic desensitization, and couples therapy.

Occupational therapists work with individuals and families to improve functioning and adaptive behavior in everyday activities as well as the individual's perceived quality of life. Anxiety disorders are always accompanied by great emotional discomfort, which impacts both the client and the family. Anxious people inevitably restrict their lives in order to accommodate the dysfunction. A parent may refuse to take family vacations because of a fear of crossing bridges or flying in an airplane. Another person may give up a satisfying job because of panic attacks. An older adult may drive away everyone in her support system with her excessive, relentless worrying. The challenge for the occupational therapist is to help the client cope and therefore function productively. Improving effectiveness may be accomplished by actually reducing the level of anxiety, or it may be achieved by teaching the client to grapple with life stresses in spite of anxiety. Both strategies involve the development of self-management skills. Empowering the client through instruction in acquiring and developing these skills can be extremely beneficial. Relaxation, assertiveness and general social skills training, community mobility, expressive craft and art activities, the functional behavior approach, education/lifestyle alterations, rational/cognitive approaches, and time management are key strategies. Anxiety often takes a chronic course and requires much adaptation. Many people with anxiety are able to live productively when given the tools to cope more effectively.

REVIEW QUESTIONS

1. What occupational therapy goals might a home health clinician establish for a homebound elderly woman who has panic attacks when she attempts to leave the house to visit friends or do daily errands?
2. What types of community programs might assist someone who has not been able to work for several years because of flashbacks that impair concentration?
3. How could an occupational therapist simultaneously address a hospitalized student's stress disorder and depression following the sudden death of a parent?
4. Which types of interventions might be most successful for adults hospitalized for trauma and PTSD?
5. What is mindfulness-based training and how would you incorporate it into occupational therapy programs?

REFERENCES

Agras, S. (1985). *Panic: Facing fears, phobias, and anxiety*. Stanford: Stanford Alumni Association.

Agras, S., & Berkowitz, R. (1994). Behavior therapy. In R. E. Hales, S. C. Udofsky, & J. A. Talbott (Eds.), *Textbook of psychiatry* (2nd ed., pp. 1061–1081). Washington, DC: American Psychiatric Press.

Alberti, R. & Emmons, M. (1990). *Your perfect right. A guide to assertive behavior*. San Luis Obispo, CA: Impact Publishers.

American Occupational Therapy Association (AOTA). (2008). Occupational therapy practice framework: Domain and process (2nd ed.). *American Journal of Occupational Therapy, 62*, 625–683.

American Psychiatric Association (APA). (2000). *Diagnostic and statistical manual of mental disorders*-Text Revision (4th ed.). Washington, DC: APA.

Anxiety Disorders Association of America. (2002). *Brief overview of anxiety disorders*. Retrieved from http://www.adaa.org/AnxietyDisorderInfor/OverviewAnxDis.cfm.

Bandura, A. (1977). Self-efficacy: Towards a unifying theory of behavioral change. *Psychological Review, 84*(2), 191–215.

Bandura, A. (1995). *Self-efficacy in changing societies*. New York: Cambridge University Press.

Bandura, A. (1997). *Self-Efficacy: The exercise of control*. New York: W. H. Freeman & Co.

Benson, H. (1976). *The relaxation response*. Boston: G. K. Hall.

Booth, R. J., & Petrie, K. (2002). Emotional expression and health changes: Can we identify biological pathways? In S. Lepore & J. Smyth (Eds.), *The writing cure* (pp. 157–175). Washington, DC: American Psychological Association.

Bourne, E. (2011). *Anxiety and phobia workbook* (5th ed.). Oakland, CA: New Harbinger.

Burns, D. D. (1999). *Ten days to self-esteem*. New York: Quill.

Champagne, T. (2011 March). Attachment, trauma, and occupational therapy practice. *OT Practice*, CE-1- CE-8.

Champagne, T., & Stromberg, N. (2004). Sensory approaches in inpatient psychiatric settings: Innovative alternatives to seclusion and restraint. *Journal of Psychosocial Nursing, 42*, 35–44.

Clark, D., Salkovskis, P., & Chalkley, A. (1985). Respiratory control as a treatment for panic attacks. *Behavior Therapy and Experimental Psychiatry, 16*(1), 23–30.

Craske, M. (2009). *Cognitive behavioral therapy*. Washington, DC: American Psychological Association.

Davidson, J. R. (2001). Recognition and treatment of posttraumatic stress disorder. *Journal of the American Medical Association, 286*(5), 584–588.

Davis, M., Eshelman, E., & McKay, M. (2008). *The relaxation and stress reduction workbook* (6th ed.). Oakland, CA: New Harbinger.

Deegan, P. E. (2001). *Recovery as a self-directed process of healing and transformation*. Retrieved from http://www.intentionalcare.org/art_re.htm

Depoy, E., & Kolodner, E. (1991). Psychological performance factors. In C. Christiansen & C. Baum (Eds.), *Occupational therapy—Overcoming human performance deficits* (pp. 304–332). Thorofare, NJ: Slack.

Dozois, D. J., & Dobson, K. S. (2004). *The prevention of anxiety and depression: Theory, research and practice*. Washington, DC: American Psychological Association.

Dryden, W. (2003). *Albert Ellis, Live!* London: Sage.

Ellis, A. (1976). *Growth through reason*. North Hollywood, CA: Wilshire.

Evans, S., Ferrandoa, S., Findlera, M., Stowella, C., Smart, C., & Haglin, D. (2008). Mindfulness-based cognitive therapy for generalized anxiety disorder. *Journal of Anxiety Disorders, 22*, 716–721.

Freeman, C., & Power, M. (2007). Handbook of evidence-based psychotherapies: A guide for research and practice. Chichester, West Sussex, England: John Wiley & Sons.

Freeman, L. W., & Lawlis, F. G. (Eds.). (2001). *Complementary & alternative medicine.* St. Louis, MO: Mosby.

Gaddis, S. (2010). Positive assertive pushback for nurses. Retrieved from http://www .CommunicationsDoctor.com.

Heller, S. (2002). *Too loud, too bright, too fast, too tight: What to do if you are sensory defensive in an overstimulating world.* New York: HarperCollins.

Hofmann, S. G., Sawyer, A. T., Witt, A. A., & Oh, D. (2010). The effect of mindfulness-based therapy on anxiety and depression: A meta-analytic review. *Journal of Consulting and Clinical Psychology, 78*(2), 169–183. Retrieved from doi: 10.1037/a0018555

Huppert, J. D., Cahill, S. P., & Foa, E. B. (2009). Anxiety disorders: Cognitive-behavioral therapy. In B. Sadock, V. Sadock, & P. Ruiz (Eds.), *Kaplan and Sadock's comprehensive textbook of psychiatry* (9th ed., pp. 1915–1926). Philadelphia: Wolters Kluwer Lippincott, Williams and Wilkins.

Jacobson, E. (1938). *Progressive relaxation.* Chicago: University of Chicago Press.

Kielhofner, G. (Ed.). (2007). *A model of human occupation: Theory and application* (4th ed.). Baltimore: Williams & Wilkins.

Kinnealey, M., & Fuiek, M. (1999). The relationship between sensory defensiveness, anxiety, and perception of pain in adults. *Occupational Therapy International, 6*(3), 195–206.

Kinnealey, M., Oliver, B., & Wilbarger, P. (1995). A phenomenological study of sensory defensiveness in adults. *American Journal of Occupational Therapy, 49*(5), 444–451.

Krisanaprakornkit, T., Piyavhatkul, N., & Laopaiboon, M. (2009). Meditation therapy for anxiety disorders. The Cochrane Collaboration, John Wiley & Sons. Retrieved from http://www .cochranelibrary.com

Krug, S. I., Scheier, I. H., & Cattell, R. B. (1976). *Handbook for the IPAT anxiety scale.* Champaign, IL: Institute for Personality and Ability Testing.

Lakein, A. (1973). *How to get control of your time and your life.* New York: David McKay.

Lazar, S., & Offenkranz, W. (2010). Psychotherapy in the treatment of posttraumatic stress disorder (pp 87–102). In S. Lazar (Ed.), *Psychotherapy, it is worth it: A comprehensive review of its cost-effectiveness.* Washington, DC: American Psychiatric Association.

Levy, R. (2008). *Miraculous health: How to heal your body by unleashing the hidden power of your mind.* New York: Atria Books.

Liebgold, H. (2000). *Curing anxiety, phobias, shyness, and OCD.* San Rafael, CA: Liebro.

Lisetti, C., Pozzo, E., Lucas, M., Hernandez, F., Silverman, W., Kurtines, B., et al. (2009). Second-life biosensors and exposure therapy for anxiety disorders. *Annual Review of Cybertherapy and Telemedicine, 7*, 19–21, 1554–8716.

Mays, J. H. (1987). The issue is: Assertiveness training for occupational therapists. *American Journal of Occupational Therapy, 41*(1), 51–53.

McClure-Tone, E. R., & Pine, D. S. (2009). *Clinical features of the anxiety disorders.* In B. Sadock, V. Sadock, & P. Ruiz (Eds.), *Kaplan and Sadock's comprehensive textbook of psychiatry* (9th ed., pp. 1844–1856). Philadelphia: Lippincott, Williams and Wilkins.

McLay, R. &, Spira, J. (2009). Use of a portable biofeedback device to improve insomnia in a combat zone: A case report. *Applied Psychophysiology Biofeedback, 34* (4), 319–321.

Merikangas, K. R., & Kalaydjian, A. E. (2009). Epidemiology of anxiety disorders. In B. Sadock, V. Sadock, & P. Ruiz (Eds.), *Kaplan and Sadock's comprehensive textbook of psychiatry* (9th ed., pp. 1856–1864). Philadelphia: Lippincott, Williams and Wilkins.

Mueser, K., Rosenberg, S., & Rosenberg, H. (2009). *Treatment of post-traumatic stress disorder in special populations: A Cognitive restructuring program.* Arlington, VA: American Psychiatric Association.

National Institute of Mental Health (NIMH). (n.d.). *Anxiety disorders.* Retrieved from http://nimh .nih.gov/health/publications/anxiety-disorders/complete-index.shtml

Pennebaker, J. (2004). Writing to heal: A guided journal for recovering from trauma and emotional upheaval. Oakland, CA: New Harbinger Publications.

Pennebaker, J. (2007). *Emotion, disclosure and health* (5th ed.). Washington, DC: American Psychological Services.

Prior, S. (1998). Determining the effectiveness of a short-term anxiety management course. *British Journal of Occupational Therapy, 61*(5), 207–213.

Ratanasiripong, P., Sverduk, K., Hayashino, D., & Prince. (2010). Setting up the next generation bio-feedback program for stress and anxiety management for college students: A simple and cost-effective approach. *College Student Journal, 44*(1), 97–100.

Ravindran, L. N., & Stein, M. B. (2009). Anxiety disorders: Somatic treatment. In B. Sadock, V. Sadock, & P. Ruiz (Eds.), *Kaplan and Sadock's comprehensive textbook of psychiatry,* (9th ed., pp. 1906–1914). Philadelphia: Lippincott, Williams and Wilkins.

Reiner, R. (2008). Integrating a portable biofeedback device into clinical practice for patient with anxiety disorders: Results of a pilot study. *Applied Psychophysiology and Biofeedback, 35,* 55–61.

Rosier, C., Williams, H., & Ryrie, I. (1998). Anxiety management groups in a community mental health team. *British Journal of Occupational Therapy, 61*(5), 203–206.

Rosenblatt, A. (2010). Psychotherapy in the treatment of anxiety disorders. In S. Lazar (Ed.), *Psychotherapy, It is worth it: A comprehensive review of its cost-effectiveness* (pp. 103–134). Washington, DC: American Psychiatric Association.

Roth, A., & Fonagy, P. (1996). *What works for whom: A critical review of psychotherapy research.* New York: Guilford.

Shapiro, F., & Maxfield, L. (2002). Eye movement desensitization and reprocessing (EMDR): Information processing in the treatment of trauma. *Journal of Clinical Psychology, 58*(8), 933–946.

Sims, A., & Snaith, P. (1988). *Anxiety in clinical practice.* New York: Wiley.

Smith, M. (1975). *When I say no, I feel guilty: How to cope using the skills of systematic assertive therapy.* New York: Bantam Books.

Smyth, J. M., Stone, A. A., Hurewitz, A., & Kaell, A. (1999). Effects of writing about stressful experiences on symptom reduction in patients with asthma or rheumatoid arthritis. *Journal of American Medical Association, 281*(14), 1304–1309.

Spector, J. (2007). Eye movement desensitisation and reprocessing (EMDR). In C. Freeman & M. Power, *Handbook of evidence-based psychotherapies: A guide for research and practice,* (pp. 93–110). Chichester, West Sussex, England: John Wiley & Sons.

Spielberger, C. D. (1983). *State-Trait Anxiety Inventory for Adults.* Redwood City, CA: Mind Garden.

Stein, D., Hollander, E., & Rothbaum, B. (2010) (Eds.). *Textbook of anxiety disorders* (2nd ed.) Arlington, VA: American Psychiatric Association.

Stein, F., & Nikolic, S. (1989). Teaching stress management techniques to a schizophrenic patient. *American Journal of Occupational Therapy, 43*(3), 162–169.

Stein, F., & Smith, J. (1989). Short-term stress management programme with acutely depressed in-patients. *Canadian Journal of Occupational Therapy, 56*(4), 185–191.

Steinglass, J., Sysko, R., Glasofer, D., Albano, A. M., Simpson, A. B., & Walsh, T. (2011). Rationale for the application of exposure and response prevention to the treatment of anorexia nervosa. *International Journal of Eating Disorders, 44*(2), 134–141. Retrieved from doi: 10.1002/eat.20784

Taylor, B., & Arnow, B. (1988). *The nature and treatment of anxiety disorders.* New York: Free Press.

Wolpe, J. (1973). *The practice of behavior therapy.* Elmsford, NY: Pergamon.

World Health Organization (WHO). (2011). *International Classification of Diseases (ICD-10).* Retrieved from http://www.who.int/classifications/icd/en/

Wright, J. H., & Beck, A. T. (1994). Cognitive therapy. In R. E. Hales, S. C. Udofsky, & J. A. Talbott (Eds.), *Textbook of psychiatry* (2nd ed., pp. 1083–1114). Washington, DC: American Psychiatric Press.

Zigmond, A., & Snaith, R. (1983). *The Hospital Anxiety and Depression Scale.* Windsor, UK: NFER Nelson.

Websites

National Institute of Mental Health:

> http://www.nimh.nih.gov/health/publications/anxiety-disorders/index.shtml

Anxiety disorders Association of America:

> http://www.adaa.org/

Surgeon General's Office:

> http://www.surgeongeneral.gov/library/mentalhealth/chapter4/sec2.html

American Psychological Association:

> http://apa.org/topics/anxiety/index.aspx

American Academy of Child and Adolescent Psychiatry:

> http://www.aacap.org/cs/AnxietyDisorders.ResourceCenter

Journal of Anxiety Disorders On-line:

> http://www.sciencedirect.com/science/journal/08876185

The Role Checklist:

> FOakley@cc.nih.gov

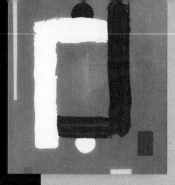

Chapter 10

Personality Disorders

Elizabeth Cara, PhD, OTR, MFT

▮▮ KEY TERMS

affective instability

dimensions

ego-syntonic

"hardwired"

mentalization

personality

splitting

traits

CHAPTER OUTLINE

Introduction

The Personality Continuum and Etiology of Personality Disorders

The *DSM-IV-TR* Personality Disorders

    Differences Between Axis I and Axis II

    Dimensions of Personality

    The ICD-10 Personality Disorders

    Cultural Controversy

    Clinical Picture

Interdisciplinary Assessment and Treatment

    Psychopharmacology

    Interpersonal Approach

Occupational Therapy Treatment Interventions

    Leisure

    Work

    Social Participation

    Self-Care

    Groups

Summary

INTRODUCTION

Personality disorders are important in contemporary society because 10 to 20 percent occur in the U.S. population and half of psychiatric patients, either in or out of institutions, have personality disorders. Therefore, they are consumers of many different community services and resources (Sadock, Sadock, & Ruiz, 2009). A recovery model dictates that treatment addresses a positive quality of life, and ability to work and love rather than simply reducing symptoms.

Diverse approaches and research have led to more specific treatment and manuals for working with those with personality disorders, primarily borderline personality disorders (Livesley, 2003, 2006; Linehan, 1992, Neacsiu, Rizvi, & Linehan, 2010). (See Table 10-1 for a description of various theories of personality disorders that guide treatment.) Also, long-term research studies (Paris, 2002, 2008b) and a better understanding of biological and genetic origins and developmental mechanisms are changing approaches to treatment and are increasing understanding of personality disorders (Livesley, 2003, 2006; Livesley & Jang, 2008; Millon, 2011). Research shows that distress caused by personality disorders can be ameliorated to some extent and there is cause for some optimism (Fonagy & Bateman, 2006; Gunderson & Gabbard, 2001; Waldinger, 2010). However, there are many methodological issues in research into personality disorders, specifically borderline personality disorder, that have to be addressed in the future that will further the treatment of those with personality disorders (Zanarini et al., 2010). It is hoped that the DSM-5 with its dimensional approach will aid in addressing the methodological issues.

Individuals with personality disorders can indeed be treated (Fonagy & Bateman, 2006; Linehan, 2010; Waldinger, 2010), and occupational therapy, with its focus on adaptive functioning and behavior in everyday life and specific new sensory approaches (Champagne, 2011; Champagne & Stromberg, 2004; LeBel & Champagne, 2010; LeBel, Champagne, Stromberg, & Coyle, 2010) can be helpful. In fact, individuals with personality disorders often are bright, charming, and creative. Although they may be described otherwise, and are sometimes considered difficult to treat because of the challenges and opportunities for self-learning that may occur in treatment, they can be rewarding and gratifying clients, particularly when adaptation not personality change is the desired goal.

Because personality disorders are Axis II diagnoses, there will usually be another Axis I condition, such as depression, post-traumatic stress, generalized anxiety, or substance addiction that brings an individual with a personality disorder into mental health treatment settings. In addition, people with personality disorders may be seen in other than mental health settings, for example, in a treatment setting for traumatic brain injury subsequent to a failed suicide attempt, in physical rehabilitation subsequent to impulsive behavior that resulted in a diving or driving accident, or in pediatric settings where a child's behavior may in part be a response to poor parenting skills or dysfunctional family relationships. Because occupational therapy focuses on adaptive function and behavior in

TABLE 10-1. Theories of Personality Disorders

Disorder	Theory
Biophysical	Anticipate that chemical deficiencies or other defects will be found that account for symptoms. Just as physical disease represents a disease of the organ system that manifests in the realm of the physical body, psychological disease reflects central nervous system disruptions that will manifest in the realm of behavior, emotions, and thought (Sadock & Sadock, 2000).
Neuropsychiatric	Recognize the influence of the neurobiological system on mood and behavioral symptoms. Neuroanatomical (functional) and neurochemical (operational) aspects are assessed to determine how they are causing or amplifying symptoms. It holds that intrinsic dispositions are modifiable by medicine, environments can be changed, and biological factors underlie some dimensions of personality disorders (Ratey, 1995).
Psychodynamic	Emphasize the impact of early experiences and past events. Early theories were based on the model of the ego, id, and superego that defined the disorder depending on which structure predominated—the id with predominant erotic behavior, the ego with narcissistic behavior, and the superego with compulsive behavior. Traits were later associated with frustrations or indulgences during the psychosexual stages. Character formations were thought to have a defensive function. Currently, Kernberg (1999) posits three levels of structural organization: psychotic, borderline, or neurotic. Those with normal personalities have a cohesive sense of self and ego-strength to remain integrated in spite of pressure from internal or external forces and have a mature internalization of social values (Millon, Meagher, & Grossman, 2001) while those with personality disorders experience disintegration of sense of self under pressure and do not fully internalize values. Contemporary theories focus on the infant-caregiver environment and a method called **mentalization**, which focuses on individuals capacities to understand their own and others' mental states in an attachment context (valued relationship) so that they can modulate their affect, regulate impulses, and function better in interpersonal relationships (Fonagy & Target, 1996; Bateman & Fonagy, 2009).
Behavioral	Emphasize environmental influences and learning from the social environment (Sadock & Sadock, 2000). Currently assess three response systems: verbal-cognitive mode, affective-physiological mode, and overt-motor response system (Millon, Meagher, & Grossman, 2001).
Cognitive	Individuals react to the world depending on their perception of it. A person's way of construing the world determines behavior. Dysfunctional feelings and behaviors reflect biased schemas and result in repetitive interpersonal errors (Millon, 1996).
Interpersonal	Personality is understood in terms of recurrent interpersonal tendencies that are the social product of interactions with significant others (Millon, Meagher, & Grossman, 2001) and shape and perpetuate styles of behavior, thought, and feeling. An individual always transacts with real others or with her or his expectations about them. All important events in life are interpersonal. There are maladaptive causal sequences between interpersonal perceptions, behavior, and others' reactions. Sequences are often activated in inappropriate situations.

TABLE 10-1. Continued

Disorder	Theory
Biopsychosocial/ Evolutionary	An interaction of biology and environment determines whether traits become disorders. In the presence of psychological risk factors such as trauma, loss, or inadequate parenting, personality traits tend to be amplified. Also called *predisposition stress theory* (Widom, Czaja, & Paris, 2009; Paris, 2010). Newer theory looks at how disorders represent maladaptive functions due to inability to relate in the environment (Millon, 1996).
Neurobiological/ Temperaments	Biological constitutional dispositions are central to understanding personality disorders. Attempt to break down constituents of temperament that underlie personality traits, for example, neurotransmitter types may relate to certain dimensions of personality. Traits or dispositions may be associated with a particular neurotransmitter system (Millon, Meagher, & Grossman, 2001).

© Cengage Learning 2013

everyday life, it is a very important aspect of treatment (Livesley, 2007). The methods and strategies grounded in occupations in environmental context provide opportunities to modify behavior. The Occupational Therapy Practice Framework's (OTPF) (AOTA, 2008) focus inclusion of emotional regulation skills and an outcome of adaptation particularly empowers occupational therapy interventions. In addition, because problems manifest in both the social and interpersonal realms, it is necessary for the therapist to be competent not only in occupational treatment methods, but also in the use of self and interpersonal communication (see also Kyler, 2008, regarding use of the relationship). Therefore, a willingness to reflect and understand oneself, including one's conscious and unconscious motivations, values, thoughts, feelings, and responses, is vitally important for the occupational therapist (see Chapter 19, "The Use of Psychosocial Methods and Interpersonal Strategies in Mental Health," for a discussion of the self and interpersonal skills).

THE PERSONALITY CONTINUUM AND ETIOLOGY OF PERSONALITY DISORDERS

A brief review of what is entailed in the concept of personality will help to clarify what is meant by a "disorder" or "dysfunction" of personality. **Personality** could be considered to comprise a person's lifelong style of relating, coping, behaving, thinking, and feeling. The concept represents a network of **traits** that emerge from a matrix of biological dispositions and experiential learning, persist over extended periods of time, and characterize the individual's distinctive manner of relating in the environment (Millon, 1996). There are regularities and consistencies in behavior and forms of experience. There is a consistency and coherence to a person's experiences. Personality is not just a collection of traits but an organization that is cohesive and coherent (Livesley, 2001).

Every individual possesses a small and distinct group of primary traits that persist and endure and that exhibit a high degree of consistency across situations. These enduring (stable) and pervasive (consistent) characteristics make up a person's personality. The personality pattern, that is, the repertoire of coping skills and adaptive flexibilities, will determine whether a person will master his or her psychosocial environments. Millon (1996) views personality as composed of three polarities: positive versus negative, self versus other, and active versus passive. These polarities represent an individual's survival mode. That is, people will be motivated by the type of reinforcement they seek, whether the pursuit of pleasure or the avoidance of pain, relying on self or others for support and nurturing, and behaving in an active and controlling, or more accommodating and reactive, way (Millon, 1996).

There are two features that distinguish a personality disorder: chronic interpersonal difficulties and problems with self and identity. Chronic interpersonal difficulties are "repetitive maladaptive patterns of thoughts, feelings and actions that occur in relationship to others" (Livesley, 2001, p. 10). Problems with self and identity include a failure to develop an integrated sense of identity during adolescence, a poorly integrated sense of self and significant others, and faulty beliefs or thoughts used to process information regarding self and others.

Those people whose personality patterns do not permit consistent mastery of the psychosocial environment can be distinguished from their normal counterparts by:

- Adaptive inflexibility and poor choices of behavior
- A tendency to foster vicious circles
- Tenuous stability under stressful conditions, that is, a tendency to decompensate during times of crisis or stress

See Table 10-2 for a description of maladaptive personality patterns.

Problems of personality thus include stable and consistent traits that are not easily changed, are exhibited inappropriately and in situations in which they are not warranted, and foster vicious cycles of behavior that are difficult to stop and perpetuate and intensify already-present difficulties (Millon, 1981). Daily life activities and interactions cause overwhelming stress. This triggers maladaptive responses, which further heighten the stress and preclude obtaining support or help from others. Thus the vicious circle is put in motion. The individual with a personality disorder lacks the flexibility to choose from a broad range of interpersonal behaviors. He or she may rigidly rely on the same interpersonal behavior or choose an extreme form of behavior that is not warranted in every situation. These poor behavioral choices in turn elicit constricted and extreme responses from others. Finally, the person with a personality disorder is unaware of his or her poor choices and does not understand how the "wrong" behaviors have elicited others' responses. Consequently, there is little awareness of responsibility for the interactions and a resultant inability to change interpersonal behavior (Kiesler, 1986).

TABLE 10-2. Maladaptive Personality Patterns

Pattern	Description
Adaptive Flexibility	Interpersonal strategies for relating to others, achieving goals, and coping with stress are limited and practiced rigidly. Choices of behavior often do not match the situation in which they are used.
Vicious Circles	Person's choices elicit similar rigid or extreme responses from others. Little understanding of poor choices and how the "wrong" behaviors have "pulled" for other's responses. Consequently, there is little awareness of responsibility for the interactions and inability to change behavior. This sets into motion additional poor choices of behavior and self-defeating sequences with others, which cause already-established difficulties not only to persist but to be aggravated further.
Tenuous Stability	Lack of resilience in conditions perceived as stressful, causing extreme susceptibility to new difficulties and disruptions and reversion to familiar, maladaptive ways of coping. There is lessened control over emotions and a tendency toward developing increasingly distorted perceptions of reality.

Adapted from Millon (1981)

An important feature in the disordered personality that complicates understanding and treatment is that what therapists consider abnormal personality traits and patterns generally are perceived as appropriate by the individual. This is often described as an **ego-syntonic** feeling (Sadock & Sadock, 2007)—it "feels right" to the individual. Most people would feel troubled if they were labile, persistently distorted reality, were involved in chaotic and troublesome interactions with others, failed to engage in or were neglected in relationships, and seemed unable to understand or express empathy for others. In these situations, most people would seek help or at least talk to someone they trusted. However, for an individual with a personality disorder, it seems that these traits and patterns are not overly disturbing, troublesome, or strange. Chaos may seem strangely untroubling and part of everyday life. This may be because an individual's strategies and behavior have been determined by haphazard and causal events in the environment to which he or she has been exposed. "The particulars and coloration of many pathological patterns have their beginnings in the offhand behaviors and attitudes to which the child is incidentally exposed" (Millon, 1996, p. 112). Moreover, some behaviors also feel as if they make sense because they are **"hardwired"** into an individual's neurological makeup (Ratey, 1995). If certain strategies and behaviors have been learned and have neurological substrates, they will tend to "feel right." In fact, some models discuss borderline personality disorder in particular as a disorder of emotional dysregulation (Koerner & Linehan, 2000; Waltz & Linehan, 1999) and the patterns of personality disorders as learned in early relationships with key figures (Benjamin & Pugh, 2001). Therefore, the behaviors not only feel right to persons with the disorder, but their behavior is the only possible choice based on biological makeup and early patterns learned in relation to significant caregivers. See Table 10-1 for other theories that discuss the etiology of personality disorders.

CASE ILLUSTRATION

Robyn—Borderline Personality Disorder with Disabling Problems

Robyn was pleased with her new love of four months, James. It seemed that this relationship was a dream come true. Since the two met they had spent almost every night together, sometimes going out, but often just spending time alone. Robyn said that she finally felt that she could trust someone.

About four months into the relationship, however, Robyn became enraged and hung up on James after he called to cancel a date because he was required to work overtime (environmental event). She refused to answer his messages or to answer calls from friends. She even started refusing to leave her apartment for a while (maladaptive coping response) and began thinking that maybe James was cheating on her (distorted thinking). Robyn began to doubt her perception of the previous four months. She experienced familiar feelings that she could only describe as painful. She began to think that cutting herself would be the only way to release the pain (further aggravation of difficulties).

Discussion

Robyn demonstrated adaptive inflexibility, poor choices of behavior, tenuous stability, and a tendency to foster vicious circles. Her problems did not necessarily feel strange or "weird" to her. In fact, her choices were the only possible ones that she knew based on her biological makeup or sensitivity (emotional dysregulation) and patterns developed in early relationships with her significant caregivers.

THE *DSM-IV-TR* PERSONALITY DISORDERS

Personality disorders are characterized by:

- Their early onset
- Their stable and persistent character
- Their influence on several different domains of behavior, such as, work, relationships, free time
- Their primary expression in an interpersonal context
- A significant degree of disturbance of the personality (Derksen & Sloore, 1999)

The *Diagnostic and Statistical Manual of Mental Disorders* (*DSM-IV-TR*) (American Psychiatric Association [APA], 2000) lists general criteria for a personality disorder and recognizes common features in some of the individual disorders. In the *DSM-IV-TR*, traits are the major unit for distinguishing the personality disorders. This categorization based on traits differs from the symptom approach that emphasizes structural problems for Axis I disorders. This difference is important because it establishes (1) the idea of continuity between normal and disordered personalities, (2) that personality disorders are a combination of traits, and (3) that a hierarchy exists of lower-order traits organized into higher-order **dimensions**, such as neuroticism or extraversion. However, a collection of traits or just extreme traits are not sufficient for the disorder. The diagnosis is applied only when traits are inflexible or maladaptive and cause extreme distress or functional impairment (Livesley, 2001, 2007). Also it is an enduring pattern and the behavior is very different from what is usually expected in the person's culture. Usually, there are problems in cognition, or how self and other people are perceived, emotional responses that are usually inappropriately intense, problems with interpersonal functioning and problems with impulse control. The patterns are not due to another disorder or to another condition.

Differences Between Axis I and Axis II

1. Axis II disorders are chronic conditions whereas Axis I disorders are episodic in nature.

2. Personality disorders reflect more basic emotional dysfunctions and are more deeply rooted than Axis I disorders.

3. Personality disorders are more complex and difficult to treat than Axis I disorders (Derksen & Sloore, 1999). In fact, personality disorders often share symptoms with Axis I disorders or with each other. This co-occurrence with other disorders is often called comorbidity (Loranger, 2000; Gelder, Lopez-Ibor, & Andreasen, 2000). Personality disorders are usually associated with other disorders such as substance abuse or addiction, eating disorders, post-traumatic stress syndrome due to childhood abuse and neglect, anxiety disorders, and a tendency for self-abuse and mutilation. Currently, information points to childhood abuse and neglect as occurring in a high percentage (59%–70%) of individuals with personality disorders. A large minority of those with eating disorders have a personality disorder, and 40% of those with a personality disorder also have bulimia. Between 36% and 76% of those with anxiety disorders are estimated to also have a personality disorder (mostly avoidant, dependent, obsessive-compulsive, schizotypal, or paranoid). In addition, some studies (listed in Ruegy & Frances, 1995) support a clinical impression that there is a connection of cluster B and chronic pain, conversion (i.e., symptoms that affect motor or sensory functioning that cannot be explained by neurological or physical conditions [APA, 2000]), and somatoform symptoms (i.e., a variety of physical complaints, such as chronic fatigue, gastrointestinal symptoms, or loss of appetite, that cannot be explained by any known physical condition [APA, 2000]).

Dimensions of Personality

The individual personality disorders can be grouped or "clustered" according to similar features according to dimensions (see Table 10-3). Although the *DSM-IV-TR* classification system is considered a categorical one, there is also another dimensional perspective. The three clusters of the *DSM-IV-TR* follow a dimensional perspective; that is, they are based on traits or dispositions—a permanent inclination to behave a certain way (Gelder, Lopez-Ibor, & Andreasen, 2000). Currently, popular dimensional models of personality disorders are based on the supposition that we all share the same personality structure but differ in our combination of traits. For example, we all have dimensions of neuroticism, extraversion, openness to experience, agreeableness, and conscientiousness, though we each may fall on different places on a continuum that represents each dimension. How we express each dimension depends on our particular combination of traits. See Table 10-3 for a brief explanation of the various traits and dimensions of popular models.

Personality disorder clusters have also been described based on other dimensions (Millon, 1996). These other clusters are also described in Table 10-4. (See Table 10-5 for a more detailed list of essential features, the clinical picture, and general interpersonal approaches for the individual disorders [Sadock, Sadock, & Ruiz, 2009] according to their *DSM-IV* clusters.)

TABLE 10-3. Dimensional Models

Five-Factor Model (Costa & MacRae)*		
Neuroticism—chronic level of emotional adjustment, includes traits of anxiety, hostility, depression, self-consciousness, impulsivity, vulnerability.		
Extraversion—quantity and intensity of preferred interpersonal interactions, activity level, need for stimulation, capacity for joy, includes traits of warmth, gregariousness, assertiveness, activity, excitement seeking, positive emotions.		
Open to experience-active seeking and appreciation of experiences for their own sake; includes the traits of fantasy, aesthetics, feelings, actions, ideas, values.		
Agreeableness—kinds of interactions a person prefers along a continuum from compassion to antagonism; includes the traits of trust, straightforwardness, altruism, compliance, modesty, tendermindedness.		
Conscientiousness—degree of organization, persistence, control, and motivation in goal-directed behavior; includes the traits of competence, order, dutifulness, achievement striving, self-discipline, deliberation.		

Three-Factor Model (Eysenck)	Four-Factor Model	Dimensional Assessment of Personality (Livesley & Walton)
Extraversion	*Harm Avoidance*	*Emotional Dysregulation*
Psychoticism	*Novelty Seeking*	*Dissocial Behavior*
Neuroticism	*Reward Dependence*	*Inhibitness*
	Persistence	*Compulsivity*

*NOTE: Models cited in Livesley, 2001, and Sadock, Sadock, & Ruiz, 2009. The popular five-factor model is described in more detail to aid in understanding the dimensional models (Costa & Widiger, 2002; Livesley, 2001).

The *ICD-10* **Personality Disorders**

The *International Classification of Diseases (ICD-10) Mental and Behavioural Disorders* definition of personality disorders is perhaps more descriptive than the *DSM-IV-TR*. The *ICD-10* established by the World Health Organization (1992) classifies personality disorders as:

> a severe disturbance in the characterological constitution and behavioural tendencies of the individual, usually involving several areas of the personality, and nearly always associated with considerable personal and social disruption. Personality disorder tends to appear in late childhood or adolescence and continues to be manifest into adulthood. It is therefore unlikely that the diagnosis of personality disorder will be appropriate before the age of 16 or 17 years.

The Diagnostic Guidelines are:

Conditions not directly attributable to gross brain damage or disease, or to another psychiatric disorder, meeting the following criteria:

(a) markedly dysharmonious attitudes and behaviour, involving usually several areas of functioning, e.g. affectivity, arousal, impulse control, ways of perceiving and thinking, and style of relating to others;

(b) the abnormal behaviour pattern is enduring, of long standing, and not limited to episodes of mental illness;

(c) the abnormal behaviour pattern is pervasive and clearly maladaptive to a broad range of personal and social situations;

(d) the above manifestations always appear during childhood or adolescence and continue into adulthood;

(e) the disorder leads to considerable personal distress but this may only become apparent late in its course;

(f) the disorder is usually, but not invariably, associated with significant problems in occupational and social performance.

For diagnosing most of the subtypes listed below, clear evidence is usually required of the presence of at least three of the traits or behaviors given in the clinical description. "A Borderline Personality Disorder is named Emotionally Unstable Personality Disorder and defined as a:

> personality disorder in which there is a marked tendency to act impulsively without consideration of the consequences, together with affective instability. The ability to plan ahead may be minimal, and outbursts of intense anger may often lead to violence or "behavioural explosions"; these are easily precipitated when impulsive acts are criticized or thwarted by others. Two variants of this personality disorder are specified, and both share this general theme of impulsiveness and lack of self-control.

They name an Impulsive type in which predominant characteristics are emotional instability and lack of impulse control. Outbursts of violence or threatening behavior are common, particularly in response to criticism by others. That includes an explosive and aggressive disorder and a Borderline type. The Borderline type is described as having

> Several of the characteristics of emotional instability... present; in addition, the patient's own self-image, aims, and internal preferences (including sexual) are often unclear or disturbed. There are usually chronic feelings of emptiness. A liability to become involved in intense and unstable relationships may cause repeated emotional crises and may be associated with excessive efforts to avoid abandonment and a series of suicidal threats or acts of self-harm (although these may occur without obvious precipitants).

Cultural Controversy

Controversies based on gender bias and cultural considerations surround some of the personality disorder diagnoses. For example, at least three times more women than men are diagnosed in inpatient samples. A continuing debate surrounds the issue of gender labeling. Some of the very negative criteria that enable one to make the diagnosis are often considered "normal" female behavior. An example is the following operative definition for inclusion in borderline personality disorder: **affective instability**, marked shifts from baseline mood to depression, irritability, or anxiety. Borderline personality characteristics are accepted as more congruent with male sex roles and therefore more tolerable in men than in women (Gibson, 1990). At the same time, personality characteristics that are more congruent with male sex roles and less so with female sex roles, such as overt aggression, are not included in personality disorders. In other words, we have a diagnosis—borderline personality disorder—that is assigned mostly to women based on impulsive behavior and labile affect, which are traits usually ascribed to females rather than males, but there is no diagnosis (such as "overaggressive personality disorder") assigned mostly to men based on aggressive behavior and angry affect, the traits usually ascribed to males.

In other countries, some of the features of personality disorders may not be considered pathological (Alarcon & Foulks, 1995). Particularly since personality disorders are, by definition, based on interpersonal function, how one is perceived to behave in the social field brings into play cultural values. For example, in countries outside the United States, the features of schizotypal, avoidant, or dependent personality may have to be much more extreme to be considered deviant. The features are more deviant in the United States, where they are embedded in a more materialistic culture with strong values of individualism. Moreover, some diagnostic criteria, such as paranoia, may be the result of enculturation. For example, members of minority groups, immigrants, and political and economic refugees may act defensively to perceived indifference. Language barriers and general lack of knowledge of the rules of the majority may create guarded behaviors that are misperceived as suspicious. Similarly, a reaction to moving from a small rural area to a large urban one may involve emotional "freezing," which could be misperceived as a schizoid symptom. Alarcon and Foulks call for recognizing cultural contextualization when working with an individual with a personality disorder. This means "to put into a local and cultural perspective each and every behavior presented by a potential patient as well as each and every evaluative technique or clinical approach" (1995, p. 5). The *ICD-10* (WHO, 1992) would also agree that culture should be carefully considered. They specify that "for different cultures it may be necessary to develop specific sets of criteria with regard to social norms, rules and obligations."

Clinical Picture

Millon (1996) describes personality types according to various other domains (see Table 10-4) that give the clinician a better idea of the features of personality disorders. Table 10-5 also describes essential features and provides clinical descriptions of

TABLE 10-4. *DSM-IV-TR* and Other Personality Disorder Clusters

DSM-IV-TR Classifications		
Cluster A (Odd-Eccentric)	**Cluster B (Dramatic-Emotional)**	**Cluster C (Anxious-Fearful)**
Paranoid	Antisocial	Avoidant
Schizoid	Borderline	Dependent
Schizotypal	Histrionic	Obsessive-compulsive
	Narcissistic	

Other Classifications			
Pleasure Deficient/ Detached	**Interpersonally Imbalanced**	**Structurally Defective**	**Intrapsychically Conflicted**
Schizoid	Dependent	Schizotypal	Obsessive-compulsive
Avoidant	Narcissistic	Borderline	
	Antisocial Histrionic	Paranoid	
Characteristic isolation from external support systems and few interpersonal sources of support; thus disposed to be increasingly isolated, preoccupied, and depressed.	Primarily oriented to others (referred to as dependent) or toward themselves and their own needs (referred to as independent). They either consistently seek out others or are oriented to behave always in their own favor.	Socially incompetent, difficult to relate to, and often isolated, confused, and hostile; thus, they are unlikely to elicit support that can help them be more effective. Personality organization and behavior mitigates against adaptation.	Split between orienting themselves toward others or self and maintaining an independent or dependent stance. Consequently, they often reverse interpersonal behaviors and feel internally divided.

NOTE: Millon (1996) groups the disorders according to dimensions that include both internal and external perspectives; that is, he views the person from what may be happening internally or intrapsychically as well as how he or she interacts with others and believes that both internal personality makeup and external interpersonal behavior combine to manifest the disorder. See Millon, 2011, for discussion of future DSM-V proposals.

Based on information from Millon (1996).

the disorders. Although the view of personality disorders may change in the DSM-V (Millon, 2011), these ideas are still pertinent for understanding and treatment.

In a treatment setting the maladaptive patterns and characteristics of people with personality disorders, particularly those diagnoses listed in cluster B (Dramatic-Emotional) can evoke predictable, similar, and troubling responses from the treating therapist or staff. Due to inflexible responses to stress, seemingly minor events may

TABLE 10-5. Essential Features, Clinical Picture, and General Approach for the Various Disorders

	Paranoid	**Schizoid**	**Schizotypal**
Essential Features	Long-standing suspicion and mistrust. Suspect that others are acting to harm or exploit them. Responsibility often refused and assigned to others.	Social withdrawal, discomfort in interactions. Eccentric, constricted emotions. Detached.	Strikingly odd and strange. Difficulty in close relationships. Closest to illusions, like schizophrenia, but not psychotic.
Clinical Picture	Very moralistic, hypersensitive. Can easily spot others' vulnerabilities. Personalize coincidental events. Hypervigilant, tense, humorless. Fear both intimacy and rejection. Emotional detachment, isolated, repeatedly check for evidence of others' malevolent intentions, pathological jealousy.	Aloof, reserved, reclusive in everyday events but may have imagined life of closeness. Solitary hobbies, lack insight and self-identity, difficulty evaluating interpersonal events.	Hypervigilant to others' feelings but not their own. Superstitious, unusual uses and meanings of words. Vague, constricted speech. Concrete thinking, avoid eye contact. Shun relationships. Diminished ability to experience pleasure.
General Approach	Courtesy, honesty, respect, serious, without defensiveness. Gain confidence, avoid early confrontations, make slow, gentle attempts to engage.	Courtesy, honesty, respect. Tolerance of silence and whatever degree of involvement they present. Initiating. Gain therapeutic alliance, sometimes social skills training.	Respect, tolerant attitude. Curiosity but not confrontation or too much fascination with strange beliefs. Careful.
	Borderline	**Narcissistic**	**Histrionic**	**Antisocial**
Essential Features	Pattern of: unstable mood, behavior, relationships, self-image, impulsivity. Affective instability, emotional dysregulation, cognitive perceptual distortions.	Lack of empathy, exaggerated sense of importance or specialness. Indifference to others' feelings. Alternate between idealizing and devaluing. Constant craving for admiration.	Flamboyant, dramatic, excitable, overemotional. Shallow relationships. Coquettish, aggressively demanding, crave novelty, and excitement.	Disregard for or violation of rights of others. Often behavior results in imprisonment or court appearance. Lack of remorse. Irresponsibility. Manipulative.

TABLE 10-5. Continued

	Borderline	Narcissistic	Histrionic	Antisocial
Clinical Picture	When in crisis may show anger, anxiety, depression, and expression of feelings of emptiness. Unpredictable behavior, self-destructive acts, dependent or hostile behavior. May perceive rejection when it isn't warranted. Difficulty being alone and desperate attachments. Easily suggestible, black-and-white thinking, 8% to 10% will succeed at suicide at the mean age of 37.	Depression not fitting to event. Immature behavior, indifference to others' feelings. Tendency to overreact with rage or shame to perceived criticism. Preoccupation with own feelings of inferiority. Sudden attachment and rejection with others. Chronic envy, anger, and resentment.	Temper tantrums, accusations. Seductive or provocative behavior, though seem unaware of it. Command the center of attention, and will be very disappointed if someone else is more noticeable. Hyperemotional and labile, suggestible, sexualize all relationships.	Seeming lack of anxiety or depression not fitting to the situation. Seem charming to the same sex, manipulative to the opposite sex. Lying, exploitive, apparent easy-going behavior may be interrupted by rage, cruelty, or violence, failure to learn from experience.
General Approach	Focus on the here and now, psychoeducational support, and reality testing in a cognitive-behavioral way. Provide calmness and consistency, without being drawn into rescuing or power struggles.	Setting firm limits, interpreting behavior or understanding and support of idealization. Consistency, matter-of-fact approach.	Identification of one's thoughts and feelings. Do not get caught up in the tendency to embellish emotions. Noncontrolling, consistency, find alternatives to acting out, therapeutic communities, direct confrontation of interpersonal behavior.	Limit setting. Group treatment with peers and self-help groups.

	Avoidant	Dependent	Obsessive-Compulsive
Essential Features	Extreme sensitivity to rejection, extreme shyness. Active isolation from social environment, desire relationships but avoid any chance of disapproval.	Tendency to subordinate one's own needs to those of others. Get others to assume responsibility for major areas of one's life.	Constricted emotions, orderliness, perseverance, stubbornness, indecisiveness and rigidity, difficulty expressing warmth. Attempt to control every uncertainty and one's own thoughts and emotions.
Clinical Picture	Intense feelings of inferiority, anxious, insecure, self-critical, distant. Lacks confidence. Uncertain, hypervigilant about rejection. May have an ingratiating, waif-like quality.	Pessimism, self-doubt, fear of expressing feelings, passive. Avoid responsibility. Easier to initiate tasks for someone else than themselves.	Preoccupation with lists, details, procedures, minor problems. Few friends, fear of making mistakes, time spent with rituals. Boring conversation. Unproductive perfectionism, lack spontaneity, controlled affect.

(Continues)

TABLE 10-5. Continued

	Avoidant	Dependent	Obsessive-Compulsive
General Approach	Respectful, honest, warm, accepting. Reinforce assertiveness and self-esteem, address cognitive distortions.	Accept initial dependency, but resist assuming responsibility. Gradually expect and require independent problem solving and actions. Use Socratic questioning method. Help to enjoy feeling of independence, social skills training, cognitive restructuring.	Accepting of frankly boring conversation. Interrupt when possible. Focus on feelings whenever possible and provide opportunities for spontaneity.

Information adapted from Carrasco & Lecic-Tosevski (2000); Sadock, Sadock, & Ruiz (2009).

be perceived as very stressful. The individual may respond to a nonexistent problem in what seems to be an immature way. This may happen repeatedly.

Because cluster B disorders may be seen in a clinic setting more often than the others, the following discussion will focus on that cluster. Individuals may display a capacity to "get under the skin" of others. People may find themselves caught up in the life of the person with a personality disorder. Others may feel "stuck" in thinking too much about the individual, all of which can lead to a sense of failure to help someone. For example, in the case of Jean, Lotus, and Casey, the occupational therapy practitioner found himself thinking about them for the rest of the afternoon. He questioned whether he should have ended the group early and if he had adequately explained why he was doing so. He wondered if his treatment was effective. He felt guilty concerning Jean, annoyed concerning Casey, and detached concerning Lotus.

In a treatment setting, the relationships with staff of a person with a personality disorder often become strained or conflicted. A parallel process may happen among the staff. This may be due to an individual's tendency to treat some staff in an idealized way, with intense admiration and complete cooperation, and to treat other staff in a denigrating way, showing disdain and avoidance and acting as if they were almost invisible. This may play into one professional's wishes to be helpful and saving or provoke rejecting behavior and attendant guilt from another for not being helpful enough. Conflict begins when unspoken feelings, such as envy, jealousy, or anger, prompt behavior in which some staff members defend a patient, while others complain about him or her. Working relationships in the staff will be disrupted, and the staff members may turn away from the client. This situation is especially likely to occur with a novice therapist due to lack of experience in understanding the situation, desire to be a "good" therapist and do the right thing, inability to examine his or her own personal motives and needs, or fear of appearing vulnerable when speaking with the other staff members.

Jean, Lotus, and Casey—Inflexible Responses to Stress

When the occupational therapy practitioner ended a group 10 minutes early due to an impromptu meeting, Jean (diagnosis: narcissistic personality disorder) became teary and angry, protesting that she was overlooked, no longer felt safe in the group, and could not possibly return. Lotus (diagnosis: schizoid personality disorder) was nonchalant, said nothing, and left unnoticed. Casey (diagnosis: obsessive-compulsive personality disorder) talked about the necessity of cleaning up and ritualistically ordered and reordered the project he had been working on.

Discussion

Jean's, Lotus's, and Casey's responses to stress were each inflexible, however, each person functioned differently in accordance with the symptoms or dimensions of his or her specific disorder.

When this situation manifests itself with more than one individual or with a staff member, it is called **splitting** (Sadock & Sadock, 2007). This can be counteracted if the staff members anticipate the splitting process, strive to understand the internal feelings of the client, and recognize that he or she is not acting in this way deliberately. (Think of an approach with the difference between "can't," implying difficulties in biological structure and operations, and "won't," implying deliberate will.) Staff members must also remain aware of their own internal feelings and discuss them openly with each other. They may also model certain responses for the client. Responses should: (1) indicate that no one is all good or bad; rather, each of us has both strengths and limitations; (2) aid the client in becoming aware of the tendency to categorize people in a black-and-white way; and (3) accept the expression of both positive and negative aspects in the client, in oneself, and in other staff members. That is, it is important not to moralize or say that behavior is unacceptable or inappropriate, and rather to provide some understanding of the client's process.

INTERDISCIPLINARY ASSESSMENT AND TREATMENT

Assessment usually consists of self-report inventories, projective techniques, and structured clinical interviews (Clark & Harrison, 2001; Sadock, Sadock, & Ruiz, 2009). Instruments assess both normal and abnormal personalities based on traits or diagnostically based instruments, and based on self-report versus interviews. (All of the following instruments are cited in Clark & Harrison, 2001.) Well-known psychological assessments that are self-report, diagnostically based measures include the Millon Clinical Multiaxial Inventory—III (MCMI–III) and the Minnesota Multiphasic Personality Inventory (MMPI-2). Clinical interviews geared to the *DSM* criteria include the Structured Clinical Interview for DSM-IV Axis II (SCID-II) and the Structured Interview for DSM Personality Disorders-IV (SIDP-IV). Trait-based measures that are self-report include the Inventory of Interpersonal Problems—Personality Disorder Scales (IIP–PD; Pilkonis et al.), NEO-Personality Inventory-Revised (NEO-PI-R; Costa & McCrae, 2008), and the Structural Analysis of Social Behavior Intrex Questionnaire (SASB-IQ; Benjamin).

Trait-based measures that are interviews include the Diagnostic Interview for Borderline Patients-Revised (CIB-R; Zanarini et al.). Personality Assessment Schedule (PASl; Tyrer), and the Structured Interview for the Five-Factor Model (SIFFM; Trull & Widiger). One inventory, the Temperament and Character Inventory (TCI) (cited in Sadock, Sadock, & Ruiz, 2009) can be self-report, interview, or peer ratings and evaluates the four dimensions for all age groups.

Occupational therapy assessments are not trait or diagnostically based but are based on occupational functioning in performance areas in contexts. Therefore, occupational therapy assessments add valuable information about individuals that may not be assessed in detail in other measurements. Individuals with personality disorders have difficulty in instrumental activities of daily living, work, leisure pursuits, and social participation, so occupational therapy's emphasis on these areas of occupation in specific environments may provide valuable information to a treatment team. In addition, occupational therapy's emphasis on process, communication and interaction skills, and performance patterns may specify areas of intervention not considered by other disciplines. Finally, the occupational therapy intervention approach of modification or adaptation fits with a major difficulty encountered by people who have personality disorders. (For further information about occupational therapy assessments, see Chapter 18, "Assessment, Evaluation, and Outcome Measurement.")

Assessments cited in the occupational therapy literature include general occupational assessments such as the Occupational Circumstance Assessment-Interview and Rating Scale (OCAIRS) (Forsyth, Deshpande, & Kielhofner, 2005) or (OCAIRS-S)-Swedish version (Falklof & Haglund, 2010), the Assessment of Life Habits (LIFE-H) version 3.1, Short Form (Lariviere, Desrosiers, Tousignant, & Boyer, 2010), and the Adult Sensory Profile (Moro, 2007). Each of these assessments was used in the context of research or intervention programs for Borderline Personality Disorder, Cluster B Personality Disorders, or the maladaptive coping strategy or emotional dysregulation involved in self-mutilation, respectively.

Recent research indicates that manualized therapy programs, particularly those created for borderline personality disorder, are successful (Paris, 2008a, 2008b) as well as intense outpatient psychotherapy, group psychotherapy, and day or therapeutic community treatment. Manualized therapy programs created from cognitive

(Koerner & Linehan, 2000; Linehan & Heard, 1992) and interpersonal (Benjamin & Pugh, 2001) models of therapy explicitly outline treatment programs of one to two years. These programs, particularly Linehan's Dialectical Behavior Therapy, have been adopted and found effective in many community mental health settings, including occupational therapy programs (Moro, 2007; Falklof & Haglund, 2010). Long-term studies of 15 and 27 years (Paris, 2002) find that active psychotherapy improves the natural process of remission seven-fold, but short-term treatment of one year may reduce behaviors such as overdosing, self-harm, and use of hospitalization. Impulsivity is often more likely to change first and emotional dysregulation may take longer to change. Interestingly, these long-term studies showed that borderline symptoms tend to reduce after 15 years, and after 27 years many of the participants did not show borderline symptoms.

Group psychotherapy based on behavioral theories includes social skills training, role playing, and reinforcement used to identify and alter maladaptive behavior. Psychodynamic group therapy clarifies and confronts ego-syntonic traits, and increases capacity to tolerate and integrate emotions, to learn about the impact of one's behavior on others, and to acquire and practice new methods of interacting (Piper & Joyce, 2001).

Day or community treatment or partial hospitalization programs are most effective when they have a high staff-to-client ratio, a minority of low-functioning clients, clear lines of communication, task-oriented groups, and a routine that everyone is expected to follow.

The aim of treatment is not to modify the personality, (in fact, one expert believes that since personality traits are enduring and not changeable that such treatment is contraindicated (Livesley, 1999) but to reverse the process by which traits are amplified to disorders. General therapy is teaching clients how to make better use of their personality traits so that traits and therefore individuals become more adaptive. Generally, techniques are designed to modulate emotions to optimal intensities, limit rigid and inappropriate behavior, expand behavior repertoires, develop more satisfying social roles, and establish more stable social networks (Paris, 1999; 2008a). General suggestions for treatment are listed in Table 10-6. Crisis situations may be precipitated by troubles in relationships and adapting to life changes and also by resultant depression, suicidal thoughts, and impulsive behavior.

Psychopharmacology

Although there have been few studies of pharmacology in those with personality disorders in the last 10 years, research and clinical trials suggest that some personality characteristics are associated with abnormalities in the central nervous system (Markovitz, 2001). About 40% to 50% of personality differences can be explained in terms of heredity (Lopez-Ibor, 2000; Paris, 1999). Furthermore, abnormalities in the central nervous system are associated with behavioral changes, and perhaps some personality traits arise from biological underpinnings. Also, severe psychosocial

TABLE 10-6. General Treatment Suggestions for Personality Disorder Clusters

Cluster A (Paranoid, Schizoid, Schizotypal)	Cluster B (Borderline, Narcissistic, Histrionic, Antisocial)	Cluster C (Avoidant, Dependent, Obsessive-Compulsive)
Nondirective cognitive therapy, support to reduce isolation, encourage expressions of emotions, social skills training. Not necessarily capable of sustained intimate relationships so need steady employment in interpersonally undemanding jobs.	Social skills training, cognitive therapy, therapeutic milieu, firm structure, psychoeducation, teach tolerance of interpersonal distress and acting less on impulses, self-management or mindfulness skills, focus on a hierarchy of targeted behaviors. Develop task orientations through employment and less demanding interpersonal contacts through social networks.	Tend to deal with anxiety by avoidance or procrastination so encourage more risks and emotional expressions. Time-limited dynamic therapies are active and confrontational.

Overall Principles: Milieu and group treatments are successful, maladaptive behavior can and should be pointed out and examined, feedback from peers is very useful, new ways of relating can and should be practiced, individuals can benefit from mindfulness training and being helpful to others.

Based on: Paris, 1999, 2008a, 2008b; Piper & Joyce, 2001; Sadock, Sadock, & Ruiz, 2009

stress may alter gene expression and life-threatening trauma may set in motion neurobiological changes that continue to affect mood, behavior, memory, and arousal throughout life. In fact, children exposed to both neglect and abuse are presumably prone to both underdevelopment of the hippocampus- and amygdala-mediated memory systems and permanent "branding" of painful memories in the cortex. In addition, they are likely to have a "kindled" nervous system, that is, one prone to overreact even to mild stimuli that happen to be reminiscent of the original trauma. (Koenigsberg et al., 2000)

Most studies have been conducted with clients who most frequently present for treatment, for example, those with borderline, antisocial, schizotypal, and avoidant personality disorders. However, the majority of studies concern borderline personality disorder (Markovitz, 2001; Tyrer, 2000). Most medications to treat borderline personality disorder are used to treat the other symptoms of major depression, anxiety, or psychotic episodes. For example, those with avoidant personality disorder may respond to antianxiety medication, with schizotypal to antipsychotics, those with poor impulse control to antidepressives with specific serotonergic action (Lopez-Ibor, 2000). Selective serotonin reuptake inhibitors (SSRIs) seem to be the most promising group of medications to reduce depression, anxiety, impulsivity, and self-injury (Markovitz, 2001). Currently, neurotransmitter studies focus on serotonin, dopamine, and norepinephrine (Ratey, 1995; Ruegy & Frances, 1995). It is believed that serotonin deficits may be implicated in suicide and impulsively violent behavior and may be linked to impulsivity in general.

In fact, drugs are given judiciously due to the potentials for suicide and poly-drug abuse. Due to the potential for staff splitting, maintaining a consistent approach and constant, clear communication between and among all treating professionals is a necessity.

Interpersonal Approach

The literature regarding personality disorders indicates that the therapeutic alliance is extremely important to treatment. The elements of a therapeutic alliance are a bond with the therapist, agreement on goals of treatment, and a sense of working together on tasks for addressing important issues. This last element is labeled the *working alliance* and has been identified as the strongest predictor of successful outcome with borderline personality disorder (Clark & Harrison, 2001).

Perhaps the concept of therapeutic alliance comes closest to occupational therapy's intervention of therapeutic use of self defined in the Occupational Therapy Practice Framework (AOTA, 2008). (However, see Chapter 19, "The Use of Psychosocial Methods and Interpersonal Strategies in Mental Health," which expands the discussion of the therapeutic use of self.)

Table 10-7 lists general interpersonal treatment approaches that are useful guides for all practitioners, including occupational therapists, when interacting with individuals with personality disorders (recognizing however, that each person and performance context is unique). These general interpersonal techniques are culled from supportive, cognitive, psychodynamic, and interpersonal models of treatment (Winston, Rosenthal, & Muran, 2001), principles of wellness (Sadock, Sadock, & Ruiz, 2009), and mindfulness training (Linehan, 1992) grounded in experience. In occupational therapy, activity and daily living groups promote a focus on here-and-now

TABLE 10-7. General Interpersonal Treatment Approaches

Useful Concepts for Interaction
Establish a collaborative stance. Establish agreement on the goals and tasks of therapy and be explicit how the tasks relate to the goals.
Communicate in a conversational style. Provide encouragement that tells the client something about herself, for example, "that took courage." Provide understanding along with advice.
Confront defensive behavior in a supportive atmosphere by focusing on the client's demonstrated behavior instead of your judgment of it.
Provide consistency in the structure of your program and behavior and in limit setting.
Encourage membership in social support groups.
Whenever possible, assist the client to think through the consequences of actions—sometimes called *anticipatory guidance and rehearsal.* That is, together move through situations hypothetically considering possibilities and suggest more appropriate or novel ways to handle the hypothetical situations.
Sincerely express pleasure and enthusiasm in the individual's attempts to change and grow.

behavior, encourage thinking sequentially and anticipating consequences, and facilitate interpersonal relating, adaptive coping, and realistic thinking. Because problems are manifested in the interpersonal realm, attention to the interpersonal approach is important.

OCCUPATIONAL THERAPY TREATMENT INTERVENTIONS

"More than 50 years ago Allport stated that 'personality is something and personality does something'" (Livesley, 2001, p. 13). Perhaps it can be said that the *DSM-IV-TR* (APA, 2000) is concerned with what the personality is, but less attention has been paid to what the personality does, to the functional aspects and adaptations of personality disorders. The adaptations can be described in terms of how people universally solve or negotiate major life tasks or problems. Tasks basic to adaptation are establishing an identity, figuring out where and to whom one belongs, negotiating loss and separation, and establishing where one fits in a hierarchy of family or society. Daily living tasks, work, and leisure are included in tasks basic to adaptation. Individuals with personality disorders have difficulty in these life tasks and treatment in general will address these universal life problems.

Research studies in occupational therapy with people who have personality disorders (Lariviere, Desrosiers, Tousignant, & Boyer, 2010), particularly cluster B, indicate that leisure and productive activities of school and work are the most problematic for the clients, while self-care is the least problematic. Examples of leisure and productive activities are paid jobs, "tourist activities" such as going to museums or traveling, and physical exercises. Likewise, other research (Falklof & Haglund, 2010) indicates that work and leisure performance areas and social relationships are difficult due to self-image or personal causation deficiencies and problems with self-regulation skills, perhaps both can be categorized as affecting motivation. Interestingly, leisure activities that were mentioned as those that people were competent to perform were those involving no other people: taking care of animals, furnishing, cooking, writing, working out, and reading. Those activities that were difficult to perform were influenced by motivation and feelings or emotional regulation. For example, a big effort to do things, hardest to get up in the morning, depends on how I feel, making plans without following them, and then feeling more anxious. Poor self-image, shame, fear of failure, and conflict with others limited relationships (Falklof & Haglund).

The occupational therapy studies (Falklof & Haglund, 2010) recommended Dialectical Behavior Treatment, particularly the modules of interpersonal effectiveness and mindfulness skills. Also recommended (Lariviere, Desrosiers, Tousignant, & Boyer, 2010) were prioritizing interventions in leisure activities, work and school, fitness, and interpersonal relationships.

As was mentioned earlier, there are manualized treatment programs that have been adopted in community mental health (Paris, 2008a, 2008b). Also, day treatment programs and social skills, psychosocial, and psychoeducational groups have proven successful for personality disorders (Bateman & Fonagy, 2009; Piper & Joyce, 2001; McKenzie, 2001; Ruiz-Sancho, Smith, & Gunderson, 2001).

There are many personality disorders, and each cluster is distinguished by certain features. Discussing expanded treatment for each individual disorder is beyond the scope of this text; however, this section will discuss treatment directed toward the cluster B disorders, which are most often encountered in treatment settings. Generally, in addition to an interpersonal approach, treatment consists of making behavioral, cognitive, and social interventions, such as practicing adaptive coping strategies, learning to think before acting, paying attention to emotional style and emotional regulation, learning to develop satisfying relationships, and developing a sense of effectiveness in the world—defined as personal causation (Kielhofner, 2007)—or sense of self-identity. These interventions correspond to the dimensions described by Millon (1996) and shown in Table 10-3 and to the domains listed in Table 10-4.

A common general purpose of an occupational therapy treatment program is to create a safe, interesting, and playful context for treatment (Barris, Kielhofner, & Watts, 1988) through collaboration and establishment of a setting that makes clear, consistent, functional demands within a specific time frame. The program should allow for spontaneity in work and play and provide a predictable setting in which to practice adult roles, explore adult values and identity, and reflect on one's thoughts, feelings, and behavior (mindfulness). Ultimately, the goal of occupational therapy is to facilitate clients' adaptation in their specific environment (performance context). The program should incorporate treatment that addresses problems in performance skills and patterns stemming from concurrent symptoms (substance abuse, self-mutilation, etc.; see also Paris, 2005) and essential features of personality disorders, particularly impulsive and rigid, maladaptive behavior patterns. Occupational therapy can address these issues in the standard occupational performance areas (Instrumental Activities of Daily Living [IADLs], education, work, and social participation).

Leisure

Some individuals with personality disorders lack the ability to gain satisfaction from recreational or leisure pursuits. This may be due to rigid, narrow interests; paranoid or fearful behavior; or fear of closeness. It may be due to a background of growing up where any spontaneous or exploratory behavior was dangerous because it was not approved of by caregivers, or it may be due to an inability to regulate pleasurable feelings or guilt that one is feeling pleasure. It may be due to simply not learning that one can enjoy recreational pursuits because recreation may have involved social activities that clients have shied away from, the pursuits may have been inherently competitive and therefore avoided, or perhaps the clients were so perfectionistic that they held back out of fear they could not meet their own standards.

In other cases, recreational/leisure activities may be one area in which people with personality disorders can feel spontaneous, enjoy some sense of worth for their achievements (Falklof & Haglund, 2010), and perhaps feel relief from a relentless inner turmoil. For example, Jamal loved words, so he looked forward to playing the game "Dictionary," whereby he realized that he was articulate and had an advanced vocabulary. In this case, leisure activities may demonstrate a strength that can be utilized in treatment. Leisure occupations may also counteract various cognitive beliefs and statements that clients tell themselves, such as, "I enjoy doing things by myself," "I don't deserve to have fun," or "I can't let my guard down." Leisure occupations may provide opportunities to plan sequentially, sustain attention, and anticipate actions.

Psychologically, leisure occupations may provide specific responses to overwhelming feelings and help clients regulate their emotions. Leisure occupations may provide ways in which clients can feel worthwhile and enjoy a sense of accomplishment and competence. In this way they may realize that indeed, some activities can be intrinsically pleasurable and can provide pleasure and meaning even though they are not based on approval. For example, Anais worked out at the gym so that she could gain approval from others. However, in the occupational therapy leisure group, when she carefully monitored her thoughts and feelings while working out, she realized that she also enjoyed the feeling she got after finishing a hard workout.

Socially, leisure occupations can provide avenues in which people can be around others, such as a scrabble, reading, tennis, gourmet cooking, or dog walking group, and develop casual relationships in a nonthreatening manner. They can relate to others in a reciprocal fashion, thereby developing a knowledge of empathy, while at the same time enjoying the opportunity to gain attention in an adaptive way.

Work

"There are some data suggesting that occupational difficulties may be associated with personality disorders. In two studies, 23% to 42% of participants with personality disorders were unemployed for 6 months to 4 years" (Mattia & Zimmerman, 2001, p. 110).

Work is often a troublesome area due to a person's shyness and paranoid or fearful behavior on the job. Work may also be troublesome due to a person's difficulties in regulating the expression of emotions while on the job. For example, in a session discussing a return to work, Jill was unable to state why she had been fired from her previous three jobs except that she had had trouble meeting deadlines due to feeling overwhelmed about a new relationship. Trouble with work may be due to difficulties meeting concrete standards of performance or problems in sequencing and anticipating consequences of actions or in utilizing logical thinking. Work situations may seem difficult due to a person's lack of empathy and therefore lack of ability to "read" situations or unwritten rules. People with personality disorders may be underemployed, have jobs for which they are seemingly overqualified, or have an erratic work history. Despite potential problems, work, like leisure, may be the one area where they may excel and learn to focus solely on objective tasks to the exclusion of other areas of life and vocational rehabilitation may be an overlooked area of intervention (Lariviere, Desrosiers, Tousignant, & Boyer, 2010). For example, cognitively, vocational activities may provide arenas in which participants can learn to anticipate consequences of their actions, problem-solve, develop frustration tolerance, and accept responsibility. Alternately, work may provide opportunities for clients to learn how to regulate emotions, the appropriate times and situations in which to express them, and how to tolerate stress from performance standards. Work activities could provide arenas in which people can learn social appropriateness and how to get along with others in the workplace.

Social Participation

Research (Paris, 2002, 2008a, 2008b) indicates that over time, relationships and social adjustment improve for those with borderline personality disorder. Surprisingly, many participants who improved tended to avoid intimate relationships and concentrate on establishing careers and social networks. In fact, "many who improve find that having less intimate friends, belonging to a social community, or having a pet provides more stability than could have been achieved through intimacy" (p. 319). Due to these findings, occupational therapists should concentrate interventions on community and family interactions and roles (Lariviere, Desrosiers, Tousignant, & Boyer, 2010), perhaps in peer-operated self-help centers (Swarbrick & Ellis, 2009).

Self-Care

Usually people with personality disorders are independent in self-care, except perhaps when undergoing acute crises. Indeed, self-care skills seem to be the least problematic for them (Lariviere, Desrosiers, Tousignant, & Boyer, 2010). They possess self-care skills, although at times, due to personality patterns such as impulsivity, they may not use them and they may display poor judgment. For example, even though Jolene had an itemized budget, she felt deprived and so spent half of her one-year student loan on a wardrobe. She rationalized that she needed to have clothes for work when she graduated. Most treatment for self-care, then, would focus on IADLs and how to utilize skills or on motivation and judgment strategies. Often this involves concrete planning and goal setting with built-in rewards or recognizing activities that are valued. It may involve learning how to handle impulsive behavior, such as simply stopping whatever one is doing, breathing deeply, or phoning a friend. More recently, occupational therapists have advocated the use of sensory processing strategies for self-mutilation behavior such as cutting or burning (Champagne, 2011; Champagne & Stromberg, 2004; Moro, 2007; see also Chapter 13, "Mental Health of Adolescents," for a discussion of self-mutilation). It may be learning how to think before acting, such as focusing on self-talk and "changing the tape." Occupational therapists may use cognitive strategies from Dialectical Behavior Therapy that replace self-denigrating thoughts with statements about the self being worthy and healthy with mindfulness strategies to understand emotions and ways of regulating emotions.

Inner self-care skills—those that concern taking care of the internal self (called the *internal environment* in other chapters of this book) in a psychological/

emotional way by utilizing a knowledge of the self and psychological skills in a social environment—may be practiced. Cognitively, an individual focuses on how to think before acting and how to anticipate events in a step-by-step manner. Psychologically, an individual may assume a self-identity, learn values and interests, and practice how to recognize what is pleasurable and interesting for its own sake through exploration and mastery. Socially, being able to work with others helps to develop a capacity for empathy for oneself and others by learning that everyone has strengths and weaknesses. For example, in a group utilizing art media in which the task was to "draw your favorite place" and then tell others about it, Robert was able to wait patiently for his turn. As others discussed their work, he realized that he had similar emotions about his favorite place and that he could understand their statements. He also realized that he valued aspects of nature that brought him tranquility.

Groups

Groups can be either nonverbal or verbal. Nonverbal groups that provide opportunities to work in the presence of others and relate in a casual way can be nonthreatening and motivating. Working in groups on concrete craft and art projects provides structured ways of utilizing one's strengths, resources, and talents while providing an engaging context in which to explore values and interests. Relaxation and restorative groups provide concrete ways to intervene in impulsive situations or when an individual has the experience of feeling overcome by overwhelming emotions. In addition, clients can explore activities that provide intrinsic pleasure. Verbal groups, particularly those that include action and then reflection on the action, can call on individual problem-solving skills, accessing and delineating of emotions, and recognition of how they interfere maladaptively (such as in work). They can also provide training in social skills and communication and in how to be empathic with others. Thus, occupational therapists provide skills training groups that may address emotional regulation, interpersonal skills, awareness of self or mindfulness, and tolerating stressful conditions or situations. Groups focus on problem solving, relationship, and skills training (Moro, 2007).

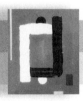

CASE ILLUSTRATION

Robyn—Treatment Course for Borderline Personality Disorder

Friends of Robyn who worked with her at a large store that sold DVDs, CDs, and classic, old records became concerned about her when she failed to show up for work for three days. When they went to her apartment, they found that she had not been eating or sleeping and that she had burned herself in two different places on her body. After evaluation in an emergency room, she agreed to psychiatric treatment.

An occupational therapy evaluation with the Allen Diagnostic Module (Earhart, Allen, & Blue, 1993) revealed cognitive functioning of 5.0 (able to cognitively explore the environment, but restricted to overt trial-and-error learning and unable to anticipate consequences). An Occupational Performance History Interview (OPHI) (Kielhofner, 2002; Kielhofner & Henry, 1988; Kielhofner, Henry, Whalens, & Rogers, 1991) revealed that Robyn perceived that she did not have control in any areas of her life, wished for a better job or career, and had a sense that she had troubled relationships. Although recently she had not engaged in hobbies or other forms of recreation, she enjoyed jewelry making and furniture refinishing and had worked out with weights. Based on this information, and in concert with her occupational therapy practitioner, Robyn chose to attend the following groups:

1. The "Coping Skills" group addressed topics such as "stamping out impulsivity," "what to do when you want to hurt yourself," and "bringing tranquility into your life." The group included education, discussion, paper-and-pencil exercises, and trying out of new behaviors while in the acute setting.

2. The "About Work" group included working on small jobs that were time limited and paid, learning about work behaviors and environments, discussing the "unwritten rules" of work, and analyzing and reflecting on each work session.

3. The "Becoming Creative with Crafts" group offered a variety of art and craft projects

that could be learned and completed in short time frames.

Robyn's chosen goals of treatment were to handle her self-mutilating and impulsive behavior, find another job and explore career options, and learn to feel better about herself. She worked individually with an occupational therapy practitioner to organize a workout schedule and further explore career options. After one week she had practiced some coping skills. Specifically, when she had the urge to burn herself, she learned that she could stop. At the same time, she began to experiment with making painted picture frames, which became popular on the unit. In the vocational group, she began to realize her problems in following through, and that she created problems in work when she became too attached to co-workers. She began to explore careers that would suit this trait, that is, she explored careers where she could complete short-term tasks instead of long-term projects and where she would not be distracted by too many co-workers.

Prior to discharge, the occupational therapy practitioner assisted Robyn in exploring options in the community for continuing her interests and anticipated how she might handle setbacks when she was alone in her own home. In a pre-discharge review, Robyn stated that she "felt better about herself." She had learned that she could follow through in the art and craft group and, in fact, that she possessed some creativity and originality. She realized that perhaps she could indeed positively affect her environment. In fact, people had asked her to make craft projects for them and she had successfully practiced moderating her impulsive behavior. She decided that she would rescue a cat from the local humane society since she could take care of this pet and enjoy loving it but it also could be independent enough to not require too much daily care. She also felt hopeful about finding a new job. Since she had explored her abilities and personality aspects in relation to her career, she realized that she could maintain more control of her own destiny and satisfaction. The occupational therapy practitioner put her in touch with the department of vocational rehabilitation so that they could open a case and assist her in further exploring her job and career interests and obtaining work.

Discussion

Robyn's course of treatment demonstrates how occupational therapy, individual and group, in all performance areas is a useful and creative aspect of treatment for a person with a personality disorder.

SUMMARY

Understanding and treating personality disorders is difficult and often daunting to new students and clinicians for various reasons, including an unclear symptomatic picture, different classifications based on personality traits, behavior that alternates between functioning and instability, and problems that involve other people. However, treatment is possible based on an understanding of personality and the therapist's willingness to reflect on his or her own responses. Recent research and detailed treatment programs indicate that those with personality disorders can be successfully treated and live healthy and happy lives.

Disabling personality patterns and traits lead to problems with adapting in most areas of life. Occupational therapy includes an interpersonal approach (for example, a collaborative stance, consistency, and understanding) and interventions in leisure, work, social, and some self-care areas. Manualized treatment programs and day treatment, both individual psychotherapy and various supportive group therapies using techniques following various treatment models—behavioral, cognitive, psychodynamic, and interpersonal—provide an optimistic picture for individuals with personality disorders.

REVIEW QUESTIONS

1. What are the new developments in research and treatment that lead to successful outcomes?
2. What are dimensional models? How do they explain personality disorders?
3. What sensory strategies are suggested for self-mutilation?

4. What are useful ways of interacting in a clinical setting with individuals with personality disorders?
5. Why are the work, leisure, and social participation areas of performance particularly important for people with personality disorders?

REFERENCES

Alarcon, R., & Foulks, E. (1995). Personality disorders and culture. *Cultural Diversity and Mental Health, 1*(1), 3–17.

American Occupational Therapy Association (AOTA). (2008). Occupational therapy practice framework: Domain and process (2nd ed.). *American Journal of Occupational Therapy, 62,* 625–683.

American Psychiatric Association (APA). (2000). *Diagnostic and statistical manual of mental disorders* (4th ed., Text rev.). Washington, DC: Author.

Barris, R., Kielhofner, G., & Watts, J. (1988). *Occupational therapy in psychosocial practice.* Thorofare, NJ: Slack.

Bateman, A., & Fonagy, P. (2009). Randomized controlled trial of outpatient metallization-based treatment versus structured clinical management for borderline personality disorder. *American Journal of Psychiatry, 166,* 12, 1355–1364. Retrieved from http://www.ajp.psychiatry online.org

Benjamin, L. S., & C. Pugh. (2001). Using interpersonal theory to select effective treatment interventions. In W. J. Livesley (Ed.), *Handbook of personality disorders: Theory, research and treatment* (pp. 414–436). New York: Guilford.

Carrasco, J. L., & Lecic-Tosevski, D. (2000). Specific types of personality disorder. In M. G. Gelder, J. J. Lopez-Ibor, & N. Andreasen (Eds.), *New Oxford textbook of psychiatry* (pp. 927–953). New York: Oxford University Press.

Champagne, T. (2011). *Sensory modulation and environment: Essential elements of occupation.* (3rd. ed.). Australia: Pearson Assessment.

Champagne, T., & Stromberg, N. (2004). Sensory approaches in inpatient psychiatric settings: Innovative alternatives to seclusion and restraint. *Journal of Psychosocial Nursing, 42,* 35–44.

Clark, L. A., & Harrison, J. A. (2001). Assessment instruments. In W. John Livesley (Ed.), *Handbook of personality disorders: Theory, research and treatment* (pp. 277–306). New York: Guilford.

Costa, P. T., & McCrae, R. R. (2008). The revised Personality Inventory (NEO-PI-R). In G. Boye, G. Matthews, & D. H. Saklofske, *The Sage handbook of personality theory and assessment, vol 2.* (p. 717). Los Angeles: Sage.

Costa, P. T. J., & Widiger, T. A. (2002). Introduction: Personality disorders and the five-factor model of personality. In J. P. T. Costa & T. H. Widiger (Eds.), *Personality disorders and the five-factor model of personality* (2nd ed., pp. 3–14). Washington, DC: American Psychological Association.

Derksen, J., & Sloore, H. (1999). Psychodiagnostics and indications for treatment in cases of personality disorder: Some pitfalls. In J. Derksen, C. Maffei, & H. Groen (Eds.), *Treatment of personality disorders.* New York: Springer.

Earhart, C. A., Allen, C. K., & Blue, T. (1993). *Allen Diagnostic Module. The manual.* Colchester, CT: S&S Worldwide.

Falklof, I., & Haglund, L. (2010). Daily Occupations and adaptation to daily life described by women suffering from Borderline Personality Disorder. *Occupational Therapy in Mental Health, 26,* 4, 354–374.

Fonagy, P. , & Target, M. (1996). Playing with reality: I. Theory of mind and the normal development of psychic reality. *International Journal of Psycho-Analysis, 77,* 217–233.

Fonagy, P., & Bateman, A. (2006). Editorial: Progress in the treatment of borderline personality disorder. *British Journal of Psychiatry, 188,* 1–3. Retrieved from doi: 10.1192/bjp.bp.105.012088

Forsyh, K., Deshpande, S., & Kielhofner, G. (2005). *The Occupational Circumstances Assessment Interview and Rating Scale (OCAIRS)* version 4. Chicago: Model of Human Occupation Clearinghouse.

Gelder, M. G., Lopez-Ibor, J. J., & Andreasen, N. (Eds.). (2000). *New Oxford textbook of psychiatry*. New York: Oxford University Press.

Gibson, D. (1990). Borderline personality disorder: Issues of etiology and gender. *Occupational Therapy in Mental Health, 10*(4), 63–77.

Gunderson, J. G., & Gabbard, G. O. (2001). Personality disorders—Introduction. In G. O. Gabbard (Ed.), *Treatment of psychiatric disorders* (pp. 2223–2225). Washington, DC: American Psychiatric Publishing.

Kernberg, O. (1999). The psychotherapeutic treatment of borderline patients. In J. Derksen, C. Maffei, & H. Groen (Eds.), *Treatment of personality disorders* (pp. 167–182) New York: Kluwer Academic/Plenum.

Kielhofner, G. (2002). *A model of human occupation: Theory and application* (3rd ed.). Baltimore: Lippincott, Williams & Wilkins.

Kielhofner, G. (2008). *A model of human occupation: Theory and application* (4th ed.). Baltimore: Lippincott, Williams & Wilkins.

Kielhofner, G., & Henry, A. D. (1988). Development and investigation of an occupational performance history interview. *American Journal of Occupational Therapy, 42*(8), 489–498.

Kielhofner, G., Henry, A., Whalens, D., & Rogers, E. S. (1991). A generalizability study of the Occupational Performance History Interview. *Occupational Therapy Journal of Research, 11*, 292–306.

Kiesler, D. J. (1986). The 1982 interpersonal circle: An analysis of DSM-III personality disorders. In T. Millon & G. Klerman (Eds.), *Contemporary directions in psychopathology: Towards the DSM-IV*. New York: Guilford.

Koenigsberg, H. W., Kernberg, O. F., Stone, M. H., Appelbaum, A. H., Yeomans, F. E., & Diamond, D. (2000). *Borderline patients: Extending the limits of treatability*. New York: Basic.

Koerner, K., & Linehan, M. (2000). Research on dialectical behavior therapy for patients with borderline personality disorder. *The Psychiatric Clinics of North America, 23*(1), 151–167.

Kyler, P. (2008). Client-centered and family-centered care: Refinement of the concepts. *Occupational Therapy in Mental Health, 24*(2), 100–120.

Lariviere, N., Desrosiers, J., Tousignant, M., & Boyer, R. (2010). Exploring social participation of people with cluster B personality disorders. *Occupational Therapy in Mental Health, 26*(4), 375–386.

LeBel, J., & Champagne, T. (2010, June). Integrating sensory and trauma-informed interventions: A Massachusetts State Initiative, Part 2. *American Occupational Therapy Association, Mental Health Special Interest Section, 33*, 2.

LeBel, J., Champagne, T., Stromberg, N., & Coyle, R. (2010, March). Integrating sensory and trauma-informed interventions: A Massachusetts State Initiative, Part 1. *American Occupational Therapy Association, Mental Health Special Interest Section, 33*, 1.

Linehan, M. M., & Heard, (1992). *Dialectical Behavior Therapy for Borderline Personality*. New York: Guilford.

Livesley, W. J. (1999). The implications of recent research on the etiology and stability of personality and personality disorder for treatment. In J. Derksen, C. Maffei, & H. Groen (Eds.), *Treatment of personality disorders* (pp. 25–38). New York: Kluwer Academic/Plenum Publishers.

Livesley, W. J. (2001). Conceptual and taxonomic issues. In W. J. Livesley (Ed.), *Handbook of personality disorders: Theory, research and treatment* (pp. 3–38). New York: Guilford.

Livesley, W. J. (2003). Diagnostic dilemmas in classifying personality disorder. Advancing DSM: Dilemmas in psychiatric diagnosis. In K. A. Phillips, M. B. First, & H. A. Pincus (Eds.), *Advancing DSM: Dilemmas in psychiatric diagnosis* (pp. 153–189). Washington, DC: American Psychiatric Association,

Livesley, W. J. (2007). An integrated approach to the treatment of personality disorder. *Journal of Mental Health, 16*(1), 131–148. Retrieved from doi: 10.1080/09638230601182086

Livesley, W. J., & Jang, K. L. (2008). The behavioral genetics of personality disorder. *Annual Review of Clinical Psychology, 4,* 247–274. Retrieved from doi: 10.1146/annurev.clinpsy.4.022007.141203

Lopez-Ibor, J. (2000). Personality disorders. In M. G. Gelder & J. J. Lopez-Ibor (Eds.), *New Oxford textbook of psychiatry* (pp. 919–923). New York: Oxford University Press.

Loranger, A. W. (2000). General clinical description of personality disorders. In M. G. Gelder, J. J. Lopez-Ibor, & N. Andreasen (Eds.), *New Oxford textbook of psychiatry* (pp. 923–926). New York: Oxford University Press.

Markovitz, P. (2001). Pharmacotherapy. In W. J. Livesley (Ed.), *Handbook of personality disorders: Theory, research and treatment* (pp. 475–493). New York: Guilford.

Mattia, J. I., & Zimmerman, M. (2001). Epidemiology. In W. J. Livesley (Ed.), *Handbook of personality disorders: Theory, research and treatment* (pp. 107–123). New York: Guilford.

McKenzie, K. R. (2001). Group psychotherapy. In W. J. Livesley (Ed.), *Handbook of personality disorders: Theory, research and treatment* (pp. 497–526). New York: Guilford.

Millon, T. (1981). *Disorders of personality: DSM-III: Axis II.* New York: Wiley.

Millon, T. (1996). *Disorders of personality: DSM-IV and beyond* (2nd ed.). New York: Wiley.

Millon, T. (2011). *Disorders of personality: Introducing a DSM/ICD spectrum from normal to abnormal.* (3rd. ed). Hoboken, NJ: Wiley.

Millon, T., Meagher, S. E., & Grossman, S. D. (2001). Theoretical perspectives. In W. J. Livesley (Ed.), *Handbook of personality disorders: Theory, research and treatment* (pp. 39–59). New York: Guilford.

Moro, C. (2007). A comprehensive literature review defining self-mutilation and occupational therapy intervention approaches: Dialectical Behavior Therapy and Sensory Integration. *Occupational Therapy in Mental Health, 23*(1), 55–67.

Neacsiu, A.D., Rizvi, S. L., & Linehan, M. M. (2010). Dialectical behavior therapy skills use as a mediator and outcome of treatment for borderline personality disorder. *Behaviour Research and Therapy, 48*(9), 832–839.

Paris, J. (1999). A multidimensional approach to personality disorders and their treatment. In J. Derksen, C. Maffei, & H. Groen (Eds.), *Treatment of personality disorders* (pp. 107–117). New York: Kluwer Academic/Plenum Publishing.

Paris, J. (2002). Implications of long term outcome research for the management of patients with borderline personality disorder. *Harvard Review of Psychiatry, 10*(6), 315–323.

Paris, J. (2005). Understanding self-mutilation in borderline personality disorder. *Harvard Review of Psychiatry, 13*(3), 179–185. doi: 10.1080/10673220591003614

Paris, J. (2008a). Clinical trials of treatment for personality disorders. *Psychiatric Clinics of North America, 31*(3), 517–526. Retrieved from http://www.sciencedirect.com

Paris, J. (2008b). *Treatment of personality disorders: A guide to evidence-based practice.* New York: Guilford Press.

Paris, J. (2010). Biopsychosocial models and psychiatric diagnosis. In T. Millon, R. Krueger, E. Simonsen (Eds.), *Contemporary directions in psychopathology: Scientific foundations of the DSM-V and ICD-11* (pp. 473–482). New York: Guilford. Retrieved from doi: 1-60623-532-X

Piper, W. E., & Joyce, A. S. (2001). Psychosocial treatment outcome. In W. J. Livesley (Ed.), *Handbook of personality disorders: Theory, research and treatment* (pp. 323–343). New York: Guilford.

Ratey, J. J. (Ed.). (1995). *Neuropsychiatry of personality disorders*. Cambridge, MA: Blackwell Science.

Ruegy, R., & Frances, A. (1995). New research in personality disorders. *Journal of Personality Disorders, 9*(1), 1–48.

Ruiz-Sancho, A. M., Smith, G. W., & Gunderson, J. (2001). Psychoeducational approaches. In W. J. Livesley (Ed.), *Handbook of personality disorders: Theory, research and treatment* (pp. 460–474). New York: Guilford.

Sadock, B., & Sadock, H. (2000). *Comprehensive Textbook of Psychiatry* (7th ed.). Baltimore: Lippincott, Williams & Wilkins.

Sadock, B., & Sadock, H. (2007). *Kaplan & Sadock's Synopsis of psychiatry: Behavioral Sciences/ Clinical Psychiatry* (10th ed.). Philadelphia: Lippincott, Williams & Wilkins.

Sadock, B., Sadock, H., & Ruiz, P. (2009). Kaplan & Sadock's *Comprehensive textbook of psychiatry, Volume II* (9th ed.). Philadelphia: Lippincott, Williams & Wilkins.

Swarbrick, M., & Ellis, J. (2009). Peer-operated self-help centers. *Occupational Therapy in Mental Health, 25,* 239–251.

Tyrer, P. (2000). Drug treatment of personality disorders. In P. Tyrer (Ed.), *Personality disorders: Diagnosis, management and course* (pp. 100–104). Boston: Butterworth-Heinemann.

Waldinger, R. J. (2010). Psychotherapy in the treatment of Borderline Personality Disorder. In S. Lazar (Ed.), *Psychotherapy is worth it: A comprehensive review of its cost-effectiveness* (pp. 61–86). Washington, DC: American Psychiatric Association.

Waltz, J., & Linehan, M. M. (1999). Functional analysis of borderline personality disorder behavioral criterion patterns. In J. Derksen, C. Maffei, & H. Groen (Eds.), *Treatment of personality disorders* (pp. 18–205). New York: Kluwer Academic/Plenum.

Widom, C., Czaja, S., & Paris, J. (2009). A prospective investigation of borderline personality disorder in abused and neglected children followed up into adulthood. *Journal of Personality Disorders, 23,* 5, 443–446. Retrieved from doi: 10.1521/pedi.2009.23.5.433

Winston, A., Rosenthal, R. N., & Muran, J. C. (2001). Supportive psychotherapy. In W. J. Livesley (Ed.), *Handbook of personality disorders: Theory, research and treatment* (pp. 344–358). New York: Guilford.

Zanarini, M., Stanley, B., Black, D., Markowitz, J., Goodman, M., Pikonis, P., et al. (2010). Methological considerations for treatment trials for persons with borderline personality disorder. *Annals of Clinical Psychiatry, 22*(2), 75–83. Retrieved from http://www.works.bepress.com/charles_sanislow/77

SUGGESTED RESOURCES

Effects of Childhood Abuse

Gil, E. (1983). *Outgrowing the pain.* San Francisco: Launch.

Herman, J. (1992). *Trauma and recovery.* New York: HarperCollins.

Miller, A. (1983). *For your own good.* Toronto: McGraw-Hill.

Williams, G., & Money, J. (1980). *Traumatic abuse and neglect of children at home* (abridged). Baltimore: Johns Hopkins University Press.

Borderline and Narcissistic Disorders

Cara, E. (1992). Neutralizing the narcissistic style: Narcissism, self-psychology and occupational therapy. *Occupational Therapy in Health Care, 8,* 2–3.

Gallop, R. (1985). The patient is splitting: Everyone knows and nothing changes. *Journal of Psychosocial Nursing, 23*(4), 6–10.

Hickey, B. (1985). The borderline experience: Subjective impressions. *Journal of Psychosocial Nursing, 23*(4), 24–26.

Kernberg, O. (1975). *Borderline conditions and pathological narcissism.* New York: Aronson.

Kohut, H. (1977). *The restoration of the self.* New York: International Universities Press.

Layton, M. (1995, May–June). Emerging from the shadows: Looking beyond the borderline diagnosis. *Networker*, (May–June), 35–41.

Miller, A. (1981). *The drama of the gifted child.* New York: Basic.

Miller, S. G. (1994). Borderline personality disorder from the patient's perspective. *Hospital and Community Psychiatry, 45*, 1215–1219.

Shapiro, D. (1965). *Neurotic styles.* New York: Basic.

Obsessive-Compulsive Personality Disorder

Rapoport, J. (1989). *The boy who couldn't stop washing.* New York: Penguin.

Treatment Strategies

Linehan, M. (1993a). *Cognitive behavioral treatment of borderline personality disorder.* New York: Guilford.

Linehan, M. (1993b). *Skills training manual for treating borderline personality disorder.* New York: Guilford.

Simon, S. (1993). *In search of values: 31 strategies for finding out what really matters most to you.* New York: Time Warner.

Tavris, C. (1982). *Anger: The misunderstood emotion.* New York: Simon & Schuster.

Literary Portraits

Allison, D. (1992). *Bastard out of Carolina.* New York: Dutton.

Middlebrook, D. (1991). *Anne Sexton: A biography.* New York: Houghton-Mifflin.

Smiley, J. (1992). *A thousand acres.* New York: Knopf.

Websites

Institutes of Health: http://www.ncbi.nlm.nih.gov/pubmedhealth/PMH0001935/

Mayo Clinic: http://www.mayoclinic.com/health/personality-disorders/DS00562

Mental Health America (formerly National Mental Health Association): http://www.nmha.org/go/information/get-info/personality-disorders

PART IV

Mental Health Across the Lifespan

Part IV includes four chapters about mental health through the lifespan focusing on typical phases: infant, child, adolescent, and older adults. New to this edition is a chapter on the mental health of infants and attachment through the lifespan. Since our last edition infant mental health programs have proliferated and become the basis for programs directed toward children, adolescents, and adults. At the same time the theory of attachment has taken hold and influenced both research and practice in psychotherapy and psychosocial approaches for all age groups. Occupational therapy practice has expanded in infant intervention and pediatrics and the American Occupational Therapy Association (AOTA) has made children and adolescents a special focus of practice. Therefore, attachment ideas can be useful for occupational therapists for all age groups, not only in mental health settings but where any psychosocial practice is important. Attachment problems can occur at any time in life.

The president's new freedom committee made explicit that health practitioners should focus on the mental health of children and adolescents. The AOTA took up this call and challenged occupational therapists to develop innovative treatment for children and adolescents. The children and adolescent chapters provide specific interventions for both individual and group and systems interventions that are contemporary and innovative. They also focus on conditions that are more prevalent for those age groups including family and societal violence, suicide, substance abuse, self-mutilation, and eating disorders to name a few.

The population is becoming older and practice in geriatric setting is increasing. At the same time changes in health care affect treatment for the older adult. As in the other chapters in this section, innovative and contemporary practice, individual, group, and systems, are presented. These chapters capture the problems and conditions that can occur throughout one's life but are more prevalent at certain times in one's life, although individuals can and do account for variety. Therefore individual differences should be taken into account throughout the lifespan.

Chapter 11

Mental Health of Infants: Attachment Through the Lifespan

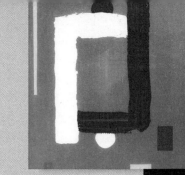

Elizabeth Cara, PhD, OTR/L, MFT
Elise Holloway, MPH, OTR/L

▪ KEY TERMS

affect regulation

attachment behaviors

attachment patterns

attachment styles

cortisol

diurnal system

ethology

evolutionary theory

HPA effect

internal working models

maternal sensitivity

non-didactic developmental
   guidance

PACE model

reactive attachment disorder

reproductive or inclusive fitness

secure base functions

Strange Situation

CHAPTER OUTLINE

Introduction
History of Attachment
What Is Attachment Exactly?
Phases of Attachment
Internal Working Models
Categories of Attachment: Evidence-Base of Attachment
      The Strange Situation
      Methods
The Patterns of Attachment
Cross-Cultural Studies
Attachment and Affect Regulation

Interpersonal Neurobiology
The HPA Effect
Attachment and Abuse and Neglect
	Foster Care and Institutionalization
	Neglect and Abuse
	Adoption
	Middle Childhood
	Children Who Are Developmentally Disabled
Clinical Programs That Focus on Attachment
	Child–Parent Psychotherapy (CPP)
	Video-Feedback Intervention to Promote Positive Parenting
	The Leiden Programs
	The UCLA Family Development Program and Minding the Baby (MTB)
	Attachment and Biobehavioral Catch-up
Occupational Therapy Treatment Guided by Programs that Promote Attachment
	Occupational Therapy Application
	Occupational Therapy Roles
	Occupational Therapy Intervention Strategies
Summary

INTRODUCTION

Last week I had the opportunity to interact with former students who graduated in our program at San Jose State in 1997. Benedict worked with emotionally disturbed teenagers in a special education program that I visited. It also included a program in early intervention. As we talked he mentioned how important the class I taught in Psychosocial Dysfunction had been to him in his work. He said he "didn't get it" in class when everything was abstract and "out there." But when he began working with teenagers, he thought, "I realized, it (psychosocial occupational therapy) is so important." It turned out that Benedict worked part time with Daneisha in a program that served a wide variety of ages. Daneisha worked with infants and their families. She joined us and as we talked Daneisha mentioned that "she sure could use some ideas about working with families, because, "it's not like you're really working with the infants, it's their parents!" Benedict and Daneisha illustrated why it is important to learn about attachment and how it infuses all of our work, no matter what setting you work in; it really is about working with infants, and their caregivers, as well as others. It is about working with the family system. Research in attachment theory has illustrated the influence of children's earliest experiences on their later development and has also shown that attachment disturbances are the root of many children's and adults' disorders.

Attachment theory is important when thinking about the family relationships with children of all ages. Research in attachment relationships has shown the connections of early attachments to one's self-regulation, sense of self, and sense of later relationships.

There has been an explosion of information about attachment theory and how it affects people throughout their lives (Cassidy & Shaver, 2008). Attachment theory has spawned much research that is now occurring in many clinical programs. The theory and its programs include many theoretical frameworks and disciplines; in fact, "it transcends theoretical frameworks" (Lieberman, 1988). Therefore, knowledge of attachment theory and research is important in clinical practice, not only in early intervention, but in middle childhood and adolescence, as well as adulthood. Indeed the research and popularity of attachment theory dictate that occupational therapists who work with all populations and in all settings have some knowledge in this exciting theory and practice. Occupational therapy purports to be a holistic field and to be client and family centered. Any client- and family-centered treatment should use the concepts of attachment to work with all members of the family. When occupational therapy practitioners work with infants and their families, they could use the attachment ideas in this chapter to work not just with infants and toddlers and not just with caregivers but with the infant–caregiver dyad that is part of the family system. Therefore, this chapter will focus primarily on infant mental health but will discuss attachment bonds throughout the lifespan.

HISTORY OF ATTACHMENT

John Bowlby was a psychoanalyst in England who in the mid twentieth century first proposed in a series of seminal papers and books (1973, 1988a, 1988b) how infants developed into social and interactional human beings. The first paper was "The Nature of a Child's Tie to His Mother" (1988b) and he elaborated in his books about attachment and loss. It was no accident that Bowlby became interested in how infants manage their emotional and psychological world and focused on the infant–caregiver dyad because he himself had been raised by a nanny who left the family's employment when he was seven. He was bereft after her loss and later realized that he possibly was more attached to his nanny than to his rather formal British parents (Bowlby, 2002).

He was influenced by contemporary psychological practice in England based on the theory of object relations, or how infants developed into self-contained emotionally and psychologically healthy young people and adults who felt self-worth, related to others, and adequately functioned in society. His beliefs about the reason for infants' ties to their mother was different than the predominant psychoanalytic beliefs at the time that infants bonded with their caregiver because they were associated with the pleasure that accompanies being fed and satiated (Cassidy, 2008). He believed that the relationship was biologically based on the proximity of the infant to the mother, which guaranteed protection and the continuation of the species.

He spoke of the attachment system, a behavioral concept from **ethology** (the study of primates in their environments and how they are influenced by their environment) and **evolutionary theory**, "species-specific system behaviours that leads to certain predictable outcomes, at least one of which contributes to reproductive fitness"

(Cassidy, 2008, p. 5). In the attachment system, proximity-seeking is activated when an infant receives information, either internally or externally generated, that a goal, the desired distance from the mother, is exceeded. The system remains activated until the goal is achieved. For example, an infant may sense that a caregiver is distracted and not tuned in when the infant needs to be soothed. Therefore, the infant may reach for the caregiver, or fidget or begin to cry. Then, the caregiver will hopefully read the infant's signals that she needs soothing, give her attention, and provide a response in tune with the infant's needs. Having received a satisfactory response, she will be soothed and the proximity-seeking behavior terminated. The attachment system will then be deactivated.

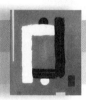

CASE ILLUSTRATION

Joey and His Mom: An Attachment System

Joey was 4 months old and had just woken up. He was wet and needed to be changed. His mother was in the room but not near him. He started to fidget but she did not respond. He began to cry and soon his mother was gazing at him, talking to him in a soothing manner, and lifting him to change him. His crying decreased and then stopped. As soon as he was changed he and his mother cooed and gazed at each other.

Discussion

Joey and his mother demonstrated attachment behavior in a system that is evolutionary and also can be found in nonhuman primates.

Bowlby was a psychoanalyst but he developed his theory of attachment based on psychoanalytic, evolutionary, and ethological ideas in an interdisciplinary manner influenced by professionals from these different fields, including people who used video to observe interactions (Cassidy & Shaver, 2008). He particularly was influenced by Rene Spitz's film, *Grief: A Peril in Infancy* (1947), James Robertson's film, *A Two-Year-Old Goes to Hospital*, Harry Harlow's films of the effects of maternal deprivation on monkeys, and films of Robert Hinde (cited in Bowlby, 1988b). This interdisciplinary perspective was important because research in ethology is naturalistic; that is, people are observed in their environments. Thus, Bowlby was aware of many rich observational studies that occurred during the 1930s and 1940s of the ill effects of prolonged institutionalization and mother-figure changes in early life on individual development (Bowlby, 1988b). (During World War II, the Germans frequently and massively bombed London. Therefore, in order to protect their children, many parents sent their infants and toddlers out of London to nurseries in the countryside where loving people, some professional nurses and therapists, cared for the infants and toddlers.

Psychoanalysts were documenting their observations of these infants and children.) These observations led to scientific research of present and real attachment (ethological research) interactions instead of reconstructing them from an adult perspective (psychoanalytic research) as had been the case previously.

Bowlby was appointed a special consultant to the World Health Organization in 1950 to contribute to a United Nations study of the needs of homeless children. He describes this opportunity as "golden" because he was able to read and discuss the literature with many other researchers (Bowlby, 1988b). He also employed a social worker, James Robertson, who had trained with Anna Freud at her nurseries and who used video to observe infants and children during separation. The result of his work was a report in a monograph titled *Maternal Care and Mental Health*. He found that the evidence "regarding the adverse influences on personality development of inadequate maternal care during early childhood and . . . the acute distress of children who find themselves separated from those they know and love [was] . . . far from negligible" (Bowlby, 1988a, p. 21).

An American psychologist, Mary Ainsworth, later collaborated with Bowlby, and it was she who developed a formal research method to research situations where infants and toddlers were separated from their caregivers, then reunited with them. This famous research study, called the **Strange Situation** (Salter Ainsworth & Bell, 1970), operationalized Bowlby's concepts about attachment and spawned many future studies of attachment in many different countries with many different age groups (Van IJzendoorn & Sagi-Schwartz, 2008). Indeed,

> [A]ttachment theory offers a set of testable hypotheses about the nature of development and . . . offers a means of systematically evaluating a variety of modes of clinical interventions . . . clearly [it] provides a new framework for observing preverbal and early representational processes and making valid inferences about the child's subjective experience on the basis of these observables. (Slade & Aber, 1992, p. 180)

Bowlby suggested that the earliest years of life are critical for later development and that infants are biologically predisposed to form relationships from which they can experience security and comfort. Very early instinctive interest in other human beings shows a baby's need for healthy relationships to feel secure. These healthy relationships influence how one will later develop good relationships and stable, regulated emotions, trust others, and value oneself. These healthy relationships, stable emotions, trust, and value of self will have an impact on how children develop cognitively and learn about the environment in which they live.

Attachment theory provides a reasonable explanation of how an attachment bond is formed, how attachment behaviors are developed and used in parenting or caregiving, and how a sense of self in relationships and interactional patterns are developed. Attachment theory provides the biological and evolutionary component of how an infant develops psychologically and becomes a healthy adult, positing attachment behaviors as evolutionarily adaptive for survival. Attachment theory and Ainsworth's later research studies of the theory delineate the types of attachments and attachment behaviors that are optimal for the infant–parent dyad, and that predict later functioning in the relationships and social world. More contemporary attachment theorists focus less on the dyad and more on multi-caregiver relationships, as well as how attachment bonds affect children, adolescents, and adults and their relationships and adaptive functioning.

WHAT IS ATTACHMENT EXACTLY?

Attachment theory states that the infant is predisposed at birth to form a selective attachment relationship with one or a few caretaking adults (Ainsworth, 1967, 1977; Ainsworth & Bell, 1970; Bowlby, 1973, 1988a, 1988b; Bretherton & Waters, 1985; Slade & Aber, 1992; Sroufe & Waters, 1977). Over the course of the phylogenic development, human and nonhuman primates evolved built-in behavioral systems that enabled attachment to occur. These systems, called **attachment behaviors**, are

> Any form of behavior that results in a person attaining or maintaining proximity to some other clearly identified individual who is conceived of as better able to cope with the world . . . that person is available and responsive and gives strong feelings of security, so encourages him to value and continue the relationship. (Bowlby, 1988b)

The attachment behaviors are those verbal gestures such as crying, cooing, laughing, and other language and those nonverbal gestures such as taking initiative, reaching, looking, smiling, approaching, and turn taking (Atkinson, Chisholm, Scott, Goldberg, Vaughn, et al., 2008). They are behaviors that indicate showing affection, seeking comfort, cooperating, asking for help, exploring, controlling, and reuniting with caregivers (Champagne, 2011). They "refer to an affective tie between infant and caregiver and to a behavioral system, flexibly operating in terms of set goals, mediated by feeling and in interaction with other behavioral systems" (Sroufe & Waters, 1977). Attachment behaviors are functionally equivalent, meaning that different behaviors can serve the same function, and one behavior can serve the same system. In other words, the type of attachment cannot be inferred from any particular behavior but must be considered according to patterns and context.

The biological goal of the attachment behavioral system is proximity to the caregiver. This establishes what Ainsworth later called the "feeling of security" or "felt security" or psychological goal. The system is a goal-corrected feedback system; when the infant is feeling secure and safe by virtue of proximity to the caregiver, the need to signal the mother, or the attachment behavioral system, is deactivated. The infant is then free to explore his or her environment. When the infant needs comfort, when there is a perception of the mother being distant or she really is distant, the attachment behavioral system is activated in the form of attachment behaviors, such as crying, crawling, and so on.

PHASES OF ATTACHMENT

There are developmental phases in attachment throughout the lifespan (Simpson & Belsky, 2008), but particularly in infancy and toddlerhood. See Table 11-1 for age-appropriate phases and behavior.

In the first phase, the infant does not show a preference for one attachment figure but is indiscriminate in attention seeking. In the second phase, the infant distinguishes caregivers and family members and prefers one attachment figure (usually mother or father). Proximity seeking behavior is directed to specific attachment figures.

In the third phase, the infant becomes more active in seeking physical proximity and social contact with the caregiver, and begins to develop internal working models or representations (beliefs, expectancies, and attitudes) of caregiver interactions. During this phase, the primary functions of the attachment system can be observed. Those functions are: proximity and maintenance of proximity, having a safe haven, and developing a secure base from which to explore. In this stage if infants are separated from the attachment figure then certain emotional responses will occur: first protest, then despair, and last detachment. In the fourth phase behaviors that signal a "goal-directed partnership" will be evident. Toddlers begin to see the world from the perspective of the caregiver; that is, they are able to recognize that the caregiver has his or her emotions, thoughts, and behaviors that are separate from infants. Toddlers can incorporate the "partners'" goals, plans, and desires into decision making. Therefore they can jointly negotiate plans and activities.

Emotions and cognitions are associated with attachment. Many emotions arise during the formation, maintenance, disruption, and renewal of attachment bonds. Positive emotions are associated with attachment and negative emotions are associated with loss of attachment; therefore, the infant may work to maintain attachments. Infants are biologically disposed to engage in this evolutionary behavior because it serves to keep infants protected, and also enables "**reproductive or inclusive fitness**" or assures that one's genes continue on in relatives (Simpson & Belsky, 2008).

The attachment system is also organized with cognitive components. The cognitive components are mental representations of the self, the attachment figure, and the

TABLE 11-1. Phases of Attachment

Chronological Age	Developmental Behavior
Birth to 2–3 months	Preference for attachment figure
2–3 months to 7 months	Discrimination for attachment figure
7 months to 3 years	More active physical proximity seeking Internal Working Models (IWMs); Functions of system appear; Stages of emotions in response to separation
3+ years	Goal-directed partnership; Aware of other's perspective; Joint activities and plans; Psychological proximity seeking

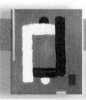

CASE ILLUSTRATION

A Mothers' Get-Together: Developmental and Attachment Behaviors in Attachment Systems

A mothers' group met each week at the local café. It was comprised of new mothers and those with toddlers. They met each week with their children but the primary purpose was to provide a social outlet to young mothers who did not work outside of the home. Jackie's daughter was 2 1/2 months, Alexandra's daughter was 2 months, Consuela's son was 6 months, Nguyen's son was 2 years, and her daughter was 3 1/2 years. Jackie and Alexandra's daughters occasionally gestured and made noises and they responded happily to any member who attended to them. Consuela's son would not stop reaching unless Consuela responded with a verbal or nonverbal affirmation. When Nguyen got up to get another latte, her son became distressed, looked for her, and began to cry, while Nguyen's daughter watched her and continued to play content with her toys.

Discussion

Each child demonstrated different attachment behavior according to stages of development.

environment and they are based on actual experiences of the infant (Cassidy, 2008). These exploratory and attachment behaviors act in a dynamic balance and the infant develops "internal working models" (IWMs) of self and others in relationship. These IWMs will then guide the developing individual throughout life.

INTERNAL WORKING MODELS

Internal working models (IWMs) are representations of past interactions and allow predicting future experience (Slade & Aber, 1992). An infant's sense of secure self and perception as self-as-worthy are derived from the attachment interaction with caregivers. If the infant comes to expect security and comfort through the caregiver's availability, the infant will internalize these expectations or, in other words, form internal mental representations of the availability of others and the worthiness of self. If the infant comes to expect that caregivers will be unavailable and/or rejecting, then IWMs or beliefs about the self, of other, and of relationships will be insecure and not worthy.

The infant relies on these IWMs to make decisions about which attachment behaviors to use in specific situations with specific persons. Thus, IWMs will influence later sense of self, interactions, and relationships, and, most importantly, one's ability to parent or develop satisfactory attachment behaviors and patterns with one's own infants. Bowlby also discussed other cognitive processes but IWMs are most prominent in his theory.

Internal working models have a "central role in adaptive human development to supportive interpersonal relationships" (Bretherton & Munholland, 2008). An important fact for occupational therapists, Bowlby was influenced by Piaget when he described IWMs as *sensorimotor*-affective representations that become increasingly complex and mentally flexible and enable simple short-term predictions and later reflection on current, past, and future relationships. He considered these representations as being developed through the senses (in early infancy) and the end result was "mental model building" (in toddlerhood, childhood, and adulthood). Bowlby stated the importance of the senses in the formation of IWMs.

> Every situation we meet with in life is construed in terms of the representational models we have of the world about us and of ourselves. Information reaching us through our sense organs is selected and interpreted in terms of those models.... On how we interpret and evaluate each situation ... turns also how we feel. (Bowlby, 1980, cited in Bretherton & Munholland, 2008, p. 103)

> Starting . . . towards the end of his first year and probably especially actively during his second and third when he acquires the powerful and extraordinary gift of language, a child is busy constructing working models of how the physical world may be expected to behave, how his mother and other significant persons may be expected to behave, how he himself may be expected to behave, and how each interacts with the other. (Bowlby, 1969/1982, cited in Bretherton & Munholland, 2008, p. 103)

In summary, IWMs are the mental representations originally developed in attachment relationships that become more cognitively complex as the infant develops. The mental models are of the interactions that an infant has with his or her caregiver and will dictate how the infant, child, or adult feels and behaves about him- or herself, others in the environment, and in romantic attachments. The IWMs will influence cognitive development and how the infants, children, and later adults will parent their own children. The IWMs are a person's psychological and social building blocks that enable secure, healthy development.

More recent studies have hypothesized that IWMs are not so internal or do not rest solely "inside the head of one person" and that IWMs are more reciprocal or depend more on the interpersonal interactions or dyad. Also, an infant may have different attachments to either parent. Thus, in this view of reciprocal relationships, IWMs may be more situational and depend more on the other person in interpersonal interactions (Cook, 2000).

CATEGORIES OF ATTACHMENT: EVIDENCE-BASE OF ATTACHMENT

John Bowlby and his colleagues provided the theory about attachment but it was his collaboration with a psychologist, Mary Ainsworth, that spawned research and identification of how infants and, later, children and adults actually are attached. The research is presented in detail here because it is the evidence for the existence of attachment styles and is known universally, as well as being a model for infant research. Therefore, occupational therapy practitioners working with infants and toddlers in any setting should be familiar and conversant with the research. Ainsworth devised a research system, called the Strange Situation (Salter Ainsworth, & Bell, 1970), that detailed the different attachment styles (individual differences) or patterns and behaviors that occur when there are consistent patterns of adequate, good-enough parenting or when there are patterns of inconsistent, inadequate, or insufficient parenting. These individual styles of attachment develop in infancy but continue as a person grows into adulthood. They are behaviors or strategies that will emerge in individuals' abilities to engage and maintain healthy relationships, to organize themselves into coherent selves, to regulate or express their emotions, to view themselves or others as worthy, to be trusting individuals, to be effective in relationships, and to explore, learn, and adapt in the world.

The Strange Situation

The aim of this experiment conducted "in the laboratory" was to assess separation and stranger anxiety, and the reaction of the infant when reunited with a caregiver (Salter Ainsworth & Bell, 1970). In the original experiment, all of the caregivers were the infants' mothers. The experimental assessment took place in a room with a one-way mirror so that observers could watch the behavior of 56 12- to 18-month-old infants with their parent or with a stranger. There were eight situations each of which was 3 minutes long. Table 11-2 lists the eight situations.

The situations were designed so that there was enough novelty so that the baby was able to explore but not strange enough that the baby would be fearful and always activate the attachment system. Also the room was set up so that there were three

TABLE 11-2. The Strange Situation

Sequential Step	Situation
1.	Mother, infant, observer enter room
2.	Mother and infant alone
3.	Stranger joins mother and infant
4.	Infant and stranger alone; mother leaves
5.	Stranger leaves; mother returns
6.	Infant alone; mother leaves
7.	Stranger returns
8.	Mother returns; stranger leaves

Adapted from http://www.simplypsychology.org/mary-ainsworth.html; information from Salter Ainsworth & Bell, 1970

chairs. At one end a baby's chair filled with toys, at another end the mother's chair and at the other end near the door the stranger's chair. Thus the baby was free to roam (and its locomotion and location marked) in a triangle of space demarcated by the three chairs (Salter Ainsworth & Bell, 1970).

The 3-minute episodes were designed so that: in # 2 the mother put the baby down, then sat in her chair unless her baby sought her attention; in # 3 the stranger entered and sat for 1 minute, then spoke for 1 minute with mother, then approached the baby showing him or her a toy; in # 4 if the baby happily engaged in play, then the stranger did not participate; if the baby was not active, the stranger attempted to engage her, whereas if the baby was distressed the stranger attempted comfort; or the situation was terminated if the baby was inconsolable. In situation # 5 the mother entered and stopped at the door so that her toddler could organize a response to her; the stranger left and when baby was happily playing then the mother left again but this time waved and said, "bye-bye." In episode #6 the baby was left alone to play but the situation was terminated if the baby was in distress. In episode # 7 the stranger entered with the same script as in episode #4, and in situation # 8, the mother returned, the stranger left, and reunion behavior took place (Salter Ainsworth & Bell, 1970).

Methods

Two observers independent of each other observed the situation and spoke about what they were observing. In the first subsample, another person took notes, and in the second subsample, the observer was recorded. Then the researchers took frequency counts of the occurrence of certain behaviors and coded for classes of behaviors using a 7-point scale. The classes of behaviors were those that we consider attachment behaviors and are listed in Table 11-3.

TABLE 11-3. Behaviors Observed in the Strange Situation

Categories of Behaviors	Examples of Behaviors
Proximity and contact seeking	Approaching, clambering up, reaching, leaning, directed cries.
Contact maintaining	Embracing, clinging, holding on, clutching, vocal protest.
Proximity and interaction avoiding	In a situation that ordinarily elicits greeting, ignoring, looking, turning, or moving away.
Contact and interaction resisting	Attempts to push away, angry screaming, throw self or toys, kicking, pouting, cranky, fussing, or petulance.
Searching	Following mother to door, opening or banging door, looking at or going to mother's chair.

Based on information from Salter Ainsworth and Bell (1970).

Results

From the results of the Strange Situation Procedure the researchers determined that there were three general **attachment styles** (1) secure, (2) ambivalent (contact-resistant) (also later named anxious-ambivalent or resistant), and (3) defensive (proximity-avoidant) (also later named anxious-avoidant or avoidant). Observations were as follows:

- In a secure attachment, infants used the caregiver as a secure base from which to explore, but cried more and explored less in an resistant pattern, and in an avoidant pattern were accepting of comfort from both the caregiver and the stranger equally.
- Separation anxiety: In a secure attachment, the infant was appropriately distressed when the caregiver left, was intensely distressed in a resistant attachment, and in an avoidant attachment was not at all distressed.
- Stranger anxiety: In a secure attachment when the caregiver was present the infant was friendly but when the caregiver was not present the infant avoided the stranger, whereas the infant feared and avoided the stranger in a resistant attachment, and in an avoidant attachment was okay with the stranger or displayed normal play behavior with the stranger.
- Reunion behavior: In a secure attachment the infant was happy and positive with the caregiver but resisted or pushed the caregiver away in a resistant attachment, and in an avoidant attachment was not interested in the caregiver.

The researchers concluded that there were three attachment styles and that the styles were determined by the caregivers' behavior (Salter Ainsworth & Bell, 1970).

Later, a student of Ainsworth, Mary Main and her colleagues, researched attachment patterns of adults. They created the Adult Attachment Interview and through this measurement were able to verify attachment patterns in adults. Therefore Bowlby's original hypothesis that early attachment is related to later behaviors was validated. Research continues that explores **attachment patterns**: of adults and which attachment patterns in adults predict attachment patterns in their children (Cassidy & Shaver, 2008).

THE PATTERNS OF ATTACHMENT

Bowlby's theory and Ainsworth's research initiated rich studies of attachment in infants, children, adolescents, and adults (Cassidy & Shaver, 2008). Generally, the secure and insecure patterns have been named somewhat differently than they originally were by Bowlby and Ainsworth and more have been delineated (see Table 11-4). Attachment concepts have permeated other fields and the significance of the attachment system and attachment behaviors is universally recognized.

TABLE 11-4. Patterns of Attachment

Patterns	Strategies
Secure	Reciprocal (proximity-seeking or attachment and exploration) interactions—Caregiver provides warm, attuned, responsive caring, and infants straightforward in eliciting protection and free to explore = positive expectations, trust, healthy selves, and relationships.
Insecure-Resistant Anxious/Ambivalent (Originally ambivalent)	Inconsistent interactions—Caregiver provides demanding, erratic caring and infants maximize behavior, resist soothing, comforting = negative expectations, distrust, depleted selves, and erratic relationships.
Insecure-Avoidant Anxious/Avoidant (Originally Defensive)	Unresponsive interactions—Caregiver provides unresponsive or over-stimulating caring, less contact and infants minimize behavior, avoid soothing and comforting = negative expectations, distrust, overly reliant selves, and empty relationships.
Disorganized	Unsafe interactions—Caregiver provides disorganized bizarre, off-cue caring and infants disorganized, fearful, coercive behavior = negative expectations, distrust, incoherent selves, and fear relationships.
Disinhibited	Indiscriminate interactions—caregiver provides no care and infants unable to selectively bond = negative expectations, incoherent, erratic selves, and socially indiscriminate relationships.
Inhibited	Failure to attach—caregiver provides no care and infants unable to bond, withdrawn = negative expectations, incoherent selves, no relationships.

Information from Berlin, Ziv, Amaya-Jackson, & Greenberg, 2005; Brandell & Ringel, 2007; Karen, 1994; Salter Ainsworth & Bell, 1970; Simpson & Belsky, 2008. Retrieved from http://www.simplypsychology.org/mary-ainsworth.html

CASE ILLUSTRATION

Father and Son—An Attachment System at Risk

Michael, an early interventionist, observed a father playing with his son. Michael noticed that the father was not quite comfortable with playing and did not understand reciprocal behavior or his son's gestures. Dad would alternately not engage in play even though his son reached for him or sometimes when his son reached for his toy, his father would grab it and show him how to play with it then press it into his hand and say, "now you do it." His son would throw the toy and turn his head and Dad would become exasperated.

Discussion

Michael was not yet attuned to his son's behavior and did not know how to play with his son. He presented conflicting behavior that was not responsive or overly responsive and his son reacted with avoidance. If this behavior developed into a pattern, his son would be at risk for an insecure-avoidant attachment.

CROSS-CULTURAL STUDIES

Mary Ainsworth (1967) first developed her classification system of attachment in Uganda in 1954–1955 where she observed mothers and their infants. Her later study in the United States (1977) was initiated to replicate this earlier one. Her first study in Africa established some important principles of attachment and raised some important cross-cultural issues. Those issues were and are: (1) the universality of the infant–mother attachment and classification system, (2) the crucial role of maternal sensitivity as an antecedent to attachment, (3) the contextual dimension of attachment, for example, in Uganda having multiple caregivers did not interfere with a secure attachment and the quality and consistency and not the number of caregivers was the crucial feature in attachment bonds. Thus, attachment theory posits that in all Western countries infants become attached to one or more specific caregiver (the universality hypothesis), the majority of infants are securely attached in Western cultures (the normativity hypothesis), secure attachment depends on the caregivers' sensitive and consistent responses (the sensitivity hypothesis), and attachment security yields differences in children's abilities to regulate their emotions, develop healthy relationships with peers, teachers, and later romantic partners, and develop cognitive competence (the competence hypothesis) (Van IJzendoorn & Sagi-Schwartz, 2008).

There have been cross-cultural studies in non-Western countries since Ainsworth's first research in Uganda (Van IJzendoorn & Sagi-Schwartz, 2008).

In Africa, research on attachment has been conducted in Uganda, Kenya, Nigeria, Mali, Botswana, Zambia, and South Africa, in both urban and hunter-gatherer societies. These studies have confirmed the maternal sensitivity and universality hypotheses, as well as the hypothesis that sensitive caregiver responses lead to independence rather than dependence. In China, where interdependence is considered a major social difference from Western societies and a social policy of only one child per family exists, research is scarcer, however, researchers have studied Chinese mothers' attitudes about attachment. These studies also confirmed the universality hypothesis, that is, although the cultural norms regarding families and children are different than those of a Western society, they subscribe to a similar definition of the attachment system and they describe an ideal child as one who is securely attached.

Although there have been few studies of attachment in Japan, the studies present different results. Japan itself can be considered a challenge to attachment research due to alternative ideas of relatedness. Specifically, in Japan there is a concept called "*amae*," which describes the attachment bond as inherently psychologically dependent unlike the claims of attachment in Western society (Van IJzendoorn & Sagi-Schwartz, 2008; Young-Bruehl & Bethelard, 2002). Therefore, it is difficult to evaluate attachment in Japan. However, this different cultural idea that is prevalent in a non-Western society provides a unique opportunity to further expand on the attachment concept.

In the two studies in Japan (Van IJzendoorn & Sagi-Schwartz, 2008), one using the same measurement as the one in China, the Attachment Q-Sort (Vaughn & Waters, 1990), found that Japanese mothers' definitions of an ideal child confirmed attachment theories ideas of a secure relationship but not *amae* and dependence. The other found that the sensitivity hypothesis was not supported.

Various studies in non-Western cultures (Van IJzendoorn & Sagi-Schwartz, 2008) have also researched the numbers of children that fall into the different attachment classifications, and some have researched maternal sensitivity, and the relationship of caregivers' attachment categories with their children's attachments. Overall, "the evidence for the cross-cultural validity of attachment theory is impressive" and "the universality hypothesis appears to be supported most strongly" (Van IJzendoorn & Sagi-Schwartz). The cross cultural studies . . . support Bowlby's . . . idea that attachment is indeed a universal phenomenon, and an evolutionary explanation seems to be warranted" (p. 897). However, the sensitivity and competence hypotheses are less supported with the most important disconfirming evidence being the Japanese studies. The three attachment categories are universal and found in every culture studied; however, the strategies are contextually different and naturally adaptive. There appears to be pressure toward general selection of a secure attachment in all cultures studied. An interesting finding that has emerged from the studies of attachment in other cultures is that there should be less of a focus on researching the dyadic attachment of one caregiver, usually mother, and one child. Other cultures have confirmed that there are multi-caregiving societies so attention in the future should be paid to social networks of caregiving (Van IJzendoorn & Sagi-Schwartz, 2008).

ATTACHMENT AND AFFECT REGULATION

An explanation of attachment that relates directly to occupational therapists is the fact that attachment allows the ability for infants and children to develop self-regulation and coping skills. An understanding of attachment and how it relates to **affect regulation** will position the occupational therapy practitioner to attend to attachment behavior in settings where infants and toddlers are treated. The quality of attachment is important for a child's sense of self and relatedness but is also important for infants and children to develop organizing and self-regulating patterns of behavior (Cassidy & Shaver, 2008). Infants develop the ability to organize emotions and to regulate their emotions within the caregiver–infant dyad.

> A securely attached child is able to use the caregiver as a safe haven when in distress (i.e., return of positive mood), and the child is then able to return to exploration of the environment. Furthermore, it is hypothesized that securely attached children internalize effective ways to cope with stress and are consequently resilient when coping with problems even in the absence of the caregiver. (Kerns, 2008, p. 375)

Although, it is hypothesized that there is a strong correlation between a quality of attachment and regulation, there are few studies of emotional regulation in childhood. The field of neurobiology, though, holds promise for explaining how emotional regulation develops.

Interpersonal Neurobiology

From birth, the developing relationship between infants and their parents help them to regulate arousal, excitement, or discomfort. It has been suggested that attachment theory is really a regulatory theory, one that reflects the plastic, experience-dependent nature of the brain (Papousek, 2011; Schore, 2000, 2010). Recent advances in the neurosciences and neuroimaging are beginning to reveal how parent–child relationships carried out during life's daily activities and based in the earliest attachment processes, are influencing brain structure and physiology. These structural and functional changes in the brain influence self-regulation and interpersonal relationships throughout life (Cozolino, 2006; Schore, 2000, 2010; Siegel, 1999). This emerging interdisciplinary field of study gives us some theory of how brain structure and function, as well as the mind, are shaped by relationship experiences. It helps us link earliest infant experiences with the lifelong ability to regulate one's emotion and to establish satisfying relationships (Cozolino, 2006; Lillas & Turnbull, 2009). The growing research in this field provides occupational therapy with a strong rationale for addressing attachment relationships, within the context of occupational therapy treatment.

The studies of affect regulation in adult attachment also attempt to explain how secure attachments help people survive bouts of distress, doubt, pain and discomfort and reestablish optimism and emotional equanimity (Mikulincer & Shaver, 2008). They also predict that attachment insecurity interferes with emotional regulation, and mental health, and that securely attached adults feel secure and confident in seeking support. Thus, attachment reinforces a person's repertoire of coping skills and capacity. Therefore, the development of coping skills and self-regulating systems is dependent on the quality of the early attachment and could be a goal of occupational therapists following the Occupational Therapy Practice Framework (AOTA, 2008) in working with infants, families, and children.

The HPA Effect

In the **HPA effect**, early stress and developmental trauma in the form of attachment disruptions caused by toxic parenting or separation influences the hypothalamic-pituitary-adrenal (HPA) system, which is responsible for regulating an individual's stress response. Essentially, the HPA regulates the production of **cortisol**, a hormone responsible for regulating stress. When trauma occurs early in one's development, the HPA is effected and it is as if the stress does not disappear. Thus, the HPA continues to manufacture cortisol even when it is not needed. This overreactive and continual response then contributes to a state of hyperarousal, in itself a state that is dysregulated. Thus neglect and trauma cause the person who is neglected or traumatized by consistent parental misattunement or separation to be in a constant state of hyperarousal and inability to regulate emotions (Corbin, 2007; Creeden, 2009).

The HPA system also is responsible for maintaining the **diurnal system** that regulates sleep and waking. For example, humans have a high level of cortisol in the morning so that they wake up and a low level at night allowing them to sleep. This diurnal system is already in place when the infant is just 6 weeks of age. Children who experience trauma and abuse at early ages have abnormal diurnal systems. Thus, sleep and rest are disturbed.

Early stress and trauma also interfere with the amygdala, the brain structure responsible for symbolic memory, both implicit (unconscious) and explicit (available to consciousness). Neglect, stress, and maltreatment influence the receptor sites in the amygdala so that inhibitory neurotransmitters are unable to modify or inhibit excited neurons. Therefore the amygdala loses its ability to calm itself. Furthermore, because the implicit memory sets rules prior to symbolic memory, it is difficult to access these memories or unconscious rules later when one is an adult. The result of this inaccessibility is the inability to modify one's implicit rules and ways of behaving. Some research indicates that a consistent, stable, attuned, and reliable caregiver or professional can assist children with early trauma and attachment disorders to become more reflective and change their patterns of implicit memories and perhaps learn to regulate emotions. Other research is less hopeful (Corbin, 2007; Creeden, 2009).

ATTACHMENT AND ABUSE AND NEGLECT

Attachment theorists suggest that abuse and particularly neglect lead to problems in attachment and later pathology. In particular, problems in attachment lead to **reactive attachment disorder** (RAD), defined in the *DSM-IV-TR* (APA, 2000). In this disorder, one may be inhibited, or withdrawn and unable to form attachments with any one person, or disinhibited, or forming attachments with any person indiscriminately regardless of attachment history (Corbin, 2007). Although it has been suggested that the types, inhibited or disinhibited, may be more fluid and perhaps this behavior is adaptive in institutions (Hardy, 2007). (For a substantial discussion of reactive attachment disorder, see also Chapter 12, "Mental Health of Children.")

Foster Care and Institutionalization

Institutionalized children face many obstacles to healthy attachment. In the United States there are over 500,000 children in foster care, and usually they are separated from caregivers due to neglect or abuse during the period when developing attachment bonds usually is most important, that is, from age zero to three years (Dozier & Rutter, 2008). Many also stay in foster care for longer than two years and over half of those return to foster care within three years. Typically, experiences prior to foster care are depriving, neglectful, or abusive. Outside of the United States many infants and toddlers have lengthy stays in orphanages and also face neglect and abuse and miss opportunities to develop attachment bonds.

Neglect and Abuse

Neglect is the failure to provide for basic safety and welfare, such as being home alone, inadequate food or shelter, and parents' inability to protect toddlers from dangerous conditions. Abuse takes the form of active physical, emotional, or sexual behavior perpetrated by adults on infants and toddlers. Those who are neglected are at risk for behavioral problems in school, difficult relationships with peers, increased anxiety, eating disorders or substance abuse, post-traumatic stress disorder, suicide and criminal activities, and, the earlier the experience, the more serious are the consequences (Dozier & Rutter, 2008).

An interesting paradox occurs if the toddler is abused by a parent: The toddler may form a selected attachment and feel connected to the parent yet typically is frightened of the very person who he looks to for survival. Therefore, resulting behavior with caregivers is odd with difficulty trusting, lack of empathy for peers who are distressed, negative attributional biases, and dissociative symptoms (Dozier & Rutter, 2008).

Adoption

Occupational therapy practitioners treat adopted infants and children and their families and therefore knowledge of the challenges that adopted children and families face may enable better practice. Some children are adopted either from the foster care system (domestic adoption) or from foreign institutions (international adoption). Those who are adopted within one year of age may be quicker to develop attachment bonds with adoptive parents than those adopted after one year of age. Although children may be adopted and provided with loving caregivers, there are still difficulties that could occur depending on the vulnerabilities of the child and the state of mind of the caregivers who adopt. Those adopted from institutions have higher rates of disorganized attachments and indiscriminate attachment behaviors and, whether from foster care or an institution, children with insecure attachment often elicit rejecting behaviors from new caregivers.

Although statistics about children from foster care and institutions can be discouraging, there is some good news, and that is that a large number of adopted children do not display the same patterns of insecure or disorganized attachment. Those who do not develop maladaptive attachments may be more resilient temperamentally, less vulnerable (for example, they were not born of a substance abusing parent), and may have been institutionalized less than six months. The children may have been placed with caregivers who have secure attachments and are also able to understand the multiple problems with attachment that their children bring, and the foster parents display a strong commitment to their adopted children (Dozier & Rutter, 2008).

As will be described later in this chapter and in Chapter 12, "Mental Health of Children," interventions may be crafted to support parents to understand and respond to their childrens' attachment signals and to assist in regulating emotions and rest and sleep. As well, interventions can aid children with RAD and attachment problems to understand appropriate behavior and to become more sensitive to others as well as to understand their own arousal needs and ways of dealing with them.

Middle Childhood

Although much has been written about attachment of parents and infants in early relationships, and research predicts later relationships and social functioning depending on quality of attachment, there has been much less information about attachment in middle childhood (Kerns & Richardson, 2005). But at this crucial period attachment security begins to be a characteristic of a person rather than of a relationship

There are other advances that are crucial in this developmental period: children become sophisticated in their thinking and how they view themselves and others (Kerns & Richardson, 2005). They now can monitor their own thinking and psychological processes such as emotions and motives, and they have more ability for self-regulation. As they become more able to think about themselves and others they also become more aware and able to perceive a self-concept and develop "global self-worth" (Harter, 1999, cited in Zionts, 2005).

Children's social worlds expand and relationships become more intense and complex. They also spend much more time in social contexts, such as sports or school, outside of the family. They become much better at perceiving the viewpoints of others and social cues and norms. They become more understanding that others including parents are different than they are and have different and unique emotions, thoughts, and motivations (Kerns, 2008; Kerns & Richardson, 2005; Mayseless, 2005).

In infancy, the attachment system promotes the development of attachment bonds in a caregiver–infant relationship. However, the attachment system in middle childhood is seen as a "safety regulating system" and the end-product is to promote not only physical but also psychological safety in close relationships. The system is activated when there is a threat, danger, or stress (either internally felt or external) to the accessibility or availability (Kerns & Richardson, 2005) of the attachment figure. The goal of attachment is felt security (affect regulation) in the context of protection in a relationship, thus the goal of the attachment system is psychological availability (Kerns & Richardson, 2005; Verschueren & Marcoen, 2005). In addition these "safe haven" and "**secure base functions**" may occur in relationships where people are not attachment figures, such as a teacher at school, or a friend in a social relationship (Mayseless, 2005). There is now a clear preference away from parents and for peers to play with.

In middle childhood the attachment behavioral system becomes more sophisticated and governed by cognitive-affective internalizations. School age children recognize that the caregiver has a point of view and can better understand their own point of view, as well as differentiate it from that of the caregiver. Children can also regulate their own emotions, relying less on the caregiver, and communicate those emotions. Therefore, there is a shift to co-regulation (AOTA, 2008; Kerns, 2008).

Children become more sophisticated also in plans that they can think about and employ and they can better articulate those plans (Kerns, 2008). Behavior also becomes more organized in terms of goals and ways to achieve the goals. Children can implement their planned goals with different people in different contexts and circumstances. Attachment behaviors also expand; strategies could include reasoning, physical distancing, not communicating, and withdrawing in addition to crying and clinging, and so on.

Studies predict the stability of attachment over time; however one study in Belgium (Verschueren & Marcoen, 2005) found that although the attachment with fathers remained the same, it increased somewhat with mothers for children from age 8 to age 11. The study explained this result by noting that children are more willing to confide in peers when younger and not so later, when they become very concerned with how peers view them. Also, children in middle childhood generally preferred their mothers over their fathers. Overall the conclusions of the study did validate the development of more differentiated perceptions of the quality of attachment with mother and father in the middle years.

In another study by the same authors cited above (Verschueren & Marcoen, 2005), higher felt security with the father was related to better social acceptance in school, adding to conclusions of a separate study (Schneider et al., cited in Verschueren & Marcoen, 2005) that felt security with the mother is predictive of children's functioning in dyadic or small group (i.e., friendship, relationships rather than social acceptance).

In middle childhood, children could bond with other figures in addition to the caregivers (Kerns & Richardson, 2005). This differentiation and diversification include different people and conditions and groups. Research (Zionts, 2005) indicates that teachers play an important role and that a high-quality teacher-student relationship may ameliorate a lower quality child–parent attachment. That is, the children who are most at risk of developing behavioral problems in school can benefit most from a close relationship with another student. These children may also be better able to adjust and succeed in school when they can form a close relationship with a teacher.

Also, responsibility for maintaining proximity, so important in the early relationships on the parents' parts, shifts to the child and the behaviors are less urgent and displayed less frequently (Kerns, 2008). Essentially, in this period there is less investment in the original attachment caregiver and a withdrawal of investment as the child prepares to refocus his or her attachment. The child begins to shift attachment investment into affectional bonds to peers and friends and, later, romantic partners (Kerns & Richardson, 2005; Mayseless, 2005).

If all goes well, children will be able to have reciprocal social interactions, develop empathy in these interactions, and display social skills. They will be able to have friendships, play and explore competently, have a sense of well-being, and show appropriate behavior in their social contexts, in addition to appropriate and adequate, if not good, school performance (Booth-LaForce, Rubin, Rose-Krasnor, Burgess, 2005). (See Chapters 10, 12, and 13 for more information about attachment disorders in children, adolescents, and adults.)

Children Who Are Developmentally Disabled

Occupational therapists often work with children on the autistic spectrum as well as others with developmental disabilities. Therefore, it is important to understand how attachment bonds are manifested in the caregiver–infant relationship for those infants or children with developmental disabilities. Research (Atkinson et al., 1999) with mixed results has been conducted of attachment in relationships with an infant or child who has a disability.

Children with autism, both preschool age and older, can develop attachments, despite social interaction deficits, however there are more insecure attachments than in those with typical development or those with other developmental disorders (Naber et al., 2007; Rutgers, Bakermans-Kranenburg, van IZjenddorn, & van Berckelaer-Onnes, 2004, 2007) . There is also a higher percentage of disorganized attachment (Naber et al.). Although these studies indicated that there is a higher percentage of insecure attachments, the parents did not report more stress than is usually associated with parenting a child with autism disorders (Rutgers et al., 2007). However, the studies were of children under the age of 3 years and it is thought that perhaps there may be more difficulties as they grow older.

Atkinson et al. (1999) studied the attachment bonds of infants and toddlers of children with Down syndrome and their caregivers. They found that overall both the child and the caregiver contributed to the relationship. Furthermore, attachment was related to the interaction of **maternal sensitivity** (response to the children's signals) and cognitive competence. The authors measured maternal sensitivity, infant and toddlers' cognitive and adaptive functioning, and attachment security in 53 infants and toddlers (31 boys and 22 girls) with Down Syndrome over a two-year period. They measured attachment with in-home observation and cognitive functioning with the Bayley Developmental Scale. They found that interaction between maternal responses to their children's signals and the children's cognitive functioning predicted attachment security. They concluded that attachment security is related to the combination of the interaction, just not children's or caregivers' individual behaviors with each other, but rather both the caregiver ability to respond and the level of cognitive functioning of their child.

Other researchers (Barnett, Butler, & Vondra, 1999) found that childhood factors such as developmental disabilities and cognitive delays (though not necessarily physical disabilities) do influence the formation of attachment patterns. Barnett et al. found that attachment patterns are shaped by a variety of other factors rather than the fact of a developmental disability or maternal sensitivity. Those factors are biological, emotional, cognitive, behavioral, and representational. Also, environment plays a crucial role in the outcome of the attachment relationship as does the social support perceived by parents (Rutgers et al., 2007).

While more research is needed to clarify if children with autism and their parents will have more difficult attachment reciprocal interactions as the children grow chronologically older, the results of these studies do indicate differences in attachment security for those with autism. Therefore, occupational therapy practitioners who work in the pediatric field can be particularly sensitive to family-centered interventions that support caregivers and interventions that promote maternal sensitivity and reciprocal social interactions (Cronin, 2004). Promotion of attachment behaviors can take place during occupational therapy interventions with families or can be suggested strategies conducted during daily life activities at home.

CLINICAL PROGRAMS THAT FOCUS ON ATTACHMENT

Research in attachment theory has illustrated the influence of children's' earliest experiences, particularly, their early relationships, on their later development and has also shown that attachment disturbances are the root of many children's and adults disorders. This research has spurred development of prevention programs in the community, in mental and public health clinics, and in prisons. It has also influenced policy (Berlin, Zeanah, & Lieberman, 2008). Occupational therapists can learn intervention strategies from the principles of these programs.

Prevention and intervention programs have been developed in the last two decades; however, they have been somewhat disparate in reaching an agreement on what works best for whom, whether long-term or short-term programs work best, which aspects of the attachment system to focus on, and what are the outcome goals (Berlin et al., 2008). Nevertheless, it has become clearer that when the outcome is attachment security, there has been moderate success, and when the outcome is improving maternal sensitivity or attachment quality, there has been much success. Also, it has become clear that for some families, a longer and intensive program is more efficacious, but for other families, a shorter, broader, and less-intense program is effective.

All of the programs' treatment strategies include one or more of three therapeutic tasks: (1) targeting the parents' IWMs, (2) targeting the parenting behavior, and (3) developing or modeling a treating professional–parent relationship (Berlin et al., 2008). In the first task, the intervener helps the caregiver gain insight into his or her own internal models of self and other with the goal of helping the parent recognize how the past strategies interfere with current interactions with his or her child. In the second task, the intervener helps the caregivers develop a capacity for reflection, particularly as it refers to interactions with their children. Thus, the parent can interpret the child's behavior differently and respond appropriately in the attachment system. Parents learn that there are two primary parenting tasks: to provide closeness as a response to the child's attachment needs and autonomy as a response to the child's exploration needs. In the third strategy, the parent learns that there could be a caring and mutual supportive relationship and therefore new attachments can develop and parents can then develop a different attachment relationship with their children. Research has supported various intense programs that last longer than one year or are of 10- to 20-week duration, and also a brief, three- to four-session program. Most of the programs utilize the three therapeutic tasks described above (Berlin et al., 2008). The programs target either the child–parent dyad or the caregiver parenting skills. Some programs are briefly explained below.

Child–Parent Psychotherapy

In child–parent psychotherapy (CPP), the patient is the infant–parent dyad and the clients are most often impoverished and traumatized families. Based on infant–parent psychotherapy developed by Selma Fraiberg (1980, 1982), it is a manualized intervention and incorporates the goals of improving caregivers' capacity for insight and reflection, and an empathic relationship, and adds a focus on the caregivers' current stressful lives and cultural values (Berlin et al., 2008). Often the therapists are masters and PhD level students who are trained rigorously in the interventions. The programs usually include weekly interventions that take place in the home or program playroom. Some are long term, over a year or more, and begin when the caregiver is pregnant. Others are briefer but just as intense and focus on didactic sessions regarding the caregivers' parenting skills and understanding of attachment and attachment behaviors, their own and their children's.

Video-Feedback Intervention to Promote Positive Parenting

A short-term program targeted to parents is the Video-feedback Intervention to Promote Positive Parenting (VIPP) (Juffer et al. cited in Rutgers et al., 2007). Such a program is an example that uses video of in-home interactions between caregiver(s) and children. Essentially, such programs provide here and now, graphic feedback reviewed with interveners that enables parents to see how their behaviors influence their toddlers and are able to modify them accordingly to promote positive attachment behaviors and reciprocal interaction. While occupational therapists will not necessarily use video-feedback of their sessions, they can access some strategies to use with caregivers to promote attachment behaviors.

The Leiden Programs

In this program, therapists visited mothers and their infants for three brief sessions lasting about two hours each. The therapists focused on mothers' sensitivity to their infants' cues and signals. In follow-up studies the mothers continued to be responsive and to be stimulating to their infants and their infants grew to be toddlers who were securely attached (Berlin et al., 2008). Such a program indicates that occupational therapists who make brief home visits can be instrumental in promoting maternal sensitivity in their sessions.

The UCLA Family Development Program and Minding the Baby (MTB)

In these programs interveners made home visits weekly during the second trimester of pregnancy through the infant's first year and then every-other-week visits in the toddler's second year. The UCLA program focuses on the mother's relationships with her family, her infant, her partner, and the intervener. The Minding the Baby (MTB) program focuses on the mother's IWMs and parenting behavior and emphasizes the mother's ability to reflect on her own behavior. Both have demonstrated successful outcomes of secure attachments and maternal sensitivity (Berlin et al., 2008).

Attachment and Biobehavioral Catch-up

This program is for foster care parents and their foster infants. Therapists make 10 visits weekly that last an hour. There are various themes in the session that address foster infants' defensive behavior, being aware of the foster parents' own histories that may predispose them to negative responses, and parenting responses. The program demonstrates successful outcomes based on the percentage of securely attached foster infants (Berlin et al., 2008).

The Circle of Security

This program consists of 20 weekly group sessions for groups of parents and focuses on "relationship capacities." These are observation skills and ability to make inferences, reflective functioning, understand the child's needs, empathy, and emotional regulation. This can be considered a psychoeducational group that also includes video of the parent–child interactions for each participant. The program demonstrates successful outcomes based on decreases in disorganized and insecure attachments (Berlin et al., 2008).

OCCUPATIONAL THERAPY TREATMENT GUIDED BY PROGRAMS THAT PROMOTE ATTACHMENT

Some useful treatment ideas that emerge in these programs and the infant–parent psychotherapy on which they are based can be incorporated by occupational therapists. In the evaluation process the infant–parent therapist uses observation skills and introspection (Lieberman & Pawl, 1993). The therapist observes how the infant functions developmentally and emotionally and how the parent experiences or responds to the infant while observing their interaction. Families who are observed usually have a negative idea of the outside bureaucracy that purports to work with them, so the therapist also reflects on the possibility of forming a therapeutic relationship (Kyler, 2008; Schultz-Krohn & Cara, 2000). Thus occupational therapists can use their own reflective and introspective skills and feelings to get an idea of how their clients might respond to their child as well as an idea of the cultural family-centered treatment that may be necessary.

Two principles of infant–parent psychotherapy can be incorporated into occupational therapy services and interactions (Lieberman & Pawl, 1993; Seligman, 1994). **Non-didactic developmental guidance** is a method that assumes caregivers are those best to use information about their child considering the relationship and emotions between the caregiver and parent. The therapist encourages the parent to view the infant's behavior in a way that interrupts viewing the infant from the parent's own negative experiences. The therapist in essence creates a "space" in which the parent can view the infant in an alternative way. This intervention is accomplished not by giving advice but by questioning or asking the caregiver's observation or experience of what is happening right then. This intervention aims to support a change in behavior as well as the caregiver's perspectives. For example, a toddler may fuss and cry and push away from a parent but the parent refuses to let the toddler go or to acknowledge the toddler because she doesn't want to "spoil the child." A therapist might question the parent by asking, what do you think will happen if you do acknowledge your child's needs? Alternatively, the therapist might remark on the active exploration and curiosity of the child. In this way, the therapist does not negate the parent's perspective and may provide a different way of thinking about the child and interaction.

Support and advocacy are activities that support the infant–caregiver relationship (Lieberman & Pawl, 1993). This support provides a role model of a caring relationship that can be emulated by the parent with the infant. These are often concrete interventions that provide relief but also hope for often bedraggled caregivers. For example, a parent may not have enough money to buy diapers so the therapist may find public health programs that are able to donate diapers. Or in a real incident, a parent was becoming agitated because she did not have a dresser. The author serendipitously found a dresser left on the street that was free for anyone to take and picked up the dresser, drove it to the client's home, and then helped the client move the dresser into her home. Although occupational therapists do not provide such concrete interventions for parents, they could provide advocacy and support in getting attention from various health care systems for an infant or toddler with a disability as well as provide an understanding of the caregivers' or family's distress.

Infant mental health strategies could be adapted for use by occupational therapists and occupational therapists could consider themselves transdisciplinary therapists. The goal of occupational therapy, like the goal of infant mental health, is to assist clients to achieve satisfactory functioning in their environment. The client in infant mental health is the caregiver and the child or their relationship. Likewise, an occupational therapist recognizes the co-occupations of caregiver and child (AOTA, 2008) and the Occupational Therapy Practice Framework addresses the interacting cultural worlds of the practitioner and family. The occupational therapist learns and uses what he or she learns about the habits, routines, and rituals of the caregiver and child (Kellegrew, 2000; Larson, 2000).

The infant mental health therapist offers support and does whatever needs to occur to bolster the infant–parent relationship. Likewise, occupational therapy's domain (AOTA, 2008) specifies advocacy as an outcome and suggests that occupational justice could be a goal of treatment. Whereas the infant mental health therapist offers non-didactic guidance, occupational therapists offer questions that result from the clinical reasoning process. Likewise, the occupational therapist uses clinical reasoning and self-reflection and introspection when working with clients (Taylor, 2008) instead of the psychoanalytic interventions that direct the infant–parent therapist. Occupational therapists also recognize their use of therapeutic self in the relationship and model the caregiver role with both caregiver and the caregiver–toddler dyad. (Schultz-Krohn & Cara, 2000).

Perhaps the concept that comes closest to working with families in infant mental health is the idea of relationship-centered care (Kyler, 2008). In relationship-centered care, the client and therapist identify strengths but also include resources of the caregiver, the community, and the environment. They understand the influence of social, economic, political, cultural, and environmental contexts. In the work in promoting attachment, the practitioner identifies the strengths of the caregiver–infant dyad and the external forces impinging on the dyad.

The infant mental health therapist pays attention to the ability of an infant to regulate their emotions and to organize their emotional responses and enlists caregivers to soothe and calm infants. The infant mental health therapist uses the various strategies mentioned above to help parents become aware of their role as regulatory agents, if you will, of their child's emotions and developing emotional coping system. Likewise, occupational therapists are mandated as part of their practice domain to work with affect regulation (client factor and coping skill) and affect regulation skill (performance skills). Thus, an occupational therapist would work in a family-centered way with parents and child, using strategies of education, therapeutic use of occupations, and self to assist parents to recognize how their infants process sensory information, and to respond in an attuned way to their sensory needs. In so doing, the occupational therapist promotes healthy affect regulation and healthy attachments.

Occupational Therapy Application

Infants and their families will not be referred to occupational therapy to promote attachment as they are in the infant–parent and other programs mentioned above. However, infants and their families will be referred to occupational therapy for eating, physical, developmental, and other problems. Within their domain of practice occupational therapy practitioners can observe and promote the attachment process while conducting occupational therapy interventions. *This then is the importance of knowing about attachment theory: it is likely that some of the clients that are referred to occupational therapy may have problems with attachment and occupational therapists can promote attachment bonds in the natural course of their treatment.* For example, some programs have been developed by or are used by occupational therapists that are sensory-integration-based, sensory modulation interventions (Champagne, 2011). Similar to therapeutic use of self, the **PACE model** developed by Daniel Hughes (2006) advocates an evidence-based approach (Becker-Weidman, 2008) that is playful, accepting, curious, and empathic. The traits advocated for caregivers or others working with foster children, in particular, can be translated into occupational therapy sensory modulation perspectives for the caregiver, such as adjusting breathing patterns to match the infant, using body positioning and language that assure attunement with each other, matching voice pace and rhythm, and using playful, exploratory, empathic, and accepting attitudes.

The following case illustrations are examples of referrals to occupational therapy in which the practitioner was able to observe and provide interventions that promoted attachment. Also, examples illustrate how it is important when working with infants and toddlers and their families to remain broad minded and open to all perspectives.

CASE ILLUSTRATION

Marisela—Concurrent Intervention: Occupational Therapy Intervention and Promoting Attachment

Marisela, a product of in vitro fertilization, was delivered at 31 weeks, gestation, weighing 3 lb, 7 ounces, to a 47-year-old mother. While she did have some respiratory distress, she never received assisted ventilation or supplemental oxygen. She had no neonatal neurological sequelae, but she did have bilateral partial congenital cataracts and underwent a partial bilateral lensectomy around 6 months of age. Afterward, she was referred to a High Risk Infant Follow-up Program. The purpose of this follow-up was to identify neurodevelopmental delays and make referrals to appropriate community-based early intervention programs.

When Marisela was 6 months 15 days old, and adjusted age 4 months 12 days, she attended her first High Risk Infant Follow-up appointment. At that time, she was noted to have somewhat decreased resting muscle tone with over-recruitment of her extensor musculature when active. Her muscle strength was moderately decreased proximally with decreased antigravity movement and continuous but consolable motor activity. Her mother, Titi, reported that the pediatrician had characterized her extremity movements as "flailing" and "purposeless." She was irritable and demonstrated limited visual responsivity as she had not yet been fitted with her contact lenses and she made no attempts to calm herself. These behaviors resulted in moderately delayed abilities in all developmental realms. Luckily, she fed from the bottle easily, enjoyed bath time, and slept all night. Marisela was referred for the local education agency's services for vision impairment and to the local early intervention agency for physical therapy (PT) and occupational therapy (OT) services.

Occupational therapy addressed sensory processing as it impacted self-regulation, parent–child interaction, and play, in addition to monitoring and promoting Marisela's transition to textured foods. During the evaluation, the OT practitioner observed Marisela, during which Titi commented that she was worried about Marisela's flailing movements and inability to stop them (a misattunement). The OT practitioner promoted attachment bonds during the interventions by interpreting Marisela's movements within a sensory modulation perspective and educating Titi about Marisela's signals of distress to her parents. She also asked Titi if it was necessary to "stop" Marisela's flailing movements when sensory treatment might ameliorate them.

Discussion

Although Marisela and her mother, Titi, were referred to occupational therapy for vision impairment and early intervention, the occupational therapist was also able to promote attachment behaviors using observation, education, and questions resulting from clinical reasoning.

Another case illustrates how occupational therapists can observe the attachment system in the course of occupational therapy evaluation and distinguish performance and attachment system difficulties.

CASE ILLUSTRATION

Marcus and Jennifer—Distinguishing Between Performance or Attachment Problems

When Marcus was referred to occupational therapy, he was 13 months old and newly diagnosed with Failure to Thrive. He was born at full term to a 36-year-old mother and had no neonatal health problems. He had always been a little small but over the past 6 months had not grown well. His mother, Jennifer, an allied health professional who had quit her job to stay home with Marcus, reported that during the past several pediatric visits the doctor had told her to "feed him more." The doctor told Jennifer that there was no other reason that Marcus was so small. She and her husband understood the significance of "failure to thrive" and were frustrated because they felt that they were doing everything they could to get Marcus to eat and that "he just doesn't want to."

Judith, the occupational therapist, visited Marcus and Jennifer in their home, a well-kept condominium, around their usual lunch time. Marcus's father worked very long hours, typically did not participate in meal times, and was unable to participate in the session. Through interview and a non-directed play session, Judith screened Marcus as being developmentally age appropriate. Marcus was vocal and playful. He spontaneously engaged with toys and Judith's testing materials. He included both his mother and therapist in his play. He easily pulled to stand and cruised along furniture, referencing his mother whenever he moved across the living room from her.

Marcus, Jennifer, and Judith then transitioned from the living room to a dining area that was connected with the kitchen. Marcus showed no resistance to being placed in his high chair at the dining table. Jennifer and Judith sat on either side of him, facing each other. He remained smiling and playful until his mother went into the kitchen to retrieve his lunch. He then cried and tried to get out of his chair, even though his mother kept either vocal or visual contact with him. He calmed when she came back to the table. Food was placed on everyone's plate. He watched with interest as both Jennifer and Judith took a few bites, even reaching out to Jennifer's face. However, he did not make any effort to pick up the same finger food to feed himself. When his mother offered the food, he would close his mouth and turn away. If mother persisted, he fussed. Whenever he wound up with some of the sauce on his face because of turning away at the wrong time, Jennifer immediately wiped his face. Judith suggested that the food be left on Marcus's tray and that the adults continue to eat. After a while, Marcus did begin to play with the food. He soon had it smeared all over his hands. Whenever his hands did become a little messy, Jennifer quickly wiped them off. Periodically, he placed a small bite of soft food in his mouth or he allowed the therapist, not mother, to give him a small spoon of chunky puree-textured food. With both textures, he demonstrated good oral-facial strength, age appropriate oral-motor skills, and timely transition of the food bolus for swallow. No coughing, choking, gagging, or respiratory changes were seen. He did not show any aversive responses to the textures in his mouth, or on his face or hands, for that matter. When Jennifer left the table to answer her phone or go back into the kitchen, Marcus cried. By the end of the meal, he had accepted more spoons of food from Judith than his mother, and did not fuss with the therapist.

Discussion

Judith had the opportunity to observe Marcus in a broader context and his feeding difficulties did not appear to have a developmental delay, oral-motor dysfunction, or sensory processing basis as the main issue. Because Judith had some knowledge of attachment theory and treatment, she recognized a disruption in the parent–child relationship; Marcus appeared not to have a secure attachment with his mother. Jennifer clearly showed significant anxiety during the lunchtime observation and while Judith wondered how much of her anxiety was due to the recent Failure to Thrive diagnosis, it did seem that Jennifer's anxiety along with Marcus's unique temperamental response to her anxious behaviors contributed to difficult feedings and limited intake.

Occupational Therapy Roles

Marisela and Marcus exemplify the range of toddlers who are treated by pediatric occupational therapists. In different ways and at different times, they each demonstrated an attachment relationship with their parents. They have developed varying abilities to discern important social cues, have had feelings elicited during their interactions with their parents and others, and have compared, contrasted and then encoded their repeated bodily and emotional feelings into their memories. Occupational therapy had a different role to play with each child, ranging from more typical developmental therapy using occupational therapy frames of reference such as sensory integration, neurodevelopmental therapy, motor control, and oral-motor/feeding treatment to developmental guidance and parent support. In each instance, occupational therapy also played a role in promoting the attachment process, which is the foundation for later development, particularly social and emotional development (Zeanah & Smyke, 2009). In the case of Marisela the occupational therapy role was more typically developmental based on sensory-processing, play, and facilitating feeding, but the occupational therapy practitioner was also able to notice a misattunement between mother and daughter. Therefore, she was able to promote attunement and attachment behaviors at the same time while she intervened with sensory modulation, play, and feeding.

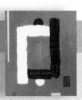

CASE ILLUSTRATION

Marisela and Titi—Collaborative Treatment: Occupational Therapy and Infant Mental Health Consultant

Marisela returned to the High Risk Infant Follow-up Program when she was 10½ months adjusted age. Since receiving contact lenses, she demonstrated markedly improved visual attention and discrimination in her play and social interactions. Her strength and quality of movement were also improved. Her overall developmental testing scores fell in the low average to mild delay range. She had begun to finger feed and had transitioned to Stage 2 puree foods but she had no interest in using the cup. She had begun to wake 1–2 times every night, crying inconsolably. Marisela's parents—Titi and her partner, Gabe— were able to attend the sessions. Her parents reported that she had significant irritable periods during which she "worked herself up to a frenzy." Her only self-soothing strategy was to suck on her wrist. They reported that she did not like to be left alone and that they believed that she had significant stranger anxiety. Both Titi and Gabe reported being ineffective in their attempts to help her cope. She was receiving vision therapy services one time per week, PT treatment two times per week, and OT treatment one time per week for continued interventions for feeding, strengthening, and play. The High Risk Infant Follow-up Program worked closely with the early intervention agency to assist Marisela's parents to access an infant mental health professional for consultation.

Her last High Risk Infant Follow-up Program appointment was when Marisela was 26 months old. Her age was no longer adjusted for prematurity, as is the community standard. Her cognitive skills were age appropriate as were her fine motor skills. Gross motor skills continued to be moderately delayed due to decreased motor control, decreased dynamic balance, and difficulties with motor planning. Her language abilities scored in the low average to mild delay range. Marisela ate "voraciously" all textures of food, using all the age-appropriate utensils. She enjoyed her bath time. She helped with tooth brushing as well as hand and face washing. Gabe and Titi reported that Marisela "loves to tidy and clean up." Routines were helpful to her. Her favorite play were activities that included her push cars and a trampoline. However, Gabe and Titi reported her to be "extremely willful" and that she would have "complete meltdowns" when her plans were interrupted. She was also described as "clingy and insecure." Marisela continued to receive vision therapy, physical therapy, and occupational therapy in addition to weekly infant mental health consultation.

Marisela's occupational therapist collaborated with her infant mental health consultant. Each discipline had a specific role to play with Marisela and her parents but both acknowledged the importance of incorporating the other discipline's strategies. The IMH consultant understood that while Marisela's sensory processing difficulties clearly played a large role in her difficulties with being calm and able to look and listen to her parents as an infant, there was now the larger context of how her primary attachment relationships with Titi and Gabe had developed. She continued to have significant self-regulatory difficulties and sought out excessive amounts of proprioceptive input to calm and organize herself. The infant mental health consultant worked with Titi and Gabe on how to read and anticipate Marisela's physical and emotional cues so that they could help her manage her feelings before she had meltdowns. She also worked with them on how they could help her pull herself together when she did fall apart. Strategies incorporated occupational therapy's interpretation of Marisela's fragile sensory modulation abilities and need for more proprioceptive input. Conversely, the occupational therapist continued to include Marisela's parents in treatment sessions rather than asking them to wait in the waiting room.

Discussion

The occupational therapist learned from the infant mental health consultant that Marisela needed her parents to emotionally assist her with her regulatory abilities; that her difficulties were not solely "sensory" in nature. Therefore, the occupational therapist included her parents in family-centered care and also adapted his communication strategies for the parents to include emotional content. Both the occupational therapist and infant mental health consultant worked together to incorporate strategies learned from each other in their respective interventions. Both became "consultants" and provided education to each other and for the parents in the infant–parent dyad.

Occupational Therapy Intervention Strategies

Occupational therapy with young children will be most effective in supporting each child's developmental progression if it consistently adapts treatment strategies to support the growing attachment relationship. This perspective suggests that the therapist:

- plans for each treatment activity to assure that the child feels safe and secure, both physically and emotionally.
- views the child's behaviors as communication and consistently responds to them.
- assists parents and other people important in the child's life to establish predictable daily rituals and routines.
- assures that the parent is involved in treatment sessions since she/he is a primary mediator of the child's emotional life.
- considers all possible explanations for a child's behaviors, that is, "clingy" behavior due to a sensory processing disorder, poor motor control, or possibly due to delayed emotional development (attachment processes).
- includes as a therapy goal that each parent and child will successfully engage in mutually rewarding interactions (Costa, 2006; Holloway, 1998; Holloway & Chandler, 2010; Landy, 2009; Williamson & Anzalone, 2001). In the case of Marcus and Titi, these strategies were demonstrated by further developments in their lives.

CASE ILLUSTRATION

Marcus and Jennifer—Examples of Occupational Therapy Strategies

Overall, it appeared to Judith that Marcus had difficulties separating from his mother (viewed his behavior as communication). Jennifer clearly was on a "short leash" in that if she left the immediate vicinity, Marcus fell apart. She reported that Marcus showed this distress throughout the day whenever she moved away from him and that it didn't matter if they were alone or with other people, including Marcus's father. The occupational therapist noted that the emotional tone of the initial lunch session was clearly heightened beyond that of when mother left Marcus's side. They both demonstrated anxiety during the mealtime, just in different ways.

Often when a young child cries or pulls away with feeding, occupational therapists theorize that he must have some degree of sensory-based oral aversion. However, occupational therapists often evaluate children's feeding skills in isolation and often this takes place in a clinical setting. The therapist then may not have the opportunity to see or appreciate the broader environmental context for mealtimes. Intervention strategies to inhibit oral aversion-type of behaviors, either from a sensory or behavioral perspective may then be the only intervention approach used.

The therapy sessions following the initial consultation consisted of guided play and snack times (assists parents to establish predictable daily rituals and routines). Therapist and mother focused on enjoying Marcus's strengths, in terms of his growing independence, increasing his ability to express his likes and dislikes, and on mother's ability to be aware of how her anxious feelings influenced the way in which she cared for, played with, and especially fed Marcus (assures that parent is involved in treatment session). Also, Judith acknowledged the stress that Jennifer must have felt as the primary feeder after hearing the Failure to Thrive diagnosis (therapeutic use of self).

While Jennifer was slowly able to adjust some of her behaviors around feeding Marcus, and did seek supportive therapy for herself, Marcus made very little change over the course of his therapy sessions in terms of overall caloric intake. Jennifer reported that they did have some enjoyable meals together at times, but that while he did not cry as much, Marcus still "just doesn't want to" eat. During the time that occupational therapy was working with Marcus and his mother, his parents decided to seek additional medical input. It was determined that he had a severe C. difficile bacterial infection in his gastrointestinal tract, which can lead to pain and feeding intolerance. Due to the severity of this infection, Marcus required a colectomy. He had this surgery about 6 months after the initial occupational therapy consultation.

Marcus's gastrointestinal recovery was quite slow. He was hospitalized several times for prolonged periods. Jennifer stayed with him in the hospital and later told Judith that once Marcus had a diagnosis and a plan of care, she felt less anxious and was able to more fully integrate some of the therapy approaches that she had used with the occupational therapist. Marcus was slowly reintroduced to foods. The slow pace served him well in that it took the pressure off of him and his parents. As his mother was now better able to help him cope with the sensations of eating, and he was no longer experiencing pain when he ate food, she was able to help him slowly progress. When she was able to see Marcus progress, her anxiety continued to lessen. When Judith last saw Marcus and Jennifer, his diet was age appropriate and his growth was getting back on track. Marcus is able to let his mother go a little and when she does leave him with familiar adults, he no longer falls apart. They were able to incorporate fun, playful routines in their day (goal of engaging in mutually rewarding activities) and they finally were able to get back on track in the attachment process.

Discussion

The therapist assisted the family in context and with a family-centered approach to improve the Marcus' attachment behaviors using strategies of targeting the parenting behavior, and modeling a professional–parent relationship. The therapist assisted Jennifer to reflect on Marcus' behavior in a different way through promoting co-occupations, and using self-reflection and introspection when working with Marcus and his mom. She also acknowledged the parent's recognition that there was still some other problem affecting the dyad when the eating behavior improved but Marcus still was not eating.

Marcus's story is a cautionary one for therapists. It reminds us that all explanations for a child's behaviors must be explored and that the foundation for some developmental, behavioral, or psychological difficulty may indeed be a medical one that then influences or facilitates the other emerging difficulties. On the other hand, Marcus' story illustrates the interplay of attachment and medical problems and the influence of parents on the self-regulation of their children.

Occupational therapy with very young children typically is related to a child's developmental delay, physical disability, or difficulties participating in family life due to dysfunction in sensory processing. Some occupational therapists may not consider themselves to be providing psychosocial occupational therapy services when working with the infant–toddler population. However, successful pediatric occupational therapy services necessarily address attachment because of its foundational role in overall development. Young children require a safe and stable caregiving environment with a warm, responsive, and consistent caregiver. At times, for parents of young children with developmental and other difficulties this is challenging to achieve. It "requires the parent to move beyond the commonly understood ways of relating to infants" (Lillas & Turnbull, 2009, p. 85) because these children may have differing types of needs and responses. The occupational therapist can assist the parent to find those alternate ways of relating that can be more successful and rewarding for both parent and child.

The following case is an example of how an occupational therapist facilitated a successful and rewarding relationship.

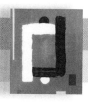

CASE ILLUSTRATION

Erik and Junko—Successful Developmental Guidance

Erik was a very small premature infant, 24 weeks' gestational age with a birth weight of 610 grams. He was hospitalized in the NICU for 5 months. He had quite a complicated neonatal history as demonstrated by his 18-page medical discharge summary. His diagnoses included: oxygen dependent bronchopulmonary dysplasia, retinopathy of prematurity with laser surgery, multiple septic episodes, renal failure, seizures treated with phenobarbital, and significant gastroesophageal reflux (GER).

Erik was discharged home on supplemental oxygen and feeding adequately by bottle. He was never able to transition to breast feeding. Within one week of his NICU discharge, he stopped accepting the bottle. His pediatrician used home health services to place and monitor a nasogastric tube for feedings. He was hypotonic with compensatory arching, exacerbated by his frequent GER and vomiting. While his laser surgery was considered successful, he ultimately was diagnosed with astigmatism and amblyopia, for which he was prescribed glasses at 14 months of age.

Early intervention services have been in place since Erik's NICU discharge. He has received OT, PT, and Infant Development services each two times per week. Erik has been developmentally delayed throughout his life, but recently, as he has neared 2½ years of age, he has begun to close the gap between his chronologic age and his developmental age in all areas. He began walking independently around 22 months' adjusted age. His receptive language has always been around age expectations while his expressive language has been delayed. He has struggled with feeding and was quite slow to transition to pureed and table foods. His overall growth has been slow as well.

Erik's father works internationally and so his mother, Junko, is a single parent for about 8 months at a time. She has worked part-time and assured that Erik consistently participated in his early intervention program as allowed by his fluctuating medical status. All of Erik's early interventionists have observed that he and Junko have a loving relationship. He is able to seek her out for comfort when upset but also is able to move away from her to explore in his immediate environment. He is cautious around new people but able to warm up to them after a period of time. From the beginning, Junko was able to read and respond to his cues: his signs of distress and calm, readiness for interaction and need for rest. She also was able to regulate her own emotional state to help Erik regulate his own. She met him where he was at, so to speak, in terms of his physiologic, motor, cognitive, communicative, and emotional needs. As he matured in these different realms, he grew in his emotional independence. Once he was able to sit independently, Erik tolerated being put down on the floor but still close to his mother. When he began using vocal signals to call to his mother, he also stopped fussing when she moved to the other side of the room. She protected him from those people who did not understand that attachment-separation processes come from the development and interaction of all developmental realms and who believed that he should be forced to separate from her to "go to the treatment room" to "learn" to separate from her. Junko did this naturally, with support and guidance from the occupational therapist. Throughout his course of therapy, the occupational therapist acknowledged Erik's emotional response to motor activities, playground play, bathing, or feeding. The occupational therapist guided Junko in observing Erik's messages, supported her in recognizing that Erik proceeded at his own pace emotionally, and planned developmental therapy activities to include and promote Erik's special relationship with his mother. As part of her treatment plan, his occupational therapist assured that Erik would feel safe, calm, and secure by incorporating his mother's presence during playful and safe occupational treatment.

Discussion

Junko used occupational therapy services during self-care and play activities and co-occupations to develop a secure attachment and self-regulation of emotions with him, despite his developmental difficulties and external pressure that urged typical age independence.

SUMMARY

This chapter discussed attachment theory, the attachment system, its origins and development, research, and cultural applications. It discussed programs that promote attachment and the relationship of those programs' principles to occupational therapy interventions. It discussed occupational therapy treatment incorporating attachment in early intervention and intensive care and principles of intervention. It advocated for occupational therapists to become knowledgeable about attachment theory, research, and recent advances in neurobiology and to address attachment in early intervention. Furthermore, it advocated that occupational therapists address psychosocial issues in early intervention.

REVIEW QUESTIONS

1. What is the importance of knowing about attachment theory?
2. What are attachment behaviors and how do they become manifested in a caregiver–child relationship in infancy and in childhood?
3. What are the primary attachment patterns? What behavior might you observe in an infant–caregiver dyad that will define each attachment pattern?
4. What are the principles and strategies of occupational therapy that are similar to the principles of infant–parent work?
5. How is attachment influenced by institutionalization and removal of a child or infant to foster care?

REFERENCES

Ainsworth, M. D. S. (1967). *Infancy in Uganda: Infant care and the growth of love.* Baltimore: Johns Hopkins University Press.

Ainsworth, M. D. S. (1977). Infant development and mother-infant interactions among Uganda and American families. In P. H. Leiderman, S. R. Tulkin, & A. H. Rosenfeld (Eds.), *Culture and infancy* (pp. 119–150). New York: Academic Press.

American Occupational Therapy Association (AOTA). (2008). The Occupational Therapy Practice Framework. *American Journal of Occupational Therapy, 62*(6), 625–683.

American Psychiatric Association (APA). (2000). *Diagnostic and statistical manual of mental disorders* (4th ed., Text rev.). Washington, DC: APA.

Atkinson, L., Chisholm, V. C., Scott, B., Goldberg, S., Vaughn, B. E., Blackwell, J., et al. (1999). Maternal sensitivity, child functional level and attachment in Down syndrome. In J. Vondra and D. Barnett (Eds.), Atypical attachment in infancy and early childhood among children at developmental risk (pp. 45–66). *Monographs of the Society for Research in Child Development, 64*(3, Serial No. 258).

Barnett, D., Butler, C. M., & Vondra, J. I. (1999). Atypical patterns of early attachment: Discussion and future directions. In J. Vondra and D. Barnett (Eds.), Atypical attachment in infancy and early childhood among children at developmental risk (pp. 172–192). *Monographs of the Society for Research in Child Development, 64*(3, Serial No. 258).

Becker-Weidman, A., & Hughes, D. (2008). Dyadic developmental psychotherapy: An evidence-based treatment for children with complex trauma and disorders of attachment. *Child and Family Social Work, 13*(3), 329-337. doi: 10.1111.1365-2206.2008.00557.x

Berlin, L. J., Zeanah, C. H., & Lieberman, A. F. (2008). Prevention and intervention programs for supporting early attachment security. In J. Cassidy and P. R. Shaver (Eds.), *Handbook of attachment: Theory, research and clinical applications* (2nd ed., pp. 745–761). New York: Guilford.

Berlin, L., Ziv, Y., Amaya-Jackson, L., & Greenberg, M. (Eds.). (2005). *Enhancing early attachments: Theory, research, intervention, and policy.* New York: Guilford.

Booth-LaForce, C., Rubin, K., Rose-Krasnor, L., & Burgess, K. (2005). Attachment and friendship: Predictors of psychosocial functioning in middle childhood and the mediating roles of social support and self-worth. In K. Kerns and R. Richardson (Eds.), *Attachment in early childhood* (pp. 161–188). New York: Guilford.

Bowlby, J. (1973). Prototypes of human sorrow. In *Attachment and loss: V. separation, anxiety and anger* (pp. 3–22). New York: Basic Books.

Bowlby, J. (1988a). Developmental psychiatry comes of age. *American Journal of Psychiatry, 145*(1), 1–10.

Bowlby, J. (1988b). *A secure base: Parent-child attachment and healthy human development* (Ch. 2, pp. 20–38). New York: Basic Books.

Bowlby, R. (March, 2002). *Attachment from early childhood through the lifespan.* Presentation at the UCLA Lifespan Learning Institute, Los Angeles, CA.

Brandell, J., & Ringel, S. (2007). *Attachment and dynamic practice: an integrative guide for social workers and other clinicians.* New York: Columbia University Press.

Bretherton, I., & Munholland, K. (2008). Internal working models in attachment relationships: Elaborating a central construct in attachment theory. In J. Cassidy and P. R. Shaver (Eds.), *Handbook of attachment: Theory, research and clinical applications* (2nd ed., pp. 102–130). New York: Guilford.

Bretherton, I., & Waters, E. (Eds.). (1985). Growing points of attachment theory and research. *Monographs of the Society for Research in Child Development, 50* (1–2; Serial No. 209).

Cassidy, J. (2008). *The nature of the child's ties.* In J. Cassidy and P. R. Shaver (Eds.), *Handbook of attachment: Theory, research and clinical applications* (2nd ed., pp. 3–22). New York: Guilford.

Cassidy, J., & Shaver, P. (Eds.) (2008). *Handbook of attachment: Theory, research, and clinical applications.* New York: Guilford.

Champagne, T. (2011). Attachment, trauma, and occupational therapy practice. *OT Practice, 16*(5), CE-1–CE-7.

Cook, W. (2000). Understanding attachment security in family context. *Journal of Personality and Social Psychology, 78*(2), 285–294.

Corbin, J. (2007). Reactive attachment disorder: A biopsychosocial disturbance of attachment. *Child and Adolescent Social Work Journal, 24,* 539–552. doi:10.1007/s10560-007-0105-x

Costa, G. (2006). Mental health principles, practices, strategies, and dynamics pertinent to early intervention practitioners. In G. M Foley & J. D. Hochman (Eds.), *Mental Health in Early Intervention: Achieving unity in principles and practice* (pp. 113–138). Baltimore, MD: Paul H. Brooks Publishing Co.

Cozolino, L. (2006) *The neuroscience of human relationships: Attachment and the developing social brain.* New York: W.W. Norton & Co.

Creeden, K. (2009). How trauma and attachment can impact neurodevelopment: Informing our understanding and treatment of sexual behavior problems. *Journal of Social Aggression, 15*(3), 261–273.

Cronin, A. (2004). Mothering a child with hidden impairments. *American Journal of Occupational Therapy, 58*(1), 83–92.

Dozier, M., & Rutter, M. (2008). Challenges to the development of attachment relationships faced by young children in foster and adoptive care. In J. Cassidy and P. R. Shaver (Eds.), *Handbook of attachment: Theory, research, and clinical applications* (pp. 698–717). New York: Guilford.

Fraiberg, S. (1980). *Clinical studies in infant mental health: The first year of life.* New York: Basic Books.

Fraiberg, S. (1982). Pathological defenses in infancy. *Psychoanalytic Quarterly, 51,* 612–615.

Hardy, L. (2007). Attachment theory and reactive attachment disorder: Theoretical perspectives and treatment implications. *Journal of Child and Adolescent Psychiatric Nursing, 20*(1), 27–39.

Holloway, E. (1998). Early emotional development and sensory processing. In J. Case-Smith (Ed.), *Pediatric Occupational Therapy and Early Intervention* (pp. 111–126). Boston, MA: Butterworth-Heinemann.

Holloway, E., & Chandler, B. E. (2010). Family-centered practice: It's all about relationships. In B. E. Chandler (Ed.), *Early childhood: Occupational therapy services for children birth to five.* (pp. 77–108). Bethesda, MD: ATOA Press.

Hughes, D. (2006). Building the bonds of attachment: Awakening love in deeply troubled children. Lanham, MD: Jason Aronson.

Karen, R. (1994). *Becoming attached: Unfolding the mystery of the infant mother bond and its impact on later life.* New York: Warner Books.

Kellegrew, D. H. (2000). Constructing daily routines: A qualitative examination of mothers with young children with disabilities. *American Journal of Occupational Therapy, 54,* 252–259.

Kerns, K. (2008) Attachment in middle childhood. In J. Cassidy and P. R. Shaver (Eds.), *Handbook of attachment: Theory, research, and clinical applications* (pp. 366–416). New York: Guilford.

Kerns, K. & Richardson, R. (Eds.). (2005). *Attachment in middle childhood.* New York: Guilford.

Kyler, P. (2008). Client-centered and family-centered care: Refinement of the concepts. *Occupational Therapy in Mental Health, 24*(2), 100–120.

Landy, S. (2009). *Pathways to competence: encouraging healthy social and emotional development in young children.* Baltimore, MD: Paul H. Brooks Publishing Co.

Larson, E. A. (2000). The orchestration of occupation: The dance of mothers. *American Journal of Occupational Therapy, 54,* 269–280.

Lieberman, A. (1988). Clinical implications of attachment theory. In J. Belsky & T. Nexzworski (Eds.), *Clinical implications of attachment* (pp. 327–351). Hillsdale, NJ: Lawrence Erlbaum Assoc.

Lieberman, A., & Pawl, J. (1993). Infant parent psychotherapy. In C. Zeanah (Ed.), *Handbook of infant mental health.* New York: Guilford Press.

Lillas C., & Turnbull, J. (2009). *Infant/child mental health, early intervention, and relationship-based therapies.* New York: W.W. Norton & Co.

Mayseless, O. (2005). Ontogeny of attachment in middle childhood: Conceptualization of normative changes. In K. Kerns and R. Richardson (Eds.), *Attachment in early childhood* (pp. 1–23). New York: Guilford.

Mikulincer, M., & Shaver, P. (2008). Adult attachment and affect regulation. In J. Cassidy and P. R. Shaver (Eds.), *Handbook of attachment: Theory, research, and clinical applications* (pp. 503–531). New York: Guilford.

Naber, F., Swinkels, S., Buitelaar, J., Bakermans-Kranenburg, M., Van IJzendoorn, M., Dietz, C., et al. (2007). Attachment in toddlers with autism and other developmental disorders. *Journal of Autism and Developmental Disorders, 37,* 1123–1138. doi:10.1007/s10803-006-0255-2

Papousek, M. (2011). Resilience, strengths, and regulatory capacities: Hidden resources in developmental disorders of infant mental health. *Infant Mental Health Journal 32*(1), 29–46.

Rutgers, A., Bakermans-Kranenburg, M., Van IJzendoorn, M., & van Berckelaer-Onnes, I. (2004). Autism and attachment: a meta-analytic review. *Journal of Child Psychology and Psychiatry, 45*(6), 1123–1134.

Rutgers, A., Van IJzendoornrn, M., Bakermans-Kranenburg, M., Swinkels, S., van Daalen, E., Dietz, C., et al. (2007). Autism, attachment and parenting: A comparison of children with autism spectrum disorder, mental retardation, language disorder, and non-clinical children. *Journal of Abnormal Psychology, 35,* 859–870. doi:10.1007.s10802-007-9129-y

Salter Ainsworth, M. D., & Bell, S. M. (1970). Attachment, exploration and separation: Illustrated by the behavior of one-year-olds in a strange situation. *Child Development, 41*(1), 49–67.

Schore, A. N. (2000). Attachment and the regulation of the right brain. *Attachment & Human Development, 2*(1), 23–47.

Schore, A. N. (2010). A neurobiological perspective on the work of Berry Brazelton. In B. M. Lester and J. D. Sparrow (Eds.), *Nurturing children and families: Building on the legacy of T. Berry Brazelton* (pp. 141–153). Malden, MA: Blackwell Publishing.

Schultz-Krohn, W., & Cara, E. (2000). Case report: Occupational therapy in early intervention: Applying concepts from infant mental health. *American Journal of Occupational Therapy, 54*(5), 550–554.

Seligman, S. (1994). Applying psychoanalysis in an unconventional context. *Psychoanalytic Study of the Child, 49*, 481–500.

Siegel, D. J. (1999). *The developing mind: How relationships and the brain interact to shape who we are.* New York: Guilford Press.

Simpson, J. A., & Belsky, J. (2008). Attachment theory within a modern evolutionary framework. In J. Cassidy and P. R. Shaver (Eds.), *Handbook of attachment: Theory, research, and clinical applications* (pp. 131–157). New York: Guilford.

Slade, A., & Aber, J. (1992). Attachments, drives and development: conflicts and convergences in theory. In J. Barron, M. Eagles, D. Wotilsky, & David, L. (Eds.), *Interface of psychoanalysis and psychology* (pp. 154–185). Washington, DC: American Psychological Association.

Sroufe, L., & Waters, E. (1977). Attachment as an organizational construct. *Child Development, 48*, 1184–1199.

Taylor, R. (2008). *The intentional relationship: Occupational therapy and the use of self.* Philadelphia: F.A. Davis.

Van IJzendoorn, M. H., & Sagi-Schwartz, A. (2008). Cross-cultural patterns of attachment: Universal and contextual dimensions. In J. Cassidy and P. Shaver (Eds.), *Handbook of attachment: Theory, research, and clinical applications* (pp. 880–905). New York: Guilford.

Vaughn, B. E., & Waters, E. (1990). Attachment behavior at home and in the laboratory: Q-sort observations and Strange Situation classifications of one-year-olds. *Child Development, 61*, 1965–1973.

Verschueren, K., & Marcoen, A. (2005). Perceived security of attachment to mother and father: Developmental differences and relations to self-worth and peer relationships at school. In K. Kerns and R. Richardson (Eds.), *Attachment in early childhood* (pp. 212–230). New York: Guilford.

Williamson, G. G., & Anzalone, M. E. (2001). *Sensory Integration and Self Regulations in Infants and Toddlers: Helping very young children interact with their environment.* Washington, DC: Zero to Three.

Young-Bruehl, E., & Bethelard, F. (2002). *Cherishment, A psychology of the heart.* New York: Simon & Schuster.

Zeanah, C. H., & Smyke, A. T. (2009). Attachment disorders. In C. H. Zeanah (Ed.), *Handbook of infant mental health* (3rd ed., pp. 421–434). New York: Guilford Press.

Zionts, L. (2005). Examining relationships between students and teachers: A potential extension of attachment theory? In K. Kerns and R. Richardson (Eds.), *Attachment in early childhood* (pp. 231–254). New York: Guilford.

SUGGESTED RESOURCES

Cohen, L.J. (2001). *Playful parenting: An exciting new approach to raising children that will help you nurture close connections, solve behavior problems, encourage confidence.* NY: Ballantine.

Hughes, D. A. (2009). *Attachment-focused parenting: Effective strategies to care for children.* NY: Norton.

Karen, R. (1998). *Becoming Attached: First Relationships and how they shape our capacity to love.* NY: Oxford University.

Mooney, C. G. (2010). *Theories of Attachment: An introduction to Bowlby, Ainsworth, Gerber, Brazelton, Kennel, and Kraus.* St. Paul, MN: Red Leaf.

Newton, R. (2008). *The Attachment Connection: Parenting a Secure and Confident Child Using the Science of Attachment Theory.* Oakland, CA: New Harbinger.

Shemmings, D., & Shemmings, Y. (2011). *Understanding disorganized attachment: Theory and practice for working with children and adults.* London: Jessica Kingsley.

Siegel, D.J., & Hartzell, M. (2003). *Parenting from the inside out: How a deeper self-understanding can help you raise children who thrive.* N.Y.: Tarcher/Penguin

Websites

John Bowlby Explains Attachment Theory:
   http://www.youtube.com/watch?v=VAAmSqv2GV8

Mary Ainsworth Strange Situation:
   http://www.youtube.com/watch?v=QTsewNrHUHU

Mary Ainsworth and Attachment:
   http://www.youtube.com/watch?v=SHP_NikTkao

Richard Bowlby on Attachment:
   http://www.youtube.com/watch?v=MrcNjFyWeWE&feature=related

James Robertson Films:
   http://www.robertsonfilms.info/

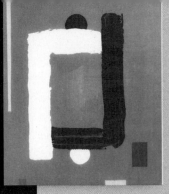

Chapter 12

Mental Health of Children

William L. Lambert, MS, OTR/L

KEY TERMS

acting out

consistency

dynamic

interpretation

latency age

nondirective play group

parallel task group

redirection

structure

time-out

CHAPTER OUTLINE

Introduction

DSM-IV-TR Diagnoses

Helpful Concepts for Treating Children

      Structure and Consistency

      Interpretation

      Time-Out

      Limit Setting

      Therapeutic Use of Self

      Team Approach and Family Involvement

      Medications

Child Settings and Programs

      School-Based Programs

      Partial Hospitalization

Implementing Programming for Children

      Evaluation and Assessment

      Intervention

Examples of Emerging Areas of Practice

      Occupational Therapy Services for a Foster Care Agency

      Foster Care Agency—Expert Witness

Foster Care Agency—Direct Service
Home-Based Occupational Therapy
Summary, Current Trends, and Recommendations

INTRODUCTION

Occupational therapy for children with emotional and behavioral disturbances has been an area of specialization within the profession for many years. Indeed, the practice of occupational therapy with children with mental and behavioral disorders requires specific knowledge of specific psychiatric and general mental health disorders and conditions, expertise in normal or typical growth and development, and practice skills unique to this population, its issues, and its concerns.

Those providing care to these children often work in collaboration with other health care professionals such as child psychiatrists, psychologists, social workers, and nurses (Hollander, 2001) or independently as consultants or contract therapists, or through a private practice. The delivery system for providing occupational therapy for this population has changed dramatically in the last two decades. In the past, the primary sites that employed therapists to provide services for children experiencing psychosocial issues were psychiatric hospitals with children's units or wards, outpatient mental health clinics, and partial hospitalization or day treatment programs (Pratt & Allen, 1989). Currently therapists who have a particular interest in working with children with emotional or behavioral problems must think outside the box—or toy box—due to the move away from medical model/hospital-based treatment. Many programs are being eliminated and clinical services reduced. Secondary to increasingly shorter lengths of stay and limited reimbursement, therapists will necessarily need to be prepared to address the mental health issues of children in school and community settings not usually thought of as psychiatric/mental health, but rather as pediatric (Argabrite, 2002; Burns & Hoagwood, 2002; Hahn, 2000; Lewis, 2002). The reader is encouraged to thoughtfully consider how to apply the concepts and information presented in this chapter in all settings where children are in need of occupational therapy services. (See also Chapter 22, "Psychosocial Occupational Therapy in the School Setting.")

This chapter presents an overview of occupational therapy practice with children who are experiencing mental health problems that are affecting their ability to function in one or more areas of their lives. Basic concepts used in providing occupational therapy to children with mental health issues are described. Occupational therapy programming is discussed based on experience and on successful interventions used in other settings (Hoffman, 1982; Llorens & Rubin, 1967). Treatment, intervention groups with examples of group protocols, and activities appropriate for this population are presented that may be used in a variety of pediatric settings.

The need to address the psychosocial needs of children in various pediatric settings began to become more prominent in occupational therapy publications

(Barnes et al., 2003; Bazyk, 2011; Case-Smith & Archer, 2008; Florey, 2003; Gray, 2005; Jackson & Arbesman, 2005; Kaplan & Telford, 1998; Lougher, 2001). The American Occupational Therapy Association Continuing Education article in *OT Practice* (AOTA, 2002) pointed out that "childhood psychosocial problems that are left untreated often become exacerbated in adolescence and young adulthood" (pp. CE4–CE6) and that children with psychosocial and other disorders must have these needs addressed in occupational therapy in pediatric settings. The article goes on to provide intervention guidelines that have long been treatment objectives in traditional psychosocial settings, such as increasing impulse control, improving frustration tolerance, tolerating transitions, and developing social interaction skills.

DSM-IV-TR DIAGNOSES

The *Diagnostic and Statistical Manual of Mental Disorders,* Fourth Edition, Text Revision (*DSM-IV-TR*, APA, 2000) lists disorders usually first diagnosed in infancy, childhood, or adolescence. Many of these disorders, such as attention deficit hyperactivity disorder (ADHD), mental retardation, and Tourette's disorder can continue to cause problems during adulthood. "Approximately one-half to two-thirds of children who have ADHD continue to have symptoms of the disorder into their teenage years and on into adulthood" (Resnick, 2005). Many disorders that are discussed in other chapters of this volume, such as schizophrenia, major depression, bipolar disorder, and post-traumatic stress disorder (PTSD) may also first be encountered in childhood (Lewis, 2002; Rutter & Taylor, 2002; Sadock & Sadock 2007). Symptoms of childhood depression include irritability, sadness, social withdrawal, and anhedonia, as well as negative feelings appearing in play (Weingarten-Dubin, 2001). Irritability is common in depression and mania in children (Harvard Mental Health Letter, May 2007). Depression has also been linked to violent behaviors (Bertucco, 2001), and children often exhibit this violent behavior with aggression or **acting out**. Acting out can be defined as the expression of thoughts and feelings through maladaptive behavior instead of recognizing and verbalizing those ideas. Children may express depressive symptoms in other ways, such as anger, as it is cognitively easier for them to be mad than sad.

A difference in the way that children with bipolar disorder present is that their moods may shift many times within the same day or same therapy session. Additionally, their "symptoms rarely follow a discrete pattern. Children, especially young children, usually do not show the adult cycle of distinct mood swings from mania to depression lasting for several months, with intervals of normal mood in between," but on the other hand, "children may also have more classic and unmistakable manic symptoms" (Harvard Mental Health Letter, May 2007). Their presentation is further complicated by frequently also meeting the criteria for ADHD and oppositional defiant disorder. "Bipolar disorder in children is especially difficult to distinguish from ADHD, since many of the symptoms—impulsiveness, distractibility, and hyperactivity—are similar" (Harvard Mental Health Letter, May 2007). A family history that includes relatives who have been diagnosed with bipolar disorder greatly assists in making this diagnosis in children. Knowing which medications were beneficial to blood relatives also makes choosing the appropriate medication for the child easier. For example, if Depakote has helped control a parent's bipolar disorder, it also may be effective with a son or daughter. Lithium and anticonvulsants are also medications frequently used to treat bipolar disorder. Figure 12-1 summarizes *DSM-IV-TR* disorders beginning in infancy and childhood.

Mental Retardation. This disorder is characterized by significantly subaverage intellectual functioning (an IQ of approximately 70 or below) with onset before age 18 years and concurrent deficits or impairments in adaptive functioning. Separate codes are provided for **Mild, Moderate, Severe,** and **Profound Mental Retardation** and for **Mental Retardation, Severity Unspecified.**

Learning Disorders. These disorders are characterized by academic function that is substantially below that expected given the person's chronological age, measured intelligence, and age-appropriate education. The specific disorders included in this section are **Reading Disorder, Mathematics Disorder, Disorder of Written Expression,** and **Learning Disorder Not Otherwise Specified.**

Motor Skills Disorder. This includes **Developmental Coordination Disorder,** which is characterized by motor coordination that is substantially below that expected given the person's chronological age and measured intelligence.

Communication Disorders. These disorders are characterized by difficulties in speech or language and include **Expressive Language Disorder, Mixed Receptive-Expressive Language Disorder, Phonological Disorder, Stuttering,** and **Communication Disorder Not Otherwise Specified.**

Pervasive Developmental Disorders. These disorders are characterized by severe deficits and pervasive impairment in multiple areas of development. These include impairment in reciprocal social interaction, impairment in communication, and the presence of stereotyped behavior, interests, and activities. The specific disorders included in this section are **Autistic Disorder, Rett's Disorder, Childhood Disintegrative Disorder, Asperger's Disorder,** and **Pervasive Developmental Disorder Not Otherwise Specified.**

Attention-Deficit and Disruptive Behavior Disorders. This section includes **Attention-Deficit/Hyperactivity Disorder,** which is characterized by prominent symptoms of inattention and/or hyperactivity-impulsivity. Subtypes are provided for specifying the predominant symptom presentation: **Predominantly Inattentive Type, Predominantly Hyperactive-Impulsive Type,** and **Combined Type.** Also included in this section are the Disruptive Behavior Disorders: **Conduct Disorder** is characterized by a pattern of behavior that violates the basic rights of others or major age-appropriate societal norms or rules; **Oppositional Defiant Disorder** is characterized by a pattern of negativistic, hostile, and defiant behavior. This section also includes two Not Otherwise Specified categories: **Attention-Deficit/Hyperactivity Disorder Not Otherwise Specified** and **Disruptive Behavior Disorder Not Otherwise Specified.**

(Continues)

FIGURE 12-1. *DSM-IV-TR* Disorders Beginning in Infancy, Childhood, or Adolescence
Information from the *Diagnostic and Statistical Manual of Mental Disorders*, 4th Edition, Text Revision (*DSM-IV-TR*, APA, 2000)

Feeding and Eating Disorders of Infancy or Early Childhood. These disorders are characterized by persistent disturbances in feeding and eating. The specific disorders included are **Pica, Rumination Disorder,** and **Feeding Disorder of Infancy or Early Childhood.** Note that Anorexia Nervosa and Bulimia Nervosa are included in the "Eating Disorders" section presented later in the DSM-IV-TR manual (p. 583).

Tic Disorders. These disorders are characterized by vocal and/or motor tics. The specific disorders included are **Tourette's Disorder, Chronic Motor or Vocal Tic Disorder, Transient Tic Disorder,** and **Tic Disorder Not Otherwise Specified.**

Elimination Disorders. This grouping includes **Encopresis,** the repeated passage of feces into inappropriate places, and **Enuresis,** the repeated voiding of urine into inappropriate places.

Other Disorders of Infancy, Childhood, or Adolescence. This grouping is for disorders that are not covered in the sections listed above. **Separation Anxiety Disorder** is characterized by developmentally inappropriate and excessive anxiety concerning separation from home or from those to whom the child is attached. **Selective Mutism** is characterized by a consistent failure to speak in specific social situations despite speaking in other situations. **Reactive Attachment Disorder of Infancy or Early Childhood** is characterized by markedly disturbed and developmentally inappropriate social relatedness that occurs inmost contexts and is associated with grossly pathogenic care. **Stereotypic Movement Disorder** is characterized by repetitive, seemingly driven, and nonfunctional motor behavior that markedly interferes with normal activities and at times may result in bodily injury. **Disorder of Infancy, Childhood, or Adolescence Not Otherwise Specified** is a residual category for coding disorders with onset in infancy, childhood, or adolescence that do not meet criteria for any specific disorder in the Classification.

FIGURE 12-1. *DSM-IV-TR* Disorders Beginning in Infancy, Childhood, or Adolescence *(Continued)*

Common diagnoses of children seen or encountered by occupational therapists in various settings include ADHD, oppositional defiant, separation anxiety, and conduct disorders. More recently attention has been focused on the occurrence and prevalence of Reactive Attachment Disorder. (For more information see Chapter 11, "Mental of Health Infants: Attachment Through the Lifespan") or Early Childhood and Autism Spectrum Disorders such as pervasive developmental disorder and Asperger's disorder in pediatric areas of practice. Autism spectrum disorders still fall under pervasive developmental disorders in the *DSM-IV-TR*; however, the former enjoys more common usage at the time of this writing. Disruptive Behavior Disorder Not Otherwise Specified (NOS), which first appeared in *DSM-IV*, provides a helpful provisional diagnosis, as the exact nature of children's mental illness is often hard to pinpoint, especially in its initial presentation.

Two prominent childhood disorders frequently receiving attention are ADHD and reactive attachment disorder (RAD). Children with ADHD often have problematic social interactions with peers, teachers, and authority figures, as well as difficulty in participating appropriately in the classroom and during extracurricular activities ("National Survey Reveals," 2002). Treatment with medications such as Ritalin, Adderall, and Metadate is often at the center of controversy and debate. These and other medications are criticized for being over-prescribed and heavily marketed to parents (Zernike & Peterson, 2001). However, to date there is no evidence of blanket adverse effects; furthermore, stimulants have been shown to be effective for hyperactivity, impulsivity, and inattention in classrooms (Fonagy, Target, Cottrell, Phillips, & Kurtz, 2002).

The specific causes for RAD are unknown; however, early experiences with caregivers of neglect and/or abuse where the parents did not address the child's basic emotional and physical needs appears to play a role and, more significantly, repeated changes in the primary caregiver or a succession of caregivers early in life (Howes & Spieker, 2008; Randolph, 1999) appears to prevent the establishment of stable, appropriate attachments. There is a high risk of this disorder for toddlers and children in foster care and orphanages. Children with attachment disorders can be frustrating to work with and to parent. They present with a high need to be in control, frequently lie without reason, and are described as having poor eye contact except when lying. Interpersonally they may be overly affectionate and inappropriately related with others including strangers or lack interest in others and do not seek attention. They may lack a conscience and deny responsibility or project blame for their actions. Frequently, they hoard or gorge on food in the absence of want. Nondirective play therapy and sensory integrative therapy have been identified as efficacious therapeutic interventions (Eshelman, 2002; Florey, 2003; Kaplan & Telford, 1998). Many treatments under the rubric of "attachment therapy" remain somewhat controversial, lack empirical support, and are thought to be antithetical to attachment theory (Dozier & Rutter, 2008). Close and ongoing collaboration with the child's family and involving parents in treatment is essential for facilitating successful outcomes. At best, therapists can attempt to assist children with RAD to form a more secure sense of self and others and to guide parents and foster parents to help regulate emotions, understand their children's signals, and provide consistent and committed care (Dozier & Rutter, 2008). (See Chapter 11, "Mental Health of Infants: Attachment Through the Lifespan," for more information on RAD and its treatment.)

CASE ILLUSTRATION

Joe—Family Intervention for a Child with Reactive Attachment Disorder

The consulting therapist for the foster care agency arrived at Joe's home and was met at the door by Joe's mother, Debbie, and his father,

Clint. Once inside, he was introduced to their adopted foster children, Danny, age 14, and Ellen, age 12, as well as Joe, a pre-adoptive foster child who is 9 years old. The reason for the referral was family difficulties arising from parenting Joe, as well as the other children. The therapist's interview with Joe's parents yielded that Joe, who has been diagnosed with reactive attachment disorder (RAD), has been stealing, hoarding food and other items in his room, and "doesn't clean up his messes," nor does he comply with directions to complete chores around the house. Interpersonally he is detached and unaffectionate with Debbie and Clint, but they remark, "he couldn't be nicer to his football coach and teachers, but it's a completely different story when it comes to us." The therapist asked what chores were assigned to each of the children and the parents replied "whatever we ask them to do—they don't do what they're told anyway, so we just end up yelling and fighting over it." When asked what the children's consequences were for not completing their chores, particularly Joe, whose behavior had generated the referral, the parents said there had not been any. The therapist suggested that perhaps a consequence for Joe might be not going to football practice or missing a game, since it was something that he valued. Debbie said, "It's too difficult to punish just Joe. All of the kids have activities after school and in the evening, so if he had to stay home, they all would have to stay home, because Clint works second shift, and I can't leave Joe home alone while I drive the others to their activities." Clint said, "Anyway, it wouldn't be fair to Joe's team. It's his responsibility to be there, and it's not the other kids' fault that Joe won't listen to us."

Intervention

The occupational therapist had a "family meeting" during the initial visit to develop and begin implementation of a family chore list. He established that the parents were in charge of this, and asked them to develop a specific list of chores for each child for the next session. Additionally, he asked the parents to develop reasonable consequences for when a child didn't complete his or her chores, and also rewards for their successful completion. The children were asked to consider what their consequences should be as well, all of which would be discussed during the next visit. The therapist then met privately with Debbie and Clint and discussed the causes and symptoms of Joe's RAD. He asked them not take Joe's behavior personally, but to put it into perspective given his diagnosis and make a list of realistic goals. He also stressed the need to reinforce Joe's positive behaviors by "catching him doing something good," as this is often difficult for parents of children who present with symptoms like Joe. Additionally he provided them with a pamphlet on the disorder to read and asked them to make a list of any questions they had for the next session. In the next session, the occupational therapist held another "family meeting" to implement the family chore list. Each child was informed of their assigned chores and the list was posted on the refrigerator, where it could remain visible and the children could easily refer to it throughout the day. All of the children agreed to give this a try, and also presented possible consequences for not completing their chores such as losing their allowance, having to go to bed early and not being able to play video games. When meeting with the parents following the meeting, the therapist further discussed with them how Joe's diagnosis affected his behavior and interactions and consequently their family and home life and discussed how to set more realistic expectations.

Discussion

Many of Joe's presenting problems were the direct result of having RAD. By providing the parents with education regarding the disorder, he guided them to make more realistic goals for a child who undoubtedly was difficult to parent, and the stress on the parent's marriage and home life improved for them, and the family as a whole. The therapist recognized the family's need for structure, consistency, and consequences for behavior is illustrated by the family meeting approach that unified the parents and established appropriate roles for them and their children through the various interventions. Parenting skills were also addressed in terms of having them consider looking at chores and other household responsibilities as opportunities to reinforce positive and extinguish negative behavior and provide rewards for compliance rather than using inconsistent punishment. Reactive attachment disorder is difficult to treat, and many of the presenting problems and symptoms displayed are not necessarily going to be resolved, as these children often change very little in terms of their personality, temperament, behavior, and interactions with their adoptive parents. Therefore, as in this example, it is necessary to treat the whole family system to affect change and bring about positive therapeutic outcomes. (For an additional case example, see "Anna" in Chapter 13, "Mental Health of Adolescents.")

Children may have more than one disorder. For example, children with ADHD may also have depression, obsessive-compulsive disorder (OCD), or all three. Children with depression may also have an anxiety disorder, and sensorimotor problems may coexist with many disorders.

The presenting problems encountered by occupational therapists treating children with emotional problems are varied (Florey, 2003; Lewis, 2002; Rutter & Taylor, 2002; Sadock & Sadock, 2007). Some may be specified by the V-codes listed in Figure 12-1. Other "typical" psychosocial stressors may include the parents' divorce; emotional, verbal, physical, and/or sexual abuse; other traumatic events, such as the death of a sibling, parent, or grandparent; and socioeconomic conditions that may be coded according to Axis V of the *DSM-IV-TR*. The child may respond to traumatic events by withdrawal, aggressive or atypical behavior, or regression to behavior expected from a younger child. Sometimes the child is confronted by a physical condition such as diabetes, which may limit the child's ability to play and eat what others are eating or require an unusually strict adherence to a medication and blood-monitoring situation (see Chapter 15, "Psychosocial Issues in Physical Disability," for further information regarding psychosocial factors in physical illness). The child may find the illness overwhelming and consequently start acting out at home or become noncompliant with the treatment of the illness in an attempt to exert control.

In other cases a dysfunctional family situation may have led to treatment. Parents sometimes lack the parenting skills required for rearing a normally developing child. In such circumstances, it may be a lack of parental supervision, an inability to set and enforce limits and rules, or the failure to distinguish and differentiate the needs of the parent from the needs of the child. In other situations, parents have placed expectations on children that the latter find overwhelming, such as a parental need to see a child excel in academics or athletics, whether or not the child values these activities. Sociological factors, such as poverty, violence, and crime, may constitute a stressful environment, resulting in depression or anxiety and leading to a need for treatment. Whatever the antecedents that lead to a child receiving professional treatment, the primary reasons are similar to many psychiatric intervention situations. These factors include the following:

- Danger of harming oneself or others
- A breakdown in role functioning, namely, appropriate behavior as a sibling, student, playmate, son, or daughter
- A decrease in obedience to, or compliance with, authority figures
- Social withdrawal
- Increase in aggression or other unacceptable or inappropriate acting-out behaviors, such as fighting, truancy, criminal activities such as theft or vandalism, fire setting, and violence directed toward pets or other animals
- Use of drugs or alcohol
- Stopping medications
- Dropping grades

Other conditions that contribute to emotional problems in children include fetal alcohol spectrum disorders (FASD) (Centers for Disease Control and Prevention [CDC], 2010). Fetal alcohol spectrum disorders include fetal alcohol syndrome (FAS), alcohol-related neurodevelopmental disorder (ARND), and alcohol-related birth defects (ARBD), ARND and ARBD formerly being described by the term fetal alcohol effects (FAE), which sometimes impair a child's ability to learn from experience or impair the usual responses to medical interventions. The offspring of mothers who used or abused alcohol or drugs during pregnancy may display a wide range of often unpredictable developmental deficits that complicate treatment and may adversely affect outcomes. These various conditions affect each child differently and can range from mild to severe.

Regardless of the unique circumstances that are part of a child's particular situation, the onset of the illness varies with each child, based on diagnosis, genetic predisposition, level of disability, and equality-of-life factors such as income level, access to health care, and stability of the family situation. Children's emotional and behavioral problems and the consequences of interpersonal and social impairments become more visible once they reach the age where they can be observed by others at day care, preschool, or the school system setting. At this time difficulties tend to become more evident and families often seek professional, clinical help.

HELPFUL CONCEPTS FOR TREATING CHILDREN

Because children are developing a self-identity and learning how to behave in their social world, concepts such as structure and consistency, interpretation, time-out, limit setting, avoidance of power struggles, modeling, and a consistent team approach are important to keep in mind when working with children. Although some of these concepts are used when working with adults, who presumably have developed some sense of identity and acceptance of social norms, they are particularly important for the developmental period when individuals are learning who they are and how to function successfully in the world.

Structure and Consistency

Two fundamental principles guiding treatment in pediatric occupational therapy addressing mental health issues are **structure** and **consistency**. For individuals with poor impulse control, attention deficits, hyperactivity, or poor response to limits and rules, increasing the amount of structure can improve their response to activity interventions, help them learn how to modulate their own emotions, and assist them in learning appropriate role behavior. The environment itself is used to provide cues to appropriate behavior similar to those used in milieu therapy or therapeutic communities.

Structure can be verbal, such as the tactic of redirection, or physical and tangible, depending on the specific activity or equipment used. **Redirection** can be defined as a verbal tactic that adds to the structure of therapy by refocusing the child on the assigned or current activity in which the child is participating and providing cues as to appropriate involvement or behavior. For example, Holly, a 9-year-old girl stops painting her sun catcher and, due to her impulsivity, leaves her seat to retrieve another one, even though she has not finished painting the first. Redirection can be provided by the therapist saying, "Holly, you are doing a beautiful job of painting your suncatcher, what color are you going to use next? Why don't you show me?" Such a statement cues Holly as to where she should be and what she should be doing in a positive way. Redirection such as in this example proves to be more effective than saying "What are you doing out of your seat?", which allows for a variety of responses on Holly's part, none of which may be the one desired by the therapist. Activities can begin with the imposition of verbal structure, such as directions and limits or rules regarding the activity. For example, the group leader or therapists may say: "Today in group we are going to share the toys in the playroom. There can be no hitting. If anyone hits someone else, he or she will have to leave the group." This instruction provides an idea or standard that can be referred to throughout the group session that provides structure, and consistency that can be established when the therapist removes a child each time he or she hits another child. For children, a poster that lists the rules of the group or activity provides an additional reference point that can be used to remind them of the structure (see Figure 12-2).

"Announcements" can be used to start a group. The children can be asked to tell something about themselves or their progress toward therapy goals. They can be encouraged to share "news" such as upcoming family events, plans for the future (following discharge from therapy), changes in their lives, activities in which they have participated, and the like. Announcements provide the therapist with useful information that may explain the child's response to therapy on that particular day. For example, if a child states, "My mom is taking me to family therapy after OT today," changes in mood or decreases in frustration tolerance might be attributed to anxiety regarding the outcome of the family therapy session later that day. This in turn may enable the therapist to make a successful interpretation that can help the child cope more effectively, learn to express feelings more adaptively, and benefit more from occupational therapy that day.

When conducting groups it is important to ensure that the group begins and ends at the designated times and follows the established routine as much as possible. Naturally, a variety of unpredictable and unavoidable circumstances can interfere with the daily course of programming. For example, a therapist may be sick or on vacation, or special events, such as holiday parties, may take temporary precedence over scheduled programming. In such cases it is important to inform clients of changes in the established consistency. This practice can prevent the eruption of acting-out behavior from a client who may otherwise feel unable to trust the adults and the therapeutic environment responsible for his or her care (see Figure 12-3).

Occupational Therapy Group Rules
1. Have Fun
2. Share
3. Listen to Staff
4. Clean Up

FIGURE 12-2. Rules Poster
© Cengage Learning 2013

1. To deal with impulsivity, never put anything on the table where you are having a group activity unless you want the children to touch it.
2. Ease transitions, which are frequently difficult for children with mental illness, with a "five-minute warning" before the group ends to prepare them for the change and deal more adaptively with endings.
3. To prevent overstimulation, provide a warm, softly lit environment that is soothing and as free from unwanted noise, disruption, and distractions as possible.
4. Children with emotional disturbances can act out often and produce a considerable amount of maladaptive behavior in therapy. "Catch them being good"—praise positive behavior as often as possible.
5. Maintain an even tone and affect while providing treatment. Your calm demeanor may influence the disruptive child's behavior—at least occasionally!
6. Sometimes groups just fall apart despite the therapist's best efforts and interventions. Don't insist that the activity occur if the children aren't ready to participate. Two effective solutions are to *end group* and *sit quietly and wait for the children to regain control.* Children learn that acting out and disruptive behavior lead to the natural consequence that they lose the opportunity to be involved in the activity. If sitting quietly lasts until the end of group time, they usually realize that their behavior prevented play and say, "Hey, we didn't do anything yet!" Gently remind them that they will need to be in control in the next session if they want the activity to happen.

FIGURE 12-3. Six Therapy Tips
© Cengage Learning 2013

A clinical example of acting-out can be seen in the case of a child, Joanie, who was not made aware of the impending absence of the therapist who normally ran her group.

CASE ILLUSTRATION

Joanie

When Joanie, 8, arrived in the therapy room, she learned that the group had been changed from an art group to a play group, which caused her to cry, kick, and scream. When an interpretation was made that the child appeared very upset, she blurted out: "I wanted to have art! I have to paint my project so I can give it to my mother!"

Discussion

Had she been informed of the change beforehand, the incident might have been averted and, instead, Joanie might have (1) been able to present her disappointment and concerns calmly, (2) been provided with options for completing her project, and (3) thereby learned how to express her internal feelings and thoughts acceptably.

A point that may be implicitly understood by occupational therapists is that another way to provide structure is through activities themselves. "The child's developmental progression is facilitated by play, games and activities, integral functions of a child's daily life" (Abramson, 1982a, p. 61). An example is making a tile mosaic project in a **parallel task group**. Structure is provided:

- When each client has his or her own project, which encourages work in a specific spot and focuses attention on a personal project.
- When an example or sample is provided that may be followed to enhance redirection to task.
- When the instructions are clear (e.g., "put tiles in the tray like this"). This encourages following the stated direction.
- When steps are graded according to therapy goals (e.g., "pick up each tile and glue it in place").

Children enjoy the structure of individual activities, which can serve as a means of exploring their abilities and skills and learn about their strengths and limitations. Puppetry, doll play, and drawing provide a technique for dramatizing and externalizing intrapsychic issues. For the older latency-age child, board games may become catalysts for communication and interpersonal relationships. "At all times, play, games and activities are active experiences, and their focus on productivity and participation offer intrinsic satisfaction for the child: To cultivate those skills necessary to fulfill life roles "(Abramson, 1982a, p. 61).

In general, in planning activities for children it should be constantly considered whether:

- The activity chosen is age-appropriate
- The activity is broken down into steps that the child can understand
- The steps are age-appropriate for a child to carry out independently
- The therapist wishes the child to carry out independently or by asking for assistance

For example, if an activity should involve a child sustaining attention to a task, perhaps a tile mosaic project involving the selection of a number of small tiles placed in a trivet is the activity of choice. If improving self-esteem is a consideration, an easy-to-do, foolproof activity such as painting a sun catcher or lacing a small coin purse may do. Where individual play skills are lacking, perhaps the creation and assembly of a toy car that the child can use independently or in conjunction with other children is the activity of choice. In any case, the activity should facilitate developmentally appropriate skills and be fun and intrinsically motivating for the child.

Although there are common considerations when choosing an activity for any person, for a child it is particularly important to be mindful of dangerous parts such as sharp edges, toxic chemicals, or toxic paints or parts that can be ingested, such as small wheels found on a toy car for toddlers. Another consideration is whether there are any items that could be used in a suicide attempt or injurious behavior, such as when knives are being used in a cooking group.

Thorough activity analysis, performing sharps counts (i.e., the number of knives, scissors, etc. used in the group), and limiting the length of string or ribbon provided are ways of ensuring safety both during therapy and afterward when projects are taken home. Depending on the participants presenting problems, copper tooling, for example, may be the wrong activity for a group of aggressive children who may not respond to the structure of the activity or may use the materials inappropriately to harm themselves or others.

Interpretation

Interpretation of, or putting words to, behavior is a therapeutic technique that provides a child with an avenue to express feelings with words, which is more often appropriate than other means such as aggression or acting out. This is often an effective way of de-escalating a child or adolescent who is displaying behavioral problems that result from an inability to use words for self-expression. In the example of Joanie, interpretation involved the therapist identifying to the child in a clear and supportive manner what she observed. Joanie could then better express the behavior's cause (whether the change in routine, a reminder of a **dynamic** within her family, or a feeling she could not identify). The identification of these issues by using interpretation clarifies the situation at hand and teaches a more adaptive coping strategy: the use of words to express feelings and reach acceptable solutions to problems. Activities can be used to provide opportunities to externalize intrapsychic issues or facilitate communication. Once issues have been externalized or communicated, interpretation helps children to understand, learn, cope, and adapt emotionally (Abramson, Hoffman, & Johns, 1979).

Time-Out

Time-out is an intervention technique that results in behavioral changes and increases the child's understanding of her role in a situation. If a child is asked to take time-out for kicking a peer while fighting over a toy, he will learn that aggression leads to the loss of the chance to play. Time-out also provides an opportunity for the adult to teach the child how to share. Thus, the child becomes better able to perceive the situation and learn from it. Similarly, if a child is removed from therapy for aggression or breaking the rules, she will become better able to think about the situation and learn from it. Time-out is the process of removing a young person from a problematic situation to a specific area away from the group and, at the same time, allowing him or her to think about the behavior that led to removal from the group.

The length of time-out should vary with the individual's age and mental capacities. For example, when a child has provoked a fight with a peer, he will be removed to a time-out chair, a "think about it" area, or another room, where he will be requested to remain for a specified amount of time. Depending on his age, he may be asked to remain in time-out until he can count to 10 or until a minute goes by on a timer. An often stated rule of thumb is one minute per year, that is, a 5-year-old would be placed on a five-minute time-out. However, what may be most effective is for the time-out not to have a specific time in minutes, but last until the child regains control and can effectively process the situation. Using this approach one can avoid situations where the child has regained control, yet had several more minutes of time-out remaining. To be consistent, the adult would have to maintain the time-out until its predetermined parameter, which may allow the child to begin acting out again and not benefit from the experience (Moffit, 1987). Immediately after the time-out the child is most amenable to positive interaction and should be engaged in the activity in a constructive way and then praised for constructive behavior. After the activity, it is important to critically analyze the incident. The child and adult should meet briefly to discuss the behavior that led to the time-out, evaluate whether the intervention was useful for the client, and develop a plan of action that will be utilized in future situations. A plan of action may involve identifying with the client alternative coping strategies (such as a self-assigned time-out) or the use of assertive responses (such as letting an adult know when he or she is feeling frustrated or agreeing on a "code word" to indicate the need for a behavior change). This process should be kept as brief as possible so that acting-out behavior is not reinforced. When used properly, a time-out can be efficacious in changing maladaptive behavior to that which is more socially appropriate. Time-out should not be conceived of as a punishment, nor should the individual taking a time-out think of it in this way but more as a consequence for problematic behavior or actions. It is important to present the time-out as a way to learn new behavior so that a positive learning experience may occur and negative or maladaptive behaviors may decrease.

Limit Setting

Limit setting involves informing others what is permissible and what is unacceptable; it lets individuals know "how far they can go." Setting limits is especially important for children because they need, and look for, limits which eventually become internalized as a set of rules that guide socially accepted behavior. The teaching of behavior such as learning to respect the property of others and not taking what doesn't belong to them begins when children are told, in effect, "Thou shall not steal" (whether this occurs at home, in school, or in a religious setting), and the rule is enforced by the parent. When consistent enforcement of the rule or limit occurs, appropriate behavior will be learned and becomes a part of that person's internal code of values, morals, or conscience. Children are protected by rules or limits, such as when adults instruct them that they may play in the yard but not in the street, or that they must be home before a certain hour. This not only teaches safety and prevents harm; it also shows children that their welfare is the concern of the parent or other adult. Limits that are thus enforced clarify the relationship between the parent (or other adult) and child and teach appropriate role behavior. Limits should be friendly but firm, short, and impersonal. Limits can be put in the context of the group rules, as when the occupational therapist says: "We must share the toys," or when a parent states, "The house rules say that fighting over what program to watch on TV leads to an early bedtime for everyone." Although setting limits may be interpreted as punishment, if stated in a protective and supportive, friendly, but firm way, it will foster more mature behavior. Naturally, the amount of limit setting depends on the needs of the child and the comfort level of the therapist (Abramson et al., 1979).

An excellent resource for shaping and modifying behavior in children between the ages of 2 and 10 years old is *1-2-3 Magic! Training Your Preschoolers and Preteens to Do What You Want* (1995) by Phelan, which develops the child's ability to follow rules and comply with adult authority. Although it is written for parents, any adult working with children who require effective behavior modification could use the concepts.

Therapeutic Use of Self

The therapeutic use of self entails the development of an individual style that works with clients in a specific way to promote change and growth and help to provide a corrective emotional experience. This is a difficult concept, or "art," to describe. "The art of occupational therapy involves captivating the child through toys, objects, and games or through the therapist's own actions so that the child becomes involved in the therapeutic process. This art is almost intangible" (Kramer & Hinojosa, 2010, p. 574). An occupational therapist responds to a child in a therapeutic manner, conveying appreciation of the child's uniqueness, kindness, love, and understanding; guiding the child through each step of occupational therapy intervention; and encouraging him or her to accomplish the task that has been chosen to meet the treatment goal. Each therapist will develop a unique and personal style or therapeutic personality for working with patients. The therapeutic use of self requires providing a new response to an old situation, which enables the client in turn to respond in a new manner that is both adaptive and appropriate. (See Chapter 19, "The Use of Psychosocial Methods and Interpersonal Strategies in Mental Health," for a further discussion of intersubjectivity and the therapeutic relationship.)

CASE ILLUSTRATION
Kay—The Therapeutic Use of Self

Kay, a client on a children's unit, could not sustain her interest or complete tasks as assigned. During a cooking group, the occupational therapist assigned her the job of chopping vegetables to be put in a salad. However, Kay did not stay with her task, and, moments later, she was in another part of the room engaging in an activity that had been assigned to another child. The young occupational therapist, in a raised voice, told Kay, "You are not where you belong," and asked what was her task. Kay said, "I'm supposed to be chopping vegetables." The therapist said, "You are driving me crazy," to which she responded, "You sound just like my mother: she always says that." At that point, the therapist realized he was not being therapeutic and was indeed responding to Kay in the same manner in which adults had always responded to her. Therefore he acknowledged that fact, apologized for sounding impatient, and redirected Kay to the task at hand (as he should have done previously).

Discussion

As demonstrated by the therapist in this case, the therapeutic use of self involves responding to clients in a way that will guide them onto a new path through developing behaviors that are appropriate and socially acceptable. This involves responding to clients in a different manner than nontherapeutic individuals in past situations.

Team Approach and Family Involvement

The team concept is particularly essential in providing services and family involvement in treatment is of utmost importance for children because of their roles as family members. Other family members should be consulted and included on the team whenever possible and be a part of treatment goals and decisions. Developmental life roles also are demonstrated to children and adolescents by other professionals such as teachers and education specialists; other therapists, such as psychologists, speech therapists, psychiatrists, or pediatricians; and activity and sports leaders, such as coaches and community activity leaders. Others who participate in a child's life should be regularly consulted. (Naturally, consultation will be with permission of the client or the responsible parent whenever possible.) Contemporary descriptions of the role of occupational therapy show that more than just sensorimotor or neuromuscular skills are being addressed for the child population. Specifically, programs are suggested that include parent-skills training, parent support and education, and facilitation of families' abilities to interact while conducting daily life occupations (Ireys, Dvet, & Sakwa, 2002; Lougher, 2001) as well as assessing play through family narratives (Burke & Schaaf, 1997).

Medications

Even though some medications, such as Ritalin, have received controversial media attention, a variety of other medications are judiciously used in the treatment of children in addition to the psychostimulants. However, there are concerns over the increase in psychotropic polypharmacy and rates are on the rise, as reported in an article titled *Pediatric Psychotropic Polypharmacy* that appeared in the August 2005 issue of *Psychiatry*. "Psychotropic Polypharmacy has been defined as the practice of prescribing two or more medications for one or more diagnosed psychiatric conditions and/ or behavioral symptoms" (Zonfrillo, Penn, & Leonard, 2005). Corresponding with this author's clinical experience, "psychiatric inpatient facilities have higher rates of polypharmacy than outpatient facilities and pediatric offices" and "in all populations, however, a stimulant co-prescribed with other drugs appears to be the most frequent form of polypharmacy. There has been an increase in the rates of prescribing atypical antipsychotics" (Zonfrillo et al., 2005).With regard to using medications to treat bipolar disorder in children, the concerns of which can be universal at this point in time, is the concern that "physicians and mental health professionals turn to pharmacological solutions because of cost-cutting pressure from insurers and HMOs" (Harvard Mental Health Letter, May 2007). In this author's inpatient experience, insurers considered medications to be "active treatment," while patients could access and participate in occupational and other therapies on an outpatient basis. In reality, medications are more readily available in most communities, especially in comparison to rural and underserved parts of the country where consumers live a distance from the urban and suburban centers where therapy services are available and accessible. Medication is often needed to assist the client in gaining control over his or her behavior or stabilizing symptoms so that she or he may more readily participate in therapy. In a clinical setting, medication is often selected after members of the interdisciplinary treatment team, including parents and guardians have been consulted and ideally the client has been observed in a variety of settings. The occupational therapist can contribute valuable observations of the client in various life roles or occupational settings following assessment of the children as they participate in therapy.

While medication is often needed to assist the client (and a psychiatrist or family physician is ultimately responsible for prescribing medications), it is important for the occupational therapist and other team members to monitor the medicated child's behaviors and physical and mental status carefully. The occupational therapist works closely with the individual and may be the first to observe emerging side effects or changes in behavior. In home, school, and outpatient settings, the same would hold true for family members, educators, and therapists working in the community. It is particularly important to monitor medications closely in young people because psychoactive medication sometimes interacts with the neurochemistry of the synapses and may interfere with development of new neuron networks and neurologically based competencies. Therefore, cognitive and behavioral approaches are usually attempted before a consideration of pharmacology.

CHILD SETTINGS AND PROGRAMS

When considering various program options, the best program will be the most normalized and balanced one, often with the goal of minimizing the need for further intervention. Children's programs may necessarily be based on a habilitative rather than a rehabilitative approach. Habilitation involves addressing skills and behaviors that were previously unlearned and undeveloped. This is opposed to the rehabilitative approach often used with adults, which focuses on the retrieval of skills clients already have or had prior to their current illness (Lambert, Moffitt, & Rose, 1989).

The role of the registered occupational therapist has been described broadly in the literature. Kent described the OTR working with children with psychosocial dysfunction as a developmental therapist with an assessment role of evaluating functioning level in skills and interests (cited in Sholle-Martin & Alessi, 1990). The OTR's role with children has been described as based on social learning, behavioral, psychoanalytic, systems analysis, and developmental models (Lougher, 2001), as well as the occupational therapy theories of Mary Reilly (1974). Evaluation emphasizes play history, temperament, family dynamics, and patterns of behavior, and treatment modalities include play, behavioral management, sensorimotor integration, values clarification, and activity groups (Reilly et al., cited in Sholle-Martin & Alessi, 1990). According to Lambert and Moffitt (1988), OTRs also implement parent–child activity groups to improve parents' ability to interact with their children (cited in Sholle-Martin & Alessi, 1990).

Inpatient hospitalization, long-term residential treatment, outpatient settings, community-based programs, partial hospitalization programs, and school-based settings may all offer opportunities for the therapist interested in providing therapy to children with mental health concerns; however, opportunities in the more traditional settings are declining. Anywhere there are children there is a possible treatment setting in which their psychosocial needs may be met. This avenue needs to be pursued if occupational therapists are to continue to use their valuable mental health skills and knowledge with children. Past developments and opportunities within the school system and occupational therapy in partial hospitalization programs are discussed here.

School-Based Programs

Following the Columbine High School shootings in April 1999, the mental health needs of children received a great deal of attention from clinicians as well as the mass media. New roles identified for occupational therapists include conducting screenings for "signs and risk factors" among students that "related to conflict and violence" and providing groups to improve appropriate expression of feelings and improving self-esteem (Johansson, 1999).

According to Hill, anger management is a critical focus (cited in Johansson, 1999, p. 9). Being part of a critical incident debriefing team in schools, working with students following a traumatic violent event, has also been identified as a role for therapists working in schools.

School districts are required to meet the special needs of their students in cases where performance in the classroom is affected. Depending on the county and the particular office of education, there may be opportunities for the occupational therapist interested in working to meet the school-aged clients' psychosocial needs. Some counties are meeting the psychosocial needs of severely emotionally disturbed (SED) students through programs offered on public school campuses. Such programs typically provide services through a special education teacher, psychiatrist, and social worker as well as teacher's aides and assistants who work with the clinical staff. Occupational therapists are included in some of these programs and may provide services including assessment, treatment, home programs, school programs, and consultation. In the school-based setting, the goal is to increase the student's function in the special education classroom with the long-term goal of participation in a regular classroom. All treatment goals should indicate progress toward this end. The occupational therapist is able to view students holistically, observe their performance in the classroom, and provide the necessary services for skill development, adaptation, and improved classroom success.

Two pertinent articles (Barnes, Beck, Grice, & Murphy, 2003; Case-Smith & Archer, 2008) illuminate the direction occupational therapy in children's mental health must move as well as present the stumbling blocks that prevent us from addressing their psychosocial, emotional, and behavioral needs. Occupational therapists working in pediatrics, from early intervention to the school systems, have been slow to provide treatment that if it were truly holistic, would include addressing all of a child's or student's presenting problems, not just those on the referral.

The school setting remains one of the largest areas of occupational therapy practice, and despite that fact, it has not yet become a noted provider of occupational therapy services that address the mental health needs of students. According to a 2008 study by Case-Smith and Archer, rather than addressing mental health issues, practitioners in school settings stated that disruptive behaviors were barriers to their treatment. They believed that these therapists perhaps did not recognize that the behavior itself could be a target for treatment and perhaps behavioral change was not part their services. Additionally, nearly two thirds of the participants in their study did not think that they were prepared to work with emotional disturbances. A 2003 study by Barnes et al. found the following obstacles to providing occupational therapy for students with emotional disturbances in the school setting according to practitioners in their study: confusion about the occupational therapy role, limited knowledge or support from the team, and bureaucratic administrative factors, among others. Other professionals believed that the role of occupational therapy was to address handwriting and sensory integration issues and that addressing the mental health needs of students was out of their purview. At the same time, therapists in this study, as in the study by Case-Smith and Archer (2008), did not believe they possessed the knowledge or preparation to provide mental health interventions. (See Chapter 22, "Psychosocial Occupational Therapy in the School Setting," for ways to overcome these barriers and to work with psychosocial issues.) These studies would lead one to believe that either we are not adequately preparing practitioners to address mental health issues or, once in the educational system, they feel confined to a narrowly defined scope of practice. The following case illustration provides examples of how a therapist working in an educational system may utilize mental health practice skills along with those required to provide services to students that address educational issues.

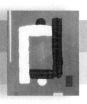

CASE ILLUSTRATION

Ryan

Ryan is a 10-year-old boy who is home schooled and receives weekly home-based occupational therapy. The therapist is working on Ryan's IEP goals of improving letter formation and spacing, visual-perceptual skills, and attention span. Following participation in a drawing activity and several games of "Connect Four" to work on improving prehensile and visual perceptual abilities and increasing his attention to tasks, which he enjoys a great deal, the therapist asks Ryan to write a sentence of his choosing on lined paper designed to improve handwriting skills, a task that has been part of his therapy sessions throughout the school year. Ryan says "I can't do that. It's too hard" and begins to lightly hit himself

in the head with his hand. The therapist, who by observation and experience knows that Ryan is not injuring himself, states "Ryan, I know that this is something that you don't enjoy doing, none the less, we are going to work on writing, which is one of the reasons we work together each week." Ryan lightly taps his forehead on the lined paper on the table and continues "I just can't!" The therapist says, "Ryan, what is something you did at your grandmother's house last weekend? I know you really enjoy going there. Maybe we could draw a picture of that after you write your sentence. Hey, maybe the sentence and the picture could be about that." Ryan stops acting out and says, "I played baseball with my cousins and my team won!" "That sounds like a lot of fun, Ryan; why don't you make that your sentence?" Ryan picks up his pencil, writes the sentence, and then draws a picture of the baseball game.

Discussion

This case illustration demonstrates how using mental health interventions such as redirection, interpretation, limit-setting, a client-centered approach, and therapeutic use of self facilitated Ryan's ability to participate in therapy. In addition to the goals in his IEP, the therapist was able to address problems that Ryan faces that impede his ability to complete his assigned school work by addressing his decreased frustration tolerance and his maladaptive coping skills.

Partial Hospitalization

Partial hospitalization programs are sometimes referred to as day treatment programs. They are another alternative designed to prevent children from entering or staying in an inpatient hospitalization setting. These programs also provide a useful service of transitioning the client from an inpatient to an outpatient setting or to provide an educational experience when the regular school cannot currently meet the needs of the child with a mental illness. These programs are sometimes affiliated with a mental health unit or residential program in the community. The clients will attend a program during typical school hours and will receive treatment groups or therapy more intensively than if they were only receiving outpatient therapy. The student may attend a program like this to avoid hospitalization or to make necessary adjustments to medication under a supervised setting. As with the school-based program and most treatment programs, the goal is to improve the clients' functioning to the degree to which they can be placed in a less intensive/restrictive environment.

IMPLEMENTING PROGRAMMING FOR CHILDREN

When developing a program of occupational therapy, it is important to assess the needs of the children, demands of the service delivery system, and structure of the program. For example, if developmental motor lags are an area of concern, sensorimotor groups may be planned. Where play skills are lacking, play groups and opportunities to develop age-appropriate play skills are of prime importance. If children in the treatment setting have difficulty expressing their thoughts and feelings appropriately, programming should address these needs (Lambert et al., 1989; Lambert & Moffitt, 1988).

The second critical step is to look at the service delivery system itself. In acute care settings there is relatively little time to provide treatment before discharge looms. Often it is the role of occupational therapy and the treatment team to begin treatment with the idea that it will be continued outside the hospital setting at school, in a partial hospitalization setting, or in an outpatient office. In a longer-term setting, treatment may be carried out entirely in one place, although because of the frequent changes in health care delivery, there may not be an extended period of time to bring about change. In terms of planning occupational therapy for an existing program, it is important to understand how therapy fits into the current program in terms of philosophy and program needs. This makes an understanding of theory important and flexibility imperative. The therapist must assume a systems approach, involving an awareness of the current program, the service delivery system, and the client's needs.

In addition to occupational therapy assessments based in specific frames of reference, groups and activities are determined by the developmental needs of individual children. For example, a child may be 12 years old chronologically but function at a 3- or 4-year-old level, with a limited ability to express feelings in words and impaired cognitive skills secondary to a diagnosis of pervasive developmental disorder or intellectual disability. Such a child may be placed in a play group that meets the needs of his or her developmental, age-appropriate level. The child's play and social behavior can be observed at the same time he or she is provided with opportunities for developmentally appropriate play activities. When a child is observed to be playing successfully at a developmentally appropriate level, he or she may then be moved up from a play group to a skills group to learn further personal and social skills (Lambert et al., 1989).

Evaluation and Assessment

General areas of assessment concern the occupational performance areas of self-care and play and also developmental milestone achievement (see Parham & Fazio, 1997, for many assessments of play). Play can be evaluated by observing a child at play and obtaining a play history concerning what toys and games the child chooses. The occupational performance mental, sensory, and movement-related functions under client factors to be assessed are primarily sensorimotor, cognitive, psychological, and social. The Child and Adolescent Functional Assessment Scale (CAFAS) is widely used (Bates, 2001; Hodges, Wong, & Latessa, 1998). Formal evaluations such as the Test of Visual Motor Skills (TVMS), the Good-Enough-Harris Draw-A-Person test, or the Erhhardt Developmental Prehension Assessment (EDPA) may further evaluate adaptive motor skills and coordination as well as a basic assessment of achievement on expected developmental milestones (cited in Asher, 2007). A useful tool for a quick assessment of many components is the Kinetic Self-Image Test (Abramson, 1982b), developed as part of the Initial Play Interview at Mount Sinai Hospital in New York. In this test, the child is asked to draw a picture of himself or herself doing something. Besides data regarding sensorimotor and cognitive functions and skills, valuable information such as interests, relationships, and self-concept can be determined. The Child Occupational Self-Assessment (COSA) and Pediatric Volitional Questionnaire (PVQ) (Kielhofner, 2007) are also some of the tools from the Model of Occupational Therapy Clearing House that determine interests (COSA) and motivating environments (PVQ).

CASE ILLUSTRATION

Josh—Kinetic Self-Image Assessment

Josh, a newly admitted boy, drew a picture of "me, my mom and Dad going for ice cream." Although the boy was 11 years old, he provided basically stick figures and a poorly drawn house. During the evaluation, Josh kept looking at the clock, and he also asked to go to the bathroom several times. When asked if he had an appointment or was waiting or looking for someone, he said, "I have a family session at 3 o'clock." However, when asked if he was leaving group to see if his parents had arrived, he angrily denied it.

Discussion

This simple assessment can be helpful in determining mental age and motor coordination, what the child is thinking about, and the quality of family or personal functioning and relationships.

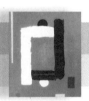

CASE ILLUSTRATION

John and Stephen—Kinetic Self-Image Assessment

John, age 10, and Stephen, age 8, were being seen for evaluation during their initial home-based therapy visit. Their parents had recently separated and the boys lived with their mother, who is a nurse. Their father had been described as having bipolar disorder and alcoholism. Divorce is probable and their mother was referred to the therapist by an outpatient child psychiatrist after he evaluated the older child. The mother, concerned with the children's reaction to the separation and pending divorce, wished to provide an outlet for the children's feelings and an arena for them to discuss their concerns. Additionally, she has concerns regarding a strong family history of bipolar disorder and alcoholism on both sides of the family and the possibility of these disorders emerging in the children. In the initial session, the Kinetic Self-Image Assessment was used to assess the boys. Each was asked to draw a picture of himself doing something. John drew a picture of "playing ball with my dad." Of note was a tall tree drawn in the center of the paper separating the boy from the father. Stephen drew a picture of "John and me playing catch." It included birds, trees, and a yellow sun.

Discussion

Clearly, John's relationship with his father and spending time with him are important and his concern about the separation is evident in the picture. For Stephen, the focus of the picture was playing with his brother and with its details and pleasant presentations indicates either a more positive approach to family dynamics or denial of the current situation.

Intervention

Play is often referred to as the work of the child; it is generally defined as the way children learn basic skills and resolve intrapersonal and interpersonal conflicts.

"From a child's play we can gain understanding of how he sees and construes the world[;] . . . play refers to a young child's activities characterized by freedom from all but personally imposed rules, . . . by fantasy involvement and by the absence of any goals outside of the activity itself" (Bettelheim, 1987, p. 15).

It is helpful to distinguish play from games because the latter are a predominant occupation of older children and adolescents. Games are usually competitive, and have agreed-upon rules that are imposed externally. Games require that the activity be pursued in a prescribed manner, without one's personal fantasy, and there is often a goal, such as winning, outside the activity (Bettelheim, 1987). With the basic acceptance of the importance of play (and later, games) as treatment (Kaplan & Telford, 1998), and also with the recognition of play as the predominant occupation of childhood, it is the primary occupation used in pediatrics and the primary activity used in pediatric groups (Abramson et al., 1979; Hoffman, 1982; Lambert & Moffitt, 1988; Parham & Fazio, 1997; Sholle-Martin & Alessi, 1990). In fact, "play therapy has become the main avenue for helping young children with their emotional difficulties" (Bettelheim, 1987, p. 15).

Play is also the primary mode of evaluating children, which is done through specific assessments and interviews and by ongoing observation. Observation, based on the broad education and the unique and specific knowledge of occupation possessed by therapists, is an excellent evaluation in and of itself. In terms of its use with children, "observation provides the opportunity to document occupation-based assessment without having to depend on youth's willingness and ability to answer questions" (Quake-Rapp, Miller, Gomathy, & En-Chi, 2008). There are various ways to initially evaluate and continue to observe play. Some useful categories to think about while observing play are (C. Grandison, personal communication, January 28, 1997):

- Developmental or stage of play, such as solitary, exploratory, parallel, project, or cooperative: A 2-year-old can be expected to engage mostly in parallel play, whereas a 10-year-old can be expected to cooperate with other children in play.

- Entrance to play: For example, does a child hesitate to play or quickly bolt toward the toys?

- Initiation toward play: That is, (1) does a child initiate play independently or wait for someone to start with, and (2) is the same pattern consistent throughout play?

- Energy level: What is the level of energy of the child at play and does it change within or over sessions? Is it the same with or without structure? Is it the same with a parent present?

- Body movement and use of space: That is, does the child know where others are? Does he or she define a small area or fill up every space? Does the child use furniture?

- Emotional tone: That is, what is the emotional tenor to the play (e.g., is it angry or sad?) and does it remain the same over time?

- Materials: What materials does the child gravitate toward and how are they used?

- Symbolic nature of play: For example, does the child use objects and play symbolically? What are the themes of play, and are they consistent throughout?

An ongoing, regularly scheduled play group also provides information as to the child's current developmental level of play as reflected in the choice of toys, games, and peers while engaged in play.

There are various play scales (Asher, 2007), play classifications (Florey, 1968), and histories that include other observations and categories. The Knox Play Scale (Knox, 1974) and the revised version (Knox, 1997), the Preschool Play Scale-Revised (PPS-R), use categories of space and material management, imitation, and type of participation. Another play observation looks at toys chosen, time of participation, quality of interaction with the toy, language, and social qualities to play. There is an emphasis on the play's developmental level (e.g., solitary, exploratory, parallel, etc.) and theme (such as aggressive, destructive, nurturing, etc.). A Parent-Teacher Play Questionnaire (Scutta & Schaaf, 1989) elicits information from others concerning a child's favorite toy, choices of toys, playmates, preferred locations for play, and any changes in the past week. The Test of Playfulness (TOP) (Bundy, 1997, 2003) observes and measures intrinsic motivation, internal control, freedom from constraints of reality, and the ability to give and read cues. It is an observational measure of play in an environment that is familiar to a child. It also measures intensity of play and play skills.

Groups

Play group is a **nondirective play group** that occurs most easily in the context of an occupational therapy playroom. A nondirective play group allows children to gravitate to and engage in the play occupations of their own choosing without the direction or suggestions for participation from the group leader. For purposes of observation and ongoing assessment, this allows for a truer picture of the child's abilities, interests and play skills, and an age-appropriate opportunity for the child to present personal and family dynamics without any leading remarks from the group leader that could bias the child's responses. On an acute inpatient unit, such a play group has been particularly efficacious for early **latency age** children. "[It] is a valuable diagnostic tool as well as a developmentally appropriate way for the children to interact with their peers and to deal with potentially stressful situations" (Abramson et al., 1979, p. 391). It also enjoys broad application to a variety of settings, particularly in outpatient therapy and in various community programs. The group's protocol is illustrated in Figure 12-4.

NAME OF GROUP: Occupational Therapy Play Group

DESCRIPTION: Play is an important part of a child's development. Children learn, express themselves, and develop interpersonal interaction skills through play. Through play, children are able to express inner feelings and conflicts in a nonthreatening way. This group's primary goal is to evaluate skills and provide an adequate environment where the children's dynamics, developmental level of play, and socialization skills can be observed and practiced.

THERAPIST NAME: William Lambert, OTR/L

TITLE: Occupational Therapist

GOALS:

1. Provide a stimulating environment where the children will be motivated to play.
2. Encourage peer interaction through play.
3. Provide insightful interpretations related to the play when appropriate.
4. Allow the children to work through dynamic issues through the play.
5. Encourage the highest developmental level of play and interpersonal interaction possible.

ENTRANCE CRITERIA:

1. Group members are selected by the OTR according to their developmental levels of play.
2. Five children is an optimal number of group members.
3. Patient has appropriate level of privileges.
4. Patient has been medically cleared by physician.

GROUP RULES:

1. Have fun
2. Share
3. Listen to staff
4. Clean up

FORMAT:

Group meets two times per week for 45 minutes with two leaders: the OTR and a member of the nursing staff.

EXIT CRITERIA:

1. Change in level of privileges.
2. Change in developmental status.
3. Discharge from the hospital.

FIGURE 12-4. Play Group Protocol
© Cengage Learning 2013

The room includes toys, water and sand play areas, dress-up clothes for fantasy play, and a table and chairs. It serves to encourage the development of play skills, which in turn facilitates the development of social skills. The play group also has the goal of providing an arena whereby children may resolve conflicts and issues that led to their current problems and dysfunction. For example, two children may use dolls to express anger at parents who abused them. They may also recreate arguments or scenes they observed in the home. For example, by using toy sharks, a child may safely and appropriately show anger or jealousy toward a sibling or peer by "eating" him or her during water play or "burying" him or her in the sandbox. A game like Sorry! helps increase frustration tolerance, and a game like Twister develops not only laterality but also the ability to practice being in close proximity to others while appropriately interacting and respecting body space. Beanbag toss games are an appropriate outlet for anger and aggression and also provide the opportunity to engage in turn taking and mild competition. Candyland and Connect Four are just a few of the many readily available childhood games that can be used or adapted to develop many different skills and prompt conversation and discussion. Inherent in many childhood games such as "Duck, Duck, Goose," "Musical Chairs," and "Dodge Ball" is a focus on developing a variety of basic abilities. "Rolling Dodge Ball" can be played in place of the conventional game. This adaptation involves rolling rather than throwing the ball at peers. This increases safety and prevents the game from becoming overly aggressive.

There are countless ways in which play can help children learn new skills and accomplish treatment goals. For example, it is more efficacious to ask children to try to clean up the entire playroom before you can count to 10 than it is to just command them to clean up the playroom because "it's time to end group." Turning an activity into a game or play, as in this example, is often more effective than other approaches. It is also congruent with the philosophy of occupational therapy and the general approach of using play as a treatment modality. The active experiences of play and the focus on productivity and participation offer intrinsic satisfaction for a child's needs. Aside from conflict resolution, play also offers children the additional ability to work on treatment goals of improving impulse control, developing cognitive skills, mastering the environment, and developing age-appropriate social interactions. Through the mastery of tasks, latency-aged children will be able to benefit from the successful interaction with objects and people in an occupational therapy group and gain mastery over themselves in the process.

Creative task groups also serve as highly effective interventions with latency-aged children. The use of tiles to make mosaics, wood projects such as creating a bookshelf or making a toy car, painting sun catchers, or participating in seasonal activities such as carving a pumpkin or baking Christmas cookies offer children rewarding experiences. In addition, the experiences teach appropriate interaction, and develop cognitive skills, such as the ability to follow directions, complete tasks, and share materials as well facilitate increased attention span and concentration. Comments made about the projects often provide a valuable additional perspective on a child's emotions and concerns. Copper tooling is a highly successful creative task project. Children frequently ask, "Can I do more than one?" or after successful completion of the project, they will ask, "Can we do copper tooling projects again?" Children have remarked, "It's fun to do—it's easy to make." Indeed, the steps of copper tooling are easy to grade according to the therapeutic purposes of the group, and the completed project reinforces self-efficacy, increases self-esteem, and validates the individual's efforts to affect positive change on the physical environment through the creation of a tangible object that may be personally enjoyed or given as a gift.

Of course, it is important to take safety precautions while completing copper tooling projects such as removing the solution (liver of sulfur) as soon as all group members have used it and conducting the group in a well-ventilated area.

Most often, creative tasks are provided as part of a parallel task group. This structure provides opportunities to develop appropriate interpersonal interactions on a limited basis, share through the use of supplies that are common to the group activity, and develop impulse control by waiting to follow the steps and to see the project through to completion.

Group goals may include learning how to follow simple, step-by-step verbal directions; sharing materials and space; interacting without being intrusive; sustaining and increasing attention span; and developing impulse control. Other information that can be gained through the use of a simple craft project includes dynamic information such as whom the gift or project is to be given and, therefore, who is important in the child's life.

Skill development group assists older children who have adequate play and social skills and need to improve problem-solving, coping, and communication skills. See the group's protocol in Figure 12-5. Group topics and discussion focus on common problems and situations that children face as well as the specific problem areas that led to treatment.

While a variety of activities can be used in the skills development group, including crafts, therapeutic board games are frequently used. "Stress Strategies" is a game used to develop coping skills, and "The Talking, Feeling, and Doing Game" (Lambert et al., 1989) facilitates the expression of thoughts and feelings. Both are examples of games that are effective in meeting treatment goals. Because they use a board game format, children are usually willing to participate and an appropriate amount of structure is provided. Children are often happy to have an outlet for their unexpressed feelings and thoughts and view the game as a safe and nonthreatening means of personal expression. See Figure 12-6 for ways to assure that the environment supports effective group and individual interventions.

NAME OF GROUP: Occupational Therapy Skill Development Group

DESCRIPTION: A developmental task group for children who have developed basic play and social skills and need to acquire skills in cognition, interpersonal interactions, and self-expression.

THERAPIST NAME: William Lambert, OTR/L

TITLE: Occupational Therapist

GOALS:
1. To improve cognitive skills such as:
   a. problem-solving
   b. organization of thoughts
   c. ability to follow directions
2. To improve interpersonal interaction skills and facilitate sharing cooperation.
3. To improve ability to express thoughts and feelings appropriately.

ENTRANCE CRITERIA:
1. Group members are selected by the OTR according to developmental need.
2. Patient should be on appropriate level of privilege to attend groups.
3. Patient is medically cleared by physician.
4. Five to seven children is the optimal number of group members.

GROUP RULES:
1. Have fun
2. Share
3. Listen to staff
4. Clean up

FORMAT:
Group meets two times per week for 45 minutes with two leaders: the OTR and a member of the nursing staff. Activities will be planned to develop specific skills through the use of games and creative tasks.

EXIT CRITERIA:
1. Change in level of privileges
2. Discharge from hospital

FIGURE 12-5. Skills Development Group Protocol
© Cengage Learning 2013

CASE ILLUSTRATION

The Talking, Feeling, and Doing Game

Seven children ages 8 to 12 years old are playing the game with the occupational therapist, a member of the nursing staff, and an OT student.

Sam rolls the dice, lands on a yellow space, and selects a "feeling" card, which reads: "Name three things that could cause a person to be angry."

He pauses and then says, "Being told to shut up, being hit, and being lied to." Dave lands on a white space and selects a "talking" card, which reads, "What kind of work does your father do? What do you think about that kind of job?" Dave answers, "He fixes trucks," although he does not mention that his father is in prison. "I'm going to race motorcycles when I grow up," he says when asked what he thinks of his father's job. Christine rolls the dice and also lands on a white space. Her card asks, "What is the best thing you can say about your family?" She replies, "They bring me candy and lots of things." John lands on a red space and picks a "doing" card, which reads, "Skip across the room and then return to your seat." He says, "I'm not doing that," but he agrees to take another card. This one asks him to pretend that he is having an argument with someone and to tell the group what it is about. "I'm arguing with Melissa. She won't share," John replies. The therapist then rolls and lands on a "feeling" space. His card reads, "When was the last time you cried?" He says, "I cried when my dad died." Then he talks about how crying is helpful in expressing feelings of sadness. Linda and Rhonda, the other adults in group, reinforce what the therapist has said. This helps the children talk about their feelings and express them appropriately.

Discussion

This game promotes, through talking, the expression of what is on children's minds. The game facilitates the expression of feelings, promotes the discussion of personal problems, and can explore family dynamics without threat and in a manner that matches the children's emotional age. It is important to have a good working knowledge of the children in the group and be familiar with their individual histories and issues to lead a game such as this effectively.

- Soft lighting to provide a calming atmosphere.
- Area rugs or carpet to play on.
- Colorful but not overstimulating room.
- Adequate tables and chairs. These do not need to be child-sized except for younger preschool-age children. Most latchkey-age children can use a conventional-sized table and chairs.
- Materials should be easy to clean.
- An area for water play and larger gross motor groups is ideal, but be adaptive! A bathtub or utility sink can do as needed or on a regular basis, depending on funding, facility, and frequency of use.
- Craft paper in large rolls can be used for many purposes—to cover the table for a craft activity, to do body tracings, to make murals and drawings, and so on. This inexpensive investment goes a long way and lasts a long time!

FIGURE 12-6. Tips for Creating an Effective Playroom or Therapy Area

There are ever-increasing numbers of blended and nontraditional families in the United States (Dozier & Rutter, 2008; Waterman, 2001). The traditional family may no longer be constituted of a biological mother and father with biological siblings. Children and adolescents may be adopted and raised by extended families, grandparents, relatives, stepparents, or family friends. Whoever the child or adolescent considers to be "family" may be permitted to join in treatment, as is often the case in the parent–child activity group (Lambert, 1990).

The parent–child activity group (Lambert, 1990) involves engaging the parents of the emotionally disturbed child in an activity with the child. It was held weekly in the occupational therapy room where families worked on a project together with the goal of completing it in one session. This group improves the parent–child interaction by engaging them together in a pleasurable, successful activity, something that may not otherwise be possible due to the child's illness. The therapist provides encouragement and support and models appropriate caregiver behavior such as setting limits on inappropriate actions and giving praise for desirable ones. The OTR assists parents in differentiating between behavior that is maladaptive and behavior that is typical for the child's developmental level. Beyond providing occupational therapy for families and their children, the OTR is able to provide those involved in the child's treatment with information about family interactive patterns, the child's response to therapy with the parents, and how well the parents are implementing what they are being taught about how to interact with their child. The parent–child activity as originally conducted expanded the scope of occupational therapy in the hospital setting to areas traditionally reserved for individual and family therapists. By providing information on the child's behavior and the therapeutic outcomes of the session, occupational therapy has enhanced the interdisciplinary treatment team's ability to see the child and family more globally and respond with more integrated treatment for both. This group can be effectively used in a variety of settings, including the home, school, or outpatient office, both with individual families or several families attending the same session. Depending upon the specific reasons for referral and the expectations of the referral source, clinical information gleaned may be shared with other clinicians involved in the case, or used by the group leader with the group participants. At the conclusion of the session the therapist may choose to process the session with all the participants present, privately with the parents/guardians or both, with both usually being the norm. Regardless, it is generally beneficial to meet with the parents/guardians apart from their children to provide opportunities for questions, discussion, and teaching or reviewing effective and appropriate parenting and intervention skills.

EXAMPLES OF EMERGING AREAS OF PRACTICE

Therapists have been challenged to follow clients into the community, to consider consulting as an alternative to direct service, and to find new sources of funding, including cash (Kautzmann, 1998; Kornblau, 1999; Learnard, 1998; Richert, 1998). Clinicians need to present occupational therapy outcomes (Richert, 1998) and market to the needs of clients and community agencies. As the location of care moves out of the hospital and lengths of stay become increasingly shorter, one arena for therapists is to go into private practice and consider private pay for reimbursement of services through community-based practice (AOTA, 2008; Dorman & Helfrich, 2001; Ramsey, Best, Merryman, Learnard, & Scheinholtz, 1998).

Following are examples of emerging areas of practice that can be implemented by using the interventions originally used in an inpatient setting described earlier in this chapter in the community through private practice. These interventions include consultation and direct service for a foster care agency and home-based therapy and are reimbursed through the therapist's private practice. Both involve a family-centered approach and a fee-for-service format for payment (cash or check). Traditional forms of reimbursement such as private insurance or managed care companies are *not* utilized or accepted. This arrangement also adds an increased measure of confidentiality and the therapist, family, or agency can determine the number of sessions.

Occupational Therapy Services for a Foster Care Agency

Providing occupational therapy services for a foster care agency brings unique and rewarding challenges and illustrates a new role for occupational therapy in the community in a nontraditional practice setting (Benoit, 2000). "Foster children exhibit diverse psychological, emotional, and behavioral problems, which have been well documented. The literature repeatedly reports that foster children have high rates of mental health, behavioral, and adaptive functioning issues" (Precin et al., 2010; see also Dozier & Rutter, 2008). The child in foster care can be assisted in adapting to various situations through occupational therapy intervention that increases the child's ability to function in an age-appropriate manner at his or her current level of development. Intervention is aimed at reducing the number of times that a child's life is interrupted so that agency goals of successful pre- and post-adoptive placements can be achieved, as well as easing a child's transition from a foster care placement to reunification with the biological parent(s) and birth family (Barney, personal communication, March 10, 2003; Derdeyn & Lamps, 2002; Nickman, 2000).

Frequently the long-term goal of foster care is to have the children reunified with their family of origin. Some states, such as California, may also pursue adoption at the same time that family reunification is attempted. Therefore, having consistent therapy that focuses on children's functioning may help them negotiate this difficult adoption or reunification situation.

CASE ILLUSTRATION

Reunification—The Rinaldo Family

Jose, age 5, lives in a large city with his mother, Rosalita, age 27. They have just successfully completed family-based therapy sessions with the occupational therapist, which was an essential piece of their reunification plan. Now Rosalita and Jose will again have Juan, Sophia, Carlos, and Jesus back in the home. Currently Juan, age 10, lives in a foster care home. Sophia, age 8; Carlos, age 6; and Jesus, age 3½ live in another foster care home. Reunification will be facilitated through two separate intervention strategies. First, parent–child activity sessions with the entire family will be conducted by the occupational therapist once a month. Second, the OTR will schedule sibling groups between the family sessions to reacquaint the brothers and sisters with each other. Rosalita and Jose arrive for their scheduled parent–child activity on Saturday morning, and join the other siblings and the OTR at the occupational therapy office. The initial intervention is for the children and mother to play together using the toys in the room, and later to make pudding to have for dessert, which will follow a lunch provided by the foster care agency. The OTR begins the activity by asking, "Juan, why don't you be a big brother and help your little sister and brothers by being in charge of pouring the milk?" This intervention occurs once the therapist notices that Rosalita appears overwhelmed and makes no attempt to organize the task. The OTR then notices Jesus

crawling for the door and retrieves him. "Sophia, will you keep an eye on Jesus so he doesn't get into trouble?" suggests the OTR. Eventually Rosalita opens the pudding package after reading the directions to the children, several of whom are not paying attention, and begins giving her children various tasks to complete. The OTR moves to the periphery of the room to facilitate the mother taking charge of the situation and to assess the parent–child interaction. Once the pudding has been spooned into cups and put in the refrigerator, the OTR cues the family to clean up the dishes. The family is given time to socialize as they wait for pizza to be delivered. The younger children fight over a toy but the mother redirects them to share. Juan, as usual, is quiet and isolative. Rosalita picks up the toddler and attempts to engage Jesus in play with nearby toys. Jose engages in spontaneous play with his younger brothers and wrestles with them. Sophia, who had been drawing, starts to cry, as she feels left out. The OTR suggests ways for her to ask her siblings to play with her, such as asking them to come draw with her or to play a game.

Discussion

Occupational therapy groups were used to facilitate reunification of several siblings living in different foster care homes with their biological mother and an additional sibling residing with her. Sibling groups based on the play-group format refamiliarize the siblings with each other during sessions employing play, games, and arts and crafts in addition to developing and building relationships and interactions among the children and provide opportunities for professional observation and assessment. The sibling groups were used in conjunction with a parent–child activity that occurred during the biological mother's scheduled monthly visit with all of her children, a vital part of the reunification process. This group used activities such as making pudding and simple meals, arts and crafts, structured play, and games designed to reinforce roles of mother, older brother, sister, younger brothers, and toddler with the therapist serving as facilitator. These groups were used to promote appropriate parent–child interactions and establish filial roles. The groups also provided a therapeutic milieu for the mother and children to meet each other in a safe setting for not only interaction but also expression of feelings regarding present and future visitation (Barney, personal communication, March 10, 2003).

The therapist provided role modeling and suggestions for improving parenting skills. He also solicited the mother's feedback as to how she perceived the reunification process to be progressing. The therapist also provided the foster care agency with ongoing reports and his assessment of family functioning and helped determine when reunification would occur. Following 21 months of occupational therapy intervention, the family was reunited and continues to live together. While therapy progressed well across time, other factors, such as the mother finding an appropriately sized home, having the home approved, and various bureaucratic requirements, lengthened the reunification process. This case illustrates how the luxury of time and many ongoing sessions can exist when traditional reimbursement sources are not used (Lambert, 2003).

Foster Care Agency—Expert Witness

In another case of family reunification, the mother failed to attend any of the scheduled parent–child activity sessions. During groups with the occupational therapist, the siblings consistently expressed their desire to remain in the preadoptive foster home and to be adopted by their foster parents. At the custody hearing, the report of the children's desire to be adopted and to have the biological mother's rights terminated to facilitate their adoption was presented to the judge and served as an objective outside opinion as well as an expert witness. In chambers, the children corroborated the therapist's testimony and the judge ruled for termination based on the children's statements, the occupational therapist's evidence, and that of others involved in the case. This evidence from various sources paved the way for adoption in an appropriate home for these children (Lambert, 2003).

Testifying in court is a unique experience (Rosen, 2002). Some suggestions when testifying are to remember to always address the judge as "your honor" and answer only the questions you are asked succinctly and specifically. The more information volunteered, the more opportunities the opposing side's attorney has to discredit your testimony.

In court hearings to involuntarily terminate parental rights of children in foster care who want to be adopted by their foster parents the responsibilities of the therapist are specific. They are to assess the children through information from interviews and therapy sessions. Then in court the therapist presents her or his clinical opinion regarding what outcome the children want, their feelings regarding the termination, and what outcome she or he recommends based on her or his area of expertise and clinical experience.

Being a witness in court includes being a developmental specialist, child advocate, and clinical expert regarding children's behavioral and emotional health through the eye and lens of occupational therapy.

Foster Care Agency—Direct Service

The occupational therapist provides other services for the foster care agency including family intervention and troubleshooting regarding developmentally appropriate rules and activities for children in foster care. This is especially important in instances where the foster parents require direction and instruction to smooth family difficulties and deal adaptively and appropriately with the children and their diverse issues, presenting problems, and diagnoses. (See the previous Case Illustration of Joe and his family earlier in this chapter.)

With the aid of occupational therapy intervention, a foster care or preadoptive home placement can remain consistent and reduce the number of times that a child's life is interrupted (Barney, personal communication, March 10, 2003). Minimizing interruptions is imperative to the mental health of children in the foster care system (Dozier & Rutter, 2008; Waterman, 2001).

Home-Based Occupational Therapy

Occupational therapists have been encouraged to develop new strategies for serving the mental health needs of children and their families (Dorman & Helfrich, 2001). Therefore, home-based intervention has been cited as a growing area of practice and uses the natural setting of the home to assess and treat areas of behavior, family dynamics, and parent–child interactions (Case-Smith & O'Brien, 2010). Interventions can include anger management, social skills training, and parent–child activities. The parent–child activity discussed previously in this chapter and in foster care case interventions above is also part of a home-based approach with the added dimension of using the family home as a treatment setting. This provides an *in vivo* environment

(Shultz et al., 2001) to observe situations and interactions that affect therapy outcomes but are not able to be observed in other settings. For example, the 24-hour television, the dog running through the house barking because of a thunderstorm, a younger sibling who intrudes on the session with his brother and steals game board pieces, dinner late or burning, and so on, provide real-life situations and stressors that can be observed and used as intervention points in therapy.

Upon referral from a child psychiatrist, occupational therapists may see children and their families in their own homes to address the variety of psychosocial deficits and problems that led the children and their families to seek professional help. Again, the duration and length of therapy is determined largely by the family and the therapist, with direction provided by the referring psychiatrist. The occupational therapist must possess an extensive background in providing psychosocial interventions to children with emotional disturbances and their families and be able to practice autonomously. An additional benefit to this practice setting is that there is rarely a missed appointment, although a family may forget about the scheduled visit. Receiving payment upon conclusion of the session eliminates the need for billing, and seeing children and their families in their homes eliminates the need for renting office space. However, it does include other incurred expenses that should be taken into account regarding billing and determining the hourly rate, such as mileage, the price of gas, and increased wear and tear on one's car. Also, like many other home health therapists, one's car becomes a clinic where supplies are kept, and for a pediatric therapist the car often becomes a traveling collection of toys, games, and other therapy supplies.

Infant mental health is a relatively new area of pediatric mental health that offers opportunities to occupational therapists (Bazyk, 2011; Jackson & Arbesman, 2005). Additionally, addressing bullying and other current problems facing young people offer opportunities for therapists wishing to address the psychosocial needs of this population. (See Chapter 11, "Mental Health of Infants: Attachment Through the Lifespan," and Chapter 13, "Mental Health of Adolescents," for more information on these topics.)

SUMMARY, CURRENT TRENDS, AND RECOMMENDATIONS

The various conditions of children with mental illnesses include *DSM IV-TR* (APA, 2000) Axis I diagnoses such as depression, bipolar, and post-traumatic stress disorders, in addition to disorders first diagnosed in infancy and childhood, such as attention deficit hyperactivity, oppositional defiant, reactive attachment, and disruptive behavior disorders. When connecting behavior and diagnosis, genetic predispositions to mental illness and the symptoms and presenting problems of the disorders should be considered as well as environmental psychosocial stressors such as family dysfunction, abuse, trauma, neglect, violence, and poverty. Developmental level and age-appropriate tasks should also be considered when working with children with emotional disturbances.

Useful concepts to consider when working with this population are structure and consistency, redirection, interpretation of behavior, time-out, a personal therapeutic style, a team approach, and the judicious use of psychotropic medications.

When implementing a programming for this population it is important to consider the needs of the consumers, the demands of the service delivery system, and the structure of the current or planned program. Various assessments, including observation, are useful tools for occupational therapists planning therapeutic interventions. Interventions for children can be based primarily on play and include nondirective play, skill development, creative tasks, and parent–child activity groups.

"Sicker and quicker" has become an often-used phrase when describing the trend toward offering less time for therapy for hospitalized children who may have very severe emotional and behavioral problems. This is currently true in settings outside of the hospital as well. As managed care often replaces traditional insurance and reimbursement programs, timeframes for therapy are becoming shorter and inpatient hospitalizations are being curtailed in favor of community-based care. Unfortunately, cost containment may also limit access to occupational therapy unless therapists make the transition from traditional hospital and medical model practice settings to emerging areas of practice and community-based care. In an attempt to bring their expertise to these other arenas of the continuum of care, therapists need to "think outside the box," or perhaps "outside of the toy box in the clinic," and explore new ways of providing therapy to this population. These new ways include, but are not limited to, foster care, home, public, and private school settings, and in exploring the possibilities extant in the unfamiliar territory of the variety of agencies and programs already in place that provide services to children with and without identified disorders who to date have not employed occupational therapists, and those who have, most notably the school systems. Looking to the community for the answers to the question of how we can serve children with mental health issues is the beginning of our journey to provide occupational therapy to what may be considered an underserved population. In addition, our unique ability to address the whole child in every way, including occupationally, needs to become an accepted and well known fact to enable us to move forward in meeting the largely unmet needs of children with mental health problems and their families.

Children in need of services to remediate mental and behavioral pathology and develop and integrate new skills can be found everywhere—in the hospital, the school, at daycare, at home, and in your neighborhood (Forness, Florey, & Greene, 1993). This is still true. As children and often their parents are not always effective self-advocates, it is incumbent upon therapists to advocate for appropriate services, including occupational therapy, for underserved populations such as children and their families who are struggling with mental health issues. Indeed the Occupational Therapy Practice Framework (AOTA, 2008) includes interventions for populations and communities, and interventions and outcomes that include advocacy and occupational justice.

In researching this third edition of this chapter, relatively few current articles on the topic of children's mental health were able to be retrieved, despite the American Occupational Therapy Association's emphasis on treatment of children and adolescents with emotional disturbances (Cotrell, 2007). Considering the ongoing discussion on expanding the role of occupational therapy in addressing the mental health of children dating back to at least Llorens and Rubin's (1967) text, *Developing Ego Functions in Disturbed Children: Occupational Therapy in Milieu* and Forness, Florey, and Green's seminal plenary session (1993), *Hidden in Plain Sight: Children with Behavior Disorder in School Systems,* at the 73rd annual conference of the American Occupational Therapy Association in Seattle, WA. it is time to include the mental and emotional health of children in occupational therapy evaluation and treatment interventions. The relative dearth of current research and publications would indicate the great need for conducting and publishing research as well as articles on current practice to add to the body of knowledge in this area for our profession. Without an evidence base for our practice in children's mental health, our continued ability to provide services to this population is placed in jeopardy. Yet occupational therapy has much to offer as evidenced by this textbook.

REVIEW QUESTIONS

1. Which childhood disorder is characterized by a lack of warmth and relatedness by the child toward his parents/caregivers that results from inconsistent parenting and caregiving during infancy and early childhood? Name two symptoms of this disorder.
2. Identify four intervention strategies that can be used to reduce acting-out or behavior problems.
3. What are two creative tasks that are effective in providing structure?
4. Identify three common games that can be used therapeutically with children with mental illness.
5. Identify two play activities that provide age-appropriate outlets for feelings and thoughts in children.

REFERENCES

Abramson, R. M. (1982a). Therapeutic activities for the hospitalized child. In L. Hoffman (Ed.), *The evaluation and care of severely disturbed children* (pp. 61–69). New York: SP Medical & Scientific Books.

Abramson, R. M. (1982b). Developmental and diagnostic assessment. In L. Hoffmann (Ed.), *The evaluation and care of severely disturbed children* (pp. 37–44). New York: SP Medical & Scientific Books.

Abramson, R. M., Hoffman, L., & Johns, C. A. (1979). Play group psychotherapy for early latency-age children on an in-patient psychiatric unit. *International Journal of Group Psychotherapy, 29,* 383–392.

American Occupational Therapy Association (AOTA). (2002, April 18). The psychosocial deficits of children with regulatory disorders. *OT Practice,* CE4–CE6.

American Occupational Therapy Association (AOTA). (2008). The occupational therapy practice framework. *American Journal of Occupational Therapy, 62*(6), 625–683.

American Psychiatric Association (APA). (2000). *Diagnostic and statistical manual of mental disorders.* (4th ed., text revision). Washington, DC: APA.

Argabrite, R. (2002, March 25). O.T. in the schools: Embracing our psychosocial roots. *OT Practice, 7*(6), 21–25.

Asher, I. E. (2007). *Occupational therapy evaluation tools: An annotated index* (3rd ed.). Bethesda, MD: American Occupational Therapy Association.

Barnes, K., Beck, K., Vogel, K., Grice, K. O., & Murphy, D. (2003). Perceptions regarding school based occupational therapy for children with emotional disturbances. *American Journal of Occupational Therapy, 57,* 337–341.

Bates, M. (2001). Child and Adolescent Functional Assessment Scale (CAFAS): Review and current status. *Clinical Child and Family Psychology Review, 4,* 1, 63–84.

Bazyk, S. (Ed.). (2011). *Mental health promotion, prevention, and intervention with children and youth: A guiding framework for occupational therapy.* Bethesda, MD: American Occupational Therapy Association.

Benoit, W. (2000). Foster Care. In B. J. Sadock & V. A. Sadock. (Eds.), *Kaplan and Sadock's comprehensive textbook of psychiatry* (7th ed., pp. 2873–2877). Philadelphia: Lippincott Williams & Wilkins.

Bertucco, M. (2001, May/June). Bad behavior. *Psychology Today,* 28.

Bettelheim, B. (1987, March). The importance of play. *Atlantic Monthly,* 35–46.

Bipolar Disorder in Children Difficult to Diagnose, Reports the Harvard Mental Health Letter. (January 01, 2007). *Health & Medicine Week, 422.*

Bundy, A. (1997). Play and playfulness: What to look for. In D. Parham and L. Fazio (Eds.), *Play in occupational therapy for children* (pp. 52–66). St. Louis, MO: Mosby.

Bundy, A. (2003). *Test of playfulness manual* (vers. 4). Sydney, Australia: University of Sydney.

Burke, J. P., & Schaaf, R. C. (1997). Family narratives and play assessment. In L. D. Parham & L. S. Fazio (Eds.), *Play in occupational therapy for children* (pp. 67–85). St. Louis, MO: Mosby.

Burns, B. J., & Hoagwood, K. (2002). *Community treatment for youth: Evidence-based interventions for severe emotional and behavioral disorders.* New York: Oxford University Press.

Case-Smith, J., & Archer, L. (2008). School-based services for students with emotional disturbance: Findings and recommendations. *OT Practice, 13*(1), 17–20.

Case-Smith, J., & O'Brien, J. (2010). *Occupational therapy for children* (6th ed.). Maryland Heights, Missouri: Mosby Elsevier.

Centers for Disease Control and Prevention (2010). Retrieved from http://www.cdc.gov/ncbddd/fasd/index.html

Cottrell, R. (2007). The new freedom initiative:-transforming mental health care: Will OT be at the table? *Occupational Therapy in Mental Health, 23,* 2, 1–25.

Derdeyn, A. P., & Lamps, C. A. (2002). Adoption. In M. L. Lewis (Ed.), *Child and adolescent psychiatry: A comprehensive textbook* (pp. 1266–1274). Philadelphia: Lippincott Williams & Wilkins.

Dorman, W., & Helfrich, C. (2001). *Psychosocial competence and its impact on function in children and youth.* Paper presented at the meeting of the American Occupational Therapy Association, Philadelphia.

Dozier, M., & Rutter, M. (2008). Challenges to the development of attachment relationships faced by young children in foster and adoptive care. In J. Cassidy & P. Shaver (Eds.), *Handbook of attachment: Theory, research and clinical applications* (2nd ed., pp. 698–717). New York: Guilford Press.

Dryfoos, J. G. (1992). Adolescents at risk. A summary of work in the field: Programs and policies. In D. Rogers & E. Ginzberg (Eds.), *Cornell University Medical College Seventh Conference on Health Policy* (pp. 128–141). Boulder: Westview.

Eshelman, L. (2002, June). *Treatment approaches.* Paper presented at the Reactive Attachment Disorder conference sponsored by the Milton S. Hershey Medical Center College of Medicine, Scranton, PA.

Florey, L. L. (1968). *A developmental classification of play.* Unpublished master's thesis, University of Southern California, Los Angeles.

Florey, L. (2003). Psychosocial dysfunction in childhood and adolescence. In E. B. Crepeau, E. S. Cohn, & B. A. B. Schell (Eds.), *Willard and Spackman's occupational therapy* (10th ed., pp. 731–744). Philadelphia: Lippincott Williams & Wilkins.

Fonagy, P., Target, M., Cottrell, D., Phillips, J., & Kurtz, Z. (2002). *What works for whom?: A critical review of treatments for children and adolescents.* New York: Guilford.

Forness, S., Florey, L., & Green, S. (1993). *Hidden in plain sight: Children with behavior disorder in school systems.* Paper presented at the 73rd annual conference of the American Occupational Therapy Association, Seattle, WA.

Gray, K. (2005). Mental illness in children and adolescents: A place for occupational therapy. *Mental Health Special Interest Section, 28*(2), 1–4.

Hahn, C. (2000, October 23). Building mental health roles into a school system practice. *OT Practice,* 14–16.

Harvard Medical School. (2007). Bipolar disorder in children. *Harvard Mental Health Letter, 23*(11).

Hodges, K., Wong, M., & Latessa, M. (1998). Use of the Child and Adolescent Functional Scale (CAFAS) as an outcome measure in clinical settings. *Journal of Behavioral Health Services and Research, 25,* 325–336.

Hoffman, L. (1982). *The evaluation and care of severely disturbed children.* New York: SP Medical & Scientific Books.

Hollander, E. (2001). *Professional handbook of psychotropic drugs.* Springhouse, PA: Springhouse.

Howes, C., & Spieker, S. (2008). Attachment relationships in the context of multiple caregivers. In J. Cassidy and P. Shaver (Eds.), *Handbook of attachment: Theory, research and clinical applications* (2nd ed., pp. 317–332). New York: Guilford Press.

Ireys, H. T., Devet, K. A., & Sakwa, D. (2002). Family support and education. In B. J. Burns & K. Hoagwood (Eds.), *Community treatment for youth: Evidence-based interventions for severe emotional and behavioral disorders* (pp. 154–175). New York: Oxford University Press.

Jackson, L., & Arbesman, M. (Eds.). (2005). *Children with behavioral and psychosocial needs.* AOTA Practice Guidelines Series. Bethesda, MD: American Occupational Therapy Association.

Johansson, C. (1999, August 5). O.T. prescription for school violence. *OT Week.*

Kaplan, C., & Telford, R. (1998). *The butterfly children: An account of non-directive play therapy.* New York: Churchill Livingstone.

Kautzmann, L. (1998). *Managed behavioral healthcare: Opportunities and challenges for practice.* Paper presented at the meeting of the American Occupational Therapy Association, Baltimore.

Kielhofner, G. (Ed.). (2007). *A model of human occupation: Theory and application* (4th ed.). Baltimore: Lippincott Williams & Wilkins.

Knox, S. (1974). A play scale. In M. Reilly (Ed.), *Play as exploratory learning* (pp. 247–266). Beverly Hills, CA: Sage.

Knox, S. (1997). Development and current use of the Knox Preschool Play Scale. In L. D. Parham & L. S. Fazio (Eds.), *Play in occupational therapy for children* (pp. 35–51). St. Louis, MO. Mosby.

Kornblau, B. (1999). *Expanding your practice in an era of health care reform.* Paper presented at the meeting of the American Occupational Therapy Association, Indianapolis, IN.

Kramer, P., & Hinojosa, J. (2010). *Frames of reference for pediatric occupational therapy* (3rd ed.). Baltimore: Lippincott Williams & Wilkins.

Lambert, W. (1990). *Parent-child activity: Assessment and treatment of families.* Paper presented at the Pennsylvania Occupational Therapy Association Annual Conference, Philadelphia.

Lambert, W. (2003). *Family-centered mental health OT with foster care children.* Paper presented at the meeting of the Pennsylvania Occupational Therapy Association, Pittsburgh, PA.

Lambert, W., & Moffitt, R. (1988). *A collaborative approach to developmental group in child psychiatry.* Paper presented at the Pennsylvania Occupational Therapy Association Annual Conference, State College, PA.

Lambert, W., Moffitt, R., & Rose, J. (1989). *Therapeutic use of toys and games in child psychiatry.* Paper presented at the Pennsylvania Occupational Therapy Association Annual Conference, Hershey, PA.

Learnard, L. T. (1998). *Occupational therapy consultation and rehabilitative services.* Paper presented at the meeting of the American Occupational Therapy Association, Baltimore.

Lewis, M. L. (Ed.). (2002). *Child and adolescent psychiatry: A comprehensive textbook.* Philadelphia: Lippincott Williams & Wilkins.

Llorens, L., & Rubin, E. (1967). *Developing ego functions in disturbed children: Occupational therapy in milieu.* Detroit: Wayne State University Press.

Lougher, L. (Ed.). (2001). *Occupational therapy for child and adolescent mental health.* New York: Churchill Livingstone.

Moffit, R. (1987). *Guidelines for reinforcing socially acceptable behaviors and extinguishing inappropriate, maladaptive behaviors.* Unpublished manuscript.

National Survey Reveals Impact of ADHD. (2002, January 28). *Advance for Occupational Therapy Practitioners,* 42.

Nickman, S. L. (2000). Adoption. In B. J. Sadock & V. A. Sadock (Eds.), *Kaplan and Sadock's comprehensive textbook of psychiatry* (7th ed., pp. 2868–2872). Philadelphia: Lippincott Williams & Wilkins.

Parham, L. D., & Fazio, L. S. (Eds.). (1997). *Play in occupational therapy for children.* St. Louis, MO: Mosby.

Phelan, T. W. (1995). *1-2-3 Magic! Getting your preschoolers and preteens to do what you want.* Glen Ellyn, IL: Child Management.

Pratt, P. N., & Allen, A. S. (1989). *Occupational therapy for children* (2nd ed.). St. Louis, MO: Mosby.

Precin, P., Timque, J., & Walsh, A. (2010). A Role for Occupational Therapy in Foster Care, *Occupational Therapy in Mental Health, 26,* 2, 151–175.

Quake-Rapp, C., Miller, B., Gomathy, A., & En-Chi, C. (2008). Direct observation as a means of assessing frequency of maladaptive behavior in youths with severe emotional and behavioral disorder (2008). *American Journal of Occupational Therapy, 62,* 2, 206–211.

Ramsey, R., Best, L., Merryman, B., Learnard, L., & Scheinholtz, M. (1998). *Payment and programming for occupational therapy in behavioral health care.* Short course presented at the meeting of the American Occupational Therapy Association, Baltimore.

Randolph, E. (1999). *Children who shock and surprise: A guide to attachment disorders* (3rd ed.). Salt Lake City, UT: RFR.

Reilly, M. (Ed.). (1974). *Play as exploratory learning.* Beverly Hills, CA: Sage.

Resnick, R. (2005). Attention deficit hyperactivity disorder in teens and adults: They don't all outgrow it. *Journal of Clinical Psychology, 61*(5), 529–533.

Richert, G. (1998). *Cutting edge response to systems change; Community-based consultation: Expanding mental health services.* Paper presented at the meeting of the American Occupational Therapy Association, Baltimore.

Rosen, D. N. (2002). Testifying in court: A trial lawyer's perspective. In M. L. Lewis (Ed.), *Child and adolescent psychiatry: A comprehensive textbook* (pp. 1309–1314). Philadelphia: Lippincott Williams & Wilkins.

Rutter, M., & Taylor, E. (Eds.). (2002). *Child and adolescent psychiatry* (4th ed.). Oxford: Blackwell Science.

Sadock, B. J., & Sadock, V. A. (Eds.). (2007). *Kaplan and Sadock's comprehensive textbook of psychiatry* (10th. ed.). Philadelphia: Lippincott Williams & Wilkins.

Scutta, C., & Schaaf, R. C. (1989, October). *A time for play?* Paper presented at the Pennsylvania Occupational Therapy Association Annual Conference, Hershey, PA.

Sholle-Martin, S., & Alessi, N. E. (1990). Formulating a role for occupational therapy in child psychiatry: A clinical application. *American Journal of Occupational Therapy, 44*(10), 871–882.

Shultz, S., et al. (2001). *Issues in specific populations and intervention strategies: Behavioral disorder practice model.* Paper presented at the meeting of the American Occupational Therapy Association, Philadelphia.

Waterman, B. (2001). Mourning the loss builds the bond: Primal communication between foster, adoptive, or stepmother and child. *Journal of Loss and Trauma, 6*, 277–300.

Weingarten-Dubin, J. (2001, May/June). More than a mood. *Psychology Today, 26*, 1663.

Zernike, K., & Peterson, M. (2001, August 19). School's backing of behavior drugs comes under fire. *New York Times National Edition, 1*, 30.

Zonfrillo, M., Penn, J., & Leonard, H. (2005). Pediatric Psychotropic Polypharmacy. *Psychiatry, 2*(8), 14–19.

SUGGESTED RESOURCES

Banus, B. S., Kent, C. A., Norton, Y., Sukiennicki, D. R., & Becker, M. L. (1982). *The developmental therapist* (2nd ed.). Thorofare, NJ: Slack.

Berger, K. S. (2008). *The developing person through the lifespan* (7th ed.). New York: Worth.

Bingham, M., Edmondson, J., & Stryker, S. (1983). *Choices: A teen women's journal for self awareness and personal planning.* Santa Barbara, CA: Advocacy.

Blake, J. (1990). *Risky times: How to be AIDS-smart and stay healthy: A guide for teenagers.* New York: Workman. (Spanish version published in 1993)

Byrne, K. (1987). *A parents' guide to anorexia and bulimia.* New York: Henry Holt.

Freud, A. (1967). *The ego and the mechanisms of defense.* New York: International Universities Press.

Gil, E. (1983). *Outgrowing the pain: A book for and about adults abused as children.* New York: Dell.

Hall, C. S. (1982). *A primer of Freudian psychology.* New York: Harper & Row.

Heron, A. (Ed.). (1994). *Twenty writings by gay and lesbian youth.* Boston: Alyson.

Hunter, M. (1990). *Abused boys: The neglected victims of sexual abuse.* New York: Ballantine.

Levy, B. (1993). *In love and in danger: A teen's guide to breaking free of abusive relationships.* Seattle: Seal.

McCoy, K., & Wibbelsman, C. (1992). *The new teenage body book.* New York: Body/Perigee.

New Games Foundation. (1976). *The new games book.* Garden City, NY: Doubleday.

Outward Bound, USA. (1981). *Learning through experience in adventure based education.* New York: Morrow.

Stein, M. B., Hyde, K. L., & Monopolis, S. J. (1991). Child and family outreach services as an adjunct to child and adolescent mental health treatment. *International Journal of Partial Hospitalization, 7*(1), 69–75.

Steiner, H. (1995). *Treating adolescents.* San Francisco: Jossey-Bass.

Vogler, R., & Bartz, W. (1992). *Teenagers and alcohol.* Philadelphia: Charles.

Child and Adolescent Websites

American Psychiatric Association: http://www.healthyminds.org/More-Info-For/Children.aspx

American Psychological Association: http://www.apa.org/pi/families/children-mental-health.aspx

Animal Assisted Therapy White Paper: http://research.vet.upenn.edu/Portals/36/media/CIAS_AAI_white_paper.pdf http://nrepp.samhsa.gov/AboutNREPP.aspx

Child/Adolescent Substance Abuse: http://www.aacap.org/cs/root/resources_for_families/child_and_adolescent_mental_illness_statistics

Images of Children's Mental Health: http://www.google.com/search?q=children's+mental+health&start=30&hl=en&sa=N&biw=1264&bih=620&prmd=ivnscm&tbm=isch&tbo=u&source=univ&ei=911BTtmYD9Kv0AGM7Z3LCQ&ved=0CGQQsAQ4Hg

Mental Health Association - Resources for Young adults and adolescents: http://www.nmha.org/go/children

NAMI—Teen and Child Focus: http://www.nami.org/template.cfm?section=child_and_teen_support

National Center for Children In Poverty Resources: http://nccp.org/publications/pub_687.html

National Federation of Families for Children's Mental Health- Family Advocacy: http://ffcmh.org/

National Institute of Health Medline Plus Library: http://www.nlm.nih.gov/medlineplus/childmentalhealth.html

National Institute of Mental Health: http://nimh.nih.gov/health/topics/child-and-adolescent-mental-health/index.shtml

Substance Abuse and Mental Health Services/Recovery: http://store.samhsa.gov/home

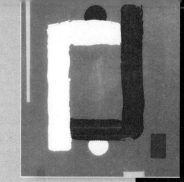

Chapter 13

Mental Health of Adolescents

William L. Lambert, MS, OTR/L
Elizabeth Carley, OTD, OTR/L

KEY TERMS

decompensation

power struggles

resiliency

self-efficacy

self-mutilation

suicide

CHAPTER OUTLINE

Introduction

Etiology of Adolescent Mental Health or Illness

    Cultural and Economic Effects on Etiology of Adolescent Mental Health or Illness

Disorders, Diagnoses, and Presenting Problems

    Presenting Problems

    Suicide

    Self-Mutilation

    Eating Disorders

Bullying and School Violence

Helpful Concepts for Treating Adolescents

    Structure and Consistency

    Limit Setting

    Avoiding Power Struggles

    Therapeutic Use of Self in Relationship

    Creating a Therapeutic Environment

    Team Approach

    Medications/Psychopharmacology

Adolescent Settings and Programs

    Traditional Settings

    Inpatient Programs

427

        Partial Hospitalization Programs
        Outpatient Therapy
        School-Based Programs
        Evidence-Based Programs
    Implementing Programs
    Evaluation
    Intervention
        Arts and Crafts
        Board Games
        Resources for Facilitating Adolescent Topical, Focus, and Psychoeducational Groups
        Creative Expression
    Summary

INTRODUCTION

What comes to mind when you think about adolescence or being a teenager? The responses could be as varied as are the lived experiences of individuals in this developmental stage. As with other stages of development across the lifespan, there may be common characteristics, but just as many differences that depend on a number of factors. We tend to think of adolescence as a period of fluctuating hormones, moodiness, and an angst-filled search for identity, all of which are true. Oftentimes adolescence is conceived of as a necessarily difficult passage, and it frequently is for those individuals having mental health issues, but most likely not more so than people of any age. Are all childhoods happy? Is midlife always met with a crisis? Do the elderly consider themselves to be living in their "golden years"? How many times has an adolescent been told that they should be enjoying themselves because "these are the best years of your life"? This romantic notion is well described by Bruce Springsteen in his song "Glory Days": "Glory days well they'll pass you by. . .", where he tells of tales of reflections of adolescent experience: "I had a friend who was a big baseball player back in high school" and "there's a girl that lives up the block back in school she could turn all the boys' heads."

Stereotypes and misconceptions may cloud our ability to see adolescents as unique individuals whose mental health problems reflect external as well as internal factors. Client-centered care would inform us to consider the individual adolescent and his or her mental health issues in context. Personal factors such as heredity, the family's structure and place on the function–dysfunction continuum, level of ability to cope, **self-efficacy**, resilience and available support systems all play a part in whether or not an adolescent will develop a mental illness. Equality of life issues such as socioeconomic status, neighborhood composition, education, access to healthcare, and availability of social participation present external factors that can play an important role in not only developing mental health problems, but also in how easily they can be resolved.

This chapter will combine the knowledge gained by the authors through decades of working in the field with adolescents with emotional, behavioral, and mental health issues with currently available data and evidence-based information to guide effective and rewarding occupational therapy intervention with this population. Thus, in keeping with the principles that run through each edition, this chapter will rely on theoretical and clinical evidence.

ETIOLOGY OF ADOLESCENT MENTAL HEALTH OR ILLNESS

Many current views of mental illness focus on heredity and genetic predisposition as probable causes, just as these factors are often taken into consideration in the development/acquisition and diagnosis of other physical conditions such as cardiac disease, certain types of cancer, diabetes, arthritis, and so on. The nature versus nurture argument is an old one, but looking at both factors together may be useful. For example an adolescent possessing a strong family history of depression suffers the loss of a parent, which in turn leads to financial problems that necessitate moving to a smaller home in a different neighborhood. The move facilitates leaving friends behind and going to a new school. The multiple losses and the consequences (i.e., loss of support system and social life) of moving experienced by this individual may lead to a major depressive episode that includes suicidal ideation, plan, and intent. However, a different teen without a family history of depression may possess enough internal resources that allow for recovery through the possession of sufficient adaptive coping skills and the ability to use family and others for support. In addition possibly the use of an antidepressant medication and/or outpatient therapy might help resolve this person's grief and loss issues. A possible diagnosis for this second individual might be Adjustment Disorder with Depressed Mood.

A variety or combination of psychosocial stressors may impact an adolescent's mental health, such as physical, sexual, or emotional abuse, experiencing a traumatic event, social isolation, and a dysfunctional family system. Just as these risk factors may increase the likelihood of an adolescent developing mental illness, certain individual strengths can act as protective barriers against the onset of mental health problems. Among these strengths are courage, hope, optimism, interpersonal skills, and perseverance. Being a part of a strong, healthy family system can also support an adolescent in their **resiliency** against mental illness. Although the two complement each other, a distinction has been made between the practices of mental illness prevention and mental health promotion. Prevention focuses on the avoidance of risk factors, while mental health promotion seeks to improve an individual's protective mechanisms, including increasing self-esteem, mastery, well-being, and social inclusion (National Research Council, 2009). Depending on the practice setting and the needs of the individual, occupational therapists can be effective in both prevention and mental health promotion with adolescents. Effective treatment often consists of concurrently reducing risk factors and promoting protective barriers to help our clients achieve and maintain their highest possible level of mental health.

Cultural and Economic Effects on Etiology of Adolescent Mental Health or Illness

The developmental tasks of adolescence are determined not only by biological and physical development, but by cultural and environmental influences. Adolescents from different ethnic and cultural backgrounds can face different expectations in their roles as teenagers. As the United States becomes increasingly diverse, children of diverse cultural backgrounds and children of immigrants enter adolescence with cultural beliefs and values that influence their identify formation and development. Children of immigrants live in families with median incomes 20% lower than the family incomes of children whose parents were born in the United States (Chaudry & Fortuny, 2010). Due to economic hardship, the children of lower income families sometimes face pressures to assist their family, which can lead to a decrease in the youth's motivation or ability to achieve academically. These pressures include parents encouraging their teenage children to work part time or full time to help the family financially or for the teenage girls to stay home and care for their younger siblings while their parents work.

Based on data from 2008, high school dropout rates for children of families in the lowest quartile of income was 16% versus only 2% among the highest earning families in the United States (U.S. Department of Commerce, 2009). There also remains a striking gap in dropout statistics between Caucasian, African American, and Latino adolescents, with African American youth dropping out at more than twice the rate of Caucasian teens, while the dropout rate of Latino high school students is more than four times that of their Caucasian peers (U.S. Department of Education, 2010). Given these statistics, it is apparent that economic and cultural factors affect adolescents, particularly in terms of educational attainment. In turn, poverty and a lack of resources correlate with more violence and higher rates of mental health needs for youth growing up in these environments.

Cultural and ethnic differences also affect the ways in which adolescents experience role identity through the transition from childhood to adulthood. Cultural experiences act as rites of passage for adolescents. Many teenagers attend school dances and begin to date and, through experiences like these, begin to develop an identity separate from that of their parents and family. For example, in many Latin American cultures, the Quinceañera, or the celebration of the fifteenth birthday, represents a girl's entrance into womanhood, and this practice has been adopted by many of Latin American descent who are living in the United States. This idea of a rite of passage can help adolescents identify a concrete point that symbolizes their "becoming an adult," although in reality this is a long process, lasting through the years of adolescence. Similar rites of passage include bar and bas mitzvahs and confirmation, although how much this is experienced as entering adulthood in modern culture is questionable with the current consideration of the period of adolescence extending beyond the teen years and into the early and mid twenties.

DISORDERS, DIAGNOSES, AND PRESENTING PROBLEMS

Mental health diagnoses are currently defined in the *Diagnostic and Statistical Manual—Part IV—Text Revision (DSM-IV-TR)*, which specifies disorders typically diagnosed in childhood or adolescence (APA, 2000). With the expected completion and publication of the DSM-5 (expected in 2013), there may be changes in symptoms, presentation, and diagnostic criteria for certain disorders. It is likely that there will also be the addition of new diagnoses, including those diagnosed during childhood or adolescence, and occupational therapists in mental health settings will need to educate themselves on these revisions, as they may affect the way in which adolescent clients should be treated or observed (see Chapter 5, "Psychological Theories and Their Treatment Methods in Mental Health Practice," for more information on the next edition of the *DSM*). Typical diagnoses vary to some degree according to the treatment setting. Two diagnoses frequently encountered in an inpatient program, where admissions are limited to those in an acute or crisis phase of their disorder, are major depression/major depressive disorders and bipolar disorder, with hospitalization facilitated by being assessed as a serious threat to self or others. Additionally, individuals whose **decompensation** includes self-mutilation or cutting, threatening physical violence, suicidal ideation, intent or plan, or a psychotic episode that may be a precursor to a formal thought disorder such as schizophrenia may also present for treatment in this setting. Other common diagnoses are conduct disorder, attention-deficit hyperactivity disorder (ADHD), personality disorder, attachment disorders, or any of the diagnoses found in the *DSM-IV-TR* that may be assigned to an adult, such as obsessive-compulsive disorder (OCD) or post-traumatic stress disorder (PTSD). Adolescents may also present with co-occurring or concomitant problems with substance abuse and eating disorders.

The diagnoses encountered in outpatient or community-based settings tend to be less acute or serious than among those who have been admitted to an inpatient hospital program. Among the most common are adjustment disorders, dysthymic disorder, disruptive behavior disorder, depressive disorder, ADHD, oppositional defiant disorder, and PTSD (see Table 13-1). These disorders can be co-occurring and may also present with substance abuse issues or eating disorders.

TABLE 13-1. Disorders That Can Be Diagnosed in Adolescence

ATTENTION-DEFICIT HYPERACTIVITY DISORDER (ADHD) AND DISRUPTIVE BEHAVIOR DISORDERS.

ADHD is a behavioral condition that makes focusing on everyday requests and routines challenging. ADHD is distinguished between two types: inattention and impulsivity. ADHD can also present as combined type, with both inattention and impulsivity.

Conduct Disorder	The individual violates rules, age-appropriate norms, or the rights of others, evidenced by aggression against people or animals, property destruction, lying or theft, or seriously violating rules. The symptoms cause impairment in job, school, or social life. Severity, such as mild, moderate, or severe, is also coded. This is a common precursor to *Antisocial Personality Disorder*.
Oppositional Defiant Disorder	Characterized by a pattern of negativistic, hostile, and defiant behaviors.

ANXIETY DISORDERS are found in adolescents and include such diagnoses as *Specific Phobia, Social Phobia, Obsessive-Compulsive Disorder (OCD),* and *Generalized Anxiety Disorder.* In adolescents, generalized anxiety disorder is often expressed as excessive worries over the quality of performance even when it is not being judged.

Post-Traumatic Stress Disorder (PTSD)	An anxiety disorder following exposure to any sort of trauma and causes disturbed thought, flashbacks, and disordered sleep.

EATING DISORDERS are severe disturbances in eating behavior. The most common disorders are *Anorexia Nervosa, Bulimia Nervosa,* and *Eating Disorder, Not Otherwise Specified.* Individuals with anorexia nervosa have disordered thought causing them to restrict food, sometimes to the point of starvation. Bulimia nervosa is marked by consuming of excessive amounts of food, then purging by making themselves vomit or using laxatives.

MOOD DISORDERS

Major Depression	Noted by a period of at least two weeks during which there is depressed mood or loss of pleasure or interest in almost all activities. Sadness is present and in adolescents there may be irritability. Also present may be hypersomnia, psychomotor retardation, and delusions.
Dysthymic Disorder	A chronic form of depression, lasting more than two years in adults, one year in children, and requires the presence of fewer symptoms than the diagnosis of major depression.
Bipolar Disorder	Characterized by both manic and mixed manic and depressive episodes. Approximately 10% to 15% of adolescents with recurrent major depressive episodes go on to develop bipolar disorder.
Cyclothymic Disorder	Characterized by numerous periods of hypomanic and depressive symptoms that do not last long enough to meet criteria for either major depressive episode or bipolar disorder. This disorder often begins in early life and is thought to reflect a temperamental disposition to other mood disorders.

SUBSTANCE-RELATED DISORDERS include disorders related to abusing chemicals, including alcohol, side effects of medication, or a toxin. In adolescents these disorders are most often divided into *Substance Use Disorder* (substance dependence and substance abuse) or *Substance-Induced Disorders* (such as substance intoxication).

Multiaxial diagnoses require occupational therapists to attend to all five axes, but for adolescents they should attend especially to Axis IV, which lists psychosocial and environmental problems.

Adapted from *DSM-IV-TR* (APA, 2000).

Presenting Problems

Changes in occupational functioning, role performance, affect, and mood often signal the development of a mental health problem. The inability to adequately perform occupations in areas of activities of daily living (ADL), instrumental activities of daily living (IADL), education, work, sleep/rest, play and leisure, and social participation that had previously been successful may indicate an evolving mental health problem. Often schizophrenia emerges during late adolescence, and a scenario such as changes in grooming, taking care of one's pet, ability to concentrate on school work, restlessness and an inability to relax, and participation in formerly rewarding free time activities such as computer games or playing golf with friends, along with emerging positive and negative symptoms, could be representative of someone developing a thought disorder. Performance for this adolescent would likely decrease in the roles of family member, student, or friend/peer, as in carrying out the role of emerging young adult who is capable of being well-groomed, appropriately dressed, and able to carry out expected responsibilities in his home, school, and community. Other clinical manifestations represented here would be possible positive symptoms of schizophrenia such as auditory hallucinations and negative symptoms such as a flattened affect and avolition (APA, 2000). The regression in the above scenario, or decompensation, illustrates how treatment for adolescents would tend toward being rehabilitative, rather than habilitative, as is often the case with children, because the adolescent would need to recover lost skills and abilities at which he or she had previously been proficient. Often it depends on the symptoms and characteristics of the diagnosis and the client factors as well as context of the adolescent. It can be useful to view mental health and/or illness as a continuum where one can move back and forth that is unique to the individual. Presenting problems may be seen in overt behavior, sometimes referred to as externalizing, while other, internalizing symptoms are dependent upon the report of the adolescent.

The presence of internalizing and externalizing behaviors and symptoms depends upon the diagnosis and the presentation of the individual. Diagnoses like depression often include feelings of sadness, social isolation or withdrawal, or symptoms that are not necessarily displayed outwardly. Oppositional defiant disorder, on the other hand, is marked by defiance toward authority figures such as teachers or parents, and is often displayed by verbal outbursts, fighting, or otherwise disruptive behaviors. The type of symptoms and behaviors being exhibited can affect the identification of mental illness. For example, those with depressive symptoms that are internalized can be viewed as the quiet or "good" kids in the classroom, and are not identified as having any issues for which they need to receive treatment or support. Those adolescents with disorders that include externalizing behaviors are more frequently identified as "the problem kid" with more referrals to the dean or principal for disrupting their class and peers. Therefore those with externalizing behaviors related to their mental illness can be much easier to identify and diagnose. Because of this, it is important that teachers and other adults who work with adolescents not ignore those individuals who are quiet and may not act out or display disruptive behaviors, so that all youth with mental illness receive the treatment and support they need. The following may be examples of the presenting problems for adolescents with mental health issues, and may signal the need for mental health services:

Changes in behavior:

- Social withdrawal
- Opposition, defiance, and lack of respect for authority figures
- School avoidance/truancy
- Decreased impulse control
- Decreased frustration tolerance
- Aggression

Changes in affect or mood:

- Anger
- Hostility
- Sadness
- Lability
- Grandiosity

Changes in relationships:

- Parent–child
- Siblings/extended family
- Peers/friends
- Teachers/religious leaders

Presenting a danger to self or others:

- Suicidal ideation, intent, or plan
- Threatening harm or death to others
- Risk-taking behaviors
- Use of drugs and alcohol (beyond teenage experimentation)

Suicide

Suicide was the third leading cause of death for young people aged 15 to 24 years of age in 2007. Statistically, women are more likely to attempt suicide than men, with men being more successful at completing a suicide attempt, specifically boys between the ages of 15 and 19 were five times more likely to commit suicide than girls (cited in U.S. Department of Health and Human Services, National Institute for Mental Health, n.d.).

Drawing a plan for suicide is a common step, for example, in high school approximately 1 in 5 and in college 1 in 10 students have written a plan. An alarming 10% of high school student have attempted suicide of which a third of those individual's required medical attention (Gutman, 2005).

A variety of factors may cause an adolescent to consider ending his or her life; for example, the antecedent for an adolescent suicide is in response to an event in the past 24 hours such as rejection-related events by a peer group or a relationship or being in trouble and facing legal or disciplinary action (Gutman, 2005). According to the National Institute for Mental Health (2011), risk factors for suicide include:

- Depression and other mental health disorders
- Prior suicide attempt
- Family history of mental illness/substance abuse
- Family history of suicide
- Family violence, physical or sexual abuse
- Firearms in the home (used in half of all suicides)
- Incarceration
- Exposure to the suicidal behavior of others

    Additional risk factors include (Brent, 2003):

- Co-occurring mental and alcohol or substance abuse disorder
- Parental psychopathology
- Hopelessness
- Impulsive and/or aggressive tendencies
- Life stressors, especially interpersonal losses and legal or disciplinary problems

Frequently it is difficult for professionals, as well as family members, peers, and others, to believe that an adolescent or any individual is seriously considering suicide. However, *all* suicidal verbalizations or gestures need to be taken seriously. The National Institute for Mental Health (2011) advises that the mere mention of suicide should not be considered an attention-seeking behavior but rather a sign of serious emotional distress. Suicide is often looked at in terms of ideation, plan, and intent.

Ideation refers to thoughts of committing suicide; *plan* as the means one would use to carry out suicide or how they one would do it, such as using a gun, by hanging or ingesting poison, and when they would do it such as, upon discharge, after Christmas, or if forced to end a relationship. An individual who has suicidal ideation is unable to reflect back on positive aspects of the past but rather focused on the current unpleasant, negative experience or thoughts. This obsessive thinking of unpleasant, negative experience or thoughts overrides one's memories and is thought by neuropsychologists to facilitate in the brain a network of memories, which can lead to suicidal ideation (Gutman, 2005). *Intent* refers to whether the person is intending to carry out the plan. It is essential that an individual who has intent and is suicidal should immediately seek mental health treatment; this should not be postponed nor should the suicidal person be left unattended (NIMH, 2011). Additional interventions include:

- Attempting to get the person to seek help from a doctor or the nearest emergency room
- Dial 911
- Eliminate access to firearms and other potential items for self-harm, including unsupervised access to medications
- Consider ideation, plan, and intent
- Taking personal responsibility as a professional to keep the individual safe (NIMH, 2011)

Prevention Programs

Prevention programs in schools that identify factors that put kids at risk for suicide can be effective strategies in deterring adolescents from suicide (Brent, 2003). Such programs serve to educate students and families about factors that may increase the risk of adolescent suicide (AOTA, 2005; Brent, 2003). Necessarily it is the role of occupational therapists practicing in settings where adolescents are to be found to develop and implement programming to address the needs of at-risk adolescents. Often such programs are in the educational system and other sites in the community (AOTA, 2004).

One prevention program identified adolescents in high schools to be peer leaders who modeled and trained their peers to identify adults they could trust, as an effort to enhance protective factors associated with reducing suicide. The intervention program increased perceptions of adult support for suicidal adolescents and increased the acceptability of asking for help (Wyman et al., 2010). Adolescents who are having suicidal ideation often do not know where to turn, and increasing their comfort in asking for help, or identifying those adults they feel they can trust could potentially save lives. Occupational therapists working with youth who are depressed and considering suicide can play this important role. Developing the rapport and the trust necessary to build an effective therapeutic relationship could also be vital in gaining the trust of a hopeless teenager, who may feel they have nowhere else to turn. It is also important that as occupational therapists we know how to access the appropriate resources in terms of therapists and crisis intervention for whom to refer suicidal youth, as these individuals may be in need of hospitalization or less restrictive environments in which to receive psychotherapy and other supportive services and possibly medication to treat their symptoms.

Other preventive measures include increasing suicide awareness among this population, their families, and the communities in which they live; developing emergency or safety plans; and focusing on medication compliance (AOTA, 2005), particularly where the medication may have unpleasant side effects. Patient education is also needed to help individuals recognize emerging symptoms and to seek immediate help (Gutman, 2005). Emergency plans, contingency plans and contracts, and specifying what to do if suicidal ideation occurs are essential (Gutman, 2005). Contracts are sometimes called a *contract for safety*. The contract for safety asks the patient to contract, or commit to telling an appropriate person or persons if he or she is having thoughts of suicide. In a hospital or other clinical settings this may be any member in the therapeutic environment. In the community this may be a parent, guardian, or other involved appropriate party with whom the client has agreed to contact in the event of relapse or decompensation.

Occupational Therapy

Occupational therapy intervention for at-risk adolescents focuses on fostering self-understanding through reality-based treatment where participants can develop social and communication skills and identify adaptive coping strategies through meaningful occupations (AOTA, 2004). Occupational therapists can assist adolescents to develop self-management skills and ways to organize the environment to decrease excess stress and pressure. With the client-centered focus that occupational therapy provides, therapists can engage clients in activities that they personally find meaningful and purposeful, and which can improve resiliency and self-esteem. These activities can also aide in decreasing feelings of hopelessness characteristic of depression (AOTA, 2004), as many individuals who attempt suicide meet the criteria for a mental health diagnosis (Gutman, 2005; NIMH, 2011). Occupations selected should teach strategies to manage suicidal thoughts and alternative activities that the adolescent can use to stop or divert them from negative thoughts or suicidal ideation. Therapeutic activities should be chosen that can provide the adolescent with hope and a future-oriented focus (AOTA, 2004) while being developmentally appropriate and satisfying as well. Helpful occupational therapy interventions, according to Gutman (2005), include:

- Patient and family education about suicide and mental health disorders
- Facilitating the ability to manage relapse and disappointment with progress with an effective plan in place

- Assist patients in making realistic choices despite feelings of hopelessness
- Reinforcing the need to remain actively involved in treatment
- Ongoing medication compliance
- Family member involvement
- Identification of support groups and other resources
- Foster understanding of and strategies to handle setbacks in the recovery process

"The first days of hospitalization and the days just prior to discharge are high risk periods for suicide" (Gutman, 2005). As people stabilize, they can experience a period where they do not appear suicidal; however, their positive mood often belies the fact that they have made the decision to kill themselves. This is commonly believed by many clinicians in the field. Patients are also often disappointed with the course of recovery as setbacks and relapses can and do occur as recovery is not always complete (Gutman, 2005).

It is difficult to listen and deal with the circumstances that lead adolescents to consider and attempt suicide. It is even more difficult to have a patient commit suicide while under your care or the care of your facility, or after they leave your treatment program. In consideration of working with at-risk youth, this must be clearly understood. The therapist needs to reach a comfort level with addressing what are literally life and death issues. Using therapeutic use of self, a "self" must be developed that can comfortably, empathically, and effectively deal with adolescents who are, have been, and may be again, suicidal, as well as those for whom treatment did not prevent them from taking their own lives. This is perhaps the most difficult treatment issue to leave at the workplace and not take home with you at the end of the day.

Self-Mutilation

Self-mutilation is defined by Favazza (1996), one of the leading researchers in this area, as "the deliberate destruction or alteration of one's body tissue without conscious suicidal intent" (pp. xviii–xix). Other names for these behaviors include "superficial-moderate self-mutilation, self-injurious behavior, parasuicide, and self-wounding" (Klonsky, Oltmanns, & Turkheimer, 2003, p. 1501), all of which are used interchangeably (Moro, 2007). It includes cutting, burning, scratching, and skin picking (Andover, Pepper, & Gibb, 2007; Favazza, 1996; Walsh, 2008). In this author's clinical experience, it has often been referred to as cutting, and those that engage in these behaviors as "cutters," a rather inappropriate client reference as opposed to the more client-centered and respectful, a person who cuts or self-mutilates. Considering that therapeutic use of self in relationship is essential in providing occupational therapy, and our responsibility to treat our clients with dignity and respect, it behooves us to not refer to individuals as their illness or condition, particularly when addressing a behavior that can leave lasting scars, both on the physical body itself, and the psyche of the individual as well.

Why Does It Occur?

Individuals who self-mutilate often have difficulty expressing their feelings and the reason for its occurrence may be that it serves as a coping strategy (Moro, 2007). Moro states "according to case studies and research, people often report a sense of rising anxiety, tension, and an extreme urge to mutilate immediately before the act. During the act, people state they seem to lose themselves . . . or to feel a sense of depersonalization or emptiness" and "immediately following the act, the prevailing mood people report is that of tension release, reduced anger, a feeling of control and security, and an overall sense of euphoria" (pp. 57–58). This "sense of depersonalization prior to the act and a relief of anxiety, tension or inner pain after the act" were also found by Williams and Bydalek (2007).

The following informal interview of a patient who engaged in self-mutilation supports Williams and Bydalek's (2007) finding. It is worth noting she clearly seemed to present that it was a coping skill that worked for her, and it illustrates how effective she believed her coping strategies to be, and how difficult the former one may be to replace with something more appropriate.

> Therapist: *Why do you participate in self-mutilation?*
>
> Client: *I do it to let out my feelings. They build up and when I cut I watch the blood flow and I feel better.*
>
> Therapist: *Does it hurt?*
>
> Client: *I don't really feel it.*

Occupational Therapy Interventions

As in most occupational therapy–based treatment the focus is on everyday functioning and the occupations that the client engages in on a daily basis. Occupations and activities related to school, relationships with friends and family, work, and socializing activities (e.g., sports, clubs, driving, and going out) are their primary focus. Therapeutic frameworks such as cognitive and sensory therapies (Kaiser, Gillette, & Spinazzola, 2010) have been found to be efficacious for those suffering from this condition. Interventions using these frameworks include self-management as it relates to stress, anger and emotional management and regulation, problem solving, and time management (Moro, 2007). Using cognitive-behavioral therapy approaches, therapists can focus on maladaptive thinking, which prevents occupational performance in daily life (Moro, 2007). Specifically, "DBT focuses on the concept that during times of extreme stress or anxiety, the 'mind-body' system shuts down. Thinking becomes concrete and focused on the here and now and this prevents the mind from calming the body. The body finds a means to calm itself, through the use of self-mutilation." Additionally the occupational therapy sessions address "problem solving, skills training, relationship strategies and contingency management" (Moro, 2007, p. 62). Also, some settings use sensory interventions, such as tactile stimulation and massage, to decrease incidents of self-mutilation. In addition, Williams and Bydalek (2007) suggested interventions such as exploring with clients what measures might be self-soothing and training in communication skills so that clients could express their feelings instead of acting them out on their bodies. In this author's clinical experience, teaching strategies that mimic the actual destruction of body tissues but cause no lasting effect, such as holding an ice cube to the skin or snapping a rubber band around the wrist, can be effective to replace self-harm behaviors when the individual is transitioning between maladaptive and adaptive coping skills.

Eating Disorders

There are few articles on the topic of eating disorders in occupational therapy literature, and only four that focused on adolescents and eating disorders. This would seem to indicate a strong need for occupational therapists to publish their work with this population to establish an evidence base and increase referrals for clients with eating disorders to occupational therapists who seem well positioned to treat them. This would also appear to be an emerging practice area for occupational therapists desiring to work in mental health in a very vital role. In fact, some occupational therapists believe that occupational therapy can provide successful interventions that focus on self-efficacy or self-concept for teens with eating disorders (Gardiner & Brown, 2010).

Eating disorders are known by their *DSM-IV-TR* diagnoses of Anorexia Nervosa, Bulimia Nervosa, and Eating Disorder, Not Otherwise Specified. Binge-eating disorder, which is classified under Eating Disorders, NOS, may be encountered by occupational therapists secondary to concomitant health problems being treated by occupational therapy (Costa, 2009). Occupational therapists working with clients with eating disorders use a variety of approaches, including psychodynamic, cognitive, developmental, behavioral, family oriented, and medical (Gardiner & Brown, 2010). Gardiner and Brown further suggest that occupational therapy practitioners are well prepared to address the needs of the eating disorder population. Occupational therapy, practitioners understand occupations, behaviors associated with those occupations, and cognitive processing; through cognitive-behavioral therapy, occupational therapists address individuals' issues. These skills complimented by psychosocial training enable the practitioner to customize interventions specific to the client using a structured symptom-focused treatment approach. Furthermore, the occupational therapist's training to use groups in all practice setting and a keen sense of the importance of psychosocial relationships mean the practitioner is able to effectively facilitate family intervention related groups as well as peer self-help groups. It has been shown that mental health treatment that involves the family is more effective in the long-term outcomes for individuals with anorexia nervosa than is individual treatment (Lock et al., 2010). Occupational therapists work with adolescents with eating disorders in inpatient and outpatient settings; however, treatment of eating disorders and concomitant altered body image concerns (Shearsmith-Farthing, 2001) is an area of specialization within adolescent mental health and mental health practice in general.

Intervention Specific to Adolescents with Eating Disorders

Treatment can include working with the individual to establish eating routines and working with the family to assist the client to understand the disorder and how the family can affect the course of the disorder. Occupational therapy practitioners commonly use groups when treating adolescences with eating disorders. Some of the groups are self-expressive, such as body image, or psychoeducational that may include stress- and anxiety- or time-management (Kloczko & Ikiugu, 2006). As mentioned previously, meaningful occupation-based groups that are very structured and objective focused are highly effective; these may include meal planning, shopping, cooking, and dining together.

Individual therapy with adolescents with anorexia nervosa can be based on psychodynamic therapy (Lock et al., 2010). Interventions based on this approach help teens to build autonomy, self-reliance, and assertiveness presumably based on self-awareness and the ability to self-reflect. Therapists working with adolescents in family-based therapy focus on a safe and reassuring environment. The ultimate goal is for the adolescent to have a healthy autonomy at meal time and the patient to feel supported and not blamed (by the family members) and to assist the parents to support and encourage healthy eating (Lock et al., 2010).

The use of activity analysis and therapists' ability to grade activities are among the unique contributions occupational therapy can make in providing treatment for this population (Gardiner & Brown, 2010). In family therapy approaches based on a highly researched and commonly used approach in recovery for those with anorexia nervosa, initial treatment necessitates that the patients or caregivers selects and prepares the food; however, over time the responsibility is shared and then the responsibility given to the adolescent (Gardiner & Brown, 2010). It is in this treatment that food-related fears and rituals need to be addressed and the graded reintroduction of food selection, food preparation, and eating in social settings, facilitated by the occupational therapist, could be vital in achieving full recovery.

The occupational therapist has the unique ability to use these occupations as a therapeutic tool by analyzing, synthesizing, adapting, grading, and using the activities in intervention as suggested by the Occupational Therapy Practice Framework (AOTA, 2008). Some examples of treatment are to facilitate engagement in appropriate levels of leisure and exercise activities, to acquire social skills, and the selection of or reintegration into vocational experiences that will support and promote mental health and recovery.

Essentially, the eating disorder is a maladaptive coping mechanism that has to be addressed and changed before adaptive behaviors emerge. The unique benefit of occupational therapy with this population is that the approach is holistic and incorporates tasks and occupation-based activities where the adolescent can practice and learn to apply healthy adaptive ways of coping in a safe and supportive environment.

It should be noted that a major lifestyle change is necessary for treatment to be successful (Costa, 2009) and that while emphasizing more appropriate behavior in terms of the health of one with an eating disorder in treatment is important, alternative ways of coping can only be adopted when the therapist understands the needs that are addressed by the disordered eating. A practitioner cannot just point out healthier eating behavior but has to acknowledge the feelings behind the eating disorder in addition to recognizing the attention the behavior promotes.

BULLYING AND SCHOOL VIOLENCE

Bullying and school violence is a growing epidemic in the United States. Since the time of the 1999 Columbine shootings, bullying has received increasing attention ("Bullying: what to do about it," 2011; Goertz et al., 2008; "Youth Violence," 2010), and continues to receive frequent media coverage. The increased awareness makes bullying a significant issue that must be addressed in school settings (Baum, 1999; Bullying, 2011). Bullying and school violence can have the negative effect of causing depression, moodiness, and an increase in the number of days adolescents miss from school (Bullying, 2011; Youth Violence, 2010). Many disciplines including education, social work, psychology, and psychiatry began to collaborate to address this issue as a result of government funding aimed at stopping school violence. Although occupational therapists were not a part of these interdisciplinary teams, for occupational therapy to start advocating becoming part of the teams addressing school violence has been considered important (Baum, 1999). A workshop entitled "Mental Health of Children and Youth: Prevention and Intervention" was presented at the annual AOTA Conference in 2001. This workshop covered the AOTA/FAST Research Project, which was funded by the Center for Mental Health Services Violence Prevention Project, Substance Abuse Mental Health Services Administration, and the U.S. Department of Health and Human Services. The goals of this project were to "create new opportunities for occupational therapy practitioners, develop evidence to support the role of OT in violence prevention and the special contribution of OT to FAST (Families and Schools Together)" (Scheinholtz, Swith, Clark, & Jaffe, 2001). The following therapists participated. Wilma Dorman presented her work as a private practitioner "to identify specific social/emotional needs in the children who enter a private practice (or could come into a private practice)" and how to "design and create programs to meet their needs" (2009). Yvonne Swith presented on "Current Trends and Perceptions of Occupational Therapists Regarding Services to Children with Behavioral and Psychosocial Problems in a School Based Setting" as part of the same workshop, and an overview of *Communities Creating Circles of Peace*, "a community-based violence prevention initiative" (Witchger Hansen, 2001) was highlighted. Despite the attention school violence received at the time, attention waned. The 2011 AOTA conference program did not include a single presentation on this subject. For whatever reason, public and professional interest in this subject spikes when incidents such as Columbine or the shootings at Virginia Tech, and most recently in Tucson, occur and then just as quickly subsides. This is not to say that interest was not sincere and well intentioned, but to point out the fact that whether it is professional organizations, the media, or the populace as a whole, it has proven difficult to sustain attention to these problems long enough to produce change and continued support to address the mental health needs of adolescents and young adults. Nonetheless, occupational therapists are well positioned to address these issues and bullying by using a holistic approach that focuses on occupation-based interventions that promote overall health and well-being with adolescents. Included in the program at the 2001 AOTA program was "Top Ten Ways to Enhance Occupational Therapist's Provision of Social-Emotional Skills" by Gloria Frolek Clark. She pointed out that while occupational therapy practitioners had education that prepared them to address students' mental health needs in the school setting, they were not perceived as such by other education professionals. Among her suggestions were that therapists should report on the mental health needs of students in team meetings to increase others' awareness of occupational therapists' skills in addressing social-emotional skills and to assess students based upon the referral, but to also assess social-emotional abilities and their impact on development and presenting problems to educate referral sources on the expertise and services we can offer in this area (Scheinholtz, Swith, Clark, & Jaffe, 2001).

Roles for occupational therapy could be to understand the occupational nature of violence, to advocate for public health concerns, and to help adolescents develop the skills needed to safely live in their environment and in fostering social skills and teaching respect for diversity (Baum, 1999; Daunhaurer & Jacobs, 2007; Goertz et al., 2008).

Community and school violence affect some adolescents' access to participation in healthy or productive occupations. In addition to bullying and violence on school campuses, for many youth, gang violence poses a serious threat. Youth growing up in inner cities are often born into a world in which they are forced to pledge allegiance to a certain neighborhood or gang for their own safety. Even if youth try to avoid the gang world, they are often caught up in the violence, by simply being born on a certain block, or by being mistaken for someone who is gang affiliated. The violence and danger in these neighborhoods seriously impede participation in those activities "typical" of high school. If a teen's neighborhood is not safe enough to walk home after dark, they will miss out on afterschool sports or dance teams, or other occupations that can be pivotal in character building or feeling occupationally fulfilled. These youth suffer not only from occupational deprivation, but often from symptoms of PTSD. Gang conflict often leads to violence and shootings, and many youth have experienced the loss or injury of a family member or friend. This loss or the witnessing of such traumatic events contributes to mental health issues including PTSD and depression among this subsection of adolescents. Occupational therapists who encounter these youth through community agencies, schools, or hospitals have the responsibility of increasing their actual and perceived levels of safety. This can be done by encouraging youth to share their experiences, and to deal with their effects. As violence is commonplace in many of these communities, without the services provided by occupational therapists and other mental health professionals, youth often do not realize that these traumas have a lasting effect on their emotional well-being and overall functioning.

HELPFUL CONCEPTS FOR TREATING ADOLESCENTS

(Also see Chapter 19 for more information on methods and strategies.)

Structure and Consistency

The teenage years are marked by transition and instability, as teens must navigate the often-chaotic path from childhood to adulthood. This is not to say that the transition is necessarily difficult. Many adolescents enjoy their teenage years and transition to adulthood with minimal difficulty. In addition to the typical transitions all adolescents' experience, those who are identified as having a mental health issue have often experienced trauma, loss, or other environmental stressors that have contributed to the development of their mental illness or presenting problems. These stressors could include a family changing residences and therefore schools frequently, the death or loss of a loved one, violence in their neighborhood, abuse, or other problems within the family system. As many teens who are receiving mental health treatment lack consistency or support within their home environments, providing this structure and consistency in the treatment setting is crucial. Consistency can be achieved in many ways, including ensuring that the mental health staff working with the youth remains constant, the time and place of the sessions are the same every week, and the structure of the session or group remains the same so that the adolescent knows what to expect. This structure will facilitate the establishment of trust in their therapist and their peers, and will allow the adolescents to disclose more and work more honestly and openly toward their treatment goals and objectives.

Limit Setting

Pushing the limits is something that comes naturally to most adolescents. Part of navigating through this period of transition is pushing and testing the limits set by authority figures to see what happens and for adolescents to test their own autonomy and maturity. Setting limits in a mental health setting ensures consistency, and makes it clear to the adolescent what to expect. Because teenagers are in the process of gaining more independence and control over their own lives, it is important to allow adolescents to take some responsibility in helping to develop the expectations and rules for the group. Most teens are more likely to follow the rules and adhere to the expectations of treatment if they were involved in their creation, instead of having rules imposed on them. Providing positive reinforcement instead of just negative consequences can be very helpful in setting limits for the participants. Adolescents, especially those with disruptive behaviors, are very accustomed to suffering negative consequences (e.g., referrals to the dean, suspension from school, etc.) and are not used to being positively affirmed for their behavior. Thus, the use of praise and positive reinforcements, including incentives, can be extremely effective in improving behavior and adherence to rules in mental health treatment settings. The "Game of Life" is one such incentive program that can be used to encourage positive behaviors and to learn consequences. The program is used in mental health groups and youth receive points for positive behaviors and participation, including volunteering to share first or assisting their peers or staff with activities. At the end of the group session or an allotted number of group sessions, the participant with the most points receives an incentive, which was decided upon by the group initially, an award, a gift card, or whatever the youth had decided upon as a motivator in the beginning of the group. When the incentives are chosen by the client, the youth are more motivated to work toward receiving these points so that they will be rewarded.

Avoiding Power Struggles

Adolescents have more life experience than children, and are usually more mature. Because of this they are more capable of negotiating with adults, as well as manipulating staff, rules, and systems. By allowing adolescent clients opportunities to make decisions and have control in the group setting, a therapist can fulfill adolescents' need to express autonomy and act independently. Engaging with youth in struggles for power within the treatment setting can be detrimental to the therapeutic process, as it can cause role confusion for the therapist and the youth, and encourages youth to perpetuate negative, challenging behaviors. The occupational therapist has to take care in allowing the adolescent client enough autonomy to not feel as though they're being "treated like a child," but provide enough structure to maintain a therapeutic environment for the clients. One effective method of avoiding **power struggles** is by providing choices. Providing choices gives the adolescent the opportunity to have a sense of control and the ability to express autonomy in an acceptable, positive manner. One study showed that "Offering choices to adolescents living in a psychiatric setting elicited a statistically significant difference in performance" and "provided evidence that choice making within parameters set by the occupational therapist can enhance performance among adolescents living in behavioral treatment facilities" (Schroeder Oxer & Kopp Miller, 2001). Examples of providing choices are:

- Allowing the adolescent to choose between two or three different types of activities that all will be effective in meeting a treatment goal. For example, it the therapist is working on the objective of increasing social interaction through a parallel task group, giving the client the choice between painting sun catchers and making a tile mosaic provides an opportunity for decision making and a sense of control over their own treatment. It is also an example of client-centered care.

- Asking a group to plan the menu for a cooking group. Ways of providing parameters that will guide them in making reasonable and appropriate selections include giving them a budget within they must stay, sample menus, a theme such as a picnic or a spaghetti dinner or "Italian Night," and a time frame for preparing, eating, and cleaning up after the meal.

- Avoiding a potentially dangerous or assaultive situation by offering an adolescent who is becoming angry and verbally threatening choices that teach adaptive coping and anger management skills through a therapeutic interpretation: "Brittany, I can see that this group is becoming frustrating and upsetting for you. Would you like to leave and take a few minutes by yourself, or would you rather step out into the hall with me and we can talk about what's bothering you?"

Therapeutic Use of Self in Relationship

Given this phase of development, where teenagers typically gravitate away from relationships with adults and the peer group becomes all-important, it is vital for the therapist to master the therapeutic use of one's self in the relationship to foster successful outcomes (AOTA, 2008). Oftentimes adolescents with mental health problems have had actual or perceived negative relationships with adults. Instances of this may include past abuse, rejection, and broken promises by adult authority figures; abandonment, real or imagined, by their family members; and interaction with law enforcement officers, school officials, and members of the community brought on by the symptoms of their particular disorders or conditions. (See Chapter 11 for more information on attachment through the lifespan.) Some key points to consider:

- Create a feeling of acceptance and worth, especially important for those with low self-esteem and poor self-concept.

- Establish and maintain trust and rapport.

- Provide a safe environment for self disclosure.

- Provide active listening and take responses seriously. Many times adolescents have been waiting for the opportunity to talk to an adult who wants to hear about their problems, symptoms, and personal issues.

- Sense of humor is essential.
- Be a reliable and available resource and confidant; however, maintain an appropriate therapeutic role by keeping in mind that you are not trying to be their friend or peer, but an adult who can be trusted.
- Don't pretend to be something you're not. Adolescents can see through any phony and insincere behavior on the part of the therapist, which will prevent trust and appropriate rapport from developing.

Creating a Therapeutic Environment

Milieu therapy as it was originally intended to be implemented is becoming less and less of an option and reality in many settings today, especially in the more traditional settings that have embraced it in the past such as impatient units in mental health facilities and general hospitals. Essentially, the concept of milieu therapy involves the establishment of a "therapeutic community" where the human and nonhuman environment are conceived of as having beneficial therapeutic qualities that aid an individual in recovering from mental illness. While programs today lack the consistency in staffing patterns, mix of clients, and a short length of stay, such a concept can possibly be carried out in the OT area, where manipulation and control of the treatment environment can occur for at least the time the client is in therapy. A "family room" type therapy setting where incandescent lighting was used instead of fluorescent overhead lighting, which provided rocking chairs, art, and furnishings and gave the appearance of a home environment, proved useful in putting adolescents at ease in this author's experience. They looked forward to coming to occupational therapy, and upon entering on their first visit would remark about how "nowhere else looks like this—this is great!" and would more easily settle into group and participate in an observably more relaxed manner.

Team Approach

There are many advantages to having the opportunity to practice in a setting that utilizes an interdisciplinary treatment team approach. In an interdisciplinary treatment team approach, clinicians from a variety of professions gather to share their observations and assessment of clients' behavior, the client's response to treatment, and their suggestions for the direction and outcome of treatment (Hussey, Sabonis-Chafee, & O'Brien, 2007). This provides valuable insights to each member of the team, including the occupational therapy practitioner, for planning intervention and working in concert with other professionals to help clients achieve their treatment goals. In the absence of working in a setting that uses this approach, it would be beneficial for the clinician to have mentors and colleagues with whom to confer to lend direction and clarity to a case and assist with troubleshooting when questions or difficulties arise.

If a psychiatrist has been the referral source, contact and discussion regarding the course of treatment can be of great benefit, especially for the therapist who is practicing autonomously, such as in private practice.

Medications/Psychopharmacology

In the current era of health care, medications are held in high esteem in the overall treatment of adolescents and others experiencing mental health problems, particularly by reimbursers in inpatient settings who deem the use of medication as "active treatment." For those practicing in such a setting, patient response to medication often carries more weight than how they are responding to occupational therapy and other services. This, of course, can be frustrating, particularly when managed care takes the position that stabilization on a medication necessarily needs to take place in the hospital, while occupational therapy and other therapy services can be accessed outside of the hospital setting. In many communities, this is not the case, especially considering how few occupational therapists are providing services in community, non-hospital settings, and how few jobs presently exist for interested therapists to do so. Despite these hurdles, appropriate use of psychotropic medication can facilitate an individual's ability to participate in therapy through the reduction of symptoms that may have previously prevented their active involvement in treatment. Occupational therapists need to have a working knowledge of currently prescribed medications to monitor the effects, side effects, and possible benefits to the adolescent. A key role occupational therapy can play is the reporting of the benefits or lack thereof of a medication on the performance of occupations and level of functioning as observed during occupational therapy, thereby assisting other health professionals in establishing a therapeutic medication regimen that enhances function and the achievement of established treatment goals. A downside to having effective medications available to treat a variety of symptoms is the client's false perception that the medication or being started on a medication is the treatment issue, and not that the condition or the personal experience of the mental illness is the focus of therapy. Given the widespread marketing and discussion of psychotropic medication, many adolescents present for treatment stating "I'm only here to get my medications adjusted" or " I have a chemical imbalance—once the meds kick in I'll be fine," ignoring or denying the many effects their illness has had on their growth and development, occupational performance, and their consequential need to learn new skills to facilitate recovery from their mental illness and the deleterious effects it has had on their lives. It is important to reinforce and remember that medications are helpful in symptom reduction, allowing for fuller participation in therapy, which ultimately enables adolescents to return to satisfying lives with new or retrieved skills that have been made possible by their participation in therapy with the benefits derived from being placed on the right medication.

CASE ILLUSTRATION

Mary—An Example of the Useful Concepts in Practice

Mary was an 18-year-old hospitalized on an inpatient adolescent unit with presenting problems of self-mutilation and suicidal thoughts, ideation, and plans. She attempted suicide prior to her admission as well as during her hospitalization. She presented with a high degree of lethality and potential for self-harm. For example, her arms and legs were covered with scars as well as recently inflicted cuts, cuts serious to put her at risk for infection. On one occasion, program staff discovered razor blades in a letter sent to her in response to the request she had made for them in a recent contact. While Mary was a patient on an acute inpatient unit, her length of stay was weeks rather than days due to her frequent attempts to kill herself, even while on suicide precautions that required a member of the nursing staff to be within an arm's length from her at all times around the clock. Once she attempted to use a washcloth to commit suicide while a female staff member was present.

Her hospitalization was an ongoing cycle of being on and off suicide precautions and earning privileges to go to meals in the cafeteria and occupational therapy groups held off the unit. Mary was a bright young woman who, despite her current problems, planned to finish high school and attend college. She responded especially well to occupational therapy, and was an active participant in groups with treatment goals for increasing Mary's self-esteem, self-concept, and self-worth, as well as developing adaptive coping skill and strategies to deal more effectively and appropriately with expressing feelings in a non-harmful manner. The therapist had established a strong rapport with her in occupational therapy, providing her with interventions that she could use currently to address her problems in a group setting, and providing her with encouragement and support regarding getting well and with a future-oriented outlook for continuing her education and transition to adulthood. After a month or two of this ongoing cycle, the treatment team was considering transfer to a state long-term care facility, as her response to the program, therapies, and medication did not appear to be producing any lasting results and improvement. Additionally, discussion focused on restricting her to the unit and not allowing her to attend occupational therapy, as the nursing staff felt she was unable to be kept safe in that environment. This presented a dilemma: Was Mary's safety a greater cause for concern than her involvement in therapy, and if so, how could her attendance in occupational therapy continue until she was transferred to a long-term care facility, where an opening could be months away? Necessarily Mary needed to be kept safe from self-harm, but she also benefited from the active treatment provided by occupational therapy. A compromise was reached that involved Mary in the decision-making process. Mary would remain on suicide precautions and be accompanied by a member of the nursing staff at all times, including while she was in occupational therapy. The therapist and nursing staff presented Mary with the choice of submitting to a body search following her return from occupational therapy to ensure her safety, or remaining on the unit until discharge. Mary chose to continue to attend occupational therapy and would comply with the body search after group. Mary remained on suicide precautions for the remainder of her hospitalization, and was an active participant in occupational therapy, which she attended without incident. Once regularly attending occupational therapy, Mary and the therapist, along with a Level II OT student, planned an adolescent program event involving all the other patients and staff based on a reality television show that Mary especially liked and watched with her peers that proved highly successful and enjoyable for the entire program one afternoon.

Discussion

Mary's case illustrates many of the concepts involved in planning and implementing appropriate care and treatment for a severely mentally ill adolescent. For the nursing staff, the primary goal is to keep Mary safe, which they accomplished through their thorough room searches for contraband and being present when Mary opened her mail or received gifts to inspect for items that could provide Mary with the means of self-harm or suicide. They carried out the protocol for suicide precautions, a written doctor's order, which prevented her from committing suicide on the unit. The psychiatrist provided ongoing assessment, prescribed antidepressant medication, and directed the interdisciplinary treatment team. The occupational therapist used therapeutic use of self in relationship and a positive, client-centered approach in providing intervention. The adolescent program offered structure and consistency to provide a framework for treatment in general and the program staff enforced limits. The interdisciplinary treatment team planned Mary's ongoing treatment with input from all of the disciplines mentioned, including social work, which provided Mary with individual, group, and family therapy. This case also illustrates the need to adjust the structure and the established program and to remain flexible and creative in order to provide treatment interventions that best meet the needs of the patient when unusual circumstances arise.

ADOLESCENT SETTINGS AND PROGRAMS

Opportunities for providing mental health interventions for adolescents exist in a variety of traditional and non-traditional settings. Traditional sites based on the medical model, such as hospitals and inpatient units, historically employed occupational therapists who wanted to practice in mental health. As mental health facilities and programs close, downsize, or reorganize, frequently to cut costs and maximize profits, occupational therapy positions have been lost, but more importantly the resulting problems in terms of access to services and a shortage of providers is interfering with the ability of adolescents to obtain proper treatment for their mental health issues (New Freedom Commission on Mental Health, 2003). This necessitates broadening our scope of treatment in settings not usually thought of as being mental health providers to address the mental health needs of adolescents where occupational therapists continue to be a presence.

Traditional Settings

Historically, the main employers of occupational therapists in mental health have been hospitals, in what have been commonly called psychiatric units, free-standing psychiatric or mental health hospitals, or what are now more commonly known as behavioral health facilities. Partial hospitalization programs and residential treatment centers are also traditional treatment settings for adolescents with mental health issues.

Inpatient Programs

Inpatient programs include hospital-based units and free-standing hospitals that provide around-the-clock nursing and medical care in the most restrictive setting for those individuals with the highest acuity or degree of lethality. These medical model programs usually are locked units with an emphasis on maintaining safety and establishing stability for program participants, usually referred to as patients. These individuals are those considered to be a risk to themselves or others, such as those who have verbalized suicidal ideation, plan, and intent or have made an actual suicide attempt. In addition to providing a safe environment where patient symptoms can be stabilized and observed on a 24-hours-a-day, seven-days-a-week basis, these programs serve the purpose of initiating and monitoring psychotropic medications used to stabilize the symptoms that led to inpatient hospitalization. Programming typically involves individual, group, and family therapies, and may include school in a classroom setting or individual basis, so that patients can continue their education despite inpatient hospitalization during the school year. The treatment team is headed by a psychiatrist who directs treatment as well as nurses, social workers, psychologists, teachers, utilization review staff (usually nurses), and occupational, recreational, art, music, and dance/movement therapists, depending on the facility.

Partial Hospitalization Programs

Partial hospitalization programs provide services similar to the inpatient program in a less restrictive environment. These programs are not locked. Participants attend during school hours for education, therapy, and medication management and are followed by a psychiatrist. Partial hospitalization can be a step down program from the hospital, or can be an alternative to regular education for adolescents requiring this level of mental health services. Day programs can be similar to partial programs.

Outpatient Therapy

Many adolescents benefit from individual, group, and/or family outpatient therapy. Typical providers are psychiatrists, psychologists, and master's prepared social workers and counselors. Occupational therapists, such as this author, have and continue to provide outpatient services through a small private practice, currently seeing adolescents in their homes upon referral from a psychiatrist, school district, or other providers. (See Chapter 12, "Mental Health of Children," for further information.)

CASE ILLUSTRATION

ANNA—Reactive Attachment Disorder and Family Treatment

Anna is a 14-year-old girl referred to an outpatient occupational therapist by a local child and adolescent psychiatrist. She has had traditional outpatient therapy in the recent past, which has proved unsuccessful, and Anna stopped attending. She has a diagnosis of reactive attachment disorder (RAD) and her presenting problems include conflictual family relationships, particularly with her adoptive mother.

Background and history

Anna born in Russia and was adopted at the age of seven by her current adoptive parents. Prior to her adoption she grew up in a home where her parents were neglectful due to their active substance abuse. Her biological parents were rarely home, and Anna was cared for by a series of neighbors and relatives who were present on an inconsistent basis. She was often left by herself, and consequently she had resorted to stealing food for sustenance. She was removed from the home at five years of age and placed in an orphanage. Her adoptive parents, Tony and Maria, are financially well off and spent a great deal of money and time arranging for Anna's adoption when they were unable to conceive. Anna was a difficult child with frequent temper tantrums who was cool and distant to her parents and frequently disobedient as she grew older. Her parents have tried numerous interventions; including taking her to a center in a major city that specializes in treating children with RAD when she was eight. Despite their best intentions and attempts at therapeutic interventions to help resolve their problems, things in the household have not changed, but actually gotten worse as Anna has entered adolescence. Additionally, the couple was able to conceive a daughter in the intervening years who is now five years old. Anna has threatened the sister and believes that the parents favor her. The therapist enters the case at this impasse.

The outpatient therapist arrived at the family home and began by interviewing Anna and completing a Kinetic Self-Drawing Assessment. Anna draws a picture of herself drawing a picture. Her goal for treatment is "I want to have a happy family." Additionally he had interviewed her parents and solicited their goals for treatment. Tony would like for Anna to "just get along with her mother. She doesn't really have a problem with me." The therapist will later discover that while she gets along well with the father, whose business keeps him away from home more than 40 hours a week, she has stolen money from his wallet, which he now has to keep locked up. As the primary family conflict appears to be with the mother, the therapist arranges a session for them to complete a mother–daughter collage about their family. The therapist notes that they work in a parallel manner, with little to no conversation, although the mother tries to initiate. Later, when processing the session, the mother remarked, "we pretty much worked on our own," and Maria said that she "hadn't really expected anything to be different. This is the way it always is." Following a subsequent individual session the mother told the therapist, "I've been able to overhear some of your sessions and I want you to know she's not telling you the truth about what happens around here. She didn't tell you about how she tried to push me down the stairs when we were arguing about her finishing the vacuuming, and our week was nothing like she described." At this point the therapist decides to have family meeting style sessions where a forum can be created to discuss family events and dynamics. Some progress is made; however, Anna, continues to be disrespectful, not follow rules, lie, and remains disrespectful, especially towards her mother. As her father and mother begin to align to reinforce consequences for negative behavior, Anna begins to be nasty and disrespectful to the father as well. Tony "just can't understand it. We give her all these great things that she could never have had in Russia and she's so ungrateful. Soon as she gets one thing, she wants something else. She's never grateful for anything." The family meetings focused on having the parents present as a united front with regard to limits, expectations, and consequences, although Tony continued to believe that "Maria is too hard on her. I think if we give her more positives, she'll come around" when Maria tried to follow through with limits and consequences. Therapy made progress initially as Tony and Maria assumed more appropriate parental roles. As their position strengthened, Anna became more oppositional, limit testing, and threatening. At home one Friday, the therapist received a call from Tony that "Anna has threatened to kill all of us." Based on her history of threats and the attempt to push the mother down the stairs, he recommended inpatient hospitalization and walked the father through the necessary steps. He asked the father to call him if he had any difficulties. At the next session it was found that the father did not follow through. At this point in the therapeutic process, the therapist contacted the referring psychiatrist for guidance. The doctor believed that the therapist was doing the right things in therapy and offered to see the family and possibly start a low dose of medication. The family did not go to the appointment, and in that week's session Tony stated "I won't have my daughter turned into a zombie" and not only re- fused to discuss the matter further, but he left the room and the session. All of the particulars of this case cannot be presented in this case illustration, but eventually the family and the therapist agreed that "we're just spinning our wheels" and that progress was no longer being made. The thera- pist reviewed the course of therapy with the par- ents, provided his interpretation that they were not able to provide consistent limits and conse- quences, that Anna, who had voiced that she did not want to live with them any longer, contin- ued to pose a threat to them and their younger daughter, and choices needed to be made regard- ing Anna remaining in the home or sent to board- ing school, as she was academically sound, had no desire to work on a relationship with them, posed a threat to the young family, and would be leaving for college in a few short years. He gave them praise for continuing to try to effect change despite what they knew about RAD and how many avenues they had tried, and offered to re- enter the case to assist in Anna's placement if that was what they chose. They thanked the therapist, stated that they had believed this was "their best chance" at improving their situation, but did not call him again.

Discussion

Unlike the outpatient, family-based case illustra- tion of "Frank" found later in this chapter, this case does not have what would appear to be a "happy ending." Of course, not all attempts at therapy do. It does however illustrate a num- ber of important points and positive outcomes.

Therapy based in the home on an outpatient basis increased Anna's involvement in therapy and provided the therapist with a truer picture of family dynamics than might have been had at an outpatient office. While the parents strength- ened their positions and roles to a degree, the fact that they could not agree on how to parent Anna effectively became clear to the therapist as well as to each other. The therapist at one point suggested marital counseling and the mother re- plied, "many have." As is always the case in pro- viding effective occupational therapy, the patient has to be a willing participant in the therapeutic process, as do the parents when working with ad- olescents. Therapy clarified relationships, barri- ers to successfully meeting treatment goals, and led the family to the point where they had to be willing to change if change was to occur. When that didn't happen, the therapist used reflection, sought guidance from the referring psychiatrist, presented the parents with options, and knew when to terminate therapy based upon the re- sponse of the parents and Anna to intervention. It is difficult to come to the decision, based on clinical reasoning that further intervention will be futile unless the participants are willing to ac- cept what is being presented and make changes accordingly. Perhaps this family was not ready to do that. Perhaps they never will be. Nonetheless, they expressed their gratitude for the therapist's attempts at trying to help them resolve their is- sues. As is the case with occupational therapy in mental health, if not other settings as well, the therapist often cannot and may never know what the ultimate outcomes of therapy actually were.

School-Based Programs

The goal of school-based occupational therapy services is to assist youth in improving their functioning specifically in the area of academic performance. (Also, see Chapter 22, Psychosocial Occupational Therapy in the School Setting for more information for school-based, psychosocial occupational therapy.) Occupational therapists who work for school districts do not typically address psychosocial needs alone, and focus more on developmental and physical issues such as handwriting and fine motor skills. Under the Individuals with Disabilities Act (IDEA), emotional disturbance is one of the 13 categories of educational disability under which youth can qualify for services. Emotional disturbance is defined as ". . . a condition exhibiting one or more of the following characteristics over a long period of time and to a marked degree that adversely affects a child's educational performance: (A) An inability to learn that cannot be explained by intellectual, sensory, or health factors, (B) An inability to build or maintain satisfactory interpersonal relationships with peers and teachers, (C) Inappropriate types of behavior or feelings under normal circumstances (e.g. fighting with peers, acting out in class, drug use), (D) A general pervasive mood of unhappiness or depression, or (E) A tendency to develop physical symptoms or fears associated with personal or school problems" (Code of Federal Regulations, Title 34, Section 300.7(c) (4) (i)).

Based on this definition of emotional disturbance as an educational disability, school-based occupational therapists should address the psychosocial needs of children and adolescents in the school settings. These youth can receive other mental health services through other mental health professionals (school psychologists, counselors, or social workers) but often end up falling through the cracks and not receiving the treatment they need, as there is a lack of mental health services in many school settings. Despite a general belief that occupational therapy can offer effective treatment for this population of students, the research evidence to demonstrate this is thin (Barnes, Beck, Vogel, Grice, & Murphy, 2003). Barnes et al. (2003) presented a study of occupational therapists treating students with emotional disturbances, in which interest and support for occupational therapy treatment of this population within the schools were expressed. The authors found that many barriers to treatment of this population existed, including a lack of education or training of therapists, decreased financial support, and a dearth of research supporting the practice. Occupational therapy's history and roots in mental health position occupational therapists to work with emotional disturbances and mental illnesses within the school district.

There are community-based organizations that attempt to fill the gaps in services to address the psychosocial needs of adolescents in some districts and schools. Few of these agencies employ occupational therapists, despite the understanding that youth referred for mental health services benefit greatly from the addition of an occupational therapist to the treatment team. An occupational therapist working for a school-based mental health agency goes into the schools and facilitates group or individual mental health sessions with youth who have been referred for mental health services.

Group Versus Individual Services

Adolescents can be seen by occupational therapists individually or in groups in their schools or clinics. Individual sessions allow occupational therapists to focus on individual areas of need more directly to build the skills necessary for the youth to meet their mental health goals. Groups allow a space for youth to connect with each other, building social skills and allowing them to accept their own issues, as they see similar issues in others as well. Groups also help adolescents build trust, by opening up to peers and adults whom they otherwise would not interact. Group dynamics are an important concept to address, as one new adolescent in the group can affect trust and disclosure (see Chapter 20, "Groups," for information on groups in mental health treatment).

There has been a recent shift from hospital and inpatient services to community-based treatment programs, as hospital stays have decreased. Therefore, community-based mental health agencies have become increasingly important to ensure adolescents are getting the treatment they need. With this shift more universal preventive programs become vital, to decrease the need for intensive inpatient mental health treatment. As hospital stays decrease, so does the average length of treatment in outpatient settings for youth. Many evidence-based programs have proven that a shorter, more intensive treatment program in outpatient mental health therapy can be more effective than a less frequent, more longitudinal method of treatment. For example, a community-based occupational therapist working in a school might begin to see her client three times per week instead of only once, and then discharge the adolescent after three months, versus previously seeing the youth once a week for a more extended period of time.

Benefits and Challenges in the School Setting

Working with youth at school has many conveniences, including easy access, as they spend the majority of their day there as well as access to teachers who offer a good source of information about behaviors in the classroom. Group members can also build relationships with one another that can turn into supportive friendships, even after their group therapy ends. In short, working in the schools allows an occupational therapist to work with a system already in place in an adolescent's life. However there are also challenges that are not encountered in an inpatient setting; youth with behavioral issues often have truancy issues with frequent absences and tardiness, and it can be difficult to locate them at times. Keeping confidentiality in the school setting can be difficult as youth are often pulled out of their classes and this makes their classmates aware that they are receiving some sort of special service. Group dynamics can also be influenced if group members know they will see each other in the hallways of the school outside of group. Adolescents may be more likely to self-disclose in a group if the other group members are not people they already know or people who they will not run into outside of the group setting. Because of this, confidentiality is key to establishing a safe, therapeutic environment in which youth feel comfortable sharing their personal information.

CASE ILLUSTRATION

Occupational Therapy in Group Settings—The Issue of Peer Confidentiality

Liz, the occupational therapist, co-led a group with a clinical social worker at a public high school with ninth graders who all have substance abuse issues. Ninth graders tend to be very self-conscious and respond greatly to the influence of their peers. Week after week various group members came to group after smoking marijuana and were asked to return to class, because they could not be present in the group while under the influence of substances. Aside from the substance use, all members were reluctant and some refused to participate in activities, because they were self-conscious around their school peers and were concerned with what they would think of them if they participated and shared private information. Over their winter break from school, the therapists decided to take them on a field trip out of the school setting to see if a change of scenery could help build rapport and establish trust within the group. Sure enough, bringing the group to our youth center and baking cookies helped to build rapport in an alternative setting, made them more comfortable, and helped them open up and share personal experiences with the group.

Discussion

The group leaders figured out how to address an issue that is prominent with teenagers in school—confidentiality with peers they see outside of the group every day in other settings. Essentially, the therapists' changing the environment and offering therapeutic occupational therapy groups in which the teenagers were more relaxed and able to develop trust and rapport with each other ultimately led to the achievement of their treatment goals.

Evidence-Based Programs

One of the foundational concepts of the New Freedom Commission on Mental Health (2003) and subsequent policy documents stress that evidence-based practice is germane to transforming the nation's mental health services system. Certainly, there is a range of what is considered efficacious evidence-based research and practice; however, practitioners, researchers, the mental health community, policy makers, and key stakeholders are closer to an agreement as to those essential items that are broadly accepted.

For example, The National Registry of Evidence-based Programs and Practices (NREPP) (http://nrepp.samhsa.gov/AboutNREPP.aspx) has established a peer-review database of programs and approaches that have been found to be effective. This site is under the jurisdiction of the Substance Abuse and Mental Health Services

Administration (SAMHSA) has an exhaustive list of programs that describe efficacious programs and program design to consumers and practitioners. There are also training material and tools to assist practitioners in the field who would like to submit their program for peer-review. Following are examples of some evidence-based programs that are used with the adolescent population, the first of which was developed by occupational therapists. The other programs were developed by psychologists, social workers, and other disciplines but have been adapted and implemented by occupational therapists for the adolescent population.

An evidence-based program developed at the Occupational Therapy Training Program (OTTP) in Los Angeles is a 20-week family therapy program called Loving Intervention for Family Enrichment (LIFE). The entire family attends weekly sessions in which the parents or guardians go through the Parent Project (Fry, Johnson, & Morgan, 2002) parenting program, which focuses on the challenges of parenting adolescents. This curriculum includes methods of discipline, including how to implement consequences, and psychoeducation on drugs and alcohol and mental health. The youth are divided by age group and participate in mental health groups co-facilitated by an occupational therapist and a clinical social worker or marriage and family therapist. All groups follow a curriculum of topics and engage in arts and craft activities, cooperative games, and psychoeducation. In the beginning and at the end of the 20 weeks the families come together for "multifamily activities" facilitated by therapists, in which the family learns to work together, bond with each other, and treat each other with love and respect.

Aggression Replacement Training (ART) (Goldstein et al., 1998) is a multimodal curriculum that includes Anger Control, Skill Streaming, and Moral Reasoning. This model was developed by other mental health professionals but is a good fit for occupational therapists because it uses a skill building curriculum to improve daily life functioning and allows for creativity and individualization (e.g., using artwork for clients to express selves). The model is very interactive and youth role play experiences from their own lives and learn to change negative behavior.

Caring for our Family–Family Connections is a multidisciplinary program in which occupational therapists can work with clinical social workers or marriage and family therapists to provide holistic services for the entire family, in the home and community (DePanfilis & Dubowitz, 2005). This program includes case management, identifying appropriate resources for the family, working with parents to improve parenting skills, and developing skills for all of the family members involved. Occupational therapists are uniquely positioned to provide services under this model as we are trained to view individuals holistically, including social and environmental influences and viewing the family as a unit that is part of a community, which is a concept central to this program.

The Seeking Safety program (Najavits, 2002) is designed for youth who have experienced trauma and/or substance abuse. The program is present focused, which makes it a good fit for occupational therapy practitioners because it does not involve processing the trauma, but instead focuses on coping with the symptoms and effects. Occupational therapists assist youth in building the skills to decrease negative symptoms and behaviors and increase positive coping.

IMPLEMENTING PROGRAMS

Occupational therapists are often called upon to develop programming when fortunate enough to have secured a position in a mental health setting. Likewise, as more and more occupational therapy practitioners will be encountering and treating adolescents with mental illness in non-psychiatric settings, or marketing their services to providers that have not included occupational therapy in the past, it will be incumbent upon the therapist to develop appropriate programming to meet the needs of the consumers in the setting. (See http://nrepp.samhsa.gov/AboutNREPP.aspx mentioned above for program standards.)

Developing a Program: "Where do I get started?"

- Complete a needs assessment for the site.
- Consider the goals that the clients need to accomplish/desired outcomes.
- Ask the consumers for their input and goals for therapy.
- Consider the needs of the primary consumers of the program: Do they need to work on anger management, life skills, coping skills, leisure interests, etc.?
- What is the typical length of stay? This information guides the type and complexity of the treatment you can provide, as well as provides a time frame in which you and your client have for completing decided upon goals.
- What resources are available for providing occupational therapy (e.g., physical space, budget, supplies, staff to assist in providing therapy)?
- Have an evaluation plan for the program.

CASE ILLUSTRATION

Development of a New Group Program

Purvi, an occupational therapist working for a community mental health agency, observed a lack of positive leisure occupations and access to outdoor activities among the low income adolescents she was working with. She conducted an informal needs assessment, discussing this with other therapists at the agency and the youth with whom she was working, and determined that they would benefit from a gardening or horticulture group program. Purvi considered her resources and was able to procure a donated plot of land in a community garden from the city. Based upon the needs of the youth and the input of her fellow therapists, Purvi created a 12-week curriculum for the gardening group, in which youth engage in group activities that include sensory experiences, learning to be responsible for the plants the youth plant in the garden, and interactive group activities promoting improved self-efficacy, confidence, and life skills.

Discussion

Innovative occupational therapy program development based on the interests and needs of the adolescent participants can provide not only effective mental health intervention, but access to resources low income youth are lacking.

EVALUATION

Evaluation methods may vary greatly from setting to setting. Oftentimes, standardized assessments are not the norm and each facility may either have their own or present the need for you to develop an appropriate assessment, which may include creating a screening tool as well. Observation often proves to be a very viable form of assessment. Astute observation that clinically analyzes body language, verbal and nonverbal communication and situational behavior is an invaluable tool to the occupational therapist working in mental health. Observation and completion of a particular assessment activity such as a magazine picture collage where adolescents are asked to represent themselves through words and pictures of their own choosing, or the Kinetic Self Image Assessment discussed in Chapter 12, may serve as initial assessments that provide information about task skills as well as dynamic information that may cast light on the internal and external issues that led to mental health or mental illness issues, thus providing the therapist with information that will be helpful in planning client-centered intervention. Observation allows for an occupational therapy practitioner to assess an adolescent in an non-confrontative manner versus a question and answer session or direct interview of an adolescent. These two assessments have proven themselves to be extremely useful and have been widely used by this author. Some standardized assessments that are discussed in the current literature as having been used with adolescents include the Child and Adolescent Functional Assessment Scale (CAFAS) (Bates, 2001), the Adolescent and Adult Sensory Profile (Brown & Dunn, 2002), the Canadian Occupational Performance Measure (COPM) (Law, Baptiste, McColl, Polatajko, & Pollock, 2005), and the PTSD Reaction Index (Steinberg, Brymer, Decker, & Pynoos, 2004).

Achenbach's Child Behavior Checklist (2001) and Youth Self-Report (Achenbach, 2001) have been used in outpatient settings, as these assessments provide comprehensive information about client's behaviors as well as their occupational performance and functioning. When used together a therapist can get both the youth's self-report and input from their parent or guardian about these areas. When administered as a pre- and post-tests, these assessments can help in developing treatment plans as well as measuring a client's progress.

INTERVENTION

Adolescents love doing. While some may balk at a given activity as childish, most readily participate in arts and crafts activities and group activities in general, which may include group games such as Pictionary, which serves to increase level of arousal and social participation, among other skills, or basketball, a familiar sport that provides a real life context.

Occupational therapists working with adolescents in an outpatient setting have many possible intervention activities to choose from. Craft activities are often used, and adolescents tend to enjoy these tasks. As school systems are experiencing budget crises and art programs are being cut from many educational curricula, especially in high schools, OT sessions can be an adolescent's only access to artistic activities. In addition to the relaxing or soothing effects arts and crafts have for many, these craft activities serve countless purposes in outpatient mental health treatment. Completing a simple craft activity can provide an opportunity for the therapist to work with their clients on life skills including problem solving, social interaction, time management, decision making, and frustration tolerance, and can be an effective intervention in increasing self-esteem and self-efficacy. One benefit of outpatient treatment for adolescents with mental health issues is the access a therapist can have to the youth's real life and environments. Engaging in these interventions in the youth's home or school can make the transfer of learned skills to their "real life" more smooth. In outpatient settings, mental health interventions with adolescents can include actual daily occupations, for instance searching for employment or seeking out other community resources. A community-based occupational therapist may take a teenage client out job searching, utilizing the tasks involved in this process as actual interventions. This intervention can be very effective, as most teenagers are motivated to gain part-time employment, as they desire their own source of income and the autonomy that comes with this. Activities such as encouraging the client to ask potential employers for job applications on their own, versus having assistance or supervision can be used as intervention in the community. Occupational therapists have experience grading occupational tasks up or down depending on the needs of a client, and can grade these real life tasks in the community as well, to appropriately challenge adolescent clients and provide opportunities to learn and grow. As in all occupational therapy settings, the most effective outpatient interventions are meaningful and culturally relevant to the adolescent client.

CASE ILLUSTRATION
Client—Centered Care

It is a cold January day in the northeastern part of the United States. A foot of snow covers the grounds of the adolescent treatment facility, which includes a basketball court. The occupational therapist asks during group what the members would like to do for occupational therapy that week. They reply that they would like to play basketball. When the therapist states the obvious, that the court is buried in snow, they ask if they could shovel the snow and then play basketball. The adolescent classroom teacher and the occupational therapist on the program offer to bring in snow shovels, and when they do, the adolescents quickly shovel the snow off the basketball court and then engage in several games, looking and behaving like typical adolescents and not individuals with severe mental health problems, several of whom had made suicide attempts in the week prior to their admission into the program.

Discussion

It is easy to dismiss the requests of clients, who in this case want to play basketball during the winter, and offer seemingly more sensible choices such as indoor activities. However, by involving the clients in the decision-making and problem-solving process, and giving them a sense of control over their environment and their treatment, the therapist in this example allowed the group to choose and execute their own activity, which provided them the opportunity to behave and interact in an age-appropriate and pleasurable manner, despite, and possibly temporarily, overcoming their considerable mental health issues through social participation in meaningful occupation that they themselves determined.

In both inpatient and outpatient settings, occupational therapists must consider safety issues and use thorough activity analysis to ensure that participation and the activities themselves can only provide positive outcomes. Successful interventions used in occupational therapy settings with adolescents are discussed in the following sections.

Arts and Crafts

Arts and crafts activities such as painting sun catchers, velvet art and other coloring sheets, tile mosaic trivets, murals, and seasonal decorations and activities have been successful in the inpatient setting. Creating a group banner or mural with a theme decided upon by the group can create camaraderie among adolescents who have just met and may only be in group together for a few sessions. One year in an inpatient setting, this concept was expanded to a door decorating contest near Christmas where roommates worked together using a variety of media. The adolescents became very invested in the activity and asked to work on the project outside of the designated OT time, which extended therapy into the milieu. Following completion, the therapist organized a panel of judges from the administration of the facility and all participants won an award of some type—"most colorful," "best use of materials," "most creative"—to be posted beside their door, and also Christmas candy. There are a great many activities that can be created from a roll of white craft paper, from this contest to drawing and designing a city. In this author's experience, having adolescents draw a city as a group project successfully increases social interaction, facilitates teamwork, improves affect, and increases level of arousal. Both the process and the end product provide interesting opportunities for conversation and discussion regarding the content of the drawing, as well as projective information about the participants through their individual contributions to the group project.

Board Games

The game Life provides an opportunity for discussion of future plans and facilitates sharing and self-disclosure, as well as providing socialization around a fun game. Pictionary has been very successful in providing a game that a large group can play in teams using white craft paper or a chalk or dry erase board that provides some competition and also a lot of humor and laughing with peers. The game Taboo offers a therapist an opportunity to work with adolescents on communication skills, social skills, as well as giving quieter or more shy youth an opportunity to overcome their insecurities and boost their self-efficacy. Games such as these can seem almost too simple to be "therapy," especially to other clinical staff who don't understand the therapeutic value that common occupations such as games possess. How valuable is a group that can make depressed adolescents smile, socialize, and laugh? Many effective resources have been developed specifically for therapy with adolescents. One such game is Talk It Out by Gordon Greenhalgh, Ph.D. (available through Western Psychological Service's Creative Therapy Store), which uses a board game format to help teenagers discuss age-related issues and values and facilitates problem-solving, self-disclosure, and discussion of adolescents' personal problems and feelings.

Resources for Facilitating Adolescent Topical, Focus, and Psychoeducational Groups

Although resources for all of the chapters in this text are to be found online, the following are mentioned here because they are so valuable for use with adolescents. The SEALS (Self-Esteem and Life Skills) series of wire-bound books of reproducible handouts available from Wellness Reproductions Publications, LLC, co-authored by occupational therapist Korb-Khalsa, Azok, and Leutenberg (1993), can be used to facilitate groups, particularly psychoeducational and focus groups, on a wide variety of topics including stress management, recovery, grief, anger management, and coping skills among many others. The easily reproducible pages, which can be copied and distributed among group members, provide structure for discussion as well as something that can be taken and used for future reference after group. A very useful book for those working with adolescents is *104 Activities That Build: Self-Esteem, Teamwork, Communication, Anger Management, Self-Discovery, and Coping Skills* by Alanna Jones (1998). This book provides six sections of ideas for group and individual activities that involve nominal cost and are very effective using game, written, verbal, and interactive formats geared for this population. One of the benefits of resources such as these is that once purchased they can be used indefinitely to create enjoyable and successful occupation-based therapy sessions that can address a wide variety of treatment goals. Some examples of successful group activities for adolescents are: cooking, beading crafts, tie-dye, mosaic tiling, competitive games, Wii, Pictionary, Taboo, and Scene It. Some examples of typical group topics are anger management, coping skills, stress management, self-esteem, goal setting, leisure and recreation, and vocational skills.

Creative Expression

Creative activities generally work well with adolescents, as they give the youth a chance to express themselves in a less threatening way than just talking and sharing personal information. Writing activities in which youth write about their experiences in the form of stories or poems can be a safe and powerful way to let youth express themselves in a way that feels safe and non-threatening. Artwork, music, drama, or any other creative expression can also be useful modalities in working with adolescents. As in any occupational therapy treatment, the intervention should be client centered and client driven; therefore, whatever modality the youth is motivated by should be used.

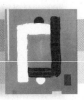

CASE ILLUSTRATION

Creative Expressive Occupational Therapy

At a community-based mental health agency, youth have the opportunity to participate in a music program as part of their treatment. For this program, an occupational therapist works with another staff member who used to be a professional music producer and the group leaders engage the youth participants in activities designed to build self-esteem, increase self-expression, and learn life skills through music. Through writing music and poetry and creating their own music and beats using state-of-the-art computer editing software, the youth create their own album. The curriculum takes clients through the full process of the music industry, including creating the music, learning about the business side (contracts, labels, negotiating, etc.), writing their own biography, and participating in a photo shoot for the cover of their album. Through this process, the occupational therapist incorporates training in life skills that are required for each step as the youth create their music. For example, communication and social skills are learned through collaborating and negotiating, and frustration tolerance is improved through what is often a challenging process for the youth.

Discussion

Through this creative, expressive process the youth learn to overcome any insecurities they may have about expressing themselves and they are able to tell their own story using music, a culturally relevant occupation.

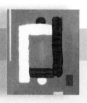

CASE ILLUSTRATION

Frank—Successful Rewarding Home-Based Occupational Therapy

Frank was a 13-year-old male at the time he was referred to an occupational therapist in private practice for home-based therapy to address depression and anger management issues. The referring psychiatrist began seeing Frank when at 12 years old when Frank began exhibiting emotional and behavioral problems following the death of his father, whom he had discovered after he had a massive heart attack. His attendance of outpatient therapy with a counselor had been poor, and eventually he refused to go.

Presenting Problems

Frank's presenting problems included isolating himself in his room at home on his computer, refusing to spend time with his family, school refusal with sporadic attendance, and angry outbursts and aggressive behaviors directed toward his mother and female siblings. He did not have any friends that he saw on any regular basis. He was frequently noncompliant with taking his prescribed antidepressant medications. Occasionally he broke household items and prior to one of the therapist's initial weekly visits he had punched a hole in a wall after a fight with his mother. When the occupational therapist suggested that Frank's mother take away his computer privileges, she refused, stating, "I'm too afraid of what he'll do." The occupational therapist interviewed Frank and his mother to establish treatment goals and establish a therapy schedule and a fee for services. Frank begrudgingly began therapy and his mother was supportive of his involvement, as well as hers in the weekly sessions.

Course of Treatment

Frank was seen for therapy for four years. Initial interventions involved working with Frank individually, which was always followed with a wrap-up and review of the session with his mother. To establish trust, the OT had established with Frank that he would keep the contents of their sessions that he wanted to remain confidential private, with the exception of any disclosures that would indicate that he was a threat to himself or others. Initially some sessions were held with the entire family, using typical board games as well as therapeutic games such as the "Ungame" to facilitate appropriate communication and interaction among family members. Later the therapist felt that enough information had been gleaned from assessing family dynamics in these family sessions, and it was determined that the best use of sessions was to meet with Frank individually. Frank's road to recovery was initially a rocky one. In some early sessions he would leave for his room in anger and swear at the therapist and his mother or siblings. Interestingly, they would swear back. On one occasion he yelled at the therapist, "and don't think you're coming up here (his room) to talk to me" and slammed the door. On prior occasions Frank had been amenable to talking, but this was clearly not one of them and the therapist respected that he was finished with therapy for that day. The volatile nature of this adolescent's mood, as well as his depressive symptoms and behavior, often presented roadblocks to therapy. Occasionally the OT would process the session on his way home or on his way to the next appointment and think to himself, "this case is going nowhere"; however he persevered. A turning point in Frank's therapy came following what ended up being a necessary change in the therapist's style, which was warm and supportive, to confrontational given the slow, uneven progress seen in the initial 18 months and Frank's resistance to change. The therapist told Frank, "Look, I'm here to help you. You are a depressed kid with a lot of problems that I'm happy to work on with you, but you have to be willing to work with me. If you're not able to do that, I don't see any point in continuing therapy." Frank thought about it for a few minutes, and then said, "All right, I'll try." From that point forward Frank worked to address issues of attending school, taking medication, responding more appropriately and without aggression or destruction when angry, developing peer relationships, and, ultimately, finding a job that would provide him with opportunities for success in meeting others, getting positive feedback for his work, and moving him in a developmentally appropriate direction as he approached his 17th birthday. Obtaining a driver's license to increase his independence and provide him with opportunities to interact with others outside his home was accomplished as well. All of these goals required a great deal of support, patience, and encouragement, but were accomplished in time. Part of the therapist's intervention was realizing and discussing with Frank that his family was a source of annoyance, and the more time he spent with peers or in a job would only benefit him. As in all cases, the goals that were worked on also had to be Frank's as well to provide client-centered and successful care. Concessions necessarily were made over issues that continued to produce power struggles instead of change.

Frank was taking his medication sporadically at best and while he would tell the occupational therapist that he had been taking his medication, in fact he had not. His mother had presented his fairly untouched medications, so improvements were being made despite his refusal to take them. The family informed the psychiatrist of this in their scheduled session, and medication compliance was dropped as a goal for treatment. When he was a senior, he continued to attend school infrequently. Frank's mother wanted him to be home-schooled as a result, but the therapist felt that attending school was a responsibility and part of the role of the adolescent, provided opportunities for social interaction, and wanted Frank to attend. The family chose to have Frank home-schooled, which was their choice, and school attendance was no longer a treatment issue. By the mutually agreed upon conclusion of Frank's therapy, he had friends with whom he hung out with at their homes and places in the community. They would have weekend sleep-overs where they brought and played games on their computers. He purchased a car and successfully worked in a restaurant, where he was eventually promoted and offered career opportunities. He began to date. He had successfully resolved his issues and recovered to a remarkable degree, ready to graduate from high school, and start considering his future. A few weeks after their last session, the therapist received an invitation to Frank's graduation party, which he attended. At the party Frank talked about his plans for the future, and when people walked up to him during their conversation, Frank would stop and say, "This is my counselor," and introduced him by name.

DISCUSSION

The flexibility of home-based therapy allowed for the family and the therapist to practice in an environment that provided an in vivo context for intervention. Client factors and activity demands could easily be worked into sessions as things progressed or regressed. In times of high levels of dysfunction, sessions could be increased to twice a week, and when considerable progress was being made, reduced to once a week or every other week, which happened frequently as Frank's mental health improved. The therapist, who was paid on a fee for service basis and not through a traditional insurance provider, allowed for the length and frequency of therapy to be determined by the client, his family, and the occupational therapist. As Frank eventually refused to take medication but did agree to continue therapy, Frank's progress and eventual recovery could be directly linked to occupational therapy intervention. Frank's family had been considerably dysfunctional, particularly in their interaction style (yelling, swearing, and "blowing up"). Therapeutic use of relationship or self was essential to the successful outcome of this case. Had the occupational therapist not worked for many years in child and adolescent mental health, where behaviors like these were frequently encountered, the foul language and high affect states that the family used as a regular part of their conversations could have been upsetting or appalling. By addressing the issues that led to referral (i.e., symptoms of depression, school refusal, and poor anger management skills) and not the family's long-standing ways of communicating in emotional reactive ways, the therapist was able to focus on the adolescent's recovery in his context, without imposing his own standards or beliefs on civility. In time, the family did interact in a more pleasant manner and the tone of the home became more placid as well. Oftentimes therapists and other clinicians do not respond in a therapeutic manner that addresses treatment issues when patients use vulgar or profane language, and say, "Now is that the way we ask for things?" (or whatever) to a swearing client, not taking into account that in that individual's home environment, context, and culture, such interaction and ways of expressing one's self may well be the norm.

The client-centered approach used by the therapist enabled Frank to feel a part of the process, giving Frank positive feedback for his accomplishments and providing the adolescent with choices and avoiding power struggles as mentioned elsewhere in this chapter, which worked effectively as demonstrated in this case. Frank's case also illustrates the qualities needed to practice effectively with adolescents, such as patience, being genuine, committed, and caring, and being able to empathize and support an individual who is still maturing—not a child but not yet an adult—and looking for guidance as they make that transition. This is not always easy when dealing with typically developing teenagers, let alone adolescents who are having great difficulty navigating this developmental phase of their lives.

SUMMARY

Until recently, the bulk of research regarding youth and adolescents with mental disorders has been focused on three main populations: (1) children with developmental delays (Landesman & Ramey, 1999; Sonnander & Claesson, 1999), (2) those who have been labeled severely emotionally disturbed (SED) (New Freedom Commission, 2003), and (3) juveniles who have already been convicted of a crime and are incarcerated within the justice system who have been diagnosed with a mental illness (Cocozza & Skowkra; 2000, Grisso, 2004). While these are important populations to address, there are also a large number of adolescents who do not fall into any of these categories who deserve the attention and mental health services that occupational therapists can offer. There continues to be a dearth of research and information on the mental health needs of adolescents within the field of occupational therapy and beyond. It is the hope of the authors that the field of occupational therapy continues to research and focus on the adolescent population, as this is a critical time of transition that requires support, specifically for adolescents with mental health concerns.

As seen in this chapter, the needs and issues surrounding adolescents are vast and depend greatly on the demands and supports of their environment, as well as their predisposition to mental health or illness. Occupational therapists can effectively provide the skills and support needed for adolescents to make it through these

Their gratitude for a listening ear

Their eagerness to discuss problems

Their candor about their circumstances

Their acceptance of others/peers (sexual orientation, race, interests, etc.)

A desire to be or return to normal

Some ability to see that things may not work out as planned

FIGURE 13-1. Rewards of Working with Adolescents in Mental Health
© Cengage Learning 2013

years of transition through the varied array of interventions appropriate to this population described in this chapter. Indeed there are many rewards of working with adolescents (see Figure 13-1).

However, those who wish to work in this very gratifying area of practice will need to conceptualize and develop new ways of meeting their mental health needs in new contexts.

With ever shorter lengths of stay and decreased funding and reimbursement for treatment of adolescents in traditional mental health settings, occupational therapists will need to address the mental health needs of adolescents in schools and other non-traditional settings, such as the OTTP program based on evidence-based practice. Emerging practice areas exist for therapists to address problems such as suicide and bullying. Private practice and community-based programs offer therapists opportunities for addressing the mental health needs of adolescents outside of traditional, medical model settings. It may be necessary to advocate for increased services for adolescents with mental health issues and market our ability to provide these services simultaneously to continue or re-establish, if not establish and create a niche for occupational therapy in working with this challenging and rewarding area of practice.

REVIEW QUESTIONS

1. Identify three changes in behavior that could be identified in a classroom that may be an indication of the presence of a mental health issue in an adolescent.
2. Explain the concept of "power struggles" and why avoiding these can be helpful in treating adolescents.
3. Identify one benefit and one challenge of working with adolescents in the school setting.
4. What are risk factors for adolescent suicide? What are some strategies for prevention?
5. What are occupational therapy interventions appropriate for adolescents experiencing mental health problems?

REFERENCES

Achenbach, T. (2001). *Child behavior checklist for ages 6–18.* Burlington, VT: ASEBA, University of Vermont.

Achenbach, T. (2001). *Youth self-report for ages 11–18.* Burlington, VT: ASEBA, University of Vermont.

American Occupational Therapy Association. (2004). *Statement on suicide prevention and youth.* Bethesda, MD: American Occupational Therapy Association, Inc.

American Occupational Therapy Association. (2005). *Statement of the American Occupational Therapy Association for the record of the U.S. Senate Committee on Indian affairs oversight hearing on youth suicide prevention.* Bethesda, MD: American Occupational Therapy Association, Inc.

American Occupational Therapy Association (AOTA). (2008). The occupational therapy practice framework. *American Journal of Occupational Therapy, 62*(6), 625–683.

American Psychiatric Association (APA). (2000). *Diagnostic and statistical manual of mental disorders*–text revision (4th ed., text revision). Washington, DC: American Psychiatric Association.

Andover, M., Pepper, C., & Gibb, B. (2007). Self-mutilation and coping strategies in a college sample. *Suicide and Life-Threatening Behavior, 37*(2), 238–243.

Barnes, K. J., Beck, A. J., Vogel, K. A., Grice, K. O., & Murphy, D. (2003). Perceptions regarding school-based occupational therapy for children with emotional disturbances. *The American Journal of Occupational Therapy, 57,* 337–341.

Bates, M. P. (2001). The Child and Adolescent Functional Assessment Scale (CAFAS): Review and current status. *Clinical Child and Family Psychology Review, 4*(1), 63–81.

Baum, C. (1999). A role for OT in preventing school violence. Retrieved from http://www.aota.org/Practitioners/PracticeAreas/Emerging/CY/PsychSoc/36225.aspx

Brown, C. & Dunn, W. (2002). *Adolescent-Adult Sensory Profile.* San Antonio, TX: Pearson.

Brent, D. (2003, June). *NAMI: Suicide in youth.* Retrieved from http://www.nami.org/Template.cfm?Section=By_Illness&Template=/TaggedPage/TaggedPageDisplay.cfm&TPLID=54&ContentID=23041.

Bullying: what to do about it. (2011). Retrieved from http://www.mentalhealthamerica.net/index.cfm?objectId=CA866CC5-1372-4D20-C890BF7CF0FDB428

Chaudry, A., & Fortuny, K. (2010). *Children of immigrants: Economic well-being.* Washington DC: Urban Institute.

Cocozza, J. J., & Skowkra, K. (2000). Youth with mental health disorders: Issues and emerging responses [Electronic version]. *Juvenile Justice, 7*(1).

Costa, D. M. (2009). Eating disorders: Occupational therapy's role. *OT Practice, 14*(11), 13.

Daunhauer, L., & Jacobs, K. (2007). OTs role in preventing youth violence. Retrieved from http://www.aota.org/Practitioners/PracticeAreas/Emerging/CY/PsychSoc/36242.aspx

DePanfilis, D., & Dubowitz, H. (2005). Family Connections: A program for preventing child neglect. *Child Maltreatment, 10,* 108–123.

Dorman, C., Lehsten, L., Woodin, M., Cohen, R., Schweitzer, J., & Tona, J. (2009). Using sensory tools for teens with behavioral and emotional problems. *OT Practice, 14*(20), 16–21.

Favazza. A. (1996). *Bodies under siege: Self-Mutilation and body modification in culture and psychiatry.* Baltimore, MD: Johns Hopkins University Press.

Fry, R., Johnson, S. M., & Morgan, R. (2002). *Parent Project Sr.: A parent workbook.* Boulder City, NV: Parent Project, Inc.

Gardiner, C., & Brown, N. (2010). Is there a role for occupational therapy within a specialist child and adolescent mental health eating disorder service? *British Journal of Occupational Therapy, 73*(1), 38–43.

Goertz, H., Benedict, B., Bui, O., Peitz, S., Ryba, R., & Cahill, S. (2008). AOTA's societal statement on youth violence. *American Journal of Occupational Therapy, 62*(6), 709–710.

Goldstein, A. P., Glick, B., & Gibbs, J. C. (1998). *Aggression replacement training.* Champaign, IL: Research Press.

Grisso, T. (2004). *Double jeopardy: Adolescent offenders with mental disorders.* Chicago: University of Chicago Press.

Gutman, S. A. (2005). Understanding suicide: What therapists should know. *Occupational Therapy in Mental Health, 21*, 55–77.

Hussey, S., Sabonis-Chafee, B., & O'Brien, J.C. (2007). *Introduction to occupational therapy.* Oxford, England: Elsevier.

Jones, A. (1998). *104 activities that build: Self-esteem, teamwork, communication, anger management, self-discovery, and coping skills.* Lusby, MD: Rec Room Publishing.

Kaiser, E., Gillette, C., & Spinazzola, J. (2010). Trauma treatment: A controlled pilot-outcome study of sensory intergration (SI) in the treatment of complex adaptation to traumatic stress. *Journal of Aggression, Maltreatment, and Trauma, 19*, 699–720.

Kloczko, E., & Ikiugu, M. (2006). The role of occupational therapy in the treatment of adolescents with eating disorders as perceived by mental health therapists. *Occupational Therapy in Mental Health, 22*(1), 63–83.

Klonsky, D., Oltmanns, T., & Turkheimer, E. (2003). Deliberate self-harm in a nonclinical population: prevalence and psychological correlates. *American Journal of Psychiatry, 160*, 1501–1508.

Korb-Khalsa, K. L., Azok, S. D., & Leutenberg, E. A. (1993). *Life management skills I: Reproducible activity handouts created for facilitators.* Beachwood, OH: Wellness Reproductions and Publishing, Inc.

Landesman, S. R., & Ramey, C. T. (1999). Early experience and early intervention for children "at-risk" for developmental delays and mental retardation. *Mental Retardation & Developmental Disabilities Research Reviews, 5*(1), 1–10.

Law, M., Baptiste, S., Carswell, A., McColl, M., Polatajko, H., & Pollock, N. (2005). *Canadian Occupational Performance (COPM).* Toronto: Canadian Association of Occupational Therapist Publications.

Lock, J., Le Grange, D., Agras, W., Moye, A., Bryson, S., & Jo, B. (2010). Randomized clinical trial comparing family-based treatment with adolescent-focused individual therapy for adolescents with anorexia nervosa. *Archives of General Psychiatry, 67*(10), 1025.

Moro, C. (2007). A comprehensive literature review defining self-mutilation and occupational therapy intervention approaches–dialectical behavior therapy and sensory integration. *Occupational Therapy in Mental Health, 23*(1), 55–67.

Najavits, L. M. (2002*). Seeking safety: A treatment manual for PTSD and substance abuse.* New York: Guilford.

National Institute for Mental Health. (2011). Retrieved from http://www.nimh.nih.gov/health/publications/suicide-in-the-us-statistics-and-prevention/index.shtml#factors

National Research Council, Institute of Medicine. (2009). *Preventing mental, emotional, and behavioral disorders among young people: Progress and possibilities.* Washington, DC: National Academies Press.

New Freedom Commission on Mental Health. (2003). *Achieving the promise: Transforming mental health care in America, Final Report.* Washington DC: U.S. Department of Health & Human Services.

Scheinholtz, M., Dorman, W., Swith, Y., Clark, G. F., & Jaffe, E. G. (2001, April). *Mental health of children and youth: Prevention and intervention.* Philadelphia.

Schroeder Oxer, S., & Kopp Miller, B. (2001). Effects of choice in an art occupation with adolescents living in residential treatment facilities. *Occupational Therapy in Mental Health, 17*(1), 39–49.

Shearsmith–Farthing, K. (2001). The management of altered body image: a role for occupational therapy. *British Journal of Occupational Therapy, 64*(8), 387–392.

Sonnander, K., & Claesson, M. (1999). Predictors of developmental delays at 18 months and later school achievement problems. *Developmental Medicine and Child Neurology, (41)*3, 195–202.

Steinberg, A. M., Brymer, M. J., Decker, K. B., & Pynoos, K. B. (2004). *The University of California at Los Angeles post-traumatic stress disorder reaction index.* New York: Springer.

U.S. Department of Commerce. (2009). *Census Bureau, Current Population Survey (CPS), October 1970 through October 2008.* Washington, DC: U.S. Department of Commerce, U.S. Census Bureau.

U.S. Department of Education, National Center for Education Statistics. (2010). *The Condition of Education 2010.* Washington, DC: U.S. Department of Education.

U.S. Department of Health and Human Services, National Institute of Mental Health. (n.d.). *Suicide in the U.S.: Statistics and prevention* (NIH Publication No. 06–4594). Retrieved from http://www.nimh.nih.gov/health/publications/suicide-in-the-us-statistics-and-prevention/index.shtml

Walsh, B. (2008). *Treating self-injury: A practical guide.* New York: Guilford Press.

Williams, K., & Bydalek, K. (2007). Adolescent self-mutilation diagnosis & treatment. *Journal of Psychosocial Nursing and Mental Health Services, 45,* 1219–1225.

Wyman, P. A., Hendricks Brown, C., LoMurray, M., Schmeelk-Cone, K., Yu, Q., et al. (2010). An outcome evaluation of the Sources of Strength suicide prevention program delivered by peer leaders in high schools. *American Journal of Public Health, 100*(9), 1653–1662.

Youth violence. (2010). Retrieved from http://www.cdc.gov/violenceprevention/pdf/YV-DataSheet-a.pdf

SUGGESTED RESOURCES

Passmore, A. (2003). The occupation of leisure: Three typologies and their influence on mental health in adolescence. *OTJR, 23*(2), 76–83.

SAMHSA's National Registry of Evidence-Based Programs and Practices (http://nrepp.samhsa.gov/AboutNREPP.aspx)—evidence based programs and standards. Tools for starting programs.

SUGGESTED WEBSITES

American Psychiatric Association:
http://www.healthyminds.org/More-Info-For/Children.aspx

American Psychological Association:
http://www.apa.org/pi/families/children-mental-health.aspx

Animal Assisted Therapy White Paper:
http://research.vet.upenn.edu/Portals/36/media/CIAS_AAI_white_paper.pdf
http://nrepp.samhsa.gov/AboutNREPP.aspx—evidence based programs and standards. Tools for starting programs.

Child/Adolescent Substance Abuse:
http://www.aacap.org/cs/root/resources_for_families/child_and_adolescent_mental_illness_statistics

Images of Chldren's Mental Health:
http://www.google.com/search?q=children's+mental+health&start=30&hl=en&sa=N&biw=1264&bih=620&prmd=ivnscm&tbm=isch&tbo=u&source=univ&ei=911BTtmYD9Kv0AGM7Z3LCQ&ved=0CGQQsAQ4Hg

Mental Health Association- Resources for Young adults and adolescents:
http://www.nmha.org/go/children

NAMI- Teen and Child Focus:
http://www.nami.org/template.cfm?section=child_and_teen_support

National Center for Children In Poverty Resources:
http://nccp.org/publications/pub_687.html

National Federation of Families for Children's Mental Health—Family Advocacy:
http://ffcmh.org/

National Institute of Health Medline Plus Library:
http://www.nlm.nih.gov/medlineplus/childmentalhealth.html

National Institute of Mental Health:
http://nimh.nih.gov/health/topics/child-and-adolescent-mental-health/index.shtml

Substance Abuse and Mental Health Services/Recovery:
http://store.samhsa.gov/home

Chapter 14

Mental Health of the Older Adult

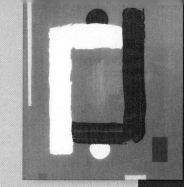

Anne MacRae, PhD, OTR/L, BCMH, FAOTA
Jerilyn (Gigi) Smith, MS, OTR/L

KEY TERMS

aging in place

delirium

dementia

elder abuse

geriatric

in vivo

lifestyle redesign

Medicare

quality of life

somatic

well elderly

CHAPTER OUTLINE

Introduction

The Demographics of Aging

Psychiatric Diagnosis

    Dementia

Mental Health Assessment

    Occupational Therapy Assessment

    Quality of Life Assessment

Occupational Therapy Intervention

    Occupation

    Environmental Support and Adaptation

    Behavioral Techniques and Humanistic Philosophy

    Prevention and Health Maintenance

Summary

INTRODUCTION

This chapter, while focusing on mental health issues that affect aging individuals, also addresses the health of the older adult from a broader perspective. The interdependence of context with physical and mental health is even more pronounced in the elderly than in the general population. Furthermore, as discussed throughout this chapter, there are several external factors that confound the ability to address psychiatric or psychological problems of this age group. Many occupational therapists have long held the belief that the medical model is insufficient to meet all of the health-related needs of the world's population. Nowhere is that more evident than in meeting the needs of the older adult. The health conditions of this population are more likely to be of a chronic nature. Many individuals have multiple medical problems that, when combined with changes that occur in the normal aging process and further superimposed with mental health issues, present a complicated case for assessment and intervention. As will be shown in this chapter, the mental as well as physical health of the older population is explicitly contingent on physical, social, and personal contexts. The medical profession has attempted to address the specific issues of aging with the development of specialties in **geriatric** medicine and psychiatry. The American Psychological Association has published a document, "Guidelines for Psychological Practice with Older Adults," that addresses attitudes, general knowledge about adult development, aging and older adults, clinical issues related to aging and psychopathology, assessment and intervention, and the need for ongoing education with respect to working with older adults with mental health issues (APA, 2004). The Guidelines stress that an interdisciplinary, coordinated care approach is essential in the treatment of this older population in order to ensure the most effective care.

THE DEMOGRAPHICS OF AGING

According to the Administration on Aging (AoA) (2009), the population of older adults (age 65+) in the United States in the year 2008 totaled 38.9 million people. This represents 12.8% of the U.S. population or more than one in every eight individuals. By the year 2030, this population is expected to more than double to 72.1 million. Minority populations are projected to increase from 8.0 million (16.3% of the elderly population) in 2010 to 12.9 million (23.6% of the elderly population) in 2020. The worldwide demographic changes are even more dramatic.

> The number of persons aged 60 years or older was estimated to be 688 million in 2006 and is projected to grow to almost 2 billion by 2050, at which time, the population of older persons will be larger than the population of children (0–4 years) for the first time in human history. (United Nations Secretariat, 2010)

This rise in numbers of older adults will have significant effects on all areas of human and societal function, particularly economics and family dynamics (Crystal, 2005). To provide effective care for this population, all health professionals will need to expand their focus beyond a medical model and become advocates for change in social, economic, and health care policies and systems.

In 2002, 17% of individuals in the United States age 64 to 75 assessed their health as fair or poor, with this number rising to 43% in those aged 85 and above (National Institute on Aging, 2007). Most older adults have at least one chronic condition and many have multiple chronic conditions. Self-report of health has repeatedly been shown in the literature to have a high correlation to disability and function (Han, 2002; National Institute on Aging, 2007). Clearly, the health care needs of this population are significant. However, these data also show that the majority of older people are healthy and are active and productive members of their communities. In 2008, 39% of community dwelling older persons rated their overall health as excellent or very good (AoA, 2009). This group is commonly referred to as the **well elderly**. Some of the factors that help the older adult stay healthy are obvious and are tied to known healthy living factors of the general population (no smoking, diet, management of preexisting health conditions, etc.). Interestingly, however, many of the factors identified in the promotion of elder health are related to the psychological and social well-being of the individual, which is discussed in this chapter.

PSYCHIATRIC DIAGNOSIS

It is widely reported in the literature that older adults have a much lower incidence of all psychiatric diagnosis, excluding cognitive disorders, than any other age group (American Geriatric Society [AGS], 2005). However, such statistics must be viewed with caution for several reasons.

1. Most older adults receive their health care through a primary physician or a general medicine clinic or institution. There is a serious lack of training and administrative support in these settings for identifying symptoms of mental illness and making appropriate referrals (AGS, 2005; Jervis, 2002).

2. There is generally a greater concern in the older population than in the general population about the stigma of mental illness and therefore treatment specified as "psychiatric" or "psychological" is often avoided (Davis, Moye, & Karel, 2002; Conner et al., 2010; Sajatovic et al., 2008).

3. The majority of older adults in the United States are at least partially dependent on **Medicare** (a government-sponsored health care payment program, primarily for those over age 65), which is woefully inadequate in reimbursement for mental health. The consequence of this is twofold: The individual avoids such treatment and the health care providers are often unwilling to diagnose and treat conditions that may not be reimbursable (AGS, 2005).

4. Presentation of psychiatric illness in the elderly is often different than in younger people and is therefore difficult to diagnose. Most notably is the tendency of the elderly to emphasize and describe **somatic** (physical) concerns rather than emotional concerns (Stewart, 2004). This often leads to both under-recognized psychiatric illness and unnecessary medical treatment.

It is estimated that there are approximately 1 million older adults in the United States with severe mental illness (SMI) and this number is expected to double by 2030 (Cohen, 2003). Older adults with SMI have complicated issues due to their psychiatric condition, lack of available, or ineffective treatment interventions and additional complications brought on by the aging process (Cummings & Kropf, 2009).

Even in cases where the individual may not meet the full criteria for a psychiatric disorder, many psychiatric symptoms may be found in the elderly population due to general medical conditions, side effects of medications, or life stressors (AGS, 2005). Many of these symptoms (described in Table 14-1) are treatable if recognized. These psychiatric symptoms are sometimes seen in **dementia**, but may also be indicative of a separate and distinct disorder that too often goes undiagnosed and therefore untreated.

TABLE 14-1. Presentation of Psychiatric Symptoms in Older Adults

Psychiatric Condition	Diagnostic Issues
Anxiety	Until a few years ago anxiety disorders were believed to decline with age. However, experts now say that anxiety is as common among the old as among the young and many older adults with an anxiety disorder had one when they were younger (ADAA, 2010). Anxiety is a common symptom that is associated with other medical and psychiatric conditions (Beattie, Pachana, & Franklin, 2010; Gum, King-Kallimanis, & Kohn, 2009), as well as changes in environment and other life stressors associated with aging. Generalized anxiety disorder (GAD) is the most common anxiety disorder in late life (Porensky et al., 2009). GAD is a chronic disorder that is unlikely to resolve without treatment (Bruce et al., 2005). New onset of anxiety in older adults may also be associated with medication side effects and drug withdrawal (Flint, 2001). Elders living alone may be more prone to a "phobic type" anxiety (Schaub & Linden, 2000). Anxiety symptoms are associated with greater disability, significant impairment in health related quality of life (Porensky et al., 2009), and greater health care usage among older adults (Hoffman, Dukes, & Wittchen, 2008). Anxiety disorders cause a great deal of distress for the elderly individual and has a significant negative impact on quality of life.
Depression	Depression in later life frequently coexists with other medical illnesses and disabilities. Late life depression is common in older individuals who have chronic or disabling medical disorders such as diabetes, cardiovascular disease, arthritis, renal disease, and stroke (Drayer et al., 2005) and often leads to increasing negative health outcomes, a worsening of self-rated health and self-perceived disability, increased somatization, higher rates of hospital and nursing home admissions, and premature mortality (Ganguli, Dodge, & Mulsant, 2002).

TABLE 14-1. Continued

Psychiatric Condition	Diagnostic Issues
Depression (Continued)	Social isolation is a significant contributor to the development of geriatric depression (Anderson, 2001). There are many factors that contribute to social isolation including mobility limitations, medical illnesses, financial constraints, loss of a spouse, significant others, and social networks. Social isolation results in impaired social engagement and decreased participation in social activities.
	Depression is not a normal part of aging, however, many believe this to be true, which contributes to it being under-recognized, under-diagnosed, and under-treated. Depression in the older population also presents itself differently than it does in younger individuals (AGS, 2005; Beattie et al., 2010; Stewart, 2004), which leads to mis- or under-diagnosis by physicians.
	A depressed or sad mood may be not be reported by the individual. More commonly reported symptoms include: anergy (lack of energy), anhedonia (absence of pleasure), loss of appetite, sleeplessness, somatic complaints (such as unexplained pain, headaches, chronic fatigue, anorexia, gastrointestinal complaints, weight loss), anxiety, apathy, withdrawal, and cognitive impairment (Alexopoulos, Schultz, & Lebowitz, 2005; Rojas-Fernandez, Miller, & Sadowski, 2010).
	Geriatric depression is a serious medical condition that can lead to a significantly compromised quality of life. Depression among the elderly can lead to suicide. Older white males have the highest rate of suicide among all age groups. Over 70% of older suicide victims visited their primary physician during the month prior to their attempt and many had depressive illness that went undetected during this visit. The majority of older adults with depression improve when they receive treatment with antidepressant medication, psychotherapy, or a combination of both (National Institute of Mental Health, 2009).
Bipolar Disorder	Diagnosis of bipolar disorder in the older adult is typically designated as early-onset (individuals who developed their illness during early adulthood) and late-onset (those who experienced their first mood episode at an older age) (Depp & Jeste, 2004). Research shows that older individuals with bipolar disorder (BD) have substantially compromised cognitive functioning, which negatively affects daily functioning and compliance with treatment (Sigfried et al., 2009). Deficits in executive functions and verbal memory are prevalent (Depp et al., 2007; Martinez-Aran et al., 2004) and when added to the changes that accompany aging in general, present a considerable challenge for the individual. This has important clinical implications in terms of determining effective intervention strategies that take into account the often significant cognitive deficits that accompany this disorder.
	Mania may also be a symptom of cognitive disorders or confused with the irritability and lability found in dementia and delirium.
Psychosis	Psychotic symptoms are associated with a myriad of different psychiatric and medical disorders, including delirium, major depression, affective illness, Alzheimer's type dementia, schizophrenia or other primary psychotic disorders, general medical conditions, and substance abuse or dependence (Kyomen & Whitfield, 2009). Psychotic features including hallucinations, thought disturbances, poverty of thinking, irrationality, delusions, and behavioral disturbance vary depending upon the etiology of the psychosis. Management of psychosis in the elderly is complicated and involves careful, multidisciplinary assessment of the individual.

(Continues)

TABLE 14-1. Continued

Psychiatric Condition	Diagnostic Issues
Substance Abuse	Alcohol and substance abuse are under-recognized in the elderly population and warning signs (such as falls, relationship conflicts, and memory impairment) may be misattributed to the aging process (Klimstra & Mahgoub, 2010). The negative effects of use, abuse, and addiction to alcohol and other substances are intensified in the older adult as a result of the aging changes, chronic disease processes, and dangerous interactions with over-the-counter and prescribed medications (Clay, 2010). Alcohol or other substance abuse is also commonly found in elders with depression and may be used as a maladaptive coping strategy. Alcohol abuse impairs memory and information processing and may go unrecognized in the early stages of dementia and yet cause significant functional deterioration. Toxicity from over-the-counter medications and combinations of prescribed medications also can cause both serious medical consequences as well as cognitive impairments that may erroneously lead to a diagnosis of early dementia (Hall, 2002). Risk factors for the initiation or exacerbation of substance abuse or addiction in elders include female sex, polypharmacy, chronic physical illness, poor health, and a history of or concurrent psychiatric or other substance use disorder (Simoni-Wastila & Yang, 2006).

© Cengage Learning 2013

CASE ILLUSTRATION

Mr. Sorensen—Differential Diagnosis: Depression and Dementia

Mr. Sorensen is a widower who lives in an elder assisted living facility. His wife of 42 years who visited him every day suddenly passed away and the family had to put their aging dog to sleep because no one was able to care for him. The staff noted that Mr. Sorensen was not eating well and was spending more time alone. He was generally noncommunicative and often appeared confused. He needed prompting to get out of bed in the morning and supervision to complete personal care.

Discussion

Grief and multiple losses are common in the elderly and can lead to depression if not addressed. The staff at the facility may not realize the magnitude of Mr. Sorensen's personal losses and dismiss his current behavior as to be expected given the recent losses in his life. Mr. Sorensen may indeed have a progressive dementia, but the life stressors he is enduring certainly warrant intervention, including counseling and/or medication, for what may be a treatable depression.

CASE ILLUSTRATION

Mrs. DeVaughn—Differential Diagnosis: Toxicity and Dementia

Mrs. DeVaughn has been displaying increased confusion, memory loss, and irritability. Her daughter, Edna, arranged for a home health care team to evaluate her safety in the home. She fully expected that a recommendation would be made for Mrs. DeVaughn to move to a supervised living situation because of what her daughter sees as deteriorating dementia. Mrs. DeVaughn refused to let the visiting nurse go over her medications with her, but agreed to let the occupational therapist help her organize her bathroom and kitchen cabinets "just to make things easier." The occupational therapist found 14 prescription medications prescribed by five different medical specialists as well as her primary care physician. She also found a plethora of over-the-counter medications as well as herbal supplements. The occupational therapist contacted the case manager nurse, who arranged with the physician to have Mrs. DeVaughn hospitalized so her medicines could either be discontinued, reduced, or changed. Within three days, Mrs. De Vaughn's mental status markedly improved and, much to her daughter's surprise, she was able to return to independent living.

Discussion

While physicians and pharmacists have increased their awareness of drug interactions and symptoms and methods for tracking medical prescriptions are much improved, the problems associated with using multiple health care providers still exists. The older adult tends to trust health care providers and is unlikely to question a prescription or offer information about other medications unless specifically asked. The occupational therapist is in an ideal position to evaluate actual medication regimens in the home by addressing daily living habits and routines and can then coordinate with the team for treatment recommendations. In any case of suspected dementia, it is vital that all other, often treatable, causes are ruled out. In the case of Mrs. DeVaughn, there may have also been a metabolic or general medical condition, such as decreased kidney function, that would increase the likelihood of toxicity (increased concentration of substances because of decreased elimination resulting in a change in mental status).

All of the symptoms and disorders listed in Table 14-1 are described in depth in various chapters of this book. However, unique to the elderly population (at least in terms of high incidence) is dementia, an emotionally, socially, and physically devastating condition, which therefore warrants further discussion.

Dementia

Dementia is a syndrome identified by the presence of multiple cognitive deficits. (For further information and definitions of cognitive deficits, see Chapter 16.) Dementia has an insidious onset, characterized by the slow onset of short-term memory loss. It is a chronic, progressive, and irreversible condition in which the individual retains normal levels of alertness. Attention and concentration are globally affected and language impairment and confabulation are common. In addition to memory impairment and other cognitive deficits, a person with a dementia demonstrates a significant decline in overall function. Dementia is irreversible in 80% to 95% of cases (Yap & Holzapfel, 2006). An estimated 2 million people in the United States suffer from severe dementia and another 1 to 5 million people experience mild to moderate dementia. Five to eight percent of people over the age of 65 have some form of dementia and the number doubles every 5 years over age 65 (Healthcommunities.com, 2011).

Dementia may be caused by a wide variety of conditions, including degenerative disorders of the central nervous system such as Parkinson's disease or Huntington's disease; cardiac disorders, which may result in vascular dementia; metabolic disorders such as diabetes that may result in vascular dementia or uncontrolled thyroid conditions; nutritional, especially vitamin, deficiencies; toxicity or drug-related, such as substance-induced dementia; brain tumors, trauma, and infections, most notably Creutzfeldt-Jacob Disease (CJD) and human immunodeficiency virus (HIV). From a medical viewpoint, it is critical to determine the underlying reason for the dementia, as many of the aforementioned conditions can be medically treated or at least controlled. However, more than half of all diagnosed dementia is caused by Alzheimer's disease, a progressive condition for which there is no known cure.

Vascular dementia and Alzheimer's disease are both strongly age-related, with the prevalence approximately doubling every five years after age 65 (Alzheimer's Disease International [ADI], 2010). The World Alzheimer Report 2010 (ADI, 2010) estimates that in 2010 there were 35.6 million people living with dementia worldwide and projects that the number of people with dementia will rise to 65.7 million by 2030 and 115.4 million by 2050. This is a dramatic increase from the estimated 18 million people who were identified with dementia in 2000. The implications of societal costs of dementia and the impact of these on families, health, and social care services are staggering.

Alzheimer's disease is progressive and often difficult to diagnose in its early stages; therefore, the diagnosis may be made retrospectively or when all other causes of the dementia have been ruled out. The relatively minor memory problems consistent with early stages of the disease may be found in any older adult and is not necessarily indicative of the relentless pending decline in function and cognition seen in Alzheimer's disease

Table 14-2 outlines the stages of the disease as described by Reisberg, Ferris, and Crook (1983) in the Global Deterioration Scale. The staging is helpful in anticipating common reactions and behaviors and adjusting intervention to address them.

TABLE 14-2. Clinical Course of Alzheimer's Disease

Stage	Description	Examples of Performance and Behaviors
Stage 1	No cognitive decline	Normal functioning—occasional lapses of memory.
Stage 2	Very mild cognitive decline	No deficits noted in occupational or social roles. However, the individual may express concern over "forgetfulness." Often forgets names or misplaces objects.
Stage 3	Mild cognitive decline	Immediate recall is impaired and agnosia may be present. Because of decreased performance in demanding employment and social situations, it is in this stage that family, friends, and coworkers may recognize a problem. Anxiety over performance is common at this stage, but there is usually significant denial as well.
Stage 4	Moderate cognitive decline	Deficits are now obvious, including poor concentration, decreased knowledge of recent and current events, and difficulties traveling alone (especially to unfamiliar places) and in handling personal finances. The individual usually remains orientated to time and familiar places and persons. There is often a withdrawal from new or challenging situations and the person generally will still be in denial of the seriousness of her or his condition.
Stage 5	Moderately severe cognitive decline	Individuals at stage 5 generally need assistance to live safely. They are likely to forget important phone numbers or emergency procedures and are frequently disoriented to time or place, but usually will remember own name and names of close friends and family. The person begins to have problems with multistep daily living activities, such as dressing, but does not need assistance with many personal care tasks such as eating or toileting.
Stage 6	Severe cognitive decline	The individual occasionally forgets spouse's name or the names of other significant people in his or her life. Retains some sketchy knowledge of past life, but is largely unaware of recent events and experiences. Disoriented to time and place. Sleep patterns are frequently disturbed. There is often marked personality/emotional changes in this stage that may include delusions, obsessiveness, anxiety, agitation, apathy, and, occasionally, violent behavior.
Stage 7	Very severe cognitive decline	Profound physical symptoms such as incontinence and limited mobility (may be unable to walk). Communication is severely impaired and may be limited to grunting. Needs assistance with all personal care.

Adapted from the *Global Deterioration Scale* by Reisberg, Ferris, & Crook, 1983.

People who exhibit symptoms of dementia may have potentially treatable conditions, such as nutritional deficits, side effects from medications, or depression, and this should be taken into careful consideration by the individual's physician.

Delirium is sometimes confused for dementia in the elderly. **Delirium** is an acute confusional state accompanied by agitation. It has an abrupt onset, fluctuating levels of alertness and variable states of orientation. Delirium affects elders primarily in acute care settings. Older adults are at an increased risk for delirium because the aging neurologic system is more vulnerable to insults caused by underlying systemic conditions (Thompson-Heisterman, 2006). Delirium is one of the most common complications of medical illness, prolonged hospital stays, or recovery from surgery among elderly individuals. Delirium is typically considered to be a short duration, temporary problem, but it may persist for months if the underlying cause is not determined and treated. Reversible causes of delirium include: drugs (especially narcotics, other pain relievers, sedatives, corticosteroids, and drugs that affect acetylcholine levels in the brain), electrolyte disturbances (dehydration and thyroid problems), lack of drugs (stopping use of long-term sedatives), infection, reduced sensory input (i.e., poor vision or hearing), urinary problems, myocardial problems, chronic obstructive lung disease, and alcohol abuse (AGS Foundation for Health and Aging, 2005). The primary goal for treatment of delirium is to identify and treat the underlying cause or causes. This includes looking at medical and environmental factors.

MENTAL HEALTH ASSESSMENT

All health care providers should be cognizant of the presence of psychiatric disorders in their elderly clients, particularly ones that are too often overlooked, such as depression and substance abuse. Simple screening tools may identify treatable conditions. The most commonly used depression screen for older adults is the Geriatric Depression Scale (GDS), originally designed by Yesavage et al. (1983) and now available in the public domain. The GDS is a 30-item self-report assessment consisting of questions related to seven common characteristics of depression in later life (somatic concern, lowered affect, cognitive impairment, feelings of discrimination, impaired motivation, lack of future orientation, and lack of self-esteem). The questions are answered with yes/no responses. The short version containing 15 questions (Shiekh & Yesavage, 1986) probably has the most widespread usage. The GDS has shown to be a reliable and cost-effective screening tool, especially when used in conjunction with other tests (Peach, Koob, & Kraus, 2001). The Short Anxiety Screening Test has been shown to be a valid tool in detecting anxiety in the elderly, especially in those with depression (Sinoff, Ore, Zlotogorsky, & Tamir, 1999). There are several screening tools used to identify geriatric alcohol abuse. One of the most popular is the Short Michigan Alcoholism Screening Test-Geriatric Version (MAST-G) (University of Michigan Alcohol Research Center, 1991). Many self-screening tools are available on the Internet and offer recommendations to the individual and their family on how to access help for the specific problem.

Given the global effects of dementia on the individual and her or his family, it is important to arrive at a working diagnosis as early as possible. There are several specific assessments to screen, diagnose, and classify the stages of Alzheimer's disease as well as other dementias. Two examples are the 7-Minute Screen (Meulen et al., 2004) and the INECO Frontal Screening Test (Torralva, Roca, Gleichgerrcht, Lopez, & Manes, 2009).

Occupational Therapy Assessment

Assessment of the overall mental health of older adults is often conducted as an interdisciplinary effort. The focus of the interdisciplinary assessment corresponds with many of the traditional domains of occupational therapy; therefore, OT assessments, especially those that focus on cognition, occupation, environment, and social relations, are valuable for this population. Figure 14-1 is a select list of assessments that focus on these areas; most, but not all, were designed by occupational therapists.

Many other assessments that are described throughout this book can also be used with the older adult population, and readers are encouraged to explore a wide variety of assessments to fit the individual needs of particular clients. A crucial contribution of occupational therapy in the assessment of the elderly individual with psychiatric illness lies in the occupational therapist's unique skill in performing functional evaluations, either through formal assessment or task analysis, *in vivo*, or in the client's natural environment. A study by Hoppes, Davis, and Thompson (2003) on the environmental effects on the assessment of people with dementia concluded that "while it may be time consuming to assess clients in specific settings of interest, this may be the only valid way to determine abilities to function in those settings" (p. 401). In Chapter 2, a case illustration was given (Uyen—Performance in Community) where the in-clinic assessment overestimated the client's functional capabilities. The next case illustration demonstrates the opposite situation.

Title of Assessment and Author(s)/Source

Activity Index & Meaningfulness of Activity Scale (Gregory, 1983).

Assessment of Communication and Interaction Skills (ACIS) (Forsyth, Salamy, Simon, & Kielhofner, available through MOHO Clearinghouse).

Assessment of Living Skills and Resources (ALSAR) (Williams et al., 1991)

Assessment of Motor and Process Skills (AMPS) (Fisher & Bray Jones, 2010; available only to therapists who have received training).

Cognitive Performance Test (CPT) (Burns, Mortimer, & Merchak, 1994).

Community Integration Measure (McColl, Davies, Carlson, Johnston, & Milnnes, 2001).

Contextual Memory Test (Toglia, available through Therapy Skill Builders).

Lowenstein Occupational Therapy Cognitive Assessment-Geriatric (LOTCA-G) (Itzkovich, Elazar, & Katz available through various sources).

Mini Mental State Exam (Folstein, Folstein, & McHugh, 1975).

Multidimensional Functional Assessment Questionnaire (Fillenbaum & Duke University, 1988).

Rivermead Behavioral Memory Test, 3rd Edition (Wilson et al., 2008).

Test of Orientation for Rehabilitation Patients (TORP) (Deitz, Tovar, Beeman, Thorn, & Trevisan, 1992).

FIGURE 14-1. Assessments for Use with Older Adults: A Selective List with a Focus on Cognition, Occupation, Environment, and Social Relations

CASE ILLUSTRATION

Mrs. Ayala—*In Vivo* Assessment

Mrs. Ayala is a 76-year-old woman with a history of vascular disease who was recently hospitalized for a transient ischemic attack (TIA). The hospital interdisciplinary team determined that she had a moderate level of dementia, most likely of the vascular type. The hospital-based occupational therapist performed a kitchen assessment in the OT clinic to determine Mrs. Ayala's safety and functional abilities in activities of daily living. During the assessment it was noted that Mrs. Ayala became quite agitated and confused. She did remember to turn off the electric range top, but then placed a plastic bowl on the burner. The occupational therapist needed to intervene to prevent the bowl from melting and then provided moderate assistance to complete the task safely.

The hospital-based team recommended that after discharge Mrs. Ayala not be allowed to stay at home alone. She lives with her daughter's family, but all family members are either at work or school during the day. The family refused to consider placement for her outside the home but did agree to home health care services.

The home health occupational therapist received the discharge notes from the hospital-based therapist. Therefore, she was quite surprised when arriving at Mrs. Ayala's home to find her in the kitchen alone successfully making Pancit (a traditional Filipino meal made of rice stick noodles, vegetables, and shrimp or meat) as well as homemade lumpia (egg rolls) for her family's dinner. When the occupational therapist expressed her concern, Mrs. Ayala laughingly replied, "I've been doing this all of my life!"

Discussion

In her own home, Mrs. Ayala demonstrated a much higher functional ability than previously seen in the hospital. She was able to perform cooking tasks that were actually much more complicated than what was asked of her during the hospital evaluation. The familiarity of the tools (such as a gas range instead of an electric one) and the layout of the kitchen often help people with memory or other cognitive deficits perform tasks automatically. The cultural familiarity with the items being prepared is also an important factor. A third, critical factor is being able to preserve an important and meaningful role as a contributing member of the family.

Quality of Life Assessment

Life satisfaction or **quality of life** assessment is now an important part of an interdisciplinary evaluation and is recognized as a desired outcome of treatment by both the World Health Organization (WHO, 2001) and the American Occupational Therapy Association (AOTA, 2010), as well as many other OT and health care organizations around the world. Despite this recent focus, there is little agreement in the literature on a definition of quality of life. According to Alzheimer's Disease International (ADI, 2000), "quality of life is a much broader concept than either health or disease. It is rather difficult to define as everyone has their own ideas" (p. 1). Some key elements identified by ADI as common elements and areas needing assessment are:

- Mobility
- Social relations
- Affording and obtaining necessities
- Living independently
- Occupations (occupying one's time)
- Comfort
- Self-esteem
- Satisfaction with daily activities
- Sources of pleasure

The important point in a quality of life assessment is to recognize the unique and subjective nature of the client's responses. Clients will have interests and priorities in

CASE ILLUSTRATION

Professor Fujiyama's Quality of Life

Dr. Fujiyama is an emeritus professor of neurobiology at a prestigious university. He is in the early to moderate stage of Alzheimer's disease. All of his adult life he took immense pride in his intellectual ability and is having great difficulty in adjusting to his memory lapses and generally decreased function. He became withdrawn and is often irritable. The home health occupational therapist wanted to engage him in self-care activities but met with great resistance. The occupational therapist decided to change her approach and offered to work with him on "cognitive" activities. She showed the doctor some interactive computer programs on biology and engaged him in several pencil and paper tasks using memory strategies. Eventually he started asking questions about cognitive rehabilitation and the theories behind her choice of activities for him. He developed an interest in using the computer and researching websites about Alzheimer's disease.

The occupational therapist would leave worksheets and suggested activities for the professor after every visit and upon her return he would confidently show the occupational therapist his completed "homework." Although Dr. Fujiyama continued to avoid most activities of daily living (ADLs) and depended on his wife or an aide to perform such tasks, his affect was brighter, he had less angry outbursts, and he appeared more engaged and interested in life.

Discussion

Although the occupational therapist was unable to engage Dr. Fujiyama in many of the traditional activities used by home health therapists, she was able to adjust her intervention to include tasks that were personally meaningful and appropriately challenging to the professor. This provided a quality of life to this client that could not be found in more "conventional" therapy.

life that may be quite different than what the therapist thinks is important. A truly client-centered approach using active listening is essential for a meaningful quality of life assessment. This information is then used to establish goals and formulate an individualized intervention plan.

Quality of life should be addressed in all occupational therapy assessments, but it has particular significance for the older adult, as the more conventional outcomes of restoration, rehabilitation, or improvement of function may not always be realistic goals for many older individuals, depending on the nature of their disability and other complicating factors. This presents one of the many challenges for occupational therapists working with the older adult, as functional "progress" is often the basis for reimbursement and conventional rehabilitation may be viewed by employers as the only OT services that should be offered. Occupational therapists need to advocate for a broadening of their role in many settings and engage in research that demonstrates the long-term cost-effectiveness of quality of life intervention.

OCCUPATIONAL THERAPY INTERVENTION

Intervention for the older adult, as with assessment, is best provided with a holistic and coordinated approach that includes professionals, family members, caregivers, and other significant individuals. However, for the purposes of this chapter, the discussion is limited to those interventions most frequently used by occupational therapists. Depending on the condition being addressed, expected outcomes may include restoration of function and rehabilitation, but goals addressing quality of life, prevention, and adaptation are also crucial for the older adult population.

Occupation

The overarching purpose of occupational therapy is to promote the "engagement in occupation to support participation" (AOTA, 2010). A study conducted by Aubin, Hachey, and Mercier (1999) suggests that "perceived competence in daily tasks and rest, and pleasure in work and rest activities are positively correlated with subjective quality of life. The influence of occupation and its meaning on quality of life, an occupational therapy assumption, is supported by these results" (p. 53). A critical review of 23 other studies concurred:

> Occupation has an important influence on health and well-being. Ranging from physiological to functional outcomes, it is clear that the performance of everyday occupations is an important part of everyday life. Withdrawal or changes in occupation for a person have a significant impact on a person's self-perceived health and well-being. (Law, Steinwender, & Leclair, 1998, pp. 89–90)

Evidence from a review of the literature from diverse sources supports the efficacy of occupational therapy intervention focusing on engagement in occupation for individuals with dementia and their caregivers (Egan, Hobson, & Fearing, 2006). The positive effects of occupation were seen both in the clients and in their caregivers as well. Hasselkus and Murray (2007) found that everyday occupation contributed to the well-being of both the caregiver and the older individual with dementia and facilitated continuity of relationships and identity for the caregiver. Successful engagement in everyday occupation by the care receiver was an important source of satisfaction for the caregiver as well. In a study conducted by Baum (1995), it was found that "individuals who remained active in occupation demonstrated fewer disturbing behaviors, required less help with basic self care, and their carers experienced less stress" (p. 59).

Although considerable research is being conducted on the effects of occupation, it is difficult to draw generalizations. In order for occupation to be effective as an intervention, it must be personally meaningful and must present an appropriate level of challenge. A task that is overly simple may be seen as demeaning, yet an overly complex task may promote feelings of failure. In order for occupation to be used as a therapeutic modality (rather than a simple diversion), it must address the goals established in the occupational therapy assessment. The occupational therapist chooses the activity or occupation in collaboration with the client. Adaptations or gradations to the activity may be necessary to meet specific goals and provide "just the right" challenge for the client. Interventions used by occupational therapists often use occupations or activities that are commonplace in daily life, which may lead to an erroneous conclusion by some that occupation-based interventions may be competently and less expensively conducted by para- or nonprofessionals. While some purely diversional activities groups are helpful and welcomed by the older adult, a groundbreaking three-year well elderly study conducted by Clark et al. (1997) concluded that "superior outcomes can be expected when an activity-centered intervention is administered by professional therapists as opposed to being conducted by nonprofessionals" (p. 1325). The occupational therapist is trained to continually assess and modify the intervention based on the client's performance to elicit outcomes that are geared toward established goal attainment. An individual untrained in occupation-based theory will not have the knowledge to make these modifications.

CASE ILLUSTRATION

The Occupations of Mr. Hatfield

Mr. Hatfield is a retired factory worker who is currently being evaluated for depression and dementia. He reports to the occupational therapist that the only thing that he ever liked doing was fishing but he can't drive his truck to the pier anymore. Through further conversation, the occupational therapist learns that Mr. Hatfield always tied his own flies for fly fishing and she asks him to teach her the craft. He wrote a shopping list of all the supplies that he needed and together they shopped for supplies and continued to tie fancy fishing flies for several sessions. Mr. Hatfield seemed to enjoy the sessions and reminisced about past great fishing trips. However, he clearly still missed his prime occupation of actually going fishing. The occupational therapist helped Mr. Hatfield contact a local volunteer organization to find a fishing companion willing and able to accompany and transport Mr. Hatfield to local

fishing spots. A successful match was made and a trip was planned for the following week. His volunteer companion also told Mr. Hatfield that there was a fly tying club over in the next town and he would be glad to take him to a meeting. Although Mr. Hatfield remained somewhat forgetful and he needed guidance to perform many tasks, his affect greatly improved.

Discussion

Although Mr. Hatfield's interests seem limited, his passion for fishing opened up possibilities for new leisure and social pursuits and provided the motivation to engage in cognitively challenging activities such as constructing a craft and shopping for supplies. The need to teach an activity (to the occupational therapist) also provided a sense of purpose and an opportunity to demonstrate mastery and competence.

Environmental Support and Adaptation

Understanding the context in which treatment is provided is critical to the occupational therapy process (see Chapter 2 for further discussion). Environment plays a vital role in both the overall functioning and the quality of life of the older adult. In the United States and in other parts of the world, the preference of older adults is to remain in their homes or communities for as long as possible. A phenomenological study conducted in Scandinavia "showed that moving to sheltered housing meant for a majority of participants that their self image changed from being self reliant and independent to becoming dependent and perceiving themselves and their care to be a burden" (Sviden, Wikstrom, & Hjortsjo-Norberg, 2002, p. 10). To meet the needs of the older population and honor their choices, facilitating **aging in place** has become a focal point of treatment both for "humanistic reasons and to minimize health care costs" (Horowitz, 2002, p. 1). As discussed in Chapter 2, occupational therapists are specifically trained in environmental adaptation that addresses the physical, social, emotional, spiritual, and cognitive contexts. Given the often complex needs of the older adult, this holistic view of the environment is essential for successful intervention. Aging in place can be facilitated through a variety of environmental interventions, including home modifications. There are many design principles, design goals, and environmental interventions designed to facilitate successful engagement in activities of daily living, however further research is needed to examine the efficacy of these interventions for individuals with mental health issues such as dementia (van Hoof, Kort, van Waarde, & Blom, 2010).

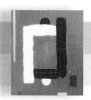

CASE ILLUSTRATION

Mrs. Christie—The Meaning of Home

Mrs. Christie lives in a large Victorian home in the city where she raised her four children. After her husband passed away, her grown children, all with families of their own, wanted her to move to a smaller home or apartment out in the suburbs, closer to them. Two of the four children also offered to have her move in with them. Although Mrs. Christie freely admits that she has slowed down "quite a bit," she still feels quite able to care for herself. Her biggest functional change has been to give up driving. She has groceries delivered or walks to the corner store and either takes a taxi or has a friend drive her to appointments. Mrs. Christie's children all agree that the house is too much work for her and they think she would be safer out of the city. Also, if she was in the suburbs they could check up on her more frequently. She steadfastly resists, stating that she would miss her friends and her garden.

Discussion

Many older adults freely choose to move to a low maintenance residence or move in with family; however, many others wish to stay in a familiar place. While the concerns expressed by Mrs. Christie's children could be realistic, they fail to take into account the personal meaning of home. In some cultures, such as the Anglo-American culture of Mrs. Christie, independence is highly prized and moving in with one's children may be seen as an imposition or failure (even if invited).

A familiar home often provides a sense of community. It is likely that Mrs. Christie knows her neighbors, grocer, church minister, and pharmacist. She has also shown the ability to be adaptive, maintaining her mobility in the community without driving. Her home is a place full of memories and favorite occupations such as gardening. Intervention geared toward helping Mrs. Christie stay as independent as possible in her own home and doing the things she likes to do, rather than encouraging her to abandon her home, would be preferable.

The social context of the environment includes the roles of caregivers, family, and the community as well as the individual client and it is often appropriate for the occupational therapist to include all or some of these others in the client's intervention program. Additionally, education, training, and support should be considered for those who make up the social context of the client. Research indicates that friends of both the older adult and the caregivers provide valuable emotional and social support (Lilly, Richards, & Buckwalter, 2003) and should be included in assessment and treatment as needed. Evaluating the needs of the caregiver and facilitating coping and caregiving strategies as well as empowering caregivers are vital roles of the occupational therapist. As an older adult declines in function, the role of the caregiver increases, thereby increasing her or his stress. If supported by outside services, including receiving necessary education to facilitate the caregiver role, the caregiver may be more effective and may be able to successfully continue in this role for a longer period of time. The cost-effectiveness of a family approach to treatment results in the older adult being able to remain in the home rather than being moved to an institutional placement.

The occupational therapist, along with the social worker, plays a critical role in reconnecting an isolated individual with her or his community by making appropriate referrals to community and social groups and by facilitating the ability to access social support systems. These community referrals may also benefit the caregiver by providing support and respite.

Although aging in place is preferred by many older adults and has many advantages, care must be taken not to assume that one's home always provides the ideal living situation. For many people the responsibility of home management is not possible or is overly stressful. According to the Administration on Aging (2009), in 2008, 72% of older men lived with their spouse, while less than one half (42%) of older women did. Additionally, older women were more than twice as likely as older men to live alone (40% and 19%, respectively). In the case of Mrs. Christie, living alone was clearly her choice and she was still actively involved in her community and had a social support network. However, for many older adults, living alone can be a frightening and lonely experience. A move to a socially active senior residence or to a family member's home may ease the loneliness as well as provide necessary support to maintain maximal well-being.

Another aspect of the environmental conditions that must be evaluated is the potential for **elder abuse**, which can occur in any setting and affects elders across all socioeconomic groups, cultures, and races. Women and "older" elders are more likely to be victimized as are seniors with dementia or other mental health and substance abuse issues.

Elder abuse can take many different forms. Physical abuse, sexual abuse, emotional or psychological abuse, neglect, abandonment, financial or material exploitation, and self-neglect (a refusal or failure to provide him- or herself with adequate food, water, clothing, shelter, personal hygiene, medication, or safety) are examples of elder abuse (National Center on Elder Abuse, 2007). According to the best available estimates, between 1 and 2 million Americans over the age of 65 have been injured, exploited, or otherwise mistreated by someone on whom they depended for care or protection (National Research Council Panel to Review Risk and Prevalence of Elder Abuse and Neglect, 2003). This may be an underestimation, as victims of elder abuse rarely report such incidences, and they are not likely to be seen in public where others may report their concerns. The older person may fear being abandoned by the very person responsible for the abuse or may be afraid of further abuse. Cognitive impairment may impede the individual's ability to report abuse.

CASE ILLUSTRATION

The Abuse of Mr. Dempsey

Mr. Dempsey is an 82-year-old former prize-fighter with Parkinson's disease and dementia. His once strong physique is now quite frail. Mr. Dempsey is unable to walk, eat, or use the toilet without assistance, and he is sometimes incontinent. Mr. Dempsey lives with his son, Charlie, in a small, run-down flat. Charlie greatly resents having to "clean up Dad's messes and put up with his babbling." However, Charlie is out of work and depends on his father's social security check for income. Charlie's resentment often turns to rage, especially when he has been drinking. On several occasions, he has punched his father, but more often, Charlie ignores his father's physical needs, sometimes forgetting to feed him or change his clothes and bedsheets.

Discussion

Elder abuse can take many forms and it is not uncommon for the abuser to financially benefit from the relationship. Victims are usually either incapable of reporting the crime or are too frightened to do so. There is also a high incidence of denial from both the abuser and victim. Assessment of potential elder abuse requires strong observation skills and an understanding of the physiology of age-related diseases. The level of force needed to injure a frail person is minimal and the consequences of improper care can lead to a myriad of serious health consequences. In the United States, it is required that all health professionals report suspected abuse to Adult Protective Services.

Behavioral Techniques and Humanistic Philosophy

Behavioral techniques used by both professionals and caregivers can greatly increase the comfort and safety of not only the older adult but also those around her or him as well. Figure 14-2 outlines helpful strategies for dealing with people with dementia. However, conflict can occur between a behavioral approach, which emphasizes safety of the older adult, and a humanistic philosophy, which emphasizes choice and respect for the older adult. The charter of principles of Alzheimer's Disease International (2000) emphasizes the importance of a humanistic, client-centered approach with the following statements: "A person with dementia continues to be a person of worth and dignity, and deserving of the same respect as any other human being" and "people with dementia should as far as possible participate in decisions affecting their daily lives and future care" (p. 1).

Dealing with troubling behaviors can be very frustrating for both the individual with dementia and the family or caregiver.

Creativity, flexibility, patience, and compassion will help the caregiver to successfully interact with and manage challenging behaviors. While we cannot change the person, we can try to accommodate the behavior rather than try to control the behavior. For example, it the person insists on sleeping on the floor, place a mattress on the floor to make him more comfortable. Changing our behavior (or the physical environment) will often result in a positive change in behavior of the individual.

Aggression & Anger
- Assure individuals who behave aggressively that they are okay—that you understand that they cannot help themselves.
- Approach the individual slowly, in full view.
- Speak in soothing, reassuring voice. Explain in short, simple statements what you are going to do, such as "I'm going to help you sit down."
- Distract the person with a snack or an activity.
- Sit or stand a little to the side rather than face them directly. You're less intimidating to them this way. Do not confront the individual with his behavior and do not try to restrain the person during a period of agitation.
- Be prepared to accept some insults and verbal abuse.
- Ask yourself if too much is being expected of them.
- Maintain structure by keeping the same routines. Keep furniture in the same place.
- Try soothing music, reading, or provide familiar, comforting smells (bread baking, potpourri).

Confusion
- Provide a nightlight to help the person see and locate familiar things and prevent falls in the dark; protect against wandering.

FIGURE 14-2. Approaches to Dealing with Challenging Behaviors

- Consider the side effects of some sedatives and cold remedies as well as prescribed drugs.
- Encourage reminiscence. Gently assist with keeping facts reasonably accurate and related to the past.
- Use communication rich in reminders, cues, gestures, and physical guiding (if appropriate) to increase personal awareness. Keep explanations simple.
- Avoid unrealistic promises.
- Keep your mood and responses consistent, provide frequent reassurance.
- Provide special personal space filled with familiar things where the confused person can go, rest, and feel safe and secure.
- Ask permission if something must be moved or changed: This helps to establish feelings of trust and control.
- Overprotection leads to feelings of helplessness and boredom. Provide reminders, directions, adequate time, and praise for self-care efforts on an adult level.
- Schedule respite care regularly in the caregiving routine so it becomes accepted and predictable.

Depression

- Respond to the impaired person with kind firmness.
- Try to rebuild self-esteem through reminiscence, participation in activities, and decisions. Notice pictures and mementos. Ask about them and listen.
- Alert the person's doctor, medications may help.
- Spend time with them. Do not ignore quiet, uncomplaining people.
- Encourage them to talk freely.
- Be familiar with the factors that predispose people to depression. They include problems with: health, living situation, losses, and a family history of depressive illness.
- A gentle touch with a reassuring smile projects a caring attitude.

Hoarding, rummaging behavior—Because of memory loss, people with dementia frequently look for something that is "missing" (e.g., rooms, clothes, personal items). These things may not look familiar so they are constantly looking for familiar things.

- Don't scold or try to rationalize with the person.
- Distract the impaired person when he/she is somewhere he/she is not supposed to be.
- Learn the impaired person's hiding places.

Incontinence

- Establish a routine for using the toilet.
- Schedule fluid intake. Limit intake in the evening before bedtime.
- Use signs to show which door leads to the bathroom.
- Use easy to remove clothing.

Repetitive Questioning

- Distraction often helps to redirect the individual to another topic.

Sleeplessness/Sundowner's syndrome—This occurs when impaired people become confused, restless, and insecure late in the afternoon and after dark.

(Continues)

FIGURE 14-2. Approaches to Dealing with Challenging Behaviors *(Continued)*

- Set up a daily routine. It will reduce anxiety about decision making and what happens next.
- Increase daytime activities, especially physical exercise.
- Alternate activity with programmed rest.
- Reduce all stimuli during rest periods.
- Strive to keep daily activities within the person's coping ability.
- Plan for afternoon and evening hours to be quiet and calm, provide structured, quiet activity such as a walk outdoors, listening to soothing music, etc.
- Turn on lights well before sunset and close the curtains at dusk. This may help reduce confusion. Keep a nightlight in the person's room, hallway, and bathroom.
- Make sure the living environment is safe—block off stairs with gates, lock doors, put away dangerous items.

Suspiciousness, distrust—Occurs most often with people with dementia when they cannot make sense of what is happening.
- Avoid grand gestures and promises that cannot be carried out.
- Do not argue about or rationally explain disappearances of the person's possessions.
- Offer to look for an item if the person says that it is missing, then distract them to another activity.
- Try nonverbal reassurances such as a gentle touch. Reassure the person that you understand their feelings.
- Learn the person's favorite hiding places.
- Explain to family members and other helpers that suspicious accusations are a part of progressive dementia.

Wandering
- Does the person need to burn off some energy by going for a walk? If so, escort them on the walk. Involve them in an exercise group. Make time for regular exercise to minimize restlessness.
- Consider the reasons that the person is walking and try to accommodate that need. Although walking may appear aimless, it most certainly has a purpose behind it, even if the person with dementia cannot explain it.
- Minimize risks, create a safe area for them to walk.
- Set up simple alarms so that the individual cannot leave the area without your knowledge.
- Use a barrier like a curtain or colored streamer to mask the door. A "stop" sign or "do not enter" sign often helps.
- Put away essential items such as coats, purses, glasses, keys. The individual may not consider going out without them.
- Divert the person from wanting to walk by giving them a clear task to perform.
- Make sure that the person has a contact phone number on him or her at all times.
- Tell neighbors and other people in advance that the person may get confused or lost.
- Always have a recent photograph of the person with dementia on hand in case he or she does wander off.

FIGURE 14-2. Approaches to Dealing with Challenging Behaviors *(Continued)*

CASE ILLUSTRATION

Mrs. Christie—One Year Later

The family arguments about Mrs. Christie living alone have escalated. In the past year she has fallen off a step stool while reaching for something in a high cabinet; gotten lost while shopping, although she was able to call a neighbor for help; and was hospitalized once for dehydration. She said the doctors told her to stop drinking so much tea and start drinking more water, which she says she now does.

Mrs. Christie's oldest daughter is especially upset by what she sees as her mother's "stubbornness" and takes the drastic move to apply to the courts to be named her conservator. After a comprehensive psychiatric and physical evaluation, the courts turn down the daughter's request, stating that Mrs. Christie is aware of the consequences of her actions and is competent to make her own decisions. The psychiatric team recommends family counseling for the mother and daughter to be able to make compromises regarding Mrs. Christie's activities and minimize the family stress.

Discussion

Mrs. Christie is asserting her right of free choice and her daughter's well-meaning, but misguided, attempts to control her mother's actions have created considerable distress. Family intervention, including psychological counseling and occupational therapy, can help this family understand the mother's needs and yet develop adaptive strategies in daily activities to ease the worry of the daughter and increase Mrs. Christie's safety in the home and community.

Prevention and Health Maintenance

A phenomenological study with elderly Swedish women (Hedelin & Strandmark, 2001) found that "the essence of mental health is the experience of confirmation, trust and confidence in the future, as well as a zest for life, development, and involvement in one's relationship to oneself and to others" (p. 9). This finding concurs with the criteria for quality of life and eloquently gives us important guidelines for prevention and health maintenance interventions for the older adult.

Although occupation is the cornerstone of occupational therapy intervention, the well elderly study by Clark et al. (1997) suggests that activity or "keeping busy" alone is insufficient for health maintenance or promotion. Rather, a systematic application of OT principles is needed, which includes highly individualized programs (even when conducted in a group setting), instruction in life management skills, and choice of occupations that are viewed as meaningful and health promoting. This study showed significant results of preventative occupational therapy in many areas, including improvement in general mental health and physical functioning as well as increased social functioning and activity, vitality, and life satisfaction. Based on this study a plethora of programs are now being developed in **lifestyle redesign**, "an intervention model that promotes quality of life in well elders" (Jackson, Mandel, Zemke, & Clark, 2001, p. 5).

Although substantial evidence that shows the effectiveness of occupational therapy in prevention and health maintenance now exists, the traditional, medically oriented model often does not allow occupational therapists to utilize their full repertoire of skills. Occupational therapists must be proactive in advocating for change in health care systems and in increasing professional recognition in order to provide necessary and meaningful intervention for the large older adult population.

SUMMARY

Over one third of occupational therapists in the United States work with older adults (AOTA, 2010). However, given the demographic data provided in this chapter, that number will continue to increase. Although the majority of older adults are well elderly, the devastating and global effects of chronic and mental illness in the older population have significant consequences for the individual, family, and society as a whole.

Occupational therapists have a unique role in preserving and fostering mental as well as physical health of the older adult. The emphasis on meaningful occupation in context that is focused on quality of life issues and prevention as well as restoration of function is a critical component of health care for the older adult.

REVIEW QUESTIONS

1. How will the expected increase in the number of older adults affect occupational therapy as a profession?
2. What difficulties are there in determining accurate psychiatric diagnosis in the older adult population?
3. Which psychiatric disorders may be mistaken for dementia?
4. How does engagement in occupation benefit the older adult?
5. What are the benefits and limitations of aging in place?

REFERENCES

Administration on Aging (AoA). (2009). *A profile of older Americans: 2009*. Department of Health and Human Services.

AGS Foundation for Health and Aging. (2005). Delirium (sudden confusion). Retrieved from http://www.healthinaging.org/agingintheknow/chapters_ch_trial.asp?ch=57

Alexopoulos, G., Schultz, S., & Lebowitz, B. (2005). Late-life depression: A model for medical classification. *Biological Psychiatry, 58,* 283–289.

Alzheimer's Disease International (ADI). (2000). Dementia: Challenge to quality of life. *World Alzheimer's Day Bulletin.* Retrieved from http://www.alz.co.uk/adi/pdf/wad2000en.pdf

Alzheimer's Disease International (ADI). (2010). World Alzheimer's Report 2010. Retrieved from http://www.alz.co.uk/research/files/WorldAlzheimerReport2010ExecutiveSummary.pdf

American Geriatric Society (AGS). (2005). Caring for older Americans: The future of geriatric medicine. *The Journal of Geriatric Society, 53*(6), 245–256.

American Occupational Therapy Association (AOTA). (2010) Scope of practice. *American Journal of Occupational Therapy, 64,* S70–S77.

American Psychological Association (APA). (2004). Guidelines for psychological practice with older adults. *American Psychologist, 59*(4), 236–260.

Anderson, D. (2001). Treating depression in old age: The reasons to be positive. *Age and Ageing, 30,* 13–17.

Anxiety Disorders Association of America (ADAA). (2010). Older adults. Retrieved from http://www.adaa.org/living-with-anxiety/older-adults

Aubin, G., Hachey, R., & Mercier, C. (1999). Meaning of daily activities and subjective quality of life in people with severe mental illness. *Scandinavian Journal of Occupational Therapy, 6,* 53–62.

Baum, C. M. (1995). The contribution of occupation to function in persons with Alzheimer's disease. *Journal of Occupational Science, 2,* 59–67.

Beattie, W., Pachana, N., & Franklin, S. (2010). Double jeopardy: Comorbid anxiety and depression in late life. *Research in Gerontological Nursing, 3*(3), 209–221.

Bruce, W., Yonkers, K., Otto, M., Eisen, J., Weisberg, R., Pagano, M., et al. (2005). Influence of psychiatric comorbidity on recovery and recurrence in generalized anxiety disorder, social phobia, and panic disorder: A 12 year prospective study. *American Journal of Psychiatry, 162,* 1179–1187.

Burns, T., Mortimer, J. A., & Merchak, P. (1994). Cognitive performance test: A new approach to functional assessment in Alzheimer's disease. *Journal of Geriatric Psychiatry and Neurology, 7*(1), 46–54.

Clark, F., Azen, S., Zemke, R., Jackson, J., Carlson, M., Mandel, D., et al. (1997). Occupational therapy for independent-living older adults: A randomized controlled study. *Journal of the American Medical Association, 278,* 1321–1326.

Clay, S. (2010). Treatment of addiction in the elderly. *Aging Health, 6*(2), 177–189.

Cohen, C. (2003). Introduction. In C. I. Cohen (Ed.), *Schizophrenia into later life.* Washington, DC: American Psychiatric Publishing.

Conner, K. O., Copeland, V., Grote, N., Koeske, G., Rosen, D., Reynolds, C. F., et al. (2010). Mental health treatment seeking among older adults with depression: The impact of stigma and race. *The American Journal of Geriatric Psychiatry, 18*(6), 531–543.

Crystal, S. (2005). The economics of an aging society. *The Gerontologist, 45*(4), 553–558.

Cummings, S., & Kropf, N. (2009). Formal and informal support for older adults with severe mental illness. *Aging and Mental Health, 13*(4), 619–627.

Davis, M. J., Moye, J., & Karel, M. J. (2002). Mental health screening of older adults in primary care. *Journal of Mental Health & Aging, 8*(2), 139–149.

Deitz, J. C., Tovar, V. S., Beeman, C., Thorn, D. W., & Trevisan, M. S. (1992). The test of orientation for rehabilitation patients: Test-retest reliability. *Occupational Therapy Journal of Research, 12*(3), 172–185.

Depp, C., & Jeste, D. (2004). Bipolar disorder in older adults: A critical review. *Bipolar Disorders, 6,* 343–367.

Depp, C., Moore, E., Sitzer, D., Palmer, B., Eyler, L., Roesch, S., et al. (2007). Neurocognitive impairment in middle-aged and older adults with bipolar disorder: Comparison to schizophrenia and normal comparison subjects. *Journal of Affective Disorders, 101,* 201–209.

Drayer, R., Mulsant, B., Lenze, E., Rollman, B., Dew, M., Kelleher, K., et al. (2005). Somatic symptoms of depression in elderly patients with medical comorbidities. *International Journal of Geriatric Psychiatry, 20*, 973–982.

Egan, M., Hobson, S., & Fearing, V. (2006). Dementia and occupation: A review of the literature. *Canadian Journal of Occupational Therapy, 73*(33), 132–140.

Fillenbaum, G., & Duke University Center for the Study of Aging and Human Development (1988). *Multidimensional functional assessment of older adults*. Hillsdale, NJ: L. Erlbaum Associates.

Fisher, A. G., & Bray Jones, K. (2010). *Assessment of motor and process skills. vol. 1: development, standardization, and administration manual* (7th ed.) Fort Collins, CO: Three Star Press.

Flint, A. J. (2001). Core concepts in geriatrics: Anxiety disorders. *Clinical Geriatrics, 9*(11), 21, 24–25, 28–30.

Folstein, M., Folstein, S., & McHugh, P. (1975). Mini mental state: A practical method for grading the cognitive state of patients for the clinician. *Journal of Psychiatric Research, 12*, 189–198.

Ganguli, M., Dodge, H., & Mulsant, B. (2002). Rates and predictors of mortality in an aging, rural, community-based cohort: The role of depression. *Archives of General Psychiatry, 59*(11), 1046–1053.

Gregory, M. D. (1983). Occupational behavior and life satisfaction among retirees. *American Journal of Occupational Therapy, 37*, 548–553.

Gum, A., King-Kallimanis, B., & Kohn, R. (2009). Prevalence of mood, anxiety, and substance-abuse disorders for older Americans in the National Comorbidity Survey-Replication. *The American Journal of Geriatric Psychiatry, 17*(9), 769–782.

Hall, C. (2002). Special considerations for the geriatric population. *Critical Care Nursing Clinics of North America, 14*(4), 427–434.

Han, B. (2002). Depressive symptoms and self-rated health in community-dwelling older adults: A longitudinal study. *Journal of the American Geriatrics Society, 50*(9), 1549–1556.

Hasselkus, B., & Murray, B. (2007). Everyday occupation, well-being, and identity: The experience of caregivers in families with dementia. *American Journal of Occupational Therapy, 61*, 9–20.

Healthcommunities.com (2011). Dementia overview, types, incidence & prevalence. Retrieved from http://www.healthcommunities.com/dementia/index.shtml

Hedelin, B., & Strandmark, M. (2001). The meaning of mental health from elderly women's perspectives: A basis for health promotion. *Perspectives in Psychiatric Care, 37*(1), 7–14.

Hoffman, D., Dukes, E., & Wittchen, H. (2008). Human and economic burden of generalized anxiety disorder. *Depression and Anxiety, 25*, 72–90.

Hoppes, S., Davis, L. A., & Thompson, D. (2003). Environmental effects on the assessment of people with dementia: A pilot study. *American Journal of Occupational Therapy, 57*(4), 396–402.

Horowitz, B. P. (2002). Occupational therapy home assessments: Supporting community living through client-centered practice. *Occupational Therapy in Mental Health, 18*(1), 1–17.

Jackson, J., Mandel, D., Zemke, R., & Clark, F. (2001). Promoting quality of life in elders: An occupation-based occupational therapy program. *World Federation of Occupational Therapists (WFOT) Bulletin, 43*, 5–12.

Jervis, L. (2002). Contending with "problem behaviors" in the nursing home. *Archives of Psychiatric Nursing, 16*(1), 32–38.

Klimstra, S., & Mahgoub, N. (2010). Alcohol and substance use disorders in the geriatric psychiatry inpatient. *Psychiatric Annals, 40*(6), 282–285.

Kyomen, H., & Whitfield, T. (2009). Psychosis in the elderly. *The American Journal of Psychiatry, 166*(2), 146–150.

Law, M., Steinwender, S., & Leclair, L. (1998). Occupation, health and well-being. *Canadian Journal of Occupational Therapy, 65*, 81–91.

Lilly, M. L., Richards, B. S., & Buckwalter, K. C. (2003). Friends and social support in dementia caregiving: Assessment and intervention. *Journal of Gerontological Nursing, 29*(1), 29–36.

Martinez-Aran, A., Vieta, E., Reinares, M., Colom, F., Torrent, C., Sanchez-Moreno, J., et al. (2004). Cognitive function across manic or hypomanic, depressed and euthymic states in bipolar disorder. *American Journal of Psychiatry, 161*, 262–270.

McColl, M. A., Davies, D., Carlson, P., Johnston, J., & Milnnes, P. (2001). The community integration measure: Development and preliminary validation. *Archives of Physical Medicine and Rehabilitation, 82*, 429–434.

Meulen, E., Schmand, B., van Campen, J., de Koning, S., Ponds, R., Scheltens, P., et al. (2004). The Seven Minute Screen: A neurocognitive screening test highly sensitive to various types of dementia. *Journal of Neurology, Neurosurgery and Psychiatry, 75*, 700–705.

National Center on Elder Abuse. (2007). Major types of elder abuse. Retrieved from http://www.ncea .aoa.gov/NCEAroot/Main_Site/FAQ/Basics/Types_Of_Abuse.aspx

National Institute of Mental Health. (2009). Depression in elderly men. Retrieved from: http://www .nimh.nih.gov/health/publications/men-and-depression/depression-in-elderly-men.shtml

National Institute on Aging. (2007). The health and retirement study: Growing older in America. NIH Publication No. 07-5757.

National Research Council Panel to Review Risk and Prevalence of Elder Abuse and Neglect. (2003). Elder mistreatment: Abuse, neglect, and exploitation in an aging America. Washington, DC.

Peach J., Koob, J. J., & Kraus, M. J. (2001). Psychometric evaluation of the Geriatric Depression Scale (GDS): Supporting its use in health care settings. *Clinical Gerontologist, 23*(3/4), 57–68.

Porensky, E., Dew M., Karp, J., Skidmore, E., Rollman, B., Shear, K., et al. (2009). The burden of late-life generalized anxiety disorder: Effects on disability, health-related quality of life, and health utilization. *The American Journal of Geriatric Psychiatry, 17*(6), 473–482.

Reisberg, B., Ferris, S. H., & Crook, T. (1983). Global Deterioration Scale. In B. Reisberg (Ed.), *A guide to Alzheimer's disease*. New York: Free Press.

Rojas-Fernandez, C., Miller, L., & Sadowski, C. (2010) Considerations in the treatment of geriatric depression: Overview of pharmacotherapeutic and psychotherapeutic treatment interventions. *Research in Gerontological Nursing, 3*(3), 176–186.

Sajatovic, M., Jenkins, J., Safavi, R., West, J., Cassidy, K., Meyer, W., et al. (2008). Personal and societal construction of illness among individuals with rapid-cycling bipolar disorder: A life-trajectory perspective. *The American Journal of Geriatric Psychiatry, 16*(9), 718–727.

Schaub, R. T., & Linden, M. (2000). Anxiety and anxiety disorders in the old and very old—Results from the Berlin Aging Study (BASE). *Comprehensive Psychiatry, 41*(2; suppl. 1), 48–54.

Shiekh, J., & Yesavage, J. (1986). Geriatric Depression Scale: Recent findings in development of a shorter version. In J. Brink (Ed.), *Clinical gerontology: A guide to assessment and intervention*. New York: Howarth.

Sigfried, N., Schouws, T., Comijs, H., Stek, M., Dekker, J., Oostervink, F., et al. (2009). Cognitive impairment in early and late bipolar disorder. *The American Journal of Geriatric Psychiatry, 17*(6), 508–514.

Simoni-Wastila, L., & Yang, H. (2006). Psychoactive drug abuse in older adults. *American Journal of Geriatric Pharmacotherapy, 4*(4), 380–394.

Sinoff, G., Ore, L., Zlotogorsky, D., & Tamir, A. (1999). Short Anxiety Screening Test—A brief instrument for detecting anxiety in the elderly. *International Journal of Geriatric Psychiatry, 14*(2), 1062–1071.

Stewart, J. (2004). Why don't physicians consider depression in the elderly? Age-related bias, atypical symptoms, and ineffective screening approaches may be at play. *Postgraduate Medicine, 115*(6), 57.

Sviden, G., Wikstrom, B. M., & Hjortsjo-Norberg, M. (2002). Elderly person's reflections on relocating to living at sheltered housing. *Scandinavian Journal of Occupational Therapy, 9*, 10–16.

Thompson-Heisterman, A. (2006). The older adult with a mental health issue. In W. K. Mohr (Ed.). *Psychiatric mental health nursing* (6th ed., pp. 811–830). Philadelphia: Lippincott, Williams & Williams.

Torralva, T., Roca, M., Gleichgerrcht, E., Lopez, P., & Manes, F. (2009). INECO Frontal Screening (IFS): A brief, sensitive, and specific tool to assess executive functions in dementia. *Journal of the International Neuropsychological Society, 15*(5), 777–786.

United Nations Secretariat. (2010). *Population ageing 2006.* United Nations, Population Division, Department of Economic and Social Affairs. (Wall Chart).

University of Michigan Alcohol Research Center. (1991). Short Michigan Alcohol Screening Test—Geriatric Version (Short MAST-G). Ann Arbor: University of Michigan.

van Hoof, J., Kort, H., van Waarde, H., & Blom, M. (2010). Environmental interventions and the design of homes for older adults with dementia: An overview. *American Journal of Alzheimer's Disease & Other Dementias, 25*(3), 202–232.

Williams, J. H., Drinka, T. J. K., Greenberg, J. R., Farrell-Holtan, J., Euhardy, R., & Schram, M. (1991). Development and testing of the assessment of living skills and resources (ALSAR) in elderly community-dwelling veterans. *Gerontologist, 31*(1), 84–91.

Wilson, B., Greenfield, E., Clare, L., Baddeley, A., Cockburn, J., Watson, P., et al. (2008). *The Rivermead Behavioral Memory Test-Third Edition (RBMT-3).* San Antonio, TX: Pearson.

World Health Organization (WHO). (2001). *International classification of functioning, disability and health* (ICF). Geneva: WHO.

Yap, E., & Holzapfel, S. (2006). Psychosocial needs of the older adult. In E. M. Varcarolis, V. B. Carson, & N. C. Shoemaker (Eds.), *Foundations of psychiatric mental health nursing: A clinical approach* (5th ed., pp. 692–715). St. Louis: Elsevier-Saunders.

Yesavage, J., Brink, T., Rose, T., Lum, O., Huang, V., Adey, M., et al. (1983). Development and validation of a geriatric depression screening scale: A preliminary report. *Journal of Psychiatric Research, 17,* 37–49.

SUGGESTED RESOURCES

Aging in Place Initiative (2011). Retrieved from http://www.aginginplaceinitiative.org/

Alzheimer's Association (2011). Alzheimer's disease. Retrieved from http://www.alz.org/index.asp

Bartels, S. J., Dums, A. R., Oxman, T. E., Schneider, L. S., Arean, P. A., Alexopoulos, G. S., et al. (2002). Evidence-based practices in geriatric mental health care. *Psychiatric Services, 53*(11), 1419–1431.

Beers, M., & Jones, T. (2008). *Merck manual of health and aging.* New York: Ballantine Books.

Bonder, B., & Dal Bello-Haas, V. (2008). *Functional performance in older adults* (3rd ed.). Philadelphia: F. A. Davis.

Coppola, S., Elliott, S., & Toto, P. (2008). *Strategies to advance gerontology excellence: Promoting best practice in occupational therapy.* Bethesda, MD: AOTA Press.

Corcoran, M. (2004). *Geriatric issues in occupational therapy: A compendium of leading research.* Bethesda, MD: American Occupational Therapy Association.

Kane, R., Ouslander, J., Abrass, I., & Resnick, B. (2008). *Essentials of clinical geriatrics* (6th ed.). Columbus, OH: McGraw-Hill Professional.

Lewis, S. C. (2003). *Elder care in occupational therapy* (2nd ed.). Thorofare, NJ: Slack.

Mandel, D., Jackson, J., Zemke, R., Nelson, L., & Clark, F. (Eds.). (1999). *Lifestyle redesign: Implementing the well elderly program.* Bethesda, MD: American Occupational Therapy Association.

MedlinePlus(2011).Seniors'Health.Retrievedfromhttp://www.nlm.nih.gov/medlineplus/seniorshealth.html

Sadavoy, J. (2004). *Comprehensive textbook of geriatric psychiatry* (3rd ed.). New York: Norton.

Mental Health with Physical Disorders

Part V includes three chapters that address psychosocial concerns across a spectrum of conditions, including a broad look at physical disability of various etiologies, brain injury, and chronic pain. Clients with dysfunction related to these conditions may or may not be seen in traditional "mental health" settings. Unfortunately, the psychosocial, cognitive, and behavioral issues discussed in these chapters are too often under-recognized or inadequately treated, yet they have been repeatedly reported to have significant impact on an individual's functional outcome with intervention.

The authors of these chapters advocate for an occupation-based approach that addresses the various psychosocial issues through assessment and intervention regardless of treatment setting. Occupational therapists are in the ideal role to both advocate for these services and educate team members and families, as our generalist background provides the holistic and comprehensive perspective to look beyond the treatment setting boundaries.

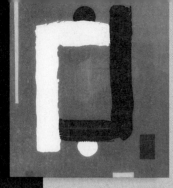

Chapter 15

Psychosocial Issues in Physical Disability

Heidi McHugh Pendleton, PhD, OTR/L, FAOTA
Winifred Schultz-Krohn, PhD, OTR/L, BCP, FAOTA

KEY TERMS

adaptation

adjustment

coping strategies

International Classification
   of Functioning, Disability,
   and Health (ICF)

life satisfaction

quality of life

self-concept

CHAPTER OUTLINE

Introduction
Occupational Therapy and the International Classification of Functioning
Cultural and Societal Factors
Concept of Self
Models of Adapting to Physical Disability
    Chronic Disabling Conditions
    Acute Onset of Disabling Conditions
Life Satisfaction and Quality of Life
Specific Psychosocial Issues with Select Disabilities
    Chronic Disorders with an Acute Onset
    Progressive Physical Disorders
    Chronic Congenital Nonprogressive Disorders
Summary

INTRODUCTION

You wake up in the morning, get out of bed, stretch, search for your glasses, and begin the process of getting ready for your day. The act of translating intention, such as getting ready for the day, into action, requires physical abilities. These physical abilities are considered a critical component of human occupation. Fisher and Kielhofner (1995) note "that merely having the desire to perform a task is not sufficient; the individual must also have the underlying capacity needed to perform" (p. 83). Understanding the importance of physical ability in the engagement in occupation and its impact on psychosocial functioning and well-being forms the foundation for this chapter. Individuals who have a physical disability may have significant problems engaging in, or resuming engagement in, personally desirable and cherished occupations. The results of this inability or decrease in ability to participate in occupation can lead to significant psychosocial problems, including depression, anxiety, poor coping ability, altered body image, decreased or altered sense of self, decreased self-esteem, and withdrawal from social interaction, to name just a few typical responses (Ackerley, Gordon, Elston, Crawford, & McPherson, 2009; Hughes, Swedlund, Petersen, & Nosek, 2001; Kemp & Kraus, 1999; Novotny, 1991; Rossi, Costa, Dantas, Ciofi-Silva, & Lopes, 2009; Tate & Forchheimer, 2001; Tzonichaki & Kleftaras, 2002).

It has been charged that many occupational therapists who are working with persons with physical disabilities seldom address psychosocial issues directly or adequately. It seems that intervention priority is given to the amelioration of the client's physical and occupational performance problems (Gutman, 2001a; Smith, 2001). It may be that the occupational therapists regard any intervention that is aimed at restoring the person's physical or functional ability to participate in occupation as simultaneously addressing her or his psychosocial problems, thus speculating that the psychosocial problems will be remediated if the individual is successful in resuming his or her occupational performance. The problem is not that simple—the psychosocial issues confronting people with physical disabilities are complex, need to be explicitly recognized by the individual as well as those working with him or her, and must be addressed directly with appropriate occupational therapy (OT) psychosocial intervention. This chapter addresses the psychosocial issues frequently encountered by a person who has a physical disability.

The **International Classification of Functioning, Disability, and Health (ICF)** is used as a framework to understand the relationship of the psychosocial issues to physical disability in this chapter. The shift in rehabilitation services over the past decade has been from "predominantly a bio-medical model to a bio-psychological approach, incorporating the individual's" perspective (Ackerley et al., 2009, p. 906). The cultural and societal factors that influence the experience of physical disability are presented, followed by a discussion of the concept of self and how it is affected in the presence of physical disability. Several models useful for understanding **adjustment** to life with physical disability are explicated and then the concept of **quality of life** with physical disability is explored.

OCCUPATIONAL THERAPY AND THE INTERNATIONAL CLASSIFICATION OF FUNCTIONING

The World Health Organization's (WHO) International Classification of Functioning (ICF) helps the occupational therapist understand the complexity of having a disability (WHO, 2001). The ICF has "moved away from being a 'consequences of disease' classification to become a 'components of health' classification"—progressing from impairment, disability, and handicap to body functions and structures, activities, and participation (WHO, 2001, p. 4). The term *body structures* refers to the anatomical parts of the body while *body functions* refers to a person's physiological and psychological functions. Also considered in this new model is the impact of environmental and personal factors as they relate to functioning. Combined, these environmental and personal factors are referred to as the *contextual factors* that influence an individual's participation in the community. The ICF has adopted a universal model that considers health along a continuum where there is a potential for everyone to have a disability.

The ICF also provides support for occupational therapists to address specifically activity and activity limitations encountered by persons with disabilities (WHO, 2001). This document also describes the importance of participation in life situations, or "domains," including learning and applying knowledge; general tasks and task demands; communication; movement; self-care; domestic life areas; interpersonal interactions; major life areas associated with work, school, and family life; and community, social, and civic life—all historically familiar areas of concern and intervention to occupational therapy. Although a physical disability may compromise a person's ability to climb stairs or dress, the ICF redirects the service provider to also consider activity limitations that may result in restricted participation in desired life situations. A problem with a person's bodily structure, such as an absent or severely contracted limb, is recognized as a potentially limiting factor but that is not the focus of intervention. The intervention is designed to foster participation in desired occupations.

Occupational therapy intervention provided for people with physical disabilities should extend beyond a focus on recovery of physical skills to address the person's engagement, or active participation, in occupations. This viewpoint is the cornerstone of the Occupational Therapy Practice Framework, Second Edition (AOTA, 2008). Such active participation in occupation is dependent upon the client's psychosocial well-being, which must be simultaneously addressed through the OT intervention. This orientation is congruent with the emphasis of the ICF.

Figure 15-1 depicts the relationships and interrelationships among cultural and societal expectations with activities, participation, and prioritized occupations

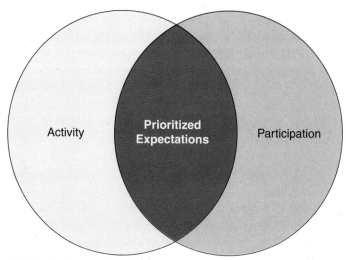

FIGURE 15-1. Cultural and Societal Expectations
© Cengage Learning 2013

as viewed through the lens of the ICF. This figure represents a synthesis of the Occupational Therapy Practice Framework and the ICF where prioritized occupations are influenced by cultural and societal expectations and occur as a product of the individual's ability to engage in an activity that promotes participation in a desired life situation.

CULTURAL AND SOCIETAL FACTORS

The process of adjusting to a physically disabling condition occurs over time and is influenced by cultural and societal expectations (Charmaz, 1995; Irvine, Davidson, Hoy, & Lowe-Strong, 2009). A person who has sustained a stroke may be willing to expend energy to propel a wheelchair but relies on others to help with meal preparation. In this situation, the person prioritizes independent mobility over independent meal preparation. The importance of independence in daily activities is heavily biased by Western cultural norms and is not a universally accepted priority (Williams & Ispa, 1999). Many cultures accommodate a person's disability by expecting family members to assume the primary caregiving role. The individual with a disabling condition is not expected to become independent because family members are responsible for the care of the person. In this cultural orientation an acceptable societal role is being dependent upon others. Not only may the dependence on others be acceptable to the society but it also may be regarded as preferable, a measure of the esteem with which the family honors the individual. Even the term *disability* has come under question when investigating how to measure disability status as reported by the individual (Schneider, 2009). Many individuals view the term *disabled* as referring to an unchangeable, mostly physical state "where a person is unable to do anything" (p. 42). When the term *disability* was used, a more accurate self-assessment of functional status and self-appraised level of participation was reported by individuals.

Culture influences a person's ability to cope or adjust to a disabling condition (Hampton & Marshall, 2000). One culture may place great importance on independence, whereas another culture is focused on group cohesiveness. The very concept of disabilities rights has been discussed as a Western perspective that may not have universal application (Bickenbach, 2009). For example, the cultural orientation of the United States is considered individualistic in nature, whereas China has a collectivistic orientation. The terms *individualistic* and *collectivistic* are often used when differentiating cultural perspectives (Brice & Campbell, 1999; Ohbuchi, Fukushima, & Tedeschi, 1999). An individualistic orientation places personal pursuits and individual achievement above group gains. A collectivistic culture emphasizes the benefit of action for the group and individual achievements are minimized. But these differing cultural orientations do not need to restrict the focus of fostering participation for the individual faced with a disabling condition (Iwama, Thomson, & MacDonald, 2009). Bickenbach (2009) argues that cultural awareness and working within cultural expectations can actually support the rights of the individual with the disabling condition to participation in the society and culture.

These differing cultural orientations can contribute to the coping methods used when an individual is faced with a disabling condition (Hampton & Marshall, 2000). Even the concept of a disability has been described as "an artifact of culture and an identity responsive to material conditions" (Frank, 2000, p. 168). Often routines and habits must be substantially revised in the face of a disabling condition. The degree to which a person is able to modify his or her routines to meet the challenge of a disability is also influenced by culture (Gallimore & Lopez, 2002).

Bonder (2001) describes a comparison of weavers from the United States and Guatemala. In Guatemala, particularly in the Mayan culture, the occupation of weaving carries a rich history and traditionally specified methods are used to engage in this activity. A Mayan woman was no longer able to sit on the floor to weave using the traditional method in this village. A suggestion was made to sit on a stool as a modification to the activity. This altered method of performing the weaving activity was rejected because it would compromise the meaning of weaving. In the United States, weaving has a personal meaning but does not carry the comparable cultural significance as in the Mayan culture in Guatemala. A woman in the United States, unable to use her left arm after a stroke, modified the activity of weaving to continue with this personally meaningful occupation.

Culture defines the features of an ideal routine (Gallimore & Lopez, 2002). The acceptability of a routine is not solely related to the end product but is also strongly rooted in cultural norms. For example, a young mother, who is physically limited by multiple sclerosis, may be very willing for her 3-year-old daughter to spend time with her mother or mother-in-law during the day but wants her daughter to be home in the evening. Although the effort of getting her daughter ready for bed may be exhausting, this is a culturally endorsed routine that defines part of this woman's role as a mother. Routines can also be severely disrupted by a surgical procedure and the rehabilitation process that follows (Fitzpatrick & Finlay, 2008). After hand surgery, individuals reported feelings of frustration with both the post-surgical limitations and the disruption in routines caused by the rehabilitation process. It has been argued that a holistic approach should be used by "attending to peoples' personal, social and practical responses beyond simply focusing in reductionist" methods to address physical function (Fitzpatrick & Finlay, 2008, p. 143).

Confounding and contributing to a person's psychosocial response to disability—depression, anxiety, decreased **self-concept**/self-worth—are the societal attitudes of those around him or her (Murray, 2009). These were undoubtedly the same views he or she once held toward those who have disability but now must be faced as referring to oneself. Noted among these views, reactions, or beliefs that society attributes to those with disabilities are that life must now be a tragedy because of having a disability, that one is now the object of pity, and even that it would be understandable if the person were to consider suicide (Hockenberry, 1995; Wright, 1983; Yerxa, 2001). The person with a disability may alternately experience being the recipient of society's stares or being invisible (Murphy, 2001; Rossi et al., 2009). For those who have a physical disability, there is almost a universal experience of being stigmatized by society (Goffman, 1963). Many also endure the beliefs of others that some personal action or attribute of the individual caused the disability. The effects of these cultural and societal responses on individuals with disabilities significantly influence self-concept, as will be explored in the following section.

CONCEPT OF SELF

A discussion of the construction of self is helpful for understanding the potential psychosocial impact of a physically disabling condition. Charmaz (2002) describes the concept of self as constructed from habits that often occur with minimal or no reflection or intention by the person. These habits are referred to as the "taken-for-granted ways" a person manages her or his daily life and how that person interacts with others in a variety of settings (p. S32). A person may engage in a habitual pattern of interacting with loved ones and this pattern may become firmly established over the years.

The pattern or habit does not necessarily serve a clear function but instead is a unique feature of that person's behavioral repertoire. The daughter who begins every conversation with her mother by saying "But Mom . . ." The son who always drops his school bag by the front door instead of taking it all the way to his room only to retrieve it later when he needs to begin his homework. The mother who can't fathom brushing her hair before she has had her first cup of coffee. The father who must read the comic pages of the newspaper before reading any other portion of the paper. These habits form the self and may be considered as a "signature of self." When this signature of self, these habitual actions or behaviors, are disrupted by illness or disease, the person may feel a disruption in the integrity of self (Charmaz, 1995). However, the concept of self may be very strongly formed and resistant to change, even when a physically disabling condition prohibits engaging in specific behaviors or habits.

Clients with chronic disabling conditions, particularly those with a progressive course, present a significant challenge to the OT practitioner. Although the occupational therapist may be able to devise clever and creative strategies to accomplish daily activities, these modifications may be viewed by a client as confirmation that the previous self is disintegrating (Charmaz, 1995).

CASE ILLUSTRATION

Ms. Kaminsky

Ms. Kaminsky is a 58-year-old woman with chronic obstructive pulmonary disorder (COPD) and severe shortness of breath. As the occupational therapist, you have made several suggestions regarding energy conservation techniques and methods to manage her daily activities. This woman would habitually blow on her tea three times before taking a sip. You suggest that after she brews the tea she allows the tea to cool slightly before drinking it or that she add a small ice cube or ice chips to cool the tea instead of blowing on it. She becomes distressed at these suggestions and refuses to drink tea.

Discussion

The habit of blowing on her tea was part of her signature of self and now that habit is no longer available to her. Although her dyspnea makes it virtually impossible for her to effectively blow on her tea to cool it, she refuses alternate methods. She actively tries to maintain previous habits to avoid reconfiguring her sense of self as a disabled person, a person with limited respiratory capacity.

For some people, at the onset of chronic physical disability it becomes clear that they will experience disruption of their daily lives and be forced to alter and redefine their sense of self (Fitzpatrick & Finlay, 2008). These individuals are likely to approach rehabilitation, including OT intervention, with motivation and resolve to maximize their remaining capabilities, learn to compensate for their disabilities, and in many instances, craft a compromise or novel concept of self. However, for many other people at the onset of physical disability, this clarity regarding changed abilities comes over a period of extended time coupled with the experience of actually "doing" or "trying" those occupations and activities that customarily contribute to their sense of self. Charmaz (2002) suggests that "until people view their daily habits as undermined and experience themselves as changed, they will maintain the concept of self established earlier" (p. S31). Many individuals with acute onset (or even progressive onset) chronic disability may not have had sufficient time to experience themselves as changed and may therefore initially view occupational therapy as irrelevant and unnecessary. In fact, as was observed by Charmaz, the very activities that commonly comprise the OT intervention confront the individual's habitualized self-concept and are experienced as negative. Shortened rehabilitation stays, lack of third-party payment for ongoing or outpatient therapy, as well as a society with limited social and temporal support contexts for people with disability may further compromise the individual's establishment of satisfactory performance of everyday occupations and resulting satisfactory self-concept.

Penny, the participant described in Clark's (1993) Slagle lecture, aptly exemplifies the aforementioned experience and, as Clark so eloquently writes, demonstrates "that rehabilitation can be experienced by the survivor as a rite of passage in which the person is moved to disability status by experts and therapists and then abandoned" (p. 1068). Following the sudden onset of a brain aneurysm, Penny, a 47-year-old professor and department chair in the school of education at a large university, experienced occupational therapy negatively. Penny described sitting in her wheelchair waiting in line for her turn for therapy, dutifully performing the routines they showed her and then being returned to the line to wait to go back to her room. She seemed to regard the OT interventions aimed at relearning self-care and other activities as comprising her customary routines as "little stuff," unchallenging, purposeless, and a waste of time. She felt "angry and resentful," wishing that "she would be able to set goals for herself so she could have a sense of progress toward something and the therapists, like personal coaches, would work with her to achieve them" (p. 1071).

Within the course of Penny's narrative Clark observes that the rehabilitation program seems to serve as a "rite of passage" to the survivor of a disabling condition, "carrying the person from one stage of life to the next" (1993, p. 1072). During this rite of passage the person is stripped of her old status (old self) and then transitions to the status of the disabled. In this transitional, or "liminal," state "one is betwixt and between, neither what one was nor what one shall become" (Moore, 1992, p. 153). When this phase is completed, the participant begins the task of reentering the world from which she has been separated (Clark, 1993, p. 1072). Penny indeed experienced this status of liminality as evidenced by her feeling disconnected from her former self—a self who was a revered academician, an accomplished skier, world traveler, gourmet cook, and treasured friend. Her experience in rehabilitation suggested that those providing treatment, regardless of their "kind and caring demeanor," supported this liminal status by seemingly stripping Penny of her prior status and relegating her to the status of the next client waiting in the line for treatment.

Once discharged, Penny felt ill-equipped with the tools to adapt to her changed self within her old familiar environment. She observed that occupations were important because they marked the new you versus the old you. During their collaboration, Clark encouraged Penny to recount her occupational history, identifying the childhood and later life occupations that had previously contributed to her success in life, that is, composing her life to that point, and then "coached" Penny in recycling these occupations to recompose her life (Clark, 1993). Penny reached back to her past, retrieving those familiar friendship strategies that were previously so adaptive for her and reestablished cherished rituals. Old friends and new friends, including Clark, facilitated Penny's concoction of a new persona, that of a proper eccentric professor, by joining her as she collected her accoutrements (including a British walking stick) and in celebrating her victories. Penny served as the primary change agent in determining her quality of life and her story of reconfiguring her self-concept using occupation is also consistent with and illustrative of other models of **adaptation** to disability, as will be evident in the following discussions.

MODELS OF ADAPTING TO PHYSICAL DISABILITY

A physically disabling condition may be chronic and relatively stable in nature, such as a congenital disorder, or, over time, the individual may be faced with a progressive loss of function. Physically disabling conditions may also occur rapidly, as is seen with a traumatic injury or accident, but then result in a chronic, and sometimes progressive, loss of function. Literature differentiates the **coping strategies** employed by persons faced with either a traumatic injury or acute illness and those faced with a chronic physically disabling condition (Charmaz, 1983, 2002; Davidhizar, 1997; Morse & O'Brien, 1995). Whether clients experience a chronic or traumatic onset of a physically disabling condition, they will require the expertise of an OT practitioner in helping them create a new sense of self regardless of the physical limitations they face.

Chronic Disabling Conditions

When a person is faced with a chronic disabling condition, particularly one associated with progressive deterioration in physical abilities, coping or adapting to the changes is an ongoing process (Charmaz, 1995). Adults and children faced with chronic physically disabling conditions must construct a sense of self with a body that does not consistently and accurately respond to their demands. This lack of reliable control over one's body is further compromised by the cultural and societal expectations that one should have control over the body (Nadeau & Tessier, 2009). Children who have cerebral palsy are at greater risk for social isolation and rejection by peers due to obvious differences in physical abilities. The lack of bowel and bladder control after the age of 2 or 3 years is considered unacceptable and yet many individuals with spina bifida, multiple sclerosis, and Parkinson's disease have incontinence (Cate, Kennedy, & Stevenson, 2002; Roe, 2000; Schultz-Krohn, Foti, & Glogoski, 2006).

Three stages have been identified in the process of adapting to a chronic physically disabling condition, but the occupational therapist should not assume that a client smoothly progresses through these stages in a linear manner. Charmaz (1995, p. 657) has described these three stages as represented in Table 15-1.

The first stage of coping is marked by the person's appreciation of his or her altered physical condition (Charmaz, 1995). Some clients fight against the experience of this new relationship between their body and their concept of self. They may reject any form of adaptive equipment because it is a symbol of an altered body. Clients may deny that previous physical abilities are no longer available to them (Katz, Fleming, Keren, Lightbody, & Hartman-Maeir, 2002). A client with severe rheumatoid arthritis may persist in attempting to wash windows in her home even though lifting her arms above her head produces severe fatigue and pain.

A chronic and progressively disabling condition requires frequent reappraisals of physical abilities. Each time a person experiences a new loss of motor control or function, such as the deterioration of fine motor skills due to the progression of multiple sclerosis or Parkinson's disease, he or she must adjust to an altered sense of bodily control (Sinnakaruppan, Macdonald, McCafferty, & Mattison, 2010). Control over the body was previously a "taken-for-granted" experience that now, with deterioration of function, requires reappraisal and revisions (Charmaz, 1995, p. 662). Initially, "people with chronic illnesses may make firm separations between their impaired bodies and their self-concepts" (p. 663). The illness or disabling condition may be viewed as an enemy that must be battled (Huttlinger et al., 1992). This stance underlies a hope for clients "to

TABLE 15-1. Adapting to a Chronic Disabling Condition

Stage and Label	Description
Stage 1: Experience and Definition of Impairment	Ongoing appraisal and acknowledgment of his or her altered physical condition.
Stage 2: Bodily Adjustment and Identity Trade-Offs	Identifies commitments and responsibilities associated with previous roles. Commitments and responsibilities are meshed with the changed physical abilities and require the person to make an identity trade-off. Creates a new identity through negotiating his or her personal needs, the expectations and needs of significant others, and the demands of the environment.
Stage 3: Surrendering to the Changed Body (Embracing the Changed Body)	Accepts the physical changes and incorporates these changes into a new concept of self. Develops respect for the limitations of the body instead of constantly trying to change the body functions.

Adapted from Charmaz, 1995.

regain their past identities" and abilities, such as complete control over their bodies to perform according to past experiences (Charmaz, 1995, p. 663). This position may be held for an extended period of time and compromises the client's ability to accept modifications and adaptations that would allow successful completion of everyday tasks.

The concept of self and the use of body should not be viewed as separate entities but as intimately connected, influencing each other to produce an integrated person (Charmaz, 2002). That does not mean a person with a disabling condition cannot achieve an integrated self, but instead, that a progressive physically disabling condition requires frequent adjustments to the relationship between the body and self. When a person experiences a progressive deterioration of physical abilities, the reliance on the use of the body is severely compromised. Each new episode or loss of function requires adjustment and often includes adjusting to a change in physical appearance. The previous model of the physical body disintegrates and a new model must be developed (Charmaz, 1995). This new body structure may be unacceptable by societal standards. Absent or severely contracted limbs as well as extraneous and involuntary movements are barely tolerated by society (Frank, 2000; Murray, 2009; Novotny, 1991; Rossi et al., 2009; Varni & Setoguchi, 1991). The person with a physical disability is expected to adjust to an undependable body, the structure and/or function of which is usually not endorsed by society.

Charmaz (1995) differentiates between struggling *against* a disorder or illness and struggling *with* a disorder or illness. A struggle against the disorder is seen as a lack of acceptance of the changed body. A struggle with the disorder reflects a degree of acceptance and an attempt to reconfigure a concept of self with an altered physical ability as was seen in Penny's successful struggle to resume her academic role with a new persona of an eccentric professor with a proper British cane. The acceptance of a changed body and efforts to mesh this body with self require energy. Occupational therapists need to be aware of the efforts expended by people with physical disabilities as they work on integrating the changed body with the concept of self. As a person reconfigures his or her concept of self integrated with a self-appraisal of the changed body, the person moves to the next stage of coping.

The second stage of coping with a physical disability requires revising identity goals due to the change in physical ability (Charmaz, 1995). This stage requires careful consideration of the social context for the person. Returning to driving after a person sustains a cerebrovascular accident (CVA) may be an important identity goal as a symbol of independence but may require substantial trade-offs to achieve this goal (Patomella, Johansson, & Tham, 2009).

For example, a young man sustained a CVA due to a ruptured aneurysm, resulting in severe loss of function of his right arm and leg. During occupational therapy he expressed a primary goal of being able to drive. He had previously driven a motorcycle and a sports car with a manual transmission. He described himself as a "biker with a hotrod" but now resigned himself to learning to drive an "old man's car" (a car with an automatic transmission) with modifications to the controls to allow him to drive using only his left hand and leg. This change in identity goals was significant for this young man. Although for his occupational therapist it was rewarding to see him regain his ability to drive, it was also important to note and address his frequent comments about his feelings of loss that he had to sell his motorcycle. He viewed himself as damaged and experienced a loss of social standing within his social network. The following example illustrates the key elements of this stage of adapting to a chronic disabling condition.

CASE ILLUSTRATION

Ms. Shapiro—Adapting to a Chronic Disabling Condition

Ms. Shapiro, a 30-year-old woman, had a clear identity of herself as a full-time professional, wife, and mother of two young children but after being diagnosed with multiple sclerosis was required to make modifications to this identity. Multiple sclerosis is chronic and progressive, marked by exacerbations and remissions of symptoms where the progression of the disease is unpredictable (Dyck, 2002). Her symptoms included weakness, visual problems, and tremors. The unpredictable nature of multiple sclerosis placed Ms. Shapiro in a position where she needed to make identity trade-offs (Charmaz, 1995). She was no longer able to work a demanding, but rewarding, full-time professional job and fulfill the expectations of caring for her children. She was faced with reducing her work hours and enlisting the help of her husband in the care of their children and with the household chores.

Mr. Choi, her husband, also a working professional, did not feel ready to accept the full responsibilities for household upkeep but did take on the responsibility of grocery shopping. He did rearrange his busy work schedule to help with the children every morning. This couple worked on a budget and they were able to hire a person to help clean the house. The interactions between this husband and wife resulted in the wife further reducing her work hours to continue as the primary caregiver for their children.

Discussion

Ms. Shapiro traded her role as a professional to continue in her role as a mother. The result of being diagnosed with multiple sclerosis and understanding the impact of the disease not only affected her identity roles but role expectations of her husband and children, necessitating trade-offs in roles and identities. These trade-offs were not made unilaterally but the decisions of which roles to relinquish and how to reconfigure identity roles were the product of interaction between this woman's priorities and the expectations of her husband and children.

The final stage of adapting to impairment requires the person to accept the physical changes brought about by the illness or disorder and to incorporate these changes into the concept of self (Charmaz, 1995, 2002; Davidhizar, 1997). This stage is not to be confused with people who become resigned to physical changes and give up hope for any positive outcomes. The hallmark of this stage is acceptance of the physical changes and a willingness to work within the confines of the changed body. Davidhizar (1997) cites several works where **life satisfaction** is not directly correlated with severity of physical disability. A person with greater physical limitations has fewer options available to engage in life situations, however, primarily due to environmental barriers.

Those with physical disabilities who stop pushing their physical body to improve find they can still exercise choice (Charmaz, 1995). The choice may be directed to different occupations that can be accomplished within the confines of the changed body. The struggle often faced by individuals during this stage is not the denial of symptoms or the false hopes of recovery, but instead, individuals are now confronted with social labels and interactions that stigmatize and restrict their choices (Dyck, 2002).

Surrendering to the changed body allows a new construction of self with routines and habits that support the new self (Charmaz, 2002). Accepting the changed body and prioritizing routines and habits appears to be expressed somewhat differently between men and women. Women tend to respond by decreasing their responsibilities to those around them and "relinquishing the super-mom image on which their self-concepts had been predicated" (p. S38). Men tend to prioritize personal relationships in routines and habits during this final stage of adapting to a changed body.

Adapting to a physical disability should not be construed as a step-by-step process whereby a client passes through one stage to another (Charmaz, 1995, 2002; Davidhizar, 1997; Dyck, 2002). Those faced with a chronic disabling condition, particularly one that is progressive in nature, may revisit any of the above stages during the course of their lifetime. The occupational therapist must be sensitive to the psychosocial support each client requires; understanding the adaptation process aids in providing meaningful OT intervention to those who have a chronic physical disability. When a person is faced with an acute onset of a physical disability, such as a spinal cord injury, traumatic brain injury, CVA, or amputation, the adaptation process is initially different from the above description due to the acute nature (Morse & O'Brien, 1995). Refer to Table 15-2 for specific details of the process of adapting to the acute onset of a physically disabling condition.

Acute Onset of Disabling Conditions

Adapting to lasting bodily changes resulting from an acute trauma has been described as a four-stage process by Morse and O'Brien (1995). The first stage was labeled as "vigilance: becoming engulfed" (p. 887). This stage occurred at the initial point of injury or acute illness and continued until the individual "relinquished self

TABLE 15-2. Adapting to Acute Onset Disabling Conditions

Stage and Label	Environmental Circumstance	Description
Stage 1: Vigilance: Becoming Engulfed	Site of onset of the acute condition, such as CVA or trauma, such as a spinal cord injury.	Encounters a separation between the experience of the body and emotions. This stage ends as the person relinquishes control to others or loses consciousness.
Stage 2: Disruption: Taking Time Out	Hospital/acute care	Experiences a disruption in reality orientation. Significant others are critical to provide an anchor to reality regarding self in the midst of the unfamiliar and disorganizing environment.
Stage 3: Enduring the Self: Confronting and Regrouping	Acute care/acute rehabilitation services	Reality orientation improves and the person becomes aware of an abrupt change in physical ability.
Stage 4: Striving to Regain Self: Merging the Old and New Reality	Rehabilitation	Tests the limits of the changed bodily functions. Revises and reformulates life goals with respect to the changed body. Creates a new sense of self.

Adapted from Morse & O'Brien, 1995.

to caregivers . . . or when they lost consciousness" (p. 887). Many of the individuals reported a separation of the subjective body and the objective body. They experienced an internal sense of calmness contrasted with their outward behavior of screaming and distress. This was often reported when severe pain was present. The stage of vigilance ended when the person surrendered care to another, often in an emergency room.

The second stage was identified as "disruption: taking time out" (Morse & O'Brien, 1995, p. 890). During this stage, individuals experienced a disruption in reality, often describing feeling as if they were in a fog. There was a great need for significant others to be present and to provide a "safe haven in a confusing nightmare" (p. 890). The role of significant others was not merely for support but served as an orienting force in a chaotic environment. Significant others were seen as the anchor for individuals who sustained an acute injury to "remind them who they were and gave them a sense of self" in the disordered world of an acute care hospital setting (p. 891).

The third stage, "enduring the self: confronting and regrouping," was marked by an improvement in reality orientation (Morse & O'Brien, 1995, p. 891). As reality orientation improved, the implications of the acute injury or illness began to be recognized. Many participants in this study experienced severe physical pain, but reported that the realization of the severity of the changed body was more difficult than the pain endured. The abrupt change signified a loss of physical control of their bodies and the environment and a dependence on others for even mundane routines. This stage was seen as the time when individuals were first faced with learning the severity of their physical limitations. One individual described how being alone produced feelings of panic and fear due to the lack of physical ability.

Those who sustained an acute injury resulting in a chronic physically disabling condition described the need for others as a support during this stage. Here the support provided was not merely as an assist to control the environment but also for encouragement. Many discussed how the encouragement from therapists and significant others helped them endure the arduous process of healing from injuries and acute illness. Several individuals described how even small gains achieved during the therapy sessions were interpreted as evidence that they could recover previous physical abilities. This also reflects the lack of acceptance of changed physical abilities (Katz et al., 2002). Although Morse and O'Brien (1995) discuss that this preserved sense of hope to reclaim previous abilities may have helped individuals with the initial healing process from burns, amputations, and spinal cord injuries, they also acknowledge that individuals "refused to accept the permanence of the damage" by holding on to the faith the medical miracles would return them to their previous selves (p. 893).

The final stage was called "striving to regain self: Merging the old and the new reality" (Morse & O'Brien, 1995, p. 893). During this stage, the rehabilitation services provided helped individuals test the limits of their newly altered bodies. Through the course of rehabilitation "the more an individual tried to do, the more he or she realized what he or she could not" do (p. 894). This stage was marked by frustration in attempting to regain previously taken-for-granted tasks such as walking and feeding oneself by using new strategies that confirm an altered body. Life goals had to be revised and reformulated due to this changed body. Many individuals reported feelings of exhaustion as they developed new routines and determined the physical limits of their newly altered bodies. Individuals who had sustained a spinal cord injury reported the amount of energy and effort they expended to complete even simple self-care tasks (Manns & Chad, 2001). The energy expenditure then limited their participation in other activities.

Individuals who sustain a traumatic injury or illness resulting in persistent physical disabilities adapt to their changed bodies and create a new sense of self. This occurs through an appraisal of their current physical capabilities. The need to decide what activities to pursue and what activities to discontinue is similar to the stage identified by Charmaz (1995) as identity trade-offs. The stages of adapting to a physically changed body, whether from an acute injury or illness or due to a chronic and often progressive condition, are provided here to help the occupational therapist understand the process of adaptation. This process should be incorporated into the intervention plan and addressed as part of the OT services provided.

LIFE SATISFACTION AND QUALITY OF LIFE

The concepts of life satisfaction and quality of life are very important when discussing the psychosocial issues of physical disabilities and adapting to limitations in body functions and structures. Life satisfaction is considered to be the subjective component of an individual's overall quality of life (Tzonichaki & Kleftaras, 2002). How satisfied an individual is with his or her life may include such factors as satisfaction with family life, engagement in leisure activities, vocational pursuits, self-care, and sexual expression. Satisfaction does not require the same level of participation from each individual but instead reflects the person's value regarding his or her level of participation in various life situations.

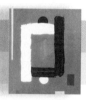

CASE ILLUSTRATION

Sam's Satisfaction in Life

Sam, a 9-year-old boy with spina bifida, used a wheelchair for mobility. He participated on a wheelchair soccer team using a large ball, had his own collection of video games, talked to other boys about how "gross" girls are, and reported being very satisfied with his life with the exception of school. Sam hated school. He had visual perceptual deficits necessitating modifications and accommodations to his educational program. Although he was unable to walk, did not have bowel and bladder control, and had visual perceptual deficits, Sam reported feeling satisfied with his overall life, particularly during summer vacation. He was quick to add that more video games would make his life better.

Discussion

Sam was able to participate in the activities he deemed important. Success in school was not a priority in Sam's life even though his parents were concerned with his performance in his educational program. Life satisfaction, from Sam's perspective, meant being able to get together with friends to play video games or wheelchair soccer. His ability to engage in these life situations was unencumbered by his diagnosis and he viewed his life as quite satisfying.

Quality of life includes life satisfaction along with overall physical and emotional health and functional status (Manns & Chad, 2001). The appraisal of quality of life is not generated solely from the individual's perspective but includes participation in activities. For example, a teenager with spastic cerebral palsy may be unable to control his arms or legs to participate in everyday activities and family members may report the need to provide assistance for dressing and bathing him (McCarthy et al., 2002). The need for others to complete basic self-care tasks for a teenager reflects the lack of physical control he experiences, thereby compromising his overall quality of life. Activity limitations and problems in participation in life situations are included when discussing the quality of life for the individual. On the other hand, Derek, a 25-year-old college senior and student body president, who has high-level quadriplegia, is unable to physically perform any activities of daily living (ADL). However, Derek is so adept at conveying his needs and preferences to his personal care attendant that at a dinner party, everyone quickly becomes unaware of the attendant's presence during the meal. In fact, Derek is in control and a very active participant in his self-care and social activity. In this instance the concept of participation is reconfigured and likely contributes positively to Derek's quality of life.

Of particular relevance to occupational therapy is what clients report as contributing to their quality of life and life satisfaction. Over 20 years ago Burnett and Yerxa (1980) found that individuals with disability, while satisfied with their performance of personal ADL, after discharge from rehabilitation felt ill prepared for functioning in the home and community. In response, Pendleton (1990) investigated occupational therapists' use of independent living skills training (ILST) and found that occupational therapists working in rehabilitation centers with clients with physical disabilities frequently placed more emphasis on therapeutic exercise and self-care training than on the skills needed for independent living and those associated with life satisfaction. These skills are often identified as the instrumental activities of daily living (IADL) but embrace more than meal preparation and time concepts. Independent living skills require the occupational therapist to include a client's participation in preferred occupations, which involves not only the environment in which these occupations take place but the socialization that supports engagement in these occupations. More recent studies indicate that those individuals with disability who report high quality of life and life satisfaction regarded socialization (friendship), leisure, and productive occupations as most responsible for their reported high quality of life and life satisfaction (Hammel, 1995; Pendleton, 1998). In fact, for the four participants in Pendleton's qualitative study of the friendships of successful women with physical disability, friendship supported participation in occupation and participation in occupation in turn facilitated their friendship.

A preponderance of the literature regarding psychosocial issues of physical disability for those with a variety of chronic disabling conditions (whether acute, progressive, or congenital onset) describes using an individual's perceived quality of life or life satisfaction as a measure of the person's success in adapting to or overcoming the emotional consequences of these diagnoses. Self-reported absence of depression, anxiety, and suicidal ideation is deemed evidence of mental health, which is frequently equated with high quality of life and life satisfaction (Kemp & Krause, 1999; Tate & Forchheimer, 2001). Adaptation to disability, and consequently satisfaction with life, is found to be related to many factors, including the individual's age, gender, cause of onset, developmental stage at onset, culture, ethnicity, religious and familial beliefs, meaning and value of the abilities lost, previous life experiences and coping styles, life stressors, and support and response of family and friends (Antonak, Livneh, & Antonak, 1993; Novotny, 1991). Also of significance is the therapeutic competence and attitudes toward disability of the health care professionals involved in their care (Novotny, 1991). One can see the importance and interrelatedness of these factors affecting psychosocial adjustment and well-being when examining the life stories of any client with a disability.

CASE ILLUSTRATION

Jenny—Age 16

Jenny has paraplegia as a result of an automobile accident she experienced at the age of 16. She was driving at the time of the accident without her parents' permission and without a driver's license. These circumstances caused Jenny guilt and anxiety and the perceived notion that the disability was a punishment for her disobedience. Furthermore, as a sophomore attending a small town high school, at an age when body image and self-concept are fragile without the challenge of disability, she did not want to return to classes, where she believed she would now be regarded negatively. Friends seemed to reinforce her beliefs when they phoned her for rides to the mall (soon after she obtained a car with hand controls) but never asked her to join them once they arrived.

Discussion

All of these factors contributed to Jenny's feelings of low self-esteem, stigma, depression, and a resulting perceived low quality of life. Factors affecting her more favorably were her loving and supportive family, her previous academic and social successes, adequate financial resources, and a comprehensive rehabilitation program at a major SCI treatment center. Regardless of the diagnosis these factors are crucial to anticipating and understanding the psychosocial ramifications of disability for a particular client like Jenny and ultimately providing the appropriate OT intervention.

SPECIFIC PSYCHOSOCIAL ISSUES WITH SELECT DISABILITIES

In the following sections the psychosocial issues common to three major categories of physical disability will be briefly discussed. Discussion will focus upon selected diagnoses from each of the categories and be illustrated by vignettes or client stories that depict real-life examples of characteristic psychosocial responses to the particular disability. An accompanying table (Table 15-3), showing expected psychosocial issues associated with specific diagnoses, commonly used assessments, and suggested OT interventions, is provided. However, this table is not intended to be an exhaustive

TABLE 15-3. Psychosocial Issues, Assessments, and Interventions

Diagnosis	Frequently Expected Psychosocial Issues	Commonly Used Assessments	Suggested Interventions
Spinal cord injury	Depression Anxiety Decreased coping Decreased self-concept Loneliness Vulnerability to abuse—especially in women	Occupational Performance History Interview (OPHI) (Kielhofner et al., 1998) Canadian Occupational Performance Measure (COPM) (Law et al., 2005) Activity Configuration (Cynkin & Robinson, 1990) Beck Depression Inventory (BDI) (Beck, Ward, Mendelson, Mock, & Erbaugh, 1961) Beck Anxiety Inventory (BAI) (Beck, Epstein, Brown, & Steer, 1988) Occupational Self-Assessment (OSA) (Baron, Kielhofner, Goldhammer, & Wolenski, 1999) Ways of Coping Questionnaire (Folkman & Lazarus, 1987)	Stress management Coping skills training Education on social connectedness Education on depression awareness Education addressing sexuality Education on the connection between occupation and emotional health
Acquired amputation	Altered body image Loss of identity/sexuality Anxiety/fear of the unknown or rejection Low self-worth Self-repulsion Phantom pain Grief Loss of sense of wholeness/decreased self-concept Depression Anger	COPE Inventory (Carver, Scheier, & Weintraub, 1989) Acceptance of Disability Scale (Linkowski, 1987). Reactions to Impairment and Disability Inventory (RIDI) (Livneh & Antonak, 1990) Prosthesis Evaluation Questionnaire (PEQ) (Legro, Smith, del Aguila, Larson, & Boone, 1998) Trinity Amputation Prosthetic Experience Scales (TAPES) (Gallagher & MacLachlan, 2000) COPM	Coping skills training Active decision making/active problem solving Education re: disability in a timely and factual manner Adequate preparation Pre-op peer discussion Peer support groups Opportunities for social involvement

TABLE 15-3. Continued

Diagnosis	Frequently Expected Psychosocial Issues	Commonly Used Assessments	Suggested Interventions
Traumatic brain injury (Also see Chapter 16)	Depression Reduced insight Denial Personality changes Decreased social competence Anger, hostility, aggressiveness, behavioral disinhibition, sex offending, impulsivity, risk taking Confusion Decreased self-awareness Decreased insight Anxiety, agitation Women—high incidence of being sexually abused pre-injury and highly vulnerable to victimization post-injury	Assessment of Communication and Interaction Skills (Forsyth, Salamy, Simon, & Kielhofner, 1998). Occupational Role History (Florey & Michelman, 1982) Role Checklist (Oakley, 1986) Life History Interview (Moorhead, 1969) OPHI OSA Glasgow Assessment Scale (GAS) (Livingston & Livingston, 1985) Portland Adaptability Inventory (PAI) (Lezak, 1987)	Education in coping strategies for both client and family Collaborative goal setting with client Intrapersonal skills groups—activity based with peer support Life skills group classes Interpersonal skills group—personal boundaries and limit setting Long-term Psychosocial Rehabilitation Groups (PSR)—club like group activities aimed at skills needed for psychosocial rehab
Cerebral vascular accident	Depression Anxiety Decreased motivation to initiate activity Isolation, loneliness Emotional lability Fear of falling	Geriatric Depression Scale (Sheikh & Yesavage, 1986) Older Adult Health and Mood Questionnaire (Kemp & Adams, 1995) Mini Mental Status (Folstein et al., 1975) Interest Checklist (Rogers, 1988) COPM	Involve client in goal setting and selecting interventions Realistic approach, particularly in setting goals Relaxation training Exploration and education in coping skills Socialization and support groups One on one discussion regarding depression, anxiety or any other observed psychosocial issue

(Continues)

TABLE 15-3. Continued

Diagnosis	Frequently Expected Psychosocial Issues	Commonly Used Assessments	Suggested Interventions
Multiple sclerosis (MS)	Depression Cognitive changes	BDI COPM OSA Expanded Disability Status Scale (EDSS) (Paty, Willoughby, & Whitaker, 1992) Fatigue Impact Scale (FIS) (Fisk, Pontefract, Ritvo, Archibald, & Murray, 1994) Multiple Sclerosis Quality of Life Inventory (MSQLI) (Ritvo et al., 1997)	Social support groups Diagnostic support groups Energy conservation
Parkinson's disease (PD)	Depression Social isolation Decreased facial expressiveness	BDI COPM OSA Unified Parkinson's Disease Rating Scale (UPDRS) (Hoehn & Yahr, 1967) Parkinson's Disease Questionnaire (PDQ-39) (Peto, Jenkinson, Fitzpatrick, & Greenhall, 1995)	Social support groups Environmental supports to facilitate control Activity/exercise groups for psycho-social support
Huntington's disease	Depression Suicide	BDI COPM OSA Unified Huntington's Disease Rating Scale (UHDRS) (Huntington Study Group, 1996)	Environmental modifications to support control Social support groups
Cerebral palsy	Dependency Behavioral problems Risk for social isolation	Pediatric Evaluation of Disability Inventory (PEDI) (Haley, Coster, Ludlow, Haltiwanger, & Andrellos, 1992) School Function Assessment (SFA) (Coster, Deeney, Haltiwanger, & Haley, 1998)	
Spina bifida	Dependency Risk for social isolation	PEDI SFA	

listing of all the possible psychosocial problems for each disability, assessments, or interventions, but rather, a simple tool to be used by the occupational therapist to inspire or jog one's thinking when confronted with the psychosocial issues experienced by clients with various diagnoses. With few exceptions, the psychosocial issue described for one diagnosis could be included with each diagnosis listed. However, for the purpose of this table, only the main problems represented repeatedly in the relevant literature are included. If, for example, working with a client with a spinal cord injury, it is hoped that the viewer of this table would peruse the categories listed for other diagnoses and consider whether any of these have implications, or applications, for her or his current client.

Chronic Disorders with an Acute Onset

By its very definition—sudden onset—psychosocial coping with this type of physical disability is experientially different than coping with progressive or congenital chronic disability. Individuals with such disability initially experience shock accompanied by high anxiety and fear for their very survival. Once survival becomes more certain their shock segues into denial of the ramifications of or the very existence of the disability (Antonak et al., 1993; Gutman, 2001a). Researchers and individuals who have written about their experience of disability point out that often it isn't until a year or more after the onset of their disability that the psychosocial issues become paramount and the search for the physical or miraculous cure recedes into a less prominent position (Gutman, 2001a; Hockenberry, 1995; Price-Lackey & Cashman, 1996). It therefore becomes a challenge to the occupational therapist to address the psychosocial issues while meeting the client's emotional readiness to contemplate such issues.

In the following sections the psychosocial issues of several diagnoses associated with acute onset will be discussed. The reader will undoubtedly note the commonalities and the differences inherent in how each psychosocial issue is experienced among the diagnoses. It is also important to keep in mind the personal, cultural, and social demographics of each client and the importance of that perspective on how each psychosocial issue might be uniquely experienced.

Spinal Cord Injury

At the onset of spinal cord injury (SCI) many individuals experience situational depression, anxiety, decreased coping skills, and altered self-concept (Angel, Kirkevold, & Pedersen, 2009; Galvin & Godfrey, 2001; Hughes, Swedlund, Petersen, & Nosek, 2001; Kemp & Kraus, 1999). Incidence of depression is increased and various studies suggest that 30% to 40% develop a depressive disorder while 20% to 25% experience anxiety. Suicide rates are two to six times higher than in the community population and substance abuse is almost twice as high for individuals with SCI (46%) than in the community population (25%), though those with SCI demonstrated a higher incidence of substance abuse prior to injury (Galvin & Godfrey, 2001). Divorce rates are significantly higher (four out of five marriages dissolve within the first two years) and there is generally a decrease in financial and employment opportunities. The incidence of depression, anxiety, and suicidal ideation four to six years after onset of injury appears to be no greater for those with SCI than for the community population. Quality of life and life satisfaction among persons with SCI were found to also mirror those of the general population with the exception of satisfaction with sexuality, physical condition, and leisure activities (Benony et al., 2002). In another study, mobility and perceived health were found to be predictors of quality of life and life satisfaction for participants with SCI (Putzke, Richards, Hicken, & De Vivo, 2002).

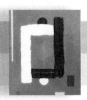

CASE ILLUSTRATION

Jim—Confronting Abrupt Change

Jim, a 30-year-old race car champion, sustained an SCI at the C6 level during a competition. Jim's concept of self is that of an athlete skilled and accomplished in a sport known for its daredevil aspects. He is also accustomed to the adulation of his fans, especially the women, who are attracted to his good looks and success. Much of his body image, self-concept, and self-esteem are dependent upon his view of himself as a physically capable race car professional. His sexuality is also highly defined by this self-concept. It is anticipated that after rehab he will use a wheelchair for mobility, be able to drive an adapted van, and accomplish most of his self-care activities using a tenodesis hand splint. Plans are for him to move back to his home where he will require part-time assistance for his bowel and bladder care, bathing, and home maintenance. He is very depressed and expresses anxiety about his social life. Next to his hospital bed he has a photo of his crashed race car and talks about his accident with visitors and rehab staff.

Discussion

Jim's concept of self is clearly being challenged, particularly with regard to his sexuality. His behavior seems consistent with that expected at the stage of adaptation previously described as "enduring the self: confronting and regrouping." While he is grappling with the abrupt changes in his physical abilities, the occupational therapist working with Jim will be challenged to help him explore his previously successful occupational strategies and reconfigure them in crafting a new self to meet his new reality.

It has been found that the longer one lives with an SCI positively correlates with an increasing feeling of life satisfaction (Kemp & Kraus, 1999). However, those who are aging with an SCI are likely to experience onset of new physical problems, including osteoporotic changes, fatigue, pain, weakness, low endurance, significantly increased incidence of heart disease (and at a significantly earlier age than their peers), and a decreased level of independence in ADL and IADL, also known as home and community skills. There is a concomitant increase in depression as individuals contemplate what these extensions of their disabilities mean for their futures. Kemp and Kraus (1999) found that these individuals reported significantly lower life satisfaction than that of their nondisabled peers or counterparts. Interestingly, the problem areas that were most responsible for their dissatisfaction with life were not primarily at the level of their body structures or routine activity performance (ADL and IADL) but rather at no longer being able to participate in valued work, social, and favored leisure occupations.

Women with SCI experience the psychosocial sequelae of disability somewhat differently than men with SCI. Tate and Forchheimer (2001) found that while women with SCI reported higher life satisfaction than men with SCI, they had lower mental health related quality of life and were likely to experience qualitatively more severe problems of poor body image, lower self-concept, and feelings of increased vulnerability, especially those women who required personal assistance. They explained that women with SCI were at higher risk for abuse, both physical (neglect) and emotional, as well as at risk for financial exploitation. They also found that the participants who had a longer time since the onset of injury reported better quality of life outcomes.

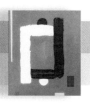

CASE ILLUSTRATION

Jenny—Age 52

Jenny, the 16-year-old girl with paraplegia described in an earlier example, is now a 52-year-old successful college professor who is happily married and typifies the problems associated with aging with an SCI. She has bilateral carpal tunnel syndrome and her shoulders are very painful after years of pushing her wheelchair and transferring to and from the bottom of a tub (which she was taught to do in occupational therapy). Her image of herself as the attractive, active, and competent woman in the sporty wheelchair is constantly being challenged as she now times her departure from the campus to coincide with that of other colleagues so that she can get a push to her car. She spent their vacation money to remodel the bathroom with a roll-in shower and purchased a van with a lift (not in her self-image either), eschewing her custom of always driving something sporty. Of most concern to Jenny is the fatigue she experiences, necessitating that she go to bed early every night and spend the weekend catching up on her rest. In order to preserve her much-loved employment she is increasingly forgoing many of her favorite leisure and social occupations and only engaging in those ADLs and IADLs that are essential. She is very anxious about what the future holds considering she is this limited at only 52. With uncharacteristic sadness she expresses that she thought she had already made the difficult adjustment when she was 16.

Discussion

Jenny's new situation is reminiscent of that described earlier in Charmaz's three-stage model of adaptation to a progressive chronic disability. Review that model with Jenny's experience in mind. Note also that Jenny's 36-year experience of SCI suggests few of the aforementioned problems of particular concern to women with SCI. However, she worries about what will happen to her should her physical and functional capabilities continue to decline or if she outlives her spouse or he becomes ill and they both require the help of a personal care attendant. If her fears are realized an older and widowed Jenny may be seeking OT intervention for help with her challenged concept of self as well as her declining physical and functional capabilities.

Acquired Amputation

Depression is a major psychosocial sequelae of acquired amputation (whether lower or upper extremity) and experienced by approximately 28% to 35% of the population (Desmond & MacLachlan, 2002; Fitzpatrick, 1999; Livneh, Antonak, & Gerhardt, 1999; Novotny, 1991; Rybarczyk, Nyenhuis, Nicholas, Cash, & Kaiser, 1995; Varni & Setoguchi, 1991; Walters & Williamson, 1998). For some individuals the failure to resume a self-perceived satisfactory life was found to have more to do with both the individual's and societal attitudes toward amputation than to the loss of the limb itself (Fitzpatrick, 1999; Murray, 2009; Rossi et al., 2009; Walters & Williamson, 1998). A study of people with lower extremity amputations found that poor body image and perceived social stigma resulting in social discomfort accounted for approximately 40% of the clinical depression experienced (Rybarczyk et al., 1995). The average length of time since amputation for their participants was 17 years, which suggested to the researchers that depression was both a short-term and a long-term adjustment problem following lower limb amputation.

Fitzpatrick (1999) observed that those individuals whose amputations are the result of a traumatic event (such as war, horrific accidents, or cancer), in which threat of death or actual death of others occurs, may be subject to post-traumatic stress disorder (PTSD). This is an anxiety disorder where the traumatic event is repeatedly relived and the emotional impact reexperienced and should be addressed before a chronic emotional disorder develops. Given the nature of the cause of many of the acute onset diagnoses it may behoove the occupational therapist to be alert to the possibility of PTSD when working with any of these clients.

Approximately 80% of persons with amputations experience the phenomenon of phantom limb (sensory perception of the amputated limb) that seldom interferes long-term with psychosocial adjustment to the changed body and eventually becomes incorporated into the individual's body image. Phantom pain, on the other hand, while experienced by fewer of this population, is a more serious problem with little or no remedy (Desmond & MacLachlan, 2002). Management of this pain is important for the person to be able to participate in important life activities and occupations such as sexual expression and was found to be associated with resuming sexual activity (Walters & Williamson, 1998). Furthermore, sexual satisfaction was found to be a predictor of quality of life and thus contributed to psychosocial adjustment for persons with amputations. Achieving social and sexual satisfaction after amputation may further imply that the individual has been able to satisfactorily incorporate his or her new body image with residual limb(s) and developed coping strategies for handling stigma (Desmond & MacLachlan, 2002).

Consider the example of a young woman who is a part-time model, athlete, and participant runner and jumper in the Para Olympics. This articulate and physically attractive woman, who has bilateral lower extremity amputations, expresses to a television audience that she regards her various prosthetic legs (running legs, modeling legs, and legs for every day) as "art," "engineering marvels," and "really beautiful." Images of her running with her black *S*-shaped metal legs ("shaped like the hind leg of a cheetah") with shoes attached, footage of her as she struts the fashion show runway in Paris, and home movies of her and her boyfriend resting after a race—her with her prostheses off and her residual limbs exposed—seem to be indicators that she has reframed her body image and society's standards of beauty into a new and satisfactory self-concept.

Traumatic Brain Injury

The psychosocial problems associated with traumatic brain injury (TBI) are not dissimilar to those of the previously discussed acute onset diagnoses but the clients' response to them is further complicated by their concomitant problems with cognition and perception (Gutman, 2001b). The average age at onset is 15 to 30 years old, with the incidence in males three times higher than in females (Bell & Pepping, 2001). There is a high incidence of depression, which may not be solely a reaction to the loss of body structures and functions or activity limitations but may also be a response to biological changes in the neuroreceptors of the temporal and frontal lobes of the brain (Antonak et al., 1993). Antonak et al. note that there is frequently a preexisting history of substance abuse and risk-taking behaviors characteristic of the males who sustain TBI. Females who sustain TBI were found to have frequently had a preinjury history of childhood sexual abuse and adult alcoholism and the resulting social and behavioral problems associated with each which need to be taken into account when coupled with the new problems (Gutman & Swarbrick, 1998). For both genders after injury there is often internalized anger caused by guilt and blaming oneself for the injury whereas externalized hostility is observed in those who blame others for their injury, although there is debate over whether the hostile behavior is organically based or an attempt at coping (Antonak et al., 1993).

An overwhelming issue is the client's decreased or unsatisfactorily altered concept of self, which is a long-term consequence of decreased social roles and social isolation. Many experience the loss of roles of dating, marriage, intimacy, and even the perceived adult role of living independently (Gutman, 2001a, 2001b). Behavioral problems frequently limit job opportunities and the resulting circumstances and environment for social interaction and friendship (Vandiver & Christofero-Snider, 2000).

Antonak et al. (1993) note that there needs to be an intellectual acceptance or acknowledgment of one's impairment and a gradual reintegration of the new body image and functioning into one's self-concept. Eventually, for most people with physical disability, there is an emotional acceptance of the disability with "integration of one's impairment into one's self concept coupled with behavioral adaptation and social reintegration into the new life situation" (p. 89). However, emotional problems are frequently not perceived by individuals with TBI, who characterize their problems as physical and cognitive, whereas family members are more likely to report the psychosocial problems as more prevalent (Antonak et al., 1993). Follow-up studies and personal accounts conducted two to seven years after onset suggest that the majority of individuals with TBI continue to have problems with psychosocial issues (Price-Lackey & Cashman, 1996; Vandiver & Christofero-Snider, 2000).

Price-Lackey and Cashman (1996) tell the compelling story of Cashman's more than five-year struggle reconfiguring her self-concept through graded participation in a previously valued occupation after a TBI. Cashman, a 30-year-old freelance journalist with an impressive eclectic academic and employment career, was driving on a mountain road when her car was backed into by a large truck. She never lost consciousness and even signed a waiver at the crash site saying that she had suffered no repercussions from the impact. Her brain injury symptoms developed later that day as she attempted to pay for her groceries at the checkout counter and had no idea what to do with the checkbook. The psychosocial issues she confronts echo those described above and one can see the significant repercussions as one by one she is unable to maintain her job, loses her house, is forced to move in with relatives, and focuses her efforts in trying to recoup some of her former skills. Though her writing never reaches its preinjury caliber, she is able to develop cognitive and coping strategies to attend graduate school in a new career trajectory that capitalizes on her current skills. (See Chapter 16 for further discussion of TBI.)

Cerebrovascular Accident

Cerebrovascular accident (CVA) is the most common physical disability diagnosis addressed by occupational therapy. There are a myriad of body structures and functions that can be affected by CVA, and each individual client may experience some or many of them to varying degrees of severity or impact on satisfactory participation in an occupation. Typical psychosocial issues may include depression, which is thought to be highly underreported, and anxiety, which is frequently associated with a fear of falling and not being able to get up—reminiscent of the onset of CVA (Smith, 2001). Other psychosocial issues include a decreased motivation to initiate activity, social isolation and loneliness, and emotional lability. Mr. Kelley's story exemplifies how the various psychosocial effects of stroke might be experienced and addressed by occupational therapy.

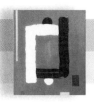

CASE ILLUSTRATION

Mr. Kelley—The Psychosocial Effects of Stroke

Mr. Kelley is an 82-year-old retired accountant who lives with his wife of 50 years in their own home close to the homes of his three grown children. Since age 62 he has "made a career out of retirement," enjoying daily golf, bowling, watching sports on television, and attending lectures and meetings of his college alumni group and a senior men's social organization. He is a master bridge player and plays couples bridge with his wife at weekly dinner/bridge games and keeps current with the tax laws so that he can volunteer to assist seniors at the local senior center in preparing their tax returns. He attends church on Sundays and drives his wife (who does not drive) to her various appointments and errands. They travel frequently and are very involved with their children and grandchildren.

While on one of their trips Mr. Kelley sustained a CVA and initially had weakness in his left side and some neglect which rather quickly resolved. After a one-week nursing home stay, where he relearned his ADL, he returned home and sat in front of TV with his exercise equipment. He confided that he felt "a little blue." His wife felt trapped in the house ("he never leaves") and fondly reminisced about the days when he left early in the morning and came home later in the afternoon ready to take her out to dinner. Fortunately the home health occupational therapist sized up the situation and together with Mr. Kelley set goals for resuming his participation in his occupational life. Mr. Kelley's depression was discussed and strategies for handling it were developed.

Additional OT intervention was aimed first at relearning the chores he customarily performed around the house. Next the occupational therapist explored his bridge and tax skills and he discovered, to his relief, that he still had those capabilities. She then referred him to a community college–based post-stroke program, where that occupational therapist worked with him on resuming his golfing and social dancing skills in time for his 50th anniversary celebration. A referral to another occupational therapist confirmed his ability to drive safely and two years after his stroke he was able to volunteer at the post-stroke program and reengage in many of his pre-stroke activities though his golfing was not at the level of proficiency he previously enjoyed—his game was now more in concert with those of his daughters and new golfing partners.

Discussion

Mr. Kelley's story exemplifies the gamut of psychosocial issues typically associated with the experience of having a CVA, including depression, decreased concept of self, and seemingly decreased motivation to initiate activity. The strategies his occupational therapist taught him to cope with his depression enabled him to practice and participate in previously loved occupations, which in turn helped to quell his anxiety and fear of falling. Repeated success in performance of his preferred occupations helped him to craft an acceptable, though changed, self-concept.

Progressive Physical Disorders

Individuals who experience a progressive loss of reliable body function through a degenerative disease process require the occupational therapist to consider how this deterioration can compromise sense of self (Charmaz, 2002). Previously established habits are no longer effective and a person is faced making continuous trade-offs as function is lost (Irvine et al., 2009). Within the general category of progressive chronic physical disorders two specific diagnoses will be described to illustrate the impact of this deterioration of function. Additionally, specific psychosocial issues are addressed.

Parkinson's Disease

Individuals with Parkinson's disease (PD) present with a progressive loss of motor control. Eventually, the person is dependent upon others for all personal care (Gaudet, 2002; Schultz-Krohn et al., 2006). The loss of physical function is associated with a degeneration of portions of the basal ganglia, resulting in a substantial reduction in neurotransmitters within the brain (Olanow, Jenner, Tatton, & Tatton, 1998).

Approximately 50% of individuals diagnosed with PD are also diagnosed with depression (Pollak, 1998). This depression is not merely reactive to the severity of symptoms or the chronic and progressive nature of the disease but appears to be related to a serotonergic deficit (Duvoisin & Sage, 1990). The depression seen in individuals with PD is similar to that in individuals without PD who have depression. An additional characteristic problem seen with individuals who have PD is decreased facial expressiveness, known as the "masked face" (Pollak, 1998). This "masked face" begins unilaterally but, as the disease progresses, there is a loss of facial expressions on both sides of the face (Duvoisin & Sage, 1990).

CASE ILLUSTRATION

The Masked Face of Mr. Sanchez

Mr. Sanchez is a 61-year-old man diagnosed with PD. He owned a small construction company but needed to retire last year due to the progression of PD. His eldest son assumed the responsibility of running the company. Mr. Sanchez has a very good relationship with all his children and they all live in the area. His children are married and he takes great pleasure in spending time with his grandchildren now that he has retired. The progression of PD, particularly the masked face, has made it very difficult for Mr. Sanchez to smile when his young grandchildren come to see him. The grandchildren interpret this lack of facial responsiveness as indifference to their presence and often ask their mother, "Why doesn't Grandpa like us?" The grandfather overheard this question and began to limit the amount of time he spent with his grandchildren to coincide with when his medications are working.

Discussion

Mr. Sanchez had experienced the loss of a worker role when he had to retire from his position as the boss of his own company. He reconfigured his sense of self to be the loving grandfather, always available to visit his grandchildren. Now that role was being revised since Mr. Sanchez's grandchildren were misinterpreting his masked face as indifference. He self-limited that role to coincide to his medication schedule, confirming how the disease process of PD was dominating his occupational configuration.

Individuals with PD often limit social participation because they are embarrassed about decreased facial expressions and movement disorders (Gaudet, 2002). The decrease in activity and participation is not just a product of the loss of motor control but the ability to adapt to the progressing loss of function and the interpretation of the loss of function by others.

Huntington's Disease

Huntington's disease (HD) is a fatal degenerative neurological disease that is characterized by progressive disorders of both voluntary and involuntary movement in addition to significant deterioration of cognitive and behavioral abilities (Phillips & Stelmach,

1996). The initial symptoms vary but are most often reported as changes in behavior, cognitive function, and unusual movements of the hands (Wiederholt, 1995). Emotional and behavioral changes are often the earliest symptoms of HD (Folstein, 1989). The movement disorder, known as chorea, is sometimes mistaken for intoxication, particularly because of the gait disturbances associated with HD. The initial cognitive changes may be seen as forgetfulness or difficulties concentrating on tasks. During the initial stages of HD, a client may experience difficulties maintaining adequate work performance. Family members often identify the initial behavioral changes seen in the person with HD as increased irritability or depression. Irritability and depression may be inappropriately attributed to the decline in work performance rather than the disease process. As HD progresses, depression often worsens and suicide is not uncommon (Wiederholt, 1995). Clients with HD are frequently hospitalized due to various psychiatric problems, including depression, emotional lability, and behavioral outbursts. Although the loss of function may contribute to the client's level of depression, depression is clearly identified as a specific characteristic of HD (Folstein, 1989).

Chronic Congenital Nonprogressive Disorders

Individuals with congenital physically disabling conditions must adapt to a body that is unable to meet cultural and societal expectations. Developmental motor skills are not attained within the expected timeframes, and for some are never attained. Congenital physically disabling conditions may be nonprogressive in nature, such as cerebral palsy and spina bifida, or progressive, such as Rett's syndrome (Rogers, 2010). The following will address two common congenital disorders that are considered nonprogressive. Even though cerebral palsy and spina bifida are considered nonprogressive in nature, as environmental demands increase in complexity, the child with either of these disorders may fall farther behind peers in performance. Of further significance is the understanding that the child with a congenital disorder is positioned within a family with expectations, hopes, and dreams. As the child grows and additional developmental milestones are unmet, families, and particularly parents, may feel socially isolated and overwhelmed by the care of the child and express loss of identity (Helitzer, Cunningham-Sabo, VanLeit, & Crowe, 2002).

Cerebral Palsy

Children with cerebral palsy (CP) present with limited motor control that can compromise mobility, self-care, and social participation (Beckung & Hagberg, 2002). These activity limitations obviously impact the child's occupational pursuits, but families are also influenced by these limitations (Helitzer et al., 2002). Children with CP were found to have a much higher frequency of behavioral problems such as disruptive behaviors and hyperactivity (McDermott et al., 1996). There was also a higher frequency of self-care dependency, surpassing what would be expected from their activity limitations due to problems with body function. The dependency frequently seen with children with CP is not solely related to problems in controlling movements. Children who have motor problems expend significant energy attempting even simple tasks such as feeding or dressing themselves.

Karen is a 12-year-old girl who has CP. The family system finds it easier to provide consistent support to help Karen dress instead of having her develop the habits to be able to dress independently. Karen has been able to complete some dressing tasks during OT intervention sessions but complains that it takes too much time. As a result of this family pattern of interacting with Karen, she has continued to be dependent on others to complete dressing tasks, past the expected age where it is culturally and socially endorsed to require assistance. This compromised her ability to attend "sleep-overs" at her friend Susie's house because of the imposition it would place on Susie's parents to dress Karen for bed and then in the morning.

Understanding the impact of limited motor control on social participation and making informed decisions regarding energy expenditures should be included in OT intervention for individuals with CP. Occupational therapy services should also address the child's developmental trajectory and prepare the child for adolescent and adult roles (King, Cathers, Polgar, MacKinnon, & Havens, 2000). King et al. interviewed 10 older adolescents with CP regarding their perceptions of success in life. These teenagers described three key features related to being successful "in life: being believed in, believing in yourself, and being accepted by others" (p. 734). The concepts of independence in self-care and control of movements were not included in the themes. These teenagers placed a much higher value on interdependence and interactions with others than on independence in personal care. Occupational therapy services provided to children and adolescents who have CP typically focus on developing independent functional skills. Unfortunately, this emphasis does not help adolescents with CP meet their goal of a successful life. King et al. argue that adolescents with CP "need opportunities to participate that will provide supportive relationships, belief in themselves, and a sense of community belonging" (p. 746).

Spina Bifida

Children with spina bifida, or myelomeningocele, have associated psychosocial issues that require careful consideration when developing an OT intervention plan (Antle, 2004). The high incidence of hydrocephalus, incontinence, sensory loss, and orthopedic surgeries is stressful for both the individual with spina bifida and the family (Cate et al., 2002). Mothers of children with spina bifida reported a compromised sense of competence as a parent and less satisfaction in their role (Hombeck et al., 1997). Appleton et al. (1997) reported that individuals with spina bifida were at a greater risk for experiencing depression, social isolation, and low self-worth.

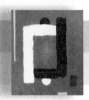

CASE ILLUSTRATION

Sandy—Social and Psychological Support

Sandy is a 15-year-old and attends a public high school. Sandy has myelomeningocele and has had over 10 surgeries, including revisions to her ventriculoperitoneal shunt placed to reduce the risk of hydrocephalus. She uses a manual wheelchair for mobility and manages her own bowel and bladder program. Sandy uses an intermittent self-catherization program and has been allowed to use the nurse's office at the school for privacy on a daily basis. She lives with both parents and her 17-year-old sister who attends the same high school. Her sister plays on the varsity soccer team and is in the marching band. Sandy is also in the marching band but to play her instrument, the flute, she requires assistance from her friend to push her wheelchair. Through the use of environmental accommodations within the school Sandy is included in many activities and is allowed to participate according to her interest level. Her one comment is that it would be nice to date but doesn't see that happening soon. She laughs and says her father is over-protective but then adds that no boys are interested in dating a girl in a wheelchair.

Discussion

The psychosocial issues faced by Sandy are common to children and adolescents with spina bifida. Borjeson and Lagergren (1990) asked teenagers with myelomeningocele to identify their concerns and half listed social and psychological issues as a greater concern than physical issues. Unfortunately, the majority of services provided these adolescents focused on the physical aspects of myelomeningocele and failed to provide the psychosocial support these teenagers needed.

SUMMARY

The experiences of the OT clients described throughout this chapter should represent a resounding call to occupational therapists to redouble their efforts to thoroughly consider and effectively address the psychosocial challenges of their clients with physical disabilities. Due to time and space limitations, many diagnoses commonly treated by occupational therapists working with clients with physical disabilities were not directly addressed. Those diagnoses that were discussed exemplify a model of how psychosocial issues associated with any physical disability diagnosis can be recognized, researched, assessed, and addressed by occupational therapy in its commitment to empower the whole person to engage in occupation to support satisfactory participation in life (AOTA, 2008).

REVIEW QUESTIONS

1. What are the differences between adapting to physical limitations that occur from a chronic illness or condition and adapting to physical limitations resulting from an acute injury or illness?
2. What is the difference between the terms *life satisfaction* and *quality of life* as is used in the literature addressing physical disabilities?
3. How do cultural and societal factors influence adaptation to a physical disability?
4. Identify three reasons for an occupational therapist to assess and provide intervention to directly address psychosocial issues for clients with physical disabilities.
5. Name three psychosocial issues of concern to those with physical disabilities and describe appropriate OT interventions to address those issues.

REFERENCES

Ackerley, S. J., Gordon, H. J., Elston, A. F., Crawford, L. M., & McPherson, K. M. (2009). Assessment of quality of life and participation within an outpatient rehabilitation setting. *Disability and Rehabilitation, 31*(11*)*, 906–915.

American Occupational Therapy Association. (2008). Occupational therapy practice framework: Domain and process (2nd ed.). *American Journal of Occupational Therapy, 62*, 625–683.

Angel, S., Kirkevold, M., & Pedersen, B. D. (2009). Rehabilitation as a fight: A narrative case study of the first year after a spinal cord injury. *International Journal of Qualitative Studies on Health and Well-being. 4*, 28–38.

Antle, B. J. (2004). Factors associated with self-worth in young people with physical disabilities. *Health & Social Work, 29*(3*)*, 167–175.

Antonak, R. F., Livneh, H., & Antonak, C. (1993). A review of research on psychosocial adjustment to impairment in persons with traumatic brain injury. *Journal of Head Trauma Rehabilitation, 8*(4), 87–100.

Appleton, P. L., Ellis, N. C., Minchom, P. E., Lawson, V., Boll, V., & Jones, P. (1997). Depressive symptoms and self-concept in young people with spina bifida. *Journal of Pediatric Psychology, 22*, 707–722.

Baron, K., Kielhofner, G., Goldhammer, V., & Wolenski, J. (1999). *The Occupational Self Assessment (OSA) (Version 1.0)*. Model of Human Occupational Clearinghouse. Chicago: University of Illinois at Chicago.

Beck, A. T., Epstein, N., Brown, G., & Steer, R. A. (1988). An inventory for measuring clinical anxiety: Psychometric properties. *Journal of Consulting and Clinical Psychology, 56*, 893–897.

Beck, A. T., Ward, C. M., Mendelson, M., Mock, J., & Erbaugh, J. (1961). An inventory for measuring depression. *Archives of General Psychiatry, 4*, 561–571.

Beckung, E., & Hagberg, G. (2002). Neuroimpairments, activity limitations, and participation restrictions in children with cerebral palsy. *Developmental Medicine and Child Neurology, 44*, 309–316.

Bell, K. R., & Pepping, M. (2001). Women and traumatic brain injury. *Physical Medicine and Rehabilitation Clinics of North America, 12*(1), 169–182.

Benony, H., Daloz, L., Bungener, C., Chahraoui, K., Frenay, C., & Auvin, J. (2002). Emotional factors and subjective quality of life in subjects with spinal cord injuries. *American Journal of Physical Medicine and Rehabilitation, 81*, 437–445.

Bickenbach, J. E. (2009). Disability, culture and the UN convention. *Disability and Rehabilitation, 31*(14), 1111–1124.

Bonder, B. (2001). Culture and occupation: A comparison of weaving in two traditions. *Canadian Journal of Occupational Therapy, 68*, 310–319.

Borjeson, M. C., & Lagergren, J. (1990). Life conditions of adolescents with myelomeningocele. *Developmental Medicine and Child Neurology, 32*, 698–706.

Brice, A., & Campbell, L. (1999). Cross-cultural communication. In R. L. Leavitt (Ed.), *Cross-cultural rehabilitation* (pp. 83–94). London: W. B. Saunders.

Burnett, S. E., & Yerxa, E. J. (1980). Community based and college based needs assessment of physically disabled persons. *American Journal of Occupational Therapy, 34*, 201–207.

Carver, C. S., Scheier, M. F., & Weintraub, J. K. (1989). Assessing coping strategies: A theoretically based approach. *Journal of Personality and Social Psychology*, 56, 267–283.

Cate, I. M. P., Kennedy, C., & Stevenson, J. (2002). Disability and quality of life in spina bifida and hydrocephalus. *Developmental Medicine and Child Neurology, 44*, 317–322.

Charmaz, K. (1983). Loss of self: A fundamental form of suffering in the chronically ill. *Sociology of Health and Illness, 5*, 168–195.

Charmaz, K. (1995). The body, identity, and self: Adapting to impairment. *Sociological Quarterly, 36*, 657–680.

Charmaz, K. (2002). The self as habit: The reconstruction of self in chronic illness. *Occupational Therapy Journal of Research, S22*, S31–S41.

Clark, F. (1993). Occupation embedded in a real life: Interweaving occupational science and occupational therapy. *American Journal of Occupational Therapy, 47*(12), 1067–1078.

Coster, W., Deeney, T., Haltiwanger, J., & Haley, S. (1998). *School Function Assessment (SFA): User's manual.* San Antonio, TX: Psychological Corporation.

Cynkin, S., & Robinson, A. M. (1990). *Occupational therapy and activities health: Toward health through activities.* Boston: Little, Brown.

Davidhizar, R. (1997). Disability does not have to be the grief that never ends: Helping patients adjust. *Rehabilitation Nursing, 22*, 32–35.

Desmond, D., & MacLachlan, M. (2002). Psychosocial issues in the field of prosthetics and orthotics. *Journal of Prosthetics and Orthotics, 14*(1), 19–22.

Duvoisin, R. C., & Sage, J. I. (1990). The spectrum of Parkinsonism. In S. Chokroverty (Ed.). *Movement disorders.* New Brunswick, NJ: PMA.

Dyck, I. (2002). Beyond the clinic: Restructuring the environment in chronic illness experience. *Occupational Therapy Journal of Research, S22*, S52–S60.

Fisher, A., & Kielhofner, G. (1995). Mind-brain-body performance subsystem. In G. Kielhofner (Ed.), *A model of human occupation theory and application* (2nd ed., pp. 83–90). Baltimore: Williams & Wilkins.

Fisk, J. D., Pontefract, A., Ritvo, P. G., Archibald, C. J., & Murray, T. J. (1994). The impact of fatigue on patients with multiple sclerosis. *Canadian Journal of Neurological Sciences, 21*, 9–14.

Fitzpatrick, M. C. (1999). The psychologic assessment and psychosocial recovery of the patient with an amputation. *Clinical Orthopaedics and Related Research, 361*, 98–107.

Fitzpatrick, N., & Finlay, L. (2008). "Frustrating disability": The lived experience of coping with the rehabilitation phase following flexor tendon surgery. *International Journal of Qualitative Studies on Health and Well-being, 3*, 143–154.

Florey, L., & Michelman, S. M. (1982). The occupational role history. *American Journal of Occupational Therapy, 36*(5), 301–308.

Folkman, S., & Lazarus, R. S. (1987). *The ways of coping questionnaire.* Palo Alto, CA: Consulting Psychologists Press.

Folstein, S. E. (1989). *Huntington's disease: A disorder of families.* Baltimore: Johns Hopkins University Press.

Folstein, M. F., Folstein, S. E., & McHugh, P. R. (1975). Mini-mental state: A practical method for grading the cognitive state of patients for the clinician. *Journal of Psychiatric Research, 12*(3), 189–198.

Forsyth, K., Salamy, M., Simon, S., & Kielhofner, G. (1998). *Assessment of communication and interaction skills*. Model of Human Occupational Clearinghouse. Chicago: University of Illinois at Chicago.

Frank, G. (2000). *Venus on wheels*. Los Angeles: University of California Press.

Gallagher, P., & MacLachlan, M. (2000). Development and psychometric evaluation of the Trinity Amputation and Prosthesis Experience Scales (TAPES). *Rehabilitation Psychology, 45*, 150–154.

Gallimore, R., & Lopez, E. M. (2002). Everyday routines, human agency, and ecocultural context: Construction and maintenance of individual habits. *Occupational Therapy Journal of Research, S22*, S70–S79.

Galvin, L. R., & Godfrey, H. P. D. (2001). The impact of coping on emotional adjustment to spinal cord injury (SCI): Review of the literature and application of a stress appraisal and coping formulation. *Spinal Cord, 39*, 615–627.

Gaudet, P. (2002). Measuring the impact of Parkinson's disease: An occupational therapy perspective. *Canadian Journal of Occupational Therapy, 69*, 104–115.

Goffman, E. (1963). *Stigma: Notes on the management of spoiled identity*. Upper Saddle River, NJ: Prentice-Hall.

Gutman, S. A. (2001a). The psychosocial sequelae of traumatic brain injury, part I: Identification. *OT Practice, 6*(3), 1–8.

Gutman, S. A. (2001b). Traumatic brain injury. In L. W. Pedretti & M. B. Early (Eds.), *Occupational therapy: Practice skills for physical dysfunction* (pp. 671–701). St. Louis, MO: Mosby.

Gutman, S. A., & Swarbrick, P. (1998). The multiple linkages between childhood sexual abuse, adult alcoholism, and traumatic brain injury in women: A set of guidelines for occupational therapy practice. *Occupational Therapy in Mental Health, 14*(3), 33–65.

Haley, S. M., Coster, W. J., Ludlow, L. H., Haltiwanger, J. T., & Andrellos, P. J. (1992). *Pediatric Evaluation of Disability Inventory (PEDI): Development, standardization and administration manual*. Boston: New England Medical Center Hospitals.

Hammel, K. W. (1995). Spinal cord injury; quality of life; occupational therapy: Is there a connection? *British Journal of Occupational Therapy, 58*(4), 151–157.

Hampton, N. Z., & Marshall, A. (2000). Culture, gender, self-efficacy, and life satisfaction: A comparison between Americans and Chinese people with spinal cord injuries. *Journal of Rehabilitation, 66*, 3–25.

Helitzer, D. L., Cunningham-Sabo, L. D., VanLeit, B., & Crowe, T. K. (2002). Perceived changes in self-image and coping strategies of mothers of children with disabilities. *Occupational Therapy Journal of Research, 22*, 25–33.

Hockenberry, J. (1995). *Moving violations: War zones, wheelchairs, and declarations of independence*. New York: Hyperion.

Hoehn, M. M., & Yahr, M. D. (1967). Parkinsonism: Onset, progression and mortality. *Neurology, 17*, 422–427.

Hombeck, G. N., Gorey-Ferguson, L., Hudson, T., Seefeldt, T., Shapera, W., Turner, J., & Uhler, J. (1997). Maternal, paternal, and marital functioning in families of preadolescents with spina bifida. *Journal of Pediatric Psychology, 22*, 167–181.

Hughes, R. B., Swedlund, N., Petersen, N., & Nosek, M. A. (2001). Depression and women with spinal cord injury. *Topics in Spinal Cord Injury Rehabilitation, 7*(1), 16–24.

Huntington Study Group. (1996). Unified Huntington's Disease Rating Scale: Reliability and consistency. *Movement Disorders, 11*, 156–142.

Huttlinger, K., Krefting, L., Drevdahl, D., Tree, P., Baca, E., & Benally, A. (1992). "Doing battle": A metaphorical analysis of diabetes mellitus among Navajo people. *American Journal of Occupational Therapy, 46*, 706–711.

Irvine, H., Davidson, C., Hoy, K., & Lowe-Strong, A. (2009). Psychosocial adjustment to multiple sclerosis: Exploration of identity redefinition. *Disability and Rehabilitation, 31*(8): 599–606.

Iwama, M. K., Thomson, N. A., & MacDonald, R.M. (2009). The Kawa model: The power of culturally responsive occupational therapy. *Disability and Rehabilitation, 31*(14), 1125–1155.

Katz, N., Fleming, J., Keren, N., Lightbody, S., & Hartman-Maeir, A. (2002). Unawareness and/or denial of disability: Implications for occupational therapy intervention. *Canadian Journal of Occupational Therapy, 69*, 281–292.

Kemp, B. J., & Adams, B. (1995). The older adult health and mood index: A new measure of depression for older persons. *Journal of Geriatric Neurology and Psychiatry, 8*, 162–167.

Kemp, B. J., & Kraus, J. S. (1999). Depression and life-satisfaction among people ageing with postpolio and spinal cord injury. *Disability and Rehabilitation, 21*(5/6), 241–249.

Kielhofner, G., Malinson, T., Crawford, C., Nowak, M., Rigby, M., Henry, A., & Walens, D. (1998). *The Occupational Performance History Interview (Version 2.0) (OPHI II)*. Model of Human Occupational Clearinghouse. Chicago: University of Illinois at Chicago.

King, G. A., Cathers, T., Polgar, J. M., MacKinnon, E., & Havens, L. (2000). Success in life for older adolescents with cerebral palsy. *Qualitative Health Research, 10*, 734–749.

Law, M., Baptiste, S., Carswell, A., McColl, M. A., Polatajko, H., & Pollock, N. (2005). *The Canadian Occupational Performance Measure* (4th ed.). Ottawa: CAOT Publications Ace.

Legro, M. W., Smith, D. G., del Aguila, M., Larson, J., & Boone, D. (1998). Prosthesis evaluation questionnaire for persons with lower limb amputations: Assessing prosthesis-related quality of life. *Archives of Physical Medicine and Rehabilitation, 79*, 931–938.

Lezak, M. D. (1987). Relationship between personality disorders, social disturbance, and physical disability following traumatic brain injury. *Journal of Head Trauma Rehabilitation, 2*(1), 57–59.

Linkowski, D. (1987). *The Acceptance of Disability Scale*. Washington, DC: George Washington University.

Livingston, M. G., & Livingston, H. M. (1985). The Glasgow Assessment Schedule (GAS): Clinical and research assessment of head injury outcome. *International Rehabilitation Medicine, 7*, 145–149.

Livneh, H., & Antonak, R. F. (1990). Reactions to disability: An empirical investigation of their nature and structure. *Journal of Applied Rehabilitation Counseling, 21*(4), 15–21.

Livneh, H., Antonak, R. F., & Gerhardt, J. (1999). Psychosocial adaptation to amputation: The role of sociodemographic variables, disability-related factors and coping strategies. *International Journal of Rehabilitation Research, 22*, 21–31.

Manns, P. J., & Chad, K. E. (2001). Components of quality of life for persons with a quadriplegic and paraplegic spinal cord injury. *Qualitative Health Research, 11*, 795–811.

McCarthy, M. L., Silberstein, C. E., Atkins, E. A., Harryman, S. E., Sponseller, P. D., & Hadley-Miller, N. A. (2002). Comparing reliability and validity of pediatric instruments for measuring health and well-being of children with spastic cerebral palsy. *Developmental Medicine and Child Neurology, 44*, 468–476.

McDermott, S., Coker, A. L., Mani, S., Krishnaaswami, S., Nagle, R. J., Barnett-Queen, L. L., et al. (1996). A population-based analysis of behavior problems in children with cerebral palsy. *Journal of Pediatric Psychology, 21*, 447–463.

Moore, A. (1992). *Cultural anthropology: The field study of human beings*. San Diego, CA: Collegiate.

Moorhead, L. (1969). The occupational history. *American Journal of Occupational Therapy, 23*, 329–334.

Morse, J. M., & O'Brien, B. (1995). Preserving self: From victim, to patient, to disabled person. *Journal of Advanced Nursing, 21*, 886–896.

Murphy, R. F. (2001). *The body silent.* New York: W. W. Norton.

Murray, C. D. (2009). Being like everybody else: the personal meanings of being a prosthesis user. *Disability and Rehabilitation, 31*(7), 573–581.

Nadeau, L., & Tessier, R. (2009). Social adjustment at school: Are children with cerebral palsy perceived more negatively by their peers than other at-risk children? *Disability and Rehabilitation, 31*(4), 302–308.

Novotny, M. P. (1991). Psychosocial issues affecting rehabilitation. *Physical Medicine and Rehabilitation, Clinics of North America, 2*(2), 373–393.

Oakley, F. M. (1986). The role checklist. *Occupational Therapy Journal of Research, 6*(3), 157–169.

Ohbuchi, K., Fukushima, O., & Tedeschi, J. T. (1999). Cultural values in conflict management. *Journal of Cross-Cultural Psychology, 30*, 51–71.

Olanow, C. W., Jenner, P., Tatton, N. A., & Tatton, W. G. (1998). Neurodegeneration and Parkinson's disease. In J. Jankovic & E. Tolosa (Eds.), *Parkinson's disease and movement disorders* (3rd ed.). Baltimore: Williams & Wilkins.

Patomella, A., Johansson, K., & Tham, K. (2009). Lived experience of driving ability following stroke. *Disability and Rehabilitation, 31*(9), 726–733.

Paty, D., Willoughby, E., & Whitaker, J. (1992). Assessing the outcome of experimental therapies in multiple sclerosis. In R. A. Rudick & D. E. Goodkin (Eds.), *Treatment of multiple sclerosis trial design, results, and future perspectives.* London: Springer-Verlag.

Pendleton, H. McH. (1990). Occupational therapists' current use of independent living skills training for adult inpatients who are physically disabled. In J. Johnson & E. Yerxa (Eds.), *Occupational science: The foundations for new models of practice* (pp. 93–108). Binghamton, NY: Haworth.

Pendleton, H. McH. (1998). *Establishment and sustainment of friendship of women with physical disability: The role of participation in occupation.* Doctoral dissertation, University of Southern California, Los Angeles. Available through UMI.

Peto, V., Jenkinson, C., Fitzpatrick, R., & Greenhall, R. (1995). The development and validation of a short measure of functioning and well-being for individuals with Parkinson's disease. *Quality of Life Research, 4*, 241–248.

Phillips, J. G., & Stelmach, G. E. (1996). Parkinson's disease and other involuntary movement disorders of the basal ganglia. In C. M. Fredericks & L. K. Saladin (Eds.), *Pathophysiology of the motor systems.* Philadelphia: F. A. Davis.

Pollak, P. (1998). Parkinson's disease and related movement disorders. In J. Bogousslasky & M. Fisher (Eds.), *Textbook of neurology.* Boston: Butterworth Heinemann.

Price-Lackey, P., & Cashman, J. (1996). Jenny's story: Reinventing oneself through occupation and narrative configuration. *American Journal of Occupational Therapy, 50*(4), 306–314.

Putzke, J. D., Richards, J. S., Hicken, B. L., & De Vivo, M. J. (2002). Predictors of life satisfaction: A spinal cord injury cohort study. *Archives of Physical Medicine and Rehabilitation, 83*, 555–561.

Ritvo, P. G., Fischer, J. S., Miller, D. M., Andrews, H., Paty, D., & LaRocca, N. G. (1997). *Multiple Sclerosis Quality of Life Inventory (MSQLI): A user's manual.* New York: National Multiple Sclerosis Society.

Roe, B. (2000). Effective and ineffective management of incontinence: Issues around illness trajectory and health care. *Qualitative Health Research, 10*, 677–690.

Rogers, J. (1988). The NPI interest checklist. In B. Hemphill (Ed.), *Mental health assessment in occupational therapy.* Thorofare, NJ: Slack.

Rogers, S. L. (2010). Common diagnosis in pediatric occupational therapy practice. In J. Case-Smith & J. C. O'Brien (Eds.), *Occupational therapy for children* (6th ed., pp. 146–192). St. Louis, MO: Mosby.

Rossi, L. A., Costa, M. C. S., Dantas, R. S., Ciofi-Silva, C. L., & Lopes, L. M. (2009). Cultural meaning of quality of life: perspectives of Brazilian burn patients. *Disability and Rehabilitation, 31*(9), 712–719.

Rybarczyk, B., Nyenhuis, D. L., Nicholas, J. J., Cash, S. M., & Kaiser, J. (1995). Body image, perceived social stigma, and the predictions of psychosocial adjustment to leg amputation. *Rehabilitation Psychology, 40*(2), 95–110.

Schneider, M. (2009). The difference a word makes: Responding to questions on 'disability' and 'difficulty' in South Africa. *Disability and Rehabilitation, 31*(1), 42–50.

Schultz-Krohn, W., Foti, D., & Glogoski, C. (2006). Degenerative diseases of the central nervous system. In H. Pendleton & W. Schultz-Krohn (Eds.), *Occupational therapy: Practice skills for physical dysfunction* (pp. 702–729). St. Louis, MO: Mosby.

Sheikh, J. I., & Yesavage, J. A. (1986). Geriatric Depression Scale (GDS): Recent evidence and development of a shorter version. *Clinical Gerontologist, 5*, 165–173.

Sinnakaruppan, I., Macdonald, K., McCafferty, A., & Mattison, P. (2010). An exploration of the relationship between perception of control, physical disability, optimism, self-efficacy and hopelessness in multiple sclerosis. *International Journal of Rehabilitation Research, 33*(1), 26–33.

Smith, J. A. (2001). *How do occupational therapists address psychosocial issues with geriatric patients?* Unpublished master's thesis, San Jose State University, San Jose, CA.

Tate, D. G., & Forchheimer, M. (2001). Health-related quality of life and life satisfaction for women with spinal cord injury. *Topics in Spinal Cord Injury Rehabilitation, 7*(1), 1–15.

Tzonichaki, I., & Kleftaras, G. (2002). Paraplegia from spinal cord injury: Self-esteem, loneliness, and life satisfaction. *Occupational Therapy Journal of Research, 22*, 96–103.

Vandiver, V. L., & Christofero-Snider, C. (2000). TBI club: A psychosocial support group for adults with traumatic brain injury. *Journal of Cognitive Rehabilitation, 18*(4), 22–27.

Varni, J. W., & Setoguchi, Y. (1991). Psychosocial factors in the management of children with limb deficiencies. *Physical Medicine and Rehabilitation Clinics of North America, 2*(2), 395–404.

Walters, A. S., & Williamson, G. M. (1998). Sexual satisfaction predicts quality of life: A study of adult amputees. *Sexuality and Disability, 16*(2), 103–115.

Wiederholt, W. (1995). Parkinson's disease and other movement disorders. In *Neurology for non-neurologists* (3rd ed.). Philadelphia: Saunders.

Williams, D., & Ispa, J. M. (1999). A comparison of the child-rearing goals of Russian and U.S. university students. *Journal of Cross-Cultural Psychology, 30*, 540–546.

World Health Organization (WHO). (2001). *International classification of functioning, disability and health (ICF)*. Geneva: Author.

Wright, B. (1983). *Physical disability: A psychosocial approach* (2nd ed.). New York: Harper & Row.

Yerxa, E. J. (2001). The social and psychological experience of having a disability: Implications for occupational therapy. In L. W. Pedretti & M. B. Early (Eds.), *Occupational therapy: Practice skills for physical dysfunction* (pp. 470–492). St. Louis, MO: Mosby.

SUGGESTED RESOURCES

Amyotrophic Lateral Sclerosis Society website: http://www.alsa.org/

Aragon, A., & Kings, J. (2010). Occupational therapy for people with Parkinson's: Best practice guidelines. Retrieved from http://www.parkinsons.org.uk/pdf/OTParkinsons_guidelines.pdf

Huntington's Disease Society of America website: http://www.hdsa.org/

National Multiple Sclerosis Society website: http://www.nationalmssociety.org

National Parkinson's Foundation website: http://www.parkinson.org/

Chapter 16

The Cognitive, Behavioral, and Psychosocial Sequelae of Brain Injury

Shawn Phipps, PhD, OTR/L, FAOTA

KEY TERMS

abstract thinking
anosognosia
confabulation
demotivational syndrome
diffuse axonal injury
disinhibition
executive function
generalization

Glasgow Coma Scale (GCS)
initiation
neuroplasticity
perseveration
post-traumatic amnesia
Rancho Los Amigos Levels of
    Cognitive Functioning

CHAPTER OUTLINE

Introduction
Diagnosis and Etiology
Prognosis for Recovery
Premorbid Psychosocial Factors
Occupational Therapy Evaluation and Intervention
Cognitive Sequelae Following Brain Injury
    Impaired Orientation
    Attention Deficits
    Impaired Memory
    Impaired Initiation and Termination of Activities
    Impaired Insight, Judgment, and Safety Awareness
    Impaired Information Processing
    Impaired Executive Functions
    Impaired Abstract Thinking and Integration of New Learning

Behavioral Sequelae Following Brain Injury
    Agitation and Aggression
    Disinhibition
    Hypersexual Behaviors
    Demotivational Syndrome
    Inappropriate Emotional Responses
Psychosocial Sequelae Following Brain Injury
    Psychiatric Disorders
    Changes in Personality and Impaired Social Pragmatics
    Impaired Coping Mechanisms
    Altered Self-Concept
    Impact of Brain Injury on Family Dynamics
Summary

INTRODUCTION

The Brain Injury Association of America (n.d.) defines *traumatic brain injury (TBI)* as "an insult to the brain, not of a degenerative or congenital nature, but caused by an external physical force, that may produce a diminished or altered state of consciousness, which results in an impairment of cognitive abilities or physical functioning." Each year, an estimated 2 million Americans sustain a TBI (Rutland-Brown, Langlois, Thomas, & Xi, 2006) and the incidence is higher in Europe and Africa (Bruns & Hauser, 2003). At least 1.4 million people sustain a TBI in the United States. Of these, about 50,000 die, 235,000 are hospitalized, 80,000 experience the onset of long-term disability, and 1.1 million are treated and released from an emergency department (Centers for Disease Control and Prevention, 2011). It has also been suggested that there is significant risk for a second or third head injury after an initial TBI, but the reports are inconsistent and the prevalence needs to be further researched. However, the literature is in agreement that a person with a TBI has at least a 15% to 20% chance of sustaining another head injury. Currently, there are an estimated 5.3 million Americans (more than 2% of the U.S. population) who are living with long-term disabilities resulting from a TBI (Centers for Disease Control and Prevention, 2003).

TBI has also been identified as the "signature injury" of the wars in Iraq and Afghanistan (Schwab, Warden, Lux, Shupenko, & Zitnay, 2007; see also Chapter 25 for further discussion). Military personnel endure TBI from gunshots or blasts and present with complex polytrauma, including posttraumatic stress disorder (PTSD) and mild TBI (MTBI) requiring extensive occupational therapy services for full participation in occupation and integration into society (Poole et al., 2007; Sayer et al., 2008; Vanderploeg et al., 2008)

The cost of TBI is estimated to be $48.3 billion annually in the United States (Centers for Disease Control and Prevention, 2003), and the emotional, behavioral, social, perceptual, and physical sequelae following brain injury are even more costly to the individuals, their families, and to society at large. In traditional rehabilitation settings, there has been a historical overemphasis on the physical impairments impacting occupational performance following brain injury, which can include hemiplegia, visual-perceptual dysfunction, and sensory disturbances. Remediative and compensatory occupational therapy approaches have traditionally focused on improving motor control, visual/perceptual skills, sensory awareness, basic (ADL) and instrumental activities of daily living (IADL), community reintegration, prevocational skills, and driving skills (McCabe et al., 2007; Rapport, Coleman Bryer, & Hanks, 2008; Tamietto et al., 2006). However, this chapter addresses the cognitive, behavioral, and psychosocial sequelae of brain injury as these are often the most disabling, challenging, and costly aspects of TBI (Cameron, Purdie, Kliewer, & McClure, 2008; Haggstrom & Lund, 2008). A client with brain injury presents with a complex clinical picture that often affects every area of occupation, including ADL and IADL, education, work, play, leisure, and social participation. In order to effectively assist the person with brain injury to reengage in daily occupations and to reintegrate into home, community, and work environments, the occupational therapist is challenged to provide holistic, client-centered care that integrates evaluation and treatment of both the physical and psychosocial dimensions of the person to support participation in the context of his or her environment (Cullen, Chundamala, Bayley, & Jutai, 2007). It is also important to consider the performance skills (e.g., motor skills, process skills, and communication/interaction skills), performance patterns (e.g., habits, routines, and roles), activity demands, and client factors (e.g., affective, cognitive, and perceptual mental functions) that impact the person's ability to participate in her or his cultural, physical, social, personal, spiritual, temporal, and/or virtual context.

DIAGNOSIS AND ETIOLOGY

Among young people, motor vehicle as well as sports and recreation accidents are among the leading causes of TBI. Although exact figures are difficult to determine, some of these accidents are a result of engaging in high-risk behaviors or due to drug or alcohol abuse. Violence, including self-inflicted gunshot wounds, accounts for at least 10% of all TBI (Bruns & Hauser, 2003). Low income has also been associated with a higher incidence of TBI, although the relationship between brain injury and socioeconomic status is not clear. Although adolescents and young adults have the highest incidence of TBI, the second largest representative group is the elderly, primarily due to falls. Older adults typically show less complete recovery from brain injury than their younger counterparts (Rothweiler, Temkin, & Dikmen, 1998).

According to the World Health Organization (2001), diagnostic information should be elicited with regard to the functioning and disability of the individual. The model of functioning and disability describes a dynamic process of evaluating impairments with body functions and structures, activity limitations, and participation restrictions, as well as personal and environmental factors that affect functioning and social participation in the fabric of daily life. For the occupational therapist evaluating a person with a brain injury, a thorough understanding of these components will strengthen the quality of the intervention plan designed to rehabilitate a person to the highest level of functioning (Fraas, Balz, & DeGrauw, 2007).

A medical diagnosis of brain injury is confirmed by specialized imaging studies using magnetic resonance imaging (MRI) and computed tomography (CT) scans, once the bruising or lesion has formed on the brain (Yudofsky & Hales, 2002). The physician is often able to predict possible cognitive, behavioral, visual-perceptual, language, and physical impairments based on the location of the lesion in the brain. However, **diffuse axonal injury**, which results from the tearing and shearing of the axons of the nerve fibers throughout the brain due to the bouncing of the brain inside the skull, is not visible on imaging studies. Therefore, the physician is required to diagnose the brain injury based on observable clinical signs and symptoms, such as the level of consciousness, cortical posturing, cognition, and behavior.

Figure 16-1 shows the six main lobes of the brain and their anatomical functions. This can also assist the occupational therapist in predicting the functional problems that may present with the client based on diagnostic and clinical information on the location of lesions to the brain. Depending on the type and amount of external force impacting the brain, one functional area, various areas, or all areas of the brain can be affected. Because each brain injury is unique, the clinical picture can vary greatly from person to person.

The most prominent impairment noted following brain injury is **post-traumatic amnesia**, or short- or long-term memory deficits resulting from concussion or head trauma. The clinician should also be aware of substance abuse, chemical dependency, or the effects of intoxication at the time of the brain injury, as the presence of substance use at the time of injury is associated with more severe cognitive impairments related to the TBI.

There are many types of brain injury with different etiologies and clinical presentations (see Table 16-1). Brain injury is typically categorized by whether the injury is acquired or the direct result of a traumatic event.

PROGNOSIS FOR RECOVERY

Prognosis for recovery following brain injury is dependent on a number of factors, such as age, the size and location of injury to the brain, substance use at the time of injury, the type of injury, the level of consciousness at the time of injury, and the length of coma if loss of consciousness has occurred (Leahy & Lam, 1998). The brain is able to recover following TBI due to its **neuroplasticity**, which enables it to reorganize alternate neuronal pathways to compensate for damaged areas. Younger age, more

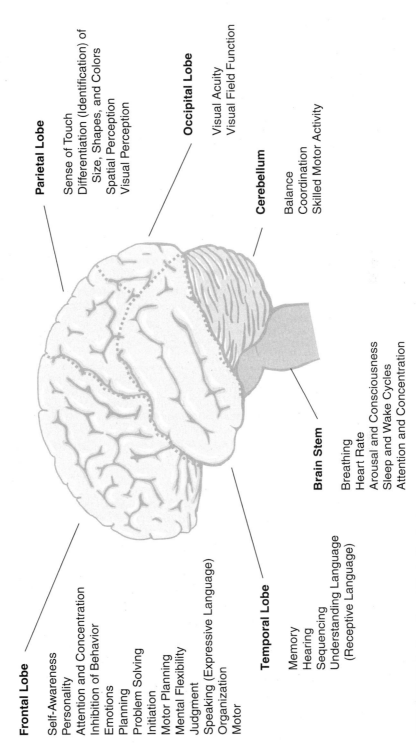

Frontal Lobe

Self-Awareness
Personality
Attention and Concentration
Inhibition of Behavior
Emotions
Planning
Problem Solving
Initiation
Motor Planning
Mental Flexibility
Judgment
Speaking (Expressive Language)
Organization
Motor

Temporal Lobe

Memory
Hearing
Sequencing
Understanding Language
(Receptive Language)

Parietal Lobe

Sense of Touch
Differentiation (Identification) of
  Size, Shapes, and Colors
Spatial Perception
Visual Perception

Occipital Lobe

Visual Acuity
Visual Field Function

Cerebellum

Balance
Coordination
Skilled Motor Activity

Brain Stem

Breathing
Heart Rate
Arousal and Consciousness
Sleep and Wake Cycles
Attention and Concentration

FIGURE 16-1. Functional Brain Anatomy
Source: Reprinted with permission of Mary Groves, OTR/L. Copyright 2003

TABLE 16-1. Types of Brain Injury

Type of Brain Injury	Definition	Etiology
Traumatic Brain Injury	Insult to the brain that may produce a diminished or altered state of consciousness, which results in an impairment of cognitive abilities or physical functioning. It can also result in the disturbance of behavioral or emotional functioning. These impairments may be either temporary or permanent and can cause partial or total functional disability or psychosocial maladjustment.	Caused by an external force; not of a degenerative or congenital natures.
Open Head Injury	Injury to the head that results in a skull fracture.	Caused by an external force that fractures the skull such as a penetrating gunshot wound.
Closed Head Injury	Impact to the head from an outside force, but the skull does not fracture or displace	Caused by an external force that does not fracture the skull
Diffuse Axonal Injury	Injury that occurs because the unmoving brain lags behind the movement of the skull, causing brain structures to tear. There is extensive tearing of nerve tissue throughout the brain. This can cause brain chemicals to be released, causing additional injury.	Caused by shaking or strong rotation of the head or by rotational forces
Concussion	The most common type of brain injury, produced by either closed or open head injuries. The brain receives trauma from an impact, a sudden momentum, or movement change. The blood vessels in the brain may stretch and cranial nerves may be damaged. A person may or may not experience a brief loss of consciousness. A concussion may or may not show up on a diagnostic imaging test.	Caused by a direct blow to the head, a gunshot wound, violent shaking of the head, or a force from a whiplash-type injury.
Contusion	Bruise or bleeding on the brain	Direct impact to the head.
Coup-Contrecoup Injury	Contusions that are both at the site of the impact and on the complete opposite side of the brain.	Occurs when the force impacting the head is not only great enough to cause a contusion at the site of impact, but also is able to move the brain and cause it to slam into the opposite side of the skull, causing an additional contusion.
Penetration Injury	Sharp object forces hair, skin, bone, and fragments from the object into the brain. A "through-and-through" injury occurs if an object enters the skull, goes through the brain, and exits the skull.	Impact of a bullet, knife, or other sharp object; mostly caused by firearms.
Shaken Baby Syndrome	Violent criminal act that causes traumatic brain injury through the whiplash-like motion.	Perpetrator aggressively shakes a baby or young child.

TABLE 16-1. Continued

Type of Brain Injury	Definition	Etiology
Acquired Brain Injury	Injury to the brain, which is not hereditary, congenital, degenerative, or induced by birth trauma, that commonly results in a change in neuronal activity, which affects the physical integrity, metabolic activity, or functional ability of the neural cell.	Anoxia, hypoxia, tumors, stroke, and/or neurotoxins, airway obstruction, near-drowning, throat swelling, choking, strangulation, crush injuries to the chest, electrical shock, vascular disruption, heart attack, stroke, arteriovenous malformation (AVM), aneurysm, intracranial surgery, infectious disease, intracranial tumors, metabolic disorders, meningitis, venereal disease, AIDS, insect-carried diseases, brain tumors, hypo- or hyperglycemia, hepatic encephalopathy, uremic encephalopathy, seizure disorders, toxic exposure, severe drug and alcohol abuse, lead poisoning, carbon monoxide poisoning, and chemotherapy.

Adapted from the Brain Injury Association of America, n.d.

focal points of injury, lack of substance use, and short episodes of loss of consciousness have been associated with a more rapid recovery.

The **Glasgow Coma Scale (GCS)** has been traditionally used to evaluate the client's level of consciousness at the scene of the accident and frequently thereafter. Table 16-2 shows the criteria for scoring the client's level of consciousness. A total score of 13 to 15 indicates a mild brain injury; a score of 9 to 12 indicates a moderate brain injury; and a total score of 8 or below indicates a severe brain injury (Zafonte et al., 1996).

The GCS has been used to quantify the severity of the brain injury and to predict long-term functional outcomes, although more recent studies have shown that the GCS is more effectively used to describe the severity of the brain injury (Bushnik, Hanks, Kreutzer, & Rosenthal, 2003; Corral et al., 2007). Therefore, severity of brain injury is not always an indicator of the long-term functional disability. For example, a person with a severe brain injury may make a significant recovery and eventually return to work (Nakase-Richardson, Yablon, & Sherer, 2007). Conversely, a person with a mild brain injury may have cognitive and psychosocial impairments that prevent him or her from resuming previous roles.

PREMORBID PSYCHOSOCIAL FACTORS

Beyond sex, age, and socioeconomic factors, premorbid psychiatric disturbances (e.g., psychotic disorders, anxiety, depression, and personality disorders) and a history of alcohol and drug abuse have all been associated with increased risk

TABLE 16-2. Glasgow Coma Scale

Examiner's Test	Patient Response	Score
EYE OPENING		
Spontaneous	Opens eyes on own	4
To speech	Opens eyes when asked to in a loud voice	3
To pain	Opens eyes when pinched	2
	Does not open eyes when pinched	3
BEST MOTOR RESPONSE		
To commands	Follows simple commands	6
To pain	Pulls examiner's hand away when pinched	5
	Pulls a part of body away when pinched	4
	Flexes body part inappropriately to pain	3
	Body becomes rigid in an extended position when examiner pinches patient (decerebrate posturing)	2
	No motor response to pinch	1
VERBAL RESPONSE		
To speech	Converses appropriately with examiner; oriented to person, place, or time	5
	Appears confused or disoriented	4
	Speaks clearly but does not make sense	3
	Makes incomprehensible sounds	2
	Makes no sound	1

Reprinted from *Introduction to Clinical Neurology, 2nd Edition* (p. 273), by D. J. Gelb, 2000, with permission from Elsevier.

of brain injury as well as increased levels of neurobehavioral disturbances post-TBI (Fann et al., 2002; Hibbard, Uysal, Kepler, Bogdany, & Silver, 1998; McGuire Burright, Williams, & Donovick, 1998; Mooney & Speed, 2001; Ruff, Camenzuli, & Mueller, 1996; Tate, Freed, Bombardier, Harter, & Brinkman, 1999). An understanding of premorbid personality features, coping mechanisms, and injury-related psychosocial stressors can assist the occupational therapist in developing an effective treatment plan.

Substance use and abuse is also a contributing factor to the occurrence and reoccurrence of TBI. Alcohol and drugs are estimated to be the primary cause of at least 50% to 75% of all TBIs in the United States. Alcohol- and drug-related TBIs are also associated with more complicated recoveries, longer hospitalizations, longer periods of agitation, and more impaired cognitive function at discharge from rehabilitation. Because so many persons with TBIs have premorbid chemical dependency issues and are not always effectively treated for these problems during rehabilitation, approximately one-third of those with substance abuse problems will return home to substance use or abuse again, which further compromises their cognitive and functional capacities. (This places the person with TBI at a much higher risk of seizures and subsequent head traumas.) It is important to educate clients with a TBI and their families on the importance of treatment for substance abuse disorders following acute rehabilitation to prevent future injuries from occurring and to promote optimal functional recovery.

CASE ILLUSTRATION

David—Premorbid Psychosocial Contributions to TBI

David is a 26-year-old man who sustained a second TBI from a motor vehicle accident. Three years ago, he had a brain injury from an assault. He has had a long history of drug and alcohol abuse. David's drugs of choice are amphetamines and alcohol. Over the past 10 years, he has been through three drug and alcohol recovery programs, but has been unable to remain sober.

Discussion

David's long history of chemical dependency has placed him at high risk for TBI. He is likely to present with more severe cognitive deficits, increased agitation levels, and a poorer functional outcome. He is also at risk for abusing substances following discharge from inpatient acute rehabilitation. In addition to treating David for his brain injury, the interdisciplinary team must place a high priority on treating the underlying substance abuse disorder and preventing a third injury. The occupational therapist plays a unique role in helping David reorganize his use of time to participate in healthy, meaningful, and purposeful activity that incorporates his unique interests, values, and roles.

OCCUPATIONAL THERAPY EVALUATION AND INTERVENTION

The occupational therapy evaluation process begins with an occupational profile that determines the TBI client's occupational history, an assessment of areas of occupation that are enabling or inhibiting the client's successful engagement in meaningful occupation, and developing a treatment plan that maximizes occupational performance in multiple contexts based on the client and family's priorities and desired outcomes (American Occupational Therapy Association, 2008). The **Rancho Los Amigos Levels of Cognitive Functioning** (Table 16-3) is a gold standard rating scale used to assist the occupational therapy practitioner in determining the client's cognitive, behavioral, and functional status following brain injury (Hagen, Malkmus, & Stenderup-Bowman, 1973). The scale has established interrater reliability and validity (Dowling, 1985; Gouvier, Blanton, LaPorte, & Nepomuceno, 1987). The eight cognitive levels include a description of the common cognitive, behavioral, and psychosocial sequelae associated with recovery from brain injury. However, because it is an ordinal scale, or a scale that ranks levels from low to high, differences between levels on the scale are not equivalent. In other words, the differences between Levels I and II on the scale are not the same as the differences between Levels II and III. Moreover, some survivors of brain injury do not always proceed through each of the levels. Some clients skip many of the levels during the recovery process, and some individuals may progress only to a certain level and no farther (Corrigan & Mysiw, 1988). The Rancho Los Amigos Levels of Cognitive Functioning provide a useful tool for evaluating the cognitive and behavioral status of the client and also aids in the treatment planning process. The Rancho Levels can also serve as an effective family education tool by helping the caregiver to understand the progression of the recovery process and effective strategies for appropriately assisting the client during recovery. Table 16-3 describes a variety of cognitive, behavioral, and psychosocial treatment strategies at each of the stages of recovery that can be implemented by the occupational therapist and through caregiver education and training.

Each person will progress differently, depending on the severity of brain damage, the length of time since the initial onset of injury, and the location of damage. Some individuals may progress through each of the eight cognitive levels, while others may progress to a certain cognitive level and no farther. It is also important to remember that each person is an individual, and each person may fit some or all of the criteria under each level.

The occupational therapy practitioner plays a critical role in assisting the person with brain injury to resume previous life roles, assume new life roles post-TBI, effectively engage in occupations that are important to him or her, and assist the person with brain injury in adapting to home, community, school, and/or work environments (Parish & Oddy, 2007; Pierce & Hanks, 2006). In the early stages of recovery, the occupational therapy practitioner may work on remediative or compensatory strategies for cognitive deficits, social skills retraining, and functional skills retraining. The task or environment may also be adapted to increase optimal functioning.

TABLE 16-3. Rancho Los Amigos Levels of Cognitive Functioning

Cognitive Level	Behavioral Characteristics	Interdisciplinary Treatment Approaches for Managing Cognitive, Behavioral, and Psychosocial Sequelae
Level I: No Response	■ Complete absence of observable change in behavior when presented with visual, auditory, tactile, proprioceptive, vestibular, or painful stimuli.	■ Explain to the individual what you are about to do. For example, "I'm going to move your leg." ■ Talk in a normal tone of voice. ■ Keep comments and questions short and simple. For example, instead of "Can you turn your head towards me?", say, "Look at me." ■ Tell the person who you are, where he is, why he is in the hospital, and what day it is. ■ Limit the number of visitors to two to three people at a time. ■ Keep the room calm and quiet. ■ Bring in favorite belongings and pictures of family members and close friends. ■ Allow the person extra time to respond, but don't expect responses to be correct. Sometimes the person may not respond at all. ■ Give the patient rest periods. They will tire more easily. ■ Engage the patient in familiar activities, such as listening to his or her favorite music, talking about family and friends, reading out loud, watching TV, combing their hair, and putting on lotion, etc. ■ The patient may understand parts of what you are saying. Therefore, be careful what you say in front of the individual.
Level II: Generalized Response	■ Demonstrates generalized reflex response to painful stimuli. ■ Responds to repeated auditory stimuli with increased or decreased activity. ■ Responds to external stimuli with physiological changes generalized, gross body movement, and/or not purposeful vocalization. ■ Responses noted above may be same regardless of type and location of stimulation. ■ Responses may be significantly delayed.	■ Same approach as for Level I.

(Continues)

TABLE 16-3. Continued

Cognitive Level	Behavioral Characteristics	Interdisciplinary Treatment Approaches for Managing Cognitive, Behavioral, and Psychosocial Sequelae
Level III: Localized Response	■ Demonstrates withdrawal or vocalization to painful stimuli. ■ Turns toward or away from auditory stimuli. ■ Blinks when strong light crosses visual field. ■ Follows moving object passed within visual field. ■ Responds to discomfort by pulling tubes or restraints. ■ Responds inconsistently to simple commands. ■ Responses directly related to type of stimulus. ■ May respond to some persons (especially family and friends), but not to others.	■ Same approach as for Levels I and II.
Level IV: Confused-Agitated	■ Alert and in a heightened state of activity. ■ May exhibit purposeful attempts to remove restraints or tubes or crawl out of bed. ■ May perform motor activities such as sitting, reaching, and walking, but without any apparent purpose. Very brief and usually nonpurposeful moments of sustained alternatives and divided attention. ■ Absent short-term memory. ■ Absent goal-directed, problem-solving, and self-monitoring behavior. ■ May cry or scream out of proportion to stimulus even after its removal. ■ May exhibit aggressive or flight behavior. ■ Mood may swing from euphoric to hostile with no apparent relationship to environmental events. ■ Unable to cooperate with treatment efforts. ■ Verbalizations are frequently incoherent and/or inappropriate to the activity or environment.	■ Tell the person where he or she is and reassure the patient that he or she is safe. ■ Bring in family pictures and personal items from home to make them feel more comfortable. ■ Allow them as much safe movement as possible. ■ Take the patient for rides in his or her wheelchair, when this has been approved by the treatment team. ■ Experiment to find familiar activities that are calming to the patient such as listening to music or eating. ■ Do not force the patient to perform activities. Instead, listen to what he or she would like to do and follow his or her lead, within safety limits. ■ Since the patient often becomes distracted, restless, or agitated, you may need to give him or her breaks and frequent changes in activities. ■ Keep the room quiet and calm. For example, turn off the television or radio, limit the amount of talking, and use a calm voice. ■ Limit the number of visitors to two to three people at a time.

TABLE 16-3. Continued

Cognitive Level	Behavioral Characteristics	Interdisciplinary Treatment Approaches for Managing Cognitive, Behavioral, and Psychosocial Sequelae
Level V: Confused-Inappropriate-Non-Agitated	▪ Alert, not agitated, but may wander randomly or with a vague intention of going home. ▪ May become agitated in response to external stimulation and/or lack of environmental structure. ▪ Not oriented to person, place, or time. ▪ Frequent brief periods of nonpurposeful sustained attention. ▪ Severely impaired recent memory, with confusion of the past and present in reaction to ongoing activity. ▪ Absent goal-directed, problem-solving, and self-monitoring behavior. ▪ Often demonstrates inappropriate use of objects without external direction. ▪ May be able to perform previously learned tasks when structure and cues are provided. ▪ Unable to learn new information. ▪ Able to respond appropriately to simple commands fairly consistently with external structures and cues. ▪ Responses to simple commands without external structure are random and nonpurposeful in relation to the command. ▪ Able to converse on a social, automatic level for brief periods of time when provided external structure and cues. ▪ Verbalizations about present events become inappropriate and confabulatory when external structure and cues are not provided.	▪ Repeat instructions as needed. Don't assume that he or she will remember what you tell him or her. ▪ Tell him or her the day, date, name and location and why he or she is in the hospital when you first arrive and before you leave. ▪ Keep comments and questions short and simple. ▪ Help him or her organize and get started on an activity. ▪ Have the family bring in pictures and personal items from home. ▪ Limit the number of visitors to two to three at a time. ▪ Give him or her frequent rest periods when he or she has problems attending.
Level VI: Confused-Appropriate	▪ Inconsistently oriented to person and place. ▪ Able to attend to highly familiar tasks in a nondistracting environment for 30 minutes with moderate redirection. ▪ Remote memory has more depth and detail than more recent memory. ▪ Vague recognition of some staff. ▪ Able to use assistive memory aids with maximal assistance. ▪ Emerging awareness of appropriate response to self, family, and basic needs.	▪ Using repetition, discuss events that have happened during the day to help the individual remember recent events and activities. ▪ He or she may need help initiating and continuing activities. ▪ Encourage the individual to participate in all therapies. He or she will not fully understand the extent of his or her problems and the benefits of therapy.

(Continues)

TABLE 16-3. Continued

Cognitive Level	Behavioral Characteristics	Interdisciplinary Treatment Approaches for Managing Cognitive, Behavioral, and Psychosocial Sequelae
	■ Emerging goal-directed behavior related to meeting basic personal needs. ■ Moderate assistance required to problem-solve barriers to task completion. ■ Supervised for old learning (e.g., self-care). ■ Shows carryover for relearned familiar tasks (e.g., self-care). ■ Maximal assistance required for new learning with little or no carryover. ■ Unaware of impairments, disabilities, and safety risks. ■ Consistently follows simple directions. ■ Verbal expressions are appropriate in highly familiar and structured situations.	
Level VII: Automatic-Appropriate	■ Consistently oriented to person and place within highly familiar environments. Moderate assistance for orientation to time required. ■ Able to attend to highly familiar tasks in a nondistracting environment for at least 30 minutes with minimal assistance to complete tasks. ■ Able to use assistive memory devices with minimal assistance. ■ Minimal supervision for new learning. ■ Demonstrates carryover of new information. ■ Initiates and carries out steps to complete familiar personal and household routines, but has shallow recall of what he or she has been doing. ■ Able to monitor accuracy and completeness of each step in routine personal and household ADL and modify plan with minimal assistance. ■ Superficial awareness of his or her condition, but unaware of specific impairments and disabilities and the limits they place on his or her ability to safely, accurately, and completely carry out his or her household, community, work, and leisure tasks. ■ Unrealistic planning for the future. ■ Unable to think about consequences of a decision or action.	■ Speak with the individual as an adult. There is no need to try to use simple words or sentences. Demonstrate respect for his or her opinion and needs when attempting to provide guidance and assistance in decision making. ■ Because the individual may misunderstand joking, teasing, or slang language, be careful to check for understanding when using humor or abstract language. ■ Encourage the individual to be as independent as possible within safety limits. Help him or her with activities when he shows problems with thinking, problem solving, and memory. Talk to him or her about these problems without criticizing. Reassure him that the problems are because of the brain injury. ■ Strongly encourage the individual to continue with therapy to increase his or her thinking, memory and physical abilities. He or she may feel completely normal. However, he or she is still making progress and may possibly benefit from continued treatment.

TABLE 16-3. Continued

Cognitive Level	Behavioral Characteristics	Interdisciplinary Treatment Approaches for Managing Cognitive, Behavioral, and Psychosocial Sequelae
	■ Overestimates abilities. ■ Unaware of others' needs and feelings. ■ Oppositional/uncooperative. ■ Unable to recognize inappropriate social interaction behavior.	■ Be sure to check with the physician on the individual's restrictions concerning driving, working, and other activities. Do not rely on the person with a brain injury for information, since he or she may feel ready to go back to their previous lifestyle. ■ Discourage him or her from drinking or using drugs. ■ Encourage him or her to use note taking as a way to help with memory problems. ■ Encourage him to carry out his self-care as independently as possible. ■ Discuss what kinds of situations make him angry and what he or she can do in these situations. ■ Talk with him about his or her feelings. ■ Learning to live with a brain injury is difficult and it may take a long time for the individual and family to adjust. The social worker and/or psychologist will provide family members and friends with information regarding counseling, resources, and support organizations.
Level VIII: Purposeful and Appropriate	■ Consistently oriented to person, place, and time. ■ Independently attends to and completes familiar tasks for one hour in a distracting environment. ■ Able to recall and integrate past and recent events. ■ Uses assistive memory devices to recall daily schedule, "to do" lists, and to record critical information for later use with stand-by assistance. ■ Initiates and carries out steps to complete familiar personal, household, community, work, and leisure routines with standby assistance, and can modify the plan when needed with minimal assistance. ■ Requires no assistance once new tasks/activities are learned.	■ Same as Level VII.

(Continues)

TABLE 16-3. Continued

Cognitive Level	Behavioral Characteristics	Interdisciplinary Treatment Approaches for Managing Cognitive, Behavioral, and Psychosocial Sequelae
	■ Aware of and acknowledges impairments and disabilities when they interfere with task completion, but requires standby assistance to take appropriate corrective action. ■ Thinks about consequences of a decision or action with minimal assistance.	
	■ Overestimates or underestimates abilities. ■ Acknowledges others' needs and feelings and responds appropriately with minimal assistance. ■ Depressed. ■ Irritable. ■ Low frustration tolerance/easily angered. ■ Argumentative. ■ Self-centered. ■ Uncharacteristically dependent/independent. ■ Able to recognize and acknowledge inappropriate social interaction behavior while it is occurring and takes corrective action with minimal assistance.	

Adapted with permission from Los Amigos Research and Educational Institute, Copyright 1975.

In the later stages of recovery, the occupational therapy practitioner uses a more client-centered approach to assist the person with brain injury to identify goals that are important to him or her and help him or her toward regaining occupational functioning in all areas of occupation, such as ADL and IADL, education, work, play, leisure, and social participation (O'Brien, 2007). Several studies have shown that persons with TBI significantly improve in their functional abilities following a client-centered and occupation-based approach to intervention (Phipps & Richardson, 2007; Teasell et al., 2007; Trombly, Radomski, & Davis, 1998; Wheeler, Lane, & McMahon, 2007; Zhu, Poon, Chan, & Chan, 2007). Client-centered assessments, such as the Canadian Occupational Performance Measure (COPM), assist the occupational therapist in tailoring treatment goals to those activities that the client needs to do or wants to do in his or her environment (Jenkinson, Ownsworth, & Shum, 2007; Law et al., 2005). The unique contribution of the occupational therapy practitioner is to assist the client in managing and adapting to the cognitive, behavioral, and psychosocial impairments by engaging in productive, meaningful, and satisfying occupations that support role performance and social participation in the context of the person's unique environment

(Phipps, 2006). The following sections outline specific client factors, including the cognitive, behavioral, and psychosocial sequelae of TBI, which should be considered during the occupational therapy evaluation and intervention process in order to maximize the TBI client's engagement in occupation.

COGNITIVE SEQUELAE FOLLOWING BRAIN INJURY

Because cognitive functions are integrated throughout all of the brain centers, all clients with brain injury will have cognitive impairment to varying degrees. The main cognitive impairments are lack of orientation, attention deficits, impaired memory, impaired initiation and termination of activities, impaired insight, impaired judgment, impaired safety awareness, decreased information-processing abilities, and impaired executive functioning and abstract thinking ability. Cognitive skills are hierarchical and successively build from lower order to higher order cognitive functions. Each area of cognition affected by brain injury is presented from lower order to higher order.

Impaired Orientation

Persons with brain injury are often in a state of confusion following their acute injuries. Affected individuals often lose a sense of the passage of time, their external environment, their situation, and even who their family and friends are. As their confusion clears and the recovery process unveils, their orientation improves (Ownsworth, Fleming, Desbois, Strong, & Kuipers, 2006).

Persons without brain injury are often oriented to who they are (person); where they are (place); what year, month, day, or time of day it is (time); and why they are in the environment they are in (reason). However, a person with brain injury can lose orientation to person, place, time, or reason. Impaired memory and topographical orientation to the environment contributes to this confusion (Sohlberg, Fickas, Hung, & Fortier, 2007). Individuals with brain injury can have difficulty remembering their identity and the identity of those around them, lose a sense of the passage of time, and have a decreased awareness of self in relation to the environment.

Attention Deficits

Attention is a complex, dynamic ability that is regulated by the arousal systems of the brain and other cerebral functions. Attention is important for maintaining concentration and focus on a relevant functional task in the environment at a particular time. It requires alertness, mental flexibility, sustained effort, and the selective ability to screen necessary and unnecessary stimulation from the environment. Attention is also imperative for higher-order information processing, such as memory and problem solving. Without attention, information cannot be coded into memory so that the individual can use this information for problem solving in future tasks. Individuals with brain injury may have minimal deficits with attention or severe attention deficits that prevent them from effectively adapting to their environment.

There are four main types of attention that are impacted following brain injury. The simplest form of attention is focused attention, which requires the ability to focus concentration on a task for a sustained period of time without external distractions. Selective attention requires the ability to sustain focus on a task while screening out distractions from the environment, such as noise and conversation. Alternating attention requires a sustained focus on a task while also attending to relevant stimulation from the environment, such as talking on the phone while boiling pasta on the stove. Divided attention is the most unconscious form of concentration that allows an individual to alternate attention between many different tasks, such as multitasking. Individuals with brain injury may be able to perform occupations using some or all types of attention, but may be impaired with their ability to sustain this attention for the required amount of time for task completion.

Impaired Memory

Impaired short-term memory is the most frequent complaint from individuals with brain injury and can often be the source of long-term disability throughout the life-span (Thickpenny-Davis & Barker-Collo, 2007). Memory requires the dynamic ability to code, store, and retrieve relevant past or present information. Memory requires sustained attention to information for temporary storage into short-term memory and encoding into long-term memory (Campbell, Wilson, McCann, Kernahan, & Rogers, 2007). Most clients with brain injury recover long-term memory, but have enduring deficits with short-term memory, which affects their ability to learn and problem-solve through new tasks and occupations.

There are many types of memory that affect an individual's ability to engage in occupation. Declarative memory is required to recall or recite information, such as personal history and experiences, people, language, and rules of social behavior (Boman, Tham, Granqvist, Bartfai, & Hemmingsson, 2007). Prospective memory requires the ability to remember future events, such as important deadlines and appointments. Because individuals with brain injury may have significant gaps in memory and are confused regarding details pertaining to time, people, and places, they may use **confabulation** to fill in the missing gaps with erroneous information. Confabulation is not an intentional process and is the result of confusion that leads the person with brain injury to unconsciously make sense out of the broken pieces of information and control his or her thought processes.

Because individuals with brain injury tend to have significant short-term memory deficits related to declarative and prospective information processing impairments, it is critical for the occupational therapy practitioner to assist the client in engaging in familiar occupations that tap into procedural memory, which is the subcortical memory of skill and task performance (Ownsworth et al., 2006). Procedural memory is responsible for assisting clients with significant memory deficits to engage in familiar tasks without cognitively recalling the steps involved. Most occupations that are performed prior to the brain injury can be accessed using procedural memory, particularly those tasks performed since early childhood.

Impaired Initiation and Termination of Activities

Survivors of brain injury tend to have difficulty initiating and terminating functional activities throughout their day. **Initiation** refers to the ability to begin an activity at an appropriate time in the day to accomplish a specific goal. This ability is impaired primarily from damage to the frontal lobe of the brain. The client may require verbal cues from caregivers to initiate an activity. Conversely, the client may have difficulty terminating an activity after starting by perseverating on a functional task that is no longer productive. **Perseveration** refers to the inability to disengage from an activity and reengage in a more appropriate activity. Perseveration may also be a constant thought pattern that permeates the individual's mind and keeps the person from engaging in more appropriate activity.

Impaired Insight, Judgment, and Safety Awareness

Individuals with frontal lobe damage from brain injury often present with impaired insight into their limitations and disabilities. Impaired insight does not result from denial as a coping mechanism. Individuals with frontal lobe damage have a cognitive impairment, also referred to as **anosognosia**, which inhibits them from recognizing or acknowledging their own deficits in cognition, perception, or mobility. Without appropriate levels of insight, the person with brain injury tends to exhibit poor judgment in decision making and self-awareness, which can lead to poor safety awareness (Goverover, Johnson, Toglia, & DeLuca, 2007). For example, an individual with poor mobility, visual neglect, and poor insight may underestimate the time required to cross a busy street or will cross without using the crosswalk.

Impaired Information Processing

Following brain injury, individuals tend to require an increased amount of time to process information during social conversations, ADL, and information from the external environment. This delayed speed in processing information is the result of a variety of factors, including decreased alertness, impaired perceptual skills, decreased attention, decreased memory, and the increased time needed for the brain to encode information before cognitively processing (Gentry, Wallace, Kvarfordt, & Lynch, 2008). It may appear as if the client is not responding or processing information at all, but with increased time, the client will often be able to answer the question or complete a functional task.

Impaired Executive Functions

Executive functions are higher-order cognitive processes that are controlled primarily by the frontal lobe (Burgess et al., 2006). Executive functions enable a person to identify a problem, plan a strategy for problem solving, develop goals for the future, and modify a plan of action based on information from the environment (Burgess et al., 1998). Individuals with brain injury tend to have difficulty, particularly in the early stages of learning, in identifying problems, planning, goal-setting, and using mental flexibility to modify a plan of action based on information received from the external environment. Impaired executive functions can often be the most disabling part of brain injury, since executive functions are essential for problem solving, planning for the future, being effective in a work environment, and managing oneself safely in the home and community. Occupational therapy evaluation and intervention centers on the utilization of individual and group therapy to challenge the client in developing planning, organization, and flexibility in a variety of unstructured tasks. For example, clients can engage in planning a group meal, where executive functions are exercised to increase problem solving and decision making around budgets, money management, shopping skills, delegation, and execution of a prepared meal.

Impaired Abstract Thinking and Integration of New Learning

Clients with brain injury tend to also have difficulty using **abstract thinking** to critically reason and use analytical methods to infer relationships between ideas and filter irrelevant details from relevant information (Burgess et al., 1998). Clients with brain injury may not be able to understand analogies, jokes, or inferences.

Because individuals with brain injury tend to think on the most concrete level, this prevents **generalization** of cognitive and functional skills to a variety of different environments, further limiting the amount of new learning that can occur. This is why it is often difficult for a client with brain injury to transfer a particular skill learned in the acute hospital environment to the home environment (Van Baalen, Odding, & Stam, 2008). It is critical for occupational therapy practitioners working with clients with brain injury to assess the environment that the client is returning to and to intervene in the client's natural environment as much as possible.

BEHAVIORAL SEQUELAE FOLLOWING BRAIN INJURY

The behavioral sequelae following brain injury are sometimes the most challenging aspects of client management. Many of the behavioral syndromes are temporary and part of the recovery process, while others can persist in some degree throughout the lifespan (Oueller & Morin, 2007). The main behavioral sequelae following brain injury are agitation, aggression, disinhibition, hypersexual behaviors, demotivational syndrome, and inappropriate emotional responses.

CASE ILLUSTRATION

Tony—Cognitive Sequelae Following TBI

Tony is a 33-year-old man who sustained a TBI from a penetrating gunshot wound to the right frontal lobe. Tony is only oriented to his own name. He is unable to recall the date, place of hospitalization, or the reason he is in the hospital. Tony also presents with a short attention span, and is only able to engage in a simple functional activity for 30 seconds before losing attention to the task. Tony has good recall of his life before the brain injury, but is unable to recall new information after a five-minute delay. Tony has difficulty initiating activity and after beginning an activity, he has difficulty transitioning to a new activity. Tony demonstrates poor safety awareness, and states that he is ready to leave the hospital. The occupational therapist has provided Tony with a memory log to help him remember important dates, people, and appointments. The occupational therapist has also structured the environment to reduce noise and distractions to assist Tony in processing information effectively and engaging in activities with a longer period of sustained attention.

Discussion

Tony demonstrates classic cognitive impairments with orientation, attention, short-term memory, initiation and termination of activity, judgment, safety awareness, and information processing. Tony will also have deficits with higher-order executive functions and abstract reasoning due to the fact that he is unable to attend to tasks for long periods of time and store information into long-term memory for effective executive functioning. His organization, time management, and planning ability will most likely be compromised due to the lower-order cognitive impairments, such as impaired orientation, attention, and memory. In addition to providing a memory log to Tony and restructuring the treatment environment, the occupational therapist can begin treatment by focusing on concrete, one-step tasks that tap into procedural memory, which is responsible for assisting clients with significant memory deficits to engage in familiar tasks without recalling the steps involved. Most occupations that are performed prior to the brain injury can be accessed using procedural memory, particularly those tasks performed since early childhood. Basic ADL, simple leisure tasks, and basic home management are examples of activities that can be used to tap into procedural memory. Each task can be upgraded or downgraded to the individual's specific cognitive level.

Agitation and Aggression

Agitation and aggression are the most common behavioral sequelae following brain injury. Agitation is typical of those clients in the Rancho Los Amigos Cognitive Level IV stage of recovery—Confused and Agitated (Hagen et al., 1973). Because of their level of confusion and inability to process sensory information from the environment correctly, clients in this stage may display decreased frustration tolerance and be socially inappropriate, restless, impulsive, verbally combative, and physically assaultive (Lombard & Zafonte, 2005). Clients in this stage can also escalate very quickly into an aggressive and combative state, and it is important to work with a team of other professionals to manage these behaviors early in the recovery process. This stage of recovery is also the most frightening for families, who often have never seen their loved one verbally or physically assault another human being. It is important to educate family members and staff that this is a normal part of the recovery process and is rarely permanent. Occupational therapy practitioners should focus on engaging the client in structured occupational performance activities and gross motor activities that expend excess energy with frequent breaks to maintain the client's attention and decrease the level of agitation from overstimulation, confusion, and fatigue (Cantor et al., 2008; Giles & Hohr, 2007; Lequerica et al., 2007).

Disinhibition

Clients with frontal lobe damage tend to also exhibit impulsive, perseveratory behavior that often disinhibits them from making inappropriate verbal remarks and causes them to participate in unsafe activities. For example, **disinhibition** is observed with a client who states that a therapist is "fat" or "ugly." The normal filters that we use to screen our behaviors in response to social norms become void. In addition, the client with brain injury may also perseverate on tasks that are nonpurposeful, inappropriate, or unsafe. It is often difficult to confront the individual, which can sometimes provoke agitation or inappropriate verbal remarks.

Hypersexual Behaviors

Individuals with brain injury can also have difficulty controlling sexual urges that can lead to inappropriate sexual advances with treatment staff, friends, and even family members. Because the therapeutic relationship between an occupational therapy practitioner and his or her client is one of respect, tolerance, and trust, some clients will misinterpret this relationship as a sexual advance on behalf of the staff member. Other times, the client purely has a sexual urge and is not able to inhibit his or her desires. Negative behaviors, such as masturbation in a public area, touching, fondling, sexual remarks, and sometimes intercourse with other clients, take place in treatment settings where there is little structure and supervision.

Demotivational Syndrome

Apathy and disinterest in previous occupations can sometimes result from frontal lobe damage following head trauma. For some clients, this **demotivational syndrome** is the result of a lack of initiation and sustained participation in activity, and for others it can be an outright refusal to participate in previously enjoyed activities. Depression can also be a contributing factor to the lack of motivation to participate in everyday activities. It is important to consult with the treatment team to differentiate between major depression and demotivational syndrome from brain injury.

Inappropriate Emotional Responses

Emotional lability, decreased affect (flat), or increased affect (euphoria) can result following brain injury. A client may laugh, cry, or scream out of proportion to the environmental stimulus. Those clients with left hemisphere damage tend to have increased levels of depression and emotional lability, from euphoric to flat (Ownsworth, 1998). It is important to note that a person may appear to be depressed, when in actuality, the

CASE ILLUSTRATION

Brad—Behavioral Sequelae Following TBI

Brad is a 19-year-old man who sustained a TBI (multiple injuries to his frontal, parietal, and temporal lobes) from an assault. He demonstrates a high level of agitation and is extremely restless. He frequently yells out profanities and is physically aggressive with staff. Brad is emotionally labile and very quickly escalates from laughing to crying and shouting out loud. Brad has also made several inappropriate sexual advances to female staff.

Discussion

Brad currently demonstrates many of the behavioral characteristics of a person recovering from brain injury at a Rancho Los Amigos Cognitive Level IV: Confused and Agitated. His behavior

is not volitional or intentional. Brad is having difficulty processing the complex information from his environment. In order to maximize Brad's recovery in this stage, the occupational therapist can engage the client in gross motor activity (such as tossing a ball or taking a walk), vestibular stimulation activities such as riding around in a wheelchair, or simple one-step activities; minimize distractions; and establish trust by providing a safe and comfortable treatment environment.

The occupational therapist may interview family members to find out which activities have provided the greatest level of comfort for the client (e.g., eating, listening to music, etc.). Do not force the client to do something he does not want to do. Instead, listen to what he wants to do and follow his lead, within safety limits. Since the client is often distractible, restless, and agitated at this phase of recovery, remember to provide frequent breaks from activity and be prepared to change activities quickly. The occupational therapist can also modify the environment to increase the client's level of comfort by having family members bring in pictures and personal items from home.

person presents with a flat, expressionless affect. Conversely, clients with right hemisphere lesions tend to have a heightened state of euphoria that is often coupled with more severe impairments in insight, emotional maturity, and perceptual awareness.

PSYCHOSOCIAL SEQUELAE FOLLOWING BRAIN INJURY

Brain injury involves a sudden onset with little preparation for the impact of various changes, unlike persistent mental illness that can develop over the course of a lifetime. One day, a person may be managing her or his own business or taking a family trip around the world, and the next day, the person may be weak on one-half of the body, unable to communicate, remember, feel, or function.

While cognition and behavior can significantly and rapidly improve during the acute stages, brain injury can have a lifelong impact on the psychosocial adjustment of the individual (Ownsworth, Fleming, Shum, Kuipers, & Strong, 2008). Thus, the psychosocial sequelae are sometimes the most devastating aspects of brain injury for the affected individual and his or her family. Changes in overall mental health, personality, coping mechanisms, self-concept, social relationships, and the family dynamic can significantly alter the person's ability to adapt and master his or her environment.

Psychiatric Disorders

Due to the chemical changes in the brain following trauma and acquired events, the individual is often susceptible to mood disorders, anxiety disorders, and perceptual dysfunction that can contribute to hallucinations and paranoia (Bornhofen & McDonald, 2008). Premorbid mental illness, particularly personality disorders and alcohol and drug abuse, can significantly impact the recovery process and the severity of the psychosocial sequelae. For example, a person who suffered from depression and also had sociopathic behaviors prior to injury may have increased levels of depressed mood, agitation, and inappropriate social behaviors. Mood disorders, chemical dependency, delirium, psychotic disorders, aggressive disorders, and anxiety disorders are among the most common psychiatric disorders following brain injury (Yudofsky & Hales, 2002). In addition, approximately one-quarter of persons with brain injury also suffer from depression and other psychiatric illnesses post-TBI, which is affected by poor premorbid social functioning and previous psychiatric disorders pre-TBI (Fedoroff et al., 1992).

Changes in Personality and Impaired Social Pragmatics

Families often report that their loved ones exhibit changes in their personality following brain injury. A variety of factors can contribute to an alteration in personality based on the severity of the damage to the areas of the brain that control premorbid personality traits, cognition, and behavior (Golden & Golden, 2003). An introverted person may suddenly become outgoing, and an outgoing person may become withdrawn and expressionless. Conversely, a person who "lived on the edge" may exhibit even more risky behaviors postinjury. Clients with TBI also tend to exhibit egocentric behaviors that interfere with their ability to participate in social activities that require turn-taking, sharing, reciprocal conversation, and other socially appropriate behaviors (Dahlberg et al., 2007). These personality changes can have a devastating effect on the ability of the person with brain injury to maintain successful relationships with partners, friends, and family members, especially when the other person does not understand the course of recovery from brain injury. As time goes on postinjury, the person with brain injury often will find close friends and family members becoming less involved in her or his life. Changes in social roles can lead to a feeling of isolation, abandonment, and depression. Building effective new relationships can also be challenged by impairments in the person's social pragmatic ability.

Impaired Coping Mechanisms

Due to impaired executive functions that inhibit problem-solving abilities and premorbid coping skills, clients with brain injury may have difficulty managing frustration, anger, and loss of function. Particularly in the later stages of recovery, the client with brain injury is required to deal with a tremendous amount of loss to his or her personality, social relationships, ability to engage in previously enjoyed occupations, and the ability to feel secure about the future. Compounding these issues are stressors including financial instability and possible legal issues postinjury. Ineffective coping strategies preinjury may also contribute to even greater impairments with coping postinjury. The client is now required to manage greater amounts of stressors in his or her life, and may or may not have the ability to learn new strategies to cope with these stressors.

Altered Self-Concept

Self-concept is the internal image one has of self regarding body image; position in the family, peer group, and community; sexual and gender identity; and personal strengths and limitations. Brain injury can result in major disfigurement due to trauma, surgical craniotomies, and scars, which impacts a person's internalized self-image. Coupled with this change are reactions from society when the person enters the community for the first time postinjury. Individuals with brain injury are usually in adolescence or early adulthood when self-concept is still forming, which impacts their ability to deal effectively with the societal expectations of beauty and attractiveness.

As individuals with brain injury recover, their long-term memory often return before their short-term memory. They often have good memory of who they were before the injury, and there is an internal conflict with having to let go of many of their goals, ambitions, and positions in society. The individual is challenged to rebuild a postinjury self-concept that is meaningful and satisfying, which can lead to an identity crisis and deep depression if they perceive to be unsuccessful in re-creating the life that has been lost (Ownsworth, 1998).

Impact of Brain Injury on Family Dynamics

Individuals with brain injury must cope with the loss of position within the family unit postinjury (Rodgers et al., 2007). The family members may also be resentful that their loved one may no longer be able to function as an effective partner, parent, or

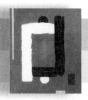

CASE ILLUSTRATION

Tammy—Psychosocial Sequelae Following TBI

Tammy is a 25-year-old who sustained a TBI from a motor vehicle accident. She also suffered multiple facial trauma from the car accident, which has left her with permanent scarring. She was diagnosed three years ago with major depression. She is currently functioning at a Rancho Los Amigos Cognitive Level VII: Automatic-Appropriate. While she has mild memory problems, her cognitive impairments are secondary to her psychosocial maladjustment to disability. Tammy demonstrates a depressed mood, a flat affect, poor frustration tolerance, and poor self-concept. She avoids social situations and prefers to be alone. She states that she is embarrassed to be around her family and friends because of her disfigurement.

Discussion

Tammy demonstrates poor psychosocial adjustment to her disability. Her major depression is magnified by the recent brain injury, which has altered her mood, coping mechanisms, self-concept, and social pragmatics. In order to work with Tammy effectively, the treatment team will need to address the underlying psychiatric disorder and assist her in developing constructive coping mechanisms, opportunities for success in task performance, graduated group interventions to work on social skills, and community reentry activities to assist her in developing acceptance of her disability.

child (Rotondi, Sinkule, Balzer, Harris, & Moldovan, 2007). Coupled with this loss is the amount of dependence the individual will have postinjury. The client will often require close supervision and assistance from family members in daily activities (Testa, Malec, Moessner, & Brown, 2006). The lost ability to live independently in the community can further reinforce the individual's perceived loss of control or mastery over his or her environment. This can create strain in the relationship between the individual with brain injury and family members (Curtiss, Klemz, & Vanderploeg, 2000; Gosling & Oddy, 1999; Lanham, Weissenburger, Schwab, & Rosner, 2000). However, a study conducted by Perlesz, Kinsella, and Crowe (2000) concluded that "many families—despite their initial traumatic experience—eventually cope well, encouraging researchers and clinicians to focus future research efforts on those families who have made good adjustments to TBI" (p. 909).

SUMMARY

Brain injury, which results from both traumatic and acquired events, is a public health concern that contributes to a high number of deaths and, for many who survive, long-term disability. Brain injury presents with a complex clinical picture because of the effects of injury on the intricate neuronal networks throughout the brain that control cognition, behavior, perception, mobility, and vital life functions.

- Cognitive sequelae following brain injury include impairments in orientation, attention, memory, initiation and termination of activities, insight, judgment, safety awareness, information processing, executive functions, abstract reasoning, and new learning.

- Behavioral sequelae following brain injury include agitation, aggression, disinhibition, hypersexual behaviors, demotivational syndrome, and inappropriate emotional responses.

- Psychosocial sequelae following brain injury include psychiatric disorders, changes in personality, impaired social pragmatics, impaired coping mechanisms, changes in self-concept, and strains on the family dynamic.

The Rancho Los Amigos Levels of Cognitive Functioning (Hagen et al., 1973) assists the occupational therapy practitioner in assessing the client's cognitive, behavioral, and psychosocial problem areas following brain injury and in planning appropriate interventions. The occupational therapy practitioner working with clients with brain injury are challenged to provide holistic, client-centered care that addresses the cognitive, behavioral, and psychosocial dimensions of the person's functioning to increase therapeutic effectiveness and to promote optimal recovery for the client.

REVIEW QUESTIONS

1. Why is it important for the occupational therapist to consider an individual's premorbid psychosocial status prior to initiating treatment?
2. How do the Glasgow Coma Scale and the Rancho Los Amigos Levels of Cognitive Functioning help the occupational therapist to predict and plan the course of intervention for a person with brain injury?
3. How do the hierarchical levels of cognition influence the individual's ability to engage in occupation?
4. How can the occupational therapy practitioner capitalize on the client's current cognitive level to maximize task performance?
5. How do behavioral factors interfere with occupational performance?
6. How could the treatment environment be structured to decrease negative behaviors?
7. How does brain injury impact the individual's self-concept, social relationships, and internal drive to master her or his environment?

REFERENCES

American Occupational Therapy Association. (2008). Occupational therapy practice framework: Domain and process (2nd ed.). *American Journal of Occupational Therapy, 62*, 625–688.

Boman, I. L., Tham, K., Granqvist., A., Bartfai, A., & Hemmingsson, H. (2007). Using electronic aids to daily living after acquired brain injury: A study of the learning process and the usability. *Disability and Rehabilitation: Assistive Technology, 2*, 23–33.

Bornhofen, C., & McDonald, S. (2008). Treating deficits in emotional perception following traumatic brain injury. *Neuropsychological Rehabilitation, 18*, 22–44.

Brain Injury Association of America. (n.d.). *Causes of brain injury.* Retrieved from http://www.biausa.org

Bruns, J., & Hauser, W. A. (2003). The epidemiology of traumatic brain injury: A review. *Epilepsia, 44*, 2–10.

Burgess, P. W., Alderman, N., Evans, J., Emslie, H., & Wilson, B. A. (1998). Ecological validity of tests of executive function. *Journal of the International Neuropsychological Society, 4*, 547.

Burgess, P. W., Alderman, N., Forbes, C., Costello, A., Coates, L. M., Dawson, D. R., et al. (2006). The case for the development and use of "ecologically valid" measures of executive function in experimental and clinical neuropsychology. *Journal of the International Neuropsychological Society, 12*, 194–209.

Bushnik, T., Hanks, R. A., Kreutzer, J., & Rosenthal, M. (2003). Etiology of traumatic brain injury: Characterization of differential outcomes up to 1 year postinjury. *Archives of Physical and Medical Rehabilitation, 84*, 255–262.

Cameron, C. M., Purdie, D. M., Kliewer, E. V., & McClure, R. J. (2008). Ten-year outcomes following traumatic brain injury: A population-based cohort. *Brain Injury, 22*, 437–449.

Campbell, L., Wilson, F. C., McCann., J., Kernahan, G., & Rogers, R. G. (2007). Single case experimental design study of Career Facilitated Errorless Learning in a patient with severe memory impairment following TBI. *NeuroRehabilitation, 22*, 325–333.

Cantor, J. B., Ashman, T., Gordon, W., Ginsberg, A., Engmann, C., Egan, M., et al. (2008). Fatigue after traumatic brain injury and its impact on participation and quality of life. *Journal of Head Trauma Rehabilitation, 23*, 41–51.

Centers for Disease Control and Prevention. (2011). *Traumatic brain injury.* Retrieved November 11, 2011, from http://www.cdc.gov/ncipc/pubres/tbi_in_us_04/tbi_ed.htm http://www.cdc.gov/TraumaticBrainInjury/index.htm

Corral, L. Ventura, J. L., Herrero, J. I., Monfort, J. L., Juncadella, M., Gabarros, A., et al. (2007). Improvement in GOS and GOSE scores 6 and 12 months after severe brain injury. *Brain Injury, 21,* 1225–1231.

Corrigan, J. D., & Mysiw, W. J. (1988). Agitation following traumatic head injury: Equivocal evidence for a discrete stage of cognitive recovery. *Archives of Physical and Medical Rehabilitation, 69,* 487–492.

Cullen, N., Chundamala, J., Bayley, M., & Jutai, J. (2007). The efficacy of acquired brain injury rehabilitation. *Brain Injury, 21,* 113–132.

Curtiss, G., Klemz, S., & Vanderploeg, R. D. (2000). Acute impact of severe traumatic brain injury on family structure and coping responses. *Journal of Head Trauma Rehabilitation, 15*(5), 1113–1122.

Dahlberg, C. A., Cusick, C. P., Hawley, L. A., Newman, J. K., Morey, C. E., Harrison-Felix, C. L., et al. (2007). Treatment efficacy of social communication skills training after traumatic brain injury: A randomized treatment and deferred treatment controlled trial. *Archives of Physical Medicine and Rehabilitation, 88,* 1561–1573.

Dowling, G. A. (1985). Levels of cognitive functioning: Evaluation of interrater reliability. *Journal of Neurosurgical Nursing, 17*(2), 129–134.

Fann, J. R., Leonetti, A., Jaffe, K., Katon, W. J., Cummings, P., & Thompson, R. S. (2002). Psychiatric illness and subsequent traumatic brain injury: A case control study. *Journal of Neurology, Neurosurgery, and Psychiatry, 72*(5), 615–620.

Fedoroff, J. P., Starkstein, S. E., Forrester, A. W., Geisler, F. H., Jorge, R. E., et al. (1992). Depression in patients with acute traumatic brain injury. *American Journal of Psychiatry, 149*(7), 918–923.

Fraas, M., Balz, M., & DeGrauw, W. (2007). Meeting the long-term needs of adults with acquired brain injury through community-based programming. *Brain Injury, 21,* 1267–1281.

Gelb, D. J. (2000). *Introduction to clinical neurology* (2nd ed.). St. Louis, MO: Elsevier Science.

Gentry, T., Wallace, J., Kvarfordt, C., & Lynch, K. B. (2008). Personal digital assistants as cognitive aids for individuals with severe traumatic brain injury: A community-based trial. *Brain Injury, 22,* 19–24.

Giles, G. M., & Hohr, J. D. (2007). Overview and inter-rater reliability of an incident-based rating scale for aggressive behavior following traumatic brain injury: The Overt Aggression Scale-Modified for Neurorehabilitation–Extended (OAS_MNR-E). *Brain Injury, 21,* 505–511.

Golden, Z., & Golden, C. J. (2003). Impact of brain injury severity on personality dysfunction. *International Journal of Neuroscience, 113*(5), 733–745.

Gosling, J., & Oddy, M. (1999). Rearranged marriages: Martial relationships after head injury. *Brain Injury, 13*(10), 785–796.

Gouvier, W. D., Blanton, P. D., LaPorte, K. K., & Nepomuceno, C. (1987). Reliability and validity of the Disability Rating Scale and Levels of Cognitive Functioning Scale in monitoring recovery from severe head injury. *Archives of Physical and Medical Rehabilitation, 68,* 94–97.

Goverover, Y., Johnson, M. V., Toglia, J., & DeLuca, J. (2007). Treatment to improve self-awareness in persons with acquired brain injury. *Brain Injury, 21,* 913–923.

Hagen, C., Malkmus, D., & Stenderup-Bowman, K. (1973). *The Rancho Levels of Cognitive Functioning* (2nd ed.). Downey, CA: Los Amigos Research and Educational Institute.

Haggstrom, A., & Lund. M. L. (2008). The complexity of participation in daily life: A qualitative study of the experiences of persons with acquired brain injury. *Journal of Rehabilitation Medicine, 40,* 89–95.

Hibbard, M. R., Uysal, S., Kepler, K., Bogdany, J., & Silver, J. (1998). Axis I psychopathology in individuals with traumatic brain injury. *Journal of Head Trauma Rehabilitation, 13*(4), 24–39.

Jenkinson, N., Ownsworth., T., & Shum, D. (2007). Utility of the Canadian Occupational Performance Measure in community-based brain injury rehabilitation. *Brain Injury, 21,* 1283–1294.

Lanham, R. A., Weissenburger, J. E., Schwab, K. A., & Rosner, M. M. (2000). A longitudinal investigation of the concordance between individuals with traumatic brain injury and family or friend ratings on the Katz adjustment scale. *Journal of Head Trauma Rehabilitation, 15*(5), 1123–1138.

Law, M., Baptiste, S., McColl, M. A., Carswell, A., Polatajko, H., & Pollock, N. (2005). *Canadian Occupational Performance Measure* (4th ed.). Ottawa, Ontario: Canadian Association of Occupational Therapists.

Leahy, B. J., & Lam, C. S. (1998). Neuropsychological testing and functional outcome for individuals with traumatic brain injury. *Brain Injury, 12*(12), 1025–1035.

Lequerica, A. H., Rapport, L. J., Loeher, K., Axelrod, B. N., Vangel, S. J., & Hanks, R. A. (2007). Agitation in acquired brain injury: Impact on acute rehabilitation therapies. *Journal of Head Trauma Rehabilitation, 22,* 177–183.

Lombard, L., & Zafonte, R. (2005). Agitation after traumatic brain injury: Considerations and treatment options. *American Journal of Physical Medicine and Rehabilitation, 84,* 797–812.

McCabe, P., Lippert, C., Weiser, M., Hilditch, M., Hartridge, C., & Villamere, J. (2007). Community reintegration following acquired brain injury. *Brain Injury, 21,* 231–257.

McGuire, L. M., Burright, R. G., Williams, R., & Donovick, P. J. (1998). Prevalence of traumatic brain injury in psychiatric and non-psychiatric subjects. *Brain Injury, 12*(3), 207–214.

Mooney, G., & Speed, J. (2001). The association between mild traumatic brain injury and psychiatric conditions. *Brain Injury, 15*(10), 865–877.

Nakase-Richardson, R., Yablon, S. A., & Sherer, M. (2007). Prospective comparison of acute confusion severity with duration of post-traumatic amnesia in predicting employment outcome after traumatic brain injury. *Journal of Neurology, Neurosurgery, and Psychiatry, 78,* 872–876.

O'Brien, L. (2007). Achieving a successful and sustainable return to the workforce after ABI: A client-centered approach. *Brain Injury, 21,* 465–478.

Oueller, M. C., & Morin, C. M. (2007). Efficacy of cognitive-behavioral therapy for insomnia associated with traumatic brain injury: A single-case experimental design. *Archives of Physical Medicine and Rehabilitation, 88,* 1481–1592.

Ownsworth, T., Fleming, J., Shum, D., Kuipers, P., & Strong, J. (2008). Comparison of individualized, group, and combined intervention formats in a randomized controlled trial for facilitating goal attainment and improving psychosocial function following acquired brain injury. *Journal of Rehabilitation Medicine, 40,* 81–88.

Ownsworth, T., Fleming, J., Desbois., J., Strong, J., & Kuipers, P. (2006). A metacognitive contextual intervention to enhance error awareness and functional outcome following traumatic brain injury: A single-case experimental design. *Journal of the International Neuropsychological Society, 12,* 54–63.

Ownsworth, T. L. (1998). Depression after traumatic brain injury. *Brain Injury, 12,* 735–751.

Parish, L., & Oddy, M. (2007). Efficacy of rehabilitation for functional skills more than 10 years after extremely severe brain injury. *Neuropsychological Rehabilitation, 17,* 230–243.

Perlesz, A., Kinsella, G., & Crowe, S. (2000). Psychological distress and family satisfaction following traumatic brain injury: Injured individuals and their primary, secondary, and tertiary caregivers. *Journal of Head Trauma, 15*(3), 909–929.

Phipps, S. (2006). Community participation. In K. M. Golisz (Ed.), *Neurorehabilitation for traumatic brain injury* (Neurorehabilitation Self-Paced Clinical Course Series, G. M. Giles, Series Senior Ed., pp. 93–134). Bethesda: MD: American Occupational Therapy Association.

Phipps, S., & Richardson, P. (2007). Occupational therapy outcomes for clients with traumatic brain injury and stroke using the Canadian Occupational Performance Measure. *American Journal of Occupational Therapy, 61*, 328–334.

Pierce, C. A., & Hanks, R. A. (2006). Life satisfaction after traumatic brain injury and the World Health Organization Model of Disability. *American Journal of Physical Medicine and Rehabilitation, 75*, 889–898.

Poole, J. H., Dahdah, M. N., Schwab, K., Lew, H. L, Warden, D. L., & Date, E. S. (2007). Long-term outcomes after traumatic brain injury in veterans: Successes and challenges. *American Journal of Physical Medicine and Rehabilitation, 86*, 333–334.

Rapport, L. J., Coleman Bryer, R., & Hanks, R. A. (2008). Driving and community integration after traumatic brain injury. *Archives of Physical Medicine and Rehabilitation, 89*, 922–930.

Rodgers, M. L., Strode, A. D., Norell, D. M., Short, R. A., Dyck, D. G., & Becker, B. (2007). Adapting multiple-family group treatment for brain and spinal cord injury intervention development and preliminary outcomes. *American Journal of Physical Medicine and Rehabilitation, 86*, 482–492.

Rothweiler, B., Temkin, N. R., & Dikmen, S. S. (1998). Aging effect on psychosocial outcome in traumatic brain injury. *Archives of Physical Medicine and Rehabilitation, 79*(8), 881–887.

Rotondi, A. J., Sinkule, J., Balzer, K., Harris, J., & Moldovan, R. (2007). A qualitative needs assessment of persons who have experienced traumatic brain injury and their primary family caregivers. *Journal of Head Trauma Rehabilitation, 22*, 14–25.

Ruff, R. M., Camenzuli, L., & Mueller, J. (1996). Miserable minority: Emotional risk factors that influence the outcome of a mild traumatic brain injury. *Brain Injury, 10*(8), 551–565.

Rutland-Brown, W., Langlois, J. A., Thomas, K. E., & Xi, Y. L. (2006). Incidence of traumatic brain injury in the United States, 2003. *Journal of Head Trauma Rehabilitation, 21*, 544–548.

Sayer, N. A., Chiros, C. E., Sigford, B., Scott, S., Clothier, B., Pickett, T., et al. (2008). Characteristics and rehabilitation outcomes among patients with blast and other injuries sustained during the global war on terror. *Archives of Physical Medicine and Rehabilitation, 89*, 163–170.

Schwab, K. A., Warden, D., Lux, W. E., Shupenko, L. A., & Zitnay, G. (2007). Defense and Veterans' Brain Injury Center: Peacetime and wartime missions. *Journal of Rehabilitation Research and Development, 44*, xiii–xxii.

Sohlberg, M. M., Fickas, S., Hung, P., & Fortier, A. (2007). A comparison of four prompt modes for route finding for community travelers with severe cognitive impairments. *Brain injury, 21*, 531–538.

Tamietto, M., Torrini, G., Adenzato, M., Pietrapiana, P., Rago, R., & Perino, C. (2006). To drive or not to drive (after TBI)? A review of the literature and its implications for rehabilitation and future research. *NeuroRehabilitation, 21*, 81–92.

Tate, P. S., Freed, D. M., Bombardier, C. H., Harter, S. L., & Brinkman, S. (1999). Traumatic brain injury: Influence of blood alcohol level on post-acute cognitive function. *Brain Injury, 13*(10), 767–784.

Teasell, R., Bayona, N., Marshall, S., Cullen, N., Bayley, M., Chundamala, J., et al. (2007). A systematic review of the rehabilitation of moderate to severe acquired brain injuries. *Brain Injury, 21*, 107–112.

Testa, J. A., Malec, J. F., Moessner, A. M., & Brown, A. W. (2006). Predicting family functioning after TBI: Impact of neurobehavioral factors. *Journal of Head Trauma Rehabilitation, 21*, 236–247.

Thickpenny-Davis, K. L., & Barker-Collo, S. L. (2007). Evaluation of a structured group format memory rehabilitation program for adults following brain injury. *Journal of Head Trauma Rehabilitation, 22*, 303–313.

Trombly, C. A., Radomski, M. V., & Davis, E. S. (1998). Achievement of self-identified goals by adults with traumatic brain injury: Phase I. *American Journal of Occupational Therapy, 52*(10), 810–818.

Van Baalen, B., Odding, E., & Stam, H. J. (2008). Cognitive status at discharge from the hospital determines discharge destination in traumatic brain injury patients. *Brain Injury, 22*, 25–32.

Vanderploeg, R. D., Schwab, K., Walker, W. C., Fraser, J. A., Sigford, B. J., Date, E. S., et al. (2008). Rehabilitation of traumatic brain injury in active duty military personnel and veterans: Defense and Veterans' Brain Injury Center randomized controlled trial of two rehabilitation approaches. *Archives of Physical Medicine and Rehabilitation, 89,* 2227–2238.

Wheeler, S. D., Lane, S. J., & McMahon, B. T. (2007). Community participation and life satisfaction following intensive, community-based rehabilitation using a life skills training approach. *OTJR: Occupation, Participation, and Health, 27,* 13–22.

World Health Organization. (2001). *International classification of functioning, disability, and health.* Geneva: World Health Organization.

Yudofsky, S. C., & Hales, R. E. (2002). *The American Psychiatric Publishing textbook of neuropsychiatry and clinical neurosciences* (4th ed.). Washington, DC: American Psychiatric Press.

Zafonte, R. D., Hammond, F. M., Mann, N. R., Wood, D. L., Black, K. L., & Millis, S. R. (1996). Relationship between Glasgow Coma Scale and functional outcome. *American Journal of Physical and Medical Rehabilitation, 75*(5), 364–369.

Zhu, X. L., Poon, W. S., Chan, C. C., & Chan, S. S. (2007). Does intensive rehabilitation improve the functional outcome of patients with traumatic brain injury (TBI)? A randomized controlled trial. *Brain Injury, 21,* 681–690.

SUGGESTED RESOURCES

Bear, M. F., Connors, L. W., & Paradiso, M. A. (2001). *Neuroscience: Exploring the brain.* Philadelphia: Lippincott Williams & Wilkins.

Crimmins, C. (2000). *Where is the mango princess?* New York: Random House.

Giles, G. M., & Clark-Wilson, J. (Eds.). (1999). *Rehabilitation of the severely brain-injured adult: A practical approach* (2nd ed.). London: Stanley Thornes.

Gutman, S. A. (2003). *Screening adult neurologic populations: A step-by-step instruction manual.* Bethesda, MD: American Occupational Therapy Association.

Yody, B. B., Schaub, C., Conway, J., Peters, S., Strauss, D., & Helsinger, S. (2000). Applied behavior management and acquired brain injury: Approaches and assessment. *Journal of Head Trauma Rehabilitation, 15*(4), 1041–1060.

SUGGESTED WEBSITES

Brain Injury Association of America http://www.biausa.org

Brain Injury Recovery Network http://www.tbirecovery.org

Brain Injury Resource Center http://www.headinjury.com

National Institute of Neurological Disorders and Stroke (NINDS) www.ninds.nih.gov/disorders/tbi/tbi.htm

Managing Pain in Occupational Therapy: Integrating the Model of Human Occupation and the Intentional Relationship Model

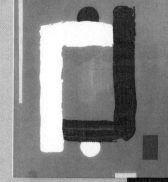

Renee R. Taylor, MA, PhD
Chia-Wei Fan, MS, OTC

KEY TERMS

acute pain

chronic pain

Model of Human Occupation

Intentional Relationship Model

CHAPTER OUTLINE

Introduction
Acute Versus Chronic Pain
Examples of Disorders Involving Chronic Pain
    Arthritis (Rheumatoid, Osteoarthritis)
    Cancer
    Central Pain Syndrome
    Peripheral Neuropathy
    Fibromyalgia
    Lower Back Pain
    Chronic Post-Surgical Pain (CPSP)
    Phantom Pain
    Complex Regional Pain Syndrome (Reflex Sympathetic Dystrophy)
    Chronic Headaches
    Chronic Pain and Depression
    Chronic Pain and Substance Abuse
Assessing Pain: An Occupational Therapy Perspective
    Clinical Interview
    Occupation-Focused Assessments
    Standardized Ratings and Assessments

Applying the Model of Human Occupation in Treatment
Effective Use of Self: The Intentional Relationship Model
Areas of Related Knowledge: The Unique Role of the Occupational Therapist
Summary

INTRODUCTION

Pain can be an intensely unwanted sensation that most people strive to avoid or escape at all costs (Taylor, 2008). In rehabilitation and other occupational therapy settings, clients receiving therapy tend to report pain frequently or silently endure it, particularly when the therapy is impairment-focused (i.e., with biomechanical or other functional goals at its apex). There are a number of aspects of occupational therapy that either precipitate or exacerbate clients' sensations of pain. Pain is one of the primary motivators for seeking medical care and the leading cause of decreased occupational productivity (Stucky, Gold, & Zhang, 2001). In 2003, the National Pain Care Policy Act was introduced in Congress to account for a significant need to make pain a priority in treatment, education, and research. Still, the extent and consistency with which various treatment providers adhere to this act vary between individuals and across settings (Cole, 2002; Keefe, Abernethy, & Campbell, 2005).

ACUTE VERSUS CHRONIC PAIN

The frequency and duration of pain can be a determining factor in the course and outcome of occupational therapy. **Acute pain** is temporary, lasting no longer than months. Acute pain begins suddenly and is felt sharply. It may signal the onset or advancement of underlying disease or it may be a consequence of injury or a medical intervention. During therapy, acute pain may be easier for clients to cope with because it is a relatively brief and self-limiting experience that is typically resolved by treating the underlying cause, by discontinuing the task, or by using a range of modalities designed to alleviate it. Most instances of acute pain disappear when the underlying cause is treated or resolved. However, there are many instances in occupational therapy settings where, due to the nature and severity of the injury or impairment, unrelieved acute pain ultimately leads to chronic pain.

Chronic pain is relentless and long-standing, lasting at least three to six months according to most definitions (Hinrichs-Rocker et al., 2009). In chronic pain situations, pain signals may remain active in the nervous system for weeks, months, or years. Psychosocial correlates and consequences may include depressed mood, irritability, anxiety, work incapacity, and activity avoidance accompanied by a fear of re-injury or post-exertional exacerbation (Berger, 2000). Clients with chronic pain are often compromised in terms of their interactions with their social and physical environments. Because of the pain, they may limit their social interactions and lose or attenuate their engagement in once-valued occupations. Anxiety associated with the pain may hinder a client's ability and motivation to return to normal work or daily activity. More immediately, chronic pain has the potential to delay, complicate, or completely interrupt occupational therapy and other rehabilitative treatments.

From a psychosocial perspective, chronic pain is tremendously frustrating to clients and providers because it continues, mostly without explanation, beyond the expected timeframe, or long after an injury has healed (Taylor, 2008). Approximately 75 to 80 million people within the United States have experienced chronic pain at any given time (Tollison, 1993). It has been found to have a significant negative impact on overall quality of life (Bay-Nielsen, Nilsson, Nordin, & Kehlet, 2004). Research has found that psychological variables and interventions may play a greater role in the experience of pain than medical ones (Block, Ohnmeiss, Guyer, Rashbaum, & Hochschuler, 2001). The influence of emotional and cognitive aspects of pain on a client's sensory experience has been shown in research examining placebo effects on pain levels (Rudy, Lieber, Boston, Gourley, & Baysal, 2003). Zalon (2004) and Taillefer et al. (2006) have both found that there is a significant correlation between chronic pain and depression. In addition, Peolsson, Vavruch, and Oberg (2006) reported that a better score on the Distress and Risk Assessment Method (an assessment designed to identify distress and evaluate the risk of poor outcome) was a critical predictor for a positive outcome regarding arm and neck pain.

People with chronic pain disorders experience high rates of depression, anxiety, and other forms of psychiatric comorbidity and psychosocial distress (Taylor, 2006). In addition to facing multiple losses in functioning and quality of life, otherwise non-disabled individuals with intractable pain are often stigmatized in health care settings (Taylor, 2006). For example, some physicians who could not find a physical cause for a client's pain simply suggested that it was imaginary. Research pointed out that clients tended to attribute most of their medical symptoms to being rooted in pain rather than depression (Sharp & Keefe, 2006). Therefore, pain among clients with depression or other psychiatric disorders is often dismissed or misdiagnosed as somatization disorder (Dewar, 2007).

Thus, it is essential that occupational therapists understand how to assess and respond to pain in the most optimal way; that is, a way that not only supports occupational engagement but also protects the psychological well-being and self-esteem of our clients.

Many occupational therapists have adopted interventions developed within other disciplines into their practice without critically considering their roles in demonstrating the efficacy of occupational therapy and the efficacy of occupation-based practice (Robinson, Kennedy, & Harmon, 2011). Therefore, this chapter focuses on the application of two occupational therapy models that are particularly relevant in assessing and treating this important and complex psychosocial issue: The **Model of Human Occupation** (Kielhofner, 2008) and the **Intentional Relationship Model** (Taylor, 2008). In tandem with other standardized pain measurements, the Model of Human Occupation (Kielhofner, 2008) can inform the assessment and treatment of a wide range of clients with chronic pain issues. Additionally, the Intentional Relationship Model (Taylor, 2008) can inform communication issues that cut across any number of occupational therapy approaches that concern pain. Both models are of particular use in situations where a practitioner's methods range from producing pain as a necessary correlate of therapy to reducing preexisting pain as a focus of intervention.

EXAMPLES OF DISORDERS INVOLVING CHRONIC PAIN

In occupational therapy, pain is oftentimes a part of practice in rehabilitation settings. Although it is not exhaustive, this section describes 12 of the more common types of chronic pain seen by occupational therapists as either primary, secondary, or comorbid to the presenting problem (Engel, 2009).

Arthritis (Rheumatoid, Osteoarthritis)

The two most common forms of arthritis include osteoarthritis and rheumatoid arthritis. Rheumatoid arthritis activates the inflammatory immune response in joints and leads to joint tissue damage. Osteoarthritis is a degenerative joint disease characterized by pain and loss of mobility, particularly in the weight-bearing joints of the body, such as the vertebrae, knees, and hips.

Cancer

Studies of inpatients and outpatients with cancer estimate pain to occur in between 57% and 80% of individuals with cancer (Beck & Falkson, 2001; Chang, Hwang, Feuerman, & Kasimis, 2000). The most common causes of pain in cancer are tumor growth, bone metastasis, post-surgical pain, pain resulting from radiation treatment, and post-chemotherapy neuropathy.

Central Pain Syndrome

Central pain syndrome occurs as a result of injury or damage to the central nervous system. This damage can be caused by stroke, multiple sclerosis, tumors, epilepsy, brain injury, spinal cord injury, or Parkinson's disease. The most commonly described type of pain associated with traumatic brain injury is headache (Sherman, Goldberg, & Bell, 2004). Additionally, over 65% of people with spinal cord injury experience pain (Cardenas, Bryce, Shem, Richards, & Elhefni, 2004). Individuals with stroke suffer shoulder pain caused by limitations in joint mobility (i.e., "frozen shoulder"), and some develop central neurogenic pain (Pain Relief Foundation, 2003).

Peripheral Neuropathy

More than 100 types of peripheral neuropathy have been identified (http://www.ninds.nih.gov). Peripheral neuropathy describes a wide range of pain syndromes that can result from damage to the large network of nerves outside of the brain and spinal cord. Sensations can include progressive numbness, tingling and pricking sensations, sensitivity to touch, and muscle weakness. In its advanced stages, sensations can include burning pain (particularly at night), paralysis and muscle wasting, and organ and gland dysfunction. Sexual dysfunction occurs, and individuals may become unable to digest food easily, maintain normal blood pressure, and sweat normally. In the most severe cases, organ failure and breathing difficulties may occur.

Fibromyalgia

Chronic, unexplained, widespread pain is the defining symptom of fibromyalgia. It occurs in 100% of individuals with this condition. To receive a diagnosis of fibromyalgia the pain must occur in all four quadrants of the body for at least three months (Wolfe, et al. 1997). Fibromyalgia pain is characterized by widespread aching in the muscles and soft tissues, pain when pressure is put on specific tender points, and pain that is usually felt in the neck, shoulders, upper back, elbows, lower back, and hip girdle.

Lower Back Pain

Chronic lower back pain is diagnosed when pain persists beyond 12 weeks. There are many potential causes of chronic lower back pain, the most common being disc protrusion and disk herniation. In cases where the extent of protrusion and herniation do not correlate with clinical symptoms and when diagnostic workup yields no structural cause, psychological and social variables are more likely to be considered (Wheeler, Stubbart, & Hicks, 2004).

Chronic Post-Surgical Pain (CPSP)

Pain is expected to follow any surgery due to the tissue damage it causes. Between 10% and 50% of people who undergo certain types of surgery go on to develop chronic post-surgical pain (CPSP) (Hinrichs-Rocker et al., 2009).

Phantom Pain

Phantom limb pain is the most common form of phantom pain. It is generally felt as pain in an absent part of the body—typically in the place where an amputated limb once existed. As many as 51% of people with upper limb amputations report phantom pain, and 64% report that this pain is moderate to severe (Kooijman, Dijkstra, Geertzen, Elzinga, & van der Schans, 2000).

Complex Regional Pain Syndrome (Reflex Sympathetic Dystrophy)

There are two subtypes of complex regional pain syndrome (CRPS). CRPS type 1 (or reflex sympathetic dystrophy) is a chronic pain state with onset due to soft tissue injury or bone injury. CRPS type 2 is a chronic pain state with onset due to nerve injury.

In addition to chronic pain, which is experienced by individuals with both subtypes of CRPS, CRPS type 2 pain is also associated with autonomic changes such as sweating, trophic changes (e.g., skin atrophy), hair loss, and joint contractures.

Chronic Headaches

There are three subtypes of chronic headaches: migraine, tension-type headache, and hemicrania continua. The chronic headache usually is diagnosed when it occurs over 15 days per month and for at least three months. Chronic migraine affects only one side of head and may result in nausea, vomiting, and sensitivity to light and sound. Tension-type headache hurts both sides of head. Its pain can radiate from the neck, eyes, to the back or other muscles in the upper body. Hemicrania causes headaches on only one side of head, which does not shift sides.

Chronic Pain and Depression

According to the American Pain Foundation, 25% to 50% of clients who complain of pain to their physician are depressed. On the other hand, 65% of depressed people also complain of pain. Pain and depression create a vicious cycle in which pain worsens the depression emotion, and then the resulting depression lowers the threshold of pain (Bair, Robinson, Katon, & Kroenke, 2003). Since chronic pain and depression involve the same nerves and neurotransmitters, antidepressants are sometimes used to treat both chronic pain and depression. Antidepressants work on reducing the perception of pain (Kroenke et al., 2009).

Chronic Pain and Substance Abuse

Medication is one of the most common modalities that have been used to treat chronic pain. However, researchers found that many medications used in pain management have potential for abuse (Serban, 2011). For example, opioids were viewed to effectively reduce acute pain and chronic pain, but physical dependence is often a natural part of the long-term use of prescribed opioids (Heit, 2003; Strassels, McNicol, & Suleman, 2005). Some possible signs for the risk of substance abuse are as follows: clients repeatedly running out of medication early, complaints about the need for additional prescriptions, unapproved use of prescribed medication to self-medicate other problems, and multiple episodes of "stolen" prescriptions (Breivik, 2005; Schneider, 2005). Therefore, clinicians should be aware of clients' histories of personal problems, such as alcohol or drug abuse. They should document medication doses and monitor clients closely for any symptoms of abuse.

It should be noted that this chapter is not intended to provide an exhaustive, systematic, or detailed review of the myriad treatment approaches to pain. Rather, a general introduction, with a focus on psychosocial interventions, is what this chapter aims to provide. When working with clients with conditions that involve pain, therapists are advised to seek out additional information about the role of pain in that specific condition or medical procedure from collaborating rehabilitation physicians, pain specialists, anesthesiologists, psychiatrists, or other mental health professionals and research-related resources.

ASSESSING PAIN: AN OCCUPATIONAL THERAPY PERSPECTIVE

As mentioned in the Occupational Therapy Practice Framework (AOTA, 2008), the process of occupational therapy includes evaluation, intervention, and outcome monitoring. The pain evaluation in occupational therapy should consist of the occupational profile and analysis of occupational performance. The occupational profile consists of information about clients' expectation and concerns about their performance. The analysis of occupational performance focuses on using assessment tools to measure factors that support or hinder clients' occupational performance. Both the profile and the performance analysis can be viewed in terms of a three-pronged approach:

1. Clinical Interview
2. Occupation-Focused Assessments
3. Standardized Ratings & Assessments

Clinical Interview

When it comes to working with pain, the more client-centered a practitioner is, the more successful any course of treatment will be. All of the assessments covered in this chapter are client-centered in that they probe for a deeper understanding of a client's pain, from the client's perspective. They look at pain as it affects various aspects of the client's daily life and his or her interactions with physical and social environments. Unlike other client-centered occupational therapy assessments, the assessments that are covered in this chapter provide a wide and in-depth range of questions, prompts, and other structures for assessing the interface between pain and occupation. Practitioners have many areas of focus and suggested lines of inquiry that they can custom-tailor to a client's needs.

Asking clients to describe their pain during one's routine clinical interview facilitates understanding, situates clients and their therapists to develop more appropriate occupational therapy interventions, and may facilitate an increased sense of perceived control among clients. Pain has been described in multiple ways. The following are common adjectives that are often used by providers and clients when discussing pain: aching, gnawing, stabbing, burning, freezing, cramping, pressing, crushing, dull, nagging, tingling, pinching, wrenching, radiating, shooting, sharp, sore, stinging, tender, throbbing, and tight. When clients are in a significant amount of pain, offering a few adjectives as examples to choose from may help give clarity to their experience.

Occupation-Focused Assessments

A conceptual framework for the assessment and management of pain should be broadly defined, addressing not only the commonly used symptom and severity variables, but also the often-overlooked occupational variables (Linton et al., 2005). The Model of Human Occupation (MOHO) (Kielhofner, 2008) is an internationally recognized and widely used practice model that provides such a framework for assessing and treating pain. In pain assessment and management, MOHO can be used to explain how pain interacts with a client's willingness to engage in occupation. Specifically, MOHO is the study of how a client's occupations are motivated, patterned, and performed (Kielhofner, 2008). For clients with chronic pain, these concepts are paramount. Pain is a profoundly draining and debilitating symptom. Therefore, the extent to which a client can identify motivating occupations and develop habitual patterns of engaging in them that are efficient and easy to perform, the better able that client will be to function and cope in everyday life.

The Occupational Performance History Interview-II (OPHI-II) is one such measure that draws upon the MOHO (Kielhofner, 2008) to support practitioners in collaboratively mapping a client's experience with pain. The OPHI-II includes three main parts. First, there is a semi-structured interview, which can be used to explore a client's life story before, during, and after pain onset. Second, the OPHI-II contains rating scales that allow therapists to evaluate clients in terms of their occupational identities, perceived competence at occupations, and facilitators/barriers in their environments. Finally, it contains a life history narrative and a place to pictorially graph the client's pain story in terms of significant events that may have predated, occurred concurrently with, or post-dated the pain.

Keponen and Kielhofner (2006) used the OPHI-II to examine how women with chronic pain experienced and organized various occupations in their lives. Using this narrative interview approach, they gained detailed knowledge about the meaning of occupations for women with chronic pain from their personal points of view (Keponen & Kielhofner, 2006). Understanding a client's unique perspective on the role of pain in his or her everyday life is fundamental in any approach to long-term pain management.

The Model of Human Occupation Screening Tool (MOHOST) (Parkinson, Forsyth, & Kielhofner, 2006) is a flexible and brief clinical assessment that was designed for practice and research by occupational therapy practitioners. It is widely used in clinical care because it allows the practitioner to incorporate the information used in screening and evaluating progress and outcomes into a scoreable, chart-note-type format. The MOHOST covers all aspects of occupational functioning including questions about a client's motivation for occupation, habitual patterns of engaging in occupation, communication skills, motor skills, process skills, and environmental supports and barriers. It is particularly applicable to pain practice and research because it provides a structured way of examining key details involving the interaction between pain and the various aspects of a client's occupational engagement.

The Occupational Self Assessment (OSA) (Baron, Kielhofner, Iyengar, Goldhammer, & Wolenski, 2006) and its companion pediatric measure, the Child Occupational Self Assessment (COSA) (Keller, Kafkes, Basu, Federico, & Kielhofner, 2005), are two additional, brief self-rating forms that measure a client's self-perceived competence at everyday occupations and the extent to which those occupations are important. In evaluating and treating pain, it is important to prioritize occupations that are volitionally gratifying to clients; that is, those occupations that clients feel competent doing and find important in their lives.

For practitioners involved with work capacity assessment and work rehabilitation, the Worker Role Interview (WRI) (Braveman et al., 2005) is a semi-structured interview that is also based on the Model of Human Occupation (Kielhofner, 2008). It is designed to assess individuals with work-related injuries with respect to MOHO concepts of personal causation (perceived competence), values, interests, habits, roles, and environmental supports. Companion measures, such as the Work Environment Impact Scale (Moore-Corner, Kielhofner, & Olson, 1998) and the Assessment of Work Performance (Sandqvist, Bjork, Gullberg, Henriksson, & Gerdle, 2009), may also be utilized to guide understanding of the roles of the environment and of the task demands in shaping an individual's pain experience during work.

Standardized Ratings and Assessments

In addition to these assessments, it is also critical that clients be asked to assign a number to their pain by rating it on a scale from 0 = "no pain" to 10 = "the most extreme pain I have ever had" (McCaffery & Beebe, 1993). These ratings may be used to track the severity of a client's pain over time. Additionally, they may be used to inform the need for medication and the effectiveness of a given medication or intervention on decreasing the pain.

There are also more comprehensive means of measuring and quantifying pain that include descriptive adjectives, visual analog scales, and pain intensity ratings. The Short-Form McGill Pain Questionnaire (Melzack, 1987) is one well-cited example used frequently in research. This questionnaire has three components. Part I (the pain rating index) lists 15 adjectives that describe pain. These adjectives are sub-classified in terms of sensory (items 1–11) and affective (items 12–15) qualities of pain. In Part II, clients rate the overall intensity of pain on an average day on a visual analog scale. The scale ranges from "no pain" to "worst possible pain." The third part of the questionnaire requires clients to make an evaluative rating of pain intensity in the present moment by choosing an appropriate word on a 0 to 5 scale. This questionnaire may be administered as homework as a baseline measure at the beginning of therapy, as a measure of progress at key points during the course of therapy, and as a measure of outcomes at the end of therapy.

APPLYING THE MODEL OF HUMAN OCCUPATION IN TREATMENT

Padilla and Bianchi (1990) argue that many medical model approaches to pain, including narcotic pharmacotherapy and surgery, run the risk of exacerbating symptoms, introducing new psychosocial problems, and impeding engagement in occupation. In part, this is due to various physical and cognitive side effects of these treatments. It is also due to the inevitable need to disrupt one's ordinary routines and limit one's social and leisure activities in order to organize one's life around following various medical directives in order to manage the pain (Padilla & Bianchi, 1990).

At the same time, purely psychobehavioral approaches to pain management, such as cognitive-behavioral therapies, relaxation, and mindfulness and meditation approaches, are equally incomplete. Critical perspectives contend that these therapies over-rely on the idea that the mind can override the physiological pain response (Padilla & Bianchi, 1990). There have been numerous studies of pharmacological, biomechanical, psychobehavioral, and interdisciplinary approaches to chronic pain management (Taylor, 2006). Despite methodological flaws, there have been decades of outcome studies on these various approaches. Although some approaches have been found to be more effective than others (e.g., interdisciplinary programs, mindfulness meditation and relaxation programs, and cognitive behavioral therapy programs), no single approach to pain management has emerged as being far superior or completely effective (Taylor, 2006).

It would make sense that no single approach could wholly account for the daunting and elusive problem of chronic pain let alone its many psychosocial comorbidities and occupational offshoots. Interdisciplinary programs strive to combine approaches so that pharmacological, biomechanical, and psychobehavioral components are all addressed. Although these programs represent an innovative step in the right direction, many lack an underlying conceptual practice model by which communication can be facilitated and services can be integrated around a theme for care. Without such an integrative and thematic approach, these kinds of programs, particularly when implemented in uncontrolled, non-research environments, run the risk of gaps in care or overlaps in care, failures in case coordination and communication, turf wars, and, in worst cases, contradictory approaches that can easily result in iatrogenic situations. Moreover, when these programs are evaluated in terms of outcomes, it is next to impossible to narrow down the mechanism of change because there is no single underlying model tying all of the interventions together (Durand, Vachon, Loisel, & Berthelette, 2003).

An integrative approach that is based on a conceptual practice model that can guide moment-to-moment clinical reasoning is needed. MOHO is a conceptual practice model that responds to this need. Padilla and Bianchi (1990) were two of the first to advocate viewing the chronic pain client from a systems perspective based on MOHO. According to this perspective, a client's motivation for occupation, habits, and performance capacity interact with facilitators and barriers in the environment. Correspondingly, they describe a three-stage occupational therapy graded activity-type program for the treatment of chronic pain in which there is a physical component, an intrapersonal component, and an interpersonal component. The physical component consists of the following:

- Relaxation training
- Adaptive equipment
- Environmental modification
- Body mechanics, work simplification, and energy conservation
- Gradual increase in time spent in productive activity

The next phase, the intrapersonal phase of the program, consists of examining how one's lifestyle, environment, and occupational roles might exacerbate or allevi-ate clients' experiences of pain (Padilla & Bianchi, 1990). Clients are then encouraged to examine their values about occupational roles and make any necessary changes in those roles in order to achieve occupational balance. Clients are also encouraged to reorganize their physical environments to better accommodate their needs. Voca-tional exploration and leisure skill development are also emphasized in this phase of the program. Additionally, this component of the program contains some elements of cognitive-behavioral therapy approaches, such as relaxation training and refuta-tion of negative automatic thoughts about the pain (for more information about cognitive-behavioral therapy, please refer to the section on related knowledge later in this chapter).

By the time clients reach the third phase of the program, they should have made the necessary changes in the areas of roles, values, activities, and environments to have achieved a sense of self-esteem and control with respect to their pain. In this phase, clients are expected to have enough control over their physical bodies and environments to enable them to face the stresses and challenges of renewed social interaction. Padilla and Bianchi (1990) point out that people close to the client, such as significant others, can engage in dysfunctional dynamics in which they either ne-glect or overprotect the client. Thus this phase focuses on communication skills and assertiveness training so that clients feel comfortable asking for appropriate levels of assistance, delegating activities when necessary, and participating in cooperative interactions in order to achieve occupational goals.

A second pain management program that relied upon MOHO as its conceptual practice model was described by Henriksson (1995a, 1995b). She studied 20 Swedish and 20 U.S. women with fibromyalgia, a condition that is usually diagnosed by tender point examination involving chronic, unexplained muscular pain in all four body quadrants. For successful pain management to occur, changes in habits, roles, ergonomic requirements, and lifestyles were necessary. Furthermore, clients required a supportive environment and comprehensive health care in order to effect these changes. The women in Sweden fared slightly better than the women in the United States due to the extra environmental support provided by the medical and legal compensation system in Sweden, which allowed the Swedish women to reduce their work hours with less consequence to their economic situations.

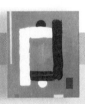

CASE ILLUSTRATION

Application of the Model of Human Occupation with a Client with Fibromyalgia

Dixie is a 42-year-old woman whose husband died in a car accident. She was driving the car and suffered multiple skin contusions and whiplash, but was wearing her seatbelt and was not critically injured. She lives with her two children. Dixie has worked as a Spanish teacher for 10 years. For the past six months, she has been experiencing chronic pain and fatigue that has limited her physical activity, and led to decreased muscle strength and endurance. After several missed days of work, Dixie consulted a rheumatologist, was diagnosed with fibromyalgia, and was referred to occupational therapy.

The occupational therapist began treatment with the Model of Human Occupation Screening Tool (MOHOST). This measure was selected to determine the extent to which fibromyalgia affected Dixie's everyday living. Then, strategies were developed to help Dixie maintain participation in her chosen activities while managing her symptoms and overall health.

Dixie's occupation participation ratings on the MOHOST indicated that she had a fair degree of occupational dysfunction (see Figure 17-1). In the areas where she made accommodations, she felt dissatisfied with herself. In the areas where she tried to keep her past routine, she failed to complete it and felt fully dissatisfied with her work. Currently, she has a low sense of control, low self-esteem, and feels unable to meet performance standards in most of her roles as a mother, friend, and teacher.

The Occupation Self Assessment (See Figure 17-2) was also administered in order to allow Dixie to indicate the importance of everyday

Motivation for Occupation				Pattern of Occupation				Communication and Interaction Skills				Process Skills				Motor Skills				Environment			
Appraisal of abilities	Expectation of success	Interest	Choices	Routine	Adaptability	Roles	Responsibility	Non-verbal skills	Conversation	Vocal expression	Relationships	Knowledge	Timing	Organization	Problem-solving	Posture & mobility	Coordination	Strength & effort	Energy	Physical space	Physical resources	Social groups	Occupational demands
F	F	F	F	F	F	F	F	F	F	F	F	F	F	F	F	F	F	F	F	F	F	F	F
A	A	A	A	A	A	A	A	A	A	A	A	A	A	A	A	A	A	A	A	A	A	A	A
I	I	I	I	I	I	I	I	I	I	I	I	I	I	I	I	I	I	I	I	I	I	I	I
R	R	R	R	R	R	R	R	R	R	R	R	R	R	R	R	R	R	R	R	R	R	R	R

Key:
F = Facilitates occupational participation
A = Allows occupational participation
I = Inhibits occupational participation
R = Restricts occupational participation

FIGURE 17-1. Dixie's Rating on the Model of Human Occupation Screening Tool (MOHOST)
© Cengage Learning 2013

occupations and set priorities for change. Together, Dixie and the therapist come up with the following goals and suggestions for her treatment process:

a. Work on values clarification to support problem-solving for her limitations.

b. Identify assistive devices or other resources that will help her with daily activities, such as housework.

c. Request reasonable accommodations at her workplace aimed at improving her ability to function at work.

Discussion

As a priority, Dixie and her therapist worked on clarifying Dixie's values so that she could be more aware of her situation and accurately identify her own limitations and impairments. Dixie was pleased when the therapist reassured her that fibromyalgia has not had a "detrimental" effect on raising her children. After hearing that, it allowed her to reduce her feelings of guilt and shame about the illness and to more actively seek assistance when necessary.

With consultation and feedback from her occupational therapist, Dixie requested a number of reasonable accommodations at work. The first was to be able to use Microsoft PowerPoint with voice activation instead of writing notes on the blackboard. By using the school's computer and projector, Dixie no longer had to bring heavy materials with her for lectures; all she needed for class was a flash drive.

Myself	Competence				Values			
	Lot of problems	Some difficulty	Well	Extremely well	Not so important	Important	Extremely important	Priority
Concentrating on my tasks.	X						X	
Physically doing what I need to do.	X					X		
Taking care of the place where I live.		X				X		
Taking care of myself.	X						X	1
Taking care of others for whom I am responsible.	X						X	2
Getting where I need to go			X			X		
Managing my finances.			X			X		
Managing my basic needs (food, medicine).		X				X		
Expressing myself to others.			X			X		
Getting along with others.		X				X		
Identifying and solving problems.		X				X		
Relaxing and enjoying myself.	X						X	
Getting done what I need to do.	X						X	
Having a satisfying routine.		X					X	
Handling my responsibilities.	X						X	3
Being involved as a student, worker, volunteer, and/or family member.	X						X	
Doing activities I like.		X			X			
Working towards my goals.	X						X	
Making decisions based on what I think is important.		X				X		
Accomplishing what I set out to do.		X				X		
Effectively using my abilities.		X					X	

FIGURE 17-2. Dixie's Ratings on the Occupation Self Assessment (OSA)
© Cengage Learning 2013

The therapist also taught Dixie several strategies of energy conservation. Dixie reported that the impairments were still affecting her life but that she had much more confidence in pacing her activities, asking for assistance, and making sure she made time for occupations that brought meaning and pleasure into her life.

EFFECTIVE USE OF SELF: THE INTENTIONAL RELATIONSHIP MODEL

Thus far, we have described how MOHO can serve as one important theoretical foundation when treating individuals with chronic pain. Equally important is effective client–practitioner communication, often referred to as *use of self* in occupational therapy (Punwar & Peloquin, 2000). Adequate information and good communication between therapist and client are a prerequisite for a successful intervention (Linton et al., 2005). In the following section, we will introduce the basic concepts of the Intentional Relationship Model (IRM) (Taylor, 2008) and its application to clients with pain.

The IRM was developed after a national study of 568 practicing occupational therapists in the United States (Taylor, Lee, Kielhofner, & Ketkar, 2007) and a qualitative exploration of 12 therapists who were nominated as exceptional in use of self by their peers (Taylor, 2008). IRM explains the concepts and skill set behind therapeutic use of self and how the relationship between therapist and client facilitates clients' occupational engagement. The model is designed to provide guidance for interpersonal reasoning and to address challenges in the day-to-day practice of occupational therapy.

IRM places the client and his or her interpersonal characteristics at the center of the therapeutic interaction. After the therapist achieves an informed understanding of the client as an interpersonal being, he or she then draws upon different aspects of his or her therapeutic personality, one-at-a-time, oftentimes sequentially, and in a deliberate and self-disciplined way. This process is referred to as *interpersonal reasoning*. It involves systematically selecting and applying one of six interpersonal modes (or aspects of the therapist's personality) based upon the client's interpersonal needs and characteristics as they interface with inevitable challenges and other key events that occur during therapy. The six interpersonal modes and a brief definition and example of each are listed in Table 17-1 (Taylor, 2008).

According to this model, the ideal is for a therapist to develop a capacity to accurately choose a single mode or a sequence of modes that best matches a client's interpersonal needs during therapy (Taylor, 2008). Additionally, the therapist should possess or develop the capacity to change modes as the client's interpersonal needs evolve over time. In addition to selecting the appropriate modes, the therapist must also utilize the modes in a way that is *emotionally congruent*. This means that the therapist's feelings and emotional intentions to use the mode must be reflected in his or her affect, body language, and tone of voice. The therapist should not hide behind a professional façade or otherwise mask his or her true feelings toward the client (unless those feelings would not serve a therapeutic purpose for the client, if revealed). The therapist who can use modes flexibly, interchangeably, and congruently is more likely to establish an open and mutually respectful and trusting relationship in therapy.

TABLE 17-1. The Six Interpersonal Modes as Applied to Clients with Pain-Related Disorder

Mode	Definition	Example
Advocating	Supporting a client's need for action, resources, or modifications to the social or physical environment, encouraging a client to express his or her needs to the therapist and to others.	Assisting a client with a chronic pain disorder in making a difficult phone call to his or her employer regarding an accommodation issue.
Collaborating	Asking a client broad and general questions so that he or she can make decisions, set goals, provide feedback, and direct his or her care, providing a client with different options from which to choose.	Asking a client experiencing acute post-surgical pain to make his or her needs known regarding what he or she would most like to get out of therapy today.
Empathizing	Striving to understand a client's perspective, validating negativity, making summary statements, mirroring a client's affect, asking gentle, value-free deepening questions.	Validating a client's reluctance to tell her partner when her pain begins to escalate during their hunting trips together.
Encouraging	Bolstering a client to improve his or her confidence, reinforcing a desired behavior through praise or reward, using humor to manage an awkward moment, entertaining a client, enjoying a moment with a client.	Praising a client with osteoarthritis for engaging in regular graded exercise as a means of improving joint range of motion and reducing pain.
Instructing	Orienting a client to the purpose and process of therapy, providing a rationale for using a specific assessment or intervention, explaining the evidence base behind what one is doing, structuring therapy so that the client knows what will happen next, explaining to a client how to do something, modeling how to perform a task, asking a rhetorical question to emphasize a point, setting a limit on a client, providing corrective feedback, providing one's professional opinion on a subject, or confronting a client about a maladaptive choice or behavior.	Educating a client with lupus-related pain about the value of energy conservation techniques, ergonomics, and assistive technologies.
Problem-solving	Asking a client strategic questions to expose and clarify his or her thinking, weighing pros and cons with a client, making lists, calendars, and plans to address a problem or dilemma.	Asking a client who is concerned about having to cancel a get-together because of a flare-up what a friend might advise him to do.

From Renee R. Taylor: *The International Relationship*. F.A. Davis, Philadelphia, © 2008, p. 147, adaption of Table 7-4, with permission.

A visual depiction of the Intentional Relationship Model is presented in Figure 17-3. There are four central elements in the model: the client, the therapist, the inevitable interpersonal events of therapy, and the occupation (Taylor, 2008). These will be discussed on the following pages as they apply to the assessment and management of pain in occupational therapy.

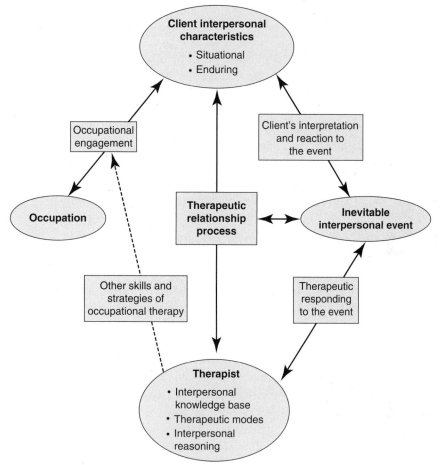

FIGURE 17-3. The Intentional Relationship Model
Source: From Renee R. Taylor: *The International Relationship.* F.A. Davis, Philadelphia, ©2008, p. 48, Figure 3-4, with permission.

1. *The client*

As described earlier, the client's interpersonal characteristics and needs drive the selection of modes and the overall application of the therapeutic reasoning process. To develop a positive relationship with the client, therapists should make every effort to know and understand the client's interpersonal characteristics from the moment that therapy begins. According to the model (Taylor, 2008), a client's interpersonal characteristics may be understood according to two dimensions.

a. Situational characteristics

b. Enduring characteristics

Situational characteristics reflect client's acute emotional reaction to an unexpected, stressful situation. For example, a newly disabled client may experience pain of a new type or severity, and as a result may express stress related to that experience by behaving in uncharacteristic ways toward others. On the other hand, enduring characteristics define a client's more stable, consistent interpersonal characteristics, and these do not vary as much across time or situation.

With respect to clients with impairments or disorders that involve pain, the model's distinction between situational and enduring characteristics becomes particularly important. This is because the stress that often accompanies pain can cause abrupt changes in a client's interpersonal behavior, causing, for example, an otherwise easygoing person to explode with anger when provided with corrective feedback during a bathing task. Alternatively, pain-related stress can exacerbate certain, difficult, interpersonal characteristics that are a more enduring part of a client's everyday personality. In either case, it is useful to understand the difference so that one does not overreact to a behavior and overpathologize it or underreact or fail to recognize a pattern that will likely continue within the relationship over time.

2. *The inevitable interpersonal events of therapy*

Interpersonal events are challenges or other occurrences within the relationship that, according to IRM, will occur inevitably during therapy. These events can create positive or negative stress and can also have a positive or negative impact on the relationship, depending on whether they are recognized and responded to in a way that is gratifying to the client. What is critical is that the therapist anticipates them, recognizes them, and responds appropriately. According to the IRM (Taylor, 2008), there are 11 categories of interpersonal events of which the expression of strong emotion is one.

For example, a client with lower back pain due to cancer-related bone metastasis may express strong emotion during the therapy, particularly if the session exacerbates the pain in some way. This client may cry, make angry statements or gestures, or lose emotional control during a therapy task or activity. Any experienced therapist working in cancer care should anticipate that this might happen, particularly if he or she is familiar with a client's interpersonal characteristics and knows that a specific intervention is likely to cause pain. The client might express strong emotion but the therapist should be prepared to respond with an interpersonal mode or set of modes that will support the client in coping with the situation.

3. *The therapist*

According to IRM (Taylor, 2008), the therapist is responsible for developing three core interpersonal capacities within therapeutic relationship.

a. A general interpersonal skill and knowledge base

b. Flexible and congruent application of the six interpersonal modes

c. A capacity for interpersonal reasoning

The therapist's interpersonal skill base is something that therapists accumulate through education in use of self, clinical supervision, and self-reflection about their experiences in clinical practice. As described earlier, the six modes define specific ways to interact with clients. Interpersonal reasoning is a stepwise process that allows the therapist to decide what to do and say in response to the inevitable interpersonal events of therapy, while taking into account the client's unique interpersonal characteristics (Taylor, 2008).

4. *The occupation*

In occupation-focused therapy approaches, the central focus of therapy is improving clients' occupational participation. Since clients' painful emotional reactions and attitudes during therapy also have the potential to influence their occupational engagement, the IRM is a supportive framework to which occupational therapists may refer. When applying the IRM in combination with existing models of practice, therapists can manage the psychosocial issues that are bound to occur in the therapy process.

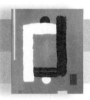

CASE ILLUSTRATION

Application of the Intentional Relationship Model

Ken is a 68-year-old man who has experienced multiple ischemic strokes affecting multiple vascular distributions, primarily the left anterior cerebral area. With the vascular distributions, he suffers from weakness on his right side and decreased alertness.

Ken has some degree of joint damage due to a pre-existing condition of osteoarthritis. When he is hospitalized, he is referred to an occupational therapist to increase mobility, to increase participation in activities of daily living (ADL), and to promote independence in self-care. However, soon after the first session involving dressing, Ken refused to participate in any further therapy sessions. He cited the severe shoulder pain he experienced while performing a one-handed dressing task. The therapist quickly realized that an interpersonal event had happened, so she decided to arrange a time for further discussion with Ken.

Discussion

Prior to her discussion with Ken, the therapist anticipated that Ken might express strong emotion during the session. Therefore, she considered beginning the session with the empathizing mode to put a significant amount of time and effort into striving to understand Ken's perspectives. As she expected, Ken disclosed his anger and frustration because the pain had continued two days after the OT session. The therapist was particularly conscious about when to talk and when to listen and, through a series of summary statements, she made sure Ken knew that she validated and supported his perspective and that she could empathize with all of the difficulties he was facing.

The therapist knew that she would have to wait before reinitiating work toward ADL training with Ken. Instead, she focused on what he wanted to talk about: his anxiety of the consequences of the stroke, his thoughts about how to live independently, and how to decrease any burden on his wife and children.

After talking about Ken's current situation, a feeling of mutual trust developed between Ken and his therapist. In time, they began to work together on ADL training. The therapist utilized the instructing mode to emphasize the educational aspects of the ADL. She started by sharing information about each strategy and breaking down the procedures step-by-step. She also demonstrated the tasks at first and physically guided Ken, providing assistance when needed. Sometimes Ken's pain and fatigue made it difficult for him to even want to try. The therapist respected his pace and shifted to the encouraging mode by frequent use of positive feedback and motivational words.

AREAS OF RELATED KNOWLEDGE: THE UNIQUE ROLE OF THE OCCUPATIONAL THERAPIST

Evidence suggests that involvement in purposeful activity may make pain easier to endure (Heck, 1988). Therefore, occupational therapists play important roles for clients with chronic pain. Engel (2009) suggests that occupational therapists may help clients with pain by applying the following methods: teaching and reinforcing socially appropriate pain expression, praising and reinforcing social interaction with issues other than pain, encouraging appropriate physical activity, introducing the patient to a support group, and teaching distraction as a method of pain management.

With respect to pain intervention and research, there are a number of areas of related knowledge that occupational therapists may explore alongside the client-centered, occupation-focused approaches described in this chapter. The most evidence-based of these approaches include interdisciplinary programs that feature cognitive-behavioral approaches as a central aspect (Taylor, 2006). The objectives of cognitive-behavioral approaches for pain clients include (Main, Sullivan, & Watson, 2007):

1. Countering demoralization by assisting patients to change their view of their pain from it being overwhelming to manageable.

2. Teaching clients the coping strategies and techniques to help them to adapt and respond to pain and its resultant problems.

3. Assisting clients in reconceptualizing themselves as active, resourceful, and competent.

4. Learning the associations between thoughts, feelings, and behavior to subsequently identify and alter automatic, maladaptive patterns.

5. Utilizing these more adaptive ways of thinking, feeling, and behaving.

6. Bolstering self-confidence and enabling clients to attribute successful outcomes to their own efforts.

7. Assisting clients in anticipating problems proactively and in generating solutions, thereby facilitating maintenance and generalization.

SUMMARY

Pain is a recurring, enduring symptom, which may cause stress and other negative emotional reactions and behaviors in clients (Taylor, 2006). Clients who receive occupation-focused, client-centered interventions may be more likely to experience positive outcomes in rehabilitation that include fewer somatic symptoms, lower perceived risk for pain, and shorter duration of pain (Jellema et al., 2006; Kielhofner, 2008). Through the application of assessments and interventions from the Model of Human Occupation (MOHO) and from the Intentional Relationship Model (IRM), therapists may achieve a more detailed clinical understanding of how to manage both the somatic and the psychosocial issues faced by clients with pain disorders. As therapists learn more about clients' experience of their symptoms and the meaning of their daily activities and behaviors, they may be able to develop increased empathy and intentionality, leading to improved therapeutic reasoning and well-planned interventions.

REVIEW QUESTIONS

1. What are the differences between acute and chronic pain?
2. What is the relationship between chronic pain and psychosocial dysfunction or mental illness?
3. Describe the Model of Human Occupation (MOHO) assessments for clients with pain.
4. What are the interpersonal modes of the Intentional Relationship Model and how does a therapist choose modes to enhance the therapeutic use of self when working with people in pain?

REFERENCES

American Occupational Therapy Association (AOTA). (2008). Occupational therapy practice framework: Domain and process (2nd ed.). *American Journal of Occupational Therapy, 62*, 625–683.

Bair, M. J., Robinson, R. L., Katon, W., & Kroenke, K. (2003). Depression and pain comorbidity: A literature review. *Archives of Internal Medicine, 163*(20), 2433–2445.

Baron, K., Kielhofner, G., Iyengar, A., Goldhammer, V., & Wolenski J. (2006). *A User's Manual for the Occupation Self Assessment (OSA)* (2.2 ed.). University of Illinois at Chicago.

Bay-Nielsen, M., Nilsson, E., Nordin, P., & Kehlet, H. (2004). Chronic pain after open mesh and sutured repair of indirect inguinal hernia in young males. *British Journal of Surgery, 91*, 1372–1376.

Beck, S. L., & Falkson, G. (2001). Prevalence and management of cancer pain in South Africa. *Pain, 94*(1), 75–84.

Berger, E. (2000). Late postoperative results in 1000 work related lumbar spine conditions. *Surgical Neurology, 54*, 101–106.

Block, A. R., Ohnmeiss, D. D., Guyer, R. D., Rashbaum, R. F., & Hochschuler, S. H. (2001). The use of presurgical psychological screening to predict the outcome of spine surgery. *Spine, 1*, 274–282.

Breivik, H. (2005). Opioids in chronic noncancer pain, indications and controversies. *European Journal of Pain, 9*(2), 127–130.

Braveman, B., Robson, M., Velozo, C., Kielhofner, G., Fisher, G. S., Forsyth, K., et al. (2005). *The Worker Role Interview (Version 10)*. Chicago, IL: Model of Human Occupation Clearinghouse: Department of Occupational Therapy.

Cardenas, D. D., Bryce, T. N., Shem, K., Richards, J. S., & Elhefni, H. (2004). Gender and minority differences in the pain experience of people with spinal cord injury. *Archives of Physical Medicine and Rehabilitation, 85*(11), 1774–1781.

Chang, V. T., Hwang, S. S., Feuerman, M., & Kasimis, B. S. (2000). Symptom and quality of life survey of medical oncology patients at a Veteran Affairs medical center: a role for symptom assessment. *Cancer, 88*(5); 1175–1183.

Cole, B. E. (2002). Pain management: Classifying, understanding, and treating pain. *Hospital Physician, 38*(6), 23–30.

Dewar, A. (2007). Chronic pain and mental illness: A double dilemma for all. *Journal of Psychosocial Nursing, 45*(7), 8–9.

Durand, M. J., Vachon, B., Loisel, P., & Berthelette, D. (2003). Constructing the program impact theory for an evidence-based work rehabilitation program for workers with low back pain. *Work, 21*, 233–242.

Engel, J. (2009). Pain management. In Crepeau, E. B., Cohn, E. S., & Boyt-Schell, B. A. (Eds.), *Willard and Spackman's occupational therapy* (11th ed.). Philadelphia: Lippincott Williams & Wilkins.

Heck, S. A. (1988). The effect of purposeful activity on pain tolerance. *American Journal of Occupational Therapy, 42*, 577–581.

Heit, H. A. (2003). Addiction, physical dependence, and tolerance: Precise definitions to help clinicians evaluate and treat chronic pain patients. *Journal of Pain and Palliative Care Pharmacotherapy, 17*(1), 15–29.

Henriksson, C. M. (1995a). Living with continuous muscular pain: Patient perspectives. Part I. *Scandinavian Journal of Caring Sciences, 9*, 67–76.

Henriksson, C. M. (1995b). Living with continuous muscular pain: Patient perspectives. Part II. *Scandinavian Journal of Caring Sciences, 9*, 77–86.

Hinrichs-Rocker, A., Schulz, K., Jarvinen, I., Lefering, R., Simanski, C., & Neugebauer, E. A. M. (2009). Psychosocial predictors and correlated for chronic post-surgical pain (CPSP)—A systematic review. *European Journal of Pain. 13*, 719–730.

Jellema, P., van der Horst, H. E., Vlaeyen, J. W., Stalman, W., Bouter, L., & van der Windt, D. (2006). Predictors of outcome in patients with (sub)acute low back pain differ across treatment groups. *Spine. 31*, 1699–1705.

Keefe, F., Abernethy, A., & Campbell, L. (2005). Psychological approaches to understanding and treating arthritis pain. *Annual Review of Psychology, 56*, 601–630.

Keller, J., Kafkes, A., Basu, S., Federico, J., & Kielhofner, G. (2005). *A User's Manual for the Child Occupational Self Assessment (COSA)* (2.1 ed.). University of Illinois at Chicago.

Keponen, R., & Kielhofner, G. (2006). Occupation and meaning in the lives of women with chronic pain. *Scandinavian Journal of Occupational Therapy, 13*, 211–220.

Kielhofner, G. (2008). *Model of human occupation: Theory and application* (4th ed.). Philadelphia: Lippincott Williams & Wilkins.

Kooijman, C. M., Dijkstra, P. U., Geertzen, J. H., Elzinga, A., & van der Schans, C. P. (2000). Phantom pain and phantom sensations in upper limb amputees: an epidemiological study. Pain, *87*(1), 33–41.

Kroenke, K., Bair, M. J., Damush, T. M., Wu, J., Hoke, S., Sutherland, J., & Tu, W. (2009). Optimized antidepressant therapy and pain self-management in primary care patients with depression and musculoskeletal pain. *Journal of the American Medical Association, 301*(20), 2099–2110.

Linton, S. J., Gross, D., Schultz, I. Z., Main, C., Côté, P., Pransky, G., et al. (2005). Prognosis and the identification of workers risking disability: Research issues and directions for future research. *Journal of Occupational Rehabilitation, 15,* 459–474.

Main, C. J., Sullivan, M. J., & Watson, P. J. (2007). *Pain management: Practical application of the biopsychosocal perspective in clinical and occupational settings* (2nd ed.). Edinburgh: Churchill Livingstone.

McCaffery, M., & Beebe, A. (1993). *Pain: Clinical manual for nursing practice.* Baltimore: C.V. Mosby Company.

Melzack, R. (1987). The Short-Form McGill Pain Questionnaire. *Pain, 30,* 191–197.

Moore-Corner, R., Kielhofner, G., & Olson, L. (1998). Work Environment Impact Scale (WEIS) (Version 2.0). Chicago, IL: Model of Human Occupation Clearinghouse: Department of Occupational Therapy.

Padilla, R., & Bianchi, E. M. (1990). Occupational therapy for chronic pain: Applying the Model of Human Occupation to clinical practice. *Occupational Therapy Practice, 1*(3), 47–52.

Pain Relief Foundation. (2003). Dealing with Pain Series: Central Post Stroke Pain. Retrieved from http://www.painrelieffoundation.org.uk/docs/painseries%20-%20cpsp.pdf

Parkinson S., Forsyth, K., & Kielhofner, G. (2006). *A User's Manual for the Model of Human Occupation Screening Tool (MOHOST)* (2.0 ed.): University of Illinois at Chicago.

Peolsson, A., Vavruch, L., & Oberg, B. (2006). Predictive factors for arm pain, neck pain, neck specific disability and health after anterior cervical decompression and fusion. *Acta Neurochirurgica, 148,* 167–173.

Punwar, J., & Peloquin, M. (2000). *Occupational therapy: Principles and practice.* Philadelphia: Lippincott Williams & Wilkins.

Robinson, K., Kennedy, N., & Harmon, D. (2011). Is occupational therapy adequately meeting the needs of people with chronic pain? *The American Journal of Occupational Therapy, 65*(1), 106–113.

Rudy, T. E., Lieber, S. J., Boston, J. R., Gourley, L. M., & Baysal, E. (2003). Psychosocial predictors of physical performance in disabled individuals with chronic pain. *The Clinical Journal of Pain. 19,* 48–30.

Sandqvist, J. L., Bjork, M. A., Gullberg, M. T., Henriksson, C. M., & Gerdle, B. U. C. (2009). Construct validity of the Assessment of Work Performance (AWP). *Work, 32,* 211–218.

Schneider, J. P. (2005). Chronic pain management in older adults: with coxibs under fire, what now? *Geriatrics, 60*(5), 30–31.

Serban, S. (2011). Drug abuse in the chronic pain patient. *International Anesthesiology Clinics, 49*(1), 135–145.

Sharp, J., & Keefe, B. (2006). Psychiatry in chronic pain: A review and update. *The Journal of Lifelong Learning in Psychiatry, 4*(4), 573–580.

Sherman, K. B., Goldberg, M., & Bell, K. R. (2004). Traumatic brain injury and pain. *Physical Medicine & Rehabilitation Clinics of North America, 17,* 473–490.

Strassels, S. A., McNicol, E., & Suleman, R. (2005). Postoperative pain management: A practice review, part 1. *American Journal of Health-System Pharmacy, 62*(18), 1904–1916.

Stucky, C. L., Gold, M.S., & Zhang, X. (2001). Mechanisms of pain. Proceedings of the *National Academy of Sciences of the United States of America, 98*(21), 11845–11846.

Taillefer, M. C., Carrier, M., Belisle, S., Levesgie, S., Lanctot, H., Boisvert, A. M., et al. (2006). Prevalence, characteristics and predictors of chronic pain following surgery: A cross-sectional study. *The Journal of Thoracic and Cardiovascular Surgery, 131*(6), 1274–1280.

Taylor, R. R. (2006). *Cognitive behavioral therapy for chronic illness and disability.* New York, NY: Springer.

Taylor, R. R. (2008). *The intentional relationship: Occupational therapy and use of self.* Philadelphia: F. A. Davis.

Taylor, R. R., Lee, S. W., Kielhofner, G., & Ketkar, M. (2007). Therapeutic use of self: A nationwide survey of practitioners' attitudes and experiences. *American Journal of Occupational Therapy, 63,* 198–207.

Tollison, C. D. (1993). Compensation status as a predictor of outcome in nonsurgically treated low back injury. *Southern Medical Journal, 86*(11), 1206–1209.

Wheeler, A. H., Stubbart, J. R., & Hicks, B. (2004). Pathophysiology of chronic back pain. eMedicine [Online]. Retrieved from http://www.emedicine.com/neuro/topic516.htm

Wolfe, F., Anderson, J., Harkness, D., Bennett, R. M., Caro, X. J., Goldenberg, D. L., Russell, I. J., & Yunus, M. B. (1997). A prospective, longitudinal, multicenter study of service utilization and costs in fibromyalgia. *Arthritis Rheum, 40*(9), 1560–1570.

Zalon, M. L. (2004). Correlates of recovery among older adults after major abdominal surgery. *Nursing Research, 53,* 99–106.

SUGGESTED RESOURCES

Taylor, R. R. (2009). Pain, fear, and avoidance: Therapeutic use of self with difficult occupational therapy populations. An online continuing education course presented for the American Occupational Therapy Association CEonCD Program. Bethesda, MD: AOTA.

Taylor, R. R. (2010). Occupation-focused interventions for people with fibromyalgia and other fatiguing conditions. An online continuing education course presented for the American Occupational Therapy Association CEonCD Program. Bethesda, MD: AOTA.

P A R T VI

Occupational Therapy Intervention in Mental Health

The three chapters in Part VI focus on the process of intervention, that is, the assessments, methods, and interpersonal strategies that practitioners use to understand and facilitate occupational engagement. The previous chapters detailed various psychosocial and developmental conditions and suggested clinical interventions specific to each condition, while these three chapters suggest the broad individual or group processes used in every intervention.

Chapter 18, "Assessment, Evaluation, and Outcome Measurement," in occupational therapy is new. This chapter emphasizes occupational engagement and prognosis, as well as the importance of collaborating with the client on meaningful and achievable goals. These ideas form the context or the background for a thorough assessment using occupational therapy tools. Chapter 19, "The Use of Psychosocial Methods and Interpersonal Strategies in Mental Health," focuses on personal methods and interpersonal strategies that are used in the context of the therapeutic relationship as well as the traditional occupational therapy processes of clinical reasoning and activity analysis used to deliver occupational therapy interventions. Chapter 19 follows and elucidates various sections of the Occupational Therapy Practice Framework.

Chapter 20, "Groups," focuses on group interventions including how to design, start, implement, and lead groups whether for individuals with various levels of function and conditions or for large communities, such as clubs or psychosocial rehabilitation programs.

Chapter 18 provides a very thorough description of the complex assessment process that is both client centered and occupation focused. The chapter also has a global focus having been written by Alison Laver-Fawcett, one of our international authors, and particularly highlights the need for understanding the terminology of evaluation and assessment, as well as understanding validity, reliability, and outcome measures.

Chapter 19 is updated to take into account the increasing emphasis on the therapeutic relationship and therapeutic use of self in treatment. Although therapeutic use of self has always been an intervention approach stressed in occupational therapy, it was not a focus of occupational therapy nor was the concept fully explored and explained. In the present chapter the concept is more fully explored. As well, while emphasizing how to develop, maintain, and use the self in a therapeutic relationship, it also discusses how to build and repair relationships.

In addition, the present chapter includes a more thorough discussion of the clinical reasoning process, particularly the ability to be attuned and mindful of our clients' and our own needs in an artful and skilled way. In addition, it discusses motivation—an implicit focus of occupational therapy in mental health settings—as a function of the clinical reasoning process.

Chapter 20, on the use of groups in occupational therapy, is updated to include large group and community treatments and psychoeducational and medical self-help groups in accordance with the Occupational Therapy Practice Framework. The chapter also discusses the contemporary paradigm of mindfulness and use of manualized therapy programs that have evidenced effective outcomes in mental health treatment.

Various research validates the existence of sensory processing disorders among people with psychiatric conditions, such as those with trauma histories and post-traumatic stress disorder (PTSD), pervasive developmental disorder (PDD), attention deficit hyperactivity disorder (ADHD), schizophrenia, or anxiety. Therefore, this chapter highlights new group sensory processing and sensory programs for mental health treatment.

Taken together the chapters provide thorough yet detailed instructions for evaluation, group, and individual treatment in occupational therapy. They also provide a thorough grounding and practical suggestions for developing, maintaining, and using the therapeutic relationship for successful treatment outcomes. Finally, they suggest evidence-based approaches in mental health care.

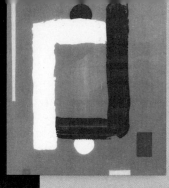

Chapter 18

Assessment, Evaluation, and Outcome Measurement

Alison Laver-Fawcett, PhD, DipCOT, OT(C), PCAP

■ KEY TERMS

assessment
carer
dynamic assessment
evaluation
goal setting
occupational profile
occupational prognosis

ongoing assessment
outcome
outcome measurement
reliability
standardized
validity

CHAPTER OUTLINE

Introduction
An Overview of Assessment
Key Concepts in Assessment and Evaluation
    What Are Standardized Tests?
    Reliability and Validity
The Assessment Process
    Problem Formulation
    Occupational Diagnosis
    Outcome Measurement
    The Complexity of Assessment
Considering the Different Purposes of Assessment
    Choosing the Best Sources of Information
    Dynamic Assessment
Summary

INTRODUCTION

The purpose of this chapter is to provide an overview of the assessment/evaluation process and discuss the importance of reliable and valid outcome measurement. Although some specific tools will be mentioned, the focus of this chapter is on the process. Much further detail on population and setting specific assessments may be found in the corresponding chapters of this book.

AN OVERVIEW OF ASSESSMENT

Occupational therapy assessment and **evaluation** should be client-centered and occupation-focused (World Federation of Occupational Therapists [WFOT], 2010). When working with people with mental illness, psychosocial distress, or who are at risk of developing related mental health problems, occupational therapists need to undertake a thorough **assessment** in order to understand the person's occupations; the psycho-emotional, sociocultural, cognitive-neurological, and physical determinants of the person's occupations (McColl et al., 2002); the person's needs, strengths, wishes, beliefs, values, habits, roles and routines; and the person's environment (physical, social, and cultural-institutional). The therapist should also consider a wide range of potential risks including risks to autonomy, medication management, relationships, risk of social isolation, loss of independence, loss of carer support, self-harm, suicide, risk of harm to others, and risk of abuse (psychological, financial, physical, sexual abuse). Information from the assessment is analyzed to understand how identified problems and risks are impacting on the person's ability to undertake desired and needed occupations and roles, and to assess his/her experience of quality of life. Figure 18-1 lists the tasks that are undertaken by the assessment therapist.

The assessment tasks listed in Figure 18-1 are not undertaken in a linear fashion. Referral information will prompt some initial thoughts about the information to be collected and the best sources and methods to use. Initial assessment data inform generation of hypotheses about the person's presentation, which in turn prompts further decisions about information required to test these hypotheses, additional sources of information to be accessed, and the most appropriate methods for data collection. Once the therapist feels that sufficient information has been collected to understand the person (i.e., his/her occupations, performance component skills/ deficits, roles, environmental contexts and risks), conclusions can be shared with the client and outcomes, aims, and goals can be negotiated to inform intervention. During intervention further information may come to light, which leads the therapist to a better understanding of the presenting problem or to the identification of additional problems that require further investigation. Ongoing assessment to review progress and the evaluation of **outcomes** will require the therapist to make further decisions about the information required and the best (i.e., the most efficient, valid, reliable, and pragmatic) sources and methods to implement.

1. Determine information required to make sound clinical decisions and clarify what information is to be collected.

2. Identify relevant sources for this information (client, carers, other professionals/staff).

3. Select assessment methods to be used to collect this information from these sources (interview, observation, questionnaires, review of client's records, dynamic assessment).

4. Choose appropriate standardized tests to support informal assessment methods (this might involve undertaking a review of the literature and/or test critique).

5. Undertake planned data collection procedures.

6. Score any standardized test data (this might involve totaling scores, converting raw scores, or plotting scores on a normative graph).

7. Analyze and synthesize data, including hypothesis generation and testing.

8. Interpret results and develop the occupational therapy diagnosis and prognosis.

9. Share/report the results, conclusions, and recommendations with the client and other stakeholders (orally and/or in writing; the therapist may be required to record summaries on to a computer database or electronic care record).

FIGURE 18-1. Assessment Tasks
Based on Laver-Fawcett (2007)

The roles of occupational therapists in psychosocial settings can vary from service to service and between countries. Whether the therapist delivers a more generic role (e.g., a mental health care coordinator in a community mental health team) or an occupational therapy specific role (such as an occupational therapist based in an occupational therapy department in an acute psychiatric hospital) will necessarily influence the scope of assessments, access to sources of information, and the selection of specific standardized assessment. For example, in the United Kingdom (UK), therapists providing more generic roles may need to undertake the FACE Core Assessment and Outcomes Package for Mental Health Services (Clifford, 2002), particularly the risk assessment within this package. There are particular issues to consider when assessing people with psychosocial problems beyond the person's ability to undertake an occupation. Therapists also need to consider the person's mental capacity, insight, and motivation to engage in occupations (e.g., a person with anorexia or depression may have the capacity, knowledge, and skills to shop and cook but may not be undertaking these). The therapist's clinical reasoning skills are critical to effective and efficient assessment and evaluation. Diagnostic reasoning (Rogers, 2004), ethical reasoning (Barnitt, 1993), and narrative reasoning (Mattingly, 1994) have particular relevance in psychosocial settings. It is very important to understand the person's lived experience and a phenomenological approach to data collection is often taken by occupational therapists working with people with mental health problems. Therapists develop through the novice to expert continuum (Higgs & Bithell, 2001) in refining interview and observation skills over time, gaining expertise in the therapeutic use of self, and administering and scoring of a range of standardized tests. (See Chapter 19 for further discussion.)

Without an effective assessment, occupational therapists are unable to develop realistic aims, collaborative and person-centered goals, and identify meaningful outcomes for intervention. Regardless of how expert a therapist is at providing interventions, there is a risk that the intervention will be useless if it is based on faulty assessment and decision-making regarding the person's needs, wishes, strengths, and problems. A valid and reliable baseline assessment is needed if the therapist wishes to measure the outcome of intervention and evaluate any changes over time. However effective the occupational therapy service is, its value is diminished if there is no evidence to support the assertion that it is an effective service. Evidence can come from service evaluation with the recipients of the occupational therapy service, their family/informal carers, and other key stakeholders (such as colleagues referring people to the service and/or colleagues who work with recipients of occupational therapy during intervention and after discharge).

One of the most important ways to demonstrate the worth of occupational therapy is by defining clear outcomes and measuring those outcomes to provide clear evidence of the effectiveness of the intervention. In many countries the drivers for **outcome measurement** are increasing. Funders of services and managers expect evidence of occupational therapy outcomes to be collected and available. Unsworth (2000) stated "current pressures to document outcomes and demonstrate the efficacy of occupational therapy intervention arise from fiscal restraints as much as from the humanitarian desire to provide the best quality health care to consumers. However, measuring outcomes is important in facilitating mutual goal setting, increasing the focus of therapy on the client, monitoring client progress, as well as demonstrating that therapy is valuable" (p. 147).

KEY CONCEPTS IN ASSESSMENT AND EVALUATION

As mentioned in the preface of this book, there are varying definitions of the terminology related to occupational therapy assessment and evaluation, which causes a dilemma for international communication in the field and for individual practitioners to communication the process. For the purposes of this chapter, the terminology presented is based on one of my previous publications and is presented in Table 18-1.

Therapists can draw on both qualitative and quantitative data using informal and/or standardized methods to make evaluative decisions. For example, a therapist might obtain self-report from clients through an informal interview to provide information on the balance of time spent across work, leisure, and self-care occupations. The therapist might combine this with a standardized interview, such as the Canadian Occupational Performance Measure (COPM) (Law et al., 2005), to explore clients' views of their performance and level of satisfaction with their occupational engagement. A standardized observational assessment, such as the Assessment of Motor Process Skills, AMPS (Fisher & Bray Jones, 2010a, 2010b), might be used to evaluate changes in a client's performance of a specific occupation, such as meal preparation. An aspect of

TABLE 18-1. Assessment, Evaluation, and Outcome Terminology

Assessment	Assessment is a process involving the selection and application of a range of informal and standardized methods (interview, observation, questionnaires, dynamic assessment, and document review) to collect information from relevant sources (the person, carers, and other staff) in order to provide an occupational profile, understand the person's skills and needs, and inform the negotiation of outcomes, setting of goals, and selection of therapeutic interventions. Assessment involves the ongoing review of the person, his/her occupations and environments, and the evaluation of the outcomes of therapeutic interventions and packages of care. Note that in the United States the Occupational Therapy Practice Framework (OTPF) (2008) defines assessment as a tool and evaluation as a process.
Evaluation	Evaluation is a component of a broader assessment process. Data is collected to inform judgments about amount, degrees or levels of a specific construct, component, or characteristic (e.g., level of independence), or to make a judgment about the degree to which an intervention has achieved the planned outcomes for a person or a group of people. Evaluation usually requires data to be collected at two time points in order to measure change over time. Evaluation may involve the translation of observations to numerical scores. Note that in the United States the Occupational Therapy Practice Framework (OTPF) (2008) defines assessment as a tool and evaluation as a process.
Outcome	An outcome is the measured or observed consequence of an action. It is of paramount importance for occupational therapists to differentiate between: a client's *desired outcome*; the *pre-determined outcomes* that a service is expected to deliver, as described in a service level agreement or commissioning contract; the *negotiated outcome* between a client and therapist, as articulated in a goal; and the *actual outcome*, which is the measured effects of a specific intervention or the effects of a multidisciplinary or interagency management plan for the client.
Outcome Measure	Outcome measurement is required to establish the effectiveness of an intervention for an individual or the effectiveness of an overall service for a population. Outcome measurement is undertaken by administering an outcome measure on at least two occasions to evaluate change over time in order to establish whether the intervention has achieved the anticipated outcome.

Adapted from Laver-Fawcett (2007)

evaluation is the formal measurement of therapeutic outcomes. The relationship between assessment, evaluation, and outcome measurement is illustrated in Figure 18-2.

There are a couple of terms in the rehabilitation literature that are used interchangeably with outcomes, these are *effects and indicators*. Law and McColl (2010) provide some clarity with their definitions of outcomes and effects. They define outcomes as "the indicators and assessments that occupational therapists use to show where occupational therapy has made a difference" (p. 2.) and they define effects as "the outcomes that occupational therapy can be successful in achieving as a result of intervention" (p. 2) and further explained that "the effects of occupational therapy are understood as an interaction of the person with the environment through the medium of occupation" (p. 5).

Problems with clients' dissatisfaction with an occupational therapy service can often arise because of unmet expectations. Part of the initial assessment process, therefore, must include establishing early on: "What are the client's desired outcomes?" Defining both the client's and the therapist's expectations has been

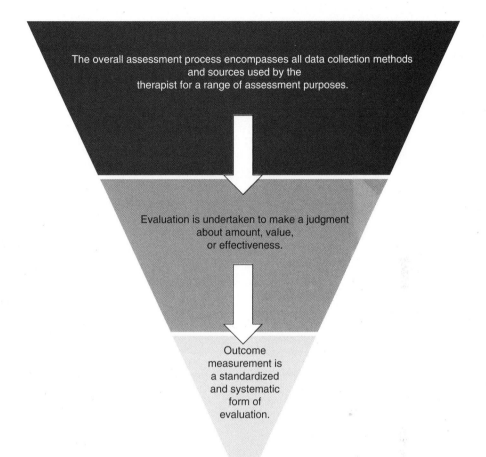

FIGURE 18-2. The Relationship Between Assessment, Evaluation, and
Outcome Measurement
Adapted from Laver-Fawcett (2007)

highlighted as an important part of "establishing a professional relationship with the
client" (Canadian Association of Occupational Therapists [CAOT], 1996, p. 86). If the
therapist believes the client's desired outcomes are unrealistic, or if some of the desired outcomes cannot be achieved within the parameters of the service the therapist
is employed to deliver, then a process of negotiation to identify and agree on more
realistic outcomes should be undertaken. Through this transaction the therapist and
client can set achievable goals for intervention and begin the intervention phase with
a shared understanding of the goal(s) and the outcome(s) they expect to achieve at
the end. Figure 18-3 summarizes the key steps for ensuring realistic outcomes are
identified, agreed, and measured.

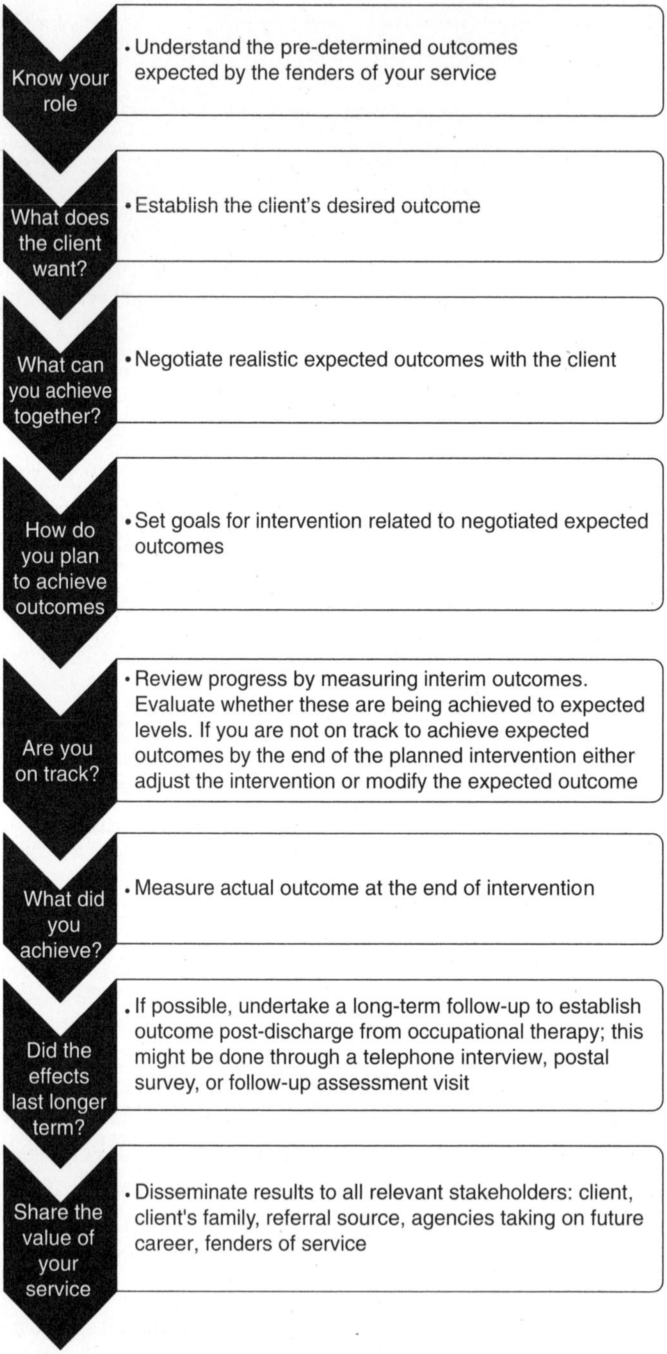

Know your role
- Understand the pre-determined outcomes expected by the fenders of your service

What does the client want?
- Establish the client's desired outcome

What can you achieve together?
- Negotiate realistic expected outcomes with the client

How do you plan to achieve outcomes
- Set goals for intervention related to negotiated expected outcomes

Are you on track?
- Review progress by measuring interim outcomes. Evaluate whether these are being achieved to expected levels. If you are not on track to achieve expected outcomes by the end of the planned intervention either adjust the intervention or modify the expected outcome

What did you achieve?
- Measure actual outcome at the end of intervention

Did the effects last longer term?
- If possible, undertake a long-term follow-up to establish outcome post-discharge from occupational therapy; this might be done through a telephone interview, postal survey, or follow-up assessment visit

Share the value of your service
- Disseminate results to all relevant stakeholders: client, client's family, referral source, agencies taking on future career, fenders of service

FIGURE 18-3. The Process of Identifying, Measuring, and Disseminating Outcomes

Cole, Finch, Gowland, and Mayo (1995) made the important point that while clinical outcome measures can be used to evaluate change over time they do not explain *why* the change has occurred. So outcome measures should not be viewed by therapists as the "be all and the end all" solution. Therapists need to interpret outcome measures in context through a wider assessment process in order to explore the mechanisms underlying a desired or observed change.

If several desired outcomes are identified it can be helpful to prioritize these (CAOT, 1996). It is often valuable to break down long-term desired outcomes such as "I want to get a full-time job" or " I want to have my own home" into a series of interim outcomes. Occupational therapists may negotiate with the client to breakdown the desired outcomes in terms of *short-, medium-,* and *long-term outcomes.* This can be particularly valuable when working with clients with psychosocial problems who will require occupational therapy input over months or years. The therapist must then work with the person to translate the outcome into goals for intervention. **Goal setting** is a very important process and helps to create "a mutual base from which to begin client-centred therapy" (Öhman & Asaba, 2009, p. 27). Sumsion (2000), following a study to agree on a definition of client-centered practice, recommended that "the client participates actively in negotiating goals which are given priority and are at the centre of assessment, intervention and evaluation" (p. 308). In order to be able to evaluate whether these goals have been achieved the therapist must articulate them so they can be measured. The SMART goal format is helpful in this regard (Griffiths & Schell, 2002, p. 232). SMART stands for:

S = Specific

M = Measurable

A = Achievable

R = Realistic

T = Time-bound

CASE ILLUSTRATION

Goal Setting with Jack

Jack is a 19-year-old man diagnosed with schizophrenia. He experienced his first episode of psychosis while studying law at university. During his illness, he moved back home with his parents. Jack's mother was a homemaker and his father worked as a lawyer. When he was first referred to the Early Intervention Team, he refused to go out of the house alone and so the occupational therapist visited Jack at home for his initial assessment. Initially, Jack was struggling to maintain a regular routine. Sometimes he did not get washed and dressed and spent the whole day in his room watching television and eating meals prepared by his mother. Jack reported he could not concentrate to read or to play video games (hobbies he previously enjoyed). Jack decided that he did not want to be a lawyer but asserted that he "wants to work towards getting a full-time job" (his desired outcome). In the past, he had undertaken a few part-time jobs in the school and during university holidays, but never had a full-time job. Jack and his occupational therapist discussed that in order to be successfully employed he needed to first work on his self-care, daily routine, social interaction, and leaving the house.

Discussion

It is important for clients to experience tangible successes on a daily and weekly basis. The therapist, therefore, developed graded goals for Jack linked to his negotiated outcomes in order to work towards Jack's long-term desired outcome of full-time employment. The short-, medium-, and long-term goals and interventions developed collaboratively with Jack are presented in Table 18-2. The therapist regularly reviewed Jack's progress with Jack and his parents by comparing what had actually been achieved during each week against his short-term goals. There was a six-month case review meeting with Jack, his parents, and the multidisciplinary team.

TABLE 18-2. Jack: Short-, Medium-, and Long-Term Goals and Interventions

Duration	Negotiated Outcomes	Intervention Goals
Short Term (first month)	By the end of the month Jack will be: ■ Getting up, washed, and showered every weekday morning. ■ Taking his prescribed medication every day. ■ Spending at least 4 hours a day outside of his bedroom.	■ Jack will get up and be showered and dressed by 12 noon at least 5 days per week. Jack's mother will record the time by which he is washed and dressed in a diary. ■ Jack is to take his prescribed medication everyday; he will be prompted and observed by his mother who will record when he takes his medication in his diary. ■ Jack will come out of his bedroom to watch television in the family room every afternoon by 1 pm for at least 2 hours. Time and duration is to be recorded by his mother in his diary.
Medium Term (months 2–5)	Within six months Jack will: ■ Be leaving the house at least five times a week. ■ Socialize with other people his own age. ■ Have improved levels of concentration and attention.	■ Jack will attend a day center for young adults with mental health problems three days per week and take an active part in individual and group activities at the day center for four months. His participation will be evaluated by self-report and staff report. ■ Jack will rejoin the local gym and exercise at least twice a week. ■ Jack will go out with a friend, or group of friends, at least once per week. ■ Jack will choose and attend an adult education class one evening per week.

TABLE 18-2. Continued

Duration	Negotiated Outcomes	Intervention Goals
Long Term (after 6 months)	■ Complete a one-year part-time course related to photography. ■ Successfully undertake a job as a volunteer at least one day per week for six months (Jack was to do this while studying part-time and attending the day center one day per week for ongoing support). ■ Successfully undertake a part-time job and hold it down for at least six months while studying part-time. ■ Secure full-time employment.	■ Develop a typed two-page curriculum vitae by (agreed date) with support from his parents and the therapist. ■ Book an appointment at the local job center and attend with one of his parents by (agreed date). ■ Seek five job advertisements of interest and draft applications to share with his parents and the therapist for feedback. Make amendments to applications based on feedback received. ■ Role play at least five interviews with the therapist, discuss feedback after each role play, and respond to feedback for improving interview technique.

They reviewed Jack's progress and his long-term goal to seek employment, rather than returning to study. Jack had achieved his short-term and medium-term outcomes, but he still wanted to seek full-time employment. To achieve success this outcome was broken down further.

What Are Standardized Tests?

A number of terms are used, often interchangeably, including *standardized test, standardized measure, standardized assessment, standardized instrument,* and *standardized tool*—the key word here is **standardized**. Testing is one method used by therapists to collect information. A standardized test provides a clear, systematic procedure for observing behavior or asking questions and describing obtained information in terms of fixed categories or a numerical scale. Standardized tests are used to collect objective, factual, and verifiable data (Asher, 2007). In some cases, the therapist's judgment is required to score and in this case clear scoring guidelines are needed to ensure inter-rater reliability. Research to develop a standardized test is a time consuming and rigorous process (Benson & Clarke, 1982). To be considered standardized, a test should be in the public domain (this could be a published test described in a journal article, purchased from a publisher, or made available by the author, perhaps through a website). The test should have a clear explanation of the specific purpose it was designed to address and the populations with which it can be used. There should be detailed instructions of how, where, and when it can be administered and a precise description of how to score the test and interpret the results. The research studies undertaken to develop the test should be described and/or referenced. For standardized tests there should be information available about the test's psychometric properties, with at least a summary of research related to the test's reliability and validity. In order for any measurement to be clinically useful it should meet two essential requirements: it must measure what the test-developers say it was designed to measure (this is known as *validity*), and this measurement must be made with a minimum of error (this is known as *reliability*). If it is a normative test then an explanation of how the normative data was obtained should be given and the norm tables should be included (Laver-Fawcett, 2007). Therapists should exercise vigilance regarding the selection and administration of tests and the ways in which they interpret and use test scores (Asher, 2007). This means therapists should have a good understanding of psychometrics and be able to critique a test and make informed judgments about its validity and reliability.

Norms have been defined by the American Occupational Therapy Association (AOTA) as "a standard, a model, or pattern for a specific group; an expected type of performance or behaviour for a particular reference group of persons" (as cited in Hopkins & Smith, 1993, p. 914). A *norm-referenced* (or normative) test, therefore, is "a test that is used to evaluate performance against the scores of a peer group whose performance has been described using a normative sample" (Laver-Fawcett, 2007, p. 423). In contrast, a *criterion-referenced* test examines performance against predefined criteria and produces raw scores that are intended to have a direct, interpretable meaning (Crocker & Algina, 1986).

Occupational therapists have a professional and ethical responsibility to remain up to date and use best evidence to support their assessment, evaluation, and the measurement of outcomes. This requires therapists to make time for continuing professional development (CPD) to review literature (e.g., studies that explore the psychometric properties of a test or the application of an existing measure in a new context or with a different population), seek training on specific measures, read test manuals, practice test administration, and develop a case to present to managers for funding to purchase tests with a strong evidence base. Recommended books and websites for these tasks are provided in the Suggested Resources at the end of the chapter.

Reliability and Validity

When tests are being standardized, research is needed to evaluate whether the test really measures what the test developer has set out to measure. This is known as **validity**. Tests also need to produce stable results over time and when used by different clinicians. This is known as **reliability**. It is critical that therapists are aware, and take into account, the reliability and validity of the standardized assessments they are using. Table 18-3 provides a summary of types of reliability and Table 18-4 is a summary of types of validity.

TABLE 18-3. DEFINITION OF KEY TERMS RELATED TO RELIABILITY

Reliability	■ Concerns how stable the results obtained on a test are under different circumstances. ■ How accurately the test scores obtained reflect the true performance of a person on the test (Ottenbacher & Tomchek, 1993). ■ Usually expressed as a correlation coefficient, percentage agreement, or level of significance (probability). ■ Perfect reliability results in a coefficient of 1.0 or 100% level of agreement and is hardly ever achieved.
Test–retest reliability	■ The correlation of scores obtained by the same person on two administrations of the same test and is the consistency of the assessment or test score over time (Anastasi, 1988). ■ Studies of test–retest reliability involve comparing scores obtained from at least two administrations of the test; the baseline administration and a retest administration (Laver-Fawcett, 2007). ■ The correlation coefficient for test–retest reliability must be at least 0.70 but for high levels of reliability 0.90 is required (Laver-Fawcett, 2007).
Parallel form reliability (equivalent/ alternative form reliability)	■ "The correlation between scores obtained for the same person on two (or more) forms of a test" (Laver-Fawcett, 2007, p. 424). ■ Coefficients ranging of at least 0.80, preferably 0.90 and above, are considered acceptable for parallel form reliability.
Inter-rater reliability	■ "The level of agreement between or among different therapists (raters) administering the test" (Laver-Fawcett, 2007, p. 422). ■ Coefficients of 0.90 or above or percentage agreement of 90% or above required for high inter-rater reliability.
Intra-rater reliability	■ "The consistency of the judgements made by the same test administrator (rater) over time" (Laver-Fawcett, 2007, p. 422). ■ Coefficients of 0.90 or above or percentage agreement of 90% or above required for high intra-rater reliability.
Internal consistency	■ "The degree to which test items all measure the same behaviour or construct" (Laver-Fawcett, 2007, p. 422). ■ Internal consistency studies explore if test items are measuring the same construct or trait and whether test items vary in difficulty.
Ceiling effect	■ "A ceiling effect occurs when the person scores the maximum possible score on a test and the test does not reflect the full extent of his/her ability" (Laver-Fawcett, 2007, p. 419).
Floor effect	■ "A floor effect occurs when a person obtains the minimum score on a test and the test does not reflect the full extent of the person's deficits" (Laver-Fawcett, 2007, p. 421).
Sensitivity	■ "The ability of a measurement or screening test to identify those who have a condition, calculated as a percentage of all cases with the condition who were judged by the test to have the condition: the 'true positive' rate" (McDowell & Newell, 1987, p. 330).
Specificity	■ "The ability of a measurement to correctly identify those who do not have the condition in question' (McDowell & Newell, 1987, p. 330).
Responsiveness to change	■ The measure of efficiency with which a test detects clinical change (Wright, Cross, & Lamb, 1998) ■ Does the test measure the amount of anticipated change in order to provide an appropriate measure of outcome?

TABLE 18-4. Definitions of Key Terms Related to Validity

Validity	■ Validity relates to the appropriateness and justifiability of the things supposed about a person's test scores and the rationale therapists have for making inferences from such scores to wider areas of functioning (Bartram, 1990). ■ Validity studies identify if the desired test domains and/or constructs are being measured (Asher, 1996). ■ Validity studies explore if test items address the desired test domains/constructs in the correct proportions (Asher, 1996).
Predictive validity	■ "The accuracy with which a measurement predicts some future event, such as mortality" (McDowell & Newell, 1987, p. 329). ■ If therapists need to make predictive judgments from the results of a test, then evidence of predictive validity is required.
Content validity (also referred to as *content relevance* or *content coverage*)	■ The degree to which a test measures what it is supposed to measure in terms of the appropriateness of its content as judged by "the comprehensiveness of an assessment and its inclusion of items that fully represent the attribute being measured" (Law, 1997, p. 431). ■ "Content validity is descriptive rather than statistically determined" (Asher, 2007, p. 19). ■ Content validity is often evaluated by a panel of people judged to be experts in the related field of assessment.
Content validity index (CVI)	■ CVI is calculated by dividing the proportion of items judged by the panel of experts to have content validity by the total number of items in that test. ■ The CVI for a specific test item is the proportion of experts who rated that item as valid. ■ For example, see study by Clemson, Fitzgerald, and Heard (1999).
Construct validity	■ "Involves the extent to which an assessment can be said to measure a theoretical construct or constructs" (Laver-Fawcett, 2007, p. 173). ■ "The ability of an assessment to perform as hypothesized (e.g. individuals discharged to an independent living situation should score higher on a self-care assessment than individuals discharged to a long-term care living situation" (Law, 1997, p. 431). ■ "Factorial validity may be considered with construct validity because it can identify the underlying structure and theoretical construct" (Asher, 1996, p. xxxi). ■ For example, see study by Baum and Edwards (1993).
Discriminative validity	■ "Relates to whether a test provides a valid measure to distinguish between individuals or groups" (Laver-Fawcett, 2007, p. 176). ■ Discriminative validity studies are undertaken for tests that have been developed to "distinguish between individuals or groups on an underlying dimension when no external criterion or gold standard is available for validating these measures" (Law, 2001, p. 287). ■ Discriminative validity study samples should be comparable in terms of significant factors (confounding variables), such as age, sex, ethnicity, educational level, and socioeconomic background (Laver-Fawcett, 2007).
Face Validity	■ Whether a test seems to measure what it is intended to measure (Asher, 2007) from the perspective of the person who is undertaking the test, the therapist administering the test, family members who may be observing the test administration, and other professionals who use the test results.

Why Is Reliability Important to Occupational Therapists?

The ability of the occupational therapist to monitor changes over time is particularly valuable. If the therapist is to be sure that any observed changes really relate to an actual change in the person (such as his/her level of independence in a particular activity), then the test used must provide stability over time as evidenced by research investigating test–retest reliability. There can be a practice effect with some of the tests that therapists use in psychosocial practice settings. In order to be sure that the change observed is not influenced by the person improving on the test from familiarity with the test items, some researchers develop two, or more, versions of the test. These versions of the same test are known as parallel (or equivalent/alternative forms). An example is the Middlesex Elderly Assessment of Mental State (MEAMS) (Golding, 1989), which has two forms (version A and B). For a therapist to feel confident about using more than one version of a test, research should show that the scores obtained by a person on one form of the test are consistent with scores obtained on the other version (parallel form reliability).

Sometimes different members of the multidisciplinary team will be responsible for assessing a person and/or the person's care may be passed between occupational therapists. Therefore, clinicians must administer a test and interpret the results in the same way so that any change obtained represents a genuine change in the person and not differences between the staff (inter-rater reliability). When the same therapist is using a standardized test across a caseload of clients or with the same person on different occasions, the way he/she administers, scores, and interprets the results of the test must be consistent and not fluctuate over time or between clients (intra-rater reliability).

A basic principle of test design is that a number of closely related observations will provide a more reliable estimate of a person's performance or behavior than just one observation (Fitzpatrick, 2004). However, for test developers there is a delicate balance to be struck between having sufficient test items to produce a reliable measure versus having so many items that people may become bored or fatigued undertaking the test, or that therapists may not use it because it is perceived to be too time consuming to administer. Internal consistency studies are undertaken to explore these issues.

Floor and ceiling effects can be a particular issue with people with learning disability or for people with dementia. It can also prove to be a problem when a test developed for one setting or population is used inappropriately in another setting or with a different population. When considering the specificity and sensitivity of a test, the therapist needs to decide whether a false positive or a false negative result will be problematic. With risk assessment it is often better to find a person does not have the identified risk rather than to have missed a risk that has been present and then leads to a hazard or incident. However, in psychosocial setting therapists should also be cognizant of the stigma that can be attached to psychiatric diagnoses and symptoms;

a false positive result that leads to an incorrect diagnosis could lead the person to experience discrimination or be provided with an incorrect intervention.

Therapists must make judgments about the acceptable amount of error that is reasonable and take the level of error indicated by evidence of reliability into account when drawing conclusions and making clinical decisions based on test results. The more critical the decisions being made (for example, about risk, capacity, or placement), the more important it is that the test being used has high levels of reliability.

Why Is Validity Important to Occupational Therapists?

In psychosocial occupational therapy many of the things occupational therapists need to assess and measure are not directly observable. In particular, therapists are interested in how people think, feel, and process experiences and information. Therapists draw upon theories and models to try to categorize and understand such internal processes. Theoretical constructs (e.g., mood, perception, pain, cognition, and volition) are, therefore, key to our understanding of human experience. Test items are developed to: elicit self-reported descriptions related to internal processes; present inputs that the person is hypothesized to respond to in particular ways; or collect proxy reports of behaviors that the theory proposes to be outward manifestations of internal process. Therapists should expect to find a clear statement explaining the underlying assumptions regarding the relationships between observations of behavior collected for the test and related concepts of function in any standardized test that uses observed behavior as an indicator of functioning related to theoretical constructs about unobservable areas of function.

It is important not to presume that tests provide data that can lead to valid predictions, and therapists should look carefully at the results of longitudinal follow-up studies to check the evidence that the test results agree with the predicted future outcome or criterion. The more important the decisions made from the results of the test, the more critical it is that research evidence supports the inferences, and related interventions and care plans, being made. This is particularly true to assessments used to assess the risk of self-harm or harm to others. Research on the Beck Scale for Suicide Ideation (SSI) (Beck, Kovacs, & Weissman, 1979) illustrates this point. Several years after the development of the SSI, Beck, Steer, Kovacs, and Garrison (1985) reported on a longitudinal study of 207 people who had been identified as suicide ideators. Their research showed that the SSI did not predict eventual suicide and the wording of the SSI items was changed to improve predictive validity. Further research found the Beck's Hopelessness Scale (Beck & Steer, 1988, revised 1993) was a better predictor of suicide risk. Asher (2007) reports that research related to the Beck's Hopelessness Scale "has supported the correlation of scores with measures of depression and suicidal intent and ideation" (p. 577) and stated that "the scale is reported to be a powerful predictor of suicide risk" (p. 577). It is noted that later research (Brown,

Beck, Steer, & Grisham, 2000) has established predictive validity of the SSI for completed suicide in patients seeking outpatient psychiatric treatment.

For discriminative tests, therapists should expect studies to ensure populations of people perform differently on the test and the test actually discriminates as expected; for example, do people with dementia obtain scores indicating a greater degree of memory deficit, than a sample of matched norms or people with depression?

While face validity is not considered a psychometric property in the technical sense (Laver-Fawcett, 2002), it is very important to occupational therapists. This is because administering a test with poor face validity can cause the person to experience test anxiety, to misunderstand the purpose of the assessment, and/or can negatively impact on rapport with the therapist. Good face validity is thought to have indirect effects on the outcome of a person's test performance; Bartram (1990) considered that facilitating rapport between the test and the test-taker could increase reliability. In addition, determining a person's motivation to engage in an assessment to the best of his/her ability is critical to obtaining valid and reliable test results because "people are more likely to take seriously activities which seem reasonable and which they feel they understand" (Bartram, 1990, p. 76).

In terms of client-centered practice, therapists should always try to select tests with good face validity and to explain thoroughly the purpose and nature of the test to their clients before testing. This is even more critical when working with people who are anxious or experiencing paranoid ideation. With these client groups it is particularly important that the testing experience is completely transparent; otherwise anxiety levels can be increased or the person might feel the therapist has a hidden motive behind the test administration. Considering that client centered practice is at the heart of the occupational therapy profession (WFOT, 2010), there is a surprising lack of face validity studies conducted to explore the face validity of occupational therapy standardized tests (Laver-Fawcett, 2007). This is an issue because occupational therapists have negatively critiqued tests that contain items perceived to lack relevance or meaning to their clients (e.g., Law, 1993). Face validity has a strong link to clinical utility.

THE ASSESSMENT PROCESS

Assessment, evaluation, and outcome measurement should be core elements of a robust occupational therapy process with any client group. For the purposes of this chapter, the occupational therapy process as described by Creek (2003) and outlined in Figure 18-4 is used as an organizational framework.

It is particularly important in psychosocial occupational therapy that the therapist explains who he/she is, his/her role within the mental health service, the purpose of the proposed assessment, how the information collected with be used, and with whom will assessment information be shared. The issue of confidentiality

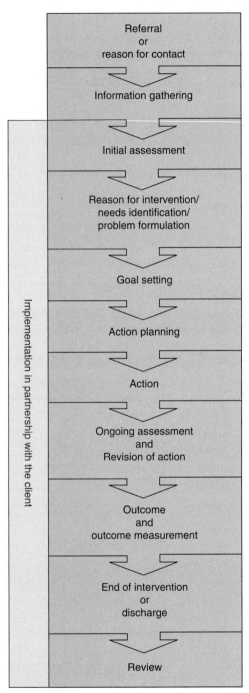

FIGURE 18-4. The Occupational Therapy Process

Reproduced from Creek, J. (2003). *Occupational therapy defined as a complex intervention* (p. 16). London: College of Occupational Therapists

should be explored openly at the outset. If relevant to the service, the therapist should seek permission to share information provided by the client with other members of the multidisciplinary team. The therapist should also explain up front that confidentiality might be broken under specific circumstances; for example, if the assessment reveals the person is contemplating suicide or self-harm or there might be a serious risk to the safety of others. Permission to involve the person's family in the assessment process and/or to share the results of the assessment with the person's family might also be sought at this point, although for some clients it may be better to develop rapport and undertake initial assessment before the subject of involving their family is broached.

Therapists should carefully plan the timing of each element of their assessment. Early on in the occupational therapy process therapists need to gather information that informs their thinking behind the approach to initial assessment. Initial assessment involves screening the referral information to assist the therapist to set some parameters around the presenting case and set the context for the presenting problem. The first contact with the person is often through an informal initial interview. The initial interview is designed to enable the therapist to build rapport with the person and start a descriptive assessment to get an overview of the person, his/her situation and the presenting problem. During the initial assessment period the therapist chooses the method for collating all the assessment information (this might be an electronic data base or electronic care record, or a data collection form developed for a specific service, or descriptive entries in the person's occupational therapy record or medical notes). The initial assessment may lead to more detailed assessment of particular areas, which can include the use of standardized tests.

An important decision to be made at the beginning of the assessment process is whether to take a "top–down" or "bottom–up" approach (Trombly, 1993). For therapists working with people with psychosocial problems and mental health diagnoses, a top–down assessment approach is usually the approach of choice. Some assessments simultaneously collect data from several levels of function, but usually an assessment tool or strategy just focuses on data at one or two levels of function. The approach will influence the order in which therapists use assessment methods and administer specific tests. For therapists referring to the ICF (WHO, 2002) as a framework for organizing assessment and evaluation, a top–down approach would involve beginning the assessment at the levels of participation, exploring the contextual and environment factors, and then considering the level of activities and body functions and structures.

The overall purpose of the assessment is to develop an **occupational profile** for the person; this provides "an understanding of the client's occupational history and experiences, patterns of daily living, interests, values, and needs . . . problems and concerns about performing occupations and daily life activities are identified, and the client's priorities are determined" (AOTA, 2008, p. 646). The client's priorities are explored in depth so the therapist can identify the person's desired outcomes. More detailed assessment helps the therapist to analyze the underlying causes of any reported dysfunction in occupational engagement, habits, routines, or roles and to define and describe the problems that are to form the focus of intervention. This often involves an assessment of some aspect of occupational performance. At this point, "actual performance is often observed in context to identify what supports performance and what hinders performance. Performance skills, performance patterns, context or contexts, activity demands, and client factors are all considered, but only selected aspects may be specifically assessed" (AOTA, 2008, p. 646). At the end of this assessment process, outcomes are negotiated between the client and the therapist and these can then form the basis for goal setting.

Problem Formulation

Opacich (1991) outlined a six-stage occupational therapy problem-oriented clinical reasoning process, which involves the therapist in:

1. Problem setting (context).
2. Framing the problem(s).
3. Delineating the problem(s).
4. Forming hypotheses.
5. Developing intervention plans.
6. Implementing treatment.

Therapists work through a problem-oriented reasoning process to analysis the complex situations and problems described by their clients and to identify the most probable underlying causes of reported or observed problems. Causation is critical to understand, as it is the driver for setting appropriate aims and goals and selecting the most effective strategy for intervention. Hypothesis generation and testing are key elements of diagnostic reasoning. In occupational therapy, diagnostic reasoning "is applied to profession-specific concepts . . . such as occupational performance" and "as diagnosticians, therapists seek to learn about a patient's functional performance and to describe it so that intervention can be initiated" (Rogers & Holm, 1989, pp. 8–9). Rogers and Holm (1991) defined a hypothesis as a tentative explanation of the cause(s) of dysfunction. The delineation of the observed/reported problem as a hypothesis involves the acquisition and interpretation of cues drawn from the assessment data. This may involve further assessment, including the administration of a standardized test.

Occupational Diagnosis

Once a thorough assessment has been undertaken, the therapist is able to synthesize the information and produce a unique occupational therapy diagnosis for the person. An occupational diagnosis is a "concise summary of a client's disruptions in occupational role that are amenable to occupational therapy" (Rogers, 2004, p. 18). It "refers to both the cognitive processes used by the occupational therapy practitioner to formulate a statement summarizing the client's occupational status, and the outcome of that process, the diagnostic statement" (p. 17). The product of diagnostic reasoning is an occupational therapy diagnosis. This is different from a medical diagnosis as it moves beyond the pathology to explain how the psychiatric diagnosis impacts on occupational performance and postulates causes of observed/reported dysfunction that may identify performance component deficits and/or contextual barriers. A diagnosis (such as hallucinations associated with schizophrenia) formulated from psychiatric assessment tells us nothing about the impact the experience of hallucinations is having on the person's ability to engage in needed and desired occupations and roles, neither does it identify the person's motivation to overcome the challenges posed by the nature of the hallucinations nor his/her level of insight.

Because many domains of concern in psychosocial occupational therapy cannot be observed in many instances the occupational diagnosis is not the definitive answer but a "best guess." Roberts (1996) acknowledged that occupational therapists cannot solve problems in the complete way that a mathematician solves a mathematical problem and stated that "there is not necessary a right answer to problems posed by humans who are ill" (p. 233). Constructing a diagnostic statement can help therapists to organize the data collected and unpackage their occupational diagnosis in a transparent and logical way. It can be useful for sharing the results of the assessment with the person, his/her family, and the multidisciplinary team.

According to Rogers (2004) the "diagnostic statement" should consist of four components: "descriptive (functional problem) + explanatory (aetiology of the problem) + cue (signs and symptoms) + pathological (medical or psychiatric)" (p. 19). The descriptive component of the diagnostic statement should describe the specific deficits identified at each level of function (i.e., participation, activities, body function, and structure) that are impacting on the person's ability to engage successfully in their chosen roles and occupations. This helps the therapist to focus on identified problems that are to be addressed through occupational therapy intervention.

The explanatory component of the diagnostic statement summarizes the therapist's hypothesis or hypotheses about the cause(s) of the problem presented in the descriptive component (Rogers, 2004). A person's problem might result from the interaction between several impairments or barriers, so there may be more than one cause identified in the explanatory component. Causes might relate to sensory impairments (e.g., visual impairment, hearing loss), physical impairment (e.g., stiffness, tremor, pain), cognitive impairment (e.g., attention deficit, short-term memory impairment), affective impairment (e.g., lack of motivation, low mood), physical environmental barriers (e.g., an unfamiliar environment or architectural hindrance), and/or social environmental barriers (e.g., the restrictive attitude of a family member, stigma).

The cue component of the diagnostic statement is where the therapist summarizes observed and reported signs and symptoms. These signs and symptoms are used to form hypotheses about the nature and cause of the identified problem. Information about psychosocial symptoms (e.g., feelings of anxiety, fear, sadness, apathy) is most often gained from the person's self-report (via interview or self-rating scales) and/or by proxy report from family members/carers.

The pathologic component of the diagnostic statement is provided to identify the pathological cause, if known, of the occupational performance deficits. This aspect of the diagnostic statement is often related to the psychiatric diagnosis). The pathologic component is a useful aspect of the diagnostic statement because "the nature of the pathology, the prognosis and pathology related contraindications establish parameters for . . . therapy interventions" (Rogers, 2004, p. 19). Occupational therapy interventions need to be developed to address the underlying cause of the problem (provided in the explanatory component) and will be influenced by a range of factors, such as whether the person has a long-term irreversible condition (e.g., a diagnosis of Alzheimer's disease) or has been diagnosed with a potentially curable illness (e.g., depression, phobia, anxiety). Table 18-5 outlines the components of the diagnostic statement as they relate to the assessment of a client with dementia.

The aims of occupational therapy intervention are clarified following assessment and will depend on the negotiated outcomes, the nature of the person's condition, and the prognosis. The aims help to identify the level of expected change and the direction of travel. The aims may involve maintenance, prevention, reduction, development and/or increase (College of Occupational Therapists [COT], 2009):

- *Improvement* in performance component skills, occupational performance, and/or engagement in roles.
- *Delayed deterioration* in performance component skills, occupational performance, and/or engagement in roles.
- *Maintenance* in performance component skills, occupational performance, and/or engagement in roles.
- *Prevention* of secondary disability/anticipatory action (e.g., through pacing techniques, provision of aids and adaptations, assistive technology, or by explaining to an employer his/her responsibilities related to mental health legislation to prevent discrimination).
- *Reduction* of symptoms or behaviors (e.g., self-harm, aggressive verbalizations, agitation, wandering, anxiety, depression) and/or reduction of environmental barriers to occupational performance (e.g., working with families, friends, and employers to reduce stigma associated with a psychiatric diagnosis).

TABLE 18-5. Application of the Diagnostic Statement

Frank is a 73-year-old gentleman with dementia. He lives at home with his wife, Joan. Frank has been referred to the occupational therapist in the community mental health team to assess his functional ability and provide education and support to his wife. Desired outcome: Frank values his privacy and dignity and wants to get dressed on his own.

Descriptive component	Frank is unable to get dressed independently. He needs verbal prompting to initiate and stay focused on the activity. He has difficulty choosing what to wear. He benefits from the visual cue of clothing laid out on his bed. His physical ability to put on clothes and doing up fastenings remains intact.
Explanatory component	Related to the following process deficits: ■ Initiation (unable to initiate dressing without verbal prompting). ■ Attention (difficulty maintaining attention on dressing activity until he has finished dressing). ■ Selecting (difficult selecting appropriate items of clothing needed to get dressed). ■ Judging (unable to judge the appropriateness of clothes for the occasion). ■ Orientation (disoriented to the season and weather outside). ■ Short-term memory impairment (unable to remember why he had entered the bedroom, unable to remember his wife's instruction to get dressed).
Cue component	As evidenced by the following descriptions provided by Joan, Frank's wife: *"I'll say to Frank, 'Well, are you going to get dressed now dear?' and he heads off to our bedroom as if he intends to get dressed and can be in there for ages, but then comes out still in his pajamas. Other times he might wander out in his underwear and start doing something completely different. Sometimes after I've reminded him several times he does get dressed but he'll be wearing completely the wrong clothes for the occasion, and then I have to get him undressed to put on more suitable clothes and he can get quite cross with me if I do that!"* As evidenced by the following self-report from an interview with Frank: Frank finds it humiliating when his wife *"tells me off for wearing the wrong stuff."* He reported: *"I do think about getting dressed but then I often get a bit distracted on the way to the bedroom, and I'll get doing something else so I forget all about getting dressed until my wife nags me again."* He reported that when he goes into the bedroom he finds it hard to choose what to wear and feels *"overwhelmed by all the clothes"* when he opens the wardrobe door, and *"anxious that I'll get it wrong again."* As evidenced by the following signs identified through observational dressing assessment: ■ Frank wanders into the bedroom, stands staring at the wardrobe for five minutes, and then walks out of the bedroom without getting dressed. ■ Frank asked the therapist *"What was I supposed to be doing?"* ■ When prompted to choose some clothes to wear, Frank selected clothes that were inappropriate for the weather (shorts and T-shirt, when it was November and very cold and icy outside). ■ When clothes were laid out on his bed and Frank was prompted to put on each item of clothing in turn, he was physically able to put on each garment.
Pathologic component	Owing to Alzheimer's disease.

- *Development* of new skills (e.g., coping skills, communication skills, social skills, relaxation techniques).

- *Increase* (e.g., level of independence in a particular activity, self-confidence, motivation, resilience, or social interaction).

Goal setting is undertaken once the therapist feels sufficient assessment data has been obtained. Goals should be negotiated with the person and, once agreed, should be linked to clearly defined outcomes. Öhman and Asaba (2009) discussed how effective goal setting can be "a demanding task, especially when the client is unsure about what he or she want . . . the client needs to be mindful of what is genuinely meaningful to him or her for the [goal setting] process to be client centred" (p. 27). Therefore, therapists may need to reflect back to the person's information provided through interviews and self-report assessments his/her identified problems, wishes, and desires and a starting point for client-centered goal setting. For appropriate goals for occupational therapy intervention to be identified, the client needs to have a clear understanding of the purpose of occupational therapy (Öhman & Asaba, 2009). Therefore, when setting goals, therapists should discuss with the person what changes may be possible for him/her to achieve through occupational therapy. This is an articulation of the occupational therapist's prognosis. The **occupational prognosis** is based on predictions of the person's likely response to occupational therapy intervention and the degree to which identified contextual facilitators and barriers may impact progress toward achieving the person's desired outcomes. In psychosocial occupational therapy, therapists may need to develop goals over several sessions in order to be sure that the most pertinent and client-centered goals are set, to prioritize these goals, and to formulate the goals in a way that allows them to be effectively evaluated. As previously discussed, the SMART goal format (Griffiths & Schell, 2002) is advised as this supports the evaluation of goals over time.

If baseline information related to these agreed outcomes has not already been obtained during the initial assessment, then baseline measures should be undertaken before the therapist moves into the planned actions necessary to provide the intervention. Initial assessment data are often used by therapists to provide a baseline. These data are then used for comparison during ongoing assessment or when measuring outcomes at the end of the intervention.

Therapists need to evaluate clients' progress during intervention through **ongoing assessment** (AOTA, 2008). It is critical that a therapist monitors how the client reacts and responds to intervention at regular points throughout the intervention process and engages the client in collaborative review of progress toward the agreed goals. This is undertaken to check whether the intervention is having the planned effect and/or whether the person's needs and goals are being adequately met. If necessary, the therapist may need to modify the planned intervention if the expected progress is not being made.

Outcome Measurement

Toward the end of the occupational therapy process, outcomes should be measured again and the actual effects of intervention achieved documented and shared with the client and key stakeholders. For some clients the therapist undertakes a follow-up assessment. It is valuable to undertake a further evaluative review after discharge in many cases. This can include further outcome measurement to ascertain longitudinal outcomes and enables the therapist to assess whether progress achieved through intervention has been maintained and whether the person's functioning has improved, deteriorated, or reached a plateau.

The Complexity of Assessment

Human beings are unique and very complex. Human function is not static and function is influenced by many factors. It is, therefore, very useful to turn theoretical models of occupational therapy and interdisciplinary models of function to aid the systematic assessment of all relevant aspects of the person and his/her functioning. Mosey (1974) proposed a biopsychosocial approach to understanding health and well-being for occupational therapists as an alternative to the medical model and other health models that were shaping therapists' practice at that time (Finlay, 2004). The biopsychosocial approach is now more widely accepted across health and social care disciplines and the World Health Organization (WHO, 2002) has proposed an "integrated biopsychosocial model of human functioning and disability" (p. 19) as the foundation for its International Classification of Functioning, Disability, and Health (ICF). Occupational therapists were involved in the development of the ICF (Brintnell, 2002) and since publication, the ICF has been adopted by some occupational therapists. As client-centered practitioners, there is a good fit between occupational therapy practice and the ICF model's mandate to place attention in health evaluation and research to insider perspectives of people with disability (McGruder, 2004; Creek, 2003). Law and Baum (2001) explored how the ICF could be applied to occupational therapy measurement, both for assessing individuals and for wider measurement contexts at a societal level when working with organizations such as schools, day care facilities, and industry. The College of Occupational Therapists (2004) explored how the ICF concepts could be embedded in the structure and process of occupational therapy practice and provided examples of standardized assessments for ICF levels. The ICF can be used by clinicians to increase effective communication and understanding (Brintnell, 2002) and the application of the ICF in occupational therapy practice "encourages a powerful dialogue with funders and managers and provides a means of communication with [clients] and their families" (McDonald, Surtees, & Wirz, 2004, p. 299).

Occupational therapy models, frames of reference, and wider models used in a particular setting, have a significant influence on therapists' choices when selecting the foci of their assessments and the standardized tests and outcome measures they utilize. Hemphill-Pearson (2008) asserted "that more than one theory and more than one frame of reference can be used to develop the patient's occupational profile" (p. 5). In clinical practice many occupational therapists describe drawing on a range of conceptual frameworks to inform their clinical reasoning and decision making. However, in some mental health settings therapists find the selection of a particular model, for example, the Model of Human Occupation (MOHO) (Kielhofner, 2008), the Person-Environment-Occupation Model (PEO) (Law et al., 1996), and the Canadian Model of Occupational Performance and Engagement (CMOP-E) (Townsend & Polatajko, 2007), to guide their assessments, interventions, and outcome measurement helps to provide a focus and coherence for their practice.

The occupational therapist needs to consider: the person's capacity and motivation to perform; how function is impacted by the demands of the task, activity, occupation, or role the person wants or needs to do; and whether functioning is being supported or restricted by a wide range of environmental actors. Facilitators of function can include family, friends, and wider social supports; societal acceptance; other people's level of understanding of mental wellness and mental health problems; and legislation to prevent discrimination against people with psychiatric diagnoses. Barriers to function can include stigma, social exclusion, institutionalization, a culture of dependency, lack of understanding, paternalistic attitudes of mental health professionals, and lack of expectations for recovery.

Given the complexity of people's occupations, roles, environments, and performance component functioning, occupational therapy assessment and evaluation are likewise complex. To be an effective, efficient, and person-centered practitioner when working with people with psychosocial problems means that the occupational therapist needs to be able to tailor the assessment, evaluation, and outcome measurement to each person and take a holistic, integrative view (Hemphill-Pearson, 2008). Therefore, occupational therapists need to develop a range of skills and a tool-kit of data collection methods and standardized tests. Therapists need to be able "to select and use assessments from a broad repertoire to achieve an integrative view of patients with emotional disorders" (Hemphill-Pearson, 2008, p. 3). Occupational therapists working with people with psychosocial needs should draw on multiple sources of information at different points in time. They need to be able to synthesize a wide variety of data in order to draw conclusions, which can be shared with their clients and with other people delivering health and social care to their clients.

Occupational therapists may work in a wide range of practice settings including more traditional clinical environments (such as hospitals, outpatient clinics, and health centers) and community settings (such as the person's home, school, supported housing, leisure club, or work environment). The practice setting(s) can have a significant influence on the nature of the assessment process, the resources available to support assessment and evaluation, and the specific standardized tests and assessment methods the therapist chooses to implement.

CONSIDERING THE DIFFERENT PURPOSES OF ASSESSMENT

Occupational therapists undertake assessment for a wide variety of reasons. It is important to know why you are undertaking an assessment at a particular point in time. Therapists should be very clear about:

- *Why* they are doing the assessment.
- *Where* is the best place to undertake the assessment.
- *When* is the best time to assess.
- *What* do they plan to do with the results from an assessment.
- *Who* will have access to the results afterward.

If the therapist is unsure of the answer to any of these questions it is helpful to think about the underlying driver for the assessment. For example: Will the assessment inform clinical decision making? Will it be used as a baseline for measuring outcomes? Will it be used to set goals for intervention? Is it required to establish final outcomes from intervention? Is it needed for review to monitor interim change and ascertain if the intervention is progressing as planned? Is the assessment needed to establish whether the client has a specific problem or diagnosis? Does the therapist need to predict level of risk, for example, to make a recommendation about safe discharge? In terms of disseminating the results of the assessment: Will the results be written up in a report or in the client's notes, or both? With whom will the assessment results be shared? his/her family? the referring doctor? other members of the multidisciplinary team? the client's health insurance company? or a lawyer for use in a legal case?

In addition, the occupational therapist uses pragmatic reasoning to choose the appropriate assessments, setting and timing. Table 18-6 discusses the criteria for selecting instruments.

Occupational therapy assessment has been categorized into different purposes. For example, the Canadian Association of Occupational Therapists (1996) divided assessment in terms of "descriptive, predictive, evaluative, programming, organizational decision-making, funding" (p. 86). In terms of client assessment, assessments can be grouped in terms of four main purposes *descriptive, predictive, discriminative, and evaluative* (Hayley, Coster, & Ludlow, 1991; Law, 1993). Table 18-7 provides explanations of each purpose. Sometimes therapists need to address just one purpose, but in psychosocial occupational therapy often several purposes need to be considered at some point during the occupational therapy process. Some standardized tests are developed to address just one purpose. However, there are a number of standardized tests, such as the COPM (Law et al., 2005), that can be used to provided a detailed descriptive assessment to inform goal setting and intervention planning and then be used to evaluate the effectiveness of the intervention. The use of tests that provide

TABLE 18-6. Criteria for Selecting Standardized Tests

Relevance	Will the test provide information that addresses the purpose of the assessment? Does the test have good face validity for this client group and service?
Feasibility	Can the test be administered with available resources (i.e., time, staff, budget, space)? Do you have the competency to undertake this test or will further training be required? Some tests take time to learn to administer and score; some may only be administered by a practitioner with particular credentials; or they may require specific equipment and materials that are costly, technical, or difficult to transport.
Utility	Who will have access to the test results and benefit from this data and how will they benefit? Is the cost worth the benefit for the clients being served and to the service? The information collected must have value, be meaningful to the client, and provide either data that inform the intervention or will evaluate outcomes. Costs to purchase the test, test materials, or consumables (e.g., food for a kitchen assessment) and/or training to administer the test need to be considered. Although there may be an initial outlay to buy a standardized test, because they are evidence based, valid, and reliable they improve the effectiveness of assessment and enable information to be collected in the most efficient way.
Reliability	How accurately do scores reflect a true performance of the individual? Is the test stable across time and raters?
Validity	Does the instrument measure what it proposes to measure? If a predictive test, does it predict what it was developed to predict? If a discriminative test, does it discriminate between the identified groups?
Role	Are there other professionals involved with the person who have undertaken assessments and what information has been obtained already? What is the therapist's role in this setting occupational therapy specialist or generic mental health worker?
Setting	Will the assessment be undertaken in the person's home or place of residence, an inpatient unit, occupational therapy department, day service, or community venue?
Model of practice	Occupation-based or skill-based? What are the assessments that have been developed to relate to the chosen model?
Age	Developmental and chronological age should be taken into account. If it is a norm-referenced test, the sample used to provide normative data should include people of the same age.
Diagnosis	You may choose a test that has been developed for people with a specific diagnosis or to aid the assessment of symptoms.
Time of day	Does the client's functioning vary depending on medication, fatigue, or time of day? Do you need to assess the person's maximum or minimum level of functioning?

data to inform more than one purpose can reduce the number of tests you need in your assessment tool kit and save time. Therefore, it is useful to be able to categorize both your informal and standardized assessment in terms of purpose and think explicitly about purpose when you are critiquing a potential standardized assessment and deciding whether it is worth purchasing and/or undertaking training to be able to use it.

The vast majority of therapists will undertake a *descriptive assessment* with their clients. An example of an assessment that provides data to support descriptive assessment is the Mayers, Lifestyle Questionnaire 2 (Mayers, 2000, 2003, 2004); this was

TABLE 18-7. Summary of Four Clinical Purposes of Assessment

Descriptive	■ Undertaken to provide a description of the person's current circumstances, past history, roles, habits, interests, level of occupational engagement, performance component skills and deficits, and desired outcomes. May be used to identify symptoms and problems to help aid diagnosis. ■ A descriptive assessment may be undertaken to gain information about environmental (physical, social, cultural-institutional) barriers and facilitators that need to be optimized or overcome to ensure a successful intervention. ■ The assessment may be undertaken on one occasion or over a period of time until sufficient information has been obtained to inform clinical decision making. ■ Data are used to inform the development of aims and goals and negotiate outcomes and lead to intervention planning. ■ Standardized descriptive tests should have adequate content, construct, and face validity. ■ If they are to be administered by more than one therapist, a high level of inter-rater reliability is also important.
Discriminative assessment	■ Used to distinguish between individuals or groups. ■ Comparisons are usually made against a normative group or another diagnostic group. ■ Discriminative assessment can be useful to refine a differential diagnosis, to assess a client against referral criteria, to prioritize referrals, to assess the person against criteria related to service provision or placement options, or when evaluating a person's level of dysfunction in relation to expectations of performance of other healthy people of that age. ■ Standardized discriminative tests should have established discriminative validity; this may include data on concurrent validity.
Predictive assessment	■ Undertaken when therapists need to make predictions about a person's future function or behavior. ■ The therapist may use the results of an assessment undertaken in one environment to predict likely function in another environment. ■ In psychosocial practice areas, therapists may undertake predictive assessment for a number of reasons, including prediction of likely function when discharged home as part of a pre-discharge assessment (e.g., level of independence, ability to safely use appliances) and risk assessment (e.g., of harm to self or others, abuse, wandering, falls). ■ Standardized predictive tests should have established predictive validity.
Evaluative assessment	■ Undertaken to evaluate changes in symptoms over time and/or the effectiveness of the intervention or management plan. ■ Needed to establish whether the level and nature of expected changes (outcomes) have been achieved. ■ Requires at least two assessments undertaken at different times. The baseline assessment data is used for comparison at the review, discharge, or when perceived significant change needs to be explored further. ■ Qualitative and/or quantitative data may be used to inform evaluative decisions. ■ Standardized evaluative tests are also known as outcome measures. ■ Standardized evaluative tests should have high levels of test–retest reliability and established responsiveness to change.

designed to enable "people with an enduring mental health problem to identify and prioritise issues affecting their quality of life" (Mayers, 2003, p. 388). Research with a sample of 33 occupational therapists and 75 clients with mental health problems found that that Mayers' Lifestyle Questionnaire 2 had good content validity, face validity, and clinical utility (Mayers, 2003).

Risk assessment to enable the prediction of types and likely levels of risk is an essential component of the assessment of people with mental health problems and is required for the effective planning or care and interventions. Occupational therapists are often required to contribute to risk assessment as members of multidisciplinary teams. Levels of risk can change very quickly in some clients and so risk assessment needs to be updated on a regular basis. The FACE Risk Profile (Clifford, 2002) is supported by predictive and concurrent validity research, and "offers clinicians a systematic approach to risk management" (Paley & McGinnis, 2003, p. 17) and a consistent method for communicating risks to clients and carers and within mental health teams.

Sometimes clinicians need to undertake discriminative assessment to distinguish between individuals or groups. *Discriminative assessment* can be useful to aid diagnosis when weighing up alternative hypotheses for the underlying cause of an observed behavior or reported symptom. For example, a test of memory could be developed to discriminate between people with dementia versus people with memory deficits associated with normal aging processes. It might also be used to discriminate between people with temporary memory problems, for example, associated with severe depression or because of confusion associated with an acute infection, as opposed to people with permanent memory impairment related to organic problems, such as dementia. An example of a discriminative assessment is the Clinical Dementia Rating (CDR) Scale (Berg, 1988), a global staging measure for dementia used to assess the influence of cognitive loss on the ability to conduct everyday activities (Meuser, 2001; Morris, 1997). Discrimination between severity levels can be useful when considering rehabilitation potential, identifying levels of care required and for research. The CDR is a structured assessment involving proxy report (semi-structured informant interview) and direct assessment of the person (semi-structured interview and observation). Information is obtained about the person's everyday performance across six domains: memory, orientation, judgment, problem solving, community affairs, and home and hobbies. People are assigned a score on a five-point scale: 0 = no cognitive impairment; 0.5 = very mild dementia; 1 = mild dementia; 2 = moderate dementia; 3 = severe dementia. Morris (1997) reported that the CDR had "become widely accepted in the clinical setting as a reliable and valid global assessment measure for DAT" (p. 173).

Evaluative assessment may be used to explore the effectiveness of intervention, but can also be useful to monitor symptoms or anticipated deterioration in function over time. People with mental health problems may need to access occupational therapy services for a long time period, for example, someone with a learning disability who is working toward moving from living with her parents to a supported housing situation. Some people may need the input of an occupational therapist at different times as the nature of their condition changes, for example, a person with vascular dementia who experiences plateaus related to level of functioning interspersed with sudden reduction of ability. Goal Attainment Scaling (GAS) (Ottenbacher & Cusick, 1990, 1993) can be a useful method of evaluation in psychosocial settings, particularly with people with learning disability or dementia (COT, 2011). An example of a well-researched and widely used assessment (Carswell et al., 2004) that can used to evaluate occupation-focused interventions is the COPM (Law et al., 2005). Chesworth, Duffy, Hodnett, and Knight (2002), reporting on research to "establish the usefulness of the COPM in measuring change in mental health clients who have undergone a course of occupational therapy" (p. 31), concluded that the "COPM is a clinically effective measure, able to detect significant changes in the levels of performance and satisfaction of clients with mental health problems" (p. 33), a finding supported by Warren (2002). The COPM has also been recommended by the British Association of Occupational Therapists (COT, 2011) for therapists working with older people.

Choosing the Best Sources of Information

Asher (2007) identifies the following methods of data collection, which may be used individually or combined: history, survey, experiment, observation, questionnaire, interview, and measurement. History taking, interview, observation, and questionnaires are the methods used most frequently to assess clients in psychosocial practice settings.

Occupational therapists have a choice to make when considering the source or sources of assessment data. Sources of information includes self-report from the client, the therapist's observations, and/or information gained from other people (proxy report) including carers and staff who are also working with the client.

Self-Report

A client-centered practitioner's self-report by the person should always be considered and included if at all possible. A range of methods can be used to obtain self-report information; these include informal or standardized interviews (open, semi-structured or structured), therapist-developed checklists, standardized questionnaires, diaries and journals, pieces of creative writing or artwork undertaken by the client, and time sheets used with clients to record activities undertaken and/or symptoms experienced. The assessment process should be a "partnership between the client and the therapist that empowers the client" (Sumsion, 2000, p. 308) to openly share his/her problems and needs, strengths and limitation, aspirations and wishes in order to identify his/her desired outcomes and goals as a focus for an intervention which will enable the client to "engage in functional performance and fulfil his or her occupational roles in a variety of environments" (p. 308). The occupational therapist should respect and partner with the person and "appreciate the person's knowledge, hopes, dreams and autonomy" (WFOT, 2010, p. 1). The results obtained from a client-centered assessment should enable "the client to make informed decisions" (Sumsion, 2000, p. 308) about his/her therapy, care, and future. Self-report helps the therapist to identify what clients want to do (desired occupations) and the things they "need or are expected to do socially and culturally" (WFOT, 2010, p. 1) (required/needed occupations). Through self-report the therapist can also seek to understand clients' attitudes toward their needed and desired occupations and their perspectives about performance and what helps or hinders their ability to participate. There is a wide choice of published self-report assessments for use in psychosocial settings. For example, there are several self-report assessments of occupational performance that are based on the Model of Human Occupation (Kielhofner, 2008), including the Occupational Self-Assessment (OSA) (Baron, Kielhofner, Iyengar, Goldhammer, & Wolenski, 2006), Occupational Circumstances Assessment Interview Rating Scale (OCAIRS) (Forsyth et al., 2005), and the Occupational Performance History Interview-II (OPHI-II) (Kielhofner et al., 2005).

Data Collected Directly by the Therapist Through Observation

Therapists may undertake observations informally, in a structured manner or by undertaking a standardized observational assessment. Inter-rater reliability and intra-rater reliability are particularly important when using observational tests and measures requiring clinical reasoning to form judgments about the client's feelings or motivations or underlying performance components. This is why some test developers stipulate that additional training is required in order for the test to be administered consistently.

In psychosocial occupational therapy we deal with a significant number of important constructs that cannot be directly observed, such as depression, anxiety, psychosis, perception, cognition, and volition, and we need to test out hypotheses and form judgments about the underlying cause of observed behavior. Reliable standardized tests can help us make these observations, and related judgments, in a rigorous and systematic way. With these constructs another psychometric property is also critical to consider; this relates to whether the test is valid.

Observational assessment is particularly useful with people with communication difficulties (such as severe learning disabilities), limited mental capacity (such as in the later stages of dementia), or younger clients. For example, Cunningham Piergrossi (2009) highlighted the importance of observational assessment with children who have mental health problems and are unable to articulate their feelings or experiences through self-report: "observed behaviour is outer and visible, but children also have an inner world of emotions, thoughts, mental images and memories. Behaviour is important; it is what the child uses to ask for help. It is the sign of discomfort, of depression, of anxiety, confusion and fear" (p. 57). Children may not always wish to cooperate with an assessment process and so setting up a likely meaningful activity linked to an age-related play task and undertaking an informal observation of the child during play can be a very useful part of the therapists' assessment process.

Informal observational assessment allows a degree of flexibility that enables therapists to use judgment and improvisation when moving from theory and hypothesis generation to an understanding of the person's unique experience and performance in a particular context. There are a number of standardized observational assessments that are appropriate for psychosocial assessment. An example of a well-researched and widely used observational assessment is the Assessment of Motor Process Skills (AMPS) (Fisher & Bray Jones, 2010a, 2010b). Hitch, Hevern, Cole, and Ferry (2007) reviewed a number of tests for application in a community mental health rehabilitation setting and adopted AMPS "because of its extensive evidence base and the detail of information it provides about the quality of performance in activities of daily living" (p. 222). Another observational assessment used in psychosocial practice is the Volitional Questionnaire (VQ) (de las Heras et al., 2007), which is an observation-based behavior rating scale of volition (goals, interests, and values) that was developed for people who cannot verbally express these concepts (Schultz-Krohn, 2007).

A limitation of observation as a method of data collection is that it only provides a snapshot at one point in time. Undertaking multiple observational assessments can be resource intensive and so therapists often need to combine observational assessment data with client self-report and/or proxy report from carers or other professionals. This helps the therapist to view the observation in a wider context and consider whether it was representative of the person's functioning/behavior at other times of day or in other environments. The synthesis of data from three or more sources is called *triangulation*.

Assessments Using Proxy Report

Proxy sources for assessment information may include:

- The person's primary caregiver (this can be an informal [usually unpaid] **carer** such as a family member, neighbor or volunteer, or a formal caregiver employed to provide care, such as a housing warden, nursing home staff, or home care staff).

- Other members of the multidisciplinary team within the service (e.g., psychiatrist, nurse, psychologist, social worker, health care assistant).

- Staff from other services who are involved with the client's care (such as their care coordinator, general practitioner, health visitor, district nurse, physiotherapist, speech and language therapist, dietitian, podiatrist).

- Other people who are supporting or working with the person (such as an employer, teacher, educator, or lawyer).

Sometimes information may be sought from more than one person, for example, both parents, several teachers and teaching assistants who support the learning of an adolescent attending secondary school, staff providing different elements of the person's care package, or the person's spouse and children. This can be useful because people's relationships and interpretations are so unique and multiple perspectives can help to provide a rich description of how the person interacts with different people and/or how occupational engagement is impacted by varying contexts and approaches.

Occupational therapists' collaboration with informal carers can occur at various stages during the occupational therapy process, not just to obtain a proxy report during an initial assessment. Carers can also provide valuable information to contribute to ongoing assessment and the evaluation of outcomes. Communication with carers should only occur if the client has previously given informed consent. There are a few cases where this may not be possible, such as when the client is a young child and the therapist is working in conjunction with his/her parents, if the person lacks capacity to provide informed consent and it is assessed that it will be in the person's best interests for the carer to be contacted, and/or the carer holds power of attorney/letter of attorney to act on the person's behalf. In addition to being a potential source of support for the person, a provider of information to enrich the assessment and collaborator in the intervention, carers have their own needs and wishes. Therefore, occupational therapists may be involved in carers' assessment; for example, to measure levels of physical and/or emotional burden or identify the carer's needs in order to signpost/refer him or her to information, education, support, and respite.

Therapists should consider a number of factors when interpreting proxy report information and considering the trustworthiness of the source, this includes: the frequency and amount of contact the proxy has with the person, the environment(s) in which the person and proxy relate, the nature of their relationship, and the degree of involvement the proxy has had regarding the person's health problem and care needs. The most frequent methods of data collection with informal proxy sources are interview (in person, over the telephone, or, more rarely, for example, when a family member lives some distance from the specialist inpatient unit, via a video call), questionnaires, and rating scales. Sometimes proxy sources are asked to keep a diary to record the frequency of behaviors or symptoms or to record when agreed goals have been met. Formal or informal caregivers might be asked to keep a record of the person's activities for a defined time period in order to gain a picture of the person's activity patterns and balance between self-care, productivity, leisure, and rest/sleep.

There are a number of useful standardized assessments that therapists can use to gain a proxy report of some aspect of the person. The Scale for Assessing Copying Skills, for example, was developed by Whelan and Speake (1979) as a proxy assessment of adolescents and adults with learning difficulties. The proxy source can be either the person's parents or a professional who knows him/her well. The Scale for

Assessing Copying Skills covers three domains: self-help, social academic, and interpersonal. The scale comprises 36 items that are described at five levels of difficulty: a = easiest level to e = most difficult level. Items are scored on two ordinal scales: a 4-point scale of whether the particular ability exists (1 = can do without help or supervision, 3 = cannot yet do, 4 = do not know whether he can do this); and an additional scale of whether the ability is adequately used or not (1 = uses this ability in an adequate amount, 7 = there is no opportunity to do this).

The Student Behavior Survey SBS (Lachar, Wingenfeld, Kline, & Gruber, 2000) is an example of a standardized proxy assessment that is designed for use with teachers "to identify school-specific behaviours that reflect socially disruptive behaviours and problems in emotional or behavioural adjustment" (Asher, 2007, p 486). The SBS assesses achievement, academic and social skills, parent cooperation, and emotional and behavioral adjustment. Teachers are asked to rate 102 items on a 4-point Likert scale covering the following domains: academic performance, academic habits, social skills, parent participation, health concerns, emotional distress, unusual behavior, social problems, verbal aggression, physical aggression, behavior problems, attention deficit hyperactivity disorder (ADHD), and oppositional defiant and conduct problems.

Some assessments enable the collection of information about the person and information about the perceived burden of the carer at the same time. An example is the Revised Memory and Behavior Problem Checklist (RMBPC) (Teri et al., 1992), which is recommended by the American Psychological Association (APA, 2011) as a reliable and valid tool for the clinical and empirical assessment of both the presence of behaviors exhibited by a person with dementia and the degree of carer subjective burden or distress related to these behaviors. The APA reports that the RMBPC has been validated for use with ethnically diverse caregivers. The original MBPC was designed by Zarit, Todd, and Zarit (1986) to obtain proxy report from carers of people with dementia. Therapists can either interview the carer or provide the MBPC in a survey format that the carer can complete on his/her own. The checklist covers items such as sleep disturbance, wandering, aggressive outbursts, and help needed with self-care. The carer's experience is assessed by asking how "upsetting" the behavior was on a Likert scale of 0 to 4 where 0 = *not at all*, 1= *a little*, 2 = *moderately*, 3 = *very much*, and 4 = *extremely*) while the frequency of observed behaviors are assessed using a Likert scale of 0 to 4 where 0 = *never occurs,* 1 = *occurs infrequently and not in the last week*, 2 = *occurred 1–2 times in the last week*, 3 = *occurred 3–6 times in the last week*, and 4 = *occurs daily or more often).* The MBPC is useful for therapists who only see the client for limited periods (e.g., therapists working in community mental health teams, crisis resolution teams, and assertive outreach teams) as it provides a broader picture of how the person is presenting in the home environment and areas where intervention for both the person with dementia and the carer would be beneficial.

An example of three linked assessments that examine carers' viewpoints and needs are the Carers Assessment of Difficulties Index (CADI), the Carers Assessment of Satisfactions Index (CASI), and the Carers Assessment of Managing Index (CAMI), which were developed by Nolan, Grant, and Keady (1998). Following a psychometric evaluation of the CADI, CASI, and CAMI, McKee et al. (2009) recommended the three assessments be used together to support in-depth work with family carers of older people. Llewellyn, Gething, Kendig, and Cant (2003) used the CADI and CAMI with parent-carers of adults with an intellectual disability. These three assessments can be undertaken together or separately and have been used in clinical practice and research. They can be used as self-rating scales or administered as an interview. There is a similar format to each assessment. The carer is presented with a series of statements and is asked to consider whether the statement applies to him/her and if so, then to rate the degree to which it is experienced. The CADI (Nolan et al., 1998) can be used to assess carers' perceptions of the difficulties associated with caregiving. The CADI comprises 30 statements to which carers rate as either "this statement does not apply to me" or if the statement applies the carer rates it as not very difficult, quite difficult, or very difficult. Items include statements such as: "The person I care for can demand too much of me," "I don't have enough private time to myself," and "I can feel helpless/not in control of the situation." This format is similar to other carers' assessments that focus on challenges and experiences of burden and reduced quality of life associated with caregiving. Examples of useful carer assessments for parents include the Parenting Stress Index (Abidin, 1995) and the Life Satisfaction Index–Parents (LSI–P) (Renwick & Reid, 1992).

The CAMI (Nolan et al., 1998) was developed to assess carer's coping strategies. The CAMI contains 37 statements describing management strategies. Carers rate strategies by choosing between "I do not use this" or "I use this and find it: not really helpful, quite helpful or very helpful." "The CAMI statements are presented on cards. This allows respondents to sort their 'very helpful' strategies in priority order and also prompts carers to tell stories about their caring and coping." (Llewellyn et al., 2003, p. 7). Another standardized proxy assessment that looks at management strategies used by carers is the Task Management Strategies Index (TMSI) (Gitlin et al., 2002). The proxy source for this assessment is family carers of people with Alzheimer's disease and related disorders who are living at home (Asher, 2007). Assessments of this nature not only help to identify current management strategies but also lead into an educational approach with carers where possible strategies are suggested by the therapist.

It is important not to presume that caregiving experiences are always burdensome, and this is why it can be useful to administer an assessment like the CASI (Nolan, Grant, & Keady, 1998). The CASI contains statements such as: "Caring has allowed to develop new skills and abilities," caring has brought me closer to the person I care for; I get pleasure from seeing the person I care for happy; and it's good to help the person I care for overcome difficulties and problems. For statements that apply to the carer, the rating scale involves the carer indicating that he/she has "no real satisfaction," "quite a lot of satisfaction," or a "great deal of satisfaction."

Dynamic Assessment

Another method of assessment which is of enormous value in psychosocial occupational therapy is **dynamic assessment** (Haywood & Lidz, 2007). Occupational therapists need to assess what the person can achieve on his/her own, but they are also interested in the extent to which performance can be improved. Dynamic assessment is useful for this purpose as it focuses on individual variations in function under different circumstances rather than comparing the person to normative data or a criterion-reference. Dynamic assessment involves the use of cues, mediation, feedback, and/or alterations of the demands of the activity during assessment to examine how changes in performance can be achieved. The therapist deliberately and systematically implements intervention techniques during the assessment and carefully observes whether, how and to what degree the person's performance changes in response. Interventions should be applied at the least intrusive level and be carefully graded. Compared to standardized tests the focus is not on the result from a single performance attempt, but is rather concerned with the process of learning and change (Toglia, Golisz, & Goverover, 2008). The dynamic assessment approach allows the therapist to explore elements of function that are not static and can be used to assess the person's ability to learn and adapt. In this approach the therapist "demonstrates strategies, provides cues, or modifies activities to improve performance (Toglia et al., 2008)This can be very useful for planning intervention approaches, providing information that facilitates function that can be shared as strategies with carers, and helping the therapist assess rehabilitation potential and the occupational prognosis. Dynamic assessment approaches have been used by occupational therapists with people with learning disabilities, schizophrenia, and dementia (e.g., see Wiedl, Schöttke, & Calero, 2001).

An example of an occupational therapy standardized assessment that uses a dynamic assessment process is the Executive Function Performance Test (EFPT) (Baum, Morrison, Hahn, & Edwards, 2007). The authors describe EFPT as a top–down functional assessment test. It was developed to assess cognitive integration and functioning in an environmental context and examines executive functions involved in task execution. The EFPT can be used for "three purposes: 1) to determine which executive functions are impaired; 2) to determine an individual's capacity for independent functioning; and 3) to determine the amount of assistance necessary for task completion" (p. 2). Baum et al. (2007) stated that "unlike other tests of function, the EFPT *does not* examine what individuals cannot do. Rather, it identifies what they can do, and how much assistance is needed for them to carry out a task. The EFPT does not simply discriminate between individuals who can do the test and those who cannot. By using a cueing system, a wider range of abilities are captured in people previously thought to be untestable" (p. 2). The person is observed performing four assessment tasks related to simple cooking, telephone use, medication management, and bill payment. Detailed cueing guidelines and cue descriptions are provided in the test manual. Cues are graded and comprise indirect verbal guidance (this is provided as a question rather than a direct instruction, such as "What should you do now?"), gestural guidance (such as pointing or miming an action), direct verbal guidance in the form of a specific one-step instruction (e.g., pick up the pen), physical assistance, and undertaking the assessment step for the person. During the assessment the therapist intervenes if the person is struggling or does not progress to the next step in the assessment task. The therapist should wait 10 seconds to observe the client and then uses the lowest level cues (indirect verbal guidance). Each cue level is given twice before the therapist tries a higher-level cue.

Another example of a standardized, norm-referenced, valid, and reliable test that incorporates dynamic assessment is the Contextual Memory Test (CMT) (Toglia, 1993). This test is used with adults with neurological or organic memory impairment. Cooke and Finkelstein Kline (2007) reported that it has been used with psychiatric patients. There are two equivalent forms of the test that enable evaluation to monitor change and reduce the potential impact of a learning effect. Results indicate how the person responds to, and benefits from, memory cues.

SUMMARY

Occupational therapists need a "tool kit" containing assessment skills and a range of standardized assessments and outcome measures. In psychosocial practice there are often shades of grey rather than black and white answers; therefore, the choices made regarding the best sources of information, timing of assessment, purposes of assessment, and methods for data collection are unique to each client and influenced by the service setting. Involving the person at the center of the assessment process is critical to obtaining information that leads to a person centered intervention. The therapist needs to obtain a clear picture of the person's desired outcomes and, if necessary, negotiate which of these can be realistically achieved through occupational therapy. Family members/carers can play a valuable role in assessment and evaluation. Therapists have an important role in assessing the carer's needs, skills, and management strategies. Valid and reliable measurement of outcomes must be undertaken in order to examine the effectiveness of intervention and demonstrate to clients, their families, and service funders the value of occupational therapy. The therapeutic use of self, interviewing, and observation skills and the ability to synthesize complex information are developed over time as the therapist transitions from a novice to an expert therapist. Continuing professional development and supervision are crucial to becoming proficient in assessment, evaluation, and outcome measurement.

REVIEW QUESTIONS

1. What is outcome measurement and why should occupational therapists measure outcomes?

2. Explain the reasons why occupational therapists should consider the reliability and validity of standardized tests? What types of reliability and validity should be considered for different purposes of assessment?

3. What factors will you need to consider when selecting relevant assessment methods and standardized tests for your area of practice?

4. What is dynamic assessment? Why is it a useful assessment method for occupational therapists?

REFERENCES

Abidin, R. R. (1995). *Parenting stress index (3rd edition) professional manual.* Odessa, FL: Psychological Assessment Resources, Inc.

American Occupational Therapy Association (AOTA). (2008). Occupational therapy practice framework: Domain and process (2nd edition). *American Journal of Occupational Therapy, 62*(6), 625–683.

American Psychological Association (APA). (2011). Revised Memory and Behavior Problem Checklist. Washington, DC: Author. Retrieved from http://www.apa.org/pi/about/publications/caregivers/practice-settings/assessment/tools/memory-behavior.aspx

Anastasi, A. (1988). *Psychological Testing* (6th ed.). New York: Macmillan.

Asher, I. E. (1996). *Occupational therapy assessment tools: An annotated index* (2nd ed.). Bethesda, MD: American Occupational Therapy Association.

Asher, I. E. (2007). *Occupational therapy assessment tools: An annotated index* (3rd ed.). Bethesda, MD: American Occupational Therapy Association.

Barnitt, R. (1993). Deeply troubling questions: The teaching of ethics in undergraduate courses. *British Journal of Occupational Therapy, 56*(11), 401–406.

Baron, K., Kielhofner, G., Iyengar, A., Goldhammer, V., & Wolenski, J. (2006). Occupational Self Assessment (OSA) version 2.2. Chicago: Model of Human Occupation Clearinghouse, University of Illinois.

Bartram, D. (1990). Reliability and validity. In J. R. Beech & L. Harding L (Eds.), *Testing people: A practical guide to psychometrics.* Windsor: NFER-Nelson.

Baum, C. M., & Edwards D. F. (1993). Cognitive performance in senile dementia of the Alzheimer Type: The Kitchen Task Assessment. *American Journal of Occupational Therapy, 47,* 431–436.

Baum, C. M., Morrison, T., Hahn, M., Edwards, D. F. (2007). Executive Function Performance Test: Test Protocol Booklet. St Louis: Program in Occupational Therapy, Washington University School of Medicine. Retrieved from http://www.rehabmeasures.org/Lists/RehabMeasures/DispForm.aspx?ID=944

Beck, A. T., Kovacs, M., & Weissman, A. (1979). Assessment of suicidal intention: The Scale for Suicide Ideation. *Journal of Consulting and Clinical Psychology, 47,* 343–352.

Beck, A. T., & Steer, R. A. (1988). *Manual for Beck Hopelessness Scale.* San Antonio, TX: The Psychological Corporation.

Beck, A. T., Steer, R. A., Kovacs, M., & Garrison, B. (1985). Hopelessness and eventual suicide: A 10-year prospective study of patients hospitalised with suicidal ideation. *American Journal of Psychiatry, 142,* 559–563.

Benson J., & Clark, F. (1982). A guide for instrument development and validation. *American Journal of Occupational Therapy, 36*(12), 789–800.

Berg, L. (1988). Clinical Dementia Rating (CDR). *Psychopharmacology Bulletin, 24*(4), 637–639.

Brintnell, S. (2002). WHO International Classification of Functioning, Disability and Health–Development and Canadian content. *World Federation of Occupational Therapists Bulletin, 45*(May), 33–37.

Brown, G. K., Beck, A. T., Steer, R. A., & Grisham, J. R. (2000). Risk factors for suicide in psychiatric outpatients: A 20-year prospective study. *Journal of Consulting and Clinical Psychology, 68,* 371–377.

Canadian Association of Occupational Therapists (CAOT). (1996). Profile of occupational therapy in Canada. *Canadian Journal of Occupational Therapy, 63*(2), 79–95.

Carswell, A., McColl, M. A., Baptiste, S., Law, M., Polatajko, H., & Pollock, N. (2004). The Canadian Occupational Performance Measure: A research and clinical literature review. *Canadian Journal of Occupational Therapy, 71*(4), 210–222.

Chesworth, C., Duffy, R., Hodnett, J., & Knight, A. (2002). Measuring clinical effectiveness in mental health: Is the Canadian Occupational Performance an appropriate measure? *British Journal of Occupational Therapy, 65*(1), 30–34.

Clemson, L., Fitzgerald, M. H., & Heard, R. (1999). Content validity of an assessment tool to identify home fall hazards: The Westmead Home Safety Assessment. *British Journal of Occupational Therapy, 62*(4), 170–179.

Clifford, P. (2002). The FACE assessment and outcome system. Nottingham: FACE Recording and Measurement Systems.

Cole, B., Finch, E., Gowland, C., & Mayo, N. (1995). *Physical rehabilitation outcome measures*. London: Williams and Wilkins.

College of Occupational Therapists (COT). (2004). *Guidance on the use of the International Classification of Functioning, Disability and Health (ICF) and the Ottawa Charter for Health Promotion in occupational therapy services*. London: COT.

College of Occupational Therapists (COT). (2009). SNOMED subsets for occupational therapists. London: COT. Retrieved from http://www.cot.co.uk/ehealth-information-management/outcome-patients-ot-subsets

College of Occupational Therapists (COT). (2011). Measuring mental wellbeing in older people. *COT/BAOT briefing 133*. London: COT.

Cooke, D. M., & Finkelstein Kline, N. (2007). Assessments of process skills and mental functions. Part 1: Cognitive assessment. In I. E. Asher (Ed.), *Occupational therapy assessment tools: An annotated index* (3rd ed.). Bethesda, MD: American Occupational Therapy Association.

Creek, J. (2003). *Occupational therapy defined as a complex intervention*. London: College of Occupational Therapists.

Crocker, L., & Algina, J. (1986). *Introduction to classical and modern test theory*. Fort Worth: Holt, Rinehart and Winston.

Cunningham Piergrossi, J. (2009). Occupational therapy and the mental health of children. *World Federation of Occupational Therapists Bulletin, 60*(Nov.), 56–58.

De las Heras, C. G., Geist, R., Kielhofner, G., & Li, Y. (2007). Volitional Questionnaire. Chicago: Model of Human Occupation Clearinghouse, University of Illinois.

Finlay, L. (2004). *The practice of psychosocial occupational therapy* (3rd ed.). Cheltenham: Nelson Thornes.

Fisher, A. G., & Bray Jones, K. (2010a). *Assessment of Motor and Process Skills Vol. 1: Development, standardization, and administration manual* (7th ed.). Fort Collins, CO: Three Star Press.

Fisher, A. G., & Bray Jones, K. (2010b). *Assessment of Motor and Process Skills. Vol. 2: User Manual* (7th ed.). Fort Collins, CO: Three Star Press.

Fitzpatrick, R. (2004). Measures of health status, health-related quality of life and patient satisfaction. In P. Pysent, Fairbank, & A. Carr (Eds.), *Outcome measures in orthopaedics and orthopaedic trauma* (2nd ed.). London: Arnold.

Forsyth. K., Deshpande, S., Kielhofner, G., Henriksson, C., Haglund, L., Olson, L., et al. (2005). Occupational Circumstance Assessment Interview Rating Scale (OCAIRS), version 4. Chicago: Model of Human Occupation Clearinghouse, University of Illinois.

Gitlin, L. N., Winter, L., Dennis, M., Corcoran, M., Schinfeld, S., & Hauck, W. (2002). Strategies used by families to simplify tasks for individuals with Alzheimer's disease and related disorders: Psychometric analysis of the task management strategy index (TMSI). *The Gerontologist, 42,* 61–69.

Golding, E. (1989). The Middlesex Elderly Assessment of Mental State (MEAMS). Suffolk: Thames Valley Test Company.

Griffiths, S., & Schell, D. (2002). Professional context. In A. Turner, M. Foster, & S. Johnson (Eds.), *Occupational therapy and physical dysfunction: Principles, skills and practice* (5th ed.). Edinburgh: Churchill Livingstone.

Hayley, S. M., Coster, W. J., & Ludlow, L. H. (1991). Pediatric functional outcome measures. *Physical Medicine and Rehabilitation Clinics of North America, 2,* 689–723.

Haywood, H. C., & Lidz, C. S. (2007). *Dynamic assessment in practice: Clinical and educational applications.* New York: Cambridge University Press.

Hemphill-Pearson, B. J. (2008). The patient's profile: An integrative approach. In B. J. Hemphill-Pearson (Ed.), *Assessment in occupational therapy mental health: An integrative approach* (2nd ed.). Thorofare, NJ: Slack.

Higgs, J., & Bithell, C. (2001). Professional expertise. In J. Higgs & A. Titchen (Eds.), *Practice knowledge and expertise in the health professions.* Oxford: Butterworth-Heinemann.

Hitch, D., Hevern, T., Cole, M., & Ferry, C. (2007). A review of the selection for occupational therapy outcome measures in a community mental health rehabilitation setting. *Australian Occupational Therapy Journal, 54,* 221–224.

Hopkins, H. L., & Smith, H. D. (Eds). (1993). *Willard and Spackman's Occupational Therapy.* Philadelphia: Lippincott Williams & Wilkins.

Kielhofner, G. (2008). *Model of Human Occupation: Theory and application* (4th ed.). Philadelphia: Lippincott Williams and Wilkins.

Kielhofner, G., Mallinson, T., Crawford, C., Nowak, M., Rigby, M., Henry, A., et al. (2005). Occupational Performance History Interview-II (OPHI-II) version 2.1. Chicago: Model of Human Occupation Clearinghouse, University of Illinois.

Lachar, D., Wingenfeld, S. A., Kline, R. B., Gruber, C. P. (2000). Student Behavior Survey (SBS). Los Angeles: Western Psychological Services.

Laver-Fawcett, A. J. (2002). Assessment. In A. Turner, M. Foster, & S. E. Johnson (Eds.), *Occupational therapy and physical dysfunction: Principles, skills and practice.* Edinburgh: Churchill Livingstone.

Laver-Fawcett, A. J. (2007). *Principles of assessment and outcome measurement for occupational therapists and physiotherapists: Theory, skills and application.* London: Wiley.

Law, M. (1993). Evaluating activities of daily living: Directions for the future. *American Journal of Occupational Therapy, 47,* 233–237.

Law, M. (1997). Self care. In J. Van Deusen & D. Brunt (Eds.), *Assessment in Occupational Therapy and Physical Therapy.* London: W.B. Saunders Company.

Law, M, (2001). Appendix 2: Outcome measures rating form guidelines. In M. Law, C. Baum, & W. Dunn (Eds.), *Measuring occupational performance: Supporting best practice in occupational therapy.* Thorofare: Slack.

Law, M., Baptiste, S., Carswell A., McColl, M., Polatojko, H., & Pollock, N. (2005). *The Canadian Occupational Performance Measure* (4th ed.). Ottawa, Canada: Canadian Association of Occupational Therapists (CAOT) Publishing.

Law, M., & Baum, C. (2001). Measurement in occupational therapy. In M. Law, C. Baum, & W. Dunn (Eds.), *Measuring occupational performance: Supporting best practice in occupational therapy.* Thorofare: Slack.

Law, M., Cooper, B., Strong S., Stewart, D., Rigby, P., & Letts, L. (1996). The person-environment-occupation model: A transactive approach to occupational performance. *Canadian Journal of Occupational Therapy, 63*(1), 9–23.

Law, M., & McColl, M. A. (2010). Occupational therapy: interventions, effects and outcomes. In M. Law & M. A. McColl (Eds.), *Interventions, effects, and outcomes in occupational therapy.* Thorofare, NJ: Slack.

Llewellyn, G., Gething, L,. Kendig, H., & Cant, R. (2003). *Invisible carers: Facing an uncertain future. A report of a study conducted with funding from the National Health and Medical Research Council 2000–2002.* Sydney: Faculty of Health Sciences and Faculty of Nursing, University of Sydney.

Mattingly, C. (1994). The narrative nature of clinical reasoning. In C. Mattingly & M. H. Flemming (Eds.), *Clinical reasoning: Forms of inquiry in a therapeutic practice.* Philadelphia: F. A. Davis.

Mayers, C. A. (2000). Quality of life: Priorities for people with enduring mental health Problems. *British Journal of Occupational Therapy, 63*(12), 591–597.

Mayers, C. A. (2003). The development and evaluation of the Mayers' Lifestyle Questionnaire (2). *British Journal of Occupational Therapy, 66*(9), 388–395.

Mayers, C. A. (2004). Mayers Lifestyle Questionnaire 2. York, UK: York St. John University. Retrieved from http://w3.yorksj.ac.uk/health/faculty-of-hls/staff--contact-details/health-staff/professor-chris-mayers.aspx

McColl, M., Law, M., Stewart, D., Doubt L., Pollock, N., & Krupa, T. (2002). *Theoretical basis of occupational therapy* (2nd ed.). Thorofare NJ: Slack.

McDonald, R., Surtees, R., & Wirz, S. (2004). The International Classification of Functioning, Disability and Health provides a model for adaptive seating interventions for children with cerebral palsy. *British Journal of Occupational Therapy, 67*(7), 293–302.

McDowell, I., & Newell, C. (1987). *Measuring health: A guide to rating scales and questionnaires.* Oxford: Oxford University Press.

McGruder, J. (2004). Disease models of mental illness and aftercare patient education: Critical observations from meta-analyses, cross-cultural practice and anthropological study. *British Journal of Occupational Therapy, 67*(7), 310–318.

McKee, K., Spazzafumo, L., Nolan, M., Wojszel, B., Lamura, G., & Bien, B. (2009). Components of the difficulties, satisfactions and management strategies of carers of older people: A principal component analysis of CADI-CASI-CAMI. *Aging & Mental Health, 13*(2), 255–264.

Meuser, T. (2001). Clinical Dementia Rating (CDR) Scale. St Louis: Alzheimer's Disease Research Center, Washington University. Retrieved from http://alzheimer.wustl.edu/cdr/PDFs/CDR_OverviewTranscript-Revised.pdf

Morris, J. C. (1997). Clinical dementia rating: A reliable and valid diagnostic and staging measure for dementia of the Alzheimer type. *International Psychogeriatrics, 9,* 173–176.

Mosey, A. (1974). An alternative: The biopsychosocial model. *American Journal of Occupational Therapy, 28,* 137–140.

Nolan, M., Grant, G., & Keady, J. (1998). *Assessing the needs of family carers: A guide for practitioners.* Brighton: Pavilion Publishing.

Öhman J. I. K., & Asaba, E. (2009). Goal setting in occupational therapy: A narrative study exploring theory and practice in psychiatry. *World Federation of Occupational Therapists Bulletin, 60*(Nov.) 22–28.

Opacich, K. J. (1991). Assessment and informed decision making. In C. Christiansen & C. Baum (Eds.), *Occupational therapy–Overcoming human performance deficits.* Thorofare: Slack.

Ottenbacher K. J., & Cusick, A. (1990). Goal attainment scaling as a method of clinical service evaluation. *American Journal of Occupational Therapy, 44*(6), 519–525.

Ottenbacher K. J., & Cusick, A. (1993). Discriminative versus evaluative assessment: some observations on goal attainment scaling: Alternative strategies for functional assessment. *American Journal of Occupational Therapy, 47*(4), 349–354.

Ottenbacher K. J., & Tomchek, S. D. (1993). Reliability analysis in therapeutic research: Practice and procedures. *American Journal of Occupational Therapy, 47*(1), 10–16.

Paley, G., & McGinnis, P. (2003). Implementing a trust-wide strategy for clinical risk assessment in mental health. *Mental Health Practice, 7*(1), 14–17.

Renwick, R. M., & Reid, D. T. (1992). *Life Satisfaction Index—Parents (LSI–P).* Toronto: Department of Occupational Therapy, University of Toronto.

Roberts, A. E. (1996). Approaches to reasoning in occupational therapy: A critical exploration. *British Journal of Occupational Therapy, 59*(5), 233–236.

Rogers, J. C. (2004). Occupational diagnosis. In M. Mollineux (Ed.), *Occupation for occupational therapists.* Oxford: Blackwell.

Rogers, J. C., & Holm, M. B. (1989). The therapist's thinking behind functional assessment I. In C. B. Royeen (Ed.), *AOTA self study series assessing function.* Rockville, MD: American Occupational Therapy Association.

Rogers, J. C., & Holm, M. B. (1991). Occupational therapy diagnostic reasoning: A component of clinical reasoning. *American Journal of Occupational Therapy, 45,* 1045–1053.

Schultz-Krohn, W. (2007). Assessments of occupational performance. In I. E. Asher (Ed,), *Occupational therapy assessment tools: An annotated index* (3rd ed.). Bethesda, MD: American Occupational Therapy Association.

Sumsion, T. (2000). A revised occupational therapy definition of client-centred practice. *British Journal of Occupational Therapy, 63*(7), 304–309.

Teri, L., Truax P., Logsdon R., Uomoto, J., Zarit, S., & Vitaliano, P. P. (1992). Assessment of behavioral problems in dementia: The Revised Memory and Behavior Problems Checklist (RMBPC). *Psychology and Aging, 7*(4), 622–631.

Toglia, J. P. (1993). *Contextual Memory Test (CMT).* San Antonio: Harcourt Assessment.

Toglia J. P., Golisz, K. M., & Goverover, Y. (2008). Evaluation and intervention for cognitive perceptual impairments. In E. B. Crepeau, B. Schell, & E. Cohn (Eds.), *Willard & Spackman's Occupational Therapy* (11th ed.). Philadelphia: Lippincott Williams & Wilkins.

Townsend, E. A., & Polatajko, H. J. (2007). *Enabling occupation II: Advancing an occupational therapy vision for health, well-being, & justice through occupation.* Ottawa: CAOT Publications ACE.

Trombly, C. (1993). Anticipating the future: Assessment of occupational function. *American Journal of Occupational Therapy, 47*(3), 253–257.

Unsworth, C. (2000). Measuring the outcome of occupational therapy: Tools and resources. *Australian Occupational Therapy Journal, 47*(4), 147–158.

Warren, A. (2002). An evaluation of the Canadian model of Occupational Performance and Engagement and the Canadian Occupational Performance Measure in mental health practice. *British Journal of Occupational Therapy, 65*(11), 515–521.

Wiedl, K. H., Schöttke, H., & Calero, M. D. (2001). Dynamic assessment of cognitive rehabilitation potential in schizophrenic persons and in old people with and without dementia. *International Journal of Psychological Assessment, 17*(2), 112–119.

Whelan, E., & Speake, B. (1979). Scale for Assessing Coping Skills. In E. Whelan & B. Speake (Eds.), *Learning to Cope.* London: Souvenir Press.

World Federation of Occupational Therapists (WFOT). (2010). Position statement on client-centredness in occupational therapy. Forrestfield, Western Australia, Australia: Author. Retrieved from http://www.wfot.org/ResourceCentre.aspx

World Health Organization (WHO). (2002). Towards a common language for functioning, disability and health ICF. Geneva: Author. Retrieved from http://www.who.int/classifications/icf/en/

Wright, J., Cross, J., & Lamb, S. (1998). Physiotherapy outcome measures for rehabilitation of elderly people: responsiveness to change of the Rivermead Mobility Index and Barthel Index. *Physiotherapy, 84*(5), 216–221.

Zarit, S. H., Todd, P. A., & Zarit, J. M. (1986). Subjective burden of husbands and wives as caregivers: A longitudinal study. *Gerontologist, 26*(3), 260–266.

SUGGESTED RESOURCES

Asher, I. E. (2007). *Occupational therapy assessment tools: An annotated index* (3rd ed.). Bethesda, MD: American Occupational Therapy Association.

This text provides an extremely useful and comprehensive overview of a very wide range of over 300 published tests useful to occupational therapists which have been reviewed by a team of international authors. One to two page succinct reviews are provided for each test.

Hemphill-Pearson, B. J. (2008). *Assessment in occupational therapy mental health: An integrative approach* (2nd ed.). Thorofare, NJ: Slack Incorporated.

Laver-Fawcett, A. J. (2007). *Principles of assessment and outcome measurement for occupational therapists and physiotherapists: Theory, skills, and application.* London: Wiley.

SUGGESTED WEBSITES

Assessment of Motor Process Skills (AMPS) document center provides information, references and training details for the AMPS, School AMPS, and the Evaluation of Social Interaction: http://www.ampsintl.com/AMPS/index.php

Canadian Occupational Performance Measure (COPM) website provides a description of COPM, references, and questions and answers about the measure and ordering information: http://www.caot.ca/copm/index.htm

Executive Function Performance Test Manual (EFPT) is available from: http://www .rehabmeasures.org/Lists/RehabMeasures/DispForm.aspx?ID=944

Information and ordering details for the FACE Core Assessment & Outcomes Package for Mental Health Services is available from the FACE Assessment and Outcome System website: www.face.eu.com. The FACE is designed to support a conversational style of interaction between the service user and practitioner. It covers physical well-being, psychological well-being, activities of daily living, social circumstances, family and carers, and carers' needs and concerns. The therapist also completes an assessment summary and rates the risks identified.

The Mayers Lifestyle Questionnaires can be obtained from Professor Chris Mayers, at the York St. John University website under the Faculty of Health and Life Sciences staff profiles at: http://w3.yorksj.ac.uk/health/faculty-of-hls/staff--contact-details/health-staff/professor-chris-mayers.aspx

The Model of Human Occupation (MOHO) clearing house website provides useful information, references, and ordering details for assessments related to MOHO (e.g., ACIS, SCOPE, COSA, OCAIRS, OPHI-II, VQ, WEIS, and WRI): http://www.uic.edu/depts/moho/

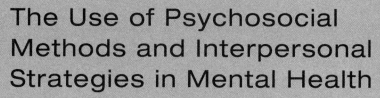
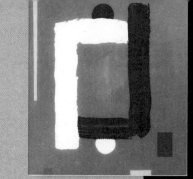

The Use of Psychosocial Methods and Interpersonal Strategies in Mental Health

Elizabeth Cara, PhD, OTR/L, MFT
Pamela R.R. Stephenson, MS, OTR/L

KEY TERMS

clinical reasoning   strategies

intersubjective process   techniques

CHAPTER OUTLINE

Introduction
Interpersonal Strategies
    Validation
    Setting Limits
    Encouragement
    Advice
    Coaching
    Confrontation
    Reframing
    Interpretation
    Metaphors
    Reality Testing
Occupational Therapy Methods
    Application—Clinical Reasoning and Motivating
    Interventions
    Therapeutic Use of Self
    Building and Repairing Relationships
    Empathy
    Therapeutic Use of Activity and Occupation
    Activity Analysis
    Activity Categorization
    Implicit and Explicit Methods
Summary

INTRODUCTION

Feeling confident in using a range of occupational therapy methods and interpersonal strategies is one of the most exciting aspects of becoming a skilled, confident practitioner. Knowing how and when to use these methods and strategies to connect with clients often makes the difference in our ability to develop client-centered practices and motivate clients to engage in treatment. Also, how an individual practitioner incorporates interpersonal strategies to match his or her individual style and specific therapeutic situation is what makes working fun! Although practitioners understand methods and general interpersonal strategies, they are uniquely applied to each client, setting, and situation that occur in practice. Deciding which strategies to use and specifically how to deliver them in each encounter is what may motivate clients and is what makes clinical practice successful as well as interesting and rewarding. Creative ways of applying methods in interpersonal strategies in mental health practice are embedded throughout this text, but this chapter introduces and explains them so that you can understand and artistically use them in your specific clinical practice.

This chapter discusses universal and specific strategies used primarily in mental health but they can also be used in physical rehabilitation, pediatric, and other practices. Indeed, Ikiugu (2010) advocates that our core psychosocial skills should be at the heart of all our therapeutic interactions, regardless of our clinical specialty. This chapter also incorporates elements of the Occupational Therapy Practice Framework (American Occupational Therapy Association [AOTA], 2008) when applicable, particularly those methods that are unique to this domain of practice and which contribute to the broader occupational therapy process.

This focus on interpersonal strategies is especially important because the therapeutic relationship is often the key element in mental health practice. Also, in mental health practice, the manifestation of symptoms and the impact of specific mental illnesses on occupational engagement vary greatly between individuals; therefore, abstract techniques assume prime importance. This chapter uses the terms *techniques* and *strategies* interchangeably according to the following definitions: **Strategies** or **techniques** include the tangible tools that are often readily identified or observed in practice. However, particularly in mental health treatment, strategies and techniques also include abstract abilities the person uses to fulfill the plan, or apply the methods, such as the style, finesse, capacity, craftsmanship, approach, or resourcefulness of the therapist. A tangible example of an occupational therapy strategy is grading an activity according to the cognitive functioning of an individual or providing just enough tools in a group so that members have to interact with each other around sharing their use. An abstract technique may include clinical reasoning about the client, which intervention may work best, and how to apply the intervention in context.

This chapter focuses on the interpersonal dimensions of strategies, such as how the occupational therapy practitioner conveys, communicates, makes contact with, relates to, proposes, and presents techniques. An example of an interpersonal emphasis may be the specific and unique way a practitioner discusses an activity with a client, including tone of voice, physicality, and gestures of the practitioner, the timing of the discussion, and how the practitioner conveys the words (including manner and speed).

INTERPERSONAL STRATEGIES

Various strategies have been identified in different ways in occupational therapy. Some are based in a model of practice (Kielhofner, 2002) while others are listed in chapters on the therapeutic use of self (Hagedorn, 2000; Peloquin, 2003). Some are explained in relationship to interactive clinical reasoning (Schwartzberg, 2002) or client-centered practice (Fearing & Clark, 2000). Whichever means have been used to explain strategies in occupational therapy, many are universal strategies used by most health professionals.

Perhaps the most important information that can be added to explanations of strategies is that they should be individualized according to the needs of the client, the practice setting, and the skills of the practitioner. These interpersonal skills are fluid and are guided by the interaction between client and practitioner, which may evolve from moment to moment. Also important is the fact that as far as possible, personal techniques should be congruent with the occupational therapy practitioner's personality. Although interpersonal strategies can be learned and practiced, and usually will deepen with clinical experience, it is nevertheless critical to be authentic and genuine. Clients in the mental health system are very attuned to practitioners' personalities and styles (even though they may not show) and can recognize when someone is not being genuine. In 1966, Yerxa (in Padilla, 2005) reminded practitioners of the importance of authenticity when interacting with clients and stressed that the authentic practitioner "is open to the client's ideas and feelings and real in responding to them" (p. 139). This assumes a genuineness in the reactions of the practitioner that is consistent with his or her personal style. However, at times, depending on the client, the setting or the technique, practitioners may need to modify their natural style in order to facilitate the therapeutic process. For example, if you tend to be upbeat and outwardly enthusiastic, you may wish to reflect on the potential impact of this when working with clients coping with acute clinical depression or with florid psychotic symptoms. The broad and universal interpersonal techniques are explained briefly and then illuminated with examples or case illustrations.

Validation

Validating is conveying respect for a client's experience or perspective, acknowledging one's understanding of a client's experience (Kielhofner & Forsyth, 2002), conveying that you value the individual (Hagedorn, 2000), and demonstrating that the client's concern is accepted (Schwartzberg, 2002). Many societies continue to perceive clients with mental health needs as individuals to be feared, if not disregarded, due to their psychiatric symptoms and frequently devalue their roles as contributing members of society. Therefore, it is essential that occupational therapy practitioners convey an understanding and acceptance of their experiences and strive to promote occupational justice within society. Validation could be verbal, such as greeting a person and saying you are glad to see him or her, or acknowledging his or her distress about talking to himself or herself around others, or it could be nonverbal, such as sitting with and listening to a person although he or she may seem to make little sense.

Setting Limits

Setting limits and personal boundaries is identifying behavior that you are unwilling to tolerate or that is inappropriate to the setting. Setting limits is a common clinical strategy in mental health, but not often explained. It is sometimes elusive to novice clinicians because it takes practice, assertiveness, knowing yourself, knowing what the client needs in that specific situation, and understanding the goals of mental health practice. To the novice practitioner, it may appear that setting limits means not caring. However, establishing behavior that you are unwilling to tolerate or accept actually conveys appropriate caring because often the client behavior that one "sets limits on" is the very behavior that is a barrier to satisfying occupational performance, roles, habits, or successful relationships.

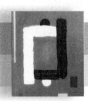

CASE ILLUSTRATION

Athena—Setting Limits

Athena attended a psychosocial treatment program based on a clubhouse model. Although she was very smart and clever, residual behaviors from her co-occurring bipolar and addictive disorders were barriers to successful occupational performance. Specifically her barbs and vicious comments directed to others often resulted in her being asked to leave jobs or terminated friendships. She had difficulty recognizing her responsibility or role in these "messy" work or relationship situations.

When she arrived at a daily group that discussed the agenda for the day, many members greeted her warmly. Having never experienced unconditional caring and believing herself unworthy, she was embarrassed and made a sarcastic remark, denigrating their warmth. The occupational therapist, who was aware of Athena's problems, immediately commented on Athena's comment by saying, "That was a pretty hurtful comment" and indicated that this was not an acceptable way to interact with peers.

She asked the other clients to tell Athena how it made them feel. Although two clients said they had no problem with the remark, two others were able to say that her sarcastic comment was somewhat hurtful.

The occupational therapist pointed out to Athena that this was the very type of comment that led to her problems with work and relationships.

Discussion

The occupational therapist understood Athena's problems and treatment needs and was able to set limits on destructive behavior, and hopefully provide some reality testing for Athena. Reality testing meant that through acknowledgment of this situation, Athena might begin to recognize and work on behaviors that were barriers to productive living and her quality of life.

Encouragement

Encouraging is providing emotional support (Kielhofner & Forsyth, 2002) and assurance for clients' actions, behaviors, or choices. In a mental health setting, encouragement is often needed for clients to engage in activities, try out new occupations or new situations, or move to the next level of treatment. In fact, it seems that encouragement is the most consistent strategy that occurs with clients in mental health. Taylor (2008) suggests that important elements of encouragement are to "instill hope, courage and the will to explore or perform a given activity" (p. 78); in other words, to assist clients to be brave and to look to the future. Perhaps encouragement implies that the therapist holds that somewhat elusive attitude of hope (Fearing & Clark, 2000; Schwartzberg, 2002) and conveys that hope through his or her encouraging. Although it seems simple and a common sense technique, it also has to be timed and specific to individual situations and clients so as not to seem that the occupational therapy practitioner is merely a cheerleader. A practitioner's desire to instill hope, whether conscious or unconscious, must be balanced with the needs of the individual client and their worldview. Sometimes, practitioners mistake encouragement for validation, or give encouragement when validation is required. The case illustration of Jocelyn provides an example of validation and encouragement.

Advice

Advising is recommending a course of action or choice and may not necessarily be consistent with client-centered, collaborative practice unless used cautiously and within a clear clinical reasoning framework. Occupational therapy practitioners may advise clients when establishing realistic goals, based on information gained through the occupational profile. Practitioners may share potential outcomes with the client and recommend how the client can reach their desired goals and outcomes. Advice is also given regularly during treatment when clients seek help to

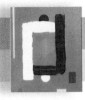

CASE ILLUSTRATION

Jocelyn—Encouragement and Validation

Jocelyn experienced depression and anxiety and attended an outpatient writing group to help alleviate her sadness and anxiety about being alone. However, she did not attend her writing group one week. The occupational therapist called her as the group started but was unable to reach her. Later, the occupational therapist e-mailed her saying that she had been missed. Jocelyn did not answer the e-mail, so the occupational therapist called her again with the same message. She reached Jocelyn on the last call and Jocelyn spoke about her distress due to a conflict she had had earlier with her only friend. The therapist listened to her story and validated that such conflicts were very difficult to handle, and must be very distressing because Jocelyn was already anxious about being alone and isolated. The therapist also stated that this conflict might have confirmed for Jocelyn that she was

not lovable. After a long conversation, she encouraged the client to come to the group, suggesting that writing about it might alleviate the distress and that the group would be helpful for suggestions on how to proceed with her friend. She also mentioned that the group members and she missed her. Jocelyn agreed to attend the next group and felt less alone.

Discussion

The occupational therapist was persistent in reaching Jocelyn and both validating Jocelyn's concerns and encouraging her to come back to the group. In this case, relying on a case-specific strategy, the therapist decided to interact with Jocelyn because she believed that Jocelyn wanted this specific response from the therapist. In other situations, she may have encouraged the group members to contact her.

accomplish their intervention program. For example, if a client wishes to pursue further education at a community college, the practitioner may advise on how to develop study or self-organizational skills. While a practitioner may wish to offer advice to discourage action that does not appear to be in the client's best interest (e.g., after leaving detox, a client wishes to meet up with substance-using friends), it is important to present this in a neutral way so that the client is able to accept or reject it, while still maintaining a working therapeutic relationship. In practice, occupational therapy practitioners may find it more helpful to utilize open questions such as "How do you feel about . . . ?" "How do you see . . . ?" "What are your thoughts about . . . ?" when discussing plans with their clients, rather than the more judgmental "You need. . . ." The latter phrase suggests that the therapist would like to control the situation or that clients are not capable of knowing their own needs. Care must be taken to assure that advice is given in a manner that conveys respect for clients and also the choices that they make.

Coaching

Coaching implies all the things that a practitioner does when she or he instructs clients during an activity. Coaching includes demonstrating, guiding, or prompting when necessary for clients to accomplish tasks. It also fosters a collaboration between the practitioner and the client and can be viewed as more supportive than an "expert" model and therefore is consistent with occupational therapy's core values. Coaching can also be a motivating factor because it redirects clients to performance aspects that may be satisfying or validating of their skills or habits (Kielhofner & Forsyth, 2002).

Confrontation

Confronting is to oppose or bring together for examination or comparison, or present for acknowledgment or contradiction. Occupational therapy practitioners may have face-to-face conversations with clients that are frank discussions of clients' behaviors, actions, skills, or performances that may be harmful or destructive. For example, an occupational therapy practitioner may confront a client who has not followed through with plans to look for a job, or may confront a client who has made denigrating remarks about other group members, and therefore has alienated herself from the group members. For example, in the case illustration of Athena, the occupational therapist set limits by confronting her behavior.

Confrontation is not carried out when the practitioner is angry, but with honesty and directness, often with an appraisal of the client's actions or behavior. In a way confrontation provides or sets limits because it is letting the client know that his or her behavior or actions are unacceptable. Confronting also conveys caring, that the practitioner cares enough about the client to notice and attempt to intervene when the client may be harming himself or herself.

Reframing

Reframing is providing alternative interpretations of behaviors, actions, performance patterns, or skills. Very often in mental health settings clients are unsure of their strengths and very knowledgeable about their weaknesses. Sometimes it is much easier for clients to see what they themselves cannot do, or what they lack, than it is to see what they themselves can do or what skills they have intact. This useful cognitive therapy technique highlights other aspects of clients' behaviors, actions, skills, or patterns when clients can only see usually negative aspects. The practitioner is able to accentuate or acknowledge the "other side of the coin" when clients only focus on one side. For example, when a client working on the computer entering a menu for the catering group complained about being too slow in typing when the practitioner seemed so much quicker, the occupational therapy practitioner noted that it was particularly important to have accurate menus and that the client seemed to be taking care to be accurate. In another instance an addict in a chemical dependency program lamented how he had "messed up his life." After validating his thoughts, the occupational therapy practitioner suggested that at least he had recognized it and could now begin to change.

Interpretation

Interpreting conveys the practitioner's understandings of the client's motivations, usually understood concurrently or intersubjectively by observation of the client's actions and verbalizations and self-observation of the practitioner's own thoughts and feelings about clients. Although interpretation is usually thought of in connection with psychotherapy or psychoanalysis, occupational therapists may interpret clients' motivations or the meaning of activities or occupations. Usually, an interpretation is offered in a timely manner and when the practitioner is absolutely sure that the interpretation will further the therapy process or performance.

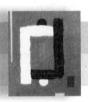

CASE ILLUSTRATION

Denny Mike—Interpretation

During an assessment, Brian, the occupational therapist, noticed that Denny Mike was seemingly interested in all activities with equal enthusiasm. As the assessment continued, Brian began to feel anxious and began to think that maybe Denny Mike was being sarcastic at best or dishonest at worst; however, Denny Mike also seemed polite and interested in the process. Brian thought that perhaps his anxiety mirrored that of the client, and perhaps Denny Mike's anxiety was driving the apparent self-report of enthusiasm for all activities. Brian offered an interpretation that maybe the client was nervous about performing well, and really did not know what he wanted, in addition to believing that to be cooperative, Denny Mike had to like everything Brian offered. Brian further stated that while he appreciated his cooperation and his courtesy, the best use of the assessment was really to find out what activities were important to him, and it was okay not to know exactly because in the process of occupational therapy he would clarify his likes and dislikes, values, and interests. Denny Mike appeared relieved and started to mention that he really did not value some interests that he had checked.

Discussion

Brian used the intersubjective experience to understand Denny Mike. Brian then was able to offer an interpretation that seemed correct because Denny Mike was visibly relieved. Also, the interpretation motivated Denny Mike to act more congruently with his desires and values and to use the assessment reliably.

Metaphors

In the language of metaphors, there is a transfer of meaning (Jones, cited in Schwartzberg, 2002) and a way of quickly grasping a concept without having to explain it in lengthy words. Using metaphors in conversations may not be a natural way of talking but can be learned and practiced (Bandler & Grinder, 1975, 1976; Lakoff, 1993; Lakoff & Johnson, 1980). Using metaphors in occupational therapy is a skill that comes with clinical experience.

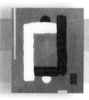

CASE ILLUSTRATION

Olivia—Use of Metaphors

After three years of practice, Tenaya, the occupational therapist, had attended many communication workshops and read many books about metaphors. When a group member, Olivia, who had many more skills that she could still learn and was not yet ready for discharge, announced that she was cured and ready to go, Tenaya used a metaphor to convey that she was not yet ready to leave. She stated that Olivia was like an ice cube that is partially on its way to being but not yet frozen. It may look like it is frozen and ready to be used, but when you put it into water, it will immediately crackle and melt. However, if you wait until the ice is completely frozen, when it is put into water, it will change the temperature of the water while it will remain intact for a long time. After listening to Tenaya, Olivia thought that she might still need to learn some skills.

Discussion

Olivia implicitly understood her own needs and changed her mind about leaving prematurely when Tenaya used a metaphor of ice cubes that conveyed her need to stay in treatment.

Reality Testing

Reality testing is offering an explanation of a situation that occurs in reality to counter obvious distortions or denials that clients may use. The understanding of what is actually happening is offered in such a way that the therapist encourages the client to think about and reflectively examine a situation. For example, in the previous case of Athena, the occupational therapist set limits around a situation that had just occurred by asking others to describe how Athena's comment had made them feel. In this situation Athena could not as easily deny the implications of her sarcastic behavior.

In addition to these universally used interpersonal strategies, the Occupational Therapy Practice Framework (AOTA, 2008) delineates methods that are unique to occupational therapy.

OCCUPATIONAL THERAPY METHODS

Broad strategies as well as methods of interventions and outcomes are specified in the Occupational Therapy Practice Framework (AOTA, 2008). The outcome of supporting health and participation in life through engagement in occupation is emphasized, but specific outcomes are also listed. This rendition of intervention makes it easier to set specific goals and to assess their outcomes. Because the practice framework defines broad strategies and methods of intervention, it also makes it easier to assess the outcomes of those strategies that you may use in practice.

Methods are: (1) to create and promote health, called health promotion; (2) to establish or restore health, called remediation or restoration; (3) to maintain health; (4) to modify, called compensation or adaptation; and (5) to prevent, called disability prevention. These broad methods are delivered through four interventions:

- Therapeutic use of self
- Therapeutic use of occupations
- Consultation
- Education

Application—Clinical Reasoning and Motivating

Perhaps because of the assumption that occupational therapy practitioners will use the Occupational Therapy Practice Framework (AOTA, 2008) in thinking and in documentation, the framework implies a clinical reasoning process. Within the framework, **clinical reasoning** is defined as a "complex multi-faceted cognitive process used by practitioners to plan, direct, perform and reflect on intervention" (p. 670) and it is viewed as a continual process that supports a client's engagement in occupation. This process includes integrating information gained from the evaluation stage along with theory, frames of reference, and evidence-based practice in order to develop and implement a collaborative intervention plan with the client. Thus, the forms of clinical reasoning always guide methods and interpersonal strategies used in practice in collaboration with the client. The clinical reasoning process (Mattingly & Fleming, 1994) forms the guide for how the practitioner will think about him/herself and the context of therapeutic interactions with the client. It enables the practitioner to plan step-by-step procedures (procedural reasoning), empathize with what is meaningful for the client (interactive reasoning), envision a past and a new future with the client (conditional reasoning), and perhaps engage in storytelling or storymaking with the client and with oneself (narrative reasoning) as a technique of facilitating the therapeutic relationship and change.

An essential element of the clinical reasoning process is reflective practice that can be described as "a deliberate, structured process involving the processing of information to assist with learning from complex situations" (Bannigan & Moores, 2009, p. 343). It requires the practitioner to reflect not only on events outside of themselves (e.g., client factors, activity demands) but also within themselves (e.g., emotions, biases, beliefs) and to critically analyze and evaluate these in order to promote professional growth. Bannigan and Moores (2009) advocate for a new model of professional thinking that integrates reflective practice with evidence-based practice, arguing that it is more inclusive and acknowledges the wide variety of contexts and environments in which occupational therapy practitioners work. The professional thinking model can be used as a framework to explore challenges or everyday events where the practitioner wishes to make sense of what has occurred in order to aid future practice.

An additional element of the clinical reasoning process is the ability to be attuned to the client's needs and our own emotions in the here and now in a mindful way. Kabat-Zahn (cited in Reid, 2009) describes mindfulness as "a means of paying attention in a particular way, on purpose, in the present moment, and in a non-judgmental way" (p. 181). This requires practitioners to be aware of their own thoughts, emotions, and reactions within the therapeutic relationship and to actively monitor these. Reid (2009) suggests that mindful occupational therapy is both a skill and an art where the practitioner puts "knowledge and skills into action while at the same time observing him- or herself in action" (p. 185). These skills can be gained through engaging in proactive systems for clinical supervision with peers, mentoring and professional development.

An intervention plan is directed by the client's priorities and the interaction of the client's performance skills, patterns, contexts, activity demands, and client factors. The process of intervention is dynamic and unpredictable and really depends moment to moment on clients' skills and patterns as they influence or are influenced by particular contexts, activities, or internal attributes. For example, clients in a psychosocial rehabilitation program may be the most skilled workers when it comes to clerical work; however, their skills may seem to deteriorate if they are required to perform the same skills in a different work environment (context), or if they have a different supervisor for the day (context), or if they are asked to complete a job with which they are not familiar (demands of the activity), or if they begin to hear voices (client factors). The context, the demands of the activity, or client factors may interfere with their ability to complete the task. Therefore, occupational therapy practitioners will use specific methods directed toward the contexts, the demands of the activity, or the client factors, and they will design specific interpersonal approaches that address the client, and most likely these approaches will motivate the client to change.

In suggesting a way of addressing motivational deficits that often accompany mental illness, Wu, Chen, and Grossman (2000) provide another useful way of thinking about the context, demands of the activity, or client factors in mental health. Essentially, they propose that a social context in which individuals' basic psychological needs are satisfied promotes intrinsic motivation. Basic psychological needs are the need for autonomy, or to determine one's own behavior; competence, or the need to experience productivity and to control outcome; and relatedness, the need to care for others. Thus an environment (context) in which a client will experience motivation will be one in which basic psychological needs (client factors) are met. Such needs can be met, and therefore intrinsic motivation can be facilitated by a combination of autonomy support, structure in activities (activity demands), and significant people being involved in therapy.

Depending on what motivates a given client, an occupational therapy practitioner may provide support, structure, and involvement in the following ways. Autonomy support can be generated by the practitioner valuing and *validating* the client's goals and interests, *encouraging* participation, providing the client with choices and abilities to make decisions, encouraging the client to act on one's own expectations rather than those of others, helping the client to take responsibility for changes rather than attribute change to the therapist, and *empathizing* with experiences of frustration due to gaps between present performance and future goals. Structure can be provided by including some challenge to clients' abilities, communicating clear expectations, providing clear feedback regarding performance, assisting clients to understand consequences of behavior (*reality testing and setting limits*), the relationship of goals and occupational therapy services, and the nature of personal gratification with one's interests versus performing for approval. Involvement may include educating, supporting, or consulting clients' significant others in the therapy process; encouraging clients' participation in group and social or community functions; or providing an empathic therapeutic relationship (Wu et al., 2000). The therapeutic relationship and therapeutic use of self will be discussed in more detail because they are methods discussed in occupational therapy's domain of practice. However, more important, they will also be discussed in a way that suggests an expanded understanding of the ideas.

No matter how a practitioner chooses to address context, activity demands, or the client implementation of an occupational therapy plan, treatment is carried out by types of interventions broadly stated as therapeutic use of self or therapeutic use of activities and occupations. Other types of interventions are consultation (identifying the problem, creating possible solutions, and trying them, and alternating if necessary), education (imparting knowledge and information about occupations, health, and participation), and advocacy (promoting occupational justice and empowering clients to seek and obtain resources), but since these are self-explanatory, they will not be discussed in this chapter.

Interventions

Occupational therapy interventions are guided by the Occupational Therapy Practice Framework's (AOTA, 2008) broad methods of therapeutic use of activity and occupations and therapeutic use of self. Under those broad categories are the techniques and methods unique to occupational therapy—activity and occupational analysis and gradation—and those techniques and methods that are borrowed or common to other practices—therapeutic use of self.

Therapeutic Use of Self

The therapeutic relationship between therapists and clients has had a significant role in the profession of occupational therapy since its inception. While the profession has fairly consistently emphasized the centrality of occupation and its relationship to health (Creek & Hughes, 2008; Meyer, 1922), it has also highlighted the importance of the relationship between therapists and clients (Frank, 1958; Mosey, 1986; Peloquin, 1991; Taylor, 2008). Therapeutic use of self is defined in the practice framework as "a practitioner's planned use of his or her personality, insights, perceptions, and judgments as part of the therapeutic process" (AOTA, 2008, p. 653). To some extent, this can be thought of as the personal approaches that a practitioner adopts in interpersonal interactions with clients, but this should also be accompanied by clear clinical reasoning for how, when, and why these approached are used. The framework advocates for client-centered practice and this is the context for employing therapeutic use of self as an intervention, in a collaborative process with clients. While the broader concept of the therapeutic relationship has been explored in the literature, there has been limited in-depth discussion of the components of therapeutic use of self and how they are used by occupational therapy practitioners until relatively recently. In a national survey of occupational therapy practitioners, Taylor, Lee, Kielhofner, and Ketkar (2009) found that more than 80% of respondents believed that "therapeutic use of self was the most important skill in their practice and the chief determinant of therapy outcomes" (p. 202). Although the practice framework provides practitioners with a working definition of therapeutic use of self (AOTA, 2008), it does not expand on how practitioners may use or evaluate this intervention in their everyday practice within the context of occupation.

Taylor (2008) notes that although the therapeutic relationship is central to the profession and has evolved over time, there has not been a "consistent conceptualization" (p. 3) of therapeutic use of self and that practitioners may have insufficient understanding of it, which subsequently impacts their ability to use it. To address this gap, Taylor has constructed the Intentional Relationship Model (Taylor, 2008), which aims to identify essential elements of therapeutic use of self and build practitioner skills within an occupational engagement perspective. Taylor identifies the four crucial elements of the model as "the client, the interpersonal events that occur during therapy, the therapist [and] the occupation" (2008, p. 47). A key component of this proactive model is for practitioners to be self-aware regarding their own personalities and therapeutic styles and how to best integrate these in the therapeutic relationship. For some practitioners, personal self-disclosure is part of employing therapeutic use of self to build the therapeutic relationship with clients. Practitioner self-disclosure has been defined as "statements that reveal something about therapists" (Hill & Knox, 2001, p. 413); however, it should be used judiciously as it may have both positive and negative effects.

Building and Repairing Relationships

Building a therapeutic relationship requires both skills and artistry on the part of the practitioner. It includes the ability to be empathic, non-judgmental, and open to working collaboratively with clients, while at the same time being mindful of setting limits and managing confrontations therapeutically. Other factors such as flexibility, humor, honesty, and humility contribute to establishing and fostering the therapeutic relationship (Haertl, 2008). When building therapeutic relationships, practitioners are required to have an awareness of the diversity of their clients and their backgrounds, experiences, and worldviews. In other words, practitioners need to become culturally competent in order to develop a client-centered practice that fits with each individual client. The impact of the therapeutic relationship has been linked to clients' functional outcomes; therefore, it is a positive investment for practitioners (Cole & McLean, 2003).

At times, challenges will arise in the therapeutic relationship and these may be client-driven, practitioner-driven, environmental/task-driven, or a combination. Practitioner-driven challenges may include issues as diverse as personal worries, workload management, or frustrations at the pace of therapy. Environmental or task-driven challenges may include lack of community facilities such as employment or housing options, which subsequently impact the interpersonal dynamics between practitioner and client. Taylor (2008) outlines several client-driven challenges including hostility, denial, disengagement, and re-emergence of symptoms. Taylor (2008) also discusses the impact that an empathic break on the part of the practitioner may have on the therapeutic relationship. She identifies this as an event that happens when the practitioner "fails to notice or understand a communication from a client or initiates a communication or behavior that is perceived by the client as hurtful or insensitive" (p. 124).

Regardless of the source, it is the practitioner's responsibility to recognize and manage the challenges in order to get the relationship back on track. As discussed previously, active clinical reasoning processes, and systems for reflection and developing self-awareness can assist in identifying the core issue and understanding how to manage it. Understanding the context of the challenge may identify potential solutions. For example, if a client's symptoms are re-emerging, then knowledge about the underlying condition and interventions may help practitioners to cope with unpredictability in interpersonal dynamics. Also, if a practitioner's frustrations about the pace of therapy or the nonresponsiveness of the client may be the challenge, the practitioner may use a self-reflective process to determine solutions. In addition, if this last practitioner challenge, in fact any of the challenges mentioned, here derail a therapeutic relationship, then seeking out consultation and supervision from an experienced practitioner is always desirable.

Empathy

Occupational therapy literature has explored the range of professional traits and approaches that practitioners may adopt in their interactions with clients (Borg & Bruce, 1997; Crepeau, Cohn, & Schell, 2003; Hagedorn, 2000; Kielhofner, 2002; Schwartzberg, 2002), with much of the emphasis focusing on empathy and trust. Both of these skills are considered essential components of the therapeutic relationship, in order to effect a client-centered approach. Peloquin (2003) identifies that empathy is multifaceted and is not only a means of establishing trust and a climate of caring within the therapeutic relationship, but also a way of recognizing the uniqueness of clients and their strengths and needs. Empathy is a professional skill that can be developed and is one ingredient of the therapeutic relationship that may effect change (based on the beliefs and theories of self-psychology, and its founder, Heinz Kohut [1971, 1977, 1985; Kohut & Elson, 1987; Siegel, 1997] and Kohut's followers [Elson, 1986; Grief, 2000; Kohut & Wolfe, 1978; Lee, 1991; Rowe, 1989; Shane, 1997]).

Contextual and Case-Specific Empathy

Empathy can be further distinguished as contextual empathy and case-specific empathy. Contextual empathy conveys caring, putting oneself in another's shoes, and the spirituality (or what Peloquin [2003] calls covenant) of "holding" a relationship sacred. An implicit aspect of each encounter in mental health is the empathic attitude that the client is valued and understood.

Case-specific empathy is used in clinical situations or therapeutic relationships by the practitioner to formulate an accurate response to an individual client in a specific context. If the therapist's responses convey empathy, then the client in turn will feel understood (Babiss, 2002) and *be more motivated to continue treatment*. So just as occupations and activities are considered the prime motivator of change in occupational therapy intervention, in mental health, the therapeutic relationship is equally important in motivating change in occupational therapy. This last statement is supported by research that finds the therapeutic relationship has proven to be important to the effectiveness of therapy (Krupnik et al., cited in Hagedorn, 2000) and is the most important aspect of psychotherapy regardless of which theory or type of therapy a practitioner espouses (Roth & Fonagy, 1996). An empathic response not only conveys caring, but also may be a response to a client's specific needs. Therefore, a case-specific response may be confronting or limit setting. It may be coaching or offering validation or reality testing. In that specific moment, the practitioner's response may not seem caring or appear to be caring, although it ultimately is because the response is exactly what is needed for the client in that specific situation. This understanding of empathy, contextual or case-specific, also demonstrates more than the therapeutic use of self.

Intersubjectivity

The use of empathy as a contextual attitude and as a case-specific response conveys that there is more than the therapeutic use of self that occurs in a therapeutic relationship; there is also therapeutic use of the other and the other-in-relationship to the practitioner. For example, empathy, empathic responses, and client progress imply that the client also has an influence on the relationship and on the therapist. While the OT practice framework emphasizes therapeutic use of self from the practitioner's perspective, which includes understanding the client's world through clinical reasoning, there is less emphasis on the fact that the client also influences the practitioner's world, until we view it from within Taylor's Intentional Relationship Model (2008). This allows us to consider that our responses and reactions as practitioners are impacted by the subjectivity of the client. Thus, particularly in a mental health setting, the intersubjective process must be emphasized (Crepeau, 1991; Stolorow, 1994; Stolorow & Atwood, 1992), as it may be contingent on how we use therapeutic use of self.

Emphasizing the **intersubjective process** means that the occupational therapy practitioner is more reflective and self-aware, or insightful (Hagedorn, 2000), in the therapeutic alliance, always reflecting on herself or himself in a self-analytical process (Stolorow, 1994). With this analytical vantage point the practitioner uses his or her thoughts and feelings to give clues about or recognize the thoughts and feelings that may be implicit with the client. Reid (2009) suggests that such "mindful practice" enables occupational therapy practitioners to "bring extra skills to their engagement with clients" because they are not only aware of external events, but also their own internal processes (p. 184). The analytical vantage point and understanding of the intersubjective nature of any therapeutic interaction or alliance then guide the occupational therapy practitioner in choosing and using various techniques or strategies on a case-specific basis. That is, the practitioner will choose strategies and techniques according to the subjective needs of each client in context. Obviously occupational therapy practitioners analyze client factors, contexts, and activities on a case-specific basis, but understanding the client's needs emerges out of awareness of the intersubjective nature of therapeutic encounters. The intersubjective nature of therapeutic encounters takes both the clients' and practitioners' factors or subjective meanings into account.

Therapeutic Use of Activity and Occupation

Although the practice framework finally defined therapeutic use of activity and occupations as the domain of occupational therapy, activities and occupations have been recognized throughout the history of occupational therapy as the core process of the profession.

There are many ways to think about and discuss activities and occupations, and there is much information regarding activity and occupational analysis in occupational therapy (Crepeau, 2003; Fidler & Velde, 1999; Hagedorn, 2000; Levine & Brayley, 1991). The practice framework (AOTA, 2008) specifically includes activity demands, and *Willard and Spackman's* 10th edition (2003) includes an occupation-based activity analysis format based on the information in the practice framework. Thus, this broad activity analysis includes categories of:

- Objects and their properties
- Space and social demands, thus attending to physical, social, and cultural contexts
- Required actions
- Required body functions and structures

However, within these broad categories, it is often difficult to ferret out which aspects of the activity demands are most useful for psychosocial purposes. Fidler and Velde (1999) note that there is still little information "regarding the inherent characteristics of activities, those elements that make up and define the nature of a given activity" (p. 1) and that "the social, cultural, and personal meanings and metaphors inherent in an activity are an essential aspect of understanding purposeful activity" (p. 3).

In addition to a perspective on activities that attends to their inherent characteristics and social, cultural, and personal meanings and metaphors, Fidler and Velde (1999) espouse another important emphasis (in Chapter 2 of her book that is written by Susan Fine) that is pertinent to mental health practice: an acknowledgment of a person's inner life. By inner life they mean mental processes that deal with thoughts and feelings and influence our behavior and that are influenced by activity and occupational performance. An apt quote captures a societal attitude that sometimes seems to be adopted by occupational therapists but that explains the significance of attending to unconscious elements of activity demands.

Acknowledging the unconscious inner life in the context of today's dynamic biopsychosocial dialectic does not commit one to the couch. It simply, and profoundly, opens the door to *a fuller understanding of how human activities at one level influence processes at another.* Exploring it is well worth the risk! (p. 13)

Because the practice framework provides essentially a broad overview of activity analysis but lacks a focus on psychosocial demands, symbolic and metaphorical meanings, or unconscious aspects that are provoked or inherent in activities, this chapter's information is based primarily on Fidler and Veldesview of activities and activity analysis. In addition, this chapter introduces another view of activity analysis that focuses on explicit and implicit methods in psychosocial activities (Eklund, 2002) because sometimes the goal in psychosocial occupational therapy is not so obvious.

Activity Analysis

The basic elements of an activity analysis are: (1) form and structure, (2) properties, (3) action processes, (4) outcome, and (5) realistic and symbolic meaning. Each of these categories is explained in more detail in the following paragraphs.

Form and Structure

Form and structure provide the rules and procedures, time to complete, and sequences that ensure predictable products or outcomes. Form and structure tell us how extensive and explicit the rules are, if the rules can be changed without significantly changing the activity, what the sequences in the activity are, and how long the activity will take to complete. A comparison of two crafts, forming a hand-built ceramic pot or constructing a wooden birdhouse, gives different structure due to the inherent pliable (clay) and nonpliable (wood) nature of the materials. Likewise, a self-grooming activity compared with completing a meal following a specific menu will provide more creativity and flexibility (self-grooming) or less creativity and flexibility (following a specific menu). The previous case illustration of Denny Mike indicated that he had difficulty expressing his unique opinions and attempted to please the therapist without thinking of his own interests. Therefore, if Denny Mike engaged in a concrete craft, it would most likely be more beneficial to give him one whose form is more pliable, so that he can experiment with fashioning his own unique design instead of following one in which he has no unique options.

Properties

Properties of an activity are the objects, materials, space, setting, equipment, and number of people required for an activity. These requirements dictate the nature of the activity and how it will impact the client. The properties of the activity form its "character" (Fidler & Velde, 1999, p. 51). For example, projects that can be accomplished by hand or with the aid of tools may convey different meanings. How might the project have different meanings depending on if it is crafted by hand or by power tool? A knitting project that is done by hand usually claims more respect (and more money) in our society than a knitting project that uses a knitting tool. Another example may be a work project that is completed in assembly line fashion. How might the project have different meanings for each of the clients that are required for the activity? How might the number of people required influence the interaction of those involved? In the case illustration of Athena, who required some limit setting due to her sarcastic comment subsequent to having difficulty accepting caring, it might be useful to engage her in a group project such as an outreach group in which members actively contact other members, or in a gardening project in which members work with each other in caring for plants.

Action Processes

Action processes identify the sensorimotor, cognitive, psychological, and interpersonal functions that the activity may demand. For example, a sports game such as flag football involves more sensorimotor processes than does watching sports, but watching sports may involve more cognitive processes than a sports game. Using the same example, the game of flag football may involve more psychological processes such as competition and aggression than cognitive processes of watching the game. Finally, the sports game may involve more interpersonal processes than watching sports if one watches a sport alone. However, if in playing the game a person only attends to his or her position and if being a spectator is a group activity, the sports viewing may include more interpersonal processes than playing the game (and many reports of superstars in baseball, such as Barry Bonds; football, such as Randy Moss; or basketball, such as Kobe Bryant, attest to isolation even while playing a game).

Outcome

The end product of activities may be a tangible product, such as a cake, or an abstract outcome, such as a decision made or a problem solved. Also, the end product may convey sociocultural meanings or meanings concerning individual values. For example, a cake might convey a cultural transition, such as in a cake celebrating graduation or a birthday, or may simply be a pleasing food item. A decision to discontinue a community vocational skills group may mean movement to the next level of work in the community or recognition that work is not important at this time in one's life or illness process.

Realistic and Symbolic Meaning

Activities and their elements have an actual, literal meaning and also have significance symbolically in personal associations or societal beliefs and cultural values. For example, maintaining a community garden may mean growing vegetables that may sustain an individual's family or psychosocial rehabilitation community by providing organic foods. Symbolically, it may mean the ability to nurture and sustain living things and to contribute in some positive way to one's community or to solving the problem of global warming. In the example of a gardening project suggested for Athena, when considering the properties of an activity, the symbolic nature of nurturing and sustaining living things and contributing to one's community may give her a way of accepting that she has the ability to nurture and care for plants, and that others may extend that same nurturing to her.

Activity Categorization

Fidler and Velde (1999) also classify activities into broad categories that can influence which activities one will use in practice according to each specific individual and context. Based on others' research (Moore & Anderson, cited in Fidler & Velde, 1999), socialization could be explained as developing from certain experiences with games and activities. Although this idea of how one develops through games and activities is readily acceptable when thinking of children, it is somehow lost when thinking of adults. However, it is no less true when thinking about adults in mental health settings, let alone adults in other settings. So this manner of categorizing activities according to the characteristic of games that contribute a socializing factor in people's lives is particularly important for individuals with mental illness whose overarching problems keep them functioning as best they can in society. These categories are listed in Table 19-1. Although activities change over time and societies, these are provided as examples of some activities that may sustain people through various life crises and changes. Readers are encouraged to think of their own interests and values and how they are related to the activities that they pursue in their own lives.

TABLE 19-1. Categories of Activities

Activity Category	Examples	Characteristics
Puzzles	Knitting, weaving, orienteering, survivor programs Learning computer software Negotiating the Internet	Contain much form and structure, predictable outcomes, clear sequences, and procedures. Performer can control and predict the outcome.
Chance	Card games—poker or solitaire Board games—Scrabble or Sequence Watching sports	Contain little form and structure, unpredictable outcomes, few rules and procedures. Performer has little control or prediction of outcomes.

TABLE 19-1. Continued

Activity Category	Examples	Characteristics
Games of strategy	Card games—bridge, hearts Board games—chess, checkers Sports participation—tennis, basketball, soccer, softball, running track	Contain some form and structure, sequences and procedures, but they depend on the other person playing—anticipation of the other's plan in conjunction with one's own plan—and are constantly and dynamically changing. Performer has some control but less prediction of outcomes.
Aesthetic	Attending concerts, museums, plays and critiquing music, art, or drama Obtaining antiques or "collectibles" Refereeing sports Performing music, art, or drama for an audience	Less defined external form and structure and rules and procedures determined by the person. Contains an evaluative element. Performer can control the process through element of making evaluative judgments or through performance. Actual performance is subject to less control of other's evaluative judgments.

© Cengage Learning 2013

CASE ILLUSTRATION

Sylvia—Characteristics of Activities

Sylvia had been hospitalized twice in her 20s because of suicide attempts after the termination of relationships that she thought were the "loves of her life." While hospitalized she had been diagnosed with major depression and borderline personality disorder. During the hospitalizations it was discovered that she also had post-traumatic stress disorder because of her mother's periodic loss of control and physical abuse, and because she often had been placed in various foster homes prior to being adopted when she was 12. While hospitalized she was unable to sustain her denial of her abusive past and to maintain the picture of her mother as someone treated unfairly by "the system."

While hospitalized and working with these issues that caused considerable stress, Sylvia worked on activities that could be categorized as puzzles. In occupational therapy, she particularly enjoyed weaving scarves on a hand-loom and finding information about Native American textiles on the Internet. She also enjoyed the occupational therapy groups in which she could discuss her feelings but in an intellectual way about various issues of daily life, including how to save money, how to have casual relationships, how to get along at work, and ways to access personal resources and develop a self-identity (see Cara [1992] for further discussion of these ideas).

After discharge Sylvia had been able to function for 10 years without rehospitalization, during which time she attended individual and group therapy. During those 10 years she had continued to have various chaotic and unhappy love relationships, most of which ended unhappily and often caused her to request extra therapy time. At these times her psychiatrist would suggest that she attend an ongoing community mental health occupational therapy group so that she could identify and pursue some new interests. Sylvia also was able to renew her interest in weaving that she had learned in the hospital, and that interest sustained her during periods of turmoil.

Now as she entered her 40s, Sylvia realized that maybe her life was satisfying without a long-term, significant relationship. She had two cats that she took care of, and she also grew plants and vegetables that she used in cooking. She had learned to cook with these natural ingredients. She had become increasingly active in a tennis league and had purchased season tickets to the ballet. In addition to supporting the ballet in a volunteer role, she also was active in Amnesty International, and felt gratified that she was able to support political prisoners.

Discussion

During acute periods of her illness and during times when she was particularly vulnerable, Sylvia engaged in activities, such as weaving, that provided much form and structure and predictable outcomes. She satisfied her nurturing desires by taking care of plants and animals, and by her volunteer roles. She also used her strength of intelligence and thought about how she felt about various instrumental activities of daily living. She began to sort out her values and interests and acquire new roles as she formed a personal identity. When she became more able to regulate her emotions, Sylvia realized that perhaps she could enjoy life although she was not attached to a man. She broadened her interests into games that included some form and structure but also some change and interactions with another person. She also broadened her interests into aesthetic activities in which each performance was less predictable and offered an element of surprise and in which she could satisfy her inquiring mind by evaluating.

Implicit and Explicit Methods

Another broad way of analyzing psychosocial interventions is placing the intervention on a continuum of explicit or implicit methods (Eklund, 2002). Although thinking in terms of explicit or implicit methods is most useful in explaining occupational therapy to those unfamiliar with it, thinking in these terms can help organize how one will deliver services. On the one hand, in an explicit method the relationship between the purpose of the activity and the end goal is clear and direct and the skill being learned is obviously necessary in an occupational performance. For example, a transportation group may be carried out because a client needs to learn how to travel to a job independently. On the other hand, in an implicit method, the purpose of the activity and the end goal are less clear and more indirect and the skill being learned is not as obviously necessary for performing a given occupation. For example, a transportation group may be carried out because a client needs to learn how to handle change, read signs, make appropriate small talk with strangers, or learn how to maintain concentration.

There are differences in various dimensions of activities that are important when thinking of using either method (Eklund, 2002). Those dimensions are: short-term goals, activities used, time required, and position in the profession. In explicit methods, the short-term goal is typically better skills in occupational performance; activities used are ADL, work, or leisure skills directly related to the goal; time required is the time it takes to master the current activity; and the methods constitute the core of occupational therapy—therapeutic use of activity. In implicit methods, the short-term goal is typically better functioning in performance components or patterns; the time required is the time it takes to master the current activity and the underlying components; and the methods are not as linked to the core of occupational therapy, but are inherent in all occupational performance.

The case of Brandon and his occupational therapist, Jackie, demonstrates the interpersonal strategies discussed in this chapter.

CASE ILLUSTRATION

Brandon—Jackie's Interpersonal Strategies

Jackie, an occupational therapist, was contacted by a local mental health agency that provides supervised and supported living environments for persons with psychiatric disabilities. She was recruited specifically to assist in the evaluation of potential tenants for the agency's new independent living apartment project that was still in the planning stage. In the development of a previous apartment program, the agency had had significant difficulty with tenants not being able to manage the demands of independent living with the level of support that had been provided. This new project would have the same level of support as the previous one and the agency wanted to ensure that they chose tenants who could successfully sustain their housing. Jackie's use of strategies with Brandon, one of the potential clients, began with evaluation although she did not know at the time that she would be working with him after the evaluation, when the apartments were built.

During the evaluation process, Jackie provided *empathic responses* to Brandon's frustrations about having mental illness, not being independent, and wanting very much to live on his own. Through the interactive clinical reasoning process she was able to gain an understanding of Brandon, his hopes, fears, dreams, and frustrations. Through *conditional reasoning* she was able to form an image of Brandon that included his past and what he might become or where he might be in the future. She encouraged Brandon to share his own personal story and *validated* his statements about himself and his situation, about his feelings toward his family, staff, and other tenants, about his frustrations when he experienced hypomania, paranoid thoughts, or hallucinations.

During the intervention process Jackie continued to provide encouragement, validation, and empathic responses. However, empathic responses did not always mean some positive statement about Brandon's behavior, choices, or feelings. For example, at times, Brandon believed that he was doing so well that he probably did not really have mental illness but was just "stressed sometimes." At those times, Jackie provided an empathic response concerning how hard it might be to accept mental illness, particularly when one seemed to be functioning so well, but that indeed she along with many others observed that he did have a mental illness and the symptoms did interfere with his life.

Because Jackie was often working in Brandon's apartment, she often encountered situations that called for *limit setting, confrontation,* and interpretation. For example, during an intervention in which the objective was making tea for a guest as the rudimentary step to having his family for dinner, Brandon stated that having her for tea really was like a date, and since she was not married and they got along so well, that maybe they should extend their "friendship" into something more serious. Jackie stated that she thought working in someone's home made it very difficult to always be aware that this work was a professional encounter. Furthermore, the type of interventions, like meal planning and hosting a dinner party that they worked on, further blurred the reality that this was a professional encounter. Nevertheless, she thought that Brandon's idea was somewhat grandiose and his grandiosity was most likely influencing him to read more into her actions and behavior than was actually there. This symptom was one of the very reasons he attended his group and for which he requested *reality testing* and she would not be doing her job if she did not let him know about it. Brandon became angry and initially accused Jackie of encouraging his romantic feelings toward her. However, Jackie *accepted* his expression of anger and continued to *confront* his denial, grandiosity, and hurt feelings. Eventually, she stated an *interpretation* that she understood that he liked, respected, and appreciated her, and perhaps it was difficult to express his feelings without "sexualizing" them. After this very difficult situation, Brandon and Jackie were able to work within professional boundaries.

At times Jackie coached Brandon, particularly when they attended the entitlement workshops, implemented the intervention plan in the supermarket, or when carrying out an objective in his plan by having tea. She often used *metaphors* and *reframing* during these times and also when Brandon reported his problems back to her after having friends or his brother and sister for breakfast (another objective in the intervention plan). After the first time he had a friend for breakfast, he reported his discouragement that he could not get everything ready at the same time. Jackie stated that this was one of the hardest, intangible aspects of cooking meals that often doesn't show up until you cook a large meal, and that he was most fortunate that it came up so early so that he could get this intangible aspect correct for the family dinner. Additionally, putting a meal together and having everything ready at the same time is like a dress rehearsal, and you want things to go wrong at the dress rehearsal not at the final performance. Brandon responded humorously that, indeed, maybe this was an example of a situation where you wished that you were a little manic!

Discussion

During evaluation and treatment Jackie used interpersonal strategies that kept the plan on track and further motivated Brandon to continue his efforts to achieve his goals.

SUMMARY

The Occupational Therapy Practice Framework (AOTA, 2008) specifies the domain and the process of occupational therapy. The occupational therapy domain is use of occupations and activities for intervention. The occupational therapy process involves clinical reasoning and interpersonal techniques and strategies to apply occupations or activities. Activity and occupational analysis and gradation are unique to occupational therapy and ways of thinking about activities in psychosocial practice (Eklund, 2002; Fidler & Velde, 1999; Wu et al., 2000) were suggested. Although interpersonal strategies are common in other fields, they are efficacious when used in occupational therapy, particularly for motivating clients to engage in treatment. An overall interpersonal approach is client-centered and grounded in empathy and trust while useful interpersonal strategies are validation, setting limits, encouragement, advice, coaching, confrontation, setting limits, reframing, use of metaphors, and reality testing.

REVIEW QUESTIONS

1. Why are limit setting and interpretation useful strategies in mental health care?
2. What is the intentional relationship? How does it relate to therapeutic use of self?
3. What is an important perspective regarding activities in a mental health practice?

4. What is intersubjectivity and why is it discussed apart from therapeutic use of self in this chapter?

5. What are the categories of activity and how do these categories define activities?

REFERENCES

American Occupational Therapy Association (AOTA). (2008). Occupational therapy practice framework: Domain and process (2nd edition). *American Journal of Occupational Therapy, 62,* 625–683.

Babiss, F. (2002). Treatment experiences: Helpful and not helpful. *Occupational Therapy in Mental Health, 18*(3/4), 39–62.

Bandler, R., & Grinder, J. (1975). *The structure of magic: A book about language and therapy* (Vol. 1). Palo Alto, CA: Science & Behavior Books.

Bandler, R., & Grinder, J. (1976). *The structure of magic, II* (Vol. 2). Palo Alto, CA: Science & Behavior Books.

Bannigan, K., & Moores, A. (2009). A model of professional thinking: Integrating reflective practice and evidence based practice. *Canadian Journal of Occupational Therapy, 76*(5), 342–350.

Borg, B., & Bruce, M. A. (1997). *Occupational therapy stories: Psychosocial interaction in practice.* Thorofare, NJ: Slack.

Cara, E. (1992). Neutralizing the narcissistic style: Narcissism, self-psychology, and occupational therapy. In S. C. Merrill (Ed.), *Occupational therapy and psychosocial dysfunction* (pp. 135–156). New York: Haworth.

Cole, M., & McLean, V. (2003). Therapeutic relationships redefined. *Occupational Therapy in Mental Health, 19*(2), 33–56.

Creek, J., & Hughes, A. (2008). Occupation and health: A review of selected literature. *British Journal of Occupational Therapy, 71*(11), 456–468.

Crepeau, E. B. (1991). Achieving intersubjective understanding: Examples from an occupational therapy treatment session. *American Journal of Occupational Therapy, 45*(11), 1016–1025.

Crepeau, E. B. (2003). Analyzing occupation and activity: A way of thinking about occupational performance. In E. B. Crepeau, E. S. Cohn, & B. A. B. Schell (Eds.), *Willard and Spackman's occupational therapy* (10th ed., pp. 189–198). Philadelphia: Lippincott Williams & Wilkins.

Crepeau, E. B., Cohn, E. S., & Schell, B. A. B. (Eds.). (2003). *Willard and Spackman's occupational therapy* (10th ed.). Philadelphia: Lippincott Williams & Wilkins.

Eklund, M. (2002). Explicit and implicit methods in psychosocial occupational therapy. *Occupational Therapy in Mental Health, 18*(2), 3–15.

Elson, M. (1986). *Self-psychology in clinical social work.* New York: Norton.

Fearing, V. G., & Clark, J. (Eds.). (2000). *Individuals in context: A practical guide to client-centered practice.* Thorofare, NJ: Slack.

Fidler, G. S., & Velde, B. P. (1999). *Activities: Reality and symbol.* Thorofare, NJ: Slack.

Frank, J. D. (1958). The therapeutic use of self. *American Journal of Occupational Therapy, 12*(4), 215–225.

Grief, G. (2000). *The tragedy of the self: Individual and social disintegration viewed through the self-psychology of Heinz Kohut.* Lanham, MD: University Press.

Haertl, K. (2008). From the roots of psychosocial practice—Therapeutic use of self in the classroom: Practical applications for occupational therapy faculty. *Occupational Therapy in Mental Health, 24*(2), 121–134.

Hagedorn, R. (2000). *Tools for practice in occupational therapy: A structured approach to core skills and processes.* Edinburgh: Churchill Livingstone.

Hill, C. E., & Knox, S. (2001). Self-disclosure. *Psychotherapy, 38*(4), 413–417.

Ikiugu, M. M. (2010). The new occupational therapy paradigm: Implications for integration of the psychosocial core of occupational therapy in all clinical specialties. *Occupational Therapy in Mental Health, 26*(4), 343–353.

Kielhofner, G. (2002). *Model of human occupation: Theory and application.* Baltimore: Lippincott Williams and Wilkins.

Kielhofner, G., & Forsyth, K. (2002). Therapeutic strategies for enabling change. In G. Kielhofner (Ed.), *Model of human occupation: Theory and application* (3rd ed., pp. 309–324). Philadelphia: Lippincott Williams & Wilkins.

Kohut, H. (1971). *The analysis of the self.* New York: International University Press.

Kohut, H. (1977). *The restoration of the self.* New York: International University Press.

Kohut, H. (Ed.). (1985). *How does analysis cure?* Chicago: University of Chicago Press.

Kohut, H., & Elson, M. (Ed.) (1987). The Kohut seminars on self psychology and psychotherapy with adolescents and young adults. New York: WW Norton & Co.

Kohut, H., & Wolfe, E. (1978). The disorders of the self and their treatment: An outline. *International Journal of Psycho-Analysis, 59,* 413.

Lakoff, G. (1993). The contemporary theory of metaphor. In A. Ortony (Ed.), *Metaphor and thought* (pp. 202–251). Cambridge: Cambridge University Press.

Lakoff, G., & Johnson, M. (1980). *Metaphors we live by.* Chicago: University of Chicago Press.

Lee, R. (1991). *Psychotherapy after Kohut: A textbook of psychotherapy.* Hillsdale, NJ: Analytic.

Levine, R. E., & Brayley, C. R. (1991). Occupation as a therapeutic medium: A contextual approach to performance interventions. In C. Christiansen & C. Baum (Eds.), *Occupational therapy: Overcoming human performance deficits.* Thorofare, NJ: Slack.

Mattingly, C., &. Fleming, M. H. (1994). *Clinical reasoning: Forms of inquiry in a therapeutic practice.* Philadelphia: F. A. Davis.

Meyer, A. (1922). The philosophy of occupational therapy. *Archives of Occupational Therapy, 1*(1), 1–10.

Mosey, A. C. (1986). *Psychosocial components of occupational therapy.* Philadelphia: Lippincott Williams & Williams.

Padilla, R. (Ed.). (2005). *A professional legacy: The Eleanor Clarke Slagle lectures in occupational therapy, 1955–2004* (2nd ed). Bethesda, MD: AOTA Press.

Peloquin, S. (1991). Occupational therapy service: Individual and collective understandings of the founders, Part 2. *American Journal of Occupational Therapy, 45*(8), 733–744.

Peloquin, S. (2003). The therapeutic relationship: Manifestations and challenges in occupational therapy. In E. B. Crepeau, E. S. Cohn, & B. A. B. Schell (Eds.), *Willard and Spackman's occupational therapy* (10th ed., pp. 157–184). Philadelphia: Lippincott Williams & Wilkins.

Reid, D. (2009). Capturing presence moments: The art of mindful practice in occupational therapy. *Canadian Journal of Occupational Therapy, 76*(3), 180–188.

Roth, A. R., & Fonagy, P. (1996). *What works for whom?: A critical review of psychotherapy research.* New York: Guilford.

Rowe, C. E. (1989*). Empathic attunement: The "technique" of psychoanalytic self-psychology.* Northvale, NJ: Jason Aronson.

Schwartzberg, S. (2002). *Interactive reasoning in the practice of occupational therapy.* Upper Saddle River, NJ: Prentice-Hall.

Shane, M. (1997). *Intimate attachments: Toward a new self-psychology.* New York: Guilford.

Siegel, C. (1997). *Heinz Kohut and the psychology of the self: The makers of modern psychotherapy.* New York: Routledge.

Stolorow, R. (1994). The intersubjective context of intrapsychic experience. In R. Stolorow, G. Atwood, & B. Brandchaft (Eds.), *The intersubjective perspective.* Northvale, NJ: Jason Aronson.

Stolorow, R., & Atwood, G. (1992). *Contexts of being: The intersubjective foundations of psychological life*. Hillsdale, NJ: Analytic.

Taylor, R. R., Lee, S. W., Kielhofner, G., & Ketkar, M. (2009). Therapeutic use of self: A nationwide survey of practitioners' attitudes and experiences. *American Journal of Occupational Therapy, 63*(2), 198–207.

Taylor, R. R. (2008). *The intentional relationship: Occupational therapy and use of self*. Philadelphia, PA: F. A. Davis.

Wu, C., Chen, S., & Grossman, J. (2000). Facilitating intrinsic motivation in clients with mental illness. *Occupational Therapy in Mental Health, 16*(1), 1–14.

Chapter 20

Groups

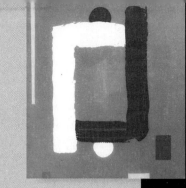

Elizabeth Cara, PhD, OTR/L, MFT

▮▮ KEY TERMS

activity group

group

group content

group dynamics

group norms

group process

group protocol

group structure

personhood skills

psychodynamic

psychoeducational

CHAPTER OUTLINE

Introduction

What Makes a Group a Group?

Advantages and Limitations of Groups

Overview of Group Therapy

    A Short History

    Models of Group Therapy

    Group Content and Structure

    Group Dynamics and Process

    Group Stages and Patterns

    The Group Roles

    Problems in Groups

    The Group Leader

Occupational Therapy Groups

    Activity Groups

    Task Groups

    Developmental Groups

    Directive Groups

    Neurodevelopmental Groups

    Sensory Intervention Groups Using Sensory Modulation Approaches

    Psychoeducational Groups

    Community and Self-Help Groups

    Other Groups

Starting a Group

The Group Protocol

Documentation and Outcome

Summary

INTRODUCTION

Occupational therapists in the psychosocial arena conduct much, if not most, of treatment in **group** settings. Group treatment can be incredibly exciting, stimulating, and interesting. It is exciting to implement or to lead groups, and it is stimulating to develop or create them. Developing and implementing groups includes both artistic and scientific elements. The science is involved in developing the **group structure**, organizing a **group protocol**, recognizing the needs of the setting and the population with whom one works, applying a knowledge of occupations and occupational skills, and utilizing good communication and interpersonal skills. The art lies in being aware of the **group process**, using oneself in a therapeutic way, and knowing, and responding to, the here-and-now needs of the individual group participants and to the participants as a group—simultaneously. Both the art and the science can be learned through acquiring knowledge and practicing experientially. This chapter discusses groups in general and how to think about occupational therapy groups so that they can be developed and implemented creatively and competently, in any setting, and with any participants.

Specifically, this chapter explains how to develop, conduct, and lead groups. It also distinguishes occupational therapy groups from other types such as psychotherapy groups that are conducted by other professionals.

WHAT MAKES A GROUP A GROUP?

There are various definitions of groups, all of which include a situation in which three or more people come together and think of themselves as a group. A group can be thought of as an intentional coming together to produce change for the members (Borg & Bruce, 1991; Hagedorn, 2000; Howe & Schwartzberg, 2001) and also as a microcosm of society, in which participants can learn about themselves and their relationships (Corey, 2008). There are common properties that characterize almost any group. These include:

- A background, history, and purpose.
- A structure imposed by the group leader, which usually consists of preparations, expectations, a composition, and arrangements.

- An interaction pattern, for example, member-to-member or member-to-leader.
- Communication or action taking place, whether verbal or nonverbal.
- Usually, a cohesion, or a "we" feeling.
- Standards or rules of acceptable behavior.

The **group norms** or standards of a group usually contribute to cohesion and a feeling of safety and trust. Norms can be explicit or implicit, verbalized or unstated, developed initially by the leader or based on the group interaction (Cole, 2005). Norms are often set and monitored by how the group leader models expected behavior and handles unwanted behavior. In addition to the leader, the environment—both physical space and how people react in and to it—and goals of the group also are responsible for the development of norms (Borg & Bruce, 1991). For example, a norm of talking to other group members and not to the leader is developed when the leader does not answer every question directed to him or her, but instead asks the group in general to answer the question. A norm of talking to, not about, each other is established when the leader asks an individual who is talking about another person in the group to direct his or her comments to the person about whom he or she is speaking. A norm of the members' acceptance and importance in the group is set when the group meets at a regular time, is held in a comfortable, distraction-free place that accommodates everyone and is identified as the space where occupational therapy happens, and supplies are made readily available. In addition, the therapist should greet participants warmly, start the group on time, and always begin and end the meeting in a similar manner. When the group leader states the clear goals of the group and the purpose for the group to each new member—or asks participants to do so—a norm is established concerning how new members will enter the group and what individuals should learn in the group is made explicit.

Common norms necessary in any group are confidentiality, a here-and-now focus, respect for each individual, and participation—though each member has a right to choose how to interact, what to disclose, and what to do in the group (Corey, 2008).

ADVANTAGES AND LIMITATIONS OF GROUPS

Practically speaking, group treatment in mental health is time and cost effective. It costs less to treat people in groups than it does to treat them on an individual basis, and they allow more people to be seen in a shorter amount of time. Group treatment facilitates personal growth by virtue of providing more people with whom to interact. Participants can learn about themselves through identifying with others; observing, and being able to compare and contrast their own experience with those of others; experiencing closeness and caring; and having opportunities to be around others in a safe or trusting context. Groups support experimentation and trying of new behavior, with a variety of feedback provided by different people (Corey, 2008). More specifically, occupational therapy groups facilitate learning new skills from others. Groups are like mini-laboratories in which one can practice skills for living in a simulated experience.

Of course, there are some limitations to group treatment. Not everyone is suited for groups. For example, an individual may be too disoriented, confused, or suspicious of others to be able to tolerate a group. A group may be too distracting or require too high a degree of abstract ability. Some clients may require individual treatment; for example, if they are inpatients in an acute care hospital, they may not be able to leave their room or setting due to precautions or illness. Last, some people may simply need the concentrated effort of individual treatment. The following section discusses some of the properties, norms, stages, and themes of groups. (For examples of specific groups see Champagne [2005] and Helfrich & Rivera [2006].)

OVERVIEW OF GROUP THERAPY

"Since humans have inhabited the earth, we have joined and been influenced by groups" (Barlow, Burlingame, & Fuhriman, 2000, p. 115). However, the history of groups has been written mostly in the beginning of the last century, and group psychotherapy has been practiced in one form or another since the early 1900s (Scheidlinger, 1994). While group therapy may bring to mind a psychoanalyst silently treating a group of adults, group therapy has been conducted by various professionals for problems ranging from psychopathology to problems in living. It has been brief to long-term and occurs in many settings. Because various disciplines have contributed to its application and theory, the history of group therapy is complex, nonlinear, and distinguished by somewhat disparate research.

A Short History

Although Europe contributes to the history, group therapy is generally thought to be an American phenomenon resulting from the energy of this open culture in the twentieth century (Barlow et al., 2000; Brabender & Fallon, 2009). "The professionally guided helping group is an American invention" (Scheidlinger, 1994, p. 197). Although early pioneers included Freud and Adler in Europe, it was Pratt in the United States who first conducted groups for individuals with tuberculosis in 1905. Shortly after Pratt, in 1909, Marsh, a minister who became a psychiatrist, gave his psychiatric clients inspirational group lectures (Scheidlinger, 1994). In the 1920s, milieu therapy and the psychoeducational method were introduced for "mental" clients. Principles of using members' influence, maintaining a here-and-now focus, and analyzing the group emerged from the group treatment of the mentally ill. Also in the first two decades of the twentieth century, Jacob Moreno founded psychodrama and began to use group action methods called sociodrama. Techniques of psychodrama that later became mainstream practice included role playing and role reversal. Drama therapy continues to have a vibrant role in occupational therapy treatment (Javaherian-Dysinger & Ebert Freire, 2010). In the 1930s, groups re-created the family, the method was introduced for children, and group leaders established credentials for leadership. These diverse applications were based on diverse theories, for example, classical psychoanalysis, existentialism, and behaviorism.

In the mid-1940s, the understanding of group process became popular as a result of World War II, which caused numerous psychiatric casualties at a time when there was a shortage of psychiatrists. Therefore, therapy in groups became a necessity. Also in the 1940s, researchers attempted to confirm the efficacy of groups and to categorize them. However, the groups were too diverse to catalogue adequately. An explosion of group practice models and outpatient groups continued throughout the 1950s. With the opening of community mental health centers in the 1960s, innovative group therapy models were developed (Scheidlinger, 1994). During the same decade research methods became more rigorous, and researchers were better able to describe various variables or factors in group therapy. Diverse aspects of groups such as therapeutic factors (hope, altruism, identification, etc.), interventions (feedback, reality-testing, role flexibility, etc.), and leader traits (directive, warm, active, etc.) were researched throughout the 1990s. Regardless of which aspects of groups have been studied, the outcomes suggest that "groups do appear to work" (Barlow et al., 2000, p. 117).

Currently, managed care and the emphasis of biology in treatment point to certain future trends. Most likely, short-term groups with one leader will proliferate, as well as large-group and community treatments and psychoeducational and medical self-help groups; also, groups will be manualized and tailored to specific client populations.

Models of Group Therapy

The increasing use of group therapy techniques has paralleled the rise in popularity of different psychological models. For example, from the concept's inception through the 1950s, groups were based on a psychoanalytic model, which was popular in the United States during this period. Today, self-help groups and brief cognitive and behaviorally oriented groups are popular because of the growth of behavioral and cognitive models and a community self-help movement grounded in the context of recovery, ". . . the process in which people are able to live, work, learn, and participate fully in their communities" (President's New Freedom Commission on Mental Health, 2003, p. 7; see also Chapters 1, 4, and 12 in this text).

Different concepts, techniques, and leadership roles will be assumed depending on which model a group is grounded. A brief explanation of various psychological models of group therapy is presented in Table 20-1. Although one may pattern a group specifically on one model, in actuality many groups are implemented utilizing various principles. Each group developer and leader will generally blend what they feel to be the most effective concepts and techniques to create a unique group (Corey, 2008).

TABLE 20-1. Models of Group Therapy

	Psychoanalytic	Humanistic	Behavioral	Cognitive-Behavioral
Philosophy Emphasis	Childhood experiences.	Self-actualization.	Changing behavior.	Changing thoughts or schemas.
	Make the unconscious conscious; mentalization.	Self-awareness.	Learning effective, eliminating maladaptive, behavior.	Learning more adaptive thinking, eliminating maladaptive thinking.
Key Concepts	Work through resistance and transference; understand early relationships.	Understanding values and discovering meaning.	Increasing effective, decreasing ineffective, behavior.	Change cognitions, thoughts, or schemas.
Goal	Insight, awareness of mental states of self and others.	Maximize climate of growth and awareness.	Change behavior.	Change thinking to influence behavior.
Role of Leader	Interpret, understand, reflect.	Keep focus in the present; model authenticity.	Organize, direct, teach new skills.	Organize, direct, teach new skills.
Techniques	Interpret and analyze, reflect.	Understanding modeling, confronting, clarifying; coaching, role modeling.	Learning principles: delineating, reinforcing, extinguishing.	Various principles: clarifying, changing or eliminating thoughts, learning schemas that influence behavior.

© Cengage Learning 2013

Group Content and Structure

The **group content** is the activity that is planned and carried out in the group (Denton, 1987) or what is said in the group (Cole, 2005; Howe & Schwartzberg, 2001). It can be either verbal or nonverbal. The way in which the activity is presented; the directions, procedures, techniques, and time arrangements; and the way in which membership is organized comprise the group structure. The content and structure of a group will naturally flow from its purpose and the style of the leader. Group content and structures have been combined in various ways to produce many types of occupational therapy groups.

Group Dynamics and Process

Group dynamics are the forces that influence the relationships of members and the group outcome (Cole, 2005). Some important dynamics of a group are the process and stages of groups, leadership styles and leader behaviors, roles that members assume, norms, and expected standards of behavior, the behavior and interaction of the group members, the group structure, and the environment in which it is held.

The group process refers to how the work of the group is carried out (Howe & Schwartzberg, 2001), including how participants relate to each other, who talks to whom, how tasks are accomplished, and how decisions are made. Group process involves two tiers (Yalom, 2005). On the first tier, it includes the here-and-now experience of the group members, who focus their attention on their feelings toward other group members, the therapist, and the group as a whole. The immediate events in the meeting take precedence. The second tier involves the group's focus on recognizing and understanding its own process. The group becomes self-reflective in looking at the here-and-now behavior that has just occurred. This two-tiered process is what facilitates learning and generalization as the group becomes a microcosm for the participants' outside lives. It becomes a personal laboratory in which to discover, study, and change one's life experience. In psychotherapy groups, "processing" about the group experience may occur during the meeting, whereby individuals may become reflective and analytical, which allows them to understand, integrate, and generalize their behavior from the group experience to their everyday life. Continual processing about the group does not usually occur as an **activity group** experience, although members may reflect and analyze their experience through the activity of the group or as it pertains to activities generally (Fidler, 1969); moreover, group leaders may—and, in fact, should—analyze and reflect on each group meeting after its completion.

CASE ILLUSTRATION

One Group's Process

Townehouse Creative Living Center was a clubhouse following the model of Fountainhouse in New York. Members who lived in board and care homes and who usually were severely and chronically mentally ill attended five days per week. All members attended groups depending on which work the group carried out. For example, the house and grounds group cleaned houses and apartments, did recycling and car washes, and conducted gardening and landscaping. The nutrition group cooked lunch daily for the members and accepted catering jobs in the community. The clerical group took on work such as stuffing envelopes, compiling and sending out mailings, and making notecards. The transitional employment program (TEP) had volunteer and paid jobs in the community that members could work at for six months at a time to gain work experience. The group also required attendance once per week at a work support group where members discussed any issues or questions that concerned work.

One of the weekly TEP groups had started and Lucius was talking about his new job at the local fast food place as the lot and lobby person. He was excited after his first day, explaining that this was the first time he had worked in 10 years. As he was talking, LaBrea came in late, dressed much fancier than usual and sexier and inappropriate for her role as a member of the day program. She said nothing and sat down. The members did not acknowledge LaBrea but all stared at her and Lucius stopped talking in mid-sentence. After a short silence of about 45 seconds, Thomas began to talk about a date that he hoped he could make when he got paid for his job on Friday. Dante began to talk boastfully about his car and how he had a girlfriend. Enrique began to talk rapidly and incoherently and Keiko then talked about a job she had years ago making pretty dresses. When Gus, the group leader, asked Lucius if he was finished, Lucius said yes and sat sulkily while LaBrea interrupted to talk about her desire for a job as a hostess in a fast food restaurant.

The content of the group started out as a discussion group where members could share their thoughts and feelings about work. Lucius verbalized his thoughts and feelings about his new job. After LaBrea arrived what was said in the group changed to discussions about dates and jobs a long time ago. The nonverbal content of the group indicated that LaBrea was dressed inappropriately and that after she arrived late, Lucius became silent and sulked, Dante became boastful,

Enrique became incoherent, and Keiko talked about work that was not meaningful to the group.

Discussion

Some hypothetical ideas about the process of the group might be:

LaBrea needed attention and achieved it by her clothes and late entrance to the group. Perhaps she was romantically interested in one of the group members and dressed and arrived late so she would be noticed. Alternatively, she may have wished to have a job as a hostess and believed that if she dressed as she thought a hostess should dress she might somehow get such a job.

Lucius was excited about his first job in a long time and was doing the work of the group by telling other members how he thought and felt about it. When interrupted by LaBrea he was hurt or angry but was unable to acknowledge that when given the opportunity by Gus.

The *other members* were influenced by LaBrea's appearance and her late entry. Thomas and Dante made associations to LaBrea's appearance and associated it with dating. Alternatively, perhaps Thomas and Dante became anxious by the interruption and LaBrea's inappropriate appearance and/or the 45-second silence but were unable to keep on track with the purpose of the group. Enrique and Keiko perhaps also became anxious and made loose associations that did not make sense for the group. Alternatively, this may be their current state and the way they participate in the group.

Group Stages and Patterns

The stages and patterns of a group can be considered as happening over a length of time in different sessions or, with the advent of shorter treatment, within one session. Stages have been described primarily with traditional psychotherapy groups in mind; however, these stages and themes can be recognized in all types of groups, including activity groups. In fact, it appears that activity groups are often nonthreatening, causing stages to occur more rapidly. Although stages are written about as if they were linear, in fact, different stages can overlap. The group process consists of the patterns or stages that groups usually go through; these are characterized by recognizable feelings and behaviors that are usually unspoken or not made explicit (Corey, 2008). Group stages have been characterized in different ways according to certain themes that arise in each stage (cited in Borg & Bruce, 1991; Cole, 2005). The themes have been described as "forming, storming, norming, and performing"; "inclusion, control, and affection"; "flight, fight, unite, and orientation"; and "conflict, harmony, and maturity." The general themes describe or explain the participants' own thoughts and feelings about the group and the other group members, including the leader. They connote the process of coming together with unknown others and involve an unknown future process: (1) wondering if one will be accepted and liked, (2) deciding on standards for the group, (3) agonizing about the degree to which one wants to be in the group and whether one can follow the norms, (4) a cohesive stage of acceptance of the self and others and investment in using the group for the work that needs to be done, and (5) an ending and consolidation of growth and learning.

Initial

In the initial stage, participants generally learn the norms and expectations, get acquainted, and attempt to determine whether they will be included or excluded. Members will decide whom they can trust and will like, how much they will be involved, and how deeply they wish to disclose. Some tasks of the group member are to begin to behave in a way that will establish trust, learn how to express feelings (especially fears, concerns, and hopes for the group), being involved in the creation of the group norms, and establishing goals for themselves. The leader functions are usually to role-model active participation, develop the rules, assist members to establish a trusting atmosphere and establish goals, and structure the group so that it will have the right balance, discouraging both excessive dependence and excessive floundering. Possible problems involving group members are the failure to participate, an unwillingness to reveal themselves, and the refusal to accept a role of advice giver or problem solver.

Transition

In the transition stage there tend to be more feelings of anxiety on the part of group members. Participants may be concerned about being accepted, how safe the group is, and the leader's competence. They may struggle with ambivalence between choosing risk taking or compliance and, possibly, control or conflict and confrontation. Tasks may include recognizing and expressing negative feelings, learning how to deal with one's own personal resistances, and overcoming conflict with others. The leader functions so as to support the group through the transition so that members will accept and resolve conflict and personal resistances. The leader provides a model of tact and directness, assists members to recognize their personal resistances and interpersonal conflicts, and encourages them to "stay with" expressing reactions that pertain to the here-and-now happenings in the group. Problems may arise if members are categorized as problem types and scapegoated, refuse to express feelings or engage in handling conflicts, or form subgroups to discuss negative reactions outside of the group but not in the presence of the group as a whole.

Working

The working stage is characterized by a high level of trust and cohesion. Members tend to participate and communicate openly in a responsible way, the group shares leadership functions, there is a willingness to take risks, conflict is recognized and handled constructively, and participants generally feel energized to change their behavior outside the group. There is a general tone of high energy and hope. Members function as independent initiators, bringing topics that they are willing to express openly to the group, offering and accepting constructive feedback, and striving to be both more challenging and more supportive of each other. The leader functions as a role model who provides a balance of support and confrontation, interprets the meaning of behavior patterns so that members can engage in a deeper level of self-exploration, explores common themes to link the work of the individual members, and encourages members to practice new skills. Possible problems include members' tendency to challenge each other, the possibility of gaining insufficient insight in the group but to understand the necessity of behavior change on the outside of the group, and the risk of becoming more anxious because of the intensity of group meetings.

Final

In the final stage group members may feel sadness and fear over the group's eventual ending, hopes and concerns for each other may be expressed, members generally ready themselves for dealing with the reality of the world outside the group, and there may be an evaluation of the group experience. Members' tasks are to deal with their feelings regarding separation, offer feedback to others, complete any unfinished business concerning others in the group, discuss changes still to be made and how to make them, and attempt to generalize what they have learned to everyday life. The leader assists the members in dealing with their feelings regarding termination, reinforces changes, and assists members to consolidate what they have learned in the group and understand how it might be applied to everyday life. Possible problems concern members' avoidance of reviewing their experience or putting it into a framework that enables generalization and the danger they may distance themselves from the other group members, thus limiting the possibility of expressing and consolidating feelings. Table 20-2 reviews group properties, norms, stages, and themes.

With the advent of shorter treatment duration, fewer groups will have the luxury of smoothly moving through the various stages to completion. Instead, groups may remain at one stage and fail to progress to the next. However, the various themes that characterize each stage may still become apparent. For example, in a short-term evaluation group, the theme of wanting to be accepted may be expressed by a group member refusing to participate in the assessment or, in a daily movement and exercise group, a member may only participate by watching from the sidelines. A theme of deciding how to be in a group may be expressed by a member attempting to take care of other group members or attempting to assume responsibility like the group leader. Harmony or affection may be achieved in a daily group that runs for a week, yet at the end some members may fail to show up for the last meeting or demean their accomplishments in the group.

The Group Roles

In addition to stages characterized by certain themes, group members may also assume certain roles that can be characterized by the group tasks that they undertake in their roles. Some roles are helpful for accomplishing the group's task while other roles help the group maintain the status quo or keep the group functioning. For example, some participants may take on a helper role, while others may seem to do the work of the

TABLE 20-2. Group Properties, Norms, Stages, and Themes

Properties	Norms
Background, history, purpose	Confidentiality
Structure	Here-and-now focus
Interaction pattern	Manner of participation
Communication	Activities
Cohesion	Individual respect
Rules and standards	

Stages	Themes
Initial	Learning expectations; Getting acquainted; Wondering about inclusion/exclusion; disclosure/involvement, trust
Transition	Wondering about acceptance/rejection; safety; leader competency Struggle with compliance versus risky behavior
Working	Trust and cohesion; Responsible communication; Constructive resolve Sharing of responsibility
Final	Evaluation of experience; Feelings of ending/separation; Completion of unfinished business; Continuing change

TABLE 20-3. Group Roles and Functions

Roles That Further Group Tasks	Function of the Roles
Initiator	Often the first to suggest solutions or ideas and sometimes literally the first person to respond to the leader's suggestions or inquiries.
Elaborator	Usually expands upon suggestions or inquiries but usually does not initiate.
Information or Opinion Seeker	Asks for clarification of facts or of participants' or the group's attitudes, values, and thoughts.
Information or Opinion Giver	Offers generalizations or facts automatically without being solicited or offers facts or opinions instead of feelings.
Coordinator	Discusses the relationship of various ideas that may organize the ideas for other participants.
Orienter	Will keep the group on track by defining how the group is keeping to or straying from the goals of the group.
Critic	Critiques the group's accomplishments or functioning as a group.
Energizer	Facilitates some action or decision making by the group.
Operator	Does things for the group following the procedures, such as putting chairs around a table or getting supplies, that help move it toward its goal but the things are not necessarily recognized because they are procedural.
Recorder	Writes down suggestions or decisions or what happens in the group.
Roles That Maintain Group Functions	**Function of the Roles**
Encourager	Praises or generally accepts the contributions of the participants.
Harmonizer	Moderates any differences among group members; usually actions are directed toward "keeping the peace."
Compromiser	Consistently changes own opinion in order to keep group harmony.
Standard Setter or Follower	Expresses the ideals to which the participants can aspire or goes along with the other group participants.
Group Observer or Commentator	Observes and comments on the group process.

Adapted from Cole (2005)

group and therefore act in accordance with the purpose or goals of the group. Table 20-3 lists some roles that have been universally identified by many theorists (Cole, 2005).

By recognizing these group roles the therapist can help members take on the roles, particularly in a task group. A successful group can be defined as one in which participants take on a variety of the roles because learning takes place as each participant experiences these roles. Also, a healthy group is usually one in which there is a balance of all of the roles. Often, participants will naturally assume these universal group roles. However, a therapist in a more structured group can explicitly assign the roles to the participants.

CASE ILLUSTRATION

Group Roles

Due to the economy, Townehouse Creative Living Center experienced a reduction in funds from the county that necessitated a cutback in the program. The staff of the clubhouse met and came to the consensus that the best way to deal with the reduction in funds was to eliminate the drop-in program that was held every day for people who did not attend regularly or consistently, but because the program was a clubhouse, members were generally not turned away. The staff presented this option to the clubhouse governing board members and the members of the club, who had been elected president, vice-president, secretary, and treasurer. The governing board agreed that eliminating the drop-in program was the best option. They also recognized that some of the drop-in members could form another vocational group based on doing clerical work. Furthermore, they thought that the drop-in members should decide among themselves who should become everyday members and who would be referred elsewhere for services. The staff followed the dictates of the governing board and planned a series of groups facilitated by a staff person for the members to form the clerical section.

At the beginning of the week, the staff facilitator, Song, informed the drop-in group of the cutback in funds and what had been recommended by both the staff and governing board. She posed a problem for the drop-in members to solve in the next few days of group. The problem was how to decide who would remain as members of a clerical section and who would be asked to seek other services. Starting the next day and for the next four days and maybe the next week she told the members that they were all welcome to join in this decision-making group. She informed the group that there were two roles that should be assigned each day, the procedural role and the recorder role, and she explained each role.

Mingus volunteered for the procedural role for the next day's group, and Aki volunteered for the recorder role for the remainder of the groups. Song thanked Aki for volunteering but wondered aloud if perhaps other members might like to share that role. Khalil spoke up and said he would like to function as the recorder, too. Dorothy agreed with Khalil and further suggested that after tomorrow members could volunteer for each role and the group would vote for the volunteers if there were more than one. Lilly followed up Dorothy's suggestion with a request that the group vote for either Aki or Khalil to be the recorder today.

After the group voted for Aki for the day's recorder the group sat in silence. Then Newton began to talk about the coffee he was drinking. Amy offered that she and Newton had gone to Peete's instead of 7-11 for their coffee in the morning and that Peete's coffee was much stronger and tasted much better. Khalil said he would be interested in going to Peete's tomorrow and asked where it was located. Silvio said that he had been to Peete's but he liked the 7-11 better because they sold donuts and had larger coffee cups.

After another silence, the leader, Song, wondered aloud if the group would like to discuss how the group members would be selected for the clerical group. Khalil suggested that they vote today on who would become the members of the clerical group. Dorothy suggested that maybe the members had different ideas and perhaps they should talk about them. Lilly agreed with Dorothy and stated that she thought the members should each have a chance to state their opinions. Rosetta stated that she, too, wanted to go to Peete's in the morning and Amy said that she would go with Rosetta. Newton stated that he would meet them there and Silvio said that he was still going to the 7-11. Etta wondered if the clubhouse would be having coffee with lunch and the group discussed if they should have coffee with lunch. The leader, Song, wondered aloud if perhaps the group was having a hard time keeping to the task because they were afraid of hurting someone's feelings.

After a silence, Khalil stated that he was afraid of being voted out of the group. Silvio thought that was not a bad idea and stated that he would vote Khalil out of the group. Khalil became angry and raised his voice as he stated that he knew Silvio did not like him since he (Khalil) had started to date LaBrea, who had been Silvio's girlfriend for a while. As both Silvio and Khalil started to argue, Newton told both Silvio and Khalil to calm down and the group members were tired of them arguing. Dorothy suggested

that they make some rules about acceptable and unacceptable group behavior. Lilly agreed and stated that arguing was not acceptable. Dorothy wondered if group members should be thrown out if they argued. Newton thought that there should be a rule against arguing, but that Silvio and Khalil should have another chance. Dorothy agreed that maybe they should have another chance, and Lilly suggested that members vote on that rule. At this point Aki wondered if she should be writing "all of this down."

The leader, Song, observed that the group seemed to have a hard time discussing how to select members of the clerical group, and wondered if Aki should be writing about everything that happened or should be writing down the rules that the group decided on. Khalil apologized for fighting and thought that Aki should be writing everything down. Dorothy wondered what they needed all of the information for, and Lilly thought that they would want all of the information because she would want to know what had happened just in case she missed a group. Dorothy changed her mind and thought that Lilly had a good idea. Newton thought that if they wrote everything down it would also include the rules so why not write everything to make sure that those who only came once or twice knew what happened. The leader, Song, suggested that perhaps what was to be recorded should be voted on by the group and the group proceeded to vote.

After the vote Song noted that it was time to stop and wondered aloud if there were any other comments or business that needed to be done. Khalil thought that they should elect a procedures person for the next day, since the chairs needed to be arranged. Dorothy suggested that the group make their own coffee in the morning and that the procedures person could be the one to make it. Lilly agreed and suggested that they vote. Newton thought that they should ask Mingus if he wanted to make the coffee and Mingus stated that he would make the coffee for the group the next day. The leader, Song, asked if Mingus needed some instructions about making coffee, but he mentioned that he had assumed that role in another group. Mingus asked if he should set up the chairs again tomorrow, and Aki then asked if she was the recorder tomorrow. No one answered but the members looked at the leader, Song.

Song wondered aloud if the group remembered that they had voted to have a person volunteer each day for the recorder. Khalil stated that he did remember voting that a person should volunteer to be the recorder each day if more than one person volunteered. Dorothy seconded Khalil, and thought that they should vote again tomorrow. Lilly wondered if anyone else wanted to be the recorder, but no one else spoke. The leader, Song,

suggested that maybe they should complete the task of choosing the recorder in the beginning of tomorrow's group and the group members agreed to do that. Amy, Newton, and Khalil stated that since Mingus was making coffee tomorrow, they would meet at Townehouse and go to Peete's another time.

Discussion

The various participants and the leader assumed different roles during the group. In this session, each of the group's participants functioned primarily in the same role throughout the group, for example, Khalil consistently initiated, Dorothy consistently elaborated, and Lilly consistently energized the group, while Newton became the harmonizer. Some of these members assumed more than one role, for example, Dorothy also became a compromiser. The leader, Song, assigned two roles to the members throughout the group, and she herself assumed the roles of information seeker, energizer, and group commentator. Song chose her roles strategically to facilitate the group process.

Problems in Groups

In addition to the roles that further the group process or maintain the group's function, theorists have also identified individuals' roles. Often the individual roles become a detriment or interfere with the movement of the group and there is a temptation to label certain people as the source of problems in groups (such as the storyteller, the avoider, the monopolizer) instead of simply labeling their behavior (Cole, 2005; Corey, 2008). It seems very human to attribute a person's behavior in a particular situation to an enduring character trait. However, this can be a danger in groups (as it is in the practice of psychiatry) due to the tendency to then consistently characterize the person by a single instance of behavior, which in reality may not occur again or may be inconsistent and only happen in certain situations. In particular, a group situation should allow for testing of behavior, and often, participants are unaware that their behavior is considered a problem. With this caveat in mind, we will now review behaviors that may interfere with the normal development of groups if allowed to persist, and that may be addressed by the group leader in fundamental ways.

Although in some instances, problematic behavior may have to do with the participant's thoughts and feelings about the group leader, in general, "problem" behavior is not usually personally directed to the leader. Often, it is mostly unconscious and unintentional. (This is a basic assumption of psychiatry.) Generally, the best procedure to use in handling "problem" behavior is to (1) attempt to understand the meaning of the behavior for that specific time, group, and group members; (2) accept the behavior in a non-defensive way and address it in a manner appropriate to the situation, the functioning of the person, and the level of disruption (disruption either in the behavior itself or to the group); and (3) allow the person to "save face" and avoid power struggles whenever possible.

Nonparticipation

A group member's nonparticipation, silence, or withdrawal is not an overt problem, but it will influence the other group members if it continues and is usually not helpful for the individual participant. Natural silences do occur in individual or group treatment, and often they may define a therapeutic moment or positive transition point. Naturally occurring silence can be distinguished from silence that is more defiant or defensive. The latter, which will be discussed here, is ongoing and noticeable as a behavior pattern, and it is not necessarily spontaneous. It may occur because the individual is not cognitively competent to handle the demands of the group or because symptoms, such as hallucinations, may be a barrier to participation. The individual may fear looking foolish or being rejected, feel unlovable and vulnerable, be paranoid or uncertain about how the group works, or not trust or want to be in the group. The leader should invite participation in the group, direct comments to the person, or make contact in some way, and if possible, he or she should directly explore what makes the person behave in that way. In an activity group, this is less problematic because clients usually will become involved. For example, a task can be adapted (e.g., graded to make the steps more simple) or the individual who does not want to participate can be asked to at least remain with the group. An extreme of nonparticipation is leaving a group before its completion. Again, the leader should consider whether the client may have been cognitively incompetent or too distracted for that specific group. Contact should be made with nonparticipants to assure their safety and let them know that their presence is valued. If appropriate, the leader should explore the reasons for departure. Sometimes clients are unable to consciously recognize or discuss their behavior. If that is the case, then the leader should either just make contact or provide a choice of reasons that they may agree to or at least think about.

Monopolizing

Monopolizing behavior is at the opposite end of the spectrum, with storytelling, questioning, advice giving, and intellectualizing somewhere in between. A person's symptoms, such as symptoms of mania, may interrupt the group or the individual may be driven by the same fears and concerns that lead to unnatural silences. Monopolistic behavior can be more problematic than silence because it demands to be addressed and will eventually cause the other members to resent the person. If the behavior is part of a person's symptoms, the leader should continually address it by interrupting the person and redirecting him or her. The behavior can be confronted by gently describing the situation, stating, for example, "I don't know if you realize that you are taking up all of the group's time. Your thoughts and feelings are important, but I think other group members would also like to participate." Alternately, the leader may attempt to deepen the person's self-understanding, as appropriate to the person and the situation, by saying, for example, "You seem to want a lot of attention, but I sense that the way you are asking for it is turning people off, which is not really what you want."

Hostility

Hostile behavior can be direct or indirect. Indirect hostility may come subtly in the form of sarcasm, jokes, seeming bored and detached, or arriving late. The individual may fear looking foolish, fear rejection, feel unlovable, be uncertain about how the group works, or not trust or want to be in the group. The person may be expressing himself or herself in a learned manner and may not recognize that this is distancing. The person may be disappointed and hurt, or he or she may be feeling angry and expressing it in an indirect way. A special case occurs often with activity groups and occupational therapists, whereby clients will denigrate an activity—or the occupational therapist who suggests it—as being too simple, childish, or totally unrelated to treatment or change. For some people, this may mean that the activity is too challenging and, perhaps, cognitively overwhelming. In that case, acknowledging the right to decline participation or changing the activity may take care of the situation. If the level of difficulty is not the apparent problem, gentle confrontation may be enough to change the behavior, such as by saying, "You seem upset today—is that so?" or "I don't know if you realize that your comment sounds somewhat angry—is that how you are feeling?" In the case of denigration of the activity, there may be different ways to approach the situation. A serious explanation of the rationale for the activity and how it may be helpful to the person will often defuse the situation. Alternately, an acceptance of the person's feelings and explanation that although the activity may appear overly simple it has additional benefits, which may defuse the hostility. Sometimes an exploration of how the person felt when engaged in the activity helps to shift or reframe the situation. In all instances of problem behavior, the leader's response will depend on the situation, the person's level of functioning, and the leader's understanding of the behavior's meaning.

CASE ILLUSTRATION

Handling Problem Behaviors in a Group

In a life skills group for young adults that met daily, participants at times discussed how to use cognitive techniques to quiet their minds and avoid distractions when asked to do group projects together with other students in their classes. They acknowledged that their anxiety, as demonstrated by obsessive and negative thoughts about themselves as individuals, often prevented them from even starting the projects. They were then labeled "lazy," ostracized from the class, and more than likely denied a grade indicative of their knowledge. After the first week of the group, Maria, the OTR, was feeling increasingly uneasy about the sessions. For the most part, the group was functioning, but two members often interfered with the process. The first, John, declined to comment when asked to share some pertinent cognitive problem or solution and often physically separated himself from the others. Most of his comments were aimed at interpreting other people's problems or offering solutions for others in the group. Another member, Louise, participated in group exercises and made comments but also often directed comments with subtle sexual innuendos to the therapist.

After careful consideration in supervision of each member's difficulties and circumstances, Maria decided to handle the two individuals in two different ways. Knowing John and observing him in other groups, she believed that he felt less intelligent than the others and feared they would find this out if he acknowledged his perceived shortcomings. Maria raised this fear as a group issue, not mentioning John but rather questioning whether others worried about rejection and acknowledging how difficult it is to reveal perceived weaknesses that have seemed hopelessly intractable. The group members, including John, were able to discuss their fears of seeming inadequate and thus to identify with, and support, each other.

Knowing Louise, the leader judged her comments to reveal a more personal issue—that Louise either liked the group leader and was expressing it in this indirect, almost unconscious, way or, perhaps, was expressing a fear about the leader's competency. She decided to discuss this with Louise personally and inquire whether Louise was aware of the nature of her comments. In fact, Louise was surprised and embarrassed to realize that she had made such comments; however, she also acknowledged her affection for Maria, who represented a healthy, strong model that Louise wished to emulate.

Discussion

Each instance of "problem behavior" meant something different for the individual participant and the group and was, therefore, handled differently. In each case, however, the therapist's reaction was congruent with her assessment of the group process, the meaning of the comment, and each person's individual process.

In addition to considering the individual's behavior as a personal problem, it is useful to consider whether one's own leadership style and manner of interacting or the group structure or content may be contributing (Howe & Schwartzberg, 2001). For example, is the activity matched with the person's ability? Is the person able to meet the demands of the group? Is the reason for the activity clear? Has the leader successfully created norms of safety and trust and interacted in a respectful and genuine manner? Has the leader assumed too much responsibility for the process of the group? Perhaps neither the leader, the interaction, nor the person is a cause of problem behavior and, instead, some outside influence has affected the group or its members. For example, was there an incident on an inpatient unit, such as a suicide attempt or theft, or was the person just notified of a workplace review by his boss or social security audit? Perhaps visitors have just left. Indeed, there can be many potential influences external to the group.

The Group Leader

The role of the group leader may change somewhat according to the type of group, but there are also general leadership aspects that define the role, communication skills that can be utilized in the role, and general **personhood skills** (which translate into leadership skills) (Corey, 2008). Every group has properties and norms and goes through stages characterized by certain themes. Table 20-4 lists ideal roles, communication skills, and personhood traits of group leaders.

Roles and Style of Leadership

Overall, the leader is the organizer of the group. He or she initiates action and interaction, directs the activities of the group, and establishes an atmosphere of trust and openness. The leader can be thought of as the "holder" of the group by virtue of his or her development, implementation, and overall investment (Yalom, 2005). Group leaders must remain aware that ongoing careful attention to the structure and content of the group through their interactions and directions continually establishes its tone and influences its success and the degree of member participation.

By establishing the norms and boundaries of a group through organization and attention, a group leader can assist members in feeling comfortable and motivated to participate. The group leader should strive to establish an "ambiance of safety." More specific aspects of the leader's role are:

- Demonstrating by example.
- Setting rules and limits, such as confidentiality, not interacting in subsets, and not interrupting.
- Providing orientation.
- Being tuned in to the mood of the group.

TABLE 20-4. The Group Leader

Role	Function
Organizer	Sets and maintains norms, boundaries, and rules. Establishes a tone, or ambiance, of safety and participation.
Role Model	Demonstrates by example. Provides orientation.
Facilitator	Determines and directs or enables the group activity and participant interactions.
Communication Skills	
Active Listening	Absorbing the content, noting a person's gestures and changes in expression, and sensing underlying messages (what a person is not saying) while simultaneously remaining fully present and concentrated in the moment for each interaction.
Reflecting	Communicating back to a person the essence of what she or he has communicated to you.
Clarifying	Recounting what a person has communicated.
Blocking	Prohibiting, either directly or by your interpretation, types of communication that are destructive to the group process or members. Examples of destructive communication are gossiping, breaking another's confidence, and invading another's privacy.
Facilitating	Inviting others to participate, that is, to express thoughts or feelings or to work on the activity of the group; to work or interact with other members or to make comments concerning other members' statements or products.
Empathizing	Providing a response to indicate you understand a person and what he or she has wished to communicate; that you can "put yourself in another person's shoes."
Personhood Skills	
Courage	The ability to admit mistakes, express fears, or act on hunches; to be direct and honest with members; to be genuine and not defensive in the face of criticism; to do what the leader expects others to do in that group situation.
Willingness	To model or exhibit behaviors that one expects of group members.
Being Present	Fully experiencing the group's activity or interactions and not being distracted from the purpose of the group.
Belief in the Group	Believing in the value of what is being done or is happening in the group.
Ability to Cope Non-defensively	Not personalizing, retaliating, or withdrawing from comments or actions that you perceiveas critical of you or your performance.
Self-Awareness	Awareness of personal goals, identity, motivations, needs, strengths and limitations, values and feelings.
Sense of Humor	The ability to laugh at yourself and to see and understand the frailty of the human condition.
Inventiveness	The capacity to be spontaneous and creative, often combined with the ability to learn from every experience in life.

Adapted from Corey & Corey (2008)

Basically, as group leader, you are a role model. Through your behavior and attitude, you model the norms you would like to create in the group (Corey, 2008; Howe & Schwartzberg, 2001; Kaplan, 1988). *This is true for all groups* whether the members only work in the presence of others or interact with each other, the content is activity-based or psychodynamic, and the structure is verbal or nonverbal. This is true even though you may perceive your role as being simply an organizer, teacher, or resource guide.

Your natural style of leadership may be broadly considered as active and directive in your involvement or as more facilitative and supportive. As a directive leader, you actively control or direct the group, usually choose the activity and direct the process, and actively direct interactions to motivate clients. A facilitative leader will remain more in the background, perhaps supporting the members as they make their own decisions and interact among themselves. Often the structure of a group may dictate the leadership style; for example, the leader may be introducing a new or novel activity, the group members cognitively may require direction, or the goal of the group may be to increase motivation or interpersonal skills. In these cases, a directive and active leadership style is required. Another example is a group whose goal is to determine community resources that support finding a job. In this task, members should be more independent and can benefit from interacting with, and supporting, each other, skills that will be required in a job. In this case, the leadership style must necessarily be facilitative. See the Case Illustration "Group Roles" for an example of a facilitative group leadership style and notice that the leader, Song, assumes the roles of organizer and role model. Notice the communication skills that Song uses in the group, and imagine the personhood skills that she must possess to be an astute and successful group leader.

Communication Skills

There are many communication skills that can be learned and become part of a group leader's repertoire of skills. Although there are many skills, some of the most important are active listening, reflecting, clarifying, blocking, facilitating, and empathizing. (These skills are explained more fully in Table 20-4.)

Personhood Skills

Other skills sometimes are more difficult to explain or acquire because they often have to do with an individual's personality, or personal traits, temperament, and experience. These can be called personality traits, but the term *personhood skills* (Corey, 2008) better conveys that these are particular traits that positively influence how one person relates to another. In occupational therapy the concept that comes closest to "personhood skills" is therapeutic use of self, defined in the Occupational Therapy Practice Framework (AOTA, 2008) as "planned use of . . . personality, insights, perceptions, and judgments as part of the therapeutic process" (p. 628). (See Chapter 19 for further discussion of these ideas.) Therapeutic use of self or personhood skills can sometimes be learned by observing the behavior of someone who has the traits and noting how he or she practices the skills in everyday life. (The personhood skills are listed and explained in Table 20-4.)

OCCUPATIONAL THERAPY GROUPS

Occupational therapy groups have much in common with groups based on other models. Often they borrow techniques, such as assertiveness training or role-playing, which originated according to other psychological models. Such a blending of methods and techniques is not uncommon in the field of mental health. However, occupational therapy groups tend to be unique in two ways. They are unique in their *focus on the activity,* which is the aspect that produces change. They are also unique in their *emphasis on occupations,* which involves changing areas of occupation and performance skills and patterns. This broad purpose can be incorporated in any occupational therapy model. Although people often erroneously assume that every group's purpose is interaction, broad categories of activity groups show that the purpose of occupational therapy groups extends far beyond simply social interaction.

Activity Groups

Activity groups have been defined in different ways in occupational therapy. A variety of activity groups are defined and practiced by occupational therapists and modeled after occupational therapy frames of reference, but no consensus has yet been reached on an inclusive, unique definition of the type of activity group employed exclusively by occupational therapists. Groups have been developed according to occupational therapy models (Kaplan, 1988; King, 1974); they generally follow the principles of other systems, especially the psychoanalytic and developmental approaches (Borg & Bruce, 1991; Fidler, 1969; Mosey, 1970, 1981); and they may delineate a specific structure (Cole, 2005; Howe & Schwartzberg, 2001; Kaplan, 1988). What they all have in common is that the content focuses on activity, emphasizes occupation, and addresses areas of occupation performance skills and patterns to aid in adaptation, improve or enhance occupational performance and quality of life, promote role competence, client satisfaction, health and wellness, prevent unhealthy lifestyle, or provide advocacy skills (AOTA, 2008). All groups also share a common structure, which de-emphasizes reflecting on the group process throughout the duration of the whole group.

Activity groups have been considered to have the properties of both psychotherapy groups and task groups (Borg & Bruce, 1991; Denton, 1987). A psychotherapy group usually emphasizes group process with a goal of resolving inter- or intrapersonal issues, whereas a task group usually emphasizes an outcome or product, which can be tangible, such as an art project, or intangible, such as a decision or recommendation and the goal of the task group is to accomplish a group task. An activity group falls somewhere in between the two types of groups. It may emphasize a group goal, yet the interaction concerning the group goal may be considered as important as the goal. Alternately, the interaction may occur through a medium of activity.

Activity groups have been defined (Howe & Schwartzberg, 2001) as those in which members are engaged in a common task directed toward occupational performance. The group focuses on function and replicates living in the community or family. The activity focuses the group's attention, and the group members learn from direct experience. The task provides form and organization and serves the needs of members in different ways, including utilizing purposeful activity in developing skills. A functional group has been proposed based on adaptation and occupation. According to this approach, groups enhance the use of occupations to help people adapt to the environment or vice versa, and groups utilize purposeful activities and active involvement (doing) so that members can maintain or develop skills in areas of occupation.

The goal of the activity group is to enable change in the areas of occupation, whether activities of daily living (ADL), instrumental activities of daily living (IADL), work, play, education, or rest and sleep; in performance skills, whether motor, process, or communication and interaction; and performance habits, whether focusing on habits, routines, roles, or rituals. Groups in mental health settings may also focus on various contexts, whether cultural, physical, social, personal, spiritual, or virtual (AOTA, 2008). Cole (2005) suggested a seven-step format for activity groups, involving introduction, the activity, sharing one's own product or experience, processing or reflecting and making sense of the experience, generalizing or summing up the responses to the activity, applying what was learned to everyday life, and summarizing the group experience. The steps can be adapted to maximize learning for any population according to the purpose of the group and the overall level of functioning of the group members.

Task Groups

In the classic task-oriented group (Fidler, 1969), a task was defined as either an end product or a service, though task accomplishment was not the purpose of the group. Instead, the task provided a shared experience whereby the participants could reflect on the relationship between behavior, thinking, and feeling and explore their impact on others. What is demonstrated in the process of participating in the task and encountering problems in doing or interacting can be observed and thus become the focus of group problem solving and trying out alternative patterns. In this way the group becomes engaged in processing behavior and then trying out more adaptive modes.

Developmental Groups

Group interaction skills have been described as a developmental sequence necessary for adaptation (Mosey, 1970, 1981, 1986). Five types of groups, from least to most developed, are (1) parallel, where tasks are done side-by-side and interaction is not required; (2) project, emphasizing task accomplishment and some interaction; (3) egocentric–cooperative, requiring more interaction and responsibility; (4) cooperative, requiring much interaction and taking care of others' needs; and (5) mature groups, where the members take on all necessary leadership roles to facilitate task accomplishment and caring for others' needs. In the hierarchy, initially task accomplishment is emphasized while interaction and meeting each other's needs are de-emphasized. At each successive level, interaction becomes more important and the role of the therapist or leader becomes less primary. At the highest level, task accomplishment is emphasized equally with meeting the needs of other group members.

Directive Groups

The directive group (Kaplan, 1986, 1988)—and also the focus group (Yalom, 1983), which was modeled on the directive group—meets the needs of the most severely and acutely mentally ill and most minimally functioning patients, representing a wide range of diagnoses, ages, and problems. The environment is actively structured in form, organization, and leadership to assure maximum participation. The directive group format is a consistent one involving orientation, introduction, a warm-up, selected activities, and a wrap-up, while the focus group format is orientation, warm-up, structured exercises, and review. The formats enable group goals of participation, interaction, attention, and initiation; within this broad range, goals can be individualized.

Neurodevelopmental Groups

Neurodevelopmental groups (King, 1974; Levy, 1974; Ross, 1987; and Ross & Bachner, 2004, cited in Cole, 2005) utilize movement activities often based on sensory integration theory and techniques. The movements are usually imitative, gross motor movements and involve tactile, kinesthetic, and proprioceptive input. The groups are designed for persons who are severely mentally ill such as those with chronic schizophrenia who have been in the mental health system for a long time. There are different terms now used for groups for those with sensory processing disorders of which sensory modulation is a subcategory and that use sensory interventions (see Beins, 2009; LeBel & Champagne, 2010; LeBel, Champagne, Stromberg, & Coyle, 2010; Moro, 2007).

Sensory Intervention Groups Using Sensory Modulation Approaches

Various research (cited in Beins, 2009) validates the existence of sensory processing disorders among people with psychiatric conditions. Therefore, interventions have evolved for children, adolescents, and adults with sensory processing disorders or with difficulty in sensory modulation (a subcategory of sensory processing disorder) or emotional regulation (AOTA, 2008) with a variety of psychiatric conditions. Such conditions may encompass those with trauma histories and post-traumatic stress disorder (PTSD), pervasive developmental disorder (PDD), attention deficit hyperactivity disorder (ADHD), schizophrenia, or anxiety. Champagne (2005, 2006) has developed sensory processing groups and sensory programs and approaches for mental health inpatient treatment and systems. She has also advocated for sensory rooms for geriatric settings as well based on principles of sensory processing and modulation. With the introduction of the Sensory Profile for Adults (Dunn, 2002), sensory deficiencies can be assessed and treatment can be planned for adolescents and adults with mental illness.

Sensory approaches are considered to be self-organizing and may be most helpful during crisis states and transitions (Champagne, 2005) or as response to trauma ("trauma sensitive work"). Essentially, they foster safety or a sense of personal control to minimize emotional distress and maintain or return to a calm state. They would address the Occupational Therapy Practice Framework (AOTA, 2008) emotional regulation and coping skills to support occupational engagement. Sensory approaches "may include direct or indirect sensory stimulation, sensorimotor activities, environmental modifications and the creation, practice and implementation of sensory diets . . . , referring to the repertoire of sensorimotor activities that appear to influence one's ability to function more optimally. . . . Examples of sensorimotor activities may be wrapping in a blanket, holding ice, biting into a lemon, performing deep breathing or isometric exercises. . . ." (Champagne, 2005, p. 2). Although treatment should be client centered and each individual client should be aided to explore what is calming and alerting to each, sensorimotor approaches and sensorimotor activities can be used in groups. Sensory modulation and regulation groups can be used in isolation or in conjunction with other groups and approaches, such as cognitive behavioral therapy or dialectical behavioral therapy (Moro, 2007), or 12-step programs.

The use of sensory intervention groups and calming rooms (Beins, 2009; Champagne, 2005, 2006) have arisen as the mental health treatment paradigm has changed from an illness approach to a recovery-based one (New Freedom Commission on Mental Health, 2003) including reducing the use of restraints and seclusion rooms. (See Chapters 1, 9, 10, and 13 for information regarding this shift.)

Mindfulness groups (Sadock, Sadock, & Ruiz, 2009) have become popular forms of evidence-based treatment for those with mental illness. A mindfulness group could be a sensory one in which the activity increases the awareness of bodily sensations and responses or facilitates bodily relaxation. Some other examples include training in progressive relaxation, tai-chi, shiatsu, yoga, karate, or other Eastern forms of movement, martial arts, and meditation.

Psychoeducational Groups

The **psychoeducational** group has a clear objective: to teach specific information or techniques to clients and their families, thus supporting clients and their families' well-being (Ruiz-Sancho, Ivanoff, & Linehan, 2001). It is typically time limited and utilizes cognitive-behavioral and social learning theory (Alonso & Swiller, 1993). For example, a group for people with eating disorders may provide facts on nutrition and the social correlates and medical consequences of eating disorders and the group may be open to those who have eating disorders and to their families or significant others. Due to the shorter duration of mental health treatment and the dictates of managed care, many professionals utilize the techniques of psychoeducation (Sadock et al., 2009).

Community and Self-Help Groups

A larger group that may occur in psychosocial rehabilitation, clubhouse, and assertive community treatment settings with particular organizations or populations (AOTA, 2008) is the community group. Such a group was explicated in the Case Illustration "One Group's Process" in the beginning of the chapter. Such groups are in line with the shift from an illness to recovery-based paradigm, particularly for those serving the severely mentally ill. In a community group, whether for clients of a large community organization or a smaller treatment unit, all members of the community of clients participate to make decisions about the organization or community. The community group could be led by elected members as was shown in the Case Illustration, or it could be facilitated by professionals but is largely the work of the clients of the community.

More self-help groups now occur in most communities (Swarbrick & Ellis, 2009). Twelve-step groups for various addictions are examples of self-help groups. Many other community self-help groups may be run by the members and offered in a public place, such as a church hall or community center. Such groups may be based on a common disorder, for example, depression, bipolar, PTSD, or eating disorder support groups or a common condition, such as survivors of domestic violence (Helfrich & Rivera, 2006). Typically, one member may facilitate the group, explain the rules of the group, such as confidentiality, and sharing or listening when others speak, and all members of the community are welcome and welcomed back.

In all these categories, the structure of the group, pattern of interaction, leader's role and methods, and techniques utilized in the group are dictated by the group developer or implementer. In one sensory group the leader may demonstrate how to stretch and have the participants practice the technique. The only verbalization may be the leader's words. In another sensory group, participants may share knowledge and demonstrate their own relaxation techniques. The leader's role may be simply as facilitator or the sessions may contain both elements.

Other Groups

Although activity groups goals are to enable change in areas of occupation, performance skills, or habits with respect to different contexts, the content of some groups may also be described by areas of occupation, performance skills, or habits with respect to different contexts. For example, some groups may be described as an ADL group, a communication group, a habit-change group, or a cultural or computer group. In these cases the activity makes up some of the content of the group and the goals of the group are really explained by the activity.

There are also other types of groups that are explained by their content and activity, but are not specific to occupational therapy, but may forward goals of occupational therapy that were mentioned previously. For example, a thematic group (Mosey, 1981, cited in Denton, 1987) is organized around a topic or theme. The aim is to help the participants change or examine attitudes or acquire knowledge and skills in certain areas. Examples of thematic group titles are "Grieving and Loss," "What Do You Say After You Say Hello?" "On Depression," "On Anger," "On Guilt," and "Recognizing Feelings."

An expressive/projective group (Denton, 1987) uses creative media to facilitate the recognition, acknowledgment, or expression of feelings and ideas. Examples of expressive groups are art or craft groups, play groups, recreation or sport activity, and music or drama (Javaherian-Dysinger & Ebert Freire, 2010) groups.

In one expressive group participants may simply sit silently together in a room, working on their own, individual crafts. The role of the leader will be to help each person initiate and follow through. Alternately, in another expressive group participants may draw themselves in a certain setting and then discuss the emotions and thoughts that the drawing evoked. In this case, the role of the group leader is more active, that is, to help members interact with each other or make connections between their drawings and their thoughts and feelings.

In a thematic group, the group leader may provide education about a topic, such as, "How Thoughts Get in Our Way." Then participants might individually write down negative things they say to themselves and when they do so. Participants may then engage in an interactive discussion facilitated by the leader.

An *ADL* group in an acute psychiatric unit may consist of learning skills for showering, personal hygiene, and grooming. The group leader may provide supplies and demonstrate the skills, while the group participants will practice skills for themselves or will help others when appropriate.

An *IADL* group on community outreach may consist of the group participants deciding who or what institution they would like to visit, discussing transportation and setting time schedules, and deciding who will use the phone book and phone to make the necessary arrangements. The group leader may facilitate by making resources available or giving advice when asked.

A *vocational* group may involve working on a clerical task on an assembly line. The role of the leader will be to set up the project, decide who will perform which roles, and monitor the work and the end products. Participants may interact and help each other or they may work only on their task.

An *education* group may include a group of residents of a board and care home identifying topics that they might be interested in and how they might obtain the information. The group together reads through adult-education brochures and pamphlets, and visits the local library and community college. The group leader obtains the pamphlets, helps the clients decide what questions they might ask, finds out from the clients if they can take public transportation or may need a van, and accompanies the clients to the institutions.

A *leisure* group in the day treatment program decides that they would like to meet other singles. They decide that they will have a dance. The group leader helps them to explore community facilities to find a low-fee rental hall. They plan the dance, including who can be invited, how they will advertise, how they will ensure safety, and what food they can have. They decide to sponsor a monthly dance.

A house and grounds section of a clubhouse spends a week learning *how to organize space and objects* for cleaning vacant apartments. The group leader is directive, bringing in tools, explaining processes, and inviting apartment managers to talk about their needs.

In preparation to attend the monthly dances, the *communication* group learns the ways people communicate with their bodies. They practice asking someone to dance and "making small talk," the rules of personal space, how to maintain gaze, and how to assume a posture that indicates warmth, openness, and interest. The group leader assigns role-plays and helps the group members to evaluate the role-plays and analyze the group process.

A 12-step group for addictive behaviors meets weekly to discuss useful *habits* that members would like to cultivate and dominating habits that they would like to eliminate. The group leader functions as a consultant, advising the group when they have questions.

A combined *spiritual/physical contexts* group of retired older people from the same community who call themselves "the transcendentalists" meet twice weekly. At the beginning of the week they discuss a physical environment, often a natural one such as the mountains or the oceans, but sometimes a man-made environment, such as a historical monument, that they wish to explore. Once they determine the environment, they plan how they will explore it. During the second meeting they explore the environment, discussing how the place affects their well-being and general sense of efficacy and comparing the places that they have visited. The group leader functions as a consultant, advising the group when they have questions or discussing the power of environments to influence people.

STARTING A GROUP

There are basic steps involved in starting a group (Rerek, 1966; see also Cole, 2005, and Egan & Joseph, 2010, for other suggestions for the steps involved in group). At each step there are questions to ask to clarify your thinking and make the group development a smooth process. If you know the steps and questions, you will know how to think about groups, and consequently, you will be able to develop and utilize groups in any setting and with any population. You will be able to work alone as a group leader, effectively and successfully, to provide meaningful treatment. Table 20-5 reviews the steps to starting a group.

TABLE 20-5. Starting a Group: Tasks and Critical Questions

Therapist Task	Critical Questions
1. Survey of client population	Who are they? What are their needs?
2. Setting	Short- or long-term? Inpatient or outpatient? Specific disorder or special services? Roles for other health professionals? Your job description?
3. Purpose	Why is this group necessary? What do you and the participants want to accomplish? What are the types of outcomes that are expected?
4. Selection criteria	How will you select participants? Who will and will not benefit? Why? Are evaluation and screening based on issues, problems, diagnosis, cognitive level, interests, gender, age?
5. Specific activities	Concrete or abstract? Simple or complex? Short or long duration? Based on a model? Easy to transport?
6. Your skills and knowledge	Are your skills adequate? Is a consultant, supervisor, or mentor available? Are you interested in this group? Is it a good fit for you?
7. Structure and logistics	Minimum and maximum allowable participants? Voluntary or required? Open or closed? When? How often? How long? Where? One or more leaders?
8. Outcome measure	How will you determine success, whether goals and purpose are being achieved?

Adapted from Rerek (1966)

The first step is to survey the client population. The questions to ask yourself are, "Who are the clients and what are their needs?" An inpatient acute setting where people of all ages stay for three days to be stabilized on medication will dictate a group setting that addresses here-and-now functioning or cognitive reorganization. An outpatient setting that provides service primarily to women who may be depressed would dictate a group for women that provides opportunities for success and mastery and addresses longer-term occupational areas or daily functioning. A setting in which intense, **psychodynamic** work is the daily focus would dictate a group that provides relaxation/restoration or recreation.

The second step is to consider the constraints of your setting. Is your setting a short-term, acute unit where people who function differently are treated together? Is it a long-term setting where people live in the community and attend four days a week? Does the setting provide treatment for a specific disorder, such as addiction, or does it provide special treatment, such as vocational services? Does the setting include many other health professionals, such as psychologists, nutritionists, social workers, recreational therapists, or movement therapists, with specific roles? Are you the only health professional with a more generalized role? Is your job description specific or are you allowed some freedom?

An important step is to establish the purpose of the group. What do you want to accomplish? What do you want the participants to accomplish? What do the participants wish to accomplish? Why is this group necessary? These questions often translate into group goals. In some groups the purpose is not to change one's life forever but rather to increase one's recognition of the internal resources needed for a transition from the structured setting or a return home. Some groups may allow people to be creative and explore the meaning of their lives, while others may help people reorganize their thinking and decrease confusion. Another type of group may be designed to improve members' personal appearance and therefore will address grooming and self-care. The purpose of a group in a day treatment setting may be to provide a sense of belonging to a community, whereas the same group in an acute care center may be intended to provide a sense of community safety and comfort.

Another step is to consider selection criteria. How will you select participants? Who will benefit from this group and who might not? Some groups will evaluate and screen participants, while others will be open to anyone who wishes to attend. Some groups may require an ability to think abstractly and will therefore screen out individuals who are actively psychotic. Some may address retirement issues and therefore will not benefit adolescents.

A step that is often dictated by the purpose and goals of the group and the nature of its membership is the consideration of what activities to use. What will be the specific activities featured? Will they be tangible or abstract? Will they be short- or long-term? Will they vary? Will they be easy to use and transport?

Stress management groups may use meditation, movement, and music or writing; ADL groups may use discussion and demonstration; and craft groups may use specific modalities, such as clay, jewelry, or leather. Some groups may be nonverbal, while others may involve a great deal of talking.

A step that has been implied in discussing group development and implementation is for the leader to consider his or her skills and knowledge. Are your skills and knowledge adequate for this group? Is there someone who can consult or mentor you? Are you excited about this group? Is it a good fit for you (does it match your personality and strengths)? Although it is important to be aware of the members' needs, which should be paramount, some of the best groups are those that interest their leaders. In fact, if you are not excited or interested in some way by a group, you should not lead it.

The structural details of the group should be well thought out. How large will the group be? Will it be voluntary, or is it required in the program? Will it be open (i.e., members may enter and leave at any time) or closed (i.e., membership remains stable for a time period)? For how long should the group meet? When and how often will it meet? Where will it meet? Will it be led by the same person or persons? Who has primary responsibility for the group? How will participants be kept informed? Often, such structural details about the group are written down in a group protocol.

A final consideration is to determine a measure of effectiveness for the group. How will you determine if this group is successful and achieves its purpose and goals? Often therapists develop and implement groups and informally assess success, usually as based on attendance or comments of the group members. If at all possible, however, a more formal evaluation of the group's success—an outcome measure—should be established. This is not a requisite in most institutions and in many fields. However, outcome measures document the usefulness and utility of your group and the profession. An ongoing formal evaluation also gives feedback about what does and does not work. It guides the therapist in providing the most useful treatment.

Formal evaluation does not have to be complicated, perplexing, or time-consuming. It could simply involve consistently taking attendance and comparing it with your institution's census to learn the percentage of patients who attend. It could involve a questionnaire about the group to be filled out by the members at various times after their attendance. It could involve questions posed before, during, and after the group experience. It could mean posing the same questions about the group after trying out different activities or techniques. A professional who engages in research (your occupational therapy professor or consultant or a psychologist on staff) will usually assist you.

THE GROUP PROTOCOL

The group content and structure are often written in a protocol. Protocols vary in form but usually include similar content. They often include the group's name, purpose, goals, content or methods, structure and logistics, method of entry, requirements, and referral criteria. They also generally cover who would and would not benefit, contraindications for membership, and name of the group leader. They often also include a short description or narrative about the group. Two examples of protocols are presented in Table 20-6. Protocols can be more extensive (Borg & Bruce, 1991; Cole, 2005; Howe & Schwartzberg, 2001) and include a more detailed description of the client population, a rationale, a frame of reference, an outline of treatment sessions, and a listing of outcome criteria.

Writing a group protocol is a way of organizing your thinking about a group. In a narrow sense, it is an aid for yourself, while in a broader sense, it is an aid for others

TABLE 20-6. Group Protocols

OCCUPATIONAL THERAPY MAC GROUP: MASTERY AND ACCOMPLISHMENT THROUGH CRAFTS

Purpose: Provide opportunities for participants to master concrete activities in a parallel group setting that is not threatening or demanding.

Goals: Long-term—Increase sense of effectiveness as demonstrated by participant self-report.

Short-term—Improve concentration and attention span and ability to plan sequentially, as demonstrated by daily assessment.

Group Content: Concrete activities (craft).

Group Structure: Therapist will present participants with crafts. Often all will be working on the same type of craft though each will have his or her own project. Crafts will be structured and graded according to Allen's Cognitive Levels (see attached). Therapist will prepare projects and client decision making will be minimal. Interaction will not be required or encouraged, although it often occurs.

Logistics:
Place: CCB 209
Number of Patients: Maximum of 8
Meeting Schedule: Daily, Monday and—Friday, 9:00–10:00 A.M.
Group Facilitator: James Lopez, OTR

OCCUPATIONAL THERAPY—LIFE SKILLS

Who:
- Those who identify areas of daily life that are problematic, disregulated, or that they would like to change.
- Those who use few coping skills or one for all situations.

Goal:
- Provide opportunities to learn a range of coping mechanisms or skills or ways of adapting.
- Provide opportunities to practice old skills of managing in new ways that are more satisfying.
- Provide opportunities to clarify values and ways of being in the world, ultimately expanding choices.

Method: Occupational therapist will provide a theme or topic regarding coping and regulation skills for each session that occurs twice a week from 7 to 9 in Room A of the community center, and will provide specific experiential exercises for the group to follow.

Contraindications: Those who are presently or those who have difficulty thinking abstractly, or are easily distracted, for example, those with psychotic or hypermanic symptoms.

Group Leader: Ahmad Wallace, OTR

with whom you work. It provides them with a brief, useful description of the group and helps them in referring people to your group and knowing what type of treatment clients are receiving. In these different ways, the group protocol contributes to the functioning of the organization for which you work, in that it also aids the institution to describe its services to prospective clients. Sometimes, the group protocol serves to demystify psychological treatment.

You may also share your protocols with your clients or members of the group, particularly on entry, as a way of explaining the group. Providing this information can relieve the fears and satisfy the curiosity of new members. Often it favorably disposes the new member to the group and aids in the rapid cohesion and integration. Group members may share protocols with their families, often giving relief to worried or curious family members and providing a basis of discussion regarding the client's difficulties and experiences, or prompting family members to join the psychoeducational groups offered for clients and families.

DOCUMENTATION AND OUTCOME

It is important to document outcomes, and group outcomes can indeed be documented. In addition to suggesting group goals or activities, the Occupational Therapy Practice Framework (AOTA, 2008) defines types of outcomes that can measure group success, such as improvement or enhancement in occupational performance, client satisfaction, or quality of life, role competence, adaptation, health and wellness, prevention, promoting healthy lifestyles, or occupational justice. A simple measurement of outcomes is self-report (Howe & Schwartzberg, 2001), whereby members are asked to evaluate a group either at the end of each session or at the end of a series of meetings. The form can be structured, providing forced choices such as "always," "sometimes," "rarely," or "never," or it can be unstructured, perhaps asking participants open-ended questions regarding their experiences.

Members can be asked to monitor their progress by filling out a behavioral assessment regarding their own behavior in the group. A behavioral observation form (Kaplan, 1988) can also be filled out by the group leaders. Assessment and observation should always tie in to the goals and the purpose of the group as a whole and the individuals in the group. This implies that an initial assessment has been performed to ascertain baseline functioning and that assumptions regarding the group and the frame of reference in which it is grounded will be explicit.

An ideal method of evaluating a group or the individual participants is goal attainment scaling (Ottenbacher & Cusick, 1990). This method employs operational goals and outcomes and explicit time sequences that are determined by the therapist, individuals, and others involved in treatment. It also includes a quantitative measurement of treatment effectiveness. It can be used both for the evaluation of group efficacy and for the evaluation of treatment efficacy for group members.

Documentation may cover the group process and content or discuss each individual in the group. It is generally written in the form of a narrative note; a more structured, problem-oriented or behavioral outcome format; or a list (Acquaviva, 1992; Borg & Bruce, 1991; Denton, 1987; Kaplan, 1988). Generally, a note regarding the group will contain a description of the activity and clients in attendance and a summary of the group experience, or what has occurred. This includes what has been accomplished, any changes since the previous group session, and any unusual occurrences. It may restate the purpose and goals of the group and whether the goals were accomplished. It may include the plan for the subsequent group meeting. A note regarding each individual in the group generally will include descriptions of the person's behavior in the group, how the person interacted and responded to interaction, how the individual participated in the activity, and changes in performance from previous group sessions. Goals may be reiterated, or the plan for an individual in the next group meeting may be stated. As with the group narrative, a baseline assessment and explicit grounding in a frame of reference are required.

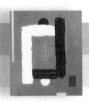

CASE ILLUSTRATION

Developing a Group, Protocol, and Plan

Janice Nyugen is an OTR in a large psychiatric hospital that treats people of all ages and diagnoses. One of her roles is as evaluator of incoming clients. After six months of evaluating six to eight clients per week, she noticed that 70% had a diagnosis of depression. Of this group, 90% were female, 60% were between the ages of 25 and 40, and about 15% had accompanying problems, such as eating disorders or addictions, for which they were attending other groups or self-help programs based on the 12 steps of Alcoholics Anonymous.

At the hospital, no groups specifically targeted people with the diagnosis of depression. Janice had been interested in this topic in school and so welcomed the opportunity to learn more. She read about depression and spoke with her supervisor about her ideas for a group. She attended case consultations and interviews and spoke with her colleagues concerning how a group for people who were depressed might fit into the program. She attended communication workshops to supplement what she learned in her occupational therapy classes and observed other people whose traits and skills of group leadership she admired. She then developed a group protocol and an explanation of the group that she had designed. Table 20-7 shows the protocol she wrote for the group. Table 20-8 delineates the group leadership, activity, process, and desired outcomes of the group.

Discussion

Janice demonstrated the correct way to go about developing a group; that is, she noticed a need and a population that were not served in her organization, she sought consultation and more knowledge, she observed other leaders' styles, she developed a logical group plan and description, and she determined how she would measure types of outcomes the group sought.

TABLE 20-7. Protocol for a Group Dealing with Depression

Name: Caring for Yourself: Dealing with Depression

Purpose: Increase opportunities for mastery and success, improve participants' strategies and tools to cope with depression, and educate participants regarding the warning signs of depression.

Goals: Given participation in the group daily for two weeks, the participants will be able to accomplish two concrete activities successfully, report improved mood as measured by the Beck Depression Inventory, state three strategies for coping with depressed mood, and state three warning signs of impending depressed mood.

Group Content: The group will include simple craft activities that can be worked on independently and finished successfully in one session, identification of thoughts and feelings relating to depressed moods, and identification of coping strategies and signs of impending depressed mood through written exercises, exploration, and discussions.

Group Structure: The leader will provide opportunities for engagement with concrete activities and assist members to complete them. The leader will actively direct written exercises and discussion and provide education regarding coping strategies and recognizing signs of impending depression. The sequence of the group is such that initially there will be little demand on the participants as they successfully complete activities, and then gradually demands will increase as exploration and discussion are introduced. However, participants do not have to initiate in this group, and interaction is initially mostly between the leader and individuals, gradually giving way to group discussion with other members, facilitated by the leader.

Who Would Benefit: This group would primarily benefit women between the ages of 25 and 50 with depressed mood who also are dealing with issues of addiction. They must be able to think abstractly and should demonstrate some capacity for self-reflection.

Who Would Not Benefit: Those who are unable to think abstractly or have psychotic thinking; those who are unable to attend to a group for at least one hour or concentrate on abstract concepts; those who are presently in a manic state.

Logistics: Monday–Friday, 9–10 A.M., 2/1–2/12.
The Rose Room, #200
Group Leader: Janice Nyugen, OTR

TABLE 20-8. Caring for Yourself: Dealing with Depression (Two-Week Process)

Day	Group Leadership	Group Activity	Group Process	Desired Outcome/ Rationale
1	Explains the group to the participants, giving them the group protocol and discussing it. Gives them self-report questionnaires to fill out concerning improvements that they seek in occupational performance, satisfaction, occupational roles, customary ways of adapting to daily situations, self-assessment of their current state of physical and mental health, and current quality of life. Solicits questions and concerns.	Reading and discussing thoughts and feelings regarding the group protocol; stating desired personal outcomes. Filling out the Beck Depression Inventory, a list of strategies each individual uses to cope with depression, and a list of behavioral and cognitive warning signs of impending depression.	The leader introduces herself or himself and members introduce themselves to each other. Most interaction is between the leader and the members.	Introduction to each other. Developing rapport with leader and members. Beginning comfort among members. Completion of evaluative measures.
2–4	Provides categories of craft activities: ceramics, jewelry, or leather. Assists members in their projects.	Craft projects.	Members work independently and individually on their chosen craft projects, with assistance from the leader when necessary. They speak casually with each other, though this is not required. They display their finished projects on the last day.	Developing rapport and comfort in the group and with each other. Increased sense of ability and mastery and therefore awareness of self-effectiveness. Beginning group participation in a nondemanding way.
5	Provides a written handout, "On Depression," that describes the symptoms of depression and theories of its cause. Directs an active discussion by asking each participant to comment on various aspects.	Group discussion with a handout about various aspects of depression.	Members read and listen to the leader's thoughts and depression. Members are asked to comment by the leader. The interaction is primarily leader-to-participant.	Beginning interaction. Education about depression. Beginning ability to identify specific, personal aspects of depression.

6	Provides written exercise, "Stressful Events." Directs participants how to do the activity. Directs a discussion of how everyday events cause more stress than one is likely to realize. Asks members to share their stress test and validates thoughts and feelings. Points out similarities with other participants.	From a list of stressful events weighted from most stressful to least stressful, chooses those that have occurred in the last year and adds up the stress score. Discusses thoughts and feelings regarding the scores and the events.	Members complete the activity individually, and share their comments, at first with the leader, then with the other members.	Recognition of stressful events. Realization of how each event may cause stress. Validation of thoughts and feelings. Decrease of isolation and guilt.
7	Provides written exercise, "Chalk Talk." Directs participants how to do the activity. Directs a discussion of how automatic negative thoughts contribute to depression. Asks each member to share their "chalk talk." Validates and points out similarities with other members. Ends with a symbolic erasure or throwing away of the negative "chalk talk," while carefully saving the positive "chalk talk."	Introduces the concept that automatic, usually negative, thoughts contribute to depression. Introduces the concept of the "chalk talk," that is, that individuals are constantly coaching themselves as they go about daily life. Members choose an event from the previous day that causes moderate stress, then list the thoughts that usually occur before, during, and after that event.	Members write their "chalk talk" individually and share their comments, at first with the leaders and then with the other members. Members begin to validate and initiate with each other.	Participants become aware of the effect of their internal, usually negative, thoughts. Participants become aware of how their thoughts interfere with behavior and occur with depression. Participants learn strategies for coping with the negative thoughts.
8	Provides written activity, "Practice." Directs participants how to do the activity. Directs a discussion of how automatic behavior contributes to depression. Asks members to share their practice routines. Validates and points out similarities with other members. Asks members to work with each other in dyads to create a new practice routine.		Members individually write their "practice routine." Members share their routine with others and validate others' comments.	Participants become aware of how their actions are automatic and can lead to depression. Participants learn new strategies to practice different behavior.

(Continues)

TABLE 20-8. Continued

Day	Group Leadership	Group Activity	Group Process	Desired Outcome/Rationale
9	Provides written activity, "Creating Positive Chalk Talk and New Practice Routines." Directs members how to do the activity. Asks members to share their thoughts and feelings. Facilitates the group working together to help each other create new talk and new routines.	Written exercises, the "Next Chalk Talk" and "Creating New Practice Routines." Leader introduces the concept of anticipating events that lead to depression. Members choose one situation/event that will evoke depression in their environment. Members create new talk and new behavior to prevent depressed mood.	Members individually choose and share the anticipated event and their automatic thoughts and behavior. Members work together designing new practice routines and chalk talks.	Members anticipate events connected to depressed mood and create mood prevention strategies. Members cooperate with each other, decrease isolation, and learn how to accept help.
10	Group leader asks members to fill out the Beck Depression Scale and a self-report of the types of outcomes concerning improvements that they sought, written during the first session, in occupational performance, satisfaction, occupational roles, customary ways of adapting to daily situations, self-assessment of their current state of physical and mental health, and current quality of life. Group leader guides the wrap-up, in which each member says good-bye and expresses a message directly to every other member.	Each member individually fills out evaluative measures and comments on them. Each member directly interacts with the other members.	Each member has a chance to express any ending thoughts or feelings about the group, each other, and what she or he had anticipated, thereby having a chance to realize a positive sense of completion.	To have comparative outcome measures so that members may recognize personal change and progress. To have comparative outcome measures regarding group goals to evaluate the efficacy of the group.

SUMMARY

Much treatment in the psychiatric arena is provided in groups. Groups are cost-effective, facilitate personal growth, and provide feedback by more than one person (though not everyone is suited for group treatment). The content, the structure, and leadership contribute to the process of the group.

Occupational therapy groups often combine principles and techniques of psychological models, but they are unique in their emphases on activity and on areas of occupation performance skills and patterns with respect to contexts. Various types and models of activity groups have been proposed for occupational therapy. A theory of activity groups is evolving; currently, occupational therapy groups can be fit into broad categories based on content.

Certain steps can be followed to successfully start a group. Starting a group involves planning and writing a group protocol. A successful group combines following the appropriate steps while assuming leadership and modeling communication skills. Group outcomes can be subsequently evaluated.

REVIEW QUESTIONS

1. What are the differences between group process and group content? How do you define each?
2. What are the stages of a group? What are the questions that group participants might have in each stage?
3. How can a leader handle monopolizing behavior in a group? Why is it important to do so?
4. What are some questions you might reflect on as you develop a group?
5. Why are sensory intervention groups using sensory modulation important for clients with mental illness?

REFERENCES

Acquaviva, J. (Ed.). (1992). *Effective documentation for occupational therapy.* Rockville, MD: American Occupational Therapy Association.

Alonso, A., & Swiller, H. (Eds.). (1993). *Group therapy in clinical practice.* Washington, DC: American Psychiatric Press.

American Occupational Therapy Association. (2008). Occupational therapy practice framework: Domain and process (2nd ed.). *American Journal of Occupational Therapy, 62,* 625–683.

Barlow, S. H., Burlingame, G. M., & Fuhriman, A. (2000). Therapeutic application of groups: From Pratt's "Thought control classes" to modern group psychotherapy. *Group Dynamics: Theory, Research and Practice, 4*(1), 115–134.

Beins, K. (2009). From clinician to consultant: Use of a sensory processing framework in mental health. *Mental Health Special Interest Section Quarterly Newsletter, 32,* 4, 1–4.

Borg, B., & Bruce, M. A. (1991). *The group system: The therapeutic activity group in occupational therapy.* Thorofare, NJ: Slack.

Brabender, V., & Fallon, A. (2009). *Group Development in Practice: Guidance for Clinicians and Researchers on Stages and Dynamics of Change.* Washington, DC: American Psychological Association.

Champagne, T. (2005). Expanding the role of sensory approaches in acute psychiatric settings. *American Occupational Therapy Association, Inc. Mental Health Special Interest Section Quarterly, 28,* 1, 1–4.

Champagne, T. (2006). Creating sensory rooms: Environmental enhancements for acute inpatient mental health settings. *American Occupational Therapy Association, Inc. Mental Health Special Interest Section Quarterly, 29,* 4, 1–3, 4.

Cole, M. B. (2005). *Group dynamics in occupational therapy* (3rd ed.) Thorofare, NJ: Slack.

Corey, G. (2008). *Groups: Process and practice* (7th ed.). Belmont, CA: Thomson Brooks/Cole.

Denton, P. L. (1987). *Psychiatric occupational therapy: A workbook of practical skills.* Boston: Little, Brown.

Dunn, W. (2002). *Adolescent Adult Sensory Profile users manual.* San Antonio, TX: Pearson Education.

Egan, B. E., & Joseph, M. (2010). Using Pierce's seven phases of the design process to understand the meaning of feeling "boxed in": A community-based group. *American Occupational Therapy Association Mental Health Special Interest Section Quarterly, 33,* 3.

Fidler, G. S. (1969). The task-oriented group as a context for treatment. *American Journal of Occupational Therapy, 23,* 43.

Hagedorn, R. (2000). *Tools for practice in occupational therapy: A structural approach to core skills and processes.* Edinburgh: Churchill Livingstone.

Helfrich, C. A., & Rivera, Y. (2006). Employment skills and domestic violence survivors: A shelter-based intervention. *Occupational Therapy in Mental Health, 22*(1), 33–48.

Howe, M., & Schwartzberg, S. L. (2001). *A functional approach to group work in occupational therapy* (3rd ed.). Philadelphia: Lippincott Williams & Wilkins.

Javaherian-Dysinger, H., & Ebert Freire, M. (2010). Drama: Still a tool for healing and understanding. *American Occupational Therapy Association, Inc. Mental Health Special Interest Section Quarterly, 33,* 4.

Kaplan, K. L. (1986). The directive group: Short term treatment for psychiatric patients with a minimal level of functioning. *American Journal of Occupational Therapy, 40,* 474–481.

Kaplan, K. L. (1988). *Directive group therapy: Innovative mental health treatment.* Thorofare, NJ: Slack.

King, L. J. (1974). A sensory integrative approach to schizophrenia. *American Journal of Occupational Therapy, 28*(9), 529–536.

LeBel, J., & Champagne, T. (2010). Integrating sensory and trauma-informed interventions: A Massachusetts state initiative, Part 2. *American Occupational Therapy Association, Inc. Mental Health Special Interest Section Quarterly, 33,* 2, 1–4.

LeBel, J., Champagne, T., Stromberg, N., & Coyle, R. (2010). Integrating sensory and trauma-informed interventions: A Massachusetts state initiative, Part 1. *American Occupational Therapy Association, Inc. Mental Health Special Interest Section Quarterly, 33,* 1, 1–4.

Levy, L. L. (1974). Movement therapy for psychiatric patients. *American Journal of Occupational therapy, 28*(6), 354–357.

Moro, C. (2007). A comprehensive literature review defining self-mutilation and occupational therapy intervention approaches: dialectical behavior therapy and sensory integration. *Occupational Therapy in Mental Health, 23,* 1, 55–67.

Mosey, A. C. (1970). The concept and use of developmental groups. *American Journal of Occupational Therapy, 24,* 272.

Mosey, A. C. (1981). *Occupational therapy: Configuration of a profession.* New York: Raven.

Mosey, A. C. (1986). *Components of psychosocial occupational therapy.* New York: Raven.

Ottenbacher, K. J., & Cusick, A. (1990). Goal attainment scaling as a method of clinical service evaluation. *American Journal of Occupational Therapy, 44*(6), 519–526.

President's New Freedom Commission on Mental Health. (2003). *Achieving the promise: Transforming mental health care in America* [Executive summary]. DHHS Publication No. SMA-03-3831. Washington, DC: Author.

Rerek, M. (1966). *The use of groups in occupational therapy.* Unpublished manuscript.

Ruiz-Sancho, A. M., Ivanoff, A. M., & Linehan, M. (2001). Psychoeducational approaches. In W. J. Livesley (Ed.), *Handbook of personality disorders: Theory, research and treatment* (pp. 460–475). New York: Guilford.

Sadock, B., Sadock, V., & Ruiz, P. (2009). *Comprehensive textbook of psychiatry* (9th ed.). Baltimore: Williams & Wilkins.

Scheidlinger, S. (1994). An overview of nine decades of group psychotherapy. *Hospital and Community Psychiatry, 45*(3), 197–225.

Swarbrick, M., & Ellis, J. (2009). Peer-operated self-help centers. *Occupational Therapy in Mental Health, 25,* 239–251.

Yalom, I. (1983). *Inpatient group psychotherapy.* New York: Basic.

Yalom, I. (2005). *The theory and practice of group psychotherapy* (5th ed.). New York: Basic.

Websites

American Society of Group Psychotherapy and Psychodrama:
www.asgpp.org

American Group Psychotherapy Association:
www.agpa.org/group/consumersguide2000.html

Group Therapy ideas and themes:
www.wilderdom.com/games/GroupTherapyIdeasThemes.htlm

Life Skills Group Manuals:
http://www.ywcatoronto.org/page.asp?pid=122
http://www.peacecorps.gov/multimedia/pdf/library/M0063_lifeskillscomplete.pdf
http://www.lifeskillshandbooks.com/sample-life-skills-sessions.html

Geared toward business but many good tips:
http://www.slideshare.net/vipinb/interpersonal-skills

Specialized Roles for Occupational Therapy in Mental Health

Just as occupational therapists treat psychiatric conditions, lifespan issues, and psychosocial consequences of physical disorders, they also intervene with psychiatric conditions within various organizational structures and through systematic treatment approaches. Chapter 21 considers psychosocial occupational therapy for those with mental illness or psychosocial distress who are incarcerated within prison systems—institutions that house an alarmingly growing population with a myriad of occupational dysfunctions. A new chapter to this edition is Chapter 22, "Psychosocial Occupational Therapy in the School Setting." Although school-based occupational therapy is well established in the United States, it is only recently that significant attention has been paid to children with mental health issues or the complex social, environmental, and behavioral problems seen in schools. Each of these chapters addresses the occupational justice issues found in the organizational structures as well as suggestions for individual and group intervention.

Although vocational programming (Chapter 23) and the treatment of substance abuse (Chapter 24) can be addressed in a wide variety of settings that employ occupational therapists, they are included in this section because many vocational and substance abuse programs are separate from mental health agencies and there are specific subsets of skills needed. These chapters present the unique perspective of occupational therapy and make the case as to how this perspective is not only beneficial to individual clients but can also enrich and enhance the effectiveness of a team approach.

Also, new to this edition is information about the military organization, our service members' experiences in Iraq and Afganistan, and common physical and psychiatric illnesses that are treated by occupational therapy practitioners. As more and more service members and returning warriors enter workplaces and educational institutions, this chapter should inform all occupational therapists who are eager to assist in reintegration from military theaters. A revised chapter on fieldwork supervision in mental health settings will be useful for occupational therapy practitioners who work in all settings. All of the chapters in this part (Chapters 21 through 26) are filled with creative and innovative programming ideas for these far reaching and much needed services.

Chapter 21

Occupational Therapy in Criminal Justice

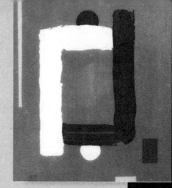

John A. White, PhD, OTR/L
Crystal Dieleman Grass, PhD, OT Reg(NS)
Toby Ballou Hamilton, PhD, MPH, OTR/L
Sandra L. Rogers, PhD, OTR/L

▬ KEY TERMS

adjudication

corrections

criminal justice

health care disparities

occupational alienation

occupational apartheid

occupational deprivation

occupational enrichment

occupational health

occupational imbalance

occupational justice

occupational restriction

Occupation-Based Self-
    Determination (OBSD)

offenders

prisonization

recidivism

reentry

therapeutic competencies

CHAPTER OUTLINE

Introduction
Overview of Criminal Justice System: Stages of Offender Involvement
Scope of Criminal Justice
Health Care in the Criminal Justice System
Mental Health in Criminal Justice and Corrections: U.S. and International Perspectives
Occupational Therapy in Criminal Justice
Occupational Justice and Injustice
Evaluation, Assessment, and Intervention
Occupation-Based Self-Determination (OBSD)
Therapeutic Competencies

Risk Assessment and Environmental Assessment
Models of Practice and Practice Knowledge Base
Models of Practice and Assessments
Interpersonal and Communication Skills
Professional and Ethical Behavior
Special Considerations for Tools and Materials
Sexuality in Forensic and Correctional Settings
Occupational Therapy Interventions in Criminal Justice and Evidence for Practice
Occupational Therapy Interventions in Criminal Justice Settings
Employment Assessment and Intervention
Prisonization and Errors in Critical Thinking
Criminal Thinking
Crime as Occupation: The Stages of the Criminal Career
An Occupational Perspective of Crime
Reentry to the Community
Summary

INTRODUCTION

Understanding the **criminal justice** system is critical for occupational therapists working in mental health and certainly for those working in correctional facilities. In this chapter we intend to show the pressing need within the criminal justice system for occupational therapists and the rewarding opportunities for practice there. We will highlight the valuable and unique perspectives of how occupationally relevant approaches can support healthier living for those incarcerated, while providing innovative programming to support successful transition for offenders as they return to community living. We will elaborate the complex factors involved in each component of the Person-Environment-Occupation interaction in OT practice for incarcerated individuals with and without mental health conditions. The opportunities and challenges of the criminal justice systems will be described with examples from our experience and from the research to provide evidence-based guidelines for practice in various levels of the criminal justice system.

Applying the principles and practices of **occupational justice**, the reader will understand how many of the problems such as criminal behavior, substance abuse, and undertreated mental health conditions are rooted in societal issues and contribute to challenges in criminal justice. Using an occupational justice approach, occupational therapists can reduce recidivism and effect system wide changes for more just circumstances and care for whole populations within the criminal justice system. This large-scale work can be integrated with more traditional OT practices with individuals to shape positive outcomes of reducing **occupational deprivation** and to provide opportunities for more productive occupational patterns, performance, and identity. By drawing on models and examples from international criminal justice research and practice, we will highlight best practices that can guide occupational therapy to proven approaches and application of occupational justice concepts.

The need for new intervention approaches that occupational therapy can offer is pressing. A recent study indicates that 14.5% of men and 31% of women entering the jails studied were found to have serious mental illnesses. The gender difference is particularly important given the rising number of women in U.S. jails. If applied to the 13 million jail admissions reported in 2007, the findings suggest that more than 2 million bookings of a person with a serious mental illness may occur annually (Steadman, Osher, Robbins, Case, & Samuels, 2009). **Offenders** with serious mental health conditions are four (for men) to six (for women) times as likely to be incarcerated as those without mental illness, and once in prison or jail are likely to spend more time incarcerated than those offenders without mental health conditions (Criminal Justice/Mental Health Consensus Project, 2002). This chapter will address a range of occupational therapy approaches applied throughout the criminal justice continuum to decrease occupational deprivation and improve occupational performance outcomes. Occupational therapy that offers a unique focus on occupation to promote development of key life skills is especially needed for offenders with mental health conditions and so will be highlighted in the theory and practice examples that follow.

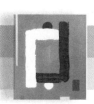

CASE ILLUSTRATION

Mary's Story

Mary is a Caucasian woman incarcerated in Oklahoma, a state that incarcerates more women than any other place in the world. Mary grew up in an impoverished family with a background of dysfunction and instability. Her mother had a history of bipolar disorder and her father abused a variety of illegal drugs. Her parents divorced when Mary was in elementary school. Mary and her brother and two sisters experienced childhood sexual and physical abuse and their father was violent at home.

Mary left home at age 16 before she finished her secondary education and married at age 19.

She experienced intimate partner violence with a series of boyfriends and her husband, never receiving abuse counseling. In her teens, her social drug use on the weekends with boyfriends and her husband soon escalated to daily drug use. By the time she was 23, she was raising three children under the age of four years old fathered by two men. Without a secondary education, Mary struggled to raise the children while working two entry-level minimum-wage jobs. Her work history was not continuous and she lost several jobs due to positive drug tests and missed workdays.

Mary was unemployed at the time of her arrest for possession of a controlled dangerous substance (CDS or illegal drugs) and forgery that supported her and her husband's drug habits. Her husband's arrest for distributing CDS occurred simultaneously. The county of their conviction exceeds the average U.S. incarceration rate by more than 300%. After four months in the county jail, a judge sentenced Mary to 36 months in prison followed by 36 months of supervision by a parole officer. The judge also required her to pay restitution of $25,000 for her forgeries.

Three of the children were placed in custody of the state and the youngest, six months, lives with Mary's mother. Mary's children have not visited her in jail or prison and she manages, despite the expense, to talk with each by phone once a month.

Discussion

Mary's childhood was marked by many of the factors (e.g., poverty, physical and sexual abuse, substance abuse, poor educational and employment history) that are typical of people who fall into criminal behaviors and who are eventually incarcerated. Despite Mary's desire to earn a living for her family, the cycle of low-paying jobs coupled with high childcare costs, exposure to negative social influences and habits brought her into the criminal justice system. However, Mary's difficulty in developing productive adaptive occupational and role performance has reinforced a downward spiral in her ability to care for herself and children. Common to many incarcerated mothers there is a strong desire to reunite with her children and resume parenting, even if from behind bars. Occupational therapy intervention can begin by helping Mary understand how her past occupational patterns have frustrated her goals of parenting and working with her to develop basic parenting skills and build her adaptive capacity to follow her recovery goals and find and keep meaningful employment.

OVERVIEW OF CRIMINAL JUSTICE SYSTEM: STAGES OF OFFENDER INVOLVEMENT

American criminal justice is a complex system through which governments at the city, county, state, and federal levels bring criminal cases through their own criminal justice jurisdictions. In general, the sequence consists of entry via law enforcement, prosecution and pretrial services, **adjudication**, sentencing and sanctions, and **corrections**. Entry into the system begins when law enforcement agents, such as police, determine the occurrence of a violation and apprehend a suspect. If sufficient evidence exists, the suspect is arrested, taken into pretrial custody, and charged with a crime. Law enforcement agents investigate the crime. If sufficient evidence or probable cause does not exist, the suspect is released.

The adjudication or courts stage begins when a magistrate or judge informs the suspect of the charges and the suspect enters a plea. If the suspect pleads guilty or accepts penalty without admitting guilt, the judge may accept the plea and sentence the offender immediately or later. Those who plead not guilty or guilty by reason of insanity are given a trial date and the right to representation by an attorney. During the trial before either a judge and jury or only a judge (bench trial), the prosecution and defense argue the evidence. If acquitted, the suspect is released. If convicted, the suspect enters the sentencing and sanctions sequence and a judge imposes a sentence. Depending on the nature of the crime, sentencing options include the death penalty, incarceration in prison or jail, or probation in which the offender is freed under certain conditions and restrictions. In addition, the offender may be required to pay fines and restitution. The offender may appeal the sentence through the court system.

The final correctional sequence begins with the offender's confinement. Those with sentences of less than one year typically serve time in city or county jails and those with longer sentences go to state or federal prisons depending on the jurisdiction. Incarcerated offenders serve time at various institutions determined by jurisdiction and appropriate level of security ranging from community, low, minimum, medium, to maximum levels. After serving a specific portion of the sentence, the inmate may be eligible for parole, a conditional release before serving the full sentence. Parole boards determine eligibility and the conditions of release and place the parolee under the supervision of a community parole officer. Parole violators may be re-incarcerated. Once released from custody, an ex-offender may re-offend (recidivate) or successfully reenter the community. Nationally, over half of all offenders recidivate, repeating the cycle (Bureau of Justice Statistics, 1997). The stages of involvement with the criminal justice system are outlined in Table 21-1 with a listing of which mental health service personnel and structures would be involved with the offender, and how these items related to the role of the occupational therapy team members.

SCOPE OF CRIMINAL JUSTICE

Beginning in the 1970s the American criminal justice system shifted its focus from re-habilitation to punishment, leading to incarceration as its primary sanction and longer sentences for crimes of all types (Haney, 2002). With less than 5% of the world's population, the United States incarcerates over 23% of those incarcerated worldwide (Hartney, 2006). Currently, 2.3 million, or 1 in every 100 adult Americans, are behind bars in prisons or jails. Another 5 million are on community-based probation and parole, accounting for 1 in every 45 American adults. Counting probationers, parolees, prisoners, and jail inmates, 1 in every 31 American adults, more than 7.3 million or over 3% of the population, are in some form of correctional control (Pew Center on the States, 2009). Incarceration rates in some individual states exceed by up to six times

TABLE 21-1. Occupational Therapy in the Criminal Justice System

Stages of the Criminal Justice System	Mental Health Service Structures	Occupational Therapy Role
Police response	Mobile crisis team	Screening regarding mental health status and service needs
	Emergency department	Assessment; referral to inpatient service
	Acute psychiatry inpatient team	Discharge planning; brokerage to community services;
Arrest	Mobile crisis team	Screening regarding mental health status and service needs
	Court diversion team	Screening; brokerage to community services
Adjudication	Entering a plea based on mental health status	Assessment of criminal responsibility/fitness to stand trial
	Mental health court	Brokerage to community services; direct provision of services
Sentencing and Sanctions	Forensic psychiatric inpatient unit/facility	Hospital-based; assessment; short- and long-term intervention
	Prison (sentences greater than 2 years)	Assessment; long-term intervention; adjustment to prison life; meeting correction plan requirements
Community Supervision	Community corrections team	Screening; brokerage to community services; direct provision of services
	General community services	Screening; brokerage to community services; direct provision of services

© Cengage Learning 2013

the rates of nations with comparable populations. Incarceration rates of four to seven times higher than other industrialized nations are explained not by more criminals or increased crime rates but by incarceration as primary sanction (Hartney, 2006). Gender and racial disparities exist, with 1 in 18 men, 1 in 45 Hispanics, and 1 in 11 blacks being in some form of custody (Pew Center on the States, 2009). The incarceration of women is even more alarming with the United States incarcerating the most women of any nation, numbering 183,400 in 2005. Comparing the number of women incarcerated in individual states to global rates, Texas ranks fourth and California seventh (Hartney, 2006). One state alone, Oklahoma, incarcerates more than double the women per capita than the other states—132 women per 100,000 population compared to the national average of 68—to lead the world in the incarceration of women (Hartney, 2006; Oklahoma Department of Corrections, 2010a; West & Sobal, 2009). The growth from 1 in 77 Americans in correctional custody 25 years ago to 1 in 31 today is the result of sentencing and correctional policies (Pew Center on the States, 2009).

HEALTH CARE IN THE CRIMINAL JUSTICE SYSTEM

The jail and prison population's health care needs are diverse. Although crime is primarily an occupation of the young, the aging of the general population and longer sentences due to "three strikes" laws that impose harsher penalties on re-cidivists result in aging offenders (Pew Center on the States, 2009). The number of prisoners 50 years and older has doubled in the last 10 years and is five times larger than 20 years ago. These offenders have more serious health care needs and increasingly need long-term care (Haugebrook, Zgoba, Maschi, Morgen, & Brown, 2010). Between 39% and 44% of American offenders in custody report chronic health problems, the most common of which are arthritis, hypertension, tuber-culosis, asthma, and heart problems. Between 60% and 68.5% of those 60 or older report current health conditions (Maruschak, 2008). Impairments in learning, speech, hearing, vision, mobility, or mental impairment are reported by 24% to 36% of incarcerated offenders with learning the most commonly reported impair-ment and 8% to 16% reporting multiple impairments. Percentages reporting im-paired hearing and vision increase with age. State and federal prisoners most likely to report impairments were homeless in the year prior to arrest, those who used needles to inject drugs, and those who reported receiving government assistance (Maruschak, 2008). State and federal offenders are more likely to report accidental injuries than fight-related injuries. Between 80% and 86% reported seeing a health care professional for injuries since admission, led by younger inmates' reports of fight-related injuries (Maruschak, 2008).

It is ironic that in the United States as the number of people not covered by health insurance grows (over 50 million in 2009) (DeNavas-Walt, Procter, & Smith, 2010), incarcerated individuals are guaranteed the provision of health services under the U.S. Constitution's Eighth Amendment preventing cruel and unusual punishment. However, the quality of that care varies considerably, especially considering the higher incidence of chronic physical and mental conditions. Though most offenders eventu-ally receive needed care, some have extended wait periods for health services, and there is wide variation in the quality of services across correctional facility types and locations (Wilper et al., 2009).

There is limited information available on the quality of mental health care in prisons; however, the Trenčín Statement on Prisons and Mental Health (World Health Organization, 2007) identifies certain principles for ensuring quality mental health care for prisoners:

1. **Inclusiveness:** Prisons should be seen as part of society and isolation from or rejection by society—for both prisoners and the staff who work with them—is crucial for successful rehabilitation and reduced recidivism.

2. **Equivalence:** Mental health care in prisons should be broadly equivalent to that available in the local community as a fundamental human right.

3. **Appropriate care and shelter:** People deprived of their liberty should be held in facilities/residences that are acceptable in basic terms of shelter, sanitation, and warmth.

4. **Good governance:** Order and accountability are needed to deliver appropriate care.

MENTAL HEALTH IN CRIMINAL JUSTICE AND CORRECTIONS: U.S. AND INTERNATIONAL PERSPECTIVES

An even greater problem exists in mental health arenas. Correctional systems have become the "new asylum" in the United States (Navasky & O'Connor, 2005). Adult offenders outnumber the 10% of the general population meeting the *Diagnostic and Statistical Manual of Mental Disorders (DSM-IV-TR)* (American Psychiatric Association, 2000) criteria for mental disorders by almost 50% (Haugebrook et al., 2010). Of the 2,760 female offenders incarcerated in the state prisons of Oklahoma at the end of 2010, 62% (N=1,707) had a history of, or were currently being treated for, mental disorder (Oklahoma Department of Corrections, 2010a).

There is international recognition that the number of people with mental illness entering the criminal justice system has been increasing, and that the prevalence of mental disorders in prisons is higher than the general population (Diamond, Wang, Holzer, Thomas, & Cruser, 2001; Elizabeth Fry Society of Mainland Nova Scotia, 2005; Sampson, Gascon, Glen, Louie, & Rosenfeldt, 2007; World Health Organization, 2007). There have been several studies on the prevalence of mental illness in jail detainees (Guy, Platt, Zwerling, & Bullock, 1985; Kal, 1977; Lamb & Grant, 1983; Monahan & McDonough, 1980; Petrich, 1976; Piotrowski, Lasacco, & Guze, 1976; Snow & Briar, 1990; Swank & Winer, 1976; Teplin, 1990; Whitmer, 1980). In 1994, a Canadian study of people admitted to the Calgary Remand Centre (Arboleda-Florez, 1994) found that 56% of men and 49.5% of women were diagnosed with a mental disorder, with the substance-related disorders being most frequent (31.7% for men, 26.1% for women). However, differences between prisons and jails limit the degree to which these findings can predict the prevalence of mental illness in prisons (Diamond et al., 2001).

Studies conducted in the United States and United Kingdom have shown significantly higher prevalence rates of schizophrenia, bipolar disorder, and major depression in prisons than the general community population (Bean, Meirson, & Pinta, 1988; California Department of Corrections, 1989; Powell, Holt, & Fondacaro, 1997; Singleton, Meltzer, & Gatward, 1998). In the United States, there is consensus that there are two to six times as many people with serious mental illness in jails and prisons than are in state mental hospitals (Fisher, Packer, Simon, & Smith, 2000; Teplin, 1990, 1994; Torrey, 1995) and it is estimated that up to 35% of offenders require mental health services (Diamond et al., 2001; James, Gregory, Jones, & Rundell, 1980).

Canadian studies of the prevalence of mental health disorders found similar results. A 1991 study (Motiuk & Porporino) randomly sampled 2,185 offenders from various prisons within the Correctional Service of Canada, including the organization's five prison hospitals, and found that approximately 20% of the general prison population had a major mental health disorder in their lifetime. A 1999 study (Brink, Doherty, & Boer, 2001) of people admitted to one regional reception center of the Correctional Service of Canada found that almost one third of study participants had a current mental illness, with mood and anxiety disorders being most frequent, and 84% of participants had experienced a mental health disorder at some point in their life. In a 2004, study of intake assessments done at reception centers throughout the Correctional Service of Canada, Bouchard (2004) found that only 3% of offenders were identified at intake as having a mental health disorder but that 14% had experienced recent psychological or psychiatric treatment prior to being incarcerated and that 21% of women and 14% of men had attempted suicide within the previous five years. In 2007, Keith Coulter, then Commissioner of the Correctional Service of Canada, stated that "there is a direct link between how well we respond to the needs of offenders with mental disorders and keeping Canadian communities safe" (Coulter, 2007, p. 3).

In the United Kingdom, mental health care in prisons is based on the principle of equivalence. That is, mental health care provided within prisons should be equivalent to the mental health care offenders would receive if they were not in prison (Wilson, 2004). Clinical in-reach teams provide services to the general population in regular prisons, including segregation, as well as those offenders housed in prison health care wings. Offenders with serious mental illness are typically moved to a prison health care wing where they may wait for months before being transferred to a community hospital (Reed & Lyne, 2000). Staff within the British prison system has begun to question the appropriateness of these prison health care wings as "alternative places" of care and the "timeliness" of waiting for months for transfer to hospital (Wilson, 2004).

In the United States, mental health services vary from state to state. A survey of prison mental health services in the state of Georgia found that "mental health services constituted a 'non-system' of care" (Elliott, 1997, p. 433). Clinical practices were left to the discretion of individual mental health staff with very little system wide direction despite the prevalence of mental health problems among offenders throughout the system.

Common challenges in providing mental health care to incarcerated offenders, such as continuity of care following transfer within a prison or release from prison, family involvement, and professional credentials among staff responsible for providing mental health services (Kerr, Roth, Courtless, & Zenoff, 1987; Ogloff, 2002; Steadman, Barbera, & Dennis, 1994), are gradually being addressed on an individualized basis. One example of this is the Harris County Jail in Texas, the third largest jail in the United States. This correctional facility has a larger mental health program than any psychiatric hospital in the state and functions as an inpatient psychiatric unit (Cruser & Diamond, 1996). Services provided include medication maintenance, counseling and nursing services, as well as follow-up care to offenders housed throughout the mega-jail. Life-skills training and group therapies address criminogenic behaviors with psychological factors, counseling is provided to inmates' families, prevocational and work programs have been developed, and dual diagnosis substance abuse programs have been formed (Cruser & Diamond, 1996). Another example is found in the National Institute of Mental Health in Angoda, Sri Lanka, where the forensic unit, "the forgotten ward," was refurbished and opened as the Forensic Psychiatry Rehabilitation Unit in July of 2010 (Ranasinghe, Gunarathne, & Alahakoon, 2011). The influence of occupational therapy in the development of this unit is clearly evident in values and beliefs guiding practice in this unit. The focus is on occupational enrichment for residents, understanding that occupational engagement is a means to mental health and well-being. Services include group sessions in art, music, creative writing, gardening and horticulture, vocational and income generating activities, meal preparation, education in reading writing and arithmetic, as well as psychoeducational groups in communication, work skills, anger management, and so on (Ranasinghe et al.).

OCCUPATIONAL THERAPY IN CRIMINAL JUSTICE

Occupational theory clearly identifies the environment as a primary influence in occupational engagement and performance (Canadian Association of Occupational Therapists [CAOT], 2002; Kielhofner, 2008; Law et al., 1996). While we often understand this in relation to the everyday life of clients, it is equally applicable to our own work as occupational therapists.

An increasing body of mental health and criminal justice literature suggests that there is value inherent in the provision of mental health care within correctional systems (Elliott, 1997; Green, Miranda, Daroowalla, & Siddique, 2005; McCoy, Roberts, Hanrahan, Clay, & Luchins, 2004; Reed & Lyne, 2000; Ruddell, 2006). However, mental health and criminal justice systems often interact in ways that create obstacles to providing care. The unique, heavily legislated environment of forensic and correctional services presents significant challenges to the provision of mental health care that can often impede the work of occupational therapists and other mental health professionals.

The mental health and criminal justice mandates are based on incompatible value structures. The mental health mandate is based on principles of psychosocial rehabilitation and recovery where professionals are responsible for providing "care" and are trained to exercise discretion in decision making. Whereas the criminal justice system is based on principles of punishment and correction in which professionals ensure "custody" requirements and are trained to conform to specific rules or procedures. When the two systems and their conflicting values interact the resulting tensions are characterized as "sickness-badness," "therapy-custody," and "treatment-punishment" dichotomies (Cruser & Diamond, 1996; Dieleman Grass, 2010). Mental health and criminal justice professionals have a tendency to operate from one value system or the other rather than considering a permutation of possibilities and making decisions based on a continuous range of options. They often blame each other for problems related to offenders with mental illness and these problems arise in part from interactions between the criminal justice and mental health systems

(Freeman & Roesch, 1989; Steadman, McCarty, & Morrissey, 1989). When staff mutually disregard or misunderstand each other's values, conflicts occur, making it difficult for mental health staff, including occupational therapists, to provide care to offenders with mental illness in the criminal justice environment (Cruser & Diamond, 1996).

OCCUPATIONAL JUSTICE AND INJUSTICE

The values inherent in an occupational justice perspective that include the right of people to have meaningful, satisfying, and healthful and equitable choices of occupation in their lives (Townsend & Wilcock, 2004; Wilcock, 1998b) provides compelling support for occupational therapy in criminal justice systems to help address the occupational injustices. With such large segments of the population being punished through incarceration and facing chronic deprivation of occupational choice along with the subsequent challenges of reentry, a claim can be made that typical criminal justice systems constitute a form of **occupational apartheid** (Muñoz et al., 2011). Occupational apartheid is the "segregation of groups of people through the [systematic] restriction or denial of access to dignified and meaningful participation in occupations of daily life" based on a characteristic shared by the members of the group (Kronenberg & Pollard, 2005, p. 67), in this case criminality. Occupational therapy actions to address such systematic denial of occupational opportunity include the provision of **occupational enrichment** (Wood, 1993) in correctional settings (Molineux & Whiteford, 1999). Enriching occupational opportunities occurs at the local level by providing sources of physical, mental, and spiritual activity that engage people's whole selves and prepare them for a life after incarceration, or in the case of long imprisonment, a more healthful institutional life. Advocacy is needed at the sociopolitical level that addresses the social, economic, and cultural factors that have led to a punishment-based versus a rehabilitative prerogative in corrections (Molineux & Whiteford, 1999).

Proper environmental and occupational enrichment must take into consideration the **occupational imbalance**, alienation (Wilcock, 1998b), and restriction (Galvaan, 2005) faced by incarcerated offenders. Occupational imbalance is a disproportionate amount of occupation leading to decreased health or well-being (Wilcock, 1998b) that is common in correctional facilities. Incarcerated individuals experience **occupational alienation** when they experience a "sense of isolation, powerlessness, frustration, loss of control, estrangement from society or self as a result of engagement in occupation which does not satisfy inner needs" (Wilcock, 1998b, p. 257). Incarceration is typically designed to isolate offenders from society, reduce or remove their power and control, and reduce sources of personal identification (e.g., uniforms, few to no personal belongings) and thus frequently creates ideal conditions for occupational alienation. Galvaan (2005) applied the concept of **occupational restriction** to domestic workers whose choices of occupation were strictly controlled and limited by their employers, but the concept also applies to incarcerated individuals. In correctional settings, offenders typically have only a few options for active engagement and the range of environments in which they pursue the limited activity choices is highly constrained.

Once adopted, an occupational justice perspective influences a practitioner's view of where action can be directed in criminal justice systems. A top-down approach will emphasize advocacy at the system (institutional, state, or national) level to influence policy and institutional practices to develop programs that improve occupational opportunities across the corrections continuum. A top-down advocacy approach can also affect societal factors that contribute to criminality and **health care disparities**. A bottom-up approach is also needed to help offenders experiencing occupational deprivation that is compounded by societal and systemic attitudes toward mental illness and criminal behavior. Applying client-centered practices ensures individual concerns and goals are factored into assessment and intervention decisions. Combining the top-down and bottom-up approaches in occupational therapy (Gutman, Mortera, Hinojosa, & Kramer, 2007) is the ideal way to combat occupational injustices that are more likely to affect people with mental health conditions who are in the criminal justice system.

Examination of the mental health and criminal justice systems' closely held values from which their policies arise can lead to enhanced models of collaborative programming and improved use of resources in both systems (Cruser & Diamond, 1996). Having different views does not preclude agreement, and may even enhance problem solving and lead to synergistic solutions when shared and shaped into common goals (Diamond, Cruser, Childs, Schnee, & Quinn, 1999). Successful provision of mental healthcare within forensic and correctional environments hinges on opening channels of communication between leaders and followers, between correctional and mental health staff, and on clarifying roles and relationships (Cruser & Diamond, 1996). Recent collaborative efforts are being made to understand both perspectives. The Oklahoma Department of Mental Health and Substance Abuse Services (2011) and the Oklahoma Department of Corrections have initiated the Justice and Mental Health Collaborative Project. Statewide cross-system training prepares probation and parole offices and community mental health workers to collaborate to provide community-based collaborative services to 300 offenders on probation or parole who are diagnosed with mental illness. The program's goal is to train 100 corrections officers and 200 community mental health workers. When values of occupational justice are included in these collaborations, significant potential for positive change in criminal justice can be realized.

An example of such collaboration in the institutional setting is shown in Figure 21-1.

EVALUATION, ASSESSMENT, AND INTERVENTION

Psychological models of community-based intervention apply to institutional and community-based corrections. Based on a living skills model for acquisition of specific living skills needed in community living (American Occupational Therapy Association [AOTA], 2003), the occupational therapist directs intervention toward

Aided by his occupational therapy student, LCDR (Lieutenant Commander) Stanley W. Bennett, MS, OTR/L of the United States Public Health Service operates a therapeutic horticulture project at a 300-bed forensic psychiatric hospital within the Federal Correctional Complex (FCC) in Butner, North Carolina. Working directly with multidisciplinary treatment teams, clients are identified from the Transitional Unit, which houses inmates who are emerging from recent acute or chronic psychological distress but require daily interactions to assess psychosocial function and safety to self and others before they can be released to the general population. Voluntary participation in the horticulture program provides not only a taste of freedom from the highly structured Transitional Unit but also a taste of good homegrown food.

After assessing horticulture participants using the Canadian Occupational Performance Measure (COPM) (Law et al., 2005), the Allen Cognitive-Level Screen (ACLS-5) (Allen et al., 2007), and the Adolescent/Adult Sensory Profile® (Brown & Dunn, 2002), LCDR Bennett helps each participant develop their own plan to recovery. The program's goal is to provide a safe and structured environment where appropriate social and work expectations are clearly defined such that meaningful and rewarding experiences can be found in the "enjoyment" of digging, pushing, pulling, caring, and realizing the fruits of their labor. It's through structured job details with daily feedback that the clients are provided the opportunity to organize their thoughts, plan ahead of time, develop insight, communicate with others, and develop job/social skills. This information is then passed along to their treatment teams to assist them in managing their plan of care in the most effective way possible.

In the horticulture garden, each participant receives a 4' x 8' plot and designs a garden of his choice to include plants such as sunflowers, herbs, cucumber, tomato, sunflowers, okra, and watermelon. In 2010, they grew 140 lb. of cucumbers alone. Participants work in the garden each morning, mindful of the photosensitive effects of some psychotropic medications and end by processing the day's work and make plans for the next day. They learn about healthy nutrition and ultimately get to enjoy their harvest in a "fellowship" setting of cooked corn, sweet pickles, and tomato sandwiches. Staff and client safety is of upmost importance given the unique situation and setting of a forensic psychiatric hospital. Therefore, contingency plans are established in case of an emergency.

FIGURE 21-1. Occupational Therapy Intervention: The Horticulture Program at the U.S. Federal Correctional Institution at Butner, North Carolina

© Cengage Learning 2013

activities of daily living (ADL) and instrumental activities of daily living (IADL) for reentry. Examples include health management and maintenance, medication management, financial management, community transportation, parenting, and communication management (especially electronic communication devices available only after release or on supervision and not widely in use before incarceration such as cell phones, smart phones, and computers with Internet connections). Table 21-2 lists examples of how IADL may appear in forensic settings and typical OT interventions to promote successful occupational performance.

OCCUPATION-BASED SELF-DETERMINATION (OBSD)

Occupation-Based Self-Determination (OBSD) developed from the Self-Determination Model and the Model of Human Occupation (MOHO) seeks to combine skills, knowledge, and beliefs to enable a person to engage in goal-directed, self-regulated, autonomous behavior (Gregitis, Gelpi, Moore, & Dees, 2010; Kielhofner, 2008; Wehmeyer, Gragoudas, & Shogren, 2006). OBSD models are uniquely

TABLE 21-2. IADL in Forensic Settings and Typical OT Interventions

IADL Occupations (AOTA, 2008a)	Examples	Forensic-Based Interventions
Care of others	Finding appropriate daycare for children or older adults.	Accessing community resources.
Child rearing	Learning how to care for and supervise children's developmental needs after parent's long absence.	Parenting classes. Childhood developmental milestones.
Communication management	Electronic devices predating incarceration and not generally allowed while incarcerated.	Using cell phones and smart phones. Using the Internet.
Community mobility	Transportation options such as public transport. Factors in people with felonies when riding in private vehicles.	Reading bus schedules. Accessing buses, taxicabs, and other public transport. Avoiding private uninsured vehicles that may contain alcohol, drugs, or weapons and drivers with felony records while on supervised release.
Financial management	Using fiscal resources. May have relied on cash due to illegal means of making money.	Using checking and savings accounts. Online banking and use of automated teller machines (ATMs). Budgeting. Maintaining financial records. Preparing tax reports.
Health management and maintenance	Developing, management, and maintaining healthy routines after period of incarceration. Making healthy decisions after a period of occupational deprivation (think of seeing TV food commercials and you have no access). Making healthy decisions without the advantages of incarceration such as ample free time and a fully equipped gym and sports teams.	Nutrition on a budget. Healthy cooking techniques. Physical fitness in community. Decreasing health behaviors through low-cost smoking cessation and weight-loss programs. Accessing free or low-cost health clinics. Maintaining a medication routine. Timely access to medication refills.
Home establishment and management	Obtaining and maintaining housing, household possessions, repair, and accessing assistance. May not have owned a home or been homeless.	Finding safe affordable housing. Acquisition and use of household tools. Routine household maintenance (unstopping a toilet, circuit breakers). Routine garden and lawn maintenance.

TABLE 21-2. Continued

IADL Occupations (AOTA, 2008a)	Examples	Forensic-Based Interventions
Meal preparation and cleanup	Providing healthy low-cost meals. Prison food is typically high in fat and low in fiber. Cooking consists of making do with microwave ovens.	Cooking is highly sequential and requires good temporal planning; skills that may be eroded or lost during incarceration.
Religious observance	Finding a meaningful set of beliefs.	Finding a welcoming spiritual community for ex-offenders.
Safety and emergency maintenance	Procedures for safe environments and unexpected situations.	Safety precautions for children and older adults. Weather precautions for new environments. Precautions for living in unsafe neighborhoods.
Shopping	Preparing lists, selecting, and completing financial transactions.	Use of online banking, automatic teller machines, and debit cards.

© Cengage Learning 2013

designed to promote self-determination performance for clients over the age of 10 for achievement of occupational performance goals. Wehmeyer et al. (2006) state "self-determined behavior refers to volitional actions that enable one to act as the primary causal agent in one's life and to maintain or improve one's quality of life" (p. 47).

This process of self-determination is coupled with an understanding of one's own strengths and limitations, and focuses on the here and now behavior (Gregitis et al., 2010; Kielhofner, 2008; Wehmeyer, 1999). The OBSD uses a "Plan, Act, Evaluate" philosophy, where planning precedes actions, and actions are followed by evaluation. The specific objectives of OBSD are to:

- Create change in occupational patterns and behaviors, to empower individuals to develop an occupational lifestyle and support system that, in turn, contribute to a health-promoting lifestyle.
- Increase development of positive habits, roles, and routines in everyday life activities (occupations) and skills.
- Set goals and take steps to achieve those goals.
- Evaluate goals.
- Engage in meaningful and satisfying occupational roles.
- Improve resilience and quality of life.

In the process of using OBSD, there is a planning phase, where clients are responsible for setting goals, planning the small steps to meet those goals, and anticipating the results. In this phase, clients are asked to be creative in solving problems, and are asked to visually rehearse action phases. In the action phase, goals are task-oriented. Clients are asked to take risks by taking action on their goals, communicate their intentions, and access resources and support systems. They develop negotiation skills, deal with conflict and potential criticism, and maintain focus and persistence. In the evaluation phase, clients compare their expected outcome to the actual outcome. Clients will compare their performance to the expected performance, and they will identify real successes, and make adjustments to begin the process anew (Gregitis et al., 2010; Wehmeyer, 1999). While research is limited with application of this approach to correctional institutions it has been successfully used with adolescents and adults with learning disabilities and substance abuse.

THERAPEUTIC COMPETENCIES

Therapeutic competencies are the skills that are essential and will support occupational therapy practitioners working in a correctional institution and include knowledge of the criminal justice setting in which they work, risk assessment (i.e., risk perception and interpretation, fundamental information, risk behaviors, and occupations), and environmental modifications that are possible within a restricted setting. Knowledge of the current models of practice in occupational therapy and knowledge of occupational science concepts (e.g., occupational justice, occupational alienation, occupational imbalance, and occupational enrichment) support the practitioner in developing client-centered and occupation-based interventions that are rich and meaningful even within a restricted environment. Other skills include knowledge of risk assessment, appropriate assessment tools, and interviewing techniques. Practitioners will be able to provide patient care in the forensic setting that is compassionate, appropriate, and effective for the treatment of psychiatric disorders. Additionally, practitioners need to demonstrate an awareness of and responsiveness to the larger context and system of health care and the ability to effectively call on system resources that are of optimal value.

Risk Assessment and Environmental Assessment

The process of choosing an assessment is based on a variety of factors: needs (condition and goals), setting, and the model of practice used are typically important aspects. An occupational therapist views every client through a lens of what they need to do, want to do, are expected to do, or a combination of one or more of these. Additionally, many of the models in practice can help to support the overall intervention strategies, for example, the Canadian Occupational Performance Measure (COPM) (Law et al., 2005) may help the client prioritize her needs while including a cognitive-behavioral approach to guide an interactional style and use of rewards to accomplish tasks as follows:

1. Demonstrate the ability to perform and document a comprehensive forensic history and examination of a forensic patient in a forensic setting, including

obtaining or conducting the following assessments, which are particularly relevant to this population:

- A violence risk assessment.

- A suicide risk assessment.

- An assessment of malingering. (Note: it is incumbent on the client-centered practitioner to examine the motivations for malingering and address the underlying issues when possible to improve occupational performance. For example, what secondary benefits does the client gain from exhibiting symptoms and how can the therapist assist the client to progress in more productive ways?)

2. Demonstrate the ability to develop and implement an appropriate treatment plan in a correctional or forensic psychiatric setting that considers the environment. Awareness of the special clinical and legal considerations in a forensic setting includes:

- Safety and security measures.

- Levels of care and therapeutic privilege.

- Collecting necessary historical and current information for the development of an appropriate treatment plan in a forensic setting, including sexual history when appropriate.

- Use of appropriate pharmacotherapy in a forensic setting.

- Use of appropriate psychotherapies in a forensic setting.

3. Demonstrate knowledge and application of the relevant legal standard(s) and development of a rational and logical forensic opinion regarding current and predicted levels of judgment and safety related to occupational performance.

Models of Practice and Practice Knowledge Base

Practitioners will be expected to be able to demonstrate medical/legal knowledge relevant to the practice of forensic occupational therapy and apply this knowledge to forensic evaluations to conduct a competent evaluation of an individual and develop a well-reasoned treatment opinion. The evaluation should include a personal interview of the offender including:

- A statement regarding limits of confidentiality, the role of the evaluator, the issues to be addressed, and the nature and scope of evaluation. The statement will include:

  - Relevant historical information.

  - A focused mental status examination.

  - A review of collateral sources of information, including collateral informants and record review.

- The use of an occupation-based, client-centered evaluation (see recommendations listed earlier in the chapter).
- Specialized interviewing techniques including Motivational Interviewing (Rollnick, Miller, & Butler, 2008).

Practitioners will need to be able to demonstrate knowledge of legal issues relevant to the practice of general and forensic occupational therapy. This knowledge typically includes:

- Basic principles of substantive and procedural law.
- Landmark mental health cases appropriate for setting.
- Correctional and mental health secure systems.
- Court systems.
- Mental health system.
- Legislative and regulatory systems.

Practitioners will need to be able to integrate evidence-based practice and appropriate models of practice into assessment and intervention and demonstrate knowledge of the appropriate models of practice, which may typically (but not exclusively) include:

- Model of Human Occupation.
- Cognitive-behavioral therapy.
- Canadian Occupational Performance Model.
- Occupation-Based Self-Determination Model.
- Occupational adaptation.

Practitioners must develop appropriate skills in obtaining up-to-date scientific and legal information to assist in the treatment and evaluation of offenders. These may include:

- Accessing legal information from relevant landmark cases, institutional regulations, attorneys, and statutes.
- Utilizing practice parameter guidelines relevant to the practice of correctional and forensic occupational therapy.
- Using information technology to access on-line medical and legal information, and support one's own education.

Models of Practice and Assessments

Many of the assessments listed in Table 21-3 would be congruent to use with other assessments in the table highlighting occupational performance areas as well.

TABLE 21-3. Models and Assessments

Model of Practice/Area of Assessment	Potential Assessments
Model of Human Occupation (MOHO)/ Occupational Engagement	<ul><li>Occupational Performance History Interview II (OPHI-II)</li><li>Occupational Self-Assessment (OSA)</li><li>Occupational Circumstances Assessment-Interview and Rating Scale (OCAIRS)</li><li>Interest Checklist</li><li>MOHO Screening Tool</li><li>Role Checklist</li><li>Volitional Questionnaire</li><li>Assessment of Communication and Interaction Skills (ACIS)</li></ul>These assessments are designed to incorporate a client's volitional and historical narrative into a more formalized assessment, which can then be used as a baseline to set goals and measure progress. These assessments are primarily self-report or semi-structured interview formats, except for the ACIS and MOHO Screening Tools, which are task based. Assessments available on the MOHO clearinghouse website located at: http://www.uic.edu/depts/moho/
Canadian Model of Occupational Performance (CMOP)/ Person Environment Occupation (PEO)/ Occupational Engagement	<ul><li>Canadian Occupational Performance Measure (COPM)</li><li>Adult Activity Card Sort (ACS) (Baum & Edwards, 2008)</li><li>Executive Function Performance Test (EFPT) (Baum, Morrison, Hahn, & Edwards, 2007)</li></ul>These assessments focus on the abilities and priorities for intervention. These assessments use a semi-structured interview or use an observation session where the client performs a single task or a series of tasks. The COPM is a semi-structured interview, which is divided into three sub-areas: self-care, productivity, and leisure. This assessment identifies a client's priorities for occupational engagement, perceived performance, and satisfaction with performance on those occupations and helps in establishing a baseline to set goals and detecting change in performance. The EFPT examines the execution of four basic tasks that are essential for self-maintenance and independent living: simple cooking, telephone use, medication management, and bill payment. The COPM website is located at: http://www.caot.ca/copm/index.htm EFPT test booklet is available at: http://www.practicechangefellows.org/documents/EFPT.pdf ACS is available at: http://myaota.aota.org/shop_aota/prodview.aspx?TYPE=D&PID=763&SKU=1247

(Continues)

TABLE 21-3. Continued

Model of Practice/Area of Assessment	Potential Assessments
Sensory Modulation/ Sensory Integration	Adult Sensory Profile is a self-questionnaire designed to provide a standardized method to evaluate the impact of sensory processing on occupational performance for people aged 11–65.
	Brown, C., & Dunn, W. (2002). *Adolescent/Adult Sensory Profile®*. Pearson PsychCorp.: San Antonio, TX.
Risk Management Model/Violence Risk Assessment	■ The HCR-20 ■ Violence Risk Scale (VRS) ■ Psychopathy Checklist-Revised (PCL-R)
	These assessments are the most broadly used and are typically based on historical and risk management and are administered by correctional staff or psychiatrist.
	The HCR-20 (Webster, Eaves, Douglas, & Wintrup, 1995, Version 1) is the most commonly used broad-band violence risk assessment instrument. HCR-20 is named from three included scales, Historical, Clinical, Risk Management, and from the number of items (20). The HCR-20 aligns risk markers into past, present, and future.
	The Violence Risk Scale (VRS), is a structured guideline designed to assess the risk of violent recidivism for institutionalized forensic clients who are going to be released to the community (Wong & Gordon, 1999).
	The Psychopathy Checklist–Revised (PCL-R), is a measure of criminal psychopathy, combining equally personality or affective-interpersonal traits (Factor 1) and behavioral or antisocial lifestyle criteria (Factor 2), based on the 16 core traits of psychopathy (Hare, 2003). Psychopathology is rated on 20 items, on a 3-point scale indicating evidence of the variable.
Psychological and Cognitive/Suicide Risk Assessment	■ Beck Depression Inventory, 2nd Edition (BDI-II) (Beck, Brown, & Steer, 1996) ■ Beck Hopelessness Scale ■ General Mental Status Exam
	Typically suicide risk assessment includes a variety of elements, including a clinical psychological or psychiatric assessment, review or relevant records, and direct questions about suicidal ideation or any risk-enhancing factors.
	Clinical questions typically include initial questions to elicit suicidal thoughts, for example: ■ Have you ever felt that life was not worth living? ■ How does the future look to you? ■ Have things ever reached the point that you thought of harming yourself?
	Brief self-report scales like the BDI-II are often used as supplements to more in-depth assessments.
	American Psychiatric Association (2003) offers practice guidelines for the assessment and treatment of patients with suicidal behaviors, and includes use of the following assessments.
	BDI-II and Hopelessness Scale are available at: www.harcourtassessment.com

TABLE 21-3. Continued

Model of Practice/Area of Assessment	Potential Assessments
Psychological and Cognitive/ Malingering Assessment	<ul><li>Criminal Forensic Evaluation</li><li>Minnesota Multiphasic Personality Inventory-2 (MMPI-2)</li><li>Structured Interview of Reported Symptoms (SIRS)</li><li>Clinical Observations</li><li>Interview</li></ul> Malingering is the intentional production of false or grossly exaggerated physical or psychological symptoms, motivated by external incentives such as avoiding military duty, avoiding work, obtaining financial compensation, evading criminal prosecution, or obtaining drugs. Psychologists and psychiatrists typically administer these assessments. The SIRS consists of 156 items developed to assess systematically deliberate distortions in the self-report of symptoms. This structured interview has eight primary scales and five scales designated as supplementary. All the scales are designed to ascertain within statistical probability whether or not the individual is attempting to malinger schizophrenia or psychosis. Individual's responses on the primary scales are classified as to being Honest, Indeterminate, Probable Malingering, or Definite Malingering. Responses on the supplementary scales are classified as whether within criteria (WC) or outside criteria (OC). An OC classification is indicative of malingering. The MMPI-2 consists of 567 items and is a self-administered standardized questionnaire. The MMPI-2 elicits a wide range of self-descriptions scored to give a quantitative measurement of an individual's level of emotional adjustment and attitude toward test taking. There are ten major scales, four validity measures, and several supplementary measures. The contents for the majority of the MMPI-2 questions are relatively obvious and deal largely with psychiatric, psychological, neurological, and physical symptoms. The MMPI-2 has direct relevance to forensic applications and includes the test's ability to measure various symptoms of psychopathology. The MMPI-2 is used in evaluations of competence to stand trial, criminal responsibly, civil competence, parental fitness, and emotional sequelae of physical and psychological trauma. The Criminal Forensic Supplement was added to the basic interpretation report. This interpretation includes critical Item listings and statements of how incarceration or pending incarceration affects basic scale scores. Assessments can be obtained at the following websites: SIRS, Western Psychological Services: http://portal.wpspublish.com/portal/page?_pageid=53,53086&_dad=portal&_schema=PORTAL MMPI-2, Pearson Assessments: http://psychcorp.pearsonassessments.com/pai/ca/cahome.htm

Interpersonal and Communication Skills

Practitioners will be able to demonstrate interpersonal and communications skills that result in effective information exchange and learning with offenders, their families, and professional associates. (See Table 21-4 for a list of slang terms. Knowing

TABLE 21-4. Slang Terms Used in Some U.S. Correctional Settings

Term	Description
Ace	Another word for "dollar."
Babydoll	Texas Syndicate slang for a Mexican Mafia member.
Back door parole	To die in prison.
Bang	A fight to the death, or shoot to kill.
Base head	Refers to a cocaine addict.
B.G.	"Baby gangster," or someone who has never shot another person.
"Blob"	Crips gang slang term for rival Blood gang members.
Boned out	Chickened out.
Boosters	Booster sessions are encouraged by case managers and treatment providers to be taken by inmates at particular risk to reoffend after release. They are part of a broad risk management strategy that includes the Stages of Change and Relapse Prevention. They are a component of the regular "aftercare" for many recently released offenders, especially offenders with mental disorders, who should receive these sessions in order to reduce the likelihood of recidivism.
Booty bandit	Incarcerated sexual predator who preys on weaker inmates, called "punks."
Breakdown	Shotgun.
Bucket	Another term for the "county jail."
Bug	Correctional staff member, such as a psychiatrist, who is deemed untrustworthy or unreliable. Inmates are cautious of "bugs" and will seldom ever mention other inmates to them.
Bug Juice	Term referring to depressant drugs, deleriants, or intoxicants.
Building Tenders	Inmates that were selected by guards to assist correctional staff. Tenders were meant to maintain order among the inmate population (often through the use of force), as well as serve as intelligence gatherers. Such people were also called "inmate guards."
Bumpin' titties	Fighting.
Busted a cap	Shot at another person.
Buster	Fraudulent gang member.
Cadillac	Inmate dorm bed or single bunk.
Cantones	Gang term for prisons.
Carnal	Term meaning "Brother," especially for RazaUnida (a Texas prison system Latino gang established in 1980s) that has exerted varying levels of control over prison drug traffic and related violence (U.S. Immigration & Customs Enforcement, 2011). http://www.ice.gov/news/releases/1109/110914corpuschristi.htm

TABLE 21-4. Continued

Term	Description
Catch a case	Getting caught, arrested, or convicted of a crime.
Catch cold	To get killed.
Chaps	Term used by the Sorenos prison gang to refer to their rivals, the Nortenos or La Nuestra Familia.
Chingasos	Hispanic gang term for fighting. Spanish for "hard hits."
Chiva	Heroin.
Chota	Police officers, or prison guards.
Chow hall	Cafeteria or dining hall.
Chuco	Texas Syndicate term for city of El Paso.
Click up	Gang term referring to getting along well with a homeboy; not looking for trouble.
Control Units	Control Units are sections of a maximum or super-maximum security facility, and most fully characterize the notion of incapacitative deterrence for the most dangerous and criminally minded offenders in the prison system. Control Units operate on a panoptical design; cells are arranged around a central security booth that lies on the ground floor. The booth's vantage point allows the constant observation of all cells at the same time through the use of security cameras and sound systems. Sometimes the security booths have computerized access to detailed case-reports of every prisoner in the unit. Prisoners are confined to their cells for 23 hours a day, and are allowed 1 hour of exercise in a tightly guarded and controlled exercise yard.
Crank	Crank is one of the many street words for methamphetamine. "Cranking up," however, is a term sometimes used in prison to refer to the administration of a substance by hypodermic needle. The hypodermic needle itself is sometimes called a "spike."
Criminogenic Need	An empirically derived, changeable risk factor present in an offender upon assessment that is used for purposes of risk assessment, prison classification, prison reclassification, treatment, and release. Criminogenic needs are also known as "dynamic needs," and include two types: stable dynamic needs, such as long-standing attitudes conducive to violence, chronic alcoholism, or a sexual preference to small male children, and acute dynamic needs, such as stress, recent divorce, hostility, or acute symptoms of drug abuse.
Croaker	A doctor or physician; someone who diagnoses illness.
Custody Rating Scale	Canadian risk scale used by Correctional Services of Canada for purposes of intake assessment and classification to custody and security level. The Custody Rating Scale consists of a variety of empirically derived risk factors, subdivided into three categories: institutional adjustment, public safety, and escape risk.
Daddies	Incarcerated sexual predators who prey on weaker inmates, called "punks."
Dancing on the blacktop	Getting stabbed.
Deuce	Prison slang for "two dollars." Also the name of a mainly youth Aboriginal prison gang operating in the Canadian prairies.
Diddler	Another term for child molester or pedophile.
Dissociation	Solitary confinement.

(Continues)

TABLE 21-4. Continued

Term	Description
Doing the Dutch	Term for committing suicide.
Fence	Refers to someone who buys and sells stolen goods.
Green Light	Prison gang term for a contract killing; also known as a "hit."
Hack	Prison guards.
Half a Yard	Prison slang for "fifty dollars."
Hole	Solitary confinement or secured housing unit (SHU).
Hooking Up	Developing a protective, sexual relationship with another inmate, which provides some resistance to the threat of being victimized by continuing rapes with more inmates. These may appear as consenting homosexual relationships to staff, but the "inmate code" often prevents prisoners from telling the truth, or "crying wolf" about their "protectors."
Horseman	Royal Canadian Mounted Police (RCMP) Officer.
Hustle	Way to earn goods or services in prison, such as reselling commissary items or trade stamps as currency; "everybody's got a hustle."
Jacket	Inmate's correctional file.
Jig and jigger	Watch for correctional officers during illegal actions or sexual activity. Jigger is the person on watch.
Jockers	Incarcerated sexual predators who prey on weaker inmates, called "punks."
Jointman	Inmate in prison who behaves like a guard.
Jug-up	Meal-time.
Killing your number	Serving one's time or getting out on parole.
Kite	A contraband letter.
Lifeboat	A pardon or commutation of sentence.
Limbo Room	An area of the prison that is reserved for or encouraging of corporal punishment.
Lugger	An inmate who smuggles in and possesses contraband and illicit substances.
Pass System	The Pass System is a Canadian program similar to a temporary absence, where inmates are allowed to leave prison, with a correctional staff escort, for humanitarian, health, rehabilitative, or medical reasons. Frequent leaves are granted for family visits, education, and employment opportunities, and recreational activities such as sports events. For those serving life in prison for committing murder, they must first be granted permission by Canada's National Parole Board. After an inmate has served six months of the sentence, he or she is eligible to leave on a temporary absence without a correctional escort. The program has a 99% success rate, although the few breaches that have occurred have proven disastrous, including murderer Daniel Gingras' "birthday" pass that allowed him to escape and kill two people.
Prison Wolf	An inmate who is sexually oriented to females on the outside, but becomes sexually oriented to males on the inside.
Psycho	Term for someone suffering from psychopathology.
Pull chain	Move from a municipal or county jail to a prison, as "we pulled chain together."

TABLE 21-4. Continued

Term	Description
Punks	Inmates subject to rape, usually white, younger, and more submissive than most inmates. The worst thing to be called in prison.
Rat	To report to correctional officers about other inmates; also the person who does so.
Red eye	Hard stare.
Ride with	Perform favors for a fellow convict, including sexual, in exchange for protection or commissary goods.
Self-report	A recently admitted inmate who is allowed to show up at reception on his or her own.
Set-tripping	To switch from one gang to another.
Shank	Term for a knife. The actual act of knifing someone is known as a "shiving."
Sharks	Correctional officers who administer mass beatings to newly admitted convicts.
Short	Nearing time for release or reentry, as in "I'm short."
Slinging rock	Selling crack cocaine.
Snitch	Inmate who informs correctional officers about other inmates. Also known as a "rat."
Soda	Cocaine.
Street newspapers	Gang term for graffiti, a communication device for gang members.
Sweet kid	Prison slang referring to an inmate who allies with an older, more experienced inmate, possibly for protection or knowledge.
Taking a nap	Short jail sentence; usually for gang members.
Tat	Tattoos.
Tecato	Term for heroin addict.
Tits-up	Term for an inmate who has died.
Topped	Term for "committed suicide." Also known as "dumped" or "knocked off." Someone who has committed suicide is said to have "topped off."
Veterano	Veteran gang member.
Wolfpacks	Wolfpacks are recent parolees that have been recruited by prison gang members sometime during their incarceration. Once released, they carry out the orders from their imprisoned commanders, who usually instruct them on generating revenue or carrying out contract killings. They are trained in prison by higher-ranking gang members, in vocabulary, symbols, hand-signals, proper dress, as well as how to profit from criminal enterprise.

© Cengage Learning 2013

insider language promotes understanding and clarity of communications as well as cultural competence in the sub-culture of incarceration.) Practioners in correctional settings need to demonstrate competence in the following communication and collaboration skills, knowledge, and behaviors:

- Develop the ability to listen to, understand, and communicate effectively with the offender.

- Effectively triangulate data sources for accuracy (e.g., records, offender interview, assessment data).
- Effectively communicate verbally with attorneys and third party agencies.
- Effectively communicate verbal opinions in testimony and/or mock trials.
- Demonstrate the ability to communicate forensic data and opinions in written format through reports and/or testimony.
- Effectively communicate with correctional officials and officers and nonmental health clinicians and others involved in disposition and management (e.g., correctional officers).
- Interact with multiple systems in a consultation role.
- Collaborate with various treatment and legal professionals in a variety of forensic and non-forensic settings.
- Utilize the "least restrictive environment" within the above system.

Professional and Ethical Behavior

The practitioner will be able to demonstrate an adequate understanding of expectations for professionalism and ethical behavior in the practice of forensic occupational therapy, including topics such as:

- Codes of ethics that apply to forensic occupational therapy such as the AOTA, CAOT, COT, and WFOT codes of ethics (American Occupational Therapy Association, 2000; Canadian Association of Occupational Therapists, 2007; College of Occupational Therapists, 2001; World Federation of Occupational Therapists, 2004).
- Legal and ethical principles relevant to the treatment and evaluation of individuals.
- Assent and consent to research in forensic subjects, including those in correctional settings.
- Sensitivity to cultural differences that may affect treatment or evaluation.
- Observation and interactions with representatives of the legal system (i.e., parole, correctional, legal representatives, etc.).

Special Considerations for Tools and Materials

A pressing concern for anyone working in a criminal justice setting is the safety and security of offenders, staff, visitors, and self. As such it is a primary responsibility for the occupational therapist to be fully apprised of the system's policies, procedures, and practices and be especially attentive to the unique safety risks and concerns related to OT interventions. Being alert to security levels in various units, locks, alarms, alerts, emergency plans, and video monitoring is vital to facility integrity and personal safety.

Therapists must be highly observant and vigilant for safety protocols within the OT area especially when tools and materials are available to offenders that could be used as weapons or used to craft weapons. Consistent communication with other staff about the status of offenders, especially those with more unpredictable behavior or history of impulsive acts, will help assure that safe and proper levels of occupational challenge are provided. The therapeutic goal is to encourage the offender to gain a sense of mastery and self-control in a safe and secure context.

For therapists with the benefit of treatment opportunities in areas such as a wood shop or kitchen, special care must be taken to assure constant monitoring of tools and utensils and to have a system in place to alert staff in case items are missing following an intervention session. Therapists must strictly adhere to safe handling practices, infection control techniques, and universal precautions in the case of blood or body fluid exposure should the need arise. See Figure 21-2 for a sample policy and procedure for tool safety and security.

For occupational therapy in high security areas, tool, utensil, or adhesive (to prevent inhalation of intoxicants) use may not be allowed and the therapist will need creativity and adaptability to employ appropriately challenging activities. By making this type of adaptation explicit, one can provide therapeutic modeling for program participants to develop adaptive skill and strategies, as well as provide opportunities for creativity and independent problem solving by the participants. In lower security settings in which tool use is allowed, strict check-out and monitoring systems must be in place and employed to assure safe use of the department and security within the facility.

GENERAL

- The OT tool room will be locked at all times and out of bounds to all inmates unless under the direct supervision of staff.
- All OT tools will be painted using assigned department color code and engraved "OT Clinic" to denote origin.
- Periodic, unscheduled searches of the entire OT clinic will be made for safety and security.

TOOL ACCOUNTABILITY

- Tools are stored in locked rooms, secured inside cabinets and on shadow boards.
- Each morning tools are inventoried.
- Tools are accounted for at the end of each group before inmates are released to their housing areas. No one is allowed to leave until all tools are accounted for.
- All inmates will be given a clothed body search for contraband before leaving the OT clinic.

USE OF TOOLS

- Inmates and OT staff are assigned a number with five corresponding numbered tags for checking out tools. For each tool used by an individual, one tag assigned to that person is placed where the tool is stored. No one will be allowed to use more than five tools at a time.
- Large floor power tools will only be used under the direct supervision of an OTR.

FIGURE 21-2. Policy and Procedures for Tool Safety and Security in a Prison-Based Occupational Therapy Clinic

People who have been incarcerated for several years may be released into a world of technology that is unfamiliar to them. Therefore it is incumbent upon the therapist to prepare the offender for the types of technology he or she is likely to encounter and help them understand its use. For example, when facilities exist and security access allows, training classes using distance learning strategies and tools, as well as other multimedia applications can familiarize offenders with common learning and employment technologies (Inciardi et al., 2007). Exploring options for accessing computers through public libraries or taking courses through community colleges can provide a way to practice newly learned skills. Directing offenders to affordable cellular phones and calling plans can provide the all-important callback phone number for potential employers and parole-related appointments.

SEXUALITY IN FORENSIC AND CORRECTIONAL SETTINGS

Sexuality is a fundamental aspect of humanity and as such has a profound influence on many aspects of occupational behavior and performance such as occupational roles, routines, social interaction, choice, and identity. The profession recognizes the critical role that sexual expression and activity play in people's daily lives and identifies sexual activity as an essential activity of daily living to be addressed in assessment and intervention across practice settings (AOTA, 2008a). The expression of one's sexuality within corrections is highly problematic due to restrictions and regulations, lack of privacy, gender-segregation, limited occupational options, and power and control issues among others. For example, in the Oklahoma Department of Corrections, all sexual contact is illegal, with the goal of protecting offenders, however, this policy resulted in a woman being sent back to prison for becoming pregnant while on probation and living in a halfway house. A relative paucity of quality studies of sexuality, sexual behavior, and sexual violence in corrections further limits the knowledge and understanding of this critical aspect of one's humanity and daily functioning (Hensley & Tewksberry, 2002; Jones & Prat, 2008) that could otherwise support occupational therapist's role and intervention. There is a need and opportunity for occupational therapists to initiate research related to sexuality in corrections to promote an understanding of the complex interaction of sexuality with occupational performance (e.g., how sexuality influences social participation, substance use and abuse, and related health behaviors).

Correctional systems, with the exception of conjugal visitation rights (usually reserved for married offenders), typically segregate offenders by gender, usually having male and female facilities geographically far apart. Except for guards and staff, offenders may go long periods without even seeing a member of the opposite sex, significantly affecting identity and social relations (Jones & Schmid, 2000). In this highly restrictive environment, sex and sexuality become distorted and used as a means of power, control, economy (e.g., sexual favors), and yet in some cases may lead to opportunities for positive affiliation and companionship that may be unrelated to one's prior sexual orientation (Hensley & Tewksberry, 2002). These positive relationships are more likely to evolve in women's correctional facilities through the creation of pairings or larger affiliations called pseudo families (groups of women who assume various family roles to fulfill needs of intimacy, affiliation, and security) (Zaitow & Thomas, 2003). However, even when sexual relationships in correctional facilities are consensual, expression of one's sexuality and sexual activity are highly constrained by constant visual and video monitoring, bed-checks, and overcrowding.

In attempting to prevent the expression of an incarcerated offender's sexuality as in the previous example from the Oklahoma Department of Corrections, a severe form of occupational deprivation can emerge in jails and prisons, which, with additional education and training, occupational therapists can effectively address. Understanding the larger context and implications of sexual expression and activity, the occupational therapist can apply models such as the Ex-PLISSIT model (Taylor & Davis, 2007), an extension of Annon's (1976) work, to support system change and healthy sexuality. The Ex-PLISSIT model provides guidelines for supporting the level of intervention by the therapist or other staff members that is appropriate to the staff member's corresponding level of knowledge and qualification. The therapist can then work at the system level to advocate for more humane treatment of offenders, and at the individual and group level to help offenders understand the implications of this chronic deprivation and develop strategies for healthy sexual expression.

Occupational therapy intervention related to sexuality should begin with a sexual history. A range of sexual histories and guidelines for applying them can be found (Association of Reproductive Health Professionals, 2002; Bartlik, Rosenfeld, & Beaton, 2005) that are designed to be used with different populations (e.g., children, adolescents, sex offenders, those who have experienced sexual abuse). All occupational therapists have the foundational education and skills to conduct a sexual history, but advanced education and training are highly recommended for therapists seeking or needing to address sexuality at more than the permission level (Annon, 1976; Taylor & Davis, 2007) to ensure quality outcomes.

Sex offenders, those incarcerated for committing rape or other sex crimes, present a special challenge for OT intervention and may often be found in correctional or mental health forensic settings. The occupational therapist needs special education and preparation to be most effective in these settings. The challenge comes in effectively balancing the sex offender's right to sexual expression and relationships with the simultaneous development of internal controls and development of healthy social and sexual behaviors. Geffner's (2004) text provides a comprehensive review of challenges, interventions, and strategies in working with a sex offender population.

Sexual coercion in correctional facilities is an ongoing concern for all involved. There are wide variations in reports of the incidence of sexual coercion from as little as 3% to as much as 45% related to variations in setting, data collection methodology, and reliability of the reporting method (Hensley & Tewksberry, 2002; Jones & Prat,

2008). A consistent feature of the results of these studies for incarcerated offenders is that over 50% of coerced sexual acts are committed by correctional staff (Beck & Harrison, 2007). Sexual coercion is often used as a means of control, demonstration of power over another individual, or both. People who have experienced sexual abuse prior to incarceration are especially vulnerable to the negative effects of sexual coercion. Blackburn, Mullings, and Marquart (2008) found in a study of over 400 incarcerated women that 68% had experienced sexual abuse prior to their prison sentence, while 17% experienced some type of sexual victimization while incarcerated. Pre-incarceration sexual abuse rates are also much higher for men than their non-incarcerated counterparts (Beck & Harrison, 2007; Hensley & Tewksberry, 2002). Although it is ideal for the occupational therapist to have advanced knowledge or certification in dealing with sexuality and the concerns unique to correctional settings, it is crucial to know which professionals within the system are well prepared to intervene so that the occupational therapist can be supportive of offenders needing advanced intervention through referral. The occupational therapist also needs to have a good foundation of understanding human sexuality and the range of sexual expression and sexual orientation in order to provide nonjudgmental and supportive services. The OT role in community transition of offenders, especially those who are leaving long-term incarceration, needs to focus on education and development of strategies for healthy expression of sexuality to support successful transition and social participation.

OCCUPATIONAL THERAPY INTERVENTIONS IN CRIMINAL JUSTICE AND EVIDENCE FOR PRACTICE

As the call for increased intervention and research in correctional institutions goes out, there is little infrastructure to support coordination efforts between levels of incarceration within countries and internationally. With growing international collaborations among occupational therapists, opportunities arise to build such coordinating structures for positive models of intervention and research in criminal justice systems. We present an overview of a representative sample of the published work to date.

Concerns about both intervention strategies and evidence for practice abound in the literature. The concerns are primarily related to the lack of coordination of services within countries and internationally and the widely varying access to services. The most frequent discussions and publications of occupational therapy in criminal justice settings come from the countries of Britain, Australia, and Canada. Duncan, Munro, and Nicol (2003) and O'Connell and Farnworth (2007) called for coordinated, multicentered, and international efforts to both decrease the isolated nature of intervention and improve research methods to systematically study the efficacy of intervention. O'Connell and Farnworth conducted a critique of the literature and found little evidence for the support of occupational therapy interventions in correctional settings, citing poor methodology and lack of current evidence as major challenges. Duncan et al. conducted a survey of therapists practicing in forensic settings and identified research priorities including development of appropriate outcome measures, developing rigorous and effective group-work programs, and use of effective risk assessment tools. Much remains to be done and their urging to both coordinate efforts and study the effects of intervention continues to be appropriate.

Therapists who provide intervention in correctional settings have only recently begun efforts to find one another and join forces. In 2002, the College of Occupational Therapists in the United Kingdom developed a strategic plan for forensic occupational therapy that may serve as a guide to other countries to coordinate efforts to both implement and study assessment and intervention (College of Occupational Therapists, 2002). An international group of researchers has begun an informal collaboration network, one outcome of which was a publication describing the application of occupational science and occupational justice to occupational therapy in corrections and associated research studies (Muñoz et al., 2011). An online network for forensic occupational therapy, based in the United Kingdom but with a growing international membership, has been operating since 2003. Through this network group clinicians, researchers, and students exchange advice, information, and resources; discuss and define the role of occupational therapy; and generate ideas for service development (Brown et al., 2010). Additionally, a program of research for occupation and mental health in forensic and prison settings was established in 2010 as a priority at the Research Centre for Occupation and Mental Health at York St. John University, UK (Grass & Farnworth, 2010).

As demonstrated in Table 21-5, there are few published studies to support occupational therapy intervention in correctional settings. Thus no clear decisions can be made based on the current evidence. This stems from the inherent challenges of the heterogeneity of the studies and offenders (including those who are in prison in specialized forensic units, jail, and community corrections) and the lack of similar outcome measures, small number of participants, and descriptive level of most of the evidence.

One of the benefits of the current evidence is the frequent use of assessment tools that include both qualitative and quantitative aspects (COPM, OPHI-II, OSA) and interventions that are occupation-based (work, education, leisure, use of ADL and IADL, social participation) and client-centered to facilitate an individualized approach to intervention.

Occupational Therapy Interventions in Criminal Justice Settings

Table 21-5 has been developed using guidelines as suggested by American Occupational Therapy Association and evidence-based medicine (AOTA, 2008b; OCEBM Table of Evidence Working Group, 2011; Sackett, Straus, Richardson, Rosenberg, & Haynes, 2000). The table provides a starting point for understanding the evidence related to occupational therapy services in the range of criminal justice settings. The reader is encouraged to seek the most recent research as the literature in the field is continually evolving. Information in the table may provide useful key search terms and lines of inquiry for new investigations.

TABLE 21-5. Evidence Related to Occupational Therapy in Criminal Justice

Intervention Purpose, Setting, and (Study Location)	Description of Intervention	Number of Participants	Amount of Intervention (Dosage)	Type of Best Evidence and Level of Evidence	Benefit to Evidence Base	Statistical Probability and Effect Size of Outcome
Description of Canadian Model of Occupational Performance (CMOP) for assessment and intervention within the context of a rehabilitation forensic hostel (Clarke, 2003). (United Kingdom)	Application of the CMOP within a context of an individualized treatment plan working on self-care, social skills, engagement in work, education, and leisure.	Residents of an intensive rehabilitation program for offenders detained in a secure forensic unit, nearing discharge.	None defined, individual for each participant.	Expert opinion.	Defined use of Canadian Occupational Performance Measure as an assessment tool and CMOP as an intervention strategy. Includes emphasis on the environment.	Not applicable.
A description of a pilot program that uses a work-based learning program within a forensic learning disability service (Smith, Petty, Oughton, & Alexander, 2010). (United Kingdom)	Pilot study, opinions of participants, and interdisciplinary team were gathered following a workplace program. Participants cleaned, refurbished, and packed equipment for shipping to hospitals, laboratories and schools in developing countries. Individualized programs were set for each participant allowing work at different skill levels. Group leaders and participants/offenders	Group participants (n = 4) were within a forensic setting for those individuals with learning disabilities. No further demographic data was provided.	Initially 1 day per week, expanding to 2 days per week. The program had been running for 45 weeks at publication date. Program was expanded to include other individuals.	Case series.	Group leaders identified benefits in social, work, literacy, and numeracy skills. Participants identified improvement in personal, work-based, mathematical, and language skills.	Not applicable.

were interviewed regarding their opinion of the program.					
Descriptive study of a community reintegration program for those incarcerated in a county jail setting (Eggers, Muñoz, Sciulli, & Crist, 2006). (United States)	The overall goal of the program is to reduce the recidivism rate by addressing the following areas: wellness, family, and support structure; skills for living; education; and employment. Individuals set goals and are successful if they meet those goals. Offenders who have 90–190 days prior to release are admitted into the program. Occupational therapy is embedded in all phases: intake, prerelease, and postrelease treatment. Occupational therapy includes: self-awareness, goal-setting, personal development, social skills, communication, and job readiness. Participant is monitored postrelease for progress toward goals.	The male inmates (n=83) within 190 days of release participated in the 8–10 week program.	Occupational therapist presents programming for 2 hours, 3 times per week for 20–40 contact hours.	Program evaluation.	Success will be measured by recidivism rates, employment rates, and improved satisfaction scores through the Occupational Self Assessment (OSA). (Baron, Kielhofner, Iyenger, Goldhammer, & Wolenski, 2006). While an 11-month review indicates success in these areas, no definitive conclusions can yet be drawn.

(Continues)

TABLE 21-5. Continued

Intervention Purpose, Setting, and (Study Location)	Description of Intervention	Number of Participants	Amount of Intervention (Dosage)	Type of Best Evidence and Level of Evidence	Benefit to Evidence Base	Statistical Probability and Effect Size of Outcome
Description of the time use of offenders in a secure forensic psychiatric facility (Farnworth, Nikitin, & Fossey, 2004). (Australia)	Participants were engaged in their typical daily routines; no intervention was provided.	Participants (n = 8) completed time diaries, and interviews (n = 5). Field notes were taken over 5 weeks, including 160 observational hours. Men ages 24–48 years. Resided at the facility for 2–24 months. All had a diagnosis of mental illness.	Not applicable.	Qualitative synthesis, case histories.	Illuminates the way inmates viewed time constructs and provides evidence for the importance of understanding occupational narratives to engage participants in a program of rehabilitation. Use of OPHI-II (Kielhofner et al., 2004).	Not applicable.
Literature and theoretical review of the application of occupational justice concepts to intervention with individuals who have been incarcerated and have a mental illness (Muñoz & Farnworth, 2009). (Australia and United States)	Information on the studies considered was located through a database search that included MEDLINE, PsychINFO, CINAHL, OTDBase, and ProQuest.	Not applicable.	Not applicable.	Expert opinion; review of literature.	Encourages the investigation of assessment tools to evaluate outcomes, and the design of intervention that utilizes occupational engagement, habits, and occupational enrichment while demonstrating effectiveness is	Not applicable.

Explored the use of a single modality—videogames with a secure forensic setting to promote leisure exploration and mastery of the environment (Gooch & Living, 2004). (United Kingdom)	Literature was reviewed related to: use of videogaming as a leisure pursuit and active leisure, limitations for exploration of mastery and coping skills in forensic settings, normalizing occupation, and "flow." No specific intervention was presented.	Not applicable, no data were collected.	Not applicable.	Expert opinion and literature review on a use of videogames as a modality in a forensic facility.	potential for a specific modality to improve productive leisure pursuits. Not applicable.
A comparison of treatment approaches for individuals with schizophrenia in a forensic hospital (Schindler, 2004a). (United States)	Investigated the effectiveness of Role Development as a guideline for practice with individuals with schizophrenia in a forensic unit. Treatment is individualized in the experimental group. Assessments were done initially, then at 4, 8, and 12 weeks. Role development intervention included a client-centered and occupation-based approach. All participants engaged in 4 hours/day of intervention; the experimental group received additional focused attention and guidance on role development.	Males (n = 84) ages 18–55 years of age, with a diagnosis of schizophrenia, with stays of a minimum of 30 days. Three groups, experimental (n = 42) and two comparison groups (n = 42 total) were conducted. Participants in the experimental group showed significant changes in scores on tasks, interpersonal skills, and social roles compared to comparison groups.	Participants received between 80 hours (at 4 weeks) and 160 hours (at 8 weeks) or 240 hours (at 12 weeks) of intervention.	Cohort Study.	Program description of the Role Development Program that addresses the development of social roles and skills that support those roles. Detailed description of the intervention, and data collection. Outcome measures included Role Functioning Scale, The Role Checklist, The Skills Scale, Interpersonal Skills Scale (Dickerson, 2008; Goodman, Sewell, Cooley, & Leavitt, 1993; Schindler, 2004b).

(Continues)

TABLE 21-5. Continued

Intervention Purpose, Setting, and (Study Location)	Description of Intervention	Number of Participants	Amount of Intervention (Dosage)	Type of Best Evidence and Level of Evidence	Benefit to Evidence Base	Statistical Probability and Effect Size of Outcome
A descriptive study of an interdisciplinary program designed to prevent substance abuse and included topics of etiology and progression and recovery of substance abuse, examination of volition, habits, routines, and leisure and vocation exploration (Tayar, 2004). (United States)	No effectiveness of the program on the offenders was measured. Students rated participation as valuable. Program is based on substance abuse programs. Each session had 10 participants but it was not the same 10 individuals each session.	Women (n = 10) in a short-term (120 days) prison setting, adults (no specification of ages given). Women resided in grouped housing.	8–12 contact hours total.	Expert opinion; case report synthesis.	Program description included descriptions of each session.	Not applicable.
Occupational therapists' perspectives of intervention needs of women incarcerated in medium security prisons (Baker & McKay, 2001). (United Kingdom)	Questionnaires were mailed to occupational therapists that are currently working with women in prison settings. The questionnaire targeted ADL, IADL, and social participation needs.	Occupational therapists (n = 45) completed the survey, with a 73% return rate.	Not applicable.	Descriptive survey study.	Allows affirmation of the needs of women who are inmates from therapists who are currently working with this population. Emphasizes need to tailor intervention specifically for population and	Not applicable.

			strive to include meaningful occupation.	Not applicable.
Explored the use of a client-centered approach in a forensic environment. (Morrow, 2008). (United Kingdom)	Observations of offenders while they engaged in 1 of 3 tasks in a secure forensic unit. Staff were also observed and completed a questionnaire.	Male offenders (n = 10) were observed. Staff (n =4) were also observed and asked to complete a questionnaire. Offenders had a variety of skill levels and mental illnesses.	Not clearly defined.	Case report.	A five-point list including; client able to evaluate work, choose goals, control learning, use the staff as facilitator and accept responsibility. Evidence for using a client-centered humanistic approach.
Descriptive pilot data on inmates' perceptions of occupational engagement in a jail program (Crist et al., 2005). (United States)	Jail inmates were invited to participate in community living skills within 6 months of their anticipated release date to support community reintegration and prevention of recidivism. As part of the participation an occupational therapist administered the OSA and those self-reports are reported (Crist et al., 2005).	Offenders (n = 67, males (n = 61) and females (n = 6). Detailed demographic data provided.	Not applicable.	Descriptive Study of self-reported perceptions.	Provides support to include environmental supports needed to maintain community living vs. skill development when developing interventions. Provided detailed demographic data. The OSA version 2.0 (Baron et al., 2006) was used to collect the data. Not applicable.

Employment Assessment and Intervention

Employment remains the most critical link to an ex-offender's successful reentry into the community (Kethineni & Falcone, 2007; Maruna, 2001). In the prisons in Chile, occupational therapists focus their efforts with prisoners on work activity. This is based on the belief that work enhances personal development, identifies and strengthens individual capabilities and potentials, personal identity, and self-esteem. Work also supports internalization of social habits that are not related to crime while promoting positive family and interpersonal relationships, initiative and creativity, skill development, and provision for one's self and one's family (Ramirez & Gonzales, 2011). This type of intervention takes various forms, as appropriate for the prisoner's skill level and security risk:

1. Dependent work—work done within the prison environment that can be understood as formal jobs provided by prison administration.

2. Independent work—work that is understood as self-employment, characterized by the manufacturing of products for sale.

3. Treatment communities—therapeutic work done in areas of the prison with lower levels of security where the approach is more on behavioral regulation and generation of habits and routines in a free environment that are pro-social.

For those at the community corrections level, finding and maintaining employment is a critical initial focus. A regular work schedule not only adds a vital societal role but also provides the structure around which all other ADL, such as sleep and personal hygiene, and IADL, such as meal preparation and community mobility, revolve. Some ex-offenders return to previous employment and others may need to fulfill requirements to reapply for suspended or revoked driver's licenses. Some, unable to return to previous employment due to their crimes, must explore new jobs and perhaps careers. Several assessments explore job interests and aptitude, including Holland's Self-Directed Search® (SDS-R) (2011) that yields personal codes used to search occupational job titles and leisure activities. Those who are initially desisting from criminal activities begin employment exploration and acquisition at the entry level. (See Chapter 23, "Vocational Programming" for more information on vocational activities in mental health settings.)

In transitional work and housing settings, such as a halfway house, obtaining employment is the key to success (Muñoz et al., 2011), and provides an excellent opportunity to implement the occupation-based self-determination (OBSD) model using the steps of Plan, Act, and Evaluate. For those unfamiliar with the job search process, the occupational therapist may begin with assessment and intervention directed to a job search of classified employment announcements. For offenders with poor to no work history, job coaching is often a successful strategy for the occupational therapist to support successful community transition. Some offenders at the community corrections level have access to computers and the Internet and those who do not use the local newspaper want ads. Table 21-6 is a brief activity analysis of using newspaper classified advertisements to assess job acquisition and cognitive skills.

TABLE 21-6. Activity Analysis for Early Steps of a Job Search

Steps in Searching Want Ads	Employment Search–Related Skills	Cognitive Skills
Searching for jobs one is qualified to do.	Using heading to find employment ads and subheadings for types of jobs. Awareness of educational levels needed for particular jobs.	Abstraction. Association and categorization. General work knowledge.
Obtaining name of company, address, and telephone number associate with a particular job.	Problem solving how to obtain missing information.	Problem solving.
Using available resources to access information.	Using telephone directory sections and guidewords to find company information. Awareness of educational levels needed for particular jobs.	Abstraction. Association and categorization.
Organizing and maintaining a list of jobs, calls, and results.	Creating and maintaining information for future reference.	Organizational skills.
Creating and practicing a script for an initial call.	Awareness of qualities the employer is seeking. Awareness of strengths and advantages of employing an offender. Self-awareness.	Self-awareness. Organizational skills.
Calling a potential employer to inquire about the position.	Awareness of qualities the employer is seeking. Self-awareness.	Receptive and expressive communication skills. Self-awareness. Memory.
Reflecting on response.	Awareness of qualities the employer is seeking. Self-awareness.	Experiential learning. Self-awareness.

The occupational therapist also assists with job acquisition activities such as completing applications, practicing responses to interview questions, and preparing grooming, dressing, and transportation routines for job interviews. In the United States, most job applications include questions about being felony charges or convictions. The generally accepted advice is to leave the "yes" or "no" boxes unchecked and to write in "will discuss at interview" so the employer can establish rapport and decide if the applicant is qualified for the job before dealing with the issue. Many applicants find it difficult to "sell" themselves by offering employers advantages of employing offenders. Those without work experience outside prison generally list prison jobs using general employment job titles. For example, an orderly position in prison generally equates to janitorial work. American employers appreciate applicants who can knowledgeably offer resources on the Work Opportunity Tax Credit program in which employers who hire ex-offenders and those in other target groups who face barriers to employment can earn tax credits (United States Department of Labor, 2010).

The quotes found in Figure 21-3 are examples of responses that employment-seeking offenders can use in interviews that cast their prison experience in a positive light and help prevent the offender from having to falsify the job application that asks about past felony convictions or incarceration.

PRISONIZATION AND ERRORS IN CRITICAL THINKING

Because correctional institutions must maintain order and safety, inmates lose rights that are often taken for granted. As occupational beings, humans require occupation for quality of life. Incarceration is a form of occupational deprivation, the lack of necessary, temporal, and meaningful occupation due to prolonged external circumstances that result in detrimental effects on health, well-being, and adaptation (Hooper, 2005; Molineux & Whiteford, 1999; Whiteford, 1997, 2000; Wilcock, 1998b). Offenders sacrifice choice, freedom, security, privacy, activity, social stimulation, structure, support, and emotional feedback while incarcerated (Molineux & Whiteford, 1999). In order to cope with incarceration, offenders adapt to the context and its inherent deprivations. The term for internalization of adaptive responses to incarceration is **prisonization**, in which the offender gradually adopts the norms of institutional life into habits, cognition, emotions, and actions (Haney, 2002). For example, fearful that others will use personal information to harm them, offenders typically do not share details of their offense or their life prior to incarceration with other offenders. Although in this sense, prisonization is a positive adaptation to prison life, the process ultimately undermines all reentry occupations (Hooper, 2005).

Three major aspects of occupational deprivation occur in correctional settings. Reasoning with the Occupational Adaptation model, occupational challenges evoke an adaptive response that can result in adaptation or mastery of the challenge or dysadaptation (Schkade & McClung, 2001). Adapting to a correctional context ideally helps an offender retain some quality of life during incarceration. However, remaining stuck or

"If I don't come to work and do my job well, I'll go back to jail or prison."
"In prison, I took courses relating to job skills you're seeking."
"One thing I learned in prison is how to get along with everyone."
"You earn a federal tax credit by employing me not more than one year after my release date."
"I learned a variety of jobs in prison and did them well."
"I offer more experience than most applicants for an entry-level position."

FIGURE 21-3. Examples of Advantages of Employing Offenders

hyperstabilized in that adaptive response during reentry into the community eventually undermines success, causes additional occupational challenges, and may lead to recidivism. Awareness of and attention to the adaptive consequences of occupational deprivation are critical to the occupational therapist's success in all forensic settings.

One of the obvious challenges of incarceration is forced powerlessness, the punitive intent of which is to restrict the offender's ability to engage in favored occupations. At a superficial level, imagine watching television and not being able to fulfill the desire to purchase and enjoy advertised goods and services. At a deeper level, institutional control of meals, rest, sleep, self-care, leisure, education, work, sexual activity, and expressions of spirituality strips privacy and choice. Offenders often note that they are told "when to eat, what to eat, when to sleep, when to wake up, and when to go to the bathroom." Two major outcomes frequently occur: The loss of ability to make decisions and choices arises from not having decisions and choices to make.

Lack of opportunity combined with reliance on institutional schedules diminishes the capacity to decide and choose. At reentry, the offender may make poor decisions, struggle with the loss of structure, and have difficulty establishing routines and schedules. The second major outcome of forced powerlessness is the erosion of self-worth. Some offenders may feel as if they deserve the humiliations of incarceration and at reentry, expect to experience degraded employment, housing, and relationships. Insidiously, forced powerlessness may mute self-initiative, independence, and self-advocacy, skills vital to adapt to community life. On reentry, this loss shows up as inability to establish realistic healthy occupational routines such as meal and bed times or sequential occupations such as laundry or cooking (Molineux & Whiteford, 1999; Whiteford, 2000).

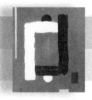

CASE ILLUSTRATION

Derek—Complete Prisonization Brings Derek Back "Inside"

Derek, a 34-year-old man with a 15-year history of depression and anxiety, had been incarcerated in federal prison for 3½ years for armed robbery. He had spent the majority of his adult life in and out of jail and this was his first federal sentence. Derek had adjusted well to the structure and routine of prison life. After serving two thirds of his sentence in maximum security, Derek was released on parole and residency at a halfway house in his home community, 275 miles from the prison. There were staff shortages at the halfway house and local community mental health services denied him service based on his criminal history. Three weeks after his release from the halfway house, Derek arrived at the front gate of the prison asking to be let back in. He reported to prison staff that he felt "lost" at the halfway house and uncertain of what to do with himself each day. He felt like he "didn't belong" there and was unable to cope, both with the everyday requirements for taking care of himself and making personal choices and with the lack of demands or expectations on him and how he used his time each day. He saw the structure and routine of prison life as being more desirable than the "freedom" of community life. Enroute to the prison, Derek traveled outside the designated area of his parole and therefore violated the conditions of his release. His parole was revoked and he was returned to prison based on this parole violation.

Discussion

There are several important occupational elements to Derek's story. First is the highly structured prison environment that determined all of Derek's occupations, preventing skill development or maintenance and the exercise of personal choice. Second is the occupational deprivation in his community life, resulting from both the paucity of occupational opportunities at the halfway house as well as the reluctance of local mental health services to work with him. The third is the response of the criminal justice system to Derek's experience and concerns. The lack of meaningful occupational engagement to prepare and assist Derek in reentering community life severely impeded his ability to establish adaptive occupational performance that would allow him to break free of the criminal justice system. Derek is experiencing occupational alienation in that his life and occupational performance has become so limited and regimented by imprisonment that he is unable to successfully cope with the choices available to him on the outside. Returning Derek to correctional custody, rather than addressing the shortcomings of services for offenders transitioning from prison to community living, reinforced his prisonization and perpetuated the cycle of occupational injustice and recidivism. Consider how the concepts related to habituation (from MOHO) and those of hyperstability and dysadaptation (from Occupational Adaptation) apply to Derek's situation.

A second challenge of incarceration is living with strict rules under continuous surveillance that results in quick and sometimes severe punishment for infractions. For some offenders, dysfunctional family backgrounds in childhood or as adults may have been similarly rule-bound, punitive, or violent. One consequence of a life governed by rules and punishment is dependency upon them, without the opportunity to develop internal controls and self-regulation. For some, incarceration reinforces and recapitulates childhood or adult trauma. For others, well-developed skills of internal control and self-regulation may atrophy during incarceration. Only at reentry may an offender's hidden internalized disorganization, distress, and fear emerge as the inability to perform occupations independently and adapt to unstructured environments and unexpected events. Many female ex-offenders express that going to the mall or a large store such as Wal-Mart was one of their greatest fears upon reentry in the community. A second consequence of a rule-bound life is that once rules and surveillance are withdrawn there are no rules at all. As a result, offenders may engage in self-destructive acts or relapse in their recovery from chronic illness, mental disorder, substance abuse, or co-occurring disorders. During her reentry, one woman analyzed that the size of the store, the display of its products, and the ease of departure as parameters affected her response. On her own, she graded her participation by attending a small county fair before the state fair and shopped in small grocery stores before progressing to supermarkets and Wal-Mart. At the time, she had not yet ventured to a mall.

A third challenge of incarceration is the ever-present possibility of personal danger and exploitation. Most offenders naturally develop a hypervigilance for threat and distrust of others. Although some limit this attitude to a select few, such as those they feel are responsible for their incarceration, or correctional officers, others extend their suspiciousness to cellmates, friends, and family. Many offenders express that they do not self-disclose or open up to others because it "can and will be used against" them, much as the Miranda rights statements frequently made during apprehension into the criminal justice system. What was once a "game face" becomes a "prison mask," a tough outer veneer of emotional overregulation and self-imposed social withdrawal. Suspicion and distrust lead to social isolation and lack of social participation. Although some isolate themselves by remaining in their cells or housing units or by seeking additional work, others may act out in expectation of placement in solitary housing units. On reentry, this social alienation appears as a diminished capacity for social participation and relationships at a crucial time for reintegration into family, friendships, and society (Haney, 2002; Harm & Phillips, 2001; Molineux & Whiteford, 1999; Travis, Soloman, & Waul, 2001; Visher, LaVigne, & Travis , 2004; Whiteford, 1997).

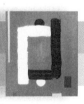

CASE ILLUSTRATION

Jean—Imprisoned by Anxiety

A woman who had developed panic attacks and agoraphobia while awaiting sentencing transferred from a large federal medical correctional center to a community halfway house in her home state. While incarcerated, she volunteered to work extra hours, admitting it to be a ploy to avoid leisure time that might require social participation. She continued to isolate herself completely in the cozier dorm-like setting of the halfway house, even eating meals alone.

Although she reportedly longed for companionship, her severe anxiety prevented her from making contact with the other women. Using a CBT approach, she practiced relaxation techniques and agreed to participate ("although terrified") in a social scavenger hunt at the request of the occupational therapist. Armed with her assignment, her task was to approach and ask women to sign her form that included items such as "Has the same number of grandchildren" or "Reads romance novels" that focused on common interests. This breakthrough intervention led to the rapid establishment of several friendships.

Discussion

Jean's story illustrates the consequences of untreated anxiety at several points in her criminal justice history. The lengthy period between the plea and sentencing phases led to occupational problems with employment and IADL, virtually imprisoning her at home, a kind of self-imposed house arrest. Once incarcerated, her anxiety exacerbated the real possibility of threat and harm and led her to use employment to avoid social participation, a self-imposed workaholism. Her social isolation became apparent at the community corrections level and the assigned CBT homework helped her break through the anxiety that kept her socially isolated and imprisoned.

A focus on particular occupational challenges of reentry and the use of the COPM to prioritize them allows the ex-offender and occupational therapist to concentrate collaboratively on the individual's most vexing challenges of reentry. Either grading exposure to challenges as in the example above or jointly addressing the most challenging issue by preparing and then accomplishing the occupation together spotlights the process of generating, evaluating, enacting, and integrating an adaption. Through postexperience analysis and application of the integration subprocess to the next most demanding occupational challenge, the ex-offender not only achieves critical reentry tasks but also adapts. Application of the Occupational Adaptation model simultaneously enhances occupational performance and occupational adaptation (Schkade & McClung, 2001).

CRIMINAL THINKING

Many have speculated on the factors that lead a person to a criminal lifestyle and career. Theories of criminal conduct dating from the 1950s to 1970s implicated factors including moral lapse, atypical response to psychological or environmental distress, a weak superego, the disparity between goals and available means, a lack of bond to the conventional social order, negative labeling, criminal self-identity, association with delinquents and criminals, need for increased levels of sensory stimulation, negative family experiences, and a rational choice of crime concluding that crime pays.

In his theory of the criminal lifestyle of repeat offenders based on his work as a clinical psychologist with the U.S. Bureau of Prisons, Walters (1990) postulated that conditions, choice, and cognition lead to specific criminal acts. He postulated that although conditions limit options, they do not determine the choice to adopt a criminal lifestyle. Walters outlined three conditional or contextual domains: physical (optimal level of sensory stimulation and an external locus of control), social (attachment, empathy, and bonding), and psychological (self-identity and role identity).

Walters theorized that fear is the offender's primary motivational factor, citing responsibility, commitment, intimacy, and failing in conventional pursuits as typical fears. In addition, he delineated four secondary motives for criminal behavior: anger/rebellion, power/control, excitement/pleasure, and greed/laziness. As extensions of normal adolescent thinking, eight distinctive criminal thinking patterns develop from conditions and the choice to engage in criminal acts, and primary and secondary motives. These thinking patterns serve to support and reinforce criminal decisions.

The combination of conditions, choice, motivation, and cognition result in four interrelated behavioral characteristics: irresponsibility, self-indulgence, learned intrusive interpersonal relationships, and chronic violations of norms, rules, and laws that define the criminal lifestyle. Clusters of criminal behavior correspond with pairs of cognitive patterns and motives to explain specific criminal events. Two cognitive patterns, blaming external circumstances (mollification) and elimination of anxiety, fear, and deterrents (through a cutoff phrase, such as "F___ it"), serve to validate motivating factors of anger and rebellion to justify breaking social rules. Two self-imposed personal exemptions to break social rules (entitlement) and intimidate or use "weak" people for personal gain (power orientation) validate the power and control issues that support intrusive interpersonal behavior. Similarly, motives of excitement and pleasure support self-indulgent behavior by presenting oneself as a basically decent person with a "soft" or "good" side (sentimentality) and overconfident superoptimism based on not getting caught for criminal acts. Irresponsibility motivated by greed and laziness is reinforced by thinking patterns of laziness and choice of the path of least resistance (cognitive indolence) and failure to focus and follow through on goals over time (discontinuity). Walters' model is summarized in Figure 21-4.

Walters (1990) concluded that change in criminal lifestyle must be based on changing patterns of thinking. In contrast, some social scientists conclude that distorted thinking and making excuses causes criminal behavior (Maruna & Mann, 2006). Regardless of whether cognitive distortion is viewed as cause or effect, the emphasis on interventions aimed at replacing an offender's cognitive distortions with realistic thinking patterns through use of cognitive behavioral therapy is widely supported in criminal justice interventions (Maruna & Mann, 2006).

The basic model of cognitive-behavioral therapy is that cognition influences emotions and behavior. In particular, one's perception of a situation, not the situation itself, determines thoughts. From experience, people form core beliefs that are global, rigid, and overgeneralized. Core beliefs are so fundamental that we rarely question them but simply accept this is how the world works or how people are. From their core beliefs, people form rules, assumptions, and attitudes apparent through their automatic thoughts. When events trigger situation-specific automatic thoughts, they evoke emotions that lead to behavior. Automatic thoughts

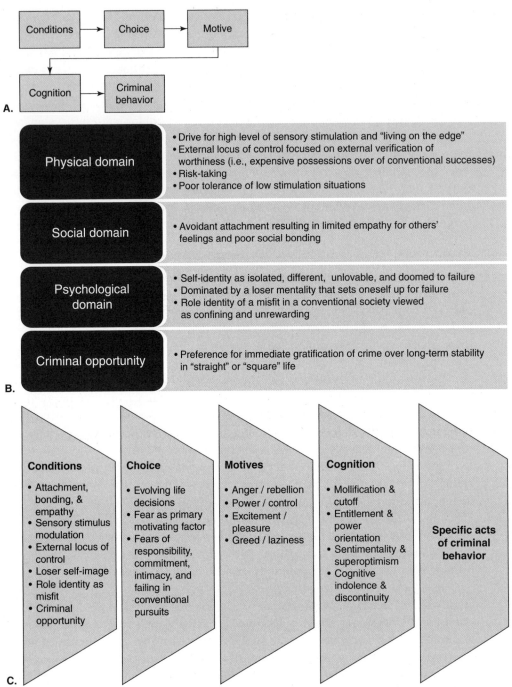

FIGURE 21-4. Graphical Representations. A. Causal Factors of the Criminal Lifestyle.
B. Conditions Associated with Criminal Lifestyle. C. Criminal Lifestyle Theory

Based on Walters, 1990.

may include distortions such as all-or-nothing thinking in which people polarize their thinking in two opposed categories rather than along a continuum as in "I'm either succeeding or failing." Another common distortion is to magnify negative input and minimize positive input. Sometimes people overgeneralize a current situation to form sweeping erroneous conclusions. Although we are generally unaware of our automatic thoughts, practice allows awareness and cognitive change (Beck, 1995) effective in reducing recidivism (MacKenzie, 2000) with people with antisocial personality disorder (Gibbon et al., 2010). However, it is of questionable value with autobiographically focused sexual offender treatment (Waldram, 2008). The reader is encouraged to explore relevant chapters in this text such as those on cognitive-behavioral therapy (see Chapter 5, "Psychological Theories and Their Treatment Methods in Mental Health Practice") and substance abuse (see Chapter 24, "Substance Abuse and Occupational Therapy").

Occupational therapists use cognitive behavioral therapy in correctional settings with individuals and psychoeducational groups to explore healthy thinking patterns, improve problem-solving, assertive communication, goal setting, social skills training, self-calming techniques, relapse prevention, and the management of anger, symptoms, and stress (Kelly, 2003). Frequently, individuals with depression and anxiety initially benefit from individual behavioral intervention, such as structured checklists and schedules, before exploring cognitive distortions or group intervention (Beck, 1995). Most occupational therapists require additional education to use the highly structured format of cognitive behavioral therapy. See Kelly for detailed group interventions, questioning methods, and resources for occupational therapy groups in criminal justice settings.

Other intervention methods in criminal justice focus on the offender's "taking responsibility" for past wrong doing as evidence of desistence and avoidance of recidivism. Shaming offenders is another principal theory in corrections aimed at making offenders assume responsibility for their crimes through "reintegrative" or punitive rituals of confession. Though widely practiced, little evidence to date supports practices aimed at internalizing responsibility for crimes (Maruna, 2001). A more therapeutic application of *post hoc* excuses is the exploring of excuses to shift intervention toward prevention. For example, an offender who offers the excuse of "being stressed" may benefit from intervention directed to improving coping skills (Maruna & Mann, 2006).

CRIME AS OCCUPATION: STAGES OF THE CRIMINAL CAREER

Walters (1990) used data to describe crime as a young man's occupation based on fear as the primary organizing motive. Though Walters used the term *occupation* more in the sense of vocation or job, the use of the term here can carry both connotations, that of job and that of occupation as a meaningful and purposeful occupation. He proposed four stages of the criminal career over which the secondary motivational factors vary.

From ages 10 to 18 years, excitement/pleasure motivates the precriminal stage. Juveniles tend to commit numerous low-level nonspecialized nuisance crimes or misdemeanors. Thrill-seeking and the desire for status, peer acceptance, and money for nonessentials motivate crimes such as auto theft to go joyriding, which is rarely seen at later stages. Thrill-seeking behaviors may be related to sensory processing issues of special interest to occupational therapists (Dunn, 2001). As the most densely populated stage, intervention at this point holds the greatest prospect for change and many opt out of a criminal lifestyle on their own.

From ages 18 through the mid-20s, the early criminal stage marks the choice to adopt a criminal lifestyle. Motivated by power/control and excitement/pleasure, this stage is further fueled by increased contact with lifestyle criminals. Although the number of crimes decrease, the severity of crimes increase and attrition occurs through death and serious injury.

Spanning the mid-20s to the early 40s, the advanced criminal stage is made up of individuals committed to a criminal lifestyle. The attrition rate is low. The loser's mentality and fear are at their peak and criminals in this stage feel and act "out of control." Therefore, gaining power or control of others predominates and individuals can be highly dangerous to self and others.

By the mid-40s, offenders reach the burn out stage, during which many opt out of the criminal lifestyle. Motivated almost equally by fear, anger/rebellion, and greed/laziness, crimes at this stage require less physicality and typically involve gambling, property crimes, and confidence games. The normal introspective turn of one's 50s influence a growing awareness that crime does not pay and fosters a new fear of growing old and dying in prison. A criminal career that began at age 11 by stealing and reselling bicycles had supported a man's criminal and violent lifestyle that resulted in partial blindness. Against his wishes, he transferred to a halfway house from prison in his 50s determined to do his time and resume his lifestyle. One morning while doing laundry with an occupational therapy student, he shared the experience of his previous sleepless night. He reported that he awoke in the middle of the night in a cold sweat, thinking how the occupational therapy staff truly believed that he would not recidivate. He described his newlyfound desistence as the realization that these expectations were so compelling that he could not return to his former lifestyle. "I don't know what I'll do now," he stated, "but I know what I won't do from now on."

AN OCCUPATIONAL PERSPECTIVE OF CRIME

These concepts of criminal lifestyle and stages of the criminal career are widely supported by the criminal justice community and anecdotal evidence. Not only does Walters' (1990) work invite occupational therapists to investigate crime as occupation and the implications of sensory preferences through the Adolescent/Adult

Sensory Profile® (Brown & Dunn, 2002), it offers occupational scientists and therapists a unique opportunity to examine criminal causes, careers, and interventions through the lens of occupational justice, occupational deprivation, prisonization, and occupational enrichment.

REENTRY TO THE COMMUNITY

In the United States, 95% of all state prisoners complete their sentences and reenter communities (Hughes & Wilson, 2002). Unfortunately, not all do so successfully or permanently. **Recidivism** is relapse to criminal behavior that is usually measured as arrest, conviction, or incarceration for a new crime within three years of release or parole (Bonczar & Glaze, 2011; Hughes & Wilson, 2002). Just over half to two thirds of all American offenders recidivate (Bonczar & Glaze, 2011; Visher, LaVigne, & Travis, 2004).

Recidivism is a complex concept and rates are often reported in relation to certain sub-groups. Among offenders released from federal prisons in Canada, one way recidivism is reported is based on type of release (Porporino, 2009): 41.6% of all those released on day parole returned to custody before the end of their sentence; 25.1% of the total number released on full parole; 46.6% of all offenders released on mandatory supervision (at two thirds of their sentence complete); and finally 23.1% of all released on other release categories. It is important to note that returns to custody include those returned for parole violations as well as those who may have committed a new crime.

Reentry challenges the newly released ex-offender to simultaneously master multiple complex occupational challenges. They must find jobs, often with incomplete secondary or vocational education or preparation; find safe, affordable housing outside of crime-ridden areas; obtain transportation; locate sources of health care and childcare on a limited budget; and manage demanding household tasks they have not performed for long periods of time. In addition, they often need to reestablish relationships with family and obtain custody of their children from whom they have been separated (Oklahoma Department of Corrections, 2010b). By simply recalling the process of facing any one of these challenges, occupational therapists can appreciate the magnitude of facing all these challenges immediately on reentry. The ex-offender must manage a combination of them simultaneously without personal, educational, or financial resources.

In order to master these occupational challenges, the ex-offender must have occupational health. **Occupational health** is the balance of physical, mental, and social well-being derived through healthy work, household management, leisure, childcare, and other activities that are socially valued and individually meaningful (Wilcock, 1998a, 1998b). American policies at the federal and state levels often make obtaining or maintaining housing, employment, licensing for jobs, and paying fines and restitution difficult or impossible. Parents face challenges with parental rights, child custody, and support. Some ex-offenders are ineligible for government assistance programs for public benefits such as financial aid for families and educational loans based on their offenses (Visher, LaVigne, & Travis, 2004). Given the effects of prisonization, these occupations prove even more challenging to many ex-offenders.

Life skills curricula addressing these occupational challenges benefit offenders who have experienced occupational deprivation and prisonization. Such programs can begin in institutional or community corrections settings. Community corrections settings maintain public safety by accounting for the offender who works in the community and lives in residential housing. Offenders may reside in a halfway house, work-release center, or at a prearranged home setting. Some offenders are monitored by global positioning devices locked onto the offender.

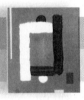

CASE ILLUSTRATION

Roberto

Roberto is a 35-year-old man who has been in and out of criminal justice system since he was 18 years old. He has been arrested and convicted multiple times for drug possession (misdemeanors), theft, and driving while under the influence (DWI). He attempted to flee when arresting officers attempt to detain him on at least two occasions. Unsure of how many times he has been arrested, released, and reconvicted, he is unable to recall details of his arrests due to being under the influence of alcohol and drugs, and more than once, he was rearrested within five days. Prior to his most recent arrest he had been clean and sober for approximately two years, when he was stopped for DWI (alcohol) and driving with a suspended license. Roberto desires a clean and sober lifestyle but describes the difficulty of staying clean and out of trouble because he knows few people who are clean and sober, with the exception of his mother and

children. He is allowed to visit his three children under supervision and while he reports enjoying them, he is not able to describe any of their skills or interests. His current plan for release is to return to a halfway house with mandatory drug testing, supervision, and curfews. He enjoys working and has found periodic work laying drywall or as a tattoo artist. He does not feel like he can talk with "regular" people, deals poorly with conflict, and has few leisure interests aside from working out with weights for 45–60 minutes three times a week. He is restricted from driving and feels this limits his employment potential. He has currently transferred from jail to the community correctional facility for the remaining 60 days of his sentence. During this 60 days he will participate in programs for the first 30 days including family participation, education, anger management, relapse prevention, and Moral Reconation Therapy (MRT). The second transition phase, lasting the remaining 30 days of the program includes working with a recovery mentor from Alcoholics Anonymous (AA) to establish employment, support groups, housing, and occupational therapy. The occupational therapist's evaluation shows the following:

Occupational Self-Assessment (OSA)	Canadian Occupational Performance Measure (COPM)
Performance 31	Total Performance Score 4.6
Volition 14	Satisfaction Score 2.4
Habituation 15	
Environment 20	

Discussion

Roberto's self-assessment shows contrasts between his sense of performance ability, but with significant challenges in volition, habituation, and environment, and as reflected in his inconsistent work history, social participation challenges, and lack of sustainable healthy routines. His COPM results show lack of satisfaction with performance of his occupational goals of connecting with his mother and his children, staying sober, exercise/working out, taking care of himself, and finding a job. Using the Model of Human Occupation orientation, much of the work in occupational therapy includes examination of developing healthy habits, roles, and routines. The Model of Human Occupation focus on habituation directs Roberto toward developing a sustainable routine, which includes work, leisure, self-care, and family activities and helping him move from a dysadaptive to adaptive mode of behavior (from Occupational Adaptation). In therapy he engages in role playing, seeks resources from the community (i.e., low cost activities he can pursue with his children), and is given assignments to follow through on some of the skills he is developing in the therapy environment using the occupation-based self-determination approach. By release, he is working part-time doing drywall (although this is only a short-term job), living in a half-way house, working with his mentor, and is regularly attending AA groups, The OT intervention includes an occupational therapist meeting him in the community for job coaching, leisure exploration (including a faith-based location that offers free gym access and AA groups), and parenting support, to promote healthy occupational routines that may end his revolving door narrative within the correctional system.

SUMMARY

The issues and challenges of occupational therapy in criminal justice systems provide excellent opportunities to apply the concepts of occupational justice. This relatively new idea in occupational therapy provides hopeful alternatives for incarcerated individuals. However, the full promise of occupational justice is how it can guide strategies and programs that can positively affect the organizational and societal factors that have created such disproportionate numbers of incarcerated populations. The scope of this chapter has focused more on the individual and organizational levels of the criminal justice system, but briefly addressed occupational justice applications to societal change for criminal justice.

Occupational therapy, with its unique understanding of the person–environment–occupation interaction, has much to offer the criminal justice system and particularly to those incarcerated or paroled individuals who also are experiencing mental illness, substance abuse issues, or both. With careful application of the limited, but growing evidence to support OT roles in corrections and forensic systems, this could be an exciting new growth area for practice. More promising still is the positive impact that an occupational justice-inspired occupational therapy practice could have on individuals and populations of people with and without mental health conditions who are part of the complex criminal justice system.

REVIEW QUESTIONS

1. Name and define the four criminal justice settings where an occupational therapy practitioner might work.
2. Define an occupational therapy practitioner's role in adjudication.
3. What are commonly used models of practice in criminal justice settings?
4. What are therapeutic/clinical competencies for occupational therapy practitioners that are specific to criminal justice settings?
5. Give examples of how engagement in instrumental activities of daily living (IADL) might differ depending on the correctional setting where an occupational therapy practitioner is employed.
6. What are the major occupational science theories that influence practice in correctional settings?

REFERENCES

Allen, C. K., Austin, S. L., David, S. K., Earhart, C. A., McCraith, D. B., & Riska-Williams, L. (2007). Allen Cognitive Level Screen-5 (ACLS-5). Camarillo, CA: ACLS and LACLS Committee.

American Occupational Therapy Association (AOTA). (2000). Occupational Therapy Code of Ethics. *American Journal of Occupational Therapy, 54*, 614–616.

American Occupational Therapy Association (AOTA). (2003). Models for Community-Based Psychosocial Practice. Online Course. C. Brown.

American Occupational Therapy Association (AOTA). (2008a). Occupational therapy practice framework: Domain and process (2nd edition). *American Journal of Occupational Therapy, 62*(6), 625–683.

American Occupational Therapy Association (AOTA). (2008b). Guidelines for evidence table. Retrieved from http://www.aota.org/DocumentVault/AJOT/Evidence-Guide.asp

American Psychiatric Association (APA). (2000). *Diagnostic and statistical manual of mental disorders* (4th ed., text rev.). Washington, DC: Author.

Annon, J. (1976). The PLISSIT Model: a proposed conceptual scheme for the behavioural treatment of sexual problems. *Journal of Sex Education & Therapy, 2*(1), 1–15.

American Psychiatric Association (APA). (2003). *Practice Guideline for the Assessment and Treatment of Patients With Suicidal Behaviors*. Arlington, VA: American Psychiatric Association.

Arboleda-Florez, J. (1994). *An epidemiological study of mental illness in a remanded population and the relationship between mental condition and criminality.* Unpublished doctoral dissertation. Calgary, Alberta: University of Calgary.

Association of Reproductive Health Professionals. (2002). Mature Sexuality Clinical Proceedings: Taking a Sexual History. *ARHP Clinical Proceedings.* Retrieved from http://www.arhp.org/ healthcareproviders/cme/onlinecme/maturecmecp/sexualhistory.cfm?ID=44

Baker, S., & McKay, E. A. (2001). Occupational therapists' perspectives of the needs of women in medium secure units. *British Journal of Occupational Therapy, 64*(9), 441–448.

Baron, K., Kielhofner, G., Lyenger, A., Goldhammer, V., & Wolenski, J. (2006). *Occupational Self Assessment (OSA)* (Version 2.2 ed.). Chicago, IL: MOHO Clearinghouse, University of Illinois.

Bartlik, B. D., Rosenfeld, S., & Beaton, C. (2005). Assessment of sexual functioning: Sexual history taking for health care practitioners. *Epilepsy & Behavior, 7,* 15–21.

Baum, C. A., Morrison, T., Hahn, M., & Edwards, D. F. (2007). *Executive Function Performance Test.* St. Louis, MO: Program in Occupational Therapy, Washington University School of Medicine.

Baum, C. M., & Edwards, D. F. (2008). *Activity Card Sort* (2nd ed.). Bethesda, MD: AOTA Press.

Bean, G., Meirson, J., & Pinta, E. (1988). *The prevalence of mental illness among inmates in the Ohio prison system* (Final report to the Department of Mental Health and the Ohio Department of Rehabilitation and Correction Interdepartmental Planning and Oversight committee for Psychiatric Services to Corrections). Columbus: Ohio State University.

Beck, A. J., & Harrison, P. M. (2007). Sexual victimization in local jails reported by inmates, 2007 (NCJ 221946). Washington, DC: Bureau of Justice Statistics. Retrieved from http://bjs.ojp.usdoj .gov/index.cfm?ty=pbdetail&iid=1148

Beck, A. T., Brown, G. K., & Steer, R. A. (Eds.). (1996). *Beck Depression Inventory Manual-II.* San Antonio: Psychological Corporation.

Beck, J. S. (1995). *Cognitive therapy: Basics and beyond* (1st ed.). New York: Guilford Press.

Blackburn, A., Mullings, J., & Marquart, J. (2008). Sexual assault in prison and beyond. *The Prison Journal, 88*(3), 351–377.

Bonczar, T. P., & Glaze, L. E. (2011). *Probation and parole in the United States, 2010.* (NCJ 236019). Washington, DC: Bureau of Justice Statistics.

Bouchard, F. (2004). A health care needs assessment of federal inmates. *Canadian Journal of Public Health, 95*(Supplement 1).

Brink, J., Doherty, D., & Boer, A. (2001). Mental disorder in federal offenders: A Canadian prevalence study. *International Journal of Law and Psychiatry, 24,* 339–356.

Brown, A., Garnett, J., Sussex, N., Watson, L. Grass, C., & Duncan, E. (2010). *Forensic occupational therapists connecting through an online community.* Poster presented at the Canadian Association of Occupational Therapists Conference, Meaningful Occupations: Enabling an Ocean of Possibilities. Halifax, NS, May 26–29.

Brown, C., & Dunn, W. (2002). *Adolescent/Adult Sensory Profile*. San Antonio, TX: Pearson PsychCorp.

Bureau of Justice Statistics. (1997). Sequence of Events in the US Criminal Justice System. Retrieved from http://www.ou.edu/oupd/cjflow.pdf

California Department of Corrections. (1989). *Current description, evaluation, and recommendations for treatment of mentally disordered offenders* (Final report submitted to the California State Legislature). San Francisco: Standard Consulting Corporation.

Canadian Association of Occupational Therapists. (CAOT). (2002). *Enabling occupation: An occupational therapy perspective.* Ottawa, ON: Canadian Association of Occupational Therapists.

Canadian Association of Occupational Therapists. (CAOT). (2007). Code of Ethics. Retrieved from http://www.caot.ca/default.asp?pageid=35

Clarke, C. (2003). Clinical application of the Canadian Model of Occupational Performance in a forensic rehabilitation hostel. *British Journal of Occupational Therapy, 66*(4), 171–174.

College of Occupational Therapists. (2001). *Code of Ethics and Professional Conduct.* Southwark, London, England: College of Occupational Therapists.

College of Occupational Therapists. (2002). *Research and development strategic vision and action plan for forensic occupational therapy.* London, England: COT.

Coulter, K. (2007). Addressing mental health needs of offenders. *Let's Talk, 32*(1), 3.

Criminal Justice/Mental Health Consensus Project. (2002). *Criminal justice-mental health consensus project report.* Retrieved from http://consensusproject.org/downloads/fact_fiscal_implications.pdf

Crist, P., Fairman, A., Muñoz, J., Hansen, A. M., Sciulli, J., & Eggers, M. (2005). Education and practice collaborations: A pilot case study between a university and county jail practitioners. *Occupational Therapy in Health Care, 19*(1), 193–210.

Cruser, D.A., & Diamond, P. (1996). An exploration of social policy and organizational culture in jail-based mental health services. *Administration and Policy in Mental Health, 24*(2), 129–148.

DeNavas-Walt, C., Proctor, B. D., & Smith, J. C. (2010). U.S. Census Bureau Current Population Reports, P60–238: *Income, Poverty, and Health Insurance Coverage in the United States: 2009.* Washington, DC: U.S. Government Printing Office.

Diamond, P., Cruser, D. A., Childs, R., Schnee, S., & Quinn, M. (1999). The impact of knowledge and opinions on the implementation of public policies for mentally ill offenders. *Administration and Policy in Mental Health, 26*(5), 329–344.

Diamond, P., Wang, E., Holzer, C., III, Thomas, C., & Cruser, D. A. (2001). The prevalence of mental illness in prison. *Administration and Policy in Mental Health, 29*(1), 21–40.

Dickerson, A. E. (2008). The role checklist. In B. Hemphill-Pearson (Ed.), *Assessment in occupational therapy mental health* (2nd ed., pp. 73–91). Thorofare, NJ: Slack.

Dieleman Grass, C. (2010). *Slow decline: The social organization of mental health care in a prison-hospital.* Unpublished doctoral dissertation. Kingston, Canada: Queen's University.

Duncan, E. A. S., Munro, K., & Nicol, M. M. (2003). Research priorities in forensic occupational therapy. *British Journal of Occupational Therapy, 66*(2), 55–64.

Dunn, W. (2001). The sensations of everyday life: Theoretical, conceptual and pragmatic considerations. *American Journal of Occupational Therapy, 55,* 608–620.

Eggers, M., Muñoz, J. P., Sciulli, J., & Crist, P. A. H. (2006). The Community Reintegration Project: occupational therapy at work in a county jail. *Occupational Therapy in Health Care, 20*(1), 17–37.

Elliott, R. (1997). Evaluating the quality of correctional mental health services: An approach to surveying a correctional mental health system. *Behavioral Sciences and the Law, 15,* 427–438.

Elizabeth Fry Society of Mainland Nova Scotia. (2005). *Women in Nova Scotia: Mental illness and the criminal justice system, a qualitative review.* Halifax, NS: Elizabeth Fry Society of Mainland Nova Scotia.

Farnworth, L., Nikitin, L., & Fossey, E. (2004). Being in a secure forensic psychiatric unit: Every day is the same, killing time or making the most of it. *British Journal of Occupational Therapy, 67*(10), 430–438.

Fisher, W., Packer, I., Simon, L., & Smith, D. (2000). Community mental health services and prevalence of severe mental illness in local jails: Are they related? *Administration and Policy in Mental Health, 27*(6), 371–382.

Freeman, R., & Roesch, R. (1989). Mental disorder and the criminal justice system: A review. *International Journal of Law and Psychiatry, 12,* 105–115.

Galvaan, R. (2005). Domestic workers' narratives: Transforming occupational practice. In F. Kronenberg, S. S. Algado, & N. Pollard (Eds.), *Occupational therapy without borders: Spirit of Survivors* (pp. 429–439). Edinburgh, Elsevier.

Geffner, R. (2004). *Identifying and treating sex offenders: Current approaches, research, and techniques.* Binghamton, NY: Haworth Maltreatment & Trauma Press.

Gibbon, S., Duggan, C., Stoffers, J., Huband, N., Vollm, B. A., Ferriter, M., et al. (2010). Psychological interventions for antisocial personality disorder [Systematic Review]. *Cochrane Database of Systematic Reviews, 6:* CD007668. Retrieved from doi:10.1002/14651858.CD007668.pub2

Gooch, P., & Living, R. (2004). The therapeutic use of videogames within secure forensic settings: a review of the literature and application to practice. *British Journal of Occupational Therapy, 67*(8), 332–341.

Goodman, S. H., Sewell, D. R., Cooley, E. L., & Leavitt, N. (1993). Assessing levels of adaptive functioning: The role functioning scale. *Community Mental Health Journal, 29,* 119–131.

Grass, C., & Farnworth, L. (2010). International launch of the Research Centre for Occupation and Mental Health, York St. John University, UK: Research program for occupation and mental health in forensic and prison settings. *15th Congress of the World Federation of Occupational Therapists,* Santiago, Chile, May 4–7.

Green, B., Miranda, J., Daroowalla, A., & Siddique, J. (2005). Trauma exposure, mental health functioning, and program needs of women in jail. *Crime & Delinquency, 51*(1), 133–151.

Gregitis, S., Gelpi, T., Moore, B., & Dees, M. (2010). Self-determination skills of adolescents enrolled in special education: An analysis of four cases. *Occupational Therapy in Mental Health, 26*(1), 67–84.

Gutman, S. A., Mortera, M. H., Hinojosa, J., & Kramer, P. (2007). The issue is: Revision of the Occupational Therapy Practice Framework. *American Journal of Occupational Therapy, 61*(1), 119–126.

Guy, E., Platt, J., Zwerling, I., & Bullock, S. (1985). Mental health status of prisoners in an urban jail. *Criminal Justice and Behaviour, 12*(1), 29–53.

Haney, C. (2002). *The psychological impact of incarceration: Implications for post-prison adjustment.* Washington, DC: U.S. Dept. of Health and Human Services.

Hare, R. D. (2003). *Hare Psychopathy Checklist-Revised (PCL-R): Second edition* [Technical Manual]. New York: Multi-Health Systems.

Harm, N. J., & Phillips, S. D. (2001). You can't go home again: Women and criminal recidivism. *Journal of Offender Rehabilitation, 32*(3), 3–21.

Hartney, C. (2006). *US rates of incarceration: A global perspective.* Oakland, CA: National Council on Crime and Delinquency.

Haugebrook, S., Zgoba, K. M., Maschi, T., Morgen, K., & Brown, D. (2010). Trauma, stress, health, and mental health issues among ethnically diverse older adult prisoners. *Journal of Correctional Health Care, 16,* 220–229.

Hensley, C., & Tewksbury, R. (2002). Inmate-to-inmate prison sexuality: A review of empirical studies. *Trauma, Violence & Abuse: A Review Journal, 3*(3), 226–243.

Holland, J. L. (2011). *Self-Directed Search® Form R: 4th Edition (SDS-R).* Lutz, FL: Psychological Assessment Resources, Inc.

Hooper, B. (2005). *From prison to community: A transitional program.* Society for the Study of Occupation: USA 5th Annual Research Conference, St. Louis, MO, SSO:USA.

Hughes, T., & Wilson, D. J. (2002). *Reentry trends in the United States.* Washington, DC: Bureau of Justice Statistics.

Inciardi, J., Surratt, H., Martin, S., O'Connell, D., Salandy, A., & Beard, R. (2007). Developing a multimedia HIV and hepatitis intervention for drug-involved offenders reentering the community. *The Prison Journal, 87*(1), 111–142.

James, J., Gregory, D., Jones, R., & Rundell, O. (1980). Psychiatric morbidity in prisons. *Hospital and Community Psychiatry, 11,* 674–677.

Jones, R. S., & Schmid, T. A. (2000). *Doing time: Prison experience and identity among first-time inmates.* Stamford, CT: JAI Press.

Jones, T., & Prat, T. (2008). The prevalence of sexual violence in prison. *International Journal of Offender Therapy and Comparative Criminology, 52*(3), 280–295.

Kal, E. (1977). Mental health in jail. *American Journal of Psychiatry, 134,* 463.

Kelly, R. (2003). Cognitive behavioural group work within forensic occupational therapy. In L. Couldrick & D. Alred (Eds.), *Forensic occupational therapy* (pp. 61–74). Philadelphia: Whurr Publishers.

Kerr, C., Roth, J., Courtless, T., & Zenoff, E. (1987). *Survey of facilities and programs for mentally ill offenders.* Department of Health and Human Services, Publication No. (ADM 86–1493). Rockville, MD: National Institute of Mental Health.

Kethineni, S., & Falcone, D. (2007). Employment and ex-offenders in the United States: Effects of legal and extra-legal factors. *Probation Journal, 54*(1), 36–51.

Kielhofner, G. (2008). *A model of human occupation: Theory and application* (4th ed.). Baltimore: Lippincott Williams & Wilkins.

Kielhofner, G., Mallinson, T., Crawford, C., Nowak, M., Rigby, M., Henry, A., et al. (2004). Occupational Performance History Interview II (OPHI-II) (Version 2.1 ed.). Chicago, IL: MOHO Clearinghouse, University of Illinois.

Kronenberg, F., & Pollard, N. (2005). Overcoming occupational apartheid: A preliminary exploration of the political nature of occupational therapy. In F. Kronenberg, S. Simi-Algado, & N. Pollard (Eds.), *Occupational therapy without borders: Learning from the spirit of survivors* (pp. 58–86). London: Elsevier Churchill Livingstone.

Lamb, H., & Grant, R. (1983). Mentally ill women in a county jail. *Archives of General Psychiatry, 40,* 363–368.

Law, M., Baptiste, S., Carswell, A., McColl, M., Polatajko, H. J., & Pollock, N. (2005). *The Canadian Occupational Performance Measure* (4th ed.). Toronto, Ontario: CAOT.

Law, M., Cooper, S., Strong, S., Stewart, D., Rigby, P., & Letts, L. (1996). The person-environment-occupational model: A transactive approach to occupational performance. *Canadian Journal of Occupational Therapy, 63*(1), 9–23.

MacKenzie, D. L. (2000). Evidence-based corrections: Identifying what works. *Crime Delinquency, 46*(4), 457–471.

Maruna, S. (2001). *Making good: How ex-convicts reform and rebuild their lives.* Washington, DC: American Psychological Association.

Maruna, S., & Mann, R. E. (2006). A fundamental attribution error? Rethinking cognitive distortions. [Article]. *Legal & Criminological Psychology, 11,* 155–177.

Maruschak, L. M. (2008). Medical problems of prisoners. (NCJ 221740). Washington, DC: Bureau of Justice Statistics. Retrieved from http://bjs.ojp.usdoj.gov/index.cfm?ty=pbdetail&iid=1097

McCoy, M., Roberts, D., Hanrahan, P., Clay, R., & Luchins, D. (2004). Jail linkage assertive community treatment services for individuals with mental illness. *Psychiatric Rehabilitation Journal, 27*(3), 243–250.

Molineux, M. L., & Whiteford, G. E. (1999). Prisons: From occupational deprivation to occupational enrichment. *Journal of Occupational Science,6*(3), 124–130.

Monahan, J., & McDonough, L. (1980). Delivering community mental health services in a county jail population: A research note. *Bulletin of the American Academy of Psychiatry and the Law, 8,* 28–32.

Morrow, T. (2008). Can a client centred approach develop autonomy and behavioural changes in male offenders attending group activities in forensic environments? *Mental Health Occupational Therapy, 13*(1), 35–39.

Motiuk, L., & Porporino, F. (1991). *The prevalence, nature and severity of mental health problems among federal male inmates in Canadian Penitentiaries.* Report No. 24, Ottawa: Research and Statistics Branch, Correctional Service Canada.

Muñoz, J. P., & Farnworth, L. (2009). An occupational and rehabilitation perspective for institutional practice. *Psychiatric Rehabilitation Journal, 32*(3), 192–198. Retrieved from doi: 10.2975/32.3.2009.192.198

Muñoz, J., Farnworth, L., Hamilton, T., Prioletti, G., Rogers, S., & White, J. A. J. (2011). Crossing borders in correctional institutions. In F. Kronenberg, N. Pollard, & D. Sakellariou (Eds.), *Occupational therapies without borders* (2nd ed., Vol. 2, pp. 235–246). London: Elsevier.

Navasky, M., & O'Connor, K. (2005). *Frontline: The new asylums* [Television broadcast]. Boston: WGBH.

O'Connell, M., & Farnworth, L. (2007). Occupational therapy in forensic psychiatry: A review of the literature and a call for a united and international response. *British Journal of Occupational Therapy, 70*(5), 184–191.

OCEBM Table of Evidence Working Group. (2011). Levels of evidence classification. Retrieved from http://www.cebm.net/index.aspx?o=1025

Ogloff, J. (2002). Identifying and accommodating the needs of mentally ill people in gaols and prisons. *Psychiatry, Psychology and the Law, 9*(1), 1–33.

Oklahoma Department of Corrections. (2010a). *Female Offender Operations FY 2010 Annual Report.* Oklahoma City. OK: Oklahoma Department of Corrections Division of Female Offender Operations.

Oklahoma Department of Corrections. (2010b). *Fiscal Year 2010 Annual Report.* Oklahoma City. OK: Oklahoma Department of Corrections.

Oklahoma Departments of Corrections and Mental Health and Substance Abuse Services. (2011). *The justice and mental health collaborative project.* Oklahoma City, OK: Oklahoma Department of Corrections.

Petrich, J. (1976). Rate of psychiatric morbidity in a metropolitan county jail population. *American Journal of Psychiatry, 133*(12), 1439–1444.

Pew Center on the States. (2009). *One in 31: The long reach of American corrections.* Washington, DC: The PEW Charitable Trusts.

Piotrowski, K., Lasacco, D., & Guze, S. (1976). Psychiatric disorders and crime: A study of pretrial psychiatric examinations. *Diseases of the Nervous System, 37,* 309–311.

Porporino, F. (2009). So you want to know the recidivism rate. *FORUM on Corrections Research.* Retrieved from http://www.csc-scc.gc.ca/text/pblct/forum/e053/e053h-eng.shtml

Powell, T., Holt, J., & Fondacaro, K. (1997). The prevalence of mental illness among inmates in a rural state. *Law and Human Behaviour, 21*(4), 427–438.

Ramirez, R., & Gonzalez, J. (2011). Occupational therapy and intervention in Chilean prisons. Unpublished annual report, CDP Santiago Sur, Gendarmerie of Chile.

Ranasinghe, K., Gunarathne, P., & Alahakoon, R. (2011). Year end report 2010 & proposed programme for 2011. Unpublished report from the Forensic Psychiatry Rehabilitation Unit, Angoda, Sri Lanka: National Institute of Mental Health.

Reed, J., & Lyne, M. (2000). In-patient care of mentally ill people in prison: results of a year's programme of semi-structured inspections. *British Medical Journal, 320,* 1031–1034.

Rollnick, S., Miller, W. R., & Butler, C. (2008*). Motivational interviewing in health care: Helping patients change behavio*r. New York: Guilford Press.

Ruddell, R. (2006). Jail interventions for inmates with mental illnesses. *Journal of Correctional Health Care, 12*(2), 118–131.

Sackett, D. L., Straus, S. E., Richardson, W. S., Rosenberg, W., & Haynes, R. B. (2000). *Evidence-based medicine: How to practice and teach EBM* (2nd ed.). Toronto, ON: Churchhill Livingstone.

Sampson, R., Gascon, S., Glen, I., Louie, C., & Rosenfeldt, S. (2007). *A roadmap to strengthening public safety: Report of the Correctional Service of Canada review panel.* Ottawa: Minister of Public Works and Government Services Canada.

Schindler, V. P. (2004a). Introduction: Social roles and schizophrenia in forensic psychiatry. *Occupational Therapy in Mental Health, 20*(3), 1–9. Retrieved from doi: 10.1300/J004v20n03_01

Schindler, V. P. (2004b). *Occupational therapy in forensic psychiatry: Role development and schizophrenia*. Binghamton, NY: Haworth Press.

Schkade, J. K., & McClung, M. (2001). *Occupational adaptation in practice: Concepts and cases*. Thorofare, NJ: Slack.

Singleton, N., Meltzer, H., & Gatward, R. (1998). *Psychiatric morbidity among prisoners in England and Wales*. London: Stationary Office.

Smith, A., Petty, M., Oughton, I., & Alexander, R. T. (2010). Establishing a work-based learning programme: Vocational rehabilitation in a forensic learning disability setting. *British Journal of Occupational Therapy, 73*(9), 431–436. Retrieved from doi: 10.4276/030802210x12839367526174.

Snow, W., & Briar, K. (1990). The convergence of the mentally disordered in the jail population. *Journal of Offender Counseling, Services and Rehabilitation, 15,* 147–162.

Steadman, H., Barbera, S., & Dennis, D. (1994). A national survey of jail diversion programs for mentally ill detainees. *Hospital and Community Psychiatry, 45*(11), 1109–1113.

Steadman, H., McCarty, D., & Morrisey, J. (1989). *The mentally ill in jail: Planning for essential services*. New York: The Guilford Press.

Steadman, H. J., Osher, F. C., Robbins, P. C., Case, B., & Samuels, S. (2009). Prevalence of serious mental illness among jail inmates. *Psychiatric Services, 60*(6), 761.

Swank, G., & Winer, D. (1976). Occurrence of psychiatric disorder in a county jail population. *American Journal of Psychiatry, 133,* 1331–1333.

Tayar, S. G. (2004). Description of a substance abuse relapse prevention programme conducted by occupational therapy and psychology graduate students in a United States women's prison. *British Journal of Occupational Therapy, 67*(4), 159–166.

Taylor, B., & Davis, S. (2007). The Extended PLISSIT Model for addressing the sexual well being of individuals with an acquired disability or chronic illness. *Sexuality and Disability, 25,* 135–139.

Teplin, L. (1990). The prevalence of severe mental disorder among urban jail detainees: Comparison with the Epidemiologic Catchment Area program. *American Journal of Public Health, 80,* 663–669.

Teplin, L. (1994). Psychiatric and substance abuse disorders among male urban jail detainees. *American Journal of Public Health, 84,* 290–293.

Torrey, E. (1995). Editorial: Jails and prisons—America's new mental hospitals. *American Journal of Public Health, 85,* 1611–1613.

Townsend, E., & Wilcock, A. A. (2004). Occupational justice. In C. H. Christiansen & E. Townsend (Eds.), *Introduction to occupation: The art and science of living* (pp. 206–225). Upper Saddle River, NJ: Prentice-Hall.

Travis, J., Solomon, A. L., & Waul, M. (2001). *From prison to home: The dimensions and consequences of prisoner reentry*. Washington, DC: The Urban Institute: Justice Policy Center.

United States Department of Labor: Employment and Training Administration. (2010). The Work Opportunity Tax Credit (WOTC): An employer-friendly benefit for hiring job seekers most in need of employment. In U.S. Department of Labor (Ed.), *Fact Sheet*. Washington, DC: U.S. Department of Labor.

United States Immigration and Customs Enforcement. (2011). Jail officials and alleged 'RadaUnida' gang member sentenced for bribery. News Release, September 14, 2011. Corpus Christi, TX. Retrieved from http://www.ice.gov/news/releases/1109/110914corpuschristi.htm

Visher, C., LaVigne, N., & Travis, J. (2004). *Returning home: Understanding the challenges of prisoner reentry*. Maryland Pilot Study: Findings from Baltimore. Washington, DC: The Urban Institute.

Waldram, J. B. (2008). The narrative challenge to cognitive behavioral treatment of sexual offenders. *Culture, Medicine and Psychiatry, 32*(3), 421–439.

Walters, G. D. (1990). *Criminal lifestyle: Patterns of serious criminal conduct.* Newbury Park, CA: Sage.

Webster, C., Eaves, D., Douglas, K. S., & Wintrup, A. (1995). *The HCR-20 Scheme: The Assessment of Dangerousness and Risk—Version 1.* Burnaby, BC: Mental Health, Law and Policy Institute, Simon Fraser University.

Wehmeyer, M. L. (1999). A functional model of self-determination: Describing development and implementing instruction. *Focus on Autism and Other Developmental Disabilities, 14*(1), 53–62.

Wehmeyer, M. L., Gragoudas, S., & Shogren, K. (2006). Self-determination, student involvement, and leadership development. In P. W. (Ed.), *Life beyond the classroom: Transition strategies for young people with disabilities* (4th ed., pp. 41–70). Baltimore, MD: Paul H. Brookes.

West, H. C., & Sobal, W. J. (2009). *Prison inmates at midyear 2008 statistical tables.* Washington, DC: Bureau of Justice Statistics.

Whiteford, G. (1997). Occupational deprivation and incarceration. *Journal of Occupational Science: Australia, 4*(3), 126–130.

Whiteford, G. (2000). Occupational deprivation: Global challenge in the new millennium. *British Journal of Occupational Therapy, 63*(5), 200–204.

Whitmer, G. (1980). From hospitals to jails: The fate of California's deinstitutionalized mentally ill. *American Journal of Orthopsychiatry, 50,* 65–75.

Wilcock, A. (1998a). Occupation for health. *British Journal of Occupational Therapy, 61*(8), 340–345.

Wilcock, A. (1998b). *An occupational perspective of health.* Thorofare, NJ: Slack.

Wilper, A. P., Woolhandler, S., Boyd, J. W., Lasser, K. E., McCormick, D., et al. (2009). The health and health care of U.S. prisoners: A nationwide survey. *American Journal of Public Health, 99*(4).

Wilson, S. (2004). The principle of equivalence and the future of mental health care in prisons. *British Journal of Psychiatry, 184,* 5–7.

Wong, S., & Gordon, A. (1999). *Violence Risk Scale.* Saskatchewan, Canada: Regional Psychiatric Centre: Research Unit.

Wood, W. (1993). Occupation and the relevance of primatology to occupational therapy. *American Journal of Occupational Therapy, 47*(6), 515–522.

World Federation of Occupational Therapists. (2004). *Code of ethics.* Retrieved from http://www.wfot .org/ResourceCentre.aspx

World Health Organization. (2007). *Trenčín statement on prisons and mental health.* Copenhagen, Denmark: World Health Organization Regional Office for Europe.

Zaitow, B. H., & Thomas, J. (2003). *Women in prison: Gender and social control.* Boulder, CO: Lynne Rienner Publishers.

SUGGESTED RESOURCES

Department of Labor: Employment & Training Administration. (2005). Reintegration of Ex-Offenders (RExO) formerly known as Prisoner Reentry Resources. In Department of Labor: Employment & Training Administration. Washington, DC: Department of Labor: Employment & Training Administration. Retrieved from: http://www.doleta.gov/RExO/ PDF/Prisoner_Reentry_Resources.pdf

Kennedy, J. (Writer), & Wilbraham, B. (Director). (2005). Finding freedom behind bars: The mindfulness prison project: a documentary: Trinity Productions.

Rollo, N. (2002). *99 days and a get up: A guide to success following release for inmates and their loved ones.* Dallas, TX: OPEN Inc.

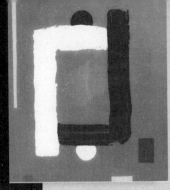

Chapter 22

Psychosocial Occupational Therapy in the School Setting

Sue Ann Folker, MS, OTR/L
Sara L. Woodward, MEd, MOT, OTR/L

■ KEY TERMS

advocacy
client-centered approach
collaborative service delivery model
environmental contexts
occupation-based interventions
occupational alienation
occupational deprivation
occupational imbalance
occupational justice

occupational marginalization
participation
positive behavioral interventions
    and supports (PBIS)
school mental health movement
three-tiered intervention approach
universal design for learning (UDL)
workload vs. caseload

CHAPTER OUTLINE

Introduction
Inclusion and Participation in the School Community: An Occupational Justice Perspective
Participation and Psychosocial Well-Being
        Who Experiences Psychosocial Issues?
School-Based Occupational Therapy: A Community-Based Practice
        Children with Identified Mental Health Disabilities
        Evaluation of Psychosocial Issues in the School Setting
        Psychosocial Occupational Therapy Interventions in the Schools
        Intervention Service Delivery Models
Actions to Address Psychosocial Issues in the School Setting
Summary

INTRODUCTION

Children's mental health is an integral part of overall health and is crucial for social and emotional well-being (American Occupational Therapy Association [AOTA], 2009). Over the last decade there has been a sustained focus regarding the promotion of healthy and safe environments in the public schools, which has contributed to an international **school mental health movement** (AOTA, 2009; Lynn, McKay, & Atkins, 2003; Svavarsdottir, 2008). Healthy and safe school environments encompass the physical, psychosocial, learning, and health-promoting environments (Jones, Fisher, Greene, Hertz, & Pritzl, 2007). Students attending schools that strive for a safe and positive physical and psychosocial environment may be less likely to experience unintentional injuries and violence, to use tobacco, alcohol, or other drugs, or to experience school failure (Jones et al., 2007).

Occupational therapy has much to offer in discussions surrounding school mental health and the prevention of mental health problems. It is crucial that occupational therapy practitioners become involved in these dialogues and actions, at both the individual school building and systemic levels, if we are to fulfill our full scope of practice in the public schools, a truly community-based setting.

When discussing children's mental health as an area of occupational therapy practice, direct services and interventions for children with diagnosed mental health disorders may immediately come to mind. However, it is important to remember that psychosocial issues affect a diverse mix of students in the public education system. These issues range from those that affect most students to those impacting students with specific mental health disabilities. Figure 22-1 illustrates some of the many psychosocial issues that are encountered by students in the school community.

Students may have psychosocial needs and differences that are influenced by a physical disability, a mental health disorder, childhood obesity, an eating disorder, abuse and/or neglect, poverty, environmental or situational stressors, homelessness, violence, suicide, and issues related to bullying or cyberbullying (Curtis, 2008; Park, Brindis, Chang, & Irwin, 2008). If psychosocial issues are not addressed with early intervening services, psychosocial problems may continue to manifest and grow, creating disparities in **participation**, social interactions, and the ability to lead a productive and meaningful life (Park et al., 2008).

Occupational therapists have a strong background in human development, as well as a thorough understanding of how **environmental contexts** impact function and participation. Using a developmental frame of reference along with theories unique to occupational therapy can help frame occupational therapy's unique contributions to school mental health.

Advocacy for psychosocial intervention by occupational therapists currently working in the school setting is necessary to bring about a change in traditional school

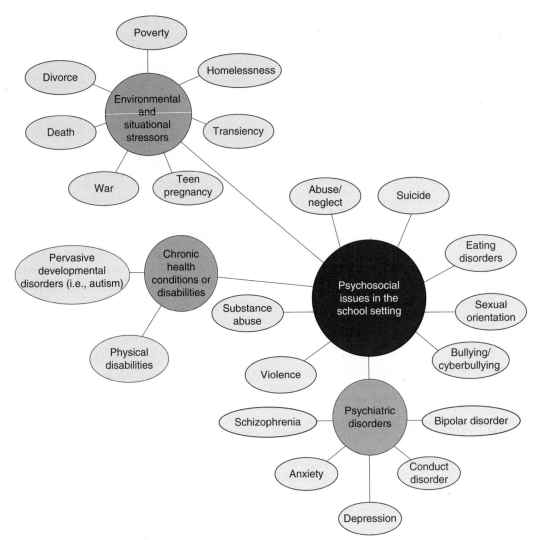

FIGURE 22-1. Psychosocial Issues in the School Setting
© Cengage Learning 2013

occupational therapy practices. Harrison and Forsyth (2005) discuss the use of theory as a means of expanding occupational therapy's role. The Model of Human Occupation (MOHO), the Canadian Model of Occupational Performance (CMOP), and the Person-Environment-Occupation (PEO) model are all important conceptual frameworks for school-based occupational therapy practitioners to utilize. They provide unique occupation-focused theory with an evidence base, embrace the complexity of human occupation, and are designed to support theory into practice (Harrison & Forsyth, 2005).

INCLUSION AND PARTICIPATION IN THE SCHOOL COMMUNITY: AN OCCUPATIONAL JUSTICE PERSPECTIVE

Students with psychosocial issues often encounter barriers to participation and engagement in meaningful occupation in the school setting (Egilson & Hemmingsson, 2009; Hemmingsson & Borell, 2002). One aspect of psychosocial occupational therapy practice in the school setting may be "righting injustices" encountered in the context of the school community to create an environment that contributes to **occupational justice** for all students (Simmons Carlson, 2009, p. 7). It is important that occupational rights be acknowledged and interpreted within the school community context. These occupational rights include: "Experiencing occupation as enriching and meaningful, developing through participation in occupations, exerting autonomy through choice in occupation, and social inclusion for participation in the typical range of occupations for a community" (Townsend & Wilcock, 2004, p. 80). An occupational justice perspective affirms a student's right to be fully included, to be a full citizen of the school community, and to engage and participate at full potential in chosen occupations rather than being "confined, barred, prohibited, undeveloped, marginalized, alienated, or otherwise restricted" (Simmons Carlsson, 2009, p. 7). Table 22-1 is based on the work of Townsend and Wilcock (2004) and describes occupational justice issues that may be encountered by students in the school community.

TABLE 22-1. Occupational Rights and Injustices in the School Setting

Occupational Right	Occupational Injustice	Example of Injustice at School
To make autonomous choices regarding occupation.	Occupational marginalization	A student is not allowed to participate in an educational program of their choice such as being denied participation in a general education environment with their peers due to their perceived level of disability by decision makers.
To "experience occupation as meaningful and enriching" (Townsend & Wilcock, 2004, p. 80).	Occupational alienation	A student is not able to participate in outings and field trips with classmates due to lack of accessible transportation.
To "participate in occupation for health and social inclusion" (p. 80).	Occupational deprivation	A student is rarely allowed to play with peers at recess because she has difficulty completing academic work and must stay in the classroom to finish the work much of the time.
To "benefit from fair privileges for diverse participation in occupations" (p. 80).	Occupational imbalance	A student who spends significant time completing homework due to a fine motor physical disability; she is not engaging in occupations that are typical of her age, such as spending time with friends or taking part in self-chosen activities.

In the public school practice occupational justice issues can be examined by looking at the access to schooling, participation in the curriculum, and participation in the social structure of school life (Simmons Carlsson, 2009). Practicing occupational therapists are particularly important to the task of incorporating the vision of occupational justice into the job descriptions, programs, guidelines, and procedures of everyday practice (Townsend, 1993). Establishing guidelines for inclusive practices will enable the school community to value all students as active participants, creating a community that values each student as a member of the school community rather than viewing some as students that present a challenge to the system. Simmons Carlsson (2009) urges school-based occupational therapists to strive for change at various levels within the organization by addressing injustices at the individual, classroom, school system, and legislative levels.

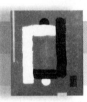

CASE ILLUSTRATION

Dominique—Occupational Deprivation in the Classroom?

Dominique is a third-grade boy whose behavioral issues are of concern to his teacher. Dominique has good academic skills and is excelling in reading. His teacher brings a list of issues that Dominique is struggling with including: disrupting the learning of other students by talking out during class, talking loudly, difficulty sitting still, and occasional outbursts of anger. His teacher reports that Dominique often needs to be sent out of the classroom during instruction so other students can learn and reports that Dominique's angry outbursts seem to be escalating. Maria, the school's occupational therapist, offers to spend time observing Dominique in the school environments. Her observations indicate that Dominique has friends and interacts with most students in a positive manner in multiple contexts, often finishes his work quickly but accurately, and then becomes bored, gets out of his seat, and moves around the room when he is listening to a discussion or is finished with his work. Dominique appears to enjoy recess and talks loudly when he is interested or enjoying an activity.

Discussion

Maria's observations indicate that Dominique demonstrates psychosocial and behavioral skills that are typical for a child his age. Dominique's cultural background is different from many of his classmates, and the teacher and Maria believes that some of the differences in his behavior are based on differing views of communication and interaction styles rather than anger or misbehavior. Maria is concerned about occupational justice issues for Dominique and other students from cultures that are different from the norm. She observed Dominique being excluded from academic and social opportunities his peers were provided with when he was sent out of the classroom during instruction and other activities. Maria talks to his teacher and diplomatically discusses her concern that Dominique is not being provided an educational experience equal to his peers. She consults with the teacher about strategies to decrease his movements in the classroom (i.e., movement breaks for the entire classroom, using an exercise ball chair, having fidgets available and cuing Dominique to use them with a discrete signal), and discusses the possibility of tolerating some of his activities as the observation data did not indicate an impact to other students' learning. She also talks to the school principal about the possibility of staff training on cultural sensitivity issues as this appears to be an issue related to lack of knowledge surrounding cultural differences rather than a behavioral issue.

PARTICIPATION AND PSYCHOSOCIAL WELL-BEING

Central to occupational therapy's founding principles is the idea of engagement in meaningful occupation. When discussing psychosocial issues in the schools we are referring to the intrapersonal, interpersonal, and social experiences that influence occupational behavior and activities (AOTA, 2004). Participation in everyday life is a crucial aspect of human development and lived experience, as well as an indicator of psychosocial well-being (AOTA, 2009; Law, 2002). Common definitions of participation include taking part or becoming involved in an activity, the state of sharing in common with others, and the act or state of receiving or having part of something (Simpson & Weiner, 2002). Thus participation in meaningful activities is an indicator of psychosocial well-being and mental health. Occupational therapists can promote mental health in the school community by "fostering participation in productive activities, fulfilling relationships with other people, and the ability to adapt to change and cope with adversity" (AOTA, 2009).

Who Experiences Psychosocial Issues?

Psychosocial issues arise when a child has difficulty engaging in participation in a range of meaningful occupations and social interaction with others for various reasons. When thinking of psychosocial issues in this light, we include children in the general student body who are experiencing situational psychosocial difficulties due to environmental stressors or trauma, children with chronic health issues and physical disabilities, and children who have identified mental health disorders. Bazyk (2007) describes how all children can benefit from school mental health interventions as summarized in Table 22-2.

In the school setting, reciprocal peer interactions are an important aspect of inclusion and participation in the school community and are one of the indicators of

TABLE 22-2. Students Who Can Benefit from Mental Health Interventions

All Students	Students Who Are "At-Risk"	Students with Psychiatric Disorders
Have been exposed to bullying or cyberbullying.	May have chronic health conditions or disabilities.	Mood disorders including: depression, bipolar disorder.
Are affected by school violence.	Have experiences of abuse or neglect.	Thought disorders including: anxiety, obsessive-compulsive disorder (OCD), post-traumatic stress disorder, schizophrenia.
Experience situational stressors at some point in time.	Are identified as having behavioral issues or are a poor fit for the classroom dynamics.	Behavior and conduct disorders.
Can benefit from school mental health policies and programs.	Who have environmental stressors (i.e., homelessness, divorce, illness, death, substance abuse, etc.).	Pervasive developmental disorders including: autism, Asperger's syndrome.

© Cengage Learning 2013

psychosocial well-being. Research indicates children with physical disabilities engage in more solitary play than their peers and display a preference for interactions with teachers and other adults over peers (Richardson, 2002). Children with high functioning autism have voiced concerns about their participation in mainstream schools, citing experiences of peer cruelty when attempting to connect with other students in an inclusive setting (Humphrey & Lewis, 2008). Children with psychiatric disorders have not historically been served by occupational therapists working in the school setting; however, these children comprise the highest percentage of students receiving education in separate off-campus educational institutions due to their level of needs or because their needs are not being met in the school (Beck, Barnes, Vogel, & Grice, 2006). These examples indicate a need for change in the physical, cultural, social, and institutional environment of the school community in order to enable participation and inclusion of all students (DeJaeghere & Zhang, 2008; Egilson & Hemmingsson, 2009; Hemmingsson & Borell, 2002).

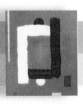

CASE ILLUSTRATION

Eduardo—Psychosocial Issues and Disability in Adolescence

Eduardo is a ninth-grade student who has a diagnosis of Duchenne muscular dystrophy. He is progressively losing muscular functions as he ages, making it difficult to continue daily life and school occupations such as self-care, eating, and school-related tasks like managing a backpack, lifting books, and writing notes quickly. Eduardo receives occupational therapy services focusing on occupational adaptations. Eduardo knows that he stands out among his peers but wants to minimize his differences as much as possible. He is not interested in using the mobile arm support or the laptop computer that has been purchased for him. Emily, his occupational therapist, thinks that Eduardo is depressed and wonders how he deals emotionally with the knowledge of his prognosis. She decides to check in with Eduardo every week and tries to build rapport through conversations and a helpful attitude. She designs client-centered interventions designed to increase his engagement in meaningful participation.

Discussion

Emily believes that engaging in meaningful occupations is important in maintaining Eduardo's health and well-being and she discusses her beliefs about the health promoting properties of occupation with his mother and teacher. She uses a **client-centered approach** with Eduardo rather than being authoritative regarding his use of adaptive equipment. A client-centered approach involves respect and welcomes a partnership with Eduardo and his family; it recognizes Eduardo's autonomy and desires for making his own choices related to occupational needs (Law, Baptiste, & Mills, 1995). In order to foster an increased sense of teamwork and community participation, Emily recommends that classroom work and projects be completed with partners or in small groups. She additionally recommends that Eduardo join an afterschool video gaming club, which Eduardo has expressed an interest in attending. Emily has offered to help with the logistics of making it possible for him to attend, such as facilitating communications between Eduardo and school staff that are coaching the gaming club and helping Eduardo negotiate transportation issues necessary for him to attend the club.

SCHOOL-BASED OCCUPATIONAL THERAPY: A COMMUNITY-BASED PRACTICE

Occupational therapists working in the public schools have an opportunity to promote occupational therapy as a community practice that contributes to the mental and physical health of students in the school community. Health promotion, prevention, and wellness are all integral to community-based practice. Health promotion and prevention includes any "planned combination of educational, political, regulatory, environmental, and organizational supports of actions and conditions of living conducive to the health of individuals, groups, or communities" (Fazio, 2008, p. 30). Many schools are currently using a **three-tiered intervention approach** to academics called Response to Intervention (RtI), which is intended to increase the number of students who benefit from early intervention services, thus decreasing the need for special education instruction for children who might benefit from shorter term intensive services or differentiated instruction that incorporates a **universal design for learning (UDL)** approach in which learning is presented and expressed through a variety of accessible modalities (Center for Applied Special Technology, 2010). The RtI model's three-tiered system operates from a premise that 80% of students can benefit from whole class universal instruction (tier one), 15% of students need targeted instruction (tier two), and 5% of students, who have not responded to tier one or two instruction, require intensive interventions (tier three) (AOTA, 2007).

Many schools are also using RtI to address behavior. The application of a three-tiered system in this area is intended to create a positive environment for all students while at the same time explicitly teaching students positive social behaviors. Similar to the three-tiered approach to academic intervention, the behavioral health promotion model or **positive behavioral interventions and supports (PBIS)** can be used to address and intervene with psychosocial issues in the school community. Figure 22-2 depicts this three-tiered intervention commonly used to address academic and behavioral instruction.

In primary prevention, or tier 1, school- and classroom-wide systems of support are in place. These systems of support are preventive in nature and apply to all students and staff members across all contexts and environments. Tier 1 supports are a proactive approach to creating a positive school environment by developing incentives for adherence to school rules and by explicitly teaching prosocial behaviors. The overall purpose of primary interventions is to reduce the number of new behavioral difficulties through strategies such as explicit behavioral instruction, clear and consistent schoolwide expectations, and clear and consistent consequences.

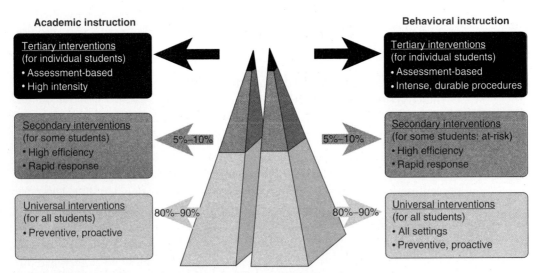

FIGURE 22-2. Designing Schoolwide Systems for Student Success

Used with permission from the OSEP Technical Assistance Center for Positive Behavior Interventions and Support (2010)

Explicit instruction can occur through curriculum adoption. Strong Kids (Merrell, Carrizales, Feuerborn, Gueldner, & Tran, 2007) is an example of a research-based social-emotional learning curriculum and has an elementary, middle, and high school component. Schools that have adopted schoolwide PBIS systems create, communicate, and review their behavioral expectations and consequences regularly with all students and staff members. Occupational therapist participation at this level involves supporting the school- and classroom-wide systems. Occupational therapists, like all other staff members, should be included in any professional development opportunities around the topic of PBIS implementation. Another way that occupational therapists could participate at this level would be participation on committees looking at curriculum adoption.

Secondary prevention, or tier 2, offers specialized group systems for students demonstrating at-risk behaviors. The main purpose of interventions at this level is to reduce the duration of existing psychosocial concerns. Identified team members, including counselors, occupational therapists, psychologists, and administrators, would complete informal behavioral assessments in order to identify the function of the problem behaviors. Tier 2 interventions are typically provided as small group instruction of students with identified risk factors and indicators of psychosocial dysfunction. These supports should supplement and not replace primary prevention. Supports at this level could also include environmental modifications. As occupational therapists are skilled in both task and environmental analysis, as well as group processes, tier 2 is well suited for occupational therapists to lend their unique lens of participation in meaningful activities.

Occupational therapist participation at tier 2 could be through the informal student assessment process that looks at the contexts and environments where the maladaptive behaviors are occurring. Occupational therapist participation at the secondary prevention level could also take place through leading small groups whereas issues of psychosocial dysfunction are addressed. Whether role playing prosocial behaviors with peers, or processing barriers to meaningful participation, occupational therapists are also a fit for tier 2 interventions.

Tertiary prevention, or tier 3, provides specialized and individualized systems for students with high-risk behaviors. The main purpose of this tier is to reduce the severity and frequency of behavioral incidents for the individual student. In this tier, students with severe and chronic psychosocial and mental health problems also undergo behavioral analysis. The analysis is likely more detailed at this tier than previous tiers resulting in individualized behavior intervention plans. As functional behavioral analyses are developed by teams, occupational therapists would not solely be responsible for their development, but would contribute to the process with their unique focus of participation through meaningful activities. Intense individualized interventions occur in tier 3. These, too, could be provided to a student by an occupational therapist.

Schoolwide systems of support for behavioral and psychosocial functioning can be addressed with a focus on prevention through a three-tiered system. Participation and intervention at all three tiers of prevention are well within the scope of occupational therapy practice. Occupational therapist participation in the PBIS system can be utilized with both student as client and system as client.

Children with Identified Mental Health Disabilities

Many mental health disorders that are described as severe emotional disturbances have their beginnings in childhood or adolescence (National Institute of Mental Health, 2010). The National Health and Nutritional Examination Survey found that 13% of children ages 8 to 15 had at least one mental disorder, such as depression, anxiety, attention deficit disorder, autism, or bipolar disorder—a rate that is comparable to diabetes, asthma, and other diseases of childhood (NIMH, 2010). Other research indicates that one in five children have a diagnosable mental health disorder such as anxiety, depression, conduct disorder, learning disability, and attention deficit hyperactivity disorder, while others experience social and emotional difficulties but do not meet diagnostic criteria (Koppelman, 2004). Of those students with mental health problems, only one in five are actually receiving needed services. Because of this, public schools are critical to the nation's mental health system. Children identified with emotional disturbances are served by the public schools more than any other agency (Beck et al., 2006).

Current practice patterns of occupational therapists working in the school system indicate that psychosocial needs of children with both emotional disturbances and physical disabilities are rarely addressed (Beck et al., 2006; Egilson & Hemmingsson, 2009; Egilson & Traustadottir, 2009). Current practice patterns of occupational therapists working in public schools, both in the United States and internationally, tend to focus on physical and sensory processing impairments and use developmental and sensory integrative frames of reference in interventions (Frolek-Clark, 2001; Simmons Carlsson, 2009; Spencer, Turkett, Vaughan, & Koenig, 2006). The founders of occupational therapy believed that engaging in occupations, the everyday activities that make life meaningful, provided an optimistic outlook for people who had physical and psychological disabilities. The founders viewed occupation as a means to addressing the holistic, mind and body needs, of individuals receiving occupational therapy (Schwartz, 2009). A paradigm shift occurred after World War II in which the profession of occupational therapy moved toward a medical model with a focus on interventions designed to remediate internal muscular and sensorimotor impairments (Schwartz, 2006). During this time a separation of physical and psychosocial practices developed and was carried over into pediatric- and school-based occupational therapy practices during the 1970s (Frolek-Clark, 2001). Practice patterns with a focus on the physical motor impairments of children have become ingrained traditions that influence the way occupational therapy is practiced in the school setting.

The introduction of documents such as the International Classification of Function (ICF) (World Health Organization, 2001) and the Occupational Therapy Practice Framework (OTPF) (AOTA, 2008) in the United States have provided guidance that promotes returning to the roots of the occupational therapy profession and integrating mind and body occupation-based intervention approaches. In the last decade the AOTA and many international occupational therapy associations and practicing bodies have sought ways to change the artificial separation of physical and mental health and promote the value of **occupation-based interventions** that are unique to our profession (Harrison & Forsyth, 2005; Miliken, Goodman, Bazyk, & Flinn, 2007). Occupational therapy has an opportunity to play a key role in education reform. Occupational therapy, as a profession, has a thorough understanding of how environmental contexts impact participation and social interactions that influence psychosocial well-being, and understands the benefits of using a student- and family-centered approach to interventions, meetings, and decision making. In addition, occupational therapy practitioners have the skills and knowledge to partner with community organizations to create innovative occupation-based programs to promote health and wellness in the school system (Maglio & McKinstry, 2008). Occupational therapy offers unique contributions to the team of school professionals who are working on school mental health issues. Occupational therapy's unique contributions to addressing psychosocial issues as part of a school mental health or academic intervention team is illustrated in Figure 22-3.

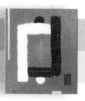

CASE ILLUSTRATION

Mikaela's Occupational Interests and Engagement

Mikaela is a student who is in a classroom for students with severe emotional and behavioral disorders. Mikaela often becomes angry, pushing over tables, stabbing herself with pencils, and ripping her clothes when she is frustrated. She has difficulty coping with situations that require problem solving or patience and gets upset when she believes somebody is making fun of her. She often has difficulty after returning from recess and her teacher and classroom staff believe her problems are due to sensory processing issues. Jonte is an occupational therapist who works with Mikaela's classroom and has become involved by setting up a classroom environment based on Mikaela's sensory profile. Jonte feels that collaboration with her teacher to support another intervention approach might offer more support for Mikaela in helping to cope with frustration.

Discussion

After attending an international occupational therapy conference, Jonte realizes the importance of occupations and occupational engagement as significant contributors to psychosocial well-being. Assessments of both the environment and Mikaela's occupational interests are important in planning client-centered interventions that will help Mikaela better cope with frustration. Mikaela can benefit from meaningful self-chosen occupation-based interventions that focus on coping skills. Jonte facilitates occupation-based interventions that can take place daily by collaborating with both Mikaela and her teacher.

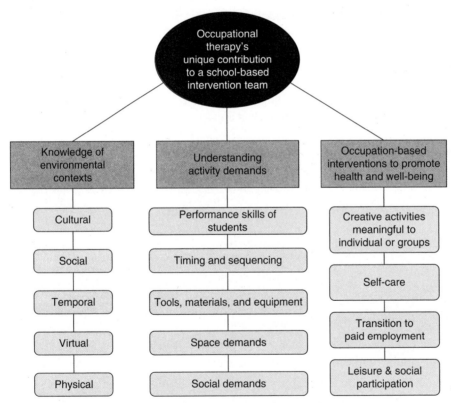

FIGURE 22-3. Occupational Therapy's Unique Contributions to a School-Based Intervention Team

© Cengage Learning 2013

Evaluation of Psychosocial Issues in the School Setting

Evaluations of students' psychosocial needs are often conducted as part of a team process and are an important part of planning tier 2 (secondary) or tier 3 (tertiary) interventions when framing the assessment from the view of a three-tiered intervention model. Assessments that are pertinent to addressing psychosocial issues in school-based practice are often used in conjunction with other school professionals and part of a collaborative team planning process, as well as a planning tool for intensive tier 3 level interventions by the school-based occupational therapist.

Occupational therapists in the school setting should strive to provide a client-centered approach to evaluation and interventions. During the assessment process it is important to involve the student, the student's family, and the child's teachers in obtaining an occupational profile. An occupational profile includes a summary of a student's occupational history, interests, strengths, and needs. Gathering information both formally and informally from stakeholders concerning their hopes, concerns, and goals is an important source of information. Occupational profile data will also provide the therapist a hypothesis regarding the reasons a student is having difficulties and assist the therapist in selecting appropriate assessments. It is also crucial to include the student in the development of meaningful goals in which they are invested in the outcome. The student's perspective is vital to developing client-centered, collaborative interventions that foster occupational engagement.

One of occupational therapy's strengths and unique contributions to a school team assessment process is the occupational therapist's skill in conducting thorough assessments of environmental contexts based on observations. Environmental assessments are a part of the analysis of occupational performance and are essential in determining the cause of many issues related to participation in academic and social activities during the school day. Interviews with students, family, and school staff in conjunction with environmental analysis are essential in determining the child's needs as they relate to the context of the environment and task. In addition, environmental analysis provides critical information to discussions related to tier 1 and tier 2 assessment and intervention of psychosocial skills at the classroom and building level.

Using the OTPF, the contexts that students encounter in the school setting can be assessed for facilitators and barriers to participation and psychosocial well-being. Occupational therapists can collaborate with the student, family, and other school professionals in helping to develop a better understandings of issues related to participation based on interrelated contextual factors that include the cultural, personal, temporal, virtual, physical, and social aspects of the environment.

Cultural

The occupational therapist can discover the cultural background of a student by asking students and/or families to participate in interviews such as the Cross Cultural Initial Interview and Observation (see Chapter 2). Increased rapport and a trusting relationship can result from developing a better understanding of a student's cultural background. Engaging the student and/or family in a discussion of their cultural values related to occupational performance lets the student know that you are interested in what is important to her or him. It is important to keep in mind that there is a great diversity in communication styles, views on time, religions, views on health and wellness, views on independence versus interdependence, views on quality of life, and views regarding meaningful participation. It is important to remember that the practitioner's views may be influencing what is deemed "in the best interest" of the student, and that the practitioner seek input from the student and their family when developing goals for the student.

Personal

It is important for occupational therapists to engage in client-centered practices that value the students' and their family's perspectives and goals. Occupational therapists have expertise in the analysis of actions and skills that comprise occupational performance in the school community. The occupational therapist can contribute to an in-depth understanding of the tasks and demands experienced in the personal context of the individual (Krupa, Fossey, Anthony, Brown, & Pitts, 2009).

Virtual

The virtual context is one of the most pervasive contexts in which adolescent students conduct their daily interactions, leading to both beneficial and damaging consequences. Computers and other technologies have provided access to materials and avenues to increased communication for students with physical and intellectual disabilities, facilitating participation in academic occupations. Cases of cyberbullying, the virtual form of bullying, are increasingly making news headlines. The rise in cyberbullying can be contributed to the rise in use of social media combined with instant text and photo messaging. It is important that school professionals are aware of the extent to which this virtual context is impacting the lives of the students in the school community and take measures to educate and provide interventions that emphasize this particular psychosocial context.

Temporal

When considering the temporal aspects of the school community contexts, it is important to understand the developmental stages of childhood and adolescence. Understanding that the preschool and early elementary years are developmentally devoted to learning through play and that adolescence is a time for learning about oneself through experiences with peers is important to understanding psychosocial issues that may be impacted by the temporal context. The school community is a group of children from ages 3 years to 21 years. Client-centered practices and assessment interviews can help to better understand the temporal context for individual students or groups of students. The occupational therapist should also assess the temporal context as it relates to valued occupations for students with disabilities. Students with disabilities may experience time differently than non-disabled peers. The expectations of time use by others in the environment (teachers, family, and peers) may need to be explored together with the student as an occupational justice issue. For example, if a student who has a physical disability impacting their fine motor skills is given excessive homework that involves writing and in-hand manipulation skills, it may take the student many hours to complete the work. This child's time is so impacted by completing homework that he or she has little time to engage in play, leisure, or health-promoting activities after school.

Physical

The physical environment consists of both the natural and built environments. The natural environment includes "geographic terrain, sensory qualities of the environment, plants and animals," while the built environment includes "buildings, furniture, tools or devices" (AOTA, 2008, p. 645). It is important for occupational therapists to be aware of these environments and how they may be contributing to participation or isolating students with and without disabilities, creating occupational disruptions and even marginalization. For example, if a student who uses a wheelchair cannot physically access areas of the school that are common for social congregation, he or she may feel isolated and left out of important peer interactions.

Social

The social environment consists of peers, teachers, and other people who are a part of the school community. Additionally the social context "is constructed by presence, relationships, and expectations of persons, organizations, and populations. Some factors affecting the social context and environment are the availability and expectations of significant individuals such as friends, teachers, caregivers, relationships with individuals, groups, or organizations, and relationships with systems (e.g., political, legal, economic, institutional) that are influential in establishing norms, role expectations, and social routines" (AOTA, 2008, p. 645). The social context can significantly impact a student's psychosocial well-being. For example, a school track coach approaches a student with a disability to be a part of the team as either a team manager or as a track and field participant, based on the students' desires. This illustrates how an influential community member seeking the student to be a valued part of the community can contribute to the child's feelings of self-esteem. In another example, a student with a disability is assigned to work with an educational assistant because the student needs help with many physical tasks. Over time this student becomes more removed from peer interactions and focuses on the interactions with the educational assistant rather than with his peer group. This student is experiencing occupational deprivation since he lacks peer friendship relationships and social interactions that are typical to childhood development. When considering the environmental contexts of the school, observation and interviews with staff, students, and families can provide a client-centered perspective of the experience of being a member of the school community. Observations by the occupational therapist as well as interviews with stakeholders can provide insightful information about the relationship between the environment and meaningful participation. Shepherd and Hanft (2008, pp. 234–236) discuss environmental contexts that are important to consider in the school setting. Figure 22-4 provides questions that can be used to guide an environmental assessment (Shepherd and Hanft, 2008, pp. 234–236).

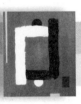

CASE ILLUSTRATION

Eduardo—Assessment of Psychosocial Issues in Adolescence

Eduardo, the ninth-grader with a diagnosis of Duchenne muscular dystrophy, faces difficulties engaging in occupations at home and at school. Eduardo is concerned about the differences between himself and his peers and has at times refused to use the adaptive equipment that has been purchased for him. Emily, his occupational therapist, is concerned about Eduardo's motivation to use the adaptive equipment and thinks that he may be depressed. It is difficult to engage him in conversation when Emily tries to talk to Eduardo about his needs. Emily thinks that Eduardo is depressed and wonders how he deals emotionally with the knowledge of his prognosis. She is not sure what to do since he is reluctant to talk with her. She decides to check in with Eduardo every week and tries to build rapport through conversations and a helpful attitude, although she is not sure that this is the best approach. She feels that she should be addressing psychosocial issues with Eduardo but she needs more information.

Discussion

Emily feels it is important to discuss her concerns about Eduardo's possible depression with his family in order to learn more about his situation and address concerns that they may be having. After discussing this situation with Eduardo's mother, Emily decides to utilize interventions that will increase the development of rapport between her and Eduardo as well as look closely at his school environment. She selects activities that will be meaningful to Eduardo and that may also solicit more expressive communication about his feelings rather than just relying on direct interviewing. She and the advisory teacher co-teach a unit called "personal culture" in order to solicit and provide opportunities for telling life stories. Following the personal culture unit, Emily meets with Eduardo individually and learns a great deal about the issues that Eduardo is experiencing (as well as those of his peers) and has some ideas for environmental considerations and occupation-based activities that she would like to share with his teacher.

In addition to environmental analysis and interviews, occupational therapists often utilize a variety of assessments that focus on psychosocial well-being in conducting an analysis of occupational performance. Table 22-3 provides descriptions of some of the assessments used to address psychosocial needs and occupational engagement in the school setting.

Psychosocial Occupational Therapy Interventions in the Schools

The use of occupation to promote health and well-being is one of occupational therapy's unique contributions to a health care intervention team, as well as a school-based academic and psychosocial intervention team. Occupational therapy is unique in its skill to look at the client, the occupation, and the environment as intertwined in the pursuit of participation and occupational engagement. Developing occupation-based interventions at all levels (tiers 1, 2, and 3) is within the scope of occupational therapists working in the school setting.

Determining occupation-based interventions is a collaborative client-centered process. Creative activities are occupation-based interventions when they are meaningful to the client due to the nature of the activity being a personally constructed individual experience (Pierce, 2001). Creative activities involve imagination and have a meaningful product, one that may either be concrete such as a piece of writing or artwork, or more abstract such as the creation of original ideas (Creek, 2002). When creative activities provide meaning and value, they provide a "versatile treatment medium with wide opportunities for choice and self-determination" (Griffiths, 2008, p. 61).

Occupation-based interventions can also focus on developing advocacy and coping skills. Individual or group activities that focus on these skills support participation and occupational engagement. Table 22-4 describes interventions that promote psychosocial well-being.

When considering the environmental contexts of the school, observation and interviews with staff, students, and families can provide a client-centered perspective of the experience of being a member of the school community. Observations by the occupational therapist as well as interviews with stakeholders can provide insightful information about the relationship between the environment and meaningful participation.

CULTURAL ENVIRONMENT

Are there activities that reflect the cultural diversity of the school?

Are there activities that reflect the cultural diversity of the classroom?

Is there acceptance of diversity in students?

Are differences in customs, ethnicity, beliefs, and values considered and respected?

Do teaching practices consider the cultural environment of the students?

Are universal behavior standards equitably applied and enforced?

SOCIAL ENVIRONMENT

Are there opportunities for peer interaction; barriers to peer interaction?

Are students provided with equal access to the social environments of the school community (recess, activities, physical access)?

What are the expectations of the student in the classroom and across school environments (rules and school routines)?

TEMPORAL ENVIRONMENT

Is the activity or routine age appropriate?

How long does the activity last?

What is the timing and sequence of the activity?

Is the time of day a factor in participation?

Is the amount of time to complete an activity a factor influencing participation in meaningful occupations?

VIRTUAL ENVIRONMENT

Do students use computers in the classroom?

In other school environments?

Are there rules about electronic device use at school such as texting and social media?

Are school materials available in electronic formats?

What types of technology are used in the classroom (interactive whiteboards, document cameras, etc.)?

Are assistive technologies needed or will universally designed technology be more appropriate?

PHYSICAL ENVIRONMENT/ACCESS

Are all areas of the school building (classroom, bathroom, gym, etc.) and grounds accessible?

Are there curb cuts, doors that can be opened at entrances?

Is the classroom space accessible?

Does the size of classroom/arrangement/number of students/classroom space impact participation? Are school materials accessible?

Is school furniture appropriately sized?

Sensory characteristics of the Physical Environment (tactile/kinesthetic, auditory, visual, movement):

Consider the lighting, acoustics, space, arrangement, noise level, extraneous noises, textures (materials, furniture, carpet, etc.), proximity to others, visual schedules, decorations in the classroom, and movement opportunities.

Do the sensory aspects of the classroom and other school environments impact participation and psychosocial well-being?

FIGURE 22-4. School Environmental Contexts: Does the Environment Support Psychosocial Well-Being?

TABLE 22-3. Psychosocial Assessments in the School Setting

Name of Assessment	Age Range	Purpose
Canadian Occupational Performance Measure, 4th Edition (COPM) (Law et al., 2005)	8 years to adult	Semi-structured interview questions used with individual students as an outcome measure. It is designed for use by occupational therapists to identify change in a student's self-perception of occupational performance over time (Canadian Association of Occupational Therapists, 2005).
Children's Assessment of Participation and Enjoyment & Preferences for Activities of Children (CAPE/PAC) (King, et al., 2004)	6–12 years	A measure designed to document how children with or without disabilities participate in everyday activities outside of school and to identify preferred activities. The CAPE/PAC can be used as a planning tool for designing after school health and activity groups.
Child Occupation Self Assessment (COSA) (Keller, Kafkes, Basu, Frederico, & Kielhofner, 2005)	Elementary through high school ages	A client-centered assessment tool that addresses dynamic social participation needs of the adolescent and allows a child to share perceptions about competence and values.
Coopersmith Self-Esteem Inventory School Form (CSEI-School Form) (Coopersmith, 2002)	8–15 years	Demonstrates the relationship of academic achievement to personal satisfaction in school life. Can be used for diagnosis, classroom screening, and pre-post evaluation.
Piers-Harris Children's Self Concept Scale, Second Edition (Piers-Harris-2) (Piers, Harris, & Herzberg, 2002)	7–18 years	Provides view of an individual's self-perception and helps identify psychosocial issues children and adolescents are experiencing in their environment. Can be used to identify specific problem areas, coping and defense mechanisms, and to facilitate the development of suitable intervention techniques.
School Setting Interview (SSI) (Hemmingsson, Egilson, Hoffman, & Kielhofner, 2005)	Middle Elementary through high school (approximately age 10 and older)	A client-centered assessment that examines the level of student-environment fit for students with physical disabilities (can be used with other groups). Facilitates planning of OT interventions in schools.
The School Function Assessment (SFA) (Coster, Deeney, Haltiwanger, & Haley, 1998)	Elementary	Measures physical, cognitive, and behavioral participation. Determines the student's ability to participate successfully in the education program using a top-down approach looking at social participation, task performance, activity performance, and functions and structures causing impairment.
Sensory Profile (Dunn, 1999); Sensory Profile School Companion (Dunn, 2006) Adolescent/Adult Sensory Profile (Brown & Dunn, 2002)	3–10 years 3–11 years 11 years and older	Questionnaires that identify responses to sensory events in a child/adolescent's daily life. Information can be used to develop goals, make accommodations, and determine appropriate modifications and interventions.

TABLE 22-4. Psychosocial Interventions in the Schools

Intervention	Purpose
OCCUPATION-BASED CREATIVE ACTIVITIES ■ Making a card and writing a letter to someone the student chooses ■ Making a collage that depicts valued roles and occupations ■ Making a timeline related to one's life ■ Creative play that involves role playing, storytelling, and acting ■ Creating rap (or other genre) songs ■ Creating a web of ideas using an electronic graphic organizer ■ Pretend play ■ Childhood play activities ■ Creative drama, arts and crafts	Creative activities are occupations when they are meaningful to the client due to the nature of the activity being a personally constructed individual experience (Pierce, 2001). When creative activities provide meaning and value they provide a "versatile treatment medium with wide opportunities for choice and self-determination" (Griffiths, 2008, p. 61).
EDUCATION/HEALTH LITERACY	Occupational therapists can provide education to students about psychosocial issues and teach students information literacy skills to access reliable and accurate information about their own health. When introduced to informational tools, students can develop confidence in managing their health and wellness.
SELF-ADVOCACY/DISABILITY IDENTITY	Children with disabilities may encounter social and occupational injustices and can benefit from developing advocacy skills to meet their needs. Children who have disabilities are often faced with a consistent focus on improving their impairments, which can erode self-confidence and feeling of values (Kielhofner, 2005). Occupational therapists can introduce students and families to literature and experiences that can facilitate the development of a positive disability identity.
SOCIAL SKILL GROUPS OR FRIENDSHIP CLUBS	Learning and practicing social skills in a supportive setting can be an important intervention for developing self-esteem and a sense of belonging. The group members can work together to choose enjoyable activities as the context for practicing the social skills. Situations where a student becomes a "reading buddy" or "art buddy" by reading books or creating art projects with younger children (or facilitating situations where younger children receive encouragement from an older "buddy" student) can promote psychosocial well-being.
SOCIAL SUPPORT GROUPS	Groups consisting of like participants or adult community member mentors can lead to increased self-esteem, better attitudes toward school and the future, acquisition of new skills, an increase in positive relationships, and increased confidence (Journey & Loukas, 2009). Occupational therapists can help to establish and facilitate mentoring programs between students and community members.

TABLE 22-4. Continued

Intervention	Purpose
OCCUPATION-BASED IN- OR AFTER-SCHOOL GROUPS ■ Walking club ■ Gardening club ■ Healthy cooking/eating club ■ Dance club ■ Language clubs ■ Knitting or crocheting club ■ Video game clubs ■ Board or card game clubs ■ Creative writing club/anime club	Occupational therapists can play a vital role and should consider collaborating with other school professionals to write grants or develop in-school or after-school programs with available funding for activities that promote school mental and physical health.

© Cengage Learning 2013

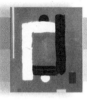

CASE ILLUSTRATION

Alex—The Experience of Multiple Psychosocial Issues

Alex is a fourth-grade student with Asperger's syndrome. He is in a classroom for highly capable students. Alex lives with his mother and two siblings and his parents have recently divorced, a situation that has been distressing to Alex. His teacher states that Alex's behavioral disruptions in the classroom and other school environment are becoming a problem. He often blurts out irrelevant information or repeats what his teacher is saying aloud. In addition, Alex has difficulty maintaining positive and rewarding relationships with peers and he has experienced bullying by peers. Alex struggles with self-image and says peers have called him fat and made fun of him because he is overweight. His mother is concerned about his safety and reports that Alex was attacked by some other students on the playground recently and came home with bruises. Lately, Alex has had difficulties riding the school bus and has gotten into fights with much younger students even when he is assigned a front row seat. There are also concerns about Alex bullying more vulnerable students and school staff have observed instances when he has become verbally abusive to students he described as "dumb."

Discussion

Several issues surrounding Alex's situation need to be addressed by the school including bullying and school violence. Proactive steps to prevent bullying and violence need to be implemented promptly by the school intervention team, which consists of administrator, counselor, psychologist, occupational therapist, speech language pathologist, nurse, classroom teacher, and special education teacher. Tier 1 interventions directed at all students need to be considered and implemented to address the bullying and violence that Alex and other students are experiencing as well as propagating. In addition, Alex would benefit from tier 2 and tier 3 interventions that are client-centered and specific to his situation. Table 22-5 describes a school intervention team approach to identifying goals to prevent school violence and bullying while also addressing Alex's specific needs.

TABLE 22-5. An Intervention Plan Focusing on Prevention and Specific Psychosocial Skills

Goal	Tier Intervention Rationale	Interventions
GOAL #1 Student will participate in classroom discussions without repeating the teacher's statements or making irrelevant comments.	Tier 3: Specially designed instruction and/or accommodations needed for this student. He has an Individual Education Plan (IEP).	Tier 3: School team, student, and family collaborate to determine appropriate classroom signals (visual cues and hand signals) to indicate to the student when a disruption is occurring. Individual sessions using role playing and social stories may be conducted by designated team members.
	Tier 2: Targeted students (not receiving specially designed instruction or accommodations) can benefit from small group instruction related to sensory processing and modulation management	Tier 2: Occupational therapist and another team member facilitate sensory processing and modulation program designed to increase awareness and management of sensory processing issues for a small group.
	Tier 1: All students can benefit from learning about sensory processing information for self-regulating techniques and better understanding of learning styles, as well as to increase understanding of other students' experiences.	Tier 1: Whole classroom activity about sensory processing can be facilitated by occupational therapist and team members such as counselor or special education teacher.
GOAL #2 Decrease incidences of bullying experienced by student.	Tier 3: Student chooses to develop a presentation on Asperger's syndrome to share with his classroom. The development of the presentation helps increase self-awareness and facilitate psychosocial well-being. Preparing the presentation using a variety of technology is an occupation that is self-chosen and meaningful to the student.	Tier 3: Occupational therapist will work with classroom teacher and student to provide 3–4 sessions in order for student to plan a classroom educational presentation designed to increase peer awareness regarding his disability.

TABLE 22-5. Continued

Goal	Tier Intervention Rationale	Interventions
	Tier 2: Classroom instruction specific to the student's situation is helpful in developing empathy	Tier 2: Occupational therapist will be part of the school team that creates activities for small groups who have engaged in bullying or experienced bullying. Groups are designed to increase empathy using occupation-based activities such as creative drama and storytelling.
	Tier 1: All students benefit from increased empathy by learning about differences. Student conducts classroom presentation about his disability.	Tier 1: Members of school team and family will work with classroom after presentation to discuss Asperger's syndrome.
GOAL #3 Decrease incidences of student bullying other children.	Tier 3: Specially designed instruction is needed to address bullying prevention with this student. This may be carried out by identified members of school team	Tier 3: Development of visual social stories and problem-solving sessions with identified members of school team to encourage empathy toward others for a period of 6–8 weeks.
	Tier 2: Some students need targeted small group work to develop increased awareness and coping skills related to bullying.	Tier 2: Inclusion in a friendship group taught by two members of the school-based intervention team.
	Tier 1: All students benefit from interventions related to bullying.	Tier 1: School team develops presentation that includes discussion and occupation-based activities (i.e., story-telling, dramatic skits) that facilitate empathy among students.
GOAL #4 Increase participation in habits and routines that promote health.	Tier 1: All students will benefit from activities that promote health.	Tier 1: School intervention team develops a schoolwide program with money received from a grant the team worked on together. Activities include: 1. Gardening project all students take part in. 2. Once a month classroom time devoted to a cooking group that focuses on healthy eating/snacks. 3. Walk to school days. 4. Building a walking track on the school grounds and starting an incentive walking club.

Intervention Service Delivery Models

When considering psychosocial interventions in the school setting, it is important to look at the job description and duties of the school-based occupational therapist. Job descriptions are important in determining the workload of the occupational therapist. Many school-based occupational therapists are trying to address the issue of **workload vs. caseload**, emphasizing the importance of the occupational therapist being available for systems interventions such as participating in early intervening service for all students rather than just the small percentage of students who receive occupational therapy services as part of their individual education program that is at the tertiary level of service (Swinth, 2008). When discussing workload vs. caseload, occupational therapists are often referring to the service delivery model as well. The workload service delivery model consists of collaborative services provided by the occupational therapist to students within the context of their natural school environments such as the classroom, cafeteria, recess, bus, and so on. The occupational therapist works closely with the student and the student's teachers to optimize the student's participation in the school environment. Participation in the school setting includes many activities, with an emphasis on academics and social and peer interactions.

In contrast, the caseload service delivery model is often practiced using a set schedule that consists of students scheduled to leave the classroom to attend occupational therapy services. This type of intervention service has been termed a pull-out service delivery model, or out of context intervention (Swinth, 2008). In this out of context service delivery model, students leave the classroom and go to a separate workspace to address their occupational therapy goals that typically consist of sensorimotor-based interventions to remediate motor skill impairments.

It is important that occupational therapists strive to develop a workload service delivery model to enable psychosocial services that are needed at a systems level. Caseloads have traditionally been based on the number of students receiving hands-on services, which provides little time for the occupational therapist to address environmental factors at the systems level that may be impacting participation of many students, contributing to psychosocial issues that go unaddressed. In contrast, the concept of workload recognizes the ways that an occupational therapist might apply their expertise to issues happening in classrooms, in school buildings, and at the educational system level (Swinth, 2008). Research indicates that a collaborative occupational therapy service delivery approach, in which the occupational therapist works with classrooms and other school environments, provides outcomes that are as effective as individual occupational therapy services provided in an out of context setting (Sayers, 2008). The provision of collaborative services as part of a school team provides an opportunity for occupational therapists to address issues at the school building level and provides for time to address psychosocial needs of students using the three-tiered intervention approach.

Striving for a workload model of service delivery is ideal; however, using caseload to determine the scope of occupational therapy services in the school setting continues to be the prevalent practice of school-based occupational therapists who are employed to work directly in the schools (Beck et al., 2006; Spencer et al., 2006). Keeping this in mind it is important to realize that if you are practicing from a caseload model, evolving to a **collaborative service delivery model**, one in which OT services are part of a team approach to intervention such as described in Table 22-5, will be a process that involves change on many levels and requires that you convince others to make this change with you. Making changes to entrenched practices can be difficult and requires a plan of action. If you are new to this practice setting tackling systemic change may seem daunting. Addressing psychosocial issues with individual students that you are already familiar with is a good place to begin adding psychosocial occupational therapy to your practice within the school community.

If you are practicing from a caseload model, you can take steps to incorporate psychosocial interventions with individual students as you plan actions for the process of making systemic changes. The case illustration of Eduardo provides an example of how an occupational therapist can begin to think about addressing psychosocial needs of an individual student as well as expanding services to a broader classroom context. The following case illustration describes an experienced occupational therapist's actions toward instituting change.

CASE ILLUSTRATION

Martin—A Plan for Change

Martin has worked as an occupational therapist in the public school system for over 10 years. He feels that he should be addressing psychosocial issues with students but is hesitant to provide occupational therapy services in this area as it is a shift from traditional school-based practices.

Historically, his job duties have been determined by his caseload, which consists of scheduled times to work individually with students who have sensorimotor impairments throughout the day. Working strictly from a caseload model is not conducive to providing preventative interventions for students not on the caseload who are experiencing psychosocial issues such as beginning signs of mental health problems, eating disorders, bullying, violence, and other psychosocial issues. Martin believes that a collaborative intervention model will allow him to engage in a primary prevention model of health care in addition to his focus on the outcomes for students on his caseload. He has read journal articles that indicate that the students he sees individually can receive equivalent positive outcomes using a collaborative intervention model and he believes that it is in the children's best interest to receive services in natural school environments.

Discussion

Collaborative intervention services involve observing students in the classroom and working with teachers and students to increase their participation both in the classroom and across the school environment. As Martin collaborates with teachers he will inevitably encounter and become familiar with students who are experiencing psychosocial issues that puts them "at risk" for negative mental health outcomes. Using a collaborative approach to intervention Martin will have the time to focus more systemically with school buildings at the primary and secondary prevention levels. Martin realizes that he needs to convince his colleagues, administrators, and families that this is an evidence-based practice idea that will benefit all involved and he develops an action plan to begin making changes. Table 22-6 illustrates the action plan to enact change.

TABLE 22-6. Steps to Change: Establishing a Focus on Psychosocial Well-Being for All Students

Action	Purpose
Find and disseminate research that supports a collaborative service model.	Increase comfort level of colleagues and administrators and demonstrate that it is an evidence-based practice.
Find and disseminate research articles that discuss psychosocial issues and interventions.	Increase the comfort level of colleagues and administrators and demonstrate the importance of utilizing the full scope of OT practice.
Start a journal club with the articles that have been collected and disseminated regarding collaboration or psychosocial issues in the schools.	Meet professional development responsibilities while providing education on evidence-based practices and best practices related to a collaborative service model that supports interventions addressing psychosocial well-being.
Discuss ideas with administrators and colleagues to make small changes that are implemented gradually regarding psychosocial OT interventions at the primary (tier 1) and secondary (tier 2). The journal club or staff meetings may be a good venue for such discussions.	Change is difficult to implement in entrenched institutional cultures. Gradual changes are often more effective and accepted.
Implement changes at one school building.	Gradual changes at one school can then be replicated in other buildings.
Become involved in interdisciplinary team meetings at the school that discuss psychosocial issues or student behaviors.	To lend a unique perspective to the school intervention team.

TABLE 22-6. Continued

Action	Purpose
Talk with the building administrator at the school where you are going to implement changes and share information about occupational therapy's unique contributions to a school-based intervention team in addressing psychosocial issues. Discuss occupational therapy's holistic perspective on health and well-being.	It is important to let others know of the benefits and unique contributions occupational therapy can bring to an intervention team. Many other professionals are not informed about the benefits of occupational therapy and it our duty to educate others if we are to be a sustainable profession.
Inform the building administrator of any change in service delivery. For example, if you are striving the change from a caseload to workload service delivery model let the administrator know your reasons for this change and why evidence supports this change.	Building administrators are responsible for everything that occurs within their building. It is important that they stay informed of any changes and they will be more supportive when there is an open line of communication.
Inform students and families of any changes to service delivery model and explain why these changes will be to their benefit.	It is important to practice client-centered occupational therapy and students and families should be involved in all decision-making regarding service delivery.
Make changes to paperwork that reflects any changes in service delivery identified in existing documents.	To remain in compliance with existing procedures and laws.
Collect data on implemented changes such as outcomes of a collaborative versus caseload service delivery model.	To document efficacy of services provided by occupational therapy.

© Cengage Learning 2013

ACTIONS TO ADDRESS PSYCHOSOCIAL ISSUES IN THE SCHOOL SETTING

There is a need for an occupational therapy presence at the systemic level of the schools to address cultural, social, physical, and institutional factors external to individuals that influence occupation and meaningful participation in the school community (Krupa et al., 2009). Occupational therapists can take actions to promote occupational justice for students in the school environment through communication, building professional relationships with colleagues, and diplomatic advocacy strategies. Occupational therapists can use an occupational justice perspective when working individually with students by incorporating client-centered interventions, teaching and encouraging self-advocacy, and providing tools to help children with physical and psychosocial disabilities with the development of a positive disability identity that affirms they are a valued member of the community (Kielhofner, 2005).

An occupational justice framework is particularly needed at the classroom, building, and organizational levels since systemic policy and procedures often inadvertently create injustices. Occupational therapists can and should take steps to implement systemic changes that encourage occupationally just practices in the school setting. Table 22-7 provides ideas for actions that can be taken to promote psychosocial well-being at the individual, classroom, building, and organizational levels within the school system.

TABLE 22-7. Actions to Promote Psychosocial Well-Being for All Students

Level	Action
Individual	Encourage students to meet their needs by engaging in self-advocacy at the organizational or legislative level. They may consider writing a letter to the special education director, the board of directors, a letter to the editor, and/or a letter or phone call to a legislator.
Classroom	Provide in-service to teachers and other school staff on issues such as the benefits of occupation-based interventions to promote health and strategies to address behavioral issues in the classroom using a sensory processing frame of reference.
Classroom/Building	Environmental observation and analysis, sharing results with school staff.
Building	■ Collaboration at multidisciplinary team meetings with the occupational therapist utilizing a top-down approach and focusing on issues related to occupation and participation rather than impairments. ■ Interdisciplinary collaboration to promote psychosocial well-being for all students, particularly for tier 1 and tier 2 interventions as described in Table 22-5. ■ Promote participation and inclusion in after school and extracurricular activities by leading an activity or collaborating with other staff to develop programs or write grants. The occupational therapist can assist with adaptations to include students with diverse physical and psychosocial needs or to problem solve ideas regarding participation of a specific student. ■ Advocate for student and family centered meetings, goals, interventions, and decision making.
Building/Organization	■ Advocate for universal design and access to building, classrooms, restrooms, computers, toys, outdoor facilities (playground/field), desks, and chairs. Universally designed environments, tools, materials, and other objects provide ease of use, accessibility, and safety (Canadian Association of Occupational Therapists, 2003). ■ Advocate to school decision makers for staff education when issues of cultural competence and sensitivity appear to be impacting a student's participation and inclusion in the school community.
Organization	■ Advocate for universal policies for behavioral supports that are implemented across school environments. Programs that support universal policies are equitable for all students since they develop a continuum of evidence-based behavior and academic interventions and supports that utilize data to make decisions and solve problems, arrange the environment to prevent the development and occurrence of problem behavior, teach and encourage prosocial skills and behaviors, and are universally and continuously implemented through screenings and collection of data (U.S. Department of Education, Office of Special Education Programs, 2010).

TABLE 22-7. Continued

Level	Action
	■ Plan and arrange meetings with district decision makers (i.e., special education director, superintendent, school board meetings) to promote the role of occupational therapy in the implementation of a district-wide adoption of a universal behavioral supports program. For example, the OTPF environmental contexts can be discussed to help others develop a better understanding of occupational therapy's expertise in environmental assessments that support a universal behavioral support program (AOTA, 2009). ■ Advocate for universal design features in new school buildings. An occupational therapist and a student with a physical disability might work together to attend planning committee meetings conducted by the school board and school district. A student or parent with a physical disability might consider writing letters to the school board, architects, and engineers involved in the design of the building. ■ Advocate for school policies that promote participation and inclusion of students with diverse needs in extracurricular activities (i.e., transportation that is physically and financially accessible). ■ Psychosocial needs of students with significant disabilities who are transitioning from the school community into the community at large need greater focus. Occupational therapists can seek opportunities to partner with community organizations to create programs that will decrease occupational disruption for these young people. It is important that these young adults have access to community venues to maintain the friendships and social supports that are currently in place in the school setting as they transition to the adult community.

© Cengage Learning 2013

SUMMARY

An important role of school-based occupational therapists is to address the psychosocial needs of students in the school community in collaboration with other school professionals, students, and families. All students encounter psychosocial issues at some point and these issues can range from environmental and situational stressors, to school violence, bullying, abuse and/or neglect, to psychiatric mental health disorders. It is crucial that occupational therapists are involved in addressing psychosocial issues at the systems level to lend the unique expertise that occupational therapy can provide. Knowledge of occupation-based interventions, knowledge of environmental factors, knowledge of activity demands as well as the knowledge of how the environment, activity, and personal factors are interrelated to influence participation and meaningful occupation are all unique contributions that occupational therapy can bring to a school-based intervention team when working with students in the school community.

Psychosocial needs can be addressed using a three-tiered model of intervention in which 80% of children can benefit from universal programs designed to elicit social and emotional well-being (primary level), 15% of children are "at-risk" for psychosocial problems and need more focused interventions (secondary level), and 5% of children, who do not respond to interventions at the primary or secondary level, need more intense interventions at the tertiary level of care. Occupational therapists can be an integral member of the school intervention team dealing with psychosocial needs of students at all levels of need and providing targeted interventions as needed.

Occupational therapists may have to start at the grassroots level and begin to advocate and take actions to make changes in current school practice to incorporate prevention and intervention of psychosocial issues in the school community. Assuming a broader scope of occupational therapy practice while using an occupational justice perspective to tackle issues at the systems level can significantly contribute to the psychosocial well-being of all children and adolescents in the school community.

REVIEW QUESTIONS

1. What are the occupational injustices that a child/student could encounter in the school community?
2. How can occupational therapists support interventions for children/students across the tiers in a school system?
3. What assessment tools are available for examining psychosocial well-being in school-aged children?
4. How can occupational therapists support psychosocial well-being of children/students at a systemic level?
5. What steps could an occupational therapy practitioner take to begin addressing the psychosocial needs of students in the school setting if this role is not currently being undertaken by occupational therapy due to the culture of the workplace?

REFERENCES

American Occupational Therapy Association (AOTA). (2004). Psychosocial aspects of occupational therapy. *American Journal of Occupational Therapy, 58,* 669–672.

American Occupational Therapy Association (AOTA). (2007). *Frequently asked questions on response to intervention for school-based occupational therapists and occupational therapy assistants.* Retrieved from http://www.aota.org/Practitioners/Practice Areas/Pediatrics/Highlights/FAQonRtI.aspx

American Occupational Therapy Association (AOTA). (2008). Occupational therapy practice framework: Domain and process (2nd ed.). *American Journal of Occupational Therapy, 62,* 625–683.

American Occupational Therapy Association (AOTA). (2009). *Raising the bar: Elevating knowledge in school mental health.* Retrieved from http://www.aota.org/Practitioners/ProfDev/CE/Aota/Webcasts/School-MH.aspx

Bazyk, S. (2007). Addressing mental health needs of children in schools. In L. Jackson (Ed.), *Occupational therapy services for children and youth under IDEA* (3rd ed., p. 99–121). Bethesda, MD: AOTA Press.

Beck, A. J., Barnes, K. J., Vogel, K. A., & Grice, K. O. (2006). The dilemma of psychosocial occupational therapy in public schools: The therapists' perceptions. *Occupational Therapy in Mental Health, 22,* 1–17.

Brown, C., & Dunn, W. (2002). *Adolescent/adult sensory profile.* San Antonio, TX: Psychological Corporation.

Canadian Association of Occupational Therapists. (2003). Canadian Association of Occupational Therapists Position Statement: Universal design and occupational therapy. *Canadian Journal of Occupational Therapy, 70*(3), 187–190.

Canadian Association of Occupational Therapists. (2005). A description of the Canadian Occupational Performance Measure. Retrieved from http://www.caot.ca/copm/description.html

Center for Applied Special Technology (CAST). (2010). *Universal design for learning.* Retrieved from http://www.cast.org/index.html

Coopersmith, S. (2002). *Revised Coopersmith self-esteem inventory manual.* Redwood, CA: Mind Garden, Inc.

Coster, W. J., Deeney, T., Haltiwanger, J., & Haley, S. M. (1998). *School Function Assessment manual.* San Antonio, TX: Psychological Corporation.

Creek, J. (2002). *Occupational therapy and mental health* (3rd ed.). Edinburgh: Churchill Livingstone.

Curtis, P. (2008). The experience of young people with obesity in secondary school: Some implications for the healthy school agenda. *Health and Social Care in the Community, 16*(4), 410–418.

DeJaeghere, J. G., & Zhang, Y. (2008). Development of intercultural competence among US American teachers: Professional development factors that enhance competence. *Intercultural Education, 19*(3), 255–268.

Dunn, W. (1999). *Sensory profile.* San Antonio, TX: Psychological Corporation.

Dunn, W. (2006). *Sensory profile school companion.* San Antonio, TX: Psychological Corporation.

Egilson, S., & Hemmingsson, H. (2009). School participation of pupils with physical and psychosocial limitations: a comparison. *British Journal of Occupational Therapy, 72*, 144–152.

Egilson, S. T., & Traustadottir, R. (2009). Participation of students with physical disabilities in the school environment. *American Journal of Occupational Therapy, 63*, 264–272.

Fazio, L. S. (2008). *Developing occupation-centered programs for the community* (2nd ed.). Upper Saddle River, Pearson Prentice Hall.

Frolek-Clark, G. (2001). Children often overlooked for occupational therapy services in educational settings. AOTA *School System Special Interest Section Quarterly, 8*(3), 1–3.

Griffiths, S. (2008). The experience of creative activity. *Journal of Mental Health, 17*(1), 49–63.

Harrison, M., & Forsyth, K. (2005). Developing a vision for the therapists working within child and adolescent mental health services: Poised or paused for action? *British Journal of Occupational Therapy, 68*(4), 181–185.

Hemmingsson, H., & Borell, L. (2002). Environmental barriers in mainstream schools. *Child Care, Health and Development, 28*, 57–63.

Hemmingsson, H., Egilson, S., Hoffman, O., & Kielhofner, G. (2005). *A user's manual for The School Setting Interview (SSI).* Version 3.0. The Swedish Association of Occupational Therapists available through the Model of Human Occupation Clearinghouse at University of Illinois at Chicago. Chicago: MOHO Clearinghouse.

Humphrey, N., & Lewis, S. (2008). 'Make me normal': The views and experiences of pupils on the autistic spectrum in mainstream secondary schools. *Autism: The International Journal of Research & Practice, 12*, 23–46.

Jones, S. E., Fisher, C., Greene, B. Z., Hertz, M. F., & Pritzl, J. (2007). Healthy and safe school environments, part I: Results from the school health policies and programs study 2006. *The Journal of School Health, 77*(8), 522–543.

Journey, B. J., & Loukas, K. M. (2009). Adolescents with disability in school-based practice: Psychosocial intervention recommendations for a successful journey to adulthood. *Journal of Occupational Therapy, Schools, & Early Intervention, 2*, 119–132.

Keller, J., Kafkes, A., Basu, S., Federico, J., & Kielhofner, G. (2005). *Child Occupational Self Assessment* (Version 2.1). Chicago: MOHO Clearinghouse.

Kielhofner, G. (2005). Rethinking disability and what to do about it: Disability studies and its implication for occupational therapy. *American Journal of Occupational Therapy, 59*(5), 487–496.

King, G., Law, M., King, S., Hurley, P., Hanna, S., Kertoy, M., Rosenbaum, P., et al. (2004). *Children's Assessment of Participation and Enjoyment (CAPE) and Preferences for Activities of Children (PAC)*. San Antonio, TX: Harcourt Assessment, Inc.

Koppelman, J. (2004). Children with mental disorders: Making sense of their needs and systems that help them. (NHPF Issue Brief No. 799). Washington, DC: National Health Policy Forum, George Washington University.

Krupa, T., Fossey, E., Anthony, W. A., & Pitts, D. B. (2009). Doing daily life: How occupational therapy can inform psychiatric rehabilitation practice. *Psychiatric Rehabilitation Journal, 32*(3), 155–161.

Law, M. (2002). Distinguished scholar lecture: Participation in the occupations of everyday life. *American Journal of Occupational Therapy, 56*, 640–649.

Law, M., Baptiste, S., Carswell, A., McColl, M. A., Polatajko, H., & Pollock, N. (2005). *Canadian Occupational Performance Measure manual* (4th ed.). Toronto, ON: CAOT Publications ACE.

Law, M., Baptiste, S., & Mills, J. (1995). Client-centered practice: What does it mean and does it make a difference? *Canadian Journal of Occupational Therapy, 62*, 250–57.

Lynn, C. J., McKay, M. M., & Atkins, M. S. (2003). School social work: Meeting the mental health needs of students through collaboration with teachers. *Children & Schools, 25*(4), 197–209.

Maglio, J., & McKinstry, C. (2008) Occupational therapy and circus: Potential partners in enhancing the health and well-being of today's youth. *Australian Occupational Therapy Journal, 55*, 287–290.

Merrell, K., Carrizales, D., Feuerborn, L., Gueldner, B., & Tran, O. (2007). *Strong kids*. Baltimore, MD: Paul H. Brooks Publishing.

Miliken, B. E., Goodman, G., Bazyk, S., & Flinn, S. (2007). Establishing a case for occupational therapy in meeting the needs of children with grief issues in school-based settings. *Occupational Therapy in Mental Health, 23*(2), 75–100.

National Institute of Mental Health (NIMH). (2010). Retrieved from http://www.nimh.nih.gov/health/topics/child-and-adolescent-mental-health/index.shtml

Park, M. J., Brindis, C. D., Chang, F., & Irwin, C. E. (2008). A midcourse review of the healthy people 2010: 21 critical health objectives for adolescent and young adults. *Journal of Adolescent Health, 42*, 329–334.

Pierce, D. (2001). Untangling activity and occupation. *American Journal of Occupational Therapy, 55*, 138–146.

Piers, E. V., Harris, D. B., & Herzberg, D. S. (2002). *Manual for the Piers-Harris children's self-concept scale* (2nd ed.). Los Angeles: Western Psychological Services.

Richardson, P. K. (2002). The school as social context: Social interaction patterns of children with physical disabilities. *American Journal of Occupational Therapy, 56*, 296–304.

Sayers, B. R. (2008). Collaboration in school settings: A critical appraisal of the topic. *Journal of Occupational Therapy, Schools & Early Intervention, 1*, 170–179.

Schwartz, K. B. (2006). History and practice trends in physical dysfunction intervention. In H. M. Pendleton & W. Schultz-Krohn (Eds.), *Pedretti's occupational therapy: Practice skills for physical dysfunction* (pp. 13–18). St. Louis, MO: Mosby.

Schwartz, K. B. (2009). Reclaiming our heritage: Connecting the *Founding Vision* to the *Centennial Vision* [Eleanor Clarke Slagle lecture]. *The American Journal of Occupational Therapy, 63*, 681–690.

Shepherd, J., & Hanft, B. (2008). Team faces and spaces. In B. Hanft & J. Shepherd (Eds.), *Collaborating for student success: A guide for school-based occupational therapy* (pp. 35–72). Bethesda, MD: The American Occupational Therapy Association, Inc.

Simmons Carlsson, C. (2009). The 2008 Frances Rutherford Lecture. Taking a stand for inclusion: Seeing beyond impairment! *New Zealand Journal of Occupational Therapy, 56*(1), 4–11.

Simpson J., & Weiner, E. (Eds.). (2002*). The Oxford English dictionary* (2nd ed.). Oxford, England: Oxford University Press.

Spencer, K. C., Turkett, A., Vaughan, R., & Koenig, S. (2006). School-based practice patterns: A survey of occupational therapists in Colorado. *American Journal of Occupational Therapy, 60*, 81–91.

Svavarsdottir, E. K. (2008). Connectedness, belonging and feelings about school among healthy and chronically ill Icelandic schoolchildren. *Scandinavian Journal of Caring Science, 22*, 463–471.

Swinth, Y. (2008). Getting into a collaborative school routine. In B. Hanft & J. Shepherd (Eds.), *Collaborating for student success: a guide for school-based occupational therapy* (pp. 139–167). Bethesda, MD: The American Occupational Therapy Association, Inc.

Townsend, E. (1993). 1993 Muriel Driver Lecture. Occupational therapy's social vision. *Canadian Journal of Occupational Therapy, 60*(4), 174–184.

Townsend, E., & Wilcock, A. (2004). Occupational justice and client-centred practice: A dialogue in progress. *Canadian Journal of Occupational Therapy, 71*(2), 75–87.

U.S. Department of Education, Office of Special Education Programs, Center on Positive Behavioral Interventions and Support. (2010). *Positive behavioral interventions and supports.* Retrieved from http://www.pbis.org

U.S. Department of Health and Human Services. (1999). *Mental health: A report of the Surgeon General.* Rockville, MD: Author. Retrieved from http://www.surgeongeneral.gov/library/mentalhealth/home.html

World Health Organization. (2001). International classification of functioning, disability and health (ICF). Geneva, Switzerland: *World Health Organization.*

SUGGESTED RESOURCES

Suggested Readings

American Occupational Therapy Association. (2006). *Transforming caseload to workload in school-based and early intervention occupational therapy services.* Retrieved from http://www.aota.org/Consumers/Professionals/WhatIsOT/CY/Fact-Sheets/38519.aspx?FT=.pdf

American Occupational Therapy Association. (2010). AOTA's principles for reauthorization of the No Child Left Behind Act (NCLB). Retrieved from http://www.aota.org/Students/Advocate/AdvocacyFact/40481.aspx

Bazyk, S. (Ed.). (2010). *Mental health promotion, prevention and intervention in children and youth: A guiding framework for occupational therapy.* Bethesda, MD: American Occupational Therapy Association.

Carter, C., Meckes, L., Pritchard, L., Swenson, S., Wittman, P. P., & Velde, B. (2004). The friendship club: An after-school program for children with Asperger syndrome. *Family and Community Health, 27*(2), 143–150.

Dunst, C. J. (2002). Family-centered practice: Birth through high school. *The Journal of Special Education, 36*(3), 139–147.

Fette, C. V., & Estes, R. I. (2009). Community participation needs of families with children with behavioral disorders: A systems of care approach. *Occupational Therapy in Mental Health, 25*, 44–61.

Franklin, C., Harris, M. B., & Allen-Meares, P. (2006). *The school services sourcebook: A guide for school-based professionals*. New York: Oxford University Press.

Individuals with Disabilities Education Improvement Act of 2004. Pub. L., 108-446, 20 U.S.C. § 1400 *et seq.*

Jackson, L. L., & Arbesman, M. (Eds.). (2005). *Occupational therapy practice guidelines for children with behavioral and psychosocial needs*. Bethesda, MD: AOTA Press.

No Child Left Behind Act of 2001, Pub. L. 107–110, 115 Stat. 1425, 20 U.S.C.§6301 *et seq.*

Rebeiro, K. L. (1998). Occupation-as-means to mental health: A review of the literature and a call for research. *Canadian Journal of Occupational Therapy, 65*(1), 12–19.

Suggested Web-Based Resources

Center for Health and Health Care in Schools, The. (n.d.). Retrieved at http://www.healthinschools.org

Democracy Center, The. (2002). *Developing Advocacy Strategy*. Retrieved at http://democracyctr.org

Positive Behavioral Interventions and Supports. (n.d.). Retrieved at http://www.pbis.org/default.aspx

SchoolMentalHealth.org. (n.d.). Retrieved at http://www.schoolmentalhealth.org/index.html

Suggested Books on Development of Disability Identity

Callahan, J. (1990). *Don't worry he won't get far on foot*. New York: Vintage.

Grandin, T. (1996). *Thinking in pictures: and other reports from my life with autism*. New York: Vintage.

Juette, M., & Berger, R. (2008). *Wheelchair warriors: Gangs, disability, and basketball*. Philadelphia: Temple University Press.

Lears, L. (2005). *Nathan's wish: a story about cerebral palsy*. Morton Grove, IL: Albert Whitman & Company.

O'Brien, M., & Kendall, G. (2003). *How I became a human being: a disabled man's quest for independence*. Madison, WI: University of Wisconsin Press.

Chapter 23

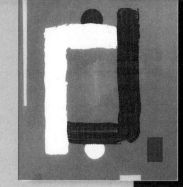

Vocational Programming

Eileen S. Auerbach, MS, OTR/L

KEY TERMS

Americans with Disabilities Act (1990)

assertive community treatment (ACT)

community support team

Individual Placement and Support (IPS) model

job coach

prevocational services

psychosocial or psychiatric rehabilitation

Role Acquisition Frame of Reference

seriously and persistently mentally ill (SMI)

supported employment (SE)

work programming

CHAPTER OUTLINE

Introduction

History of Work Programming in Occupational Therapy

Expanding Roles of Occupational Therapists

Knowing Your Customers—New Alliances
    Internal Allies
    Community Allies

Implementation of Occupational Therapy Services
    Assessment
    Forms of Intervention

Summary

INTRODUCTION

A primary goal of occupational therapists working in community mental health is to support independent living. Assisting someone to enter or reenter the workforce provides a real and meaningful context in which both the occupational therapist and the client can address issues of daily living. The work arena becomes the backdrop for occupational therapy interventions aimed at assisting an individual to reestablish his or her age-appropriate balance in work, play, and leisure.

Providing occupational therapy within a community context requires the recognition that one is truly operating in an open, dynamic system with many players. Maintaining sensitivity to the community context ensures that the activities pursued are both personally and socially meaningful. Figure 23-1 depicts the multiple levels of collaboration necessary when operating in a dynamic community context and shows how the vocational approach is the most useful and meaningful model for clients and therapists.

HISTORY OF WORK PROGRAMMING IN OCCUPATIONAL THERAPY

Occupation involves engaging with clear intent in activity that nourishes and sustains one's relationship to oneself (body, mind, and spirit) and one's relationship to the community. The value of work—that is, productive activity—has always been key to the philosophical basis of the profession. The roots of occupational therapy come from moral treatment, an approach that was used in the early 1900s for humane treatment of the mentally ill. During World War I, occupational therapy assisted disabled soldiers to regain their self-discipline, build their morale, and obtain training for reentering the civilian workforce. Operating from a holistic perspective, occupational therapy continued to be actively involved in the work adjustment of soldiers through the early 1900s during the immediate post–World War I period. During that same period, the Vocational Rehabilitation Act (Smith-Fess Act, Public Law 66–236) of 1920 established rehabilitation as a necessary service benefit for disabled individuals to enable them to return to remunerative employment (Flexor & Solomon, 1993). Occupational therapists actively developed **prevocational services** through the 1930s, and in 1943, with the passage of the Vocational Rehabilitation Amendment (Barder-La Follete Act/Public Law 78–113), people with psychiatric and developmental disabilities became eligible for such benefits. During this time, occupational therapists, including those in mental health, were actively involved with work adjustment programming.

Despite the clear need and opportunity for occupational therapists to continue and expand their roles within work programming during the post–World War II era, there was a decline in professional interest during the 1950s. However, during the 1960s the profession saw a resurgence in this area with the emergence of evaluation practices in industrial therapy.

Only from the 1980s to the present has **work programming** begun to progress beyond being seen as a specialty within community mental health practice and

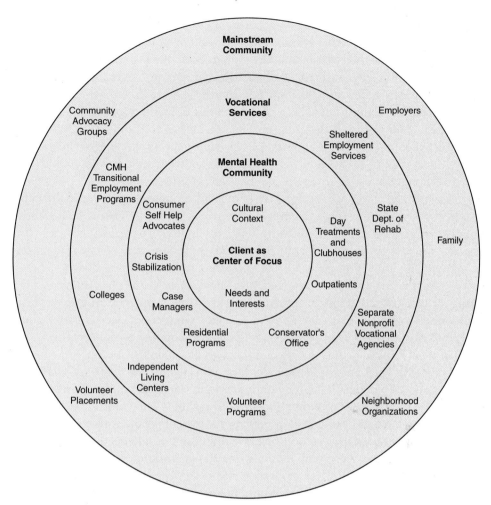

FIGURE 23-1. Levels of Collaboration
© Cengage Learning 2013

have occupational therapists begun to practice work-related interventions as part of their expected role. If occupational therapy began as a forerunner in this arena in clear alignment with rehabilitation, what contributed to the shifting paradigm? With respect to work programming, some noteworthy occurrences during the 1950s and 1960s had a significant impact in shaping the direction of mental health occupational therapy and the changes it is making today.

A phenomenon that was most prevalent in the 1950s was the adoption of the medical model of diagnosis and treatment that prevailed in all arenas of health care, including psychiatry. Occupational therapy was no exception. Embracing the medical model, occupational therapy shifted away from its holistic perspectives and adopted the more popular scientific, reductionist perspectives (Lang, 1991). This philosophical perspective viewed human behavior as purely a result of biological and physiological, mechanical function. Like a machine, the human could be dismantled and reduced and then understood by examining its structural parts. Hence, humans were considered separate from nature and the mind considered separate from the body. This perspective manifested itself in medicine as specialties in practice emerged. Emphasis was placed on developing expertise in specific modalities and techniques. While occupational therapists in physical disabilities became experts at adaptive equipment, occupational therapists in mental health became experts at craft modalities and projective techniques for supporting the psychoanalytic process.

Although the 1960s was also the era of deinstitutionalization, it was marked by greater focus on occupational therapy practice to assist the individual to "process" feelings through activity. The therapeutic focus was limited to a part of the client—the psyche—without a visibly meaningful link to the whole client as a center of focus for community function. That is not to say occupational therapy did not address function, but within the medical model, function had a biomechanical meaning. For instance, occupational therapeutic interventions were aimed at structuring medication management, with the end goal being to alleviate symptoms. Given the prevailing viewpoint of the era—that people with mental illness could never improve—achieving maintenance and stability of the condition was considered achieving function.

Ironically, while the medical model took precedence, the 1950s also saw the emergence of the psychosocial rehabilitation programs in community mental health. Hallmark agencies such as Fountain House and Thresholds were established throughout the country with the mission of improving the lives of people with mental illness by providing a supportive environment for learning skills and encouraging mastery through community membership and activity. The goal of the **psychosocial or psychiatric rehabilitation** model is to ensure that the person with a psychiatric disability can perform those physical, emotional, social, and intellectual skills needed to live, learn, and work in the community with the least amount of professional support necessary (Anthony & Liberman, 1992). The specific professional grounding of psychiatric rehabilitation was in vocational rehabilitation, and, although the concept of psychiatric rehabilitation has more recently expanded to include domains of social and community functioning, the area of work remains its primary focus. Its two main intervention strategies are client skill development and environmental resource development. As in occupational therapy's Role Acquisition Frame of Reference, the conceptual framework of this model relies upon skill development in expected social roles in the expected environment.

It was not until the late 1960s that the occupational therapy profession expressed concern over the paucity of work programming in mental health, and it was not until the late 1970s and early 1980s that occupational therapy began to increase its involvement with work programming for people with psychiatric disabilities.

Occupational therapists began to recognize that the psychosocial rehabilitation perspective was similar philosophically to the perspective held by the profession of occupational therapy. Indeed, the following principles are common to both:

- There can be no health without meaningful occupation.
- People can change themselves by their own efforts, and they have the choice—and responsibility—to do so.
- To effect change requires enlisting client choice and engaging in activities that promote skill building, exploration, education, and community role development.

The two fields share common interests, philosophies, and modes of treatment. Although it is possible to regard the two areas as competitive, most now consider occupational therapists to be full practitioners of psychiatric rehabilitation, albeit with their own developed practice framework.

An example is occupational therapy's **Role Acquisition Frame of Reference**, which is concerned with the learning of social roles required of the individual in an expected environment (Mosey, 1996). Decisions about areas of focus in treatment are determined in the context of the individual's society and cultural group, the person's current and expected environment, and conceptualized role categories. The types of roles and the ways the individual adapts to them are affected by that person's interests and goals. The assumption is that behavior is influenced by the environment, that areas of function are discrete and can be addressed separately, and that adaptive behavior is learned directly by experience in the expected environment. Purposeful activities of meaning to the individual are viewed as practical paths to learning skills and developing the abilities that form the basis of a life role like that of worker.

Acquisitional frames of reference utilize learning theories and behavioral approaches (Falk-Kessler, 1998; Mosey, 1996). Once a desired social role, such as that of worker, is prioritized, those task and interpersonal skills needed to maintain that role are acquired by practice and repetition in a reinforcing environment. It is assumed that individuals have a need to explore their environment and become competent, and the acquisitional models rely on client motivation and collaboration. There is an emphasis on doing; the person is aware and consciously learning; reality is stressed and, although activity may at first be simulated, as soon as possible there is a shift to natural activities.

In the Role Acquisition Frame of Reference, treatment to learn the adaptive behavior required by a social role would begin with task skills and interpersonal skills in the context of temporal adaptation. Behavioral change regarding social roles is acquired through activities that are designed to elicit the desired behavior. These learning activities would be of interest to the individual, would stimulate exploration and accomplishment, and would provide learning partners and role models.

EXPANDING ROLES OF OCCUPATIONAL THERAPISTS

The present trends in health care provide numerous opportunities for occupational therapists to creatively carve out new roles and perspectives. As psychotropic medications have become more effective, many disabling symptoms of **seriously and persistently mentally ill (SMI)** clients are being reduced, permitting their subsequent discharge from locked facilities back into their communities. It is the job of the **community support team** to assist these individuals in their reintegration back into community life by helping them identify and learn the skills necessary to survive. Among these skills are those needed for their new roles, such as that of worker.

But when is a person with SMI ready to return to work? And when the person experiences problems on a job, what factors need to be addressed? The occupational therapist, trained to perform task analysis in the field and to analyze the components that comprise occupational performance, is able to analyze the factors that contribute to individual performance. The occupational therapist can recommend and carry out targeted skill development for the client and can influence change in environmental factors for the severely mentally ill worker that may enhance the milieu for the rest of the workforce, disabled or not. The occupational therapist providing employment supports is able to apply knowledge of the **Americans with Disabilities Act (1990)** to facilitate compliance in such areas as reasonable accommodations, job analysis, and identification of essential functions for jobs. People with histories of severe mental illness may avoid disclosure and subsequently miss out on important job accommodations through fear of stigma and discrimination. These fears are not unfounded. Employers have ranked their level of comfort in working with the mentally ill second to last of all different disability groups (U.S. Congress, 1994). Workers with severe mental illness benefit greatly from supports in all these areas. The needs of severely mentally ill clients who wish to enter the workforce have opened up a wide variety of opportunities for occupational therapists, who can utilize their unique practice skills in **supported employment (SE)** (Arbesman & Logsdon, 2011) and education programs, assertive community treatment teams, and psychosocial clubhouses as service providers, program development consultants, and community-based advocates and educators.

KNOWING YOUR CUSTOMERS—NEW ALLIANCES

In the current health care environment, high-quality, cost-effective service within the community is a priority. For the occupational therapist, providing service in a larger public arena can mean expanding one's definition of the customer. In this instance, customers include not only those who receive direct services, but also those who fund the services—and thus indirectly benefit. These customers can become important allies.

Clearly, the most important customers are the clients served and their family members and significant others. When clients value services, their message and active support carry weight in the clinic, community, and political arenas. Family members and significant others are also significant advocates representing a powerful voice about which services are critical to the health of their loved ones.

Internal Allies

Intragency as well as interagency coordination often provides a vehicle for education within the provider community. Services that assist clients to attain functional outcomes, such as school or paid employment, demonstrate concretely to professional peers, administrators, policy makers, and community organizations the value of including occupational therapists in the multidisciplinary community team.

Community Allies

The needs and concerns of the business community are important because it is this community group that holds and creates the jobs. A core role of the employment specialist is advocacy for the client with the employer. Additional services can include troubleshooting when symptoms interfere with job performance, analysis, and recommendations to facilitate an optimal worksite environment, and collaboration on relationships with employer and coworkers. Suggestions regarding reasonable accommodations may include such areas as workstation setup, modification of schedules, assignment sharing, and need for targeted sick leave to manage therapy appointments. Employers in general avoid risk in hiring practices. Because entry-level and low-skill jobs routinely attract unreliable applicants, employers may be experienced with quirky, undependable, or slow workplace behaviors and used to spending extra time training many people with poor employment histories. Especially appealing to employers is knowing that they have a highly motivated job candidate who is supported by an employment specialist who will maintain contact with the employer, help with job skill training, facilitate good work habits, and assist in work adjustment and problem solving (Auerbach, 2001b; Marrone, Gandolfo, Gold, & Hoff, 1998).

IMPLEMENTATION OF OCCUPATIONAL THERAPY SERVICES

An occupational therapist is a facilitator at all levels of occupational therapy service and all phases of service implementation. As a facilitator, the occupational therapist's action and goals are directed by the original needs and interests expressed by clients.

Assessment

Studies (Bond, 1998; Bond, Drake, Mueser, & Becker, 1997) have repeatedly demonstrated that lengthy assessment followed by experience in treatment facility–based or transitional jobs only serve to prolong the pre-employment phase of treatment, delaying entry into paid, mainstream employment. Although clients are placed in various alternative work environments, such as treatment center-based jobs, sheltered employment, or transitional employment for many other reasons, including dealing with apprehension about loss of benefits, workplace anxiety, a stated client preference for a gradual approach into work, and unstable behaviors (Auerbach, 2001a; Auerbach & Richardson, 2005; Rogers, Anthony, Cohen, & Davies, 1997), the benefits of using these types of graduated, step wise entries into the workplace as useful means of assessing performance and predicting success have been largely discounted (Anthony, 1994; Anthony & Jansen, 1984). Instead, there has been a more recent focus on the advantages of supported employment, which places the individual in a job of that client's choice, then provides intensive supports, including on-the-job training and ongoing assessment in the actual workplace context for as long as the client needs it (Becker & Drake, 1993; Bond, 1998). There is significant evidence of the advantages of time-unlimited support and assessment in community-based, integrated employment, with this model of employment services, variously called Place-Then-Train, Choose-Get-Keep, and the **Individual Placement and Support (IPS) model** (Arbesman & Logsdon, 2011; Danley, Sciarappa, & MacDonald-Wilson, 1992; Drake, 1998). IPS is particularly effective when combined with cognitive and social skills training. However, systems of care can be slow to change, especially when there is a need for reallocation of resources. So, at this time many mental health providers continue to refer clients to a variety of more traditional pre-employment experiences. However, while clients wait for referrals to be accepted, this time can be used to address issues of clients considered to be resistant, avoidant, or otherwise not work-ready. Prevocational exposure to cognitive and psychosocial rehabilitation, including computerized cognitive training programs and skills training, can target deficits and symptoms associated with failure to succeed in workplace integration. Selective attention, short- and long-term memory, executive function, verbal fluency, and the effects of negative symptoms are all correlated with employment problems (Rouleau et al., 2009). Skills training can include finding and keeping a job, problem solving, and managing work-related social interactions. Evidence-based training aids and modules are available to use as therapeutic adjuncts (Tsang & Pearson, 2001; UCLA Social and Independent Living Skills Series, 1990). Although it is commonly accepted that, for persons with severe mental illness, skills do not readily transfer from one context to another, it has been found that workplace-related social skills can carry over into the workplace when there is regular follow-up support once the client is working, even as infrequently as once a month or over the phone (Tsang & Pearson, 2001).

Some pre-employment placements are brokered by contract agencies offering rehabilitation services, which often are more or less separate from the treatment team. Clients are evaluated and assigned to different types of training jobs prior to receiving assistance with job search, placement, and support in mainstream employment (Auerbach, 2001a; Marrone, 1993). Among these types of experiences are the following:

- Sheltered employment: Training and employment are limited to specific disability groups, including persons with developmental and psychiatric disabilities. Work is done in segregated environments on subcontracted jobs from outside industry (Bond, 1992). Payment is pro-rated according to productivity, with the center usually having a subminimum wage certificate. Sheltered settings have not proved to be an effective conduit to mainstream employment, but they do provide a work experience and a modified income to persons unable to perform in a regular, competitive work setting without intensive, continuing supervision.

- In-house jobs: These may include work-oriented day treatment programs and psychosocial rehabilitation clubhouses, such as Fountain House in New York, Thresholds in Chicago, or Towne House Creative Living Center in Oakland (Marrone, 1993). In these settings, the day activity is work, performed by both clients and staff. Staff both supervise and model appropriate workplace behaviors, teaching in the context of the job itself and also in more formalized skills training groups. Supported employment in community-based settings may also be offered in these programs after a specified period of time, in the form of assistance with job development, coaching, and continuing follow-along for a period of time.

- Transitional employment: This approach refers to "temporary community jobs employing clients under an arrangement between a psychosocial rehabilitation agency and a community employer" (Bond, 1992, p. 248). These jobs are established to be appropriate to the members' abilities and endurance, designed to help them adjust to work, enhance their self-confidence, and offer job experiences for their résumés (Bond et al., 1997).

Mental health treatment teams in acute settings such as hospitals, in longer-term settings such as locked facilities, day treatment, or behavioral health facilities, or in other longer-term settings such as outpatient and case management programs seek a definitive predictor of whether a given client will succeed in a job before they invest resources in that person's vocational rehabilitation. Despite differing opinions about clear-cut indicators of success, there are certain qualities that have been associated with positive outcomes in work-related rehabilitation efforts (Arbesman & Logsdon, 2011; Bond et al., 1997; Stauffer, 1986). We do know that persons with a work history are more likely to work again (Anthony, 1994; Anthony & Jansen, 1984). We have observed that clients' motivation to work plays a significant role in their job tenure, taking the form of their repeatedly seeking assistance to solve problems and in their general resilience (Auerbach, 2001b, Auerbach & Richardson, 2005;

Braitman et al., 1995). Also associated with success in the workplace is seeking entrance to a vocational program, ability to get along with others, level of self-esteem, and working in a job and an environment that the person likes (Anthony, 1994; Kirsh, 2000a, 2000b). Many studies demonstrate that the best clinical predictors of future work performance are ratings of a person's work adjustment skills made in a workshop setting or sheltered job site (Anthony, 1994; Anthony & Jansen, 1984). Assessment of work adjustment skills is a traditional area of expertise of the occupational therapist, and one that bears a closer look (Chan, Tsang, & Li, 2009; Kirsh et al., 2006).

From the OT perspective, the usefulness of pre-employment evaluation has less to do with anticipating success or failure on the job than with supplying information for the mental health team members who will be providing the job supports. Once the mental health treatment providers—and this may include the outpatient therapist, case manager, occupational therapist, psychiatric rehabilitation counselor, job coach, or psychiatrist—know the client's deficits or weak areas, they are in a better position to anticipate difficulties in certain workplace situations, they can tailor support strategies with the client in advance, and, earlier in the process, they can offer problem-solving assistance to client and employer, before a small disturbance or issue on a job escalates into a big problem and the client is fired or quits.

What is the purpose of an initial assessment of occupational performance? The occupational therapist is usually called in to determine competence in specific areas of daily life skills and to make a decision about the person's readiness for rehabilitation. There are several approaches to an initial occupational profile, including an unstructured or semi-structured interview (Auerbach, 2002; Henry & Mallinson, 1999; Hunter, 1999; Page, 1999); a structured checklist of information, such as Mosey's survey of task skills (Mosey, 1996, p. 453); rating scales, such as Ethridge's Pre-vocational Evaluation of Rehabilitation Potential (Ethridge, 1968); work samples, such as the Valpar series (Valpar International Corporation), which are now generally seen as too time-consuming, with equivalent information available more readily in simple observation during clinic or workshop task performance samples; and cognitive assessments, such as the Allen Cognitive Level Test (Allen, Earhart, & Blue, 1992) or Screen (Allen et al., 2009). Studies in the psychiatric rehabilitation literature for years have cited a particular rating scale, the Pre-Vocational Evaluation of Rehabilitation Potential developed by an occupational therapist (Ethridge, 1968) and considered a valid and reliable tool to assess work adjustment. This rating scale uses a 4-point scale: (1) very poor performance, (2) poor performance, (3) average or acceptable performance, and (4) excellent performance. Ethridge describes a score of 60 or above indicating good work adjustment and a score of below 60 indicating relatively poor work adjustment (p. 162).

The Program for Assertive Community Treatment, considered a model of the integration of employment and treatment services for persons with severe and persistent mental illness, initially assesses clients through a structured interview. Included are a work history and description of work interests, skills, and abilities; ratings of social functioning and psychological and illness factors, including a description of types of support needed; and relevant social-environmental factors, such as physical obstacles (e.g., transportation) or entitlement disincentives (Frey & Godfrey, 1991). As with the IPS model, PACT's vocational assessment is ongoing, with data gathered in the competitive work environment.

Occupational therapists use a variety of other tests, only some of which are designed by occupational therapists. Examples of these are the Jacobs Prevocational Skills Assessment (Jacobs, 1991), the Work Environment Impact Scale (WEIS) (Moore-Corner, Kielhofner, & Olson, 1998), the Worker Role Interview (Braveman et al., 2005), and a variety of tests to explore vocational interest areas, such as the California Occupational Preference Survey (COPS, 1971) or the Strong Interest Inventory (1994). In cases where there are mixed diagnoses, such as head injuries resulting in cognitive and physical deficits, it may be important to collaborate with practitioners in other service areas to evaluate functioning. Because occupational therapists have a broad educational background covering neurological and physical dysfunction, their scope of practice covers other areas of disability and permits them to incorporate evaluation tools with a broader emphasis than psychosocial rehabilitation.

Figure 23-2, The Occupational Profile Worksheet, is an example of a client's self-report questionnaire used as the basis of a structured interview to develop an occupational profile. The information sought is comprehensive, covering all areas of occupation, only a part of which concerns work.

All in all, in deciding the type of assessment to use, it is helpful to consider the predicted length of stay in the treatment or vocational program, the purpose for the evaluation, and whether the client is self-selected for vocational services—that is, whether it is possible to gauge in advance the client's level of motivation.

Depending on the setting, the depth, extent, and value of vocational assessment can often be tailored to meet the needs of consumers at various levels of care. The process is often determined by the consumer's level of focus and expressed desire to consider work activity. The occupational therapist may find that, at the very least, this expressed interest can be an opening for dialogue and short-term interventions. Dialogue can be particularly useful when the identified barriers to working are related to disability management issues (e.g., medication compliance, self-medication with substances).

Note that the vocational counselor may be the same person as the occupational therapist. It is also likely that the occupational therapist may work in a consultative role. The choices and decisions made regarding the vocational plan of action are determined jointly by the client and the practitioner, often within the context of

Date: _____

Team: _____

Case Manager: _____

ID#: _____

Occupational Profile

1. Client Information

Name _____ Date of Birth _____ Age _____

Address_____ Zip _____ Phone _____

Social Security No. _____ Marital Status _____

Where did you grow up?

Where is your family of origin now?

Describe your present living situation (type of housing and with whom):

Children's ages (if any):

Current source of income:

2. Education

Highest level of school completed:

Where: High School:

     College, Trade, or Vocational School:

Do you have any degrees, licenses, or certificates?

     Specify which type, date, and where received:

Have you ever had any special problems in school (e.g., learning disabilities, attention deficits)? Please describe:

Which were your favorite subjects?

Which were your least favorite subjects?

Do you plan to return to school?_____ Area of study? _____

3. Who in your household does these chores?

Grocery shopping: Laundry:

Cooking: Housecleaning:

Dishes: Bill paying:

Do you think the household tasks are shared in a fair way? _____

FIGURE 23-2. Sample Occupational Profile

Name: _____

ID#: _____

4. Work experience

Usual Occupation: _____

What are the last three jobs you have held (starting with the most recent):

	Job Title	Dates of employment	Types of Duties	Reasons for leaving
a.				
b.				
c.				

Which was your favorite job of all you've done?

Which was your least favorite job?

What are your plans for returning to work?

What would you like to be doing a year from now?

Could you benefit from vocational counseling? _____

5. Individual activities, social and leisure time

List your special interests and hobbies:

_____

_____

What other things would you like to do in your spare time?

Do you like to read? What do you usually read? _____

Have you had any trouble concentrating lately?

_____

Do you generally spend your free time ❑ alone or ❑ with others

What kinds of things have you done with friends?

(Continues)

FIGURE 23-2. Sample Occupational Profile *(Continued)*

Name: _____

ID#: _____

6. Health and fitness

Have you ever participated in physical exercise ❑, active sports ❑, or have a fitness routine ❑?

Please describe:

What could you do to be more physically fit?

Do you have any physical problems that could prevent you from participating fully in such activities as bowling, stretching exercises, dance, movement, swimming, walking, etc.? (please describe)

❑ Blood pressure problems _____

❑ Back pain _____

❑ Cardiac or circulation problems _____

❑ Seizures _____

❑ Vision problems _____

❑ Joint Problems (e.g., arthritis) _____

❑ Other _____

Do you have a special diet? Please describe:

Do you feel best when you are active and productive? (please check ✓) ❑

  Or resting and unoccupied? ❑

7. Your typical day

List the activities in your daily routine (e.g., meals, work, recreation or leisure activities, therapy appointments or programs, housekeeping or child care responsibilities, shopping):

Morning:

_____

_____

(time you usually get up: _____)

(time you usually eat breakfast: _____)

_____

_____

(time you usually eat lunch: _____)

Afternoon:

_____

_____

time you usually eat dinner: _____)

Evening:

_____

_____

(time you usually go to bed: _____)

FIGURE 23-2. Sample Occupational Profile *(Continued)*

Name: _____

ID#: _____

8. Activities of Daily Living

Are you satisfied with how you are managing your daily self-care tasks?

I'm doing:	ok	not ok	Please explain
Eating well			
Food shopping			
Cooking meals or eating in restaurants			
Shopping for clothes and personal items			
Personal cleanliness and hygiene (e.g., teeth, hair, showering, laundry)			Teeth: Hair: Showers/baths: Shaving: Laundry:
Housekeeping (e.g., dusting, cleaning kitchen, bathroom, vacuuming)			
Money managing (e.g., budgeting, cashing checks, paying bills)			
Taking care of business (e.g., filling out forms, keeping appointments, etc.)			
Transportation (e.g., ❑ walking ❑ MUNI ❑ BART ❑ car ❑ bike)			
Ability to concentrate			

9. What would you like to be doing one year from now? (e.g., any changes in work, school, social life, leisure activities, other activities of daily living, or areas of self-care?)

FIGURE 23-2. Sample Occupational Profile *(Continued)*

Adapted from Auerbach, 2002.

the treatment team. The client can choose to adopt or reject the recommendations of the practitioner. Service options can include job-seeking skills groups, time management and stress management skills training, social security benefits counseling, referral assistance to enter employment training programs or educational programs, and job development or work adjustment follow-along, depending on the desired goal. Kirsh, Cockburn, and Gewirtz (2006), in a meta-analysis of 39 articles describing models of care for persons with mental illness, identified 12 key characteristics that appeared to positively influence vocational outcomes across models of care. These characteristics are:

1. A specific focus on work, including offering employment services to all clients, even if they did not specifically express initial interest.

2. The inclusion of a vocational or employment specialist on the treatment team, especially a dedicated specialist with no other program responsibilities.

3. Job matching, choice, and attention to client preferences.

4. Ongoing, available supports.

5. Rapid placement and on-the-job training versus extended periods of evaluation and off-site training.

6. A problem-solving approach to work and daily living, including skills training in such areas as money management, symptom management, use of public transit, knowing how to dress, and workplace social skills.

7. Pay for work, which has been shown to correlate directly with increased participation in work and subsequently with reduced symptomatology and improved quality of life outcomes.

8. Attention to the work environment.

9. A team approach, especially when treatment is coordinated among staff, family, and caretaking friends.

10. Support and education for employers and coworkers, especially emphasizing active interaction with employers to understand needs and establish trust.

11. A range of services that are available and accessible.

12. Integrated services and systems.

Once the client is engaged in training or on the job, situational assessments are done to evaluate progress. These are done on the worksite while the person is performing the job or during telephone or in-person check-in before or after work. The following case illustration is an example of the evaluation process.

CASE ILLUSTRATION

Charlotte—Occupational Therapy Evaluation

Charlotte is a 56-year-old woman diagnosed with chronic paranoid schizophrenia who expressed interest in paid transitional work experience in the community. She was referred by a San Francisco mental health program to a vocational rehabilitation agency in San Francisco. Charlotte was specifically interested in the Clerical Program because her previous work history was in the secretarial field. After the initial intake interview, Charlotte was referred by the projects coordinator to occupational therapy for the vocational evaluation and assessment. The client was administered a battery of tasks designed to assess performance in specific work-related areas. Cognitive abilities, learning styles, strengths and limitations with respect to employment, social and communication skills, safety awareness, and special needs with respect to ability and disability were evaluated. Functional activities of daily living (ADL) skills, sensory perception and motor functioning, physical endurance, self-concept, and judgment were also assessed. A baseline for understanding the client's current skill level and work readiness was established to assist Charlotte, the occupational therapist, and the vocational counselors in determining appropriate job placement in the community.

As a short-term goal, Charlotte wanted to receive clerical training and transitional work experience from the Clerical Program for approximately three to four hours per day, three days per week. Her long-term educational and vocational goals were to learn computer skills for data entry and to find a part-time clerical job in the community.

From the assessment, it was determined that Charlotte had the following difficulties:

1. Poor problem-solving skills.
2. Poor short-term memory.
3. Difficulty making decisions and self-correcting work.
4. Difficulty planning with foresight and accuracy.
5. Decreased activity tolerance (two hours).
6. Need for increased time to learn new tasks.
7. Poor stress and frustration tolerance.

From the assessment, it was also determined that Charlotte had the following assets:

1. Very motivated to work and to learn computer skills.
2. Previous work experience.
3. Clear, legible penmanship.
4. Able to initiate questions when needing clarification of instruction.
5. Strong sorting and filing skills.
6. Excellent telephone-answering skills.
7. Good self-care habits.
8. Daily living routines consistent with desired goals.

From the results of the assessment, the following functional requirements were identified:

1. A very structured environment.
2. Clearly defined tasks.
3. Increased time to learn new tasks.
4. Both written and verbal instruction.
5. Compensatory techniques (e.g., lists).
6. Feedback from supervisors and coworkers regarding task performance and decision making.
7. Opportunities to practice problem-solving behavior in familiar settings with familiar people and with simple tasks in simple situations.
8. A break every two hours until activity tolerance increases.

After completing the Clerical Program five months later, Charlotte was placed in a paid transitional secretarial position at a human service agency. She did very well in her secretarial position and was referred to the job developer three months later to begin searching for permanent employment in the community.

Forms of Intervention

Client choices often determine the nature, timing, and context for occupational therapy interventions. The arena varies from the treatment or agency site to the community and the workplace. Regular assessment and/or intervention can occur at the training or work sites. The occupational therapist can often work with the training supervisors to adapt the training or work process.

Group or Individual Counseling

Counseling takes the form of problem solving as opposed to psychotherapeutic sessions. The stated objective is to support the individual in learning how to manage situations that arise within a day-to-day context. The focus is on the immediate situation, learning from the present moment, and developing personal resiliency for the future. The therapeutic value lies in consumer/client empowerment—empowering the client in his or her ability to make decisions, act on them, and learn from the experiences.

Problem solving occurs most often while assisting people to build interpersonal and communication skills. Often, uncertainty results from not knowing how to interpret an interaction. The cognitive stress from perceptions based on incomplete information or misinterpreted nonverbal cues is often the source of stress and difficulties in getting along with others (Chan et al., 2009).

People have greater motivation to take in new information and apply what they learn when they are concurrently engaged in work they like. The day-to-day issues can provide concrete incentives for addressing specific issues or to learn skills that relate directly to one's job or role.

The following case describes an example of **assertive community treatment (ACT)** by OT staff delivering first treatment center–based then community-based employment services to a client with co-occurring diagnoses.

CASE ILLUSTRATION

Mr. T.—A Gradualist Approach to Vocational Programming

Mr. T., a longtime client of a mental health day treatment center, was admitted to a newly formed assertive community treatment (ACT) program. He had an Axis I diagnosis of psychotic disorder with delusions, secondary to a left arteriovenous malformation resection, that is, a brain injury after surgery to correct a cerebrovascular abnormality, which left him with neurological deficits, including recurrent episodes of paranoid delusions of religiosity. In addition, Mr. T. had right hemiparesis, expressive and some receptive aphasia, and a seizure disorder. Because of his difficulty with word-finding and his inability to grasp effectively with his right hand, it was very difficult to develop a job for him, and he worked in treatment center–based sheltered employment for several years.

Occupational Therapy

Initial evaluation of Mr. T's functional performance showed that because he was highly motivated to achieve and had a positive attitude toward task accomplishment, he was able to compensate for many impairments. He attempted whatever arts and crafts were offered in the Individual Projects OT group, participated fully in the Living Skills Class activities, began working on the Popcorn Project during prevocational OT groups, and regularly attended the Vocational Issues Group to fulfill his desire to work. Mr. T. eventually settled into one of the day treatment center's prevocational OT jobs working on a team that made and bagged popcorn to sell in the center.

Volunteer Employment

The next step for Mr. T. was a referral to the city's transitional volunteer center, where he was assigned to the Recreation and Parks Department as a volunteer in a short-term six-month job, watering plants in the nursery. OT staff helped him and his supervisor manage some of the problems he had, such as ways he could deal with how wet his feet were getting and how to adapt the watering can. In the past, leaving Mr. T. to struggle alone with these types of problems would precipitate suspicion and paranoia toward his boss or coworkers.

Transitional Employment

After the time-limited job ended, OT staff referred Mr. T. to a vocational rehabilitation services agency that contracts with his county's Department of Community Mental Health Services to provide housing and jobs to its clients. Again, this job was categorized as transitional, that is, a temporary training job owned by the agency. Mr. T. was paid a minimum wage to mop, vacuum, and dust at a support services hotel. Despite the limited mobility of his right lower extremity, Mr. T. was assigned to work on the stairs. He reported an inability to mop the bathroom as the door kept shutting on him. OT staff made a site visit to advocate that he have limited vacuuming assignments on stairs, and provided a doorstop to keep the restroom door open for him. He was shown how to wrap his affected hand around the mop and broom handles to stabilize the implement. He worked for over the allotted nine months on this assignment.

Despite this assistance, however, the vocational rehabilitation services staff to which he had been referred determined that, although he had successfully completed this limited-tenure transitional job, he was too slow to be productive enough to compete for community-based jobs in integrated settings.

Sheltered Employment

The vocational rehabilitation services agency's job developer, an occupational therapist, did not think Mr. T. could be placed, and she recommended that he apply to the state Department of Rehabilitation for training funds to send him to a sheltered workshop. This organization gave him a packaging assignment with adapted tools at subminimum wage. He worked at this job for over a year. However, the sameness of the job

eventually bored Mr. T., and he worried that his thoughts were becoming morbid while working in this warehouse-like setting with other mentally ill and developmentally disabled workers. Although OT staff persuaded the owner to vary the work assignments, this intervention was not sufficient to keep Mr. T. in the job. The tasks involved repetitive assembly of kits while seated in a row of work stations, silent and isolated.

Competitive, Community-Based, Integrated Employment

An OT student next accompanied Mr. T. to a job fair advertised at the local fitness center. The fitness center was looking for a part-time attendant for light cleaning and to serve as a benign security presence in the locker room. Mr. T. was highly motivated to move to a more stimulating work environment with regular wages. The OT student accompanied him to the interviews, and provided the fitness center with information on the Private Industry Council (PIC), which offers assistance to employers in qualifying for tax incentives, as well as the tax credit forms for employers hiring disabled individuals who live in enterprise zones.

The fitness center employed Mr. T. and coached him through the training phase with occupational therapy consultation. He required assistance to solve simple logistical and equipment problems such as his needing a different handle length on the dustpan and larger rubber gloves for his hands. Because of Mr. T.'s aphasia, he had difficulty communicating his needs to his employer and understanding his employer's expectations and instructions. The

OT student helped him solve problems with his supervisor regarding his initial need for frequent breaks, and developed a written checklist to help him organize a task and break routine. The client's psychosocial needs were addressed through problem-solving discussions regarding his misinterpretation of constructive criticism. He gradually learned that evaluation was not rejection or a potential firing, or that his work was not valued, but simply meant that he was to do things slightly differently. Further, the OT student educated the employer regarding the client's problem with recording his hours, as he had difficulty expressing numbers verbally and in writing because of his aphasia.

Discussion

In the past, without this intensive outreach and support, Mr. T. would have succumbed to paranoia, and would have or did walk off the job or quit. The occupational therapy staff and students, with a grounding in both physical and psychosocial deficits, ability to do task analysis, and environmental modification at the job site, were prepared to help him manage work using both the gradualist and the direct entry approaches.

Money Management Skills

As individuals begin earning wages, money management and decision-making skills are developed concretely through learning how to calculate social security withholdings, report earnings, maintain records, and make decisions about increasing hours and jobs. Counseling and support are given throughout to assist the person to address the fears surrounding the loss of cash and medical benefits. Given the confusing nature of social security work incentives, it is only through continuous review of the information, support, and actual experience over time that a person can learn and gain confidence over money management. One example of a Social Security work incentive with which a client may need help in reporting is an Impairment Related Work Expense (IRWE) (Social Security Administration, 2010). A person who has special needs in order to work may deduct these expenses from the earnings reported to the Social Security Administration. A person with a mental illness or cognitive impairments may need to pay for the assistance of a travel trainer to instruct in learning the route to work or with a **job coach** to train skills related to job duties.

When an individual on supplemental security income (SSI) reaches a point when he or she has set a specific employment objective and determined the specific equipment or training needs to achieve that goal, the occupational therapist can assist in developing a Plan for Achieving Self-Support (PASS) to set aside income funds for the long-term goal. An example of a PASS plan would be setting aside 10% of one's monthly wages over a year's time to pay for a computer, to be used to develop the person's career. This investment would lower the level of the person's income, and permit fewer dollars to be deducted from the individual's monthly Social Security checks.

The Ticket to Work program of the Social Security Administration is being slowly implemented nationally, and will increase the rehabilitation and vocational choices of people receiving assistance to get to work. It is not yet clear how this program will affect specific programs in the future. But it is certain that occupational therapists providing employment supports will benefit from keeping current on this program to better inform their clients and to be certain their services are of high quality so that they may qualify to be approved providers of these services (Social Security Administration, 2010). Again, the responsibility of decision-making and choice returns to the client and is directly experienced as such.

Applying the Skills in the Community

There are numerous opportunities to assist the client to practice communication skills, stress management, and organizational skills when the practitioner accompanies the client to outside community offices such as the local Social Security office, the local Employment Development Department office or hiring hall for job searches, the public library for vocational resources, the local community college campus or training site, or local neighborhoods or businesses to explore the types of job opportunities to be found there and to actually observe people at work. The occupational therapist can assist the client to anticipate questions and role-play the situation beforehand. After the visit, reviewing what happened reinforces learning and the client's sense of mastery. Regardless of the type of community-based activity, learning and adaptation are considered part of a growth process. Failure is reframed as a lesson learned to be added to one's stock of experience, reminding individuals that they are gaining their vocational maturity much in the same way that others have.

Interventions with the Community

As an advocate, educator, or consultant, the occupational therapist often works with several types of communities and groups. Such groups may include businesses and the organizations that support them, like the local chamber of commerce and Private Industry Council, consumer advocates, and other mental health and rehabilitation providers from either county or state and private sectors. The therapist can also practice the same concept of learning and adaptation for himself or herself when planning to work with community agencies, employers, and the local community at large.

It is often to the occupational therapist's benefit to research and identify the community or group audience with regard to values, attitudes, and culture. This can be part of a needs assessment done before the occupational therapist goes in to present information or education at a particular site. For instance, when working with an employment site, the workplace culture and practices can be identified and explored with the employees to facilitate the new employees' integration on the job as well as provide support services within or outside the workplace context (see Figure 23-4).

Community Mental Health	Local Community	Business Community
Consult/Educate Mental Health Providers Regarding: ■ Work readiness ■ Program planning ■ ADA ■ System policy and service design ■ Supervision of consumer staff	Educate/Inform Members of the Community: ■ Mental illness ■ Support with symptom management ■ Resisting stigma	Consult/Educate Employers, Supervisors, Employees: ■ ADA ■ Mental illness ■ Supervising employees with mental illness ■ Staff education ■ Diversity awareness
Types of forums for these interventions can be as follows:		
Consult/Educate Mental Health Providers Regarding: ■ In-service presentations ■ Outreach	Educate/Inform Members of the Community: ■ Outreach ■ Community service education	Consult/Educate Employers, Supervisors, Employees: ■ Educational ■ Sensitivity training ■ Community outreach

FIGURE 23-3. Types of Interventions Within Different Communities
© Cengage Learning 2013

Interventions When the Employer Is Involved

Understanding the workplace culture assists to establish a dialogue with employers. An ideal situation would be an employer educated in the needs of mental health clients who would be receptive to hiring them as part of a diverse workforce and to providing the supports they might need. Employers of low-skill entry-level workers may have seen a range of performance and social behaviors in the past and found ways to draw out their best efforts. In developing an approach to informing the employer, it may be less helpful for the employer to understand all the dynamics of an individual's mental illness, and offering a great deal of technical information may even alarm or intimidate the employer. Instead, the employment specialist can explore the workplace environment, talk with the employer or coworkers, and try to identify areas where a supportive intervention could ease stress and solve problems (Marrone et al., 1998). When a job is a good fit for the client, with shared values and a positive workplace culture, the employer, therapist, and client can form a team to analyze and resolve difficult situations (Kirsh, 2000a, 2000b). Many employers are unaware of how the Americans with Disabilities Act applies to such individuals. For an occupational therapist, adaptations made at the worksite are then considered reasonable accommodations for a qualified individual who can perform the essential functions of the job with certain modifications in either the job, the environment, or the supervisory process (Mancuso, 1993) (see Figure 23-3, Types of Interventions within Different Communities).

Support is given to the employer throughout to address work issues that may arise. In the best-case scenario, an employer can appreciate certain accommodations as making good business sense for *all* employees. However, this does not always serve to eliminate the discrimination and stigma that an individual may fear or experience from others.

Interventions When the Employer Is Not Involved

When clients choose not to disclose their diagnoses, the decision must be respected and supportive interventions are done offsite. Coaching occurs in the preparation before and after the job interview, on the telephone during working hours while on break, before or after work, and/or during lunch. Accommodations are rarely explicitly presented and often are worked out by the employee independently or with coaching. See Figure 23-4 for types of reasonable accommodations.

Support takes whatever form the client perceives would be helpful, whether a peer support group, a peer counselor, a community group affiliation, a mental health agency affiliation, or family and friends for therapeutic or socialization purposes.

The Context of Services

It is important to acknowledge that the extent, nature, and depth of occupational therapeutic intervention are driven, not only by customer choices and needs but also by the setting in which the occupational therapist works. The variety of settings where

Types of Reasonable Accommodations	
Modifications can be made to:	
The Job	▪ Job sharing, trading duties between workers
Physical Environment	▪ Partitions ▪ Rearranging/positioning location of work area in office ▪ Changing fluorescent lighting
Assistive Aids or Technology	▪ Tape recorders ▪ Day organizers ▪ Handheld organizers (PDAs)
Schedule Modifications	▪ Change break times ▪ Shift scheduled hours earlier/later ▪ Work or paid/unpaid leave
Supervising Structure	▪ Additions or adaptations of supervision schedule/style ▪ Mentor/buddy ▪ Adapting mode of instruction/training
Policy and Work Culture	▪ Diversity training and education ▪ Mental health days

FIGURE 23-4. Reasonable Accommodations

© Cengage Learning 2013

Instrumental Activities of Daily Living Addressed Include:		
▪ Money Management		
▪ Transportation		
▪ Stress Management		
▪ Time Management		
▪ Physical Health Self Care		
▪ Communication Skills		
Skills Learning and Building Can Begin Within the Mental Health Community	**Skills Application Can Occur in Vocational Settings**	**Skills Refinement Can Be Ongoing Within the Mainstream Community**
▪ Partial Hospitalization		
▪ Vocational Programs		
▪ Community-Based Employment		
▪ ACT or Case Management Programs		
▪ Day Treatment		
▪ Volunteering		
▪ Education		
▪ Clubhouse Programs		
▪ Transitional Employment Programs		

FIGURE 23-5. Continuum for Occupational Therapy Assistance with Skills
© Cengage Learning 2013

occupational therapists work offer opportunities to develop programming to address varying levels of vocational and self-care needs of clients. Depending on the setting, the occupational therapist may focus on skills learning and building, skills application, or skills refinement and/or adaptation (see Figure 23-5 for occupational therapy assistance with skills).

CASE ILLUSTRATION

Lorelei—Direct Entry into Supported Employment

Lorelei is a 38-year-old woman with a diagnosis of bipolar disorder mixed, recurrent, with psychotic features. Her residential counselor suggested that she apply for a deli position at a local supermarket, and, to her surprise, she was hired. Her case manager at her assertive community treatment (ACT) program is an occupational therapist who regularly checks on her well-being on her job, and provides employment supports for Lorelei when she needs them. Because the ACT program offers long-term community support, these services are time unlimited. The two have worked on reality testing, anger management, problem-solving techniques, and assertive communications with her job supervisors, coworkers, and union representatives, including requesting reasonable accommodations for herself.

When she first started, Lorelei was thrilled to have a real community-based job in a regular integrated setting. However, issues arose that required some thinking-through. Lorelei had an excitable temperament and needed help in problem solving so that she could maintain control and achieve resolution of issues without blowing up or walking off the job. One of the occupational therapist/case manager's resources was a teaching technique found in the UCLA Social and Independent Living Skills Series, the problem-solving technique (UCLA, 1990), also described by Corrigan, Schade, and Liberman (1992). The client is assisted to understand the elements of the problem situation; a list of reasonable alternative solutions is developed and analyzed to determine feasibility; and the client decides which solution to try. Once the person has implemented the solution, the results are analyzed to determine their effectiveness. On several occasions, Lorelei had been told to close down and clean the rotisserie too late in her shift, and, because this was a big, heavy job that took her a long time, she felt she was being set up to work extra unpaid time. Was her boss trying to indicate that she was too slow? Was he exploiting her? Lorelei was able to analyze the predicament with the occupational therapist/case manager, and eventually she decided to meet with her boss. She successfully negotiated

extra time to complete the rotisserie cleanup to both their satisfaction and still be able to finish her shift on time.

Another issue resulted in a more active occupational therapist/case manager intervention to assist her in disclosing her disability. Lorelei had been hired to work the swing shift at the deli; however, after a few months she was asked to work an A.M. shift one day, a swing shift the next, followed immediately by another A.M. shift. The result was an inadequate night's sleep between the swing shift and the next morning's A.M. shift. Lorelei's situation was delicate because her psychiatric condition, bipolar disorder, can be aggravated by irregular sleep patterns. The occupational therapist/case manager drafted a letter to the employer on the ACT program's letterhead stationery, which was co-signed by Lorelei's psychiatrist, requesting that she be allowed the reasonable accommodation of working the same shift throughout the work week to help prevent relapse. Her boss was understanding and readily agreed to this request.

When Lorelei moved to her next job as cashier at a drugstore, she was confronted with a new situation that required some on-site job coaching on the part of the occupational therapist/case manager. Lorelei was complaining of back strain, and the occupational therapist met with her for an on-site activity analysis at the drugstore, where she could observe Lorelei's work tasks firsthand. She was able to help Lorelei use back-saving biomechanics. First they worked on postural alignment. Then they practiced safe lifting techniques, first sliding the heavy purchases across the counter to be held close to her body before trying to lift them, as a way to reduce the torque on her back. These interventions readily cleared up her back strain, and she was successful in continuing the new job.

Discussion

Job-related issues come up on a regular basis, and consistent support in her employment has helped Lorelei manage her symptoms, develop her problem-solving skills, and fully utilize all the resources she has available to her.

SUMMARY

Occupational therapists who work in vocational rehabilitation may find themselves operating simultaneously within multiple arenas of service provision. Rather than considering it as a specialty, occupational therapy can be reframed to identify how services can directly contribute to a person's functional goals. Regardless of the number of arenas and where one stands in the system of care (see Figure 23-1), client choice can become both the central driving force and the compass for all aspects of service. The occupational therapist becomes primarily the navigator and facilitator.

Operating in a system of care requires continuous communication, negotiation, and adaptation. Such an arena is rich with experiences in which, much like the clients, occupational therapists can constantly challenge themselves to learn and adapt professionally in order to provide effective, evidence-based services.

To practice effectively in the community, many occupational therapists want to understand the total picture of health care and the community at large. Occupational therapy in work programming is not so much a specialty as it is a different, and perhaps renewed, commitment to reintegration of the severely mentally ill client into the community.

REVIEW QUESTIONS

1. Name one occupational therapy frame of reference that closely reflects psychiatric rehabilitation's philosophy.
2. What are some unique contributions of the occupational therapist as a member of the community support team?
3. What types of assessment can an occupational therapist utilize in a work program?
4. What are some examples of workplace accommodations that may be available for workers with psychiatric disabilities?
5. How can the employment specialist help the worker make decisions about disclosure of disability to an employer?

REFERENCES

Allen, C. K., Austin, S. L., David, S. K., Earhart, C. A., McCraith, D. B., & Riska-Williams, L. (2009). *Allen Cognitive Level Screen-5 (ACLS-5) and Large Allen Cognitive Level Screen-5 (LACLS-5).* ACLS and LACLS Committee, Camarillo, CA, USA; Copyright 2007. Retrieved from http://www.allencognitivelevelscreen.org/web09ACLS-5Handoutpg2.pdf

Allen, C. K., Earhart, C. A., & Blue, T. (1992). Allen Cognitive Level Test, 1990. *Occupational therapy treatment goals for the physically and cognitively disabled.* Bethesda, MD: American Occupational Therapy Association.

Anthony, W. A. (1994). Characteristics of people with psychiatric disabilities that are predictive of entry into the rehabilitation process and successful employment. *Psychosocial Rehabilitation Journal, 17*(3), 3–13.

Anthony, W. A., & Jansen, M. A. (1984). Predicting the vocational capacity of the chronically mentally ill, research and policy implications. *American Psychologist, 39*(5), 537–544.

Anthony, W. A., & Liberman, R. P. (1992). Principles and practice of psychiatric rehabilitation. In A. P. Goldstein & L. Krasner (Series Eds.) & R. P. Liberman (Vol. Ed.), *General psychology series: Vol. 166. Handbook of psychiatric rehabilitation* (pp. 1–29). Boston: Allyn & Bacon.

Arbesman, M., & Logsdon, D. (2011). Occupational therapy interventions for employment and education for adults with serious mental illness: A systematic review. *American Journal of Occupational Therapy, 65*(3), 238–246. doi: 10.5014/ajot.2011.001289

Auerbach, E. (2001a). The individual placement and support model vs. the menu approach to supported employment: Where does occupational therapy fit in? *Occupational Therapy in Mental Health, 17*(2), 1–19.

Auerbach, E. (2001b). *The long term work experiences of persons with severe and persistent mental illness.* Unpublished master's thesis, San Jose State University, San Jose, CA.

Auerbach, E. (2002). *Occupational Profile.* Unpublished self-report questionnaire. (Available from Eileen Auerbach, 611 Frederick Street, San Francisco, CA 94117; e-mail address: EenieA@aol.com.)

Auerbach, E. S., & Richardson, P. (2005). The long term work experiences of persons with severe and persistent mental illness. *Psychiatric Rehabilitation Journal, 28*(3), 267–273.

Becker, D. R., & Drake, R. E. (1993). *A working life: The individual placement and support (IPS) program.* Hanover: New Hampshire-Dartmouth Psychiatric Research Center.

Bond, G. R. (1992). Vocational rehabilitation. In A. P. Goldstein & L. Krasner (Series Eds.) & R. P. Liberman (Vol. Ed.), *General psychology series: Vol. 166. Handbook of psychiatric rehabilitation* (pp. 244–275). Boston: Allyn & Bacon.

Bond, G. R. (1998). Principles of the individual placement and support model. *Psychiatric Rehabilitation Journal, 22,* 11–23.

Bond, G. R., Drake, R. E., Mueser, K. T., & Becker, D. R. (1997). An update on supported employment for people with severe mental illness. *Psychiatric Services, 48*(3), 335–345.

Braitman, A., Counts, P., Davenport, R., Zurlinden, B., Rogers, M., Clauss, J., et al. (1995). Comparison of barriers to employment for unemployed and employed clients in a case management program: An exploratory study. *Psychiatric Rehabilitation Journal, 19*(1), 3–8.

Braveman, B., Robson, M., Velozo, C., Kielhofner, G., Fisher, G., Forsyth, K., et al. (2005). *Worker Role Interview (WRI) (Version 10.0).* Retrieved from http://www.moho.uic.edu/assess/wri.html

California Occupational Preference Survey (COPS). (1971). San Diego: Educational and Industrial Testing Service.

Chan, A. S. M., Tsang, H. W. H., & Li, S. M. Y. (2009). Case report of integrated supported employment for a person with severe mental illness. *American Journal of Occupational Therapy, 63,* 238–244.

Corrigan, P. W., Schade, M. L., & Liberman, R. P. (1992). Social skills training. In A. P. Goldstein & L. Krasner (Series Eds.) & R. P. Liberman (Vol. Ed.), *General psychology series: Vol. 166, Handbook of psychiatric rehabilitation* (pp. 95–126). Boston: Allyn & Bacon.

Danley, K. S., Sciarappa, K., & MacDonald-Wilson, K. (1992). Choose-Get-Keep: A psychiatric rehabilitation approach to supported employment. In H. R. Lamb (Series Ed.) & R. P. Liberman (Vol. Ed.), *New directions for mental health services: Vol. 53, Effective psychiatric rehabilitation* (pp. 87–96). San Francisco: Jossey-Bass.

Drake, R. E. (1998). A brief history of the individual placement and support model. *Psychiatric Rehabilitation Journal, 22,* 3–7.

Ethridge, D. A. (1968). Pre-vocational assessment of rehabilitation potential of psychiatric patients. *American Journal of Occupational Therapy, 22*(3), 161–167.

Falk-Kessler, J. (1998). Occupational therapy models: Acquisitional frame of reference. In A. MacRae & E. Cara (Eds.), *Psychosocial occupational therapy in clinical practice* (pp. 115–119). Clifton Park, NY: Delmar, Cengage Learning.

Flexor, R. W., & Solomon, P. L. (1993). Introduction to psychiatric rehabilitation in practice. In R. W. Flexor & P. L. Solomon (Eds.), *Psychiatric rehabilitation in practice* (pp. xiii–xvii). Boston: Andover.

Frey, J. L., & Godfrey, M. (1991). A comprehensive clinical vocational assessment: The PACT approach. *Journal of Applied Rehabilitation Counseling, 22*(2), 25–28.

Henry, A. D., & Mallinson, T. (1999). The occupational performance history interview. In B. J. Hemphill-Pearson (Ed.), *Assessments in occupational therapy mental health: An integrative approach* (pp. 59–70). Thorofare, NJ: Slack.

Hunter, M. L. (1999). The prevocational assessment process in mental health occupational therapy. In B. J. Hemphill-Pearson (Ed.), *Assessments in occupational therapy mental health: An integrative approach* (pp. 109–115). Thorofare, NJ: Slack.

Jacobs, K. (1991). *Occupational therapy: Work-related programs & assessments* (2nd ed.). Boston: Little, Brown.

Kirsh, B. (2000a). Factors associated with employment for mental health consumers. *Psychiatric Rehabilitation Journal, 24*(1), 13–21.

Kirsh, B. (2000b). Organizational culture, climate and person-environment fit: Relationships with employment outcomes for mental health consumers. *Work, 14,* 109–122.

Kirsh, B., Cockburn, L., & Gewurtz, R. (2006). Best practice in occupational therapy: Program characteristics that influence vocational outcomes for people with serious mental illnesses. *The Canadian Journal of Occupational Therapy, 72*(5), 265–279.

Lang, S. (1991). Perspectives—Work for psychiatrically disabled clients. In K. Jacobs (Ed.), *Work: A journal of prevention, assessment, and rehabilitation* (pp. 6–10). Boston: Andover.

Mancuso, L. (1993). *Case studies on reasonable accommodations for workers with psychiatric disabilities.* Study funded by the Community Support Program at the Center for Mental Health Services of the U.S. Department of Health and Human Services, Substance Abuse and Mental Health Administration.

Marrone, J. (1993). Creating positive vocational outcomes for people with severe mental illness. *Psychosocial Rehabilitation Journal, 17*(2), 43–62.

Marrone, J., Gandolfo, C., Gold, M., & Hoff, D. (1998). Just doing it: Helping people with mental illness get good jobs. *Journal of Applied Rehabilitation Counseling, 29*(1), 37–48.

Moore-Corner, R., Kielhofner, G., & Olson, L. (1998). *Work Environment Impact Scale (WEIS) Version 2.0.* Retrieved from http://www.uic.edu/depts/moho/assess/weis.html

Mosey, A. C. (1996). *Psychosocial components of occupational therapy* (rev. ed.). Philadelphia: Lippincott-Raven.

Page, M. (1999). Interviewing as an assessment tool in occupational therapy. In B. J. Hemphill-Pearson (Ed.), *Assessments in occupational therapy mental health: An integrative approach* (pp. 19–39). Thorofare, NJ: Slack.

Rogers, E. S., Anthony, W. A., Cohen, M., & Davies, R. R. (1997). Prediction of vocational outcome based on clinical and demographic indicators among vocationally ready clients. *Community Mental Health Journal, 33*(2), 99–112.

Rouleau, S., Saint-Jean, M., Stip, E., & Fortier, P. (2009). The impact of a pre-vocational program on cognition, symptoms, and work re-integration in schizophrenia. *Occupational Therapy in Mental Health, 25*(1), 26–43.

Social Security Administration. (2010). The red book: A guide to work incentives. SSA Publication No. 64-030 (2010 Red Book), January 2010, ICN 436900. Retrieved from http://www.socialsecurity.gov/redbook/

Stauffer, D. (1986). Predicting successful employment in the community for people with a history of chronic mental illness. *Occupational Therapy in Mental Health, 6*(2), 31–49.

Strong Interest Inventory. (1994). Palo Alto, CA: Stanford University Press.

Tsang, H. W. H., & Pearson, V. (2001). Work-related social skills training for people with schizophrenia in Hong Kong. *Schizophrenia Bulletin, 27*, 139–148.

UCLA Social and Independent Living Skills Series. (1990). Available from dissemination coordinator, Psychiatric Rehabilitation Consultants, PO Box 2867, Camarillo, CA 93011-2867, Phone: (805) 484-5663, Fax: (805) 484-0735. Retrieved from http://www.psychrehab.com/

U.S. Congress. (1994, March). *Psychiatric disabilities, employment, and the Americans with Disabilities Act* (Office of Technology Assessment Report). Technology Assessment Board of the 103rd U.S. Congress.

Valpar International Corporation, P. O. Box 5767, Tucson, AZ 85703.

SUGGESTED RESOURCES

American Occupational Therapy Association. (2008). Occupational therapy practice framework: Domain and process (2nd ed.). *American Journal of Occupational Therapy, 62*, 625–683.

Asher, I. E. (1996). *Occupational therapy evaluation tools: An annotated index* (2nd ed.). Bethesda, MD: American Occupational Therapy Association.

Bailey, E. L., Ricketts, S. K., Becker, D. R., Xai, H., & Drake, R. E. (1998). Do long term day treatment clients benefit from supported employment? *Psychiatric Rehabilitation Journal, 22*, 24–29.

Crist, P., & Stoffel, V. (1992). The Americans with Disabilities Act of 1990 and employees with mental impairments: Personal efficacy and the environment. *American Journal of Occupational Therapy, 46*(5), 434–443.

www.Fountainhouse.org: Fountain House is a community dedicated to the recovery of men and women with mental illness by providing opportunities for members to live, work, and learn, while contributing their talents through mutual support.

Harnois, G., & Gabriel, P. (2000). *Mental health and work: Impact, issues and good practices.* Geneva: World Health Organization (document WHO/MSD/MPS/00.2). Retrieved from http://www.who.int/mental_health/media/en/73.pdf

Harvey-Krefting, L. (1985). The concept of work in occupational therapy: A historical review. *American Journal of Occupational Therapy, 39*, 301–307.

Lang, S., & Cara, E. (1989). Vocational integration for the psychiatrically disabled. *Hospital and Community Psychiatry, 40*(9), 890–892.

www.Thresholds.org: Thresholds is a psychosocial rehabilitation program for people with severe and persistent mental illness that has innovative, effective models of care.

Torrey, W. C., Bebout, R., Kline, J., Becker, D. R., Alverson, M., & Drake, R. E. (1998). Practice guidelines for clinicians working in programs providing integrated vocational and clinical services for persons with severe mental disorders. *Psychiatric Rehabilitation Journal, 21*(4), 388–393.

Unger, K. (1990, Summer). Supported postsecondary education for people with mental illness. *American Rehabilitation,* 10–14.

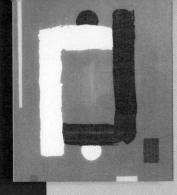

Chapter 24

Substance Abuse and Occupational Therapy

Steve Hoppes, PhD,OTR/L
Helen R. Bryce, MA, OTR/L
Suzanne M. Peloquin, PhD, OTR, FAOTA

▮▬ KEY TERMS

12-step programs

addiction

biopsychosocialspiritual model

cognitive-behavioral therapy (CBT)

harm reduction

lifestyle redesign

Living Skills Development Group

Self-Development Group

solution-focused brief therapy (SFBT)

substance abuse

CHAPTER OUTLINE

Introduction
Use, Abuse, and Dependence
    Scope of the Problem
    Are Substance Abuse and Addiction Choices, Habits, or a Disease?
Treatment Approaches
    12-Step Programs
    Cognitive-Behavioral Therapy
    Comparing Outcomes of CBT and 12-Step Programs
Rationale for Inclusion of Occupational Therapy
Occupation-Based Intervention Programming in Recovery Programs
    Screening and Evaluation Process
    Interventions
    Discontinuation of Services

Occupational Therapy at the Alcohol and Drug Abuse Center
    Client Perceptions of the Challenge
    Programming at ADA House
    Occupational Therapy Programming
    Implementing Group Interventions
    Supportive Residential Programming: Individualized Living Skills
    Student Participation
Advice
Summary

> *O God, that men should put an enemy in their mouths to steal away their brains! That we should, with joy, pleasance, revel, and applause, transform ourselves into beasts!* ~William Shakespeare, *Othello*

INTRODUCTION

Why do individuals consume illicit drugs and alcohol to the point of addiction, which unfailingly "steals away their brains" causing physical, emotional, social, and occupational devastation? What are the best pathways to recovery from substance abuse and addiction? Substance abuse is a perplexing, prevalent, and catastrophic issue in our society. But it is also true that effective, evidence-based approaches to treatment and recovery help countless individuals recover from addiction to return to healthy and richer lives. Occupational therapists hold a valuable piece of the recovery puzzle: occupational engagement.

It can appear that individuals with substance-use disorders freely choose repeated and reckless intoxication over responsible sobriety. Blaming these individuals is common in society and even in healthcare systems; compassion and understanding for substance abuse are often in short supply. A truer picture is more complex. "We're not bad people," a client said. "We just have a horrible addiction that we need help with. We need compassion to get better."

In this chapter, we'll explore the nature of alcohol and drug use, abuse, and dependence; we'll consider the scope of the problems of alcohol and drug abuse in the United States; we'll examine the question of whether substance abuse is a choice, a habit, or a disease; we'll discuss the treatment approaches with the greatest clinical support and best evidence bases; we'll explore occupation-based assessments and interventions; and we'll take you inside of an occupational therapy program at an alcohol and drug treatment facility in Texas. We'll also hear clients' advice about what therapists who work in this area need to know. The authors of this chapter have found this work immensely gratifying. We've found that, as occupational therapists, we make a difference with our clients with substance-use disorders—a big difference. We hope to pass along our enthusiasm for this work to you.

USE, ABUSE, AND DEPENDENCE

When does the use of alcohol and drugs become abuse and dependence? Because use, abuse, and dependence are on a continuum, and not discretely demarcated, definitions offer only a starting point in answering this question. **Substance abuse** refers to "the harmful or hazardous use of psychoactive substances, including alcohol and illicit drugs" (World Health Organization, n.d.). **Addiction** is "a compulsive and maladaptive dependence on a substance or behavior" (Venes, 2009).

Guidelines for abuse and dependence have been established for alcohol but are less clear for other drugs due to various types and dosages. The National Institute on Alcohol Abuse and Alcoholism (NIAAA) classifies drinking patterns by the number of drinks per day and week. In this model, one drink contains about 0.6 ounce or 14 grams of pure alcohol, which is equivalent to the alcohol content of one 12 ounce beer, 5 ounces of table wine, or 1.5 ounces of 80-proof spirits (NIAAA, n.d.).

- *"Low Risk" Drinking.* According to the National Institutes of Health, 2% of individuals who follow these guidelines develop alcoholism or alcohol abuse.
    - *Men:* no more than four drinks per day, and no more than 14 drinks per week
    - *Women:* no more than three drinks per day, and no more than seven drinks per week
- *"At Risk" or "Heavy" Drinking.* Those who exceed the "low risk drinking" guidelines fall into this category. About one in four drinkers in this category already have alcoholism or alcohol abuse, and the rest are at risk for developing these problems. The NIAAA offers this guideline: "Too much plus too often equals too risky" (NIAAA, n.d.).
- *Dependence on Alcohol or Other Drugs.* Dependence is marked by tolerance; withdrawal; drinking or using larger amounts over a longer period of time than intended; persistent desire or unsuccessful efforts to cut down; disruption of social, recreational, and occupational pursuits; and continuing drinking despite awareness of the physical and psychological problems that this causes (American Psychiatric Association [APA], 2000).

Scope of the Problem

The prevalence and social consequences of substance-use disorders are staggering. In 2009, an estimated 22.5 million persons aged 12 or older were classified with substance dependence or abuse in the past year, constituting 8.9% of the U.S. population aged 12 or older (SAMHSA, 2010). Alcohol plays a role in approximately 20% of admissions to intensive care units and 55% of fatal driving accidents; 40% of Americans experience an alcohol-related accident at some point in their lives (APA, 2000).

Addictions to illicit drugs and alcohol cost the United States more than $360 billion annually in health- and crime-related costs and losses in productivity

(Harwood, 2000; Office of National Drug Control Policy, 2004). A study by the Centers for Disease Control and Prevention (CDC, 2001) found that more than 60% of state and federal prisoners tested positive for at least one illicit drug at the time of their arrests.

Are Substance Abuse and Addiction Choices, Habits, or a Disease?

The etiology of addiction has long been debated. Is it a genetic defect, a moral short-coming, a disease, a learned behavior, or a combination of these? Any approach to an-swering this question tends to be based in assumptions about the human condition rather than evidence. While a definitive answer is not possible, assumptions about this issue guide intervention. While it may appear that individuals freely choose to use substances that inflict widespread personal, physical, emotional, social, and occupational damage, closer study reveals a more complex picture. With near con-sensus, the treatment community has come to view substance abuse and addiction as a disease. The U.S. Department of Health and Human Services (2008a) answers the question about the nature of addiction in this way: "Addiction is a chronic, often re-lapsing brain disease that causes compulsive drug seeking and use despite the harm-ful consequences to the individual who is addicted and to those around them" (p. 1).

While some people can experiment with alcohol and drugs and then stop or use them infrequently, others become addicted due to interactions of biological, environmental, and developmental factors. Addiction then leads to changes in the brain's structure and function by disrupting communication between nerve cells (U.S. Department of Health and Human Services, 2008a).

Dr. Alan I. Leshner, former director of the National Institute on Drug Abuse, wrote that drug addiction is

> a brain disease that develops over time as a result of the initially voluntary behavior of using drugs. The consequence is virtually uncontrollable com-pulsive drug craving, seeking, and use that interferes with, if not destroys, an individual's functioning in the family and in society. This medical con-dition demands formal treatment. . . . For many people these behaviors are truly uncontrollable, just like the behavioral expression of any other brain disease. . . . No matter how one develops an illness, once one has it, one is in the diseased state and needs treatment. (Leshner, 2001)

Risk factors for addiction have been identified. Alcoholism runs in families (Cotton, 1979; Goodwin et al., 1974). Based on studies of twins and adopted children, researchers estimate that half or more of the risk for alcohol dependence is based on genetics (Galanter & Kleber, 2008). Other risk factors influencing the course of alco-hol and drug use include gender (males use alcohol and drugs at higher rates than females); the presence of other mental health issues; and environmental factors such as socioeconomic status, peer pressure, physical and sexual abuse, stress, and paren-tal involvement. Developmental factors also play a role: adolescents are particularly vulnerable to risky use due to less mature decision-making, judgment, and self-control (SAMHSA, 2010; U.S. Department of Health and Human Services, 2008a).

TREATMENT APPROACHES

Because pathways into substance abuse and addiction are complex, individualized, and not fully understood, there is no "one-size-fits-all" pathway out. Any number of approaches to treating substance abuse have gathered both clinical and research support including acupuncture, meditation, psychotherapy, pharmacotherapy, motivational interviewing, contingency management, and others (Dakwar & Levin, 2009; Lowinson, Ruiz, Millman, & Langrod, 2005; Rotgers, 2003). Treatment approaches are presented in a wide variety of settings and formats and are often used in combination.

An exhaustive review of treatment approaches is beyond the scope of this chapter. The purpose of this section is to familiarize therapists with the two most common approaches for treating substance abuse and addiction, which are built on the most extensive and specific foundations of theory, research evidence, and clinical support: **12-step programs** and **cognitive-behavioral therapy (CBT)**. The section concludes with implications for occupational therapists.

12-Step Programs

Only a small percentage of individuals with substance-abuse disorders, perhaps less than 10%, seek help. When they do, the vast majority turns to 12-step programs (Hasin & Grant, 1995; Moss, Chen, & Yi, 2007). 12-step programs are based on the principles of Alcoholics Anonymous; due to their popularity, the programs have been applied to other addictive disorders, including drug **addiction** (Narcotics Anonymous), eating disorders (Overeaters Anonymous), and gambling (Gamblers Anonymous). It is safe to say that if you work in a substance-abuse program, you will encounter 12-step treatment approaches. While Alcoholic Anonymous programs are autonomous and meet in a variety of community settings, 12-step programs have been integrated into most established public and private substance treatment programs.

The 12-step explanation of addiction has been called a **biopsychosocial-spiritual model** (Wallace, 2003). Because addiction has a significant and deleterious impact on physical, psychological, social, and spiritual facets of being human, each of these must be addressed in treatment. This model frames addiction as an entrapping, interlocking set of four vicious cycles.

Physically, alcohol and drugs have been shown to produce profound changes on important neuromodulators, neurotransmitters, and neurohormones involved in the brain's transmission of information (Wallace, 2003). When alcohol and drugs alter brain chemistry, feelings of euphoria, alertness, relaxation, or well-being can result, and it is these pleasurable feelings that individuals with addictions seek. When addiction inevitably leads to overuse or attempts to withdraw, adverse changes in brain chemistry lead to negative moods, feelings of fatigue, depression, paranoia, irritation, or agitation. The insidious and escalating cycle of addiction leads to further pleasure-seeking and entrapment between repetitive positive and negative reinforcers.

Psychologically, addiction is marked by low self-esteem, anger, grandiosity, resentments, denial, minimization of difficulties, hostility, excessive self-pity, low self-confidence, low frustration tolerance, various phobias, and other neuroses (Wallace, 2003). These problems trigger a self-perpetuating cycle of increasing substance usage to relieve the suffering caused by these psychological states; in turn, increased usage exacerbates the suffering.

Social cycles operate as well. Alcohol and other drugs are often seen as a "social lubricant," useful for reducing social inhibition. While this may be effective at times for individuals who are not at risk for addiction, at-risk individuals play with fire when they rely on addictive substances to socialize. Inevitably, usage leads to an under-developed and limited social repertoire, which, in turn, leads to further social difficulties and usage as a substitute for intimacy. Families are deeply affected by addiction. Partners of individuals with addictions often develop maladaptive patterns for dealing with relationship issues. Children become tangled in the stress and discord of a parent's addiction, resulting in social and emotional problems, including excessive fears, acting out at home and school, learning difficulties, truancy, sexual experimentation, low self-confidence, and drinking and drug problems of their own (Wallace, 1987). Other common social difficulties of individuals with addictions include employment, education, and career problems; conflicted relationships with friends; legal and financial distress; arrests and incarcerations; and loss of social status (Wallace, 2003).

Spirituality is the fourth component of the biopsychosocialspiritual model. 12-step literature does not specifically define *spirituality*, preferring more general descriptions: "a willingness to believe in a Power greater than ourselves" (Alcoholics Anonymous World Services, Inc., 2011, chapter 4). Emphasis is placed on one's own conception of constructs such as Higher Power, God, or spirituality. Occupational therapy's understanding of spirituality augments that of 12-step programs and may be useful when considering shaping occupation-based interventions that address this component of the model. *Spirituality* is defined as

> the personal quest for understanding answers to ultimate questions about life, about meaning, and about relationship with the sacred or transcendent, which may (or may not) lead to or arise from the development of religious rituals and the formation of community. (American Occupational Therapy Association [AOTA], 2008, p. 675)

Addiction often leads to feelings of meaninglessness, purposelessness, isolation, and alienation. Cyclic behavior occurs within this dimension as well. Feelings of spiritual emptiness lead to substance abuse, which in turn leads to further emptiness and despair, and repeated desires to soothe the pain.

Although addiction destroys physical, psychological, social, and spiritual well-being, individuals caught in these cycles are generally ambivalent and often resistant to seeking help. While they may long to be free of the negatives of usage, they become quite attached to the fleeting and illusory pleasures and escape that alcohol and drugs bring.

12-step programs do not offer a "cure" for addiction, which is seen as a life-long disease. While the disease of addiction cannot be cured, it can be treated successfully. 12-step programs support abstinence as the only way to find release and recovery from the devastating cycles of addiction. The 12-step therapeutic processes include attending group meetings for the purpose of studying the 12 steps, one-to-one guidance from a senior member (a "sponsor"), and "working the steps."

In Step 1 of the program, participants come to accept that they cannot control their usage through conscious, deliberate effort. In Step 2, participants adopt beliefs that only a power greater than themselves can free them from substance-dependence. In Step 3, participants surrender to an undefined "Higher Power" (left to individual interpretation as God, the group itself, love, spirituality, awareness, etc.). In Step 4, participants take a "moral inventory" of their fears, anger, sadness, guilt, and resentments that trigger and influence addiction. In Step 5, participants share their self-analyses with their higher power and another person (often the sponsor). Steps 6 and 7 emphasize letting go of inner struggles, resentments, and guilt associated with perceived character faults. In Steps 8 and 9, participants identify individuals who have been harmed by their addictive behaviors and make "direct amends" to them. Step 10 involves acknowledging responsibility for one's mistakes. In Step 11, participants seek to strengthen contact with their higher power through prayer and meditation. Step 12 invites participants to share the benefits of their "spiritual awakening" with other individuals with addictions. The steps are seen as a set of tools that supports happiness, peace, and sobriety; "working the steps" is a life-long process that one never perfects.

It would be difficult to find a program for the treatment of addiction that has not been influenced by the 12-step model. Treatment outcome studies have found that individuals who participate in 12-step programs are more likely to experience reduced drinking and improved psychological health than those who do not participate in such programs (Emrick, 2004). Further consideration of evidence supporting 12-step programs will be considered after a discussion of CBT.

Cognitive-Behavioral Therapy

CBT refers to a family of treatment approaches that includes rational behavior therapy, cognitive therapy, and dialectic behavior therapy. These approaches are based on the premise that disordered thoughts cause disordered feelings and behaviors. For example, thoughts of worthlessness may lead to depression and, in turn, lead to drinking alcohol or using drugs in hopes of feeling better. Once such a pattern of thoughts is established, it can become habitual and unquestioned.

CBT is based on similar and different assumptions than 12-step programs. While 12-step programs are based on an assumption that addiction is brain disease with physical, psychological, social, and spiritual ramifications, CBT assumes that addiction is a learned habit acquired through classical conditioning, instrumental learning, modeling, and cognitive mediation (Gorman, 2001; Parks, Marlatt, & Anderson, 2004; Rotgers, 2003). In this view, addictions are maladaptive coping mechanisms strengthened by both positive reinforcement (feelings of pleasure) and negative reinforcement (removal of pain or anxiety). Viewing addiction as a habit, rather than a disease, does not discount its power or resistance to change because over-learned habits can become virtually involuntary and subconscious (Parks et al., 2004).

CBT, a biopsychosocial model, shares common ground with 12-step programs in its explanation of the development of addiction as a result of biological, psychological, and social vulnerabilities (Parks et al., 2004). These complex and interactive factors bear on the development and treatment of addiction.

CBT addresses habit change with three strategies: functional analysis of disordered thinking, skills training to increase adaptive coping responses, and relapse prevention (NAMI, 2003; Ouimette, Finney, & Moos, 1997; Rotgers, 2003; U.S. Department of Health and Human Services, 2008b). For the treatment of addiction, functional analysis includes detailed examination of thoughts, feelings, and contexts before, during, and after usage. Once disordered patterns of thinking are exposed, therapists and clients collaborate to replace them with healthier thinking, skills, behaviors, and habits leading to recovery. The final task of CBT is to identify strategies to cope with future temptations that can cause relapse into addiction. Clients are taught how to think about and address potential slips and relapses to lessen their severity.

12-step programs teach that abstinence and addiction have a dualistic relationship. In this view, abstinence is a prerequisite for successful treatment and once addicted, an individual can never successfully return to even limited usage. CBT approaches tend to reject this belief, and suggest that it is more useful to consider abstinence and addiction as opposite ends of a continuum. CBT therapists will typically work with individuals who are actively using drugs or drinking to help them move toward abstinence if that is the client's preference. CBT approaches tend to hold that individuals can transform addictions into moderate use with proper analysis of disordered thinking, skills training, and relapse prevention (Rotgers, 2003). A version of this approach is called "**harm reduction**" (Kishline, 1996; Marlatt & Tapert, 1993). Harm reduction acknowledges the difficulty of abruptly stopping usage and lifelong abstinence. If a therapist and client determine that terminating usage is unlikely, small steps are introduced to reduce usage and harm to physical, mental, and social functioning. Harm reduction views any changes that lead to reduced usage as positive and healthy (Rotgers, 2003).

While the 12-step "addiction-as-disease" model and CBT's "addiction-as-maladaptive-habits" model may seem incompatible, in practice many therapists integrate these approaches. Bristow-Braitman (1995) wrote, "The ability to apply psychological knowledge to the spiritual, and spiritual understandings to the psychological, can only enhance our work as helping professionals" (p. 417).

CBT has an impressive evidence-base supporting its effectiveness with a wide variety of problems, including depression, anxiety disorders, social phobia, obsessive-compulsive disorder, posttraumatic stress disorder, anger, sexual offending, schizophrenia, bulimia nervosa, and chronic pain (Najavits, Liese, & Harned, 2005). Empirical support of CBT in the treatment of substance abuse is less well-established but has been receiving more attention recently (Butler, Chapman, Forman, & Beck, 2006). Hester and Miller (1995) reviewed outcome studies of alcohol treatment and listed the top 10 interventions with the strongest research support; 6 of these are CBT techniques: social skills training, community reinforcement, behavioral contracting, aversion therapy, relapse prevention, and cognitive therapy.

Comparing Outcomes of CBT and 12-Step Programs

Several studies have shown outcomes of CBT and 12-step programs to be comparable. Morgenstern, Blanchard, Morgan, Labouvie, and Hayaki (2001) evaluated the effectiveness of CBT for substance abuse in comparison to 12-step programs with 252 participants in a community-based treatment facility. They wrote, "Until recently, it was assumed that science-based interventions [such as CBT] would prove superior to 12-step-oriented approaches" (p. 1014). Their study found that both CBT and 12-step programming significantly reduced substance abuse and increased abstinence, and that "outcomes were not significantly different across conditions" (p. 1014). Similarly, Wells, Peterson, Gainey, Hawkins, and Catalano (1994), in a study of 110 participants in outpatient treatment, found "no significant differences between these two treatments [CBT and 12-steps] in their ability to retain clients, in the degree to which they resulted in increased skill levels, or in their impact on cocaine or marijuana use 6 months following treatment" (p. 14). Ouimette et al. (1997) studied the effectiveness of CBT, 12-step programs, and mixed 12-step/CBT programs for 3,018 patients from U.S. Department of Veterans Affairs Medical Centers. They concluded the three approaches were "equally effective in reducing patients' substance use, psychological symptoms, and increasing the proportion of patients who avoided legal problems and were not incarcerated or homeless. . . . No differences were found on outcomes in patients who were in the purest 12-step and CB treatment programs" (p. 236).

RATIONALE FOR INCLUSION OF OCCUPATIONAL THERAPY

As occupational therapists, we apply occupation-based interventions to improve occupational performance. It may be tempting to view treatment approaches such as 12 steps or CBT as outside of our domain and not particularly relevant to our work. However, substance abuse and addictions have widespread impact on occupation and the unique occupational therapy perspective complements these models. We have found that it is to our advantage and our clients' and colleagues' advantage if we are conversant with the basic elements of the entire treatment program. A close analogy might be that of a tourist in a foreign country who wishes to fully interact with the people and culture. Learning a bit of the language and working to understand the customs enables communication and purposeful interaction. In the process, the experience becomes more meaningful, coherent, and enjoyable. Conversely, it is the occupational therapist's role to educate other members of the team as to how occupational therapy fits the overall treatment approach.

One factor to be considered in the composition of a substance-abuse treatment team is the recovery status of team members. While there is much value in having staff that has a personal understanding of the experiences of recovery, we believe that a diverse team can best meet the client's needs. Nevertheless, this is an issue that often arises from clients and must be addressed. Figure 24-1 includes comments of clients as well as the authors' views of sharing their own experiences and perspective.

We also advocate for the inclusion of occupational therapy in substance abuse treatment for the benefit of the profession as a whole. As previously discussed, substance abuse is a widespread phenomenon affecting all segments of the population. As a consequence, there is no doubt that occupational therapy practitioners will encounter clients with addiction in every treatment setting. A firm basis in the treatment approaches discussed in this chapter, both theoretically in the classroom and experientially through practicums and internships, facilitates effective interventions in all settings and clarifies the unique contributions of the profession to this field. Figure 24-2 highlights one occupational therapist's story of how her internship in a substance-abuse treatment setting informed her current practice. (Also, see Chapter 26, "Fieldwork Supervision in the Mental Health Setting," for more information from fieldwork interns' perspectives.)

OCCUPATION-BASED INTERVENTION PROGRAMMING IN RECOVERY PROGRAMS

Professional staffing patterns in traditional 12-step recovery programs typically do not support occupational therapy as a core service. Occupational therapy practitioners have had to change with the profession's paradigm shift from the medical model to more client-, family-, community-, and population-centered models of practice (AOTA, 2010a, 2010b; White, Meade, & Hadar, 2007). Consequently, occupational

Clients in recovery will raise this question, in some form, for all who would presume to help them: Are you in recovery yourself?

Our clients addressed their concerns about this issue:

- "It helps you relax to know that a therapist has been where you've been and they're not judging you."
- "Is it possible for a therapist who is not in recovery to do this work? It's definitely possible. You would have to be very spiritually connected, though. When you are spiritually connected you know how to help others who can't help themselves or who are lost. If you're spiritually connected, you have that understanding and want to do that and you won't judge . . . you'll be open."

It will be to your advantage to be prepared to answer the question, whether you're personally in recovery or not. Here is how we answer the question:

Suzanne Peloquin, who has not experienced substance dependence

The women know that I totally support them. They know that although I am not myself in recovery, I have faced life challenges that qualify me to understand pain and heartache. I always answer any question that I ask the women to answer in discussion, noting that I would not ask them to do something that I myself would not do. I tell them that I have family members who have problems with addiction, that some of them have been in AA for years, that some of them are still struggling. They know that I am in tune with them but that I also hold them to the high expectations that they must meet in the "world out there."

Steve Hoppes, who has been in recovery from substance dependence for 30 years

The fact that I'm in recovery has inalterably shaped my personality, insights, perceptions, and judgment, and in turn, my therapeutic use of self. Being able to say, "Me, too" when the conversation is about recovery is a quick entrée into my clients' trust. I use that when I believe it is to their benefit.

As occupational therapists, we use everything we have—our personalities, our knowledge, our skills, our values, our beliefs, our mistakes, and our successes—regardless of where they came from, to benefit our clients. I accept my history of substance dependence and I accept the fact that I am in recovery, one day at a time, just like my clients. Both my past mistakes and my work in recovery help me to offer the trusting, empathetic, and accepting relationships that clients with substance-abuse disorders need. I cherish this work. My clients and I understand that we're in this together and that we support each other's recovery.

Helen Bryce, who has not experienced substance dependence

I had been an occupational therapist for close to 20 years in many areas of practice when I had to hit the ground running to establish an occupational therapy program in a traditional 12-step inpatient program. How does a nonaddict or nonalcoholic work with and relate to individuals in recovery from substance use? Returning to my OT roots, I dug up some old friends—nonjudgment, compassion, and respect for the person and scooped them into my gardening basket filled with fertilizer for a therapeutic alliance, seeds of inquiry for individuals' preferences and goals, and the precise amount of water to fuel hope. Repurposing these tools to a new practice environment fueled my journey of program development, recruitment, sustainability, but most important, of connection to the persons being served to support them in creating a life of meaning.

FIGURE 24-1. Are You in Recovery Yourself?

Clinical fieldwork at an alcohol and drug treatment facility marked one of the most daunting challenges of my occupational therapy career. I found that developing therapeutic relationships with patients with substance abuse disorders required time, patience, and confidence.

I grew up in a happy suburban home and had never so much as received a speeding ticket. Most of my clients had difficulty relating to my rather sheltered lifestyle, and I to theirs. During group sessions led by a licensed counselor, I heard stories of trauma, abuse, and turmoil that nobody should ever endure. I could not help but wonder if my upbringing had been similar to that of many of my clients, would I have resorted to drugs and alcohol? These questions brought significant sadness. I was ashamed of my privileged life, which resulted in barriers between my clients and me.

Fortunately, somewhere in my eight-week rotation, I realized that feeling shame or sorrow for my clients was not working for either of us. My fortunate lifestyle was not something to feel guilty about. As an intelligent and driven student, I was a valuable asset for my clients. I was an expert on setting and achieving goals as well as living a balanced life. I knew how to apply for, achieve, and maintain a job. I could explain how to use a computer and search the Internet, a necessity for a job seeker in today's world. I knew how to submit an application for college and apply for financial aid. These objectives were relevant to my clients; through my own daily occupations, I had found an "in" with my clients as well as a way to influence their occupations. Occupational therapists are experts at developing healthy habits, defining roles, and solidifying routines through occupation. I helped clients identify and practice occupations that carried over to the real world they'd enter after discharge.

As an occupational therapist, you will cross paths with people with substance-abuse disorders. This disease affects a cross-section of your patients as well as the parents of your pediatric patients. Because I know how to design goals, interventions, and treatment plans for individuals with substance-abuse disorders, I know I can help these individuals.

FIGURE 24-2. A Student's Perspective, by Katie E. Warne, OTR/L
Reprinted by permission of Katie E. Warne, OTR/L

therapy services may not be reimbursed as such or may fall under the purview of the per diem rate. Nevertheless, the profession's unique ability to analyze occupational performance and participation to craft a relevant plan of interventions to return the individual to a meaningful life arguably has a fit in recovery programs. Individuals in recovery may voice a desire to improve role performance as a student or employee, care of self and others, money management, time and routine management, and to articulate and attain goals (Davies & Cameron, 2010).

Quality intervention begins with appropriate assessment. Drug and alcohol counselors have standardized instruments such as the Alcohol Severity Index (ASI). Appleby (1997) noted that this widely used instrument's drug and alcohol scales correlated with other substance use assessments. Occupational therapy does not have instruments that are specifically designed to address substance-related disorders; however, several occupational therapy instruments address problems of living and may apply, more specifically, to living with a substance use disorder. Occupational performance, self-efficacy, role competence, work readiness, coping strategies, and healthy leisure pursuits are some of the areas appropriate to assess with an individual in a recovery program.

Screening and Evaluation Process

As a profession with a rich history, occupational therapy is not lacking assessment instruments. In the profession's infancy, assessment was grounded in skilled observation, group process, and projective techniques. As the profession developed, the demand for evidence in practice gave rise to the emergence of a greater number of instruments with sound psychometric properties. While several instruments may have application for individuals in substance recovery, no one, perfect, occupation-centered instrument exists for this population.

An overview of selected, evidenced-based instruments with sound psychometric properties that complement the environment of drug and alcohol recovery centers for adults is presented in Table 24-1. Occupational therapy practitioners and students are advised to use their clinical judgment in considering their population of

TABLE 24-1. Selecting Appropriate Evaluation Instruments for Persons in Recovery

Instrument	Description	Application	Clinical Considerations
Canadian Occupational Performance Measure (COPM), 4th edition (Law et al, 2005)	A semi-structured interview in three areas: self-care, productivity, and leisure. Client scores his performance and satisfaction with identified occupational performance challenges.	Adults Older adults Across settings	Averages 30–40 minutes to complete. Useful for goal setting, intervention planning, and measuring outcomes.
Model of Human Occupation Screening Tool (MOHOST), version 2.0, (Parkinson, Forsyth, & Kielhofner, 2006)	A screening tool that offers a broad perspective of the persons' occupational performance. Helps determine if occupational therapy services are necessary and if more detailed assessment would be fruitful.	Adults Older adults Variety of settings	Relatively quick to use. Data gathered from the client and team. May be used at regular intervals for documentation toward goal attainment.
Occupational Performance History Interview II (OPHI-II), version 2.1, (Kielhofner et al., 2004)	A semi-structured interview focusing on occupational adaptation in three areas: occupational identity, occupational competence, and impact of occupational behavior environment.	Adults Older adults	Averages 60 minutes to complete—may be done in one comprehensive interview or two shorter interviews. Client must be able to participate in an in-depth interview. Generates a life history narrative. Keys developed for each of the three OPHI-II scales allow the therapist to obtain interval measures instantly.

TABLE 24-1. Continued

Instrument	Description	Application	Clinical Considerations
Occupational Self Assessment (OSA), version 2.2, (Baron, Kielhofner, Iyenger, Goldhammer, & Wolenski, 2006)	A self-report measure in two parts that identifies clients' problem areas in occupations, their competence in the occupation and the level of importance they assign to them.	Adults Older adults	Takes 10–20 minutes to complete. Goal setting based upon results. OSA may be used as an outcome measure.
Role Checklist (Oakley, 1984; Oakley, Kielhofner, Barris, & Reichler, 1986)	A two-part checklist that requires the client to mark if she or he has participated in the role in the past, does at present, or strives to in the future and the value she or he places on the role.	Adults Older adults Physical or psychosocial dysfunction	Based on the MOHO. Takes an average of 15 minutes to complete. Useful for intervention planning. An accessible version can be downloaded from the MOHO Clearinghouse website.
Work Environment Impact Scale (WEIS), Version 2.0, (Moore-Corner, Kielhofner, & Olson, 1998)	A semi-structured interview and rating scale, the WEIS gathers information on clients' perception of the workplace environment, the degree it supports or inhibits performance, and the "fit" between workers and their skills and the environment.	Adults with physical or psychosocial dysfunction or work difficulty or interruption	Does not apply to persons who have been unemployed for extended periods. Takes 30 minutes to complete and 10–15 minutes to complete the summary.

individuals in treatment for recovery, the treatment environment, and best practices when selecting evaluation procedures and assessment instruments.

Some therapists may choose to design their own occupational history interview tool or simply use what the treatment environment requires to develop an occupational profile. Asking key questions and listening actively can help the therapist arrive at the heart of the occupational issues the individual in recovery wants to address. For individuals whose self-esteem has been damaged with loss of roles, relationships, employment, and other valued aspects of living with purpose, a strength-based approach to therapist-client interaction may be useful (Brun & Rapp, 2001; Rapp, Siegal, & Fisher, 1992). If designing a form, thinking about organizing topics or content in terms of strengths and liabilities or barriers may be useful to the therapist.

Interventions

After constructing the client's occupational profile and collaborating to establish meaningful goals realistic in light of temporal and contextual constraints, the occupational therapist outlines therapeutic interventions for goal attainment. Prioritizing goals is paramount to success because in-patient time is tightly scheduled and occupational therapy sessions may number few as a result. For this reason brief therapy may provide an appropriate framework when treatment time is limited.

Developed by de Shazer and Berg, **solution-focused brief therapy (SFBT)** focuses on using clients' strengths to gather resources for goal achievement (de Shazer, 1985). The number of sessions may range from one to five with an average of three sessions. With each contact, the client is supported to move toward autonomy. Each session, the therapist provides feedback on how close the client or consumer is to the goal and what it will take to reach it, emphasizing the client's assets and strengths used in the process (Bannink, 2007). Attention is focused in SFBT on envisioning the goal, hope, or dream and directing resources to that end (Iveson, 2002). SFBT is considered a form of CBT as the client, not the therapist, is the expert in changing his cognitions and building resources to create his desired future life (Bannink, 2007).

An SFBT approach to occupational therapy intervention can be a natural fit in a time- and resource-limited treatment environment. How wonderful when a consumer pops in to occupational therapy and announces with urgency, "I just need to . . ."; the immediacy of her need lends itself to a client-centered and client-led approach to generating solutions to her occupational need.

CASE ILLUSTRATION

Janice—SFBT at Work

Janice's counselor was "on her case" to get a job if she wanted to get a room in the halfway house portion of the inpatient facility. Janice wanted to "just do 3 things": (1) develop a resume, (2) upload to three employers who were advertising openings; and (3) figure out the bus route to the temp agency by day after tomorrow.

Discussion

Here was an organic, teachable moment primed for a good outcome and goal accomplishment. Frequently the immediate goal articulated can be reached in three visits or less. Janice's goals were realistic. To her credit, she had a good work skill set and no history or felony convictions standing in her way. She was on her way.

For clients with co-occurring disorders, achieving goals may take longer as their issues may be more complex. Shorter individual or group sessions or scheduled breaks to manage anxiety, shortened attention, or frustration tolerance may be beneficial for some consumers.

Dagobert Runes stated that "work is man's most natural form of relaxation," and for many individuals in recovery, work is vitally important for re-designing healthy habits and routines for a satisfying life. People with addiction tend to be intelligent, creative individuals. For some, however, their entrepreneurial work choices are not always suitable for listing on a resume. Some who have a legal record or a history of incarceration may have significant gaps in employment. Occupational therapy can offer the unique contribution of a creative, yet truthful approach to constructing a functional, skills- and strength-based resume for such a consumer.

If the therapist allows that the point in time when an individual's addiction begins is when other developmental tasks and skills cease maturing, then one could consider consumers with addictions as having developmental delays—in social, cognitive, spiritual, and emotional skills. In this vein, it follows that they may never have learned life skills that pertain to securing meaningful employment and for maintaining employment for protracted periods of time. The intrinsic desire for meaningful work is not limited to individuals without substance use disorders or co-occurring disorders. Occupational therapy SFBT interactions for a consumer with a co-occurring disorder might look something like the following Case Illustration.

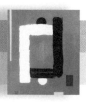

CASE ILLUSTRATION

Yosef—Gathering the Occupational Profile

Yosef is a self-described "jack of all trades, master of none" who has held several jobs, albeit for short duration, while living with co-occurring disorder, substance addiction, and bipolar disorder. When deeply depressed, Yosef uses cocaine to get going, and when manic, he uses marijuana to "even out." His drug and alcohol counselor wants him to consider applying for SSDI (Social Security Disability Insurance) due to the challenges of helping Yosef manage his diseases and his medication, but Yosef wants occupational therapy referral for help with life skills for job development. His family prides themselves on not "taking handouts," and SSDI is his last resort. He expresses a desire to find work and keep it for several years.

His occupational therapist takes a strength-based approach to engaging Yosef in evaluation. She acknowledges his goal of finding lasting employment, and points out her role of advocate and coach to help him with decisional balance as he explores the dynamic tension between his desire for employment and his counselor's recommendation to apply for SSDI instead of full-time work. She offers that while helping him to list his assets, she also will help him identify barriers to reaching his goal, employment, so they can determine if and how those barriers can be knocked down on his path to a successful, satisfying life in recovery.

Discussion

The occupational therapist knows that Yosef values work and family. She asks Yosef some initial interview questions, building on this knowledge. "What job have you most enjoyed and why?" "What have bosses told you that you do well?" "What is getting in the way of you going to work (or school)?" "What do you dream about doing or trying?" "What do you want for your child?" "What goals have you and your counselor set?"

She realizes that because of Yosef's long history of mental illness and substance abuse, he has "developmental delays" when it comes to organizing a job search. While an inpatient he will need help with several tasks, which she will break down into more manageable bits for his ensured success. He will need the following resources to get started: (1) phone message system with his voice on it (not the switchboard operator's voice), (2) bus money and knowledge of the public transportation system, (3) free email account to send resumes to prospective employers; and (4) knowledge of electronic file management to store job searches and work samples, to name just a few.

Together they discuss some of his prior challenge areas: frustration tolerance, persevering with a task to completion, and attention to detail and how those tendencies relate to securing and retaining employment. The occupational therapist gives him "homework," an occupational challenge, and asks him to return in a specified number of days to report on how well it went for him. Together they discuss what "went right" and use these positive aspects of each experience attempted to move him forward in his goals, one item on his goal "to-do list" at a time.

Intervention activities and approaches are customized to the client's preference, needs, and goals with respect to the demands of the timing of treatment and the anticipated return environment. Some areas for intervention may include educational pursuits, job exploration, leisure exploration, stress management, and resource development. Table 24-2 highlights sample life skills classes.

With an SFBT approach to occupational therapy intervention in drug and alcohol rehabilitation services, documenting consumers' progress toward their goals can be straightforward as the consumer directs his energies to what is most important to him.

Discontinuation of Services

Consumers are discontinued from occupational therapy when goals are achieved due to the brief nature of service delivery in this environment. Depending on her length of stay, she may be referred to occupational therapy again at a later point in

TABLE 24-2. Sample Life Skills Class Offerings

Life Skill Offering	Session 1	Session 2	Session 3	Session 4
CLOTHES MAKE THE MAN OR WOMAN; TAKE CARE OF THEM	**SEW WHAT** Sew on button, hook and eye, minor repairs.	**HEMMING AND HAWING** Hem up pants, skirt, or sleeves (no staples or duct tape allowed!).	**PUMPING IRON** Iron a shirt or blouse, paying attention to fabric care instructions.	**GET IT TOGETHER** Assemble an interview outfit on a budget. Dress to cover tattoos, electronic monitoring devices, etc.
GET A JOB	**ASSESSING STRENGTHS, LIABILITIES, APTITUDES, LIFE EXPERIENCES** Tap into dreams while addressing short-term goals for reducing debt, paying rent, etc.	**CHRONICLE YOUR WORK (OCCUPATIONAL) HISTORY.** Recreate your work, volunteer, and caregiving history to fold into a resume, job application, or training application.	**RESUME 101** Build a functional resume, industry-specific resume, or resume template.	**GETTING IT OUT THERE** Uploading, emailing, or hand delivering your resume.
POWERING UP FOR THE INTERVIEW	**PUTTING YOUR BEST FACE FORWARD** Individually or in small peer group, address oral hygiene (smoker's breath, tooth decay, or missing teeth from substance use) and its impact on one's presentation. Review resources for dental care, dentures, partials, or implants.	**DEALING WITH DIFFICULT QUESTIONS** Role play with therapist or small peer group how to respond to tough questions such as gaps in employment or felony conviction, responding in an honest way while playing to one's strengths and skills. Give and receive feedback.	**ACTIONS SPEAK LOUDER** With therapist or small group, practice strategies to manage behaviors resulting from heavy substance use, such as tics, non-essential tremors, jaw activity, bruxism, etc. Breathing exercises, progressive relaxation, guided imagery and positive visualization, and other mindfulness techniques can be offered.	**ANTICIPATE SUCCESS** Use an appropriately firm handshake. Establish and main comfortable eye contact. Research the company and comment or ask questions based on what you learned. Have your list of references ready. Ask when they will make their decision. Do you need to follow up with them? Send a hand-written thank you note to the person(s) who interviewed you.

(Continues)

TABLE 24-2. Continued

Life Skill Offering	Session 1	Session 2	Session 3	Session 4
GETTING IN SCHOOL; STAYING IN SCHOOL	**WHAT WAS YOUR FAVORITE SUBJECT?** Assessing learning and academic strengths, liabilities, and aptitudes and how they related to present and future goals.	**GETTING TO THE NEXT STEP** Local resources for GED, HS diploma completion; community college or vocational/technical school admission; bachelor's or other degree completion, etc.	**PAPERWORK— BRING IT ON!** Navigating the FAFSA and other forms—online, on paper, or in person.	**FINANCING THE DREAM** Applying for student aid, grants, loans, scholarship, and work-study. Tapping into opportunities such as programs for first-generation college students, minority students, veterans, persons with low income, etc.
BUILDING YOUR HOUSE: LIFE ARCHITECTURE 101 (For anyone, especially mothers, trying to regain parenting rights)	**IT'S A 911** Creating an emergency contact number list for the refrigerator (Creative component involved in constructing a personal magnet)	**LIFE HAPPENS. HAVE A PLAN.** Draw emergency egress routes for fire and a shelter area for tornado. Consider best locations for placement of smoke alarms, carbon monoxide monitors. Look up local resources for household lead and asbestos testing.	**KEEP IT SAFE** Assemble an emergency kit for power outage: 3 days of canned food, water, medicine, batteries, blankets, footwear, etc. Select child- and eco-friendly cleaning supplies. Identify safe storage place at home.	**IF YOU FIX IT, THEY WILL COME** Discuss and practice basic home repairs: running toilet, plugged up sink; replacing light bulbs; caulking around windows and doors; caulking around sinks, showers, tubs; replacing air filters; checking furnace, A/C, fireplace; cleaning dryer vents to prevent fires.
MONEY MATTERS	**DEVELOPING A MONTHLY BUDGET** Insert the "have-to" items: rent, food, medicine. Plan for emergency items: doctor visit, car repair, home repair. Fold in some "want to" items: leisure and other discretionary spending.	**SEASONS AND SALES** Identify which months are the best times to purchase certain household items (appliances, linens, clothing, electronics, etc.) and plan for purchases.	**PLAN NOW, SAVE LATER** Outline a week's worth of meals based on grocery ads, coupons, and sales. Compare savings for prepared foods versus foods you prepare.	**GROWING MONEY, SHRINKING DEBT** Identify local Consumer Credit Counseling service (sponsored by the United Way, not by a predatory lender). Pay yourself first. Apply the power of compound interest. If paid every two weeks, save the additional two paychecks each year.

TABLE 24-2. Continued

Life Skill Offering	Session 1	Session 2	Session 3	Session 4
IT TAKES A VILLAGE Who are two or three people you trust with your child? Can you trade hours for child-care coverage (sick days, personal appointments, job search time, etc.)? Could you trade a cooked meal, sewing, or yard work for child care? Be creative! We all need help at times.	**BARTERING FOR BABYSITTING** Develop your list of "trades." Make an addition to your Family Notebook.	**I'M BORED** Develop a list of local no cost, low cost recreation and leisure activities for your family. Create a personalized notebook that allows for future additions to be inserted.	**DEVELOPING DREAMERS, PROMOTING PROBLEM-SOLVERS** Explore no cost and low cost hobbies, crafts, and games to do with children to develop the whole child. Make additions to your Family Notebook with activities you and your child select together: Scouts, Boys and Girls Clubs, library activities, seasonal fairs, farmers' markets, etc. Weaving the past and positive future together: Create a weaving for the home (ribbon, yarn, cloth, colored paper) that represents a healthy family life in recovery.	**PICTURING THE FUTURE** Using resources you have identified, begin a scrapbook, photo album, photo CD, or other memory collection with your child to represent the positive future you are creating for yourselves. Have your children take turns planning the Family Night each week. The "lead child" gets to pick the game, craft, meal, or activity, "teaching" the rest of the family how it is done.
FOR THE HEALTH OF IT: TAKING CARE OF MY MIND, BODY, AND SPIRIT	**KNOWING YOUR PAST, ORGANIZING YOUR FUTURE** Erect a medical history file for you and each family member. Include routine medications, surgeries or procedures and dates, and shot records. Set up a medication (vitamin, supplement) routine (can use a notebook, pill organizer, or spread sheet if complicated) for each family member, especially those with chronic conditions such as asthma, depression, etc. Place it in the Family Medical Health binder.	**IT'S ALL ABOUT ME** Develop some "Prescription for Happiness" index cards. Write out a few cards for each area to be a healthier person (and parent)— physical activities, hobby, exercise, stress management, leisure, etc. Give yourself one "homework" index card (even if it is simply five minutes for yourself with the bathroom door closed) to nurture yourself each day.	**AN APPLE A DAY** Add one simple health prevention activity to daily routine. Tie health prevention and maintenance activities to existing routines. Focus on ownership for health; securing low cost routine health prevention, screenings, and care.	**BE QUIET, FIND PEACE** Find a few moments each day to connect to yourself. What is your body telling you? Do you need to slow down and reflect? Do you need to quiet your mind and not let yourself ruminate over "old stuff" or rehearse whatever you are dreading for tomorrow? Create a Balance of Satisfying Activities chart. What does your chart tell you? If not satisfied, what is one thing you can change? Be gentle with yourself; you are a work in progress.

her recovery program when she is ready to address another occupational challenge. Other external factors influence this timing as well. Occupational therapy services may be on hold if a client or consumer is moved to another level in the program, has a medical procedure, or has other scheduled consultations. If, for example, the client relapses, she may be abruptly discharge from the facility. The same consequence is handed down when a consumer violates the rules after failing a behavioral contract. Additionally, probation officers can unexpectedly terminate or extend treatment services.

Occupational therapy professionals' role in working with individuals in recovery may vary depending on who is sitting in front of us and what their return environment requires of them. No one professional, not drug and alcohol counselors, case managers, or occupational therapists, can meet individuals' every need, despite the team's best efforts. Because some individuals may be in treatment for only 3 to 4 weeks, they are just getting a handle on their recovery, one that takes more than 28 days to solidify. Community resources and supports, in addition to 12-step meetings for some, help individuals make more successful transitions back to community life. Table 24-3 contains a potential list of community, state, or federal resources to aid clients. Assisting individuals in developing their own contextually relevant information and referral list of resources is a powerful symbol of hope for their continued recovery journey that will endure with them long after the discontinuation of occupational therapy services.

TABLE 24-3. Resources to Help in Rehabilitation and After Service Discontinuation

WORK DEVELOPMENT NEEDS
- Department of Rehabilitation Services, Vocational Rehabilitation
- Workforce Development System
- Social Security Administration's Ticket to Work program (individuals with disabilities)
- Goodwill Industries (training and case management)
- YWCA Women's Resource Centers
- Veterans Administration (VA)
- Tribal entities (Native American) for training, education, employment, and entrepreneurial opportunities
- Employee Assistance Programs (EAP) at workplaces

LIFE SKILLS DEVELOPMENT NEEDS
- Free application for Federal Student Aid (FAFSA student loans)
- Community colleges (some have special programs for persons in recovery)
- General Educational Development (GED) testing centers
- Vocational and technical schools (service- and industry-specific education and training)
- English as a Second Language (ESL) or English Language Learners (ELL) programs

TABLE 24-3. Continued

PERSONAL CARE NEEDS
- Community closets for professional and work clothes
- Lion's Club—vision screening, glasses
- Free or sliding scale dental clinics
- Free or sliding scale medical clinics
- Food assistance programs
- Prescription medication assistance programs

HOUSING, SECURITY, AND TRANSPORTATION NEEDS
- Sober living houses or communities
- Safe, affordable housing for persons with mental illness
- Quality, affordable child care resources
- Head Start and early childhood programs
- Public transportation options
- Transportation for persons with disabilities

LEISURE, RECREATION, AND SPIRITUAL NEEDS
- Community recreations centers, YMCA, YWCA, exercise facilities, dance centers
- Public libraries, reading rooms, book discussion clubs
- Enrichment and cultural activities: museums, concert halls, theatres, fine arts centers
- Organizations for religious or spiritual development, support, and expression

© Cengage Learning 2013

OCCUPATIONAL THERAPY AT THE ALCOHOL AND DRUG ABUSE CENTER
Client Perceptions of the Challenge

Women in recovery can have good insight, and a person-centered occupational therapist considers that insight. A dozen women at the Alcohol and Drug Abuse (ADA) Center for women in recovery in Galveston, Texas, thoughtfully considered my question, "What might be helpful for others to know about women in recovery?" Their responses captured similar themes. One young woman said, "You know, addiction affects many people that society holds in high regard. The possibility of addiction spares no one." Others agreed, noting that the insidiousness of dependence on painkillers and the encroachment of a disease process in those prone to addiction are factors that many critics disregard.

Besides the nature of addiction, another theme that emerged was the work of recovery. One woman said, "Our days are disciplined. We do daily chores. We're up by 6:00 and down by 10:00." The women described the challenge of self-discovery at ADA, with one saying, "The changes that we have to make in life are scary. Using becomes a part of your life. You have to relearn how to live your life." One woman nodded, adding, "Some people think that we come here to be fixed. But you can't just fix this. You need tools—life skills—to go back and work at being successful."

The last theme was that of hope. "I am hoping that I will be able to go back," said one woman, "not just to acquire what I had before, but to go back a better person, a better mother." Another reflected, "There's so much support here from staff, counselors, and other women. It's 24-7 support. Because of that support, we have a lot of hope."

The women of ADA are wives, mothers, grandmothers, sisters, and daughters, each linked to others in communal bonds and roles. Many once held solid and respectable jobs. They feel sorrow, guilt, and shame. When asked how others might think of them, they do not ask that we dismiss their behaviors. They ask instead that we understand the power of addiction, that we appreciate the *work* of recovery, and that we hope for their futures.

Programming at ADA House

The Intensive Residential Program at ADA Center, better known locally as ADA House, was designed to provide 14 women with services that help them work at their recovery for 4 to 6 weeks. These include: individual sessions with certified counselors, some in recovery themselves; daily Alcoholics Anonymous (AA) and/or Narcotics Anonymous (NA) meetings in the community; group therapy with counselors; structured daily routines of household maintenance chores; weekend family therapy groups; public health education, educational videos on addiction; weekly volunteer services in the community; exercise and recreational activities led by staff; weekly alumnae meetings; and weekly occupational therapy groups.

Additionally as needed, counselors refer the women for mental health care through the Gulf Coast Mental Health and Mental Retardation (MHMR) Center; vocational financial assistance through the Department of Assistive Rehab Services (DARS); and medical/dental care through Galveston County Coordinated Community Clinics (4Cs clinics). State funding through the Department of State Health Services supports treatment for all women admitted to ADA.

Occupational Therapy Programming

Occupational therapy groups within ADA's Intensive Residential Program address substance dependence and recovery as these actions interface with the constructs of person, environment, and occupation (PEO) elaborated by Law et al. (1996). The PEO model's systems dynamic is well suited for a population within which personal and neurological factors interface with contextual influences in such a way that seeking and using become dominant occupations (American Psychiatric Association, 2000). As individuals in recovery note, lifestyle changes become a crucial focus.

Occupational therapy's use of skills for daily living is a hallmark practice. The profession's history of helping individuals establish or reclaim healthy and satisfying daily lives dates back to Slagle's habit training principles and to even older moral treatment routines (Brigham, 1847; Peloquin, 1994; Vaux, 1929). More recently, the phrase **lifestyle redesign** characterizes occupational therapy for those striving to make life-changes that are healthy, meaningful, and satisfying (Jackson, Carlson, Mandel, Zemke, & Clark, 1998; Moyers & Stoffel, 2001). For years, community and living skills training has associated with mental health practice in occupational therapy (Bickes, De Loache, Dicer, & Miller, 2001; Howe, Weaver, & Dulay, 1981). There is similar logic in helping women in recovery to master vital life skills.

The use in occupational therapy of activities in general and crafts in particular also has a longstanding tradition endorsed by founders Barton (1914) and Dunton (1921) among others. Although craft work has waxed and waned in practice, endorsement of activity groups as a powerful method for those facing psychosocial challenges is strong (Fidler & Fidler, 1978; Griffiths, 2008; Thompson & Blair, 1998; Reynolds, 2000). Contemporary theorists argue the benefits of occupation and the therapeutic factors of groups (Sundsteigen, Eklund, & Dahlin-Ivanoff, 2009; Webster & Schwartzberg, 1992). Therapeutic factors noted by clients in OT groups have included acceptance by others, successful interactions, use of creativity, experience of a client-centered focus, and the emergence of hope (Sundsteigen et al., 2009; Webster & Schwartzberg, 1992). Sundsteigen et al. (2009) have also argued that OT groups have helped clients both "manage" and "dare" to make occupational changes. (For more information regarding occupational therapy programming and groups, see Chapter 19, "The Use of Psychosocial Methods and Interpersonal Strategies in Mental Health," and Chapter 20, "Groups.")

Two group types structure occupational therapy at ADA, each drawing support from the literature. The **Self-Development Group** targets the capacity for self-discovery, self-expression, and self-management, through exploration of personal factors integrated into an occupation-based theme. Discussion occurs in tandem with completion of an art or craft activity that supports the theme. The **Living Skills Development Group** targets mastery in diverse activities of daily living to include competence in underlying communication, cognitive, and coping capacities. The desired outcome is competence in the requisite attitudes and skills that structure the women's anticipated roles and that support sobriety.

Program development for ADA also included a consideration of the evidence-based inquiry published by Stoffel and Moyers (2004), within which four intervention types emerged as effective: (1) brief interventions—whether phone, face-to-face, or workbook encounters—aimed at exploring the dependence problem and motivating the person to address it; (2) cognitive-behavioral approaches that modify thought patterns and emphasize coping behaviors, (3) motivational strategies such as empathic and client-centered exchanges to support change; and (4) 12-step self-help programs such as AA and NA. Consideration of these intervention types reinforced the use of brief discussions within activity groups and helped set the interactional tone as empathic, motivational, and educational.

Interventions across both OT groups address the following general goals:

- Developing coping skills to handle personal, occupational, and environmental challenges and frustrations (Bonaguro, Nalette, & Seibert, 2002; Moyers & Stoffel, 1999, 2001).

- Increasing the sense of self as capable of insight, change, mastery, and self-direction (Miller, Zweben, DiClemente, & Rychtarik,1992; Moyers & Stoffel, 2001).

- Handling typical and more unique stresses inherent in daily life and the recovery process (Moyers & Stoffel, 2001).

- Identifying, appreciating, and engaging in meaningful and healthy substance-free activities (Bonaguro et al., 2002; Jackson et al., 1998; Moyers, 1997).

- Enhancing life skills that enable the establishment and maintenance of healthy lifestyle patterns of activities of daily living, education, work, rest, and leisure (Jackson et al., 1998; Stoffel, 1994; Stoffel & Moyers, 1997).

- Cultivating problem-solving and cognitive-behavioral strategies that support life satisfaction, social participation, and sobriety (Beck, 1991; Gagne, White, & Anthony, 2007; Moyers & Stoffel, 2001).

- Enhancing communication, self-expression, and self-management skills to meet personal needs and interact effectively (Gagne et al., 2007; Hester, 1995).

Implementing Group Interventions

ADA House is a small house in a neighborhood, and therapy groups occur in its various rooms. Occupational therapy groups occur within a combined kitchen-dining room. The women engage best in this tight space when facing one another around two long tables rather than sitting with their backs to some as they do when dining. Each occupational therapy session has the women shifting their chairs from circle-work to table-work, changing both pace and place at predictable and pleasant intervals.

The 90-minute Self-Development Group consists of four segments: (1) introduction and thematic overview; (2) motivational/didactic work and discussion (Alcoholics Anonymous, 1976; Alcoholics Anonymous World Services, 2005; Miller et al., 1992); (3) crafts/expressive media on the day's theme; and (4) relaxation and stress-management exercises. The introduction applauds the commitment to sobriety; invites self-introductions; presents occupational therapy as an *occupation of minds, bodies, and spirits that supports recovery*; and highlights the norms of mutual respect and conservation of limited craft supplies. Specific therapeutic objectives are elaborated through reference to ever-present occupational therapy posters framed and affixed to a nearby wall.

Presentation of the thematic overview co-occurs with showing a sample of the art or craft of the day as occupational metaphor and motivator (Moyers & Stoffel, 2001). One session's theme, for example, is "Holding on, letting go." The subject of reflection and discussion on this day is the habitual actions or occupational patterns that the women deem either positive or negative. The thematic question targets daily patterns at ADA that the women need to retain as contrasted with any prior patterns that they must relinquish. The craft metaphor is a colorfully painted and detailed pair of wooden spring action clothespins (that hold on and let go) to become magnet or paper clip reminders of the discussion.

After the thematic overview, the women spend 25 minutes on a written psycho-educational exercise that triggers discussion. Some exercises are adaptations of those addressing recovery themes in the Life Management Skills series by Korb, Azok, and Leutenberg (1989), but most are my own design. Many incorporate the brief motivational and educational strategies supported in the literature, with an occupational emphasis (Moyers & Stoffel, 2001). Many prompt sound reasoning, cognitive reframing, and exploring a deeper sense of meaning in life (Alcoholics Anonymous, 1976; Brown, 1990; Moyers & Stoffel, 2001).

One written task, for example, asks the women to identify five common myths that magazine ads or sitcoms ask women to "buy" about womanhood. They are then asked to contrast those myths with more solidly grounded beliefs about what constitutes a woman of character in daily situations. Discussion after this exercise is animated. The challenge then follows to roll paper beads from magazine wedges and for a necklace or bracelet representing being a "real" woman.

Directions, precautions, and hints for success precede all craft work, with an emphasis on honing the same living skills required at home or on the job. Rather than tossing any materials resulting from personal accident or error, the women are encouraged to "make it right" or "make it work." The tight space demands cooperative interactions, frustration tolerance, and problem solving as women access supplies, navigate around furniture and one another, and work elbow to elbow. The work atmosphere varies with the nature of the craft. The room can be silent with intense concentration or filled with boisterous laughter. Craft and clean-up time together last about 45 minutes. If time allows, a discussion occurs of task or interpersonal problems encountered and solved, of ways in which the women made things work or made them right, with parallels made to roles and responsibilities outside of ADA House.

The last group segment consists of 5–7 minutes of a sampling of relaxation strategies that include stretching, progressive muscle relaxation, self-massage, deep breathing, and/or brief visual imagery and meditative exercises. The women are encouraged to use the exercises that work best for them throughout the week. As a final task, the women complete an anonymous survey of their satisfaction and achievement of general group goals. The weekly results help me assess outcome achievement and redirect my efforts. A tally of the results becomes part of a narrative group note entered in a state-based computerized medical record at day's end. Figure 24-3 shows the percentage of positive responses to an overarching question about satisfaction with the day's group. Most women report satisfaction most of the time.

Overall, I was satisfied with this occupational therapy group
Self development group: Across 42 consecutive sessions
    21/42 sessions: 90%–100% of clients strongly agree
    9/42 sessions: 80%–90% strongly agree
    5/42 sessions: 70%–79% strongly agree
    6/42 sessions: 60%–69% strongly agree

Overall, I was satisfied with this occupational therapy group
Skills development group: Across 42 consecutive sessions
    11/42 sessions: 90%–100% of clients strongly agree
    10/42 sessions: 80%–90% strongly agree
    6/42 sessions: 70%–79% strongly agree
    5/42 sessions: 60%–69% strongly agree
    10/42 sessions: 50%–59% strongly agree

FIGURE 24-3. Client Responses to the Satisfaction Question on Outcomes Surveys
Based on information from *OT Practice*. Copyright 2011 by the American Occupational Therapy Association.

Most women spontaneously express gratitude for the session. On one particular day, a woman about to be discharged gave me this message on a sheet of note paper she had produced in occupational therapy the previous week: "Thank you, Ma'am, for your time and effort to make our stay here a creative one. It was very nice knowing you and it was very enjoyable. Thanks for also reminding me to mind my manners. I love you for that."

The Living Skills Group within the Intensive Residential program has not been reestablished since Hurricane Ike and the depressed economy hit Galveston Island concurrently in 2008, but plans are in place to restore it. The Living Skills Group typically lasts 60 minutes, with the initial introduction and final relaxation steps similar to those in the Self-Development Group. Central work in this group is the development of skills identified as important by clients and staff during initial program planning (see Figure 24-4). Client engagement consists of brief paper–pencil tasks modified from resources such as the Life Management Skills series (Korb et al., 1989) or exercises that I have developed. These exercises are paired with applied discussions, role plays, actual tasks, or game-like activities that tap or teach the skill in question.

Time management	Household management
Setting priorities	Organization
Stress management	Letter writing and phone use
Relaxation techniques	Problem solving
Leisure exploration	Budgeting
Values clarification	Goal setting
Meal preparation	Child care
Effective communication	Anger management

FIGURE 24-4. Living Skills Targeted by Clients and Staff
Based on information from *OT Practice*. Copyright 2011 by American Occupational Therapy Association.

One skill during one session might be gathering economical and helpful hints for various activities of daily living. Each woman selects a folder with information sheets prepared from a variety of resources and entitled *personal hygiene, parenting, skin care, laundry, shopping, home maintenance, yard care, automotive care, personal health,* etc. She then spends quiet time taking notes that she deems most helpful. The women then share in the large group two to three of these hints. Additional hints emerge based on life experiences. The women seeming pleased to offer helpful ideas that may reduce stress while saving time and money.

Supportive Residential Programming: Individualized Living Skills

Following assessment of their readiness by counselors who monitor their daily progress, some women stay at ADA House for another 3 months as they establish themselves in a job. The Department of Assistive Rehab Services (DARS) offers help with the writing of resumes and the conducting of mock interviews. The women at this time transition to the Supportive Residential (SR) program within which occupational therapy is key. Occupational therapy's Individualized Livings Skills program consists of a woman's completion of written weekly living skills work. Each woman meets with me to discuss her living skills needs. I review guidelines for the program and equip her with a cluster of 50 life skill exercises assembled into a binder that becomes her OT workbook. Each woman self-directs her effort at completing three exercises weekly, based on her perceived need. Exercises address all of the living skills represented in Figure 24-4. A typical exercise may involve planning a schedule for a work day so as to meet all of her personal and work obligations as well as her obligations at ADA.

Each woman rates her effort for each exercise and reflects on its level of difficulty, noting these on the back of each completed exercise. She then writes a reflection that notes major lessons learned across all exercises and serves as a synthesis of important thoughts and reactions. I collect this written work, review it, and make notes, supportive comments, and suggestions. The women in the SR program meet with me weekly for 30 minutes, often at 7:00 a.m. before they leave for work or at 6:00 p.m. after they return. They each share reflections and discuss their progress. If two or three women are in the SR program simultaneously, we meet in small groups. I write individual notes about their weekly performance in the state-based documentation system.

Women in the SR program are strongly encouraged to use "real life" challenges as exercises in occupational therapy. Instead of a written exercise from the workbook, a woman may submit a completed draft of a 1040 form, a letter written to a landlord, or the draft of wording that might be used to secure a raise. I encourage the women to make occupational therapy "work" for them, hoping that they will "manage" and "dare" as Sundsteigen et al. (2009) argue that they can. The women also meet every other week with their counselors and weekly with their AA/NA sponsors.

After a physical assault experienced while returning from work, one woman wrote a poem, produced a collage, and crafted a reflection entitled "Feelings and What I Will Do With Them." I had asked her to find ways to self-manage, consider the steps that she might take to cope with her assault, and identify resources that she would need in order to do so. She later shared this work with a counselor in a local crisis center. She told me that she did the assignment as she did because it was "the OT way." In her reflection she explained:

> As far as steps taken and lessons learned, I believe that this is the first real situation that I have ever analyzed and learned from. Thank you so much. This really was the most productive thing for me in my recovery, and I appreciate you for caring enough to help me.

Student Participation

Academic courses supporting partnerships between the community and university have allowed students to plan and conduct OT sessions at ADA, under therapist supervision. We have used differing models for such service learning, ranging from interventions conducted across a semester to more intensive interventions across one week. Each student involved has reported that the learning had been deep and significant.

In one year, eight students worked across four weeks, planning and conducting two sessions weekly as partners. Highly diverse responses to an open-ended question that asked them to note the most memorable, significant, or meaningful aspect of their learning included these:

> Rich discussions allowed us to see that clients made the anticipated links between the craft activities and their daily lives.
>
> The happiness I felt seeing the women engage in activities that they loved.
>
> Observing positive changes in clients and having my passion for being an occupational therapist reaffirmed.
>
> The gratitude expressed by the women.
>
> Insight into myself and my leadership style in action.
>
> Clear understanding of the visible benefits of occupational therapy for this population.

The work of occupational therapy is a good fit within this setting. Clients know that their success in recovery depends on their reclaiming sober and satisfying lives one day at a time. Occupational therapy has become a valued part of the work of ADA House, a source of learning, support, and hope for women seeking sober lives.

ADVICE

We asked both clients and therapists to share their advice for therapists who are new to working with clients with substance-abuse issues. *Clients* gave us this verbatim advice (unedited to capture the reality of our work):

- "The therapists who are most effective are very up-front and honest, no holds barred. They get right in there and call you on your "bullshit." It doesn't do me much good for you to tip-toe around the subject or for you to go light with me and try to sugar coat things. It's not going to get me anywhere. It's a lot better for you to just call me out and come at me straightforward."

- "Therapists need to know that everybody is different, every situation is different and that there's some crazy stuff that goes on: heroin junkies living on the streets, selling your body for dope, leaving your baby behind so you can continue to get high. It's just a very, very nasty disease and it doesn't care who it takes. Just remember to be caring and also that you have to be stern."

Experienced therapists gave us this advice:

- "Self-care is really important in this work. Do not let your job become who you are, have things outside of work that you enjoy doing, and really set boundaries."

- "Be honest with clients without being confrontational. If you're not honest, they won't benefit; if you're confrontational they're not going to hear anything you say. Being able to walk that thin line is really important."

- "When you're very passionate about what you do, that can be very inspiring to clients. But you can't work harder than they are and care more about their recovery than they do."

Honesty, assertiveness, compassion, and maintaining good boundaries and self-care are all keys to being successful in the immensely rewarding work of helping individuals recovering from substance abuse construct healthy occupational lives.

SUMMARY

Because substance abuse is marked by occupational loss, the need for occupational therapy as a component of intervention is clear. According to the American Occupational Therapy Association, "occupational therapy is an underutilized service for people with . . . substance abuse disorders that can meet and address independent living and recovery needs. This limited access . . . is often due to a lack of understanding about how occupational therapy can help. . . ." (AOTA, 2007). Helping other health-care professionals and clients understand who we are as occupational therapists and the power of occupation is a familiar role for us. With background knowledge of the nature of substance abuse and addiction coupled with grounding in occupation, we can help clients find their unique pathways toward recovery and fully satisfying and effective occupational lives.

REVIEW QUESTIONS

1. A client who is early in recovery reflects about the nature of her years-long, daily, and increasing use of methamphetamine: "I think I just picked up a bad habit and really, I could stop anytime I wanted to. But in one of our groups, they talk like this is a disease that I will never recover from. That doesn't sound right to me. I'd like to think that once I break my bad habits, I could have a drink and party with my friends every once in a while. What do you think?" What do you tell her?

2. You work at an in-patient rehabilitation facility and one of your clients is a 75-year-old man who has undergone a hip replacement. He confides to you that he fractured his hip after falling because he had been drinking. "I've always had three or four drinks—sometimes more—every night after dinner. Maybe it's time to stop, but I'm not sure how to do that. Are there certain treatment approaches that are better than others? What would you recommend?" What do you tell him?

3. As part of a grant-funded project, you begin working with clients at a treatment center for individuals in recovery from substance abuse and addiction. On the first morning at the facility, you meet a licensed alcohol and drug counselor who is unfamiliar with occupational therapy in general and with occupational therapy's role with individuals in recovery in particular. She welcomes you to the treatment team, and then says, "Help me understand occupational therapy's goals with individuals in recovery. What types of assessments and intervention will you use? What outcomes do you expect?" What do you tell her?

4. One of your clients in recovery hasn't held a legal job in many years. He understands that a key to his recovery and independence is securing productive employment. He says to you, "I know I need to find a job, but I really don't know what I could do or where to look. Even if I found a job opening, I suppose that would involve an interview, and that makes me nervous. Can you help me?" You assure him that you can. What specific steps will you take to help him meet his goal of employment?

5. How would you design a Self-Development Group for individuals early in recovery? What would be the goals of this group? How would you design a Living Skills Development group, and what would be the goals for this group?

REFERENCES

Alcoholics Anonymous. (1976). *Alcoholics Anonymous: The story of how many thousands of men and women have recovered from alcoholism* (3rd ed.). New York: A. A. World Services.

Alcoholics Anonymous World Services. (2005). *Twelve steps and twelve traditions.* (2005). New York, NY: Author.

Alcoholics Anonymous World Services, Inc. (2011). *The big book online* (4th ed.). Retrieved from http://www.aa.org/bigbookonline/

American Occupational Therapy Association (AOTA). (2007). Statement for the record committee on education and labor hearing on "The Paul Wellstone Mental Health and Addiction Equity Act of 2007 (H.R. 1424). Retrieved from http://www.aota.org/Practitioners/Advocacy/Federal/Testimony/2007/40333.aspx?FT5.pdf

American Occupational Therapy Association (AOTA). (2008). Occupational therapy practice framework: Domain and process (2nd ed.). *American Journal of Occupational Therapy, 62,* 625–683.

American Occupational Therapy Association (AOTA). (2010a). Specialized knowledge and skills in mental health promotion, prevention, and intervention in occupational therapy practice. Retrieved from http://www.aota.org/Practitioners/Official/Skills/Mental-Health-KS.aspx

American Occupational Therapy Association (AOTA). (2010b). Statement: Occupational therapy services in the promotion of psychological and social aspects of mental health. Retrieved from http://www.aota.org/Practitioners/Official/Statements/40878.aspx

American Psychiatric Association (APA). (2000). *Diagnostic and Statistical Manual of Mental Disorders* (4th ed., text rev.). Washington, DC: Author.

Appleby, L. (1997). Assessing substance use in multiproblem patients: Reliability and validity of the alcohol severity index in a mental hospital setting. *Journal of Nervous and Mental Disease, 85*(3), 159–165.

Bannink, F. P. (2007). Solution-focused brief therapy. *Journal of Contemporary Psychotherapy, 37*(2), 87–94. Retrieved from http://www.springerlink.com/content/p5t4j74g8nj826m3/

Baron, K., Kielhofner, G., Iyender, A., Goldhammer, V., & Wolenski, J. (2006). *The occupational self assessment (OSA), version 2.2.* Chicago, IL: Model of Human Occupation Clearinghouse. User's manual available from http://www.moho.uic.edu/assess/osa.html

Barton, G. E. (1914). A view of invalid occupations. *Trained Nurse and Hospital Review, 52,* 327–330.

Beck, A. T. (1991). Cognitive therapy: A 30-year retrospective. *American Psychologist, 46*(4), 368–375.

Bickes, M. B., DeLoache, S. N., Dicer, J. R., & Miller, S. C. (2001). Effectiveness of experiential and verbal occupational therapy groups in a community mental health setting. *Occupational Therapy in Mental Health, 17*(1), 51–72.

Bonaguro, J. A., Nalette, E., & Seibert, M. L. (2002). The role of allied health professionals in substance abuse education. In M. R. Hack & H. Adger (Eds.), *Strategic plan for interdisciplinary faculty development: Arming the nation's health professional workforce for a new approach to substance use disorders* (pp. 169–184). Providence, RI: Association for Medical Education and Research in Substance Abuse.

Brigham, A. (1847). The moral treatment of insanity. *American Journal of Insanity, 4,* 1.

Bristow-Braitman, A. (1995). Addiction recovery: 12-step programs and cognitive-behavioral psychology. *Journal of Counseling & Development, 73,* 414–418.

Brown, H. P., Jr. (1990). Values and recovery from alcoholism through Alcoholics Anonymous. *Counseling and Values, 35,* 63–68.

Brun, C., & Rapp, R. C. (2001). Strengths-based case management: Individuals' perspective on strengths and the case manager relationship. *Social Work, 46*(3), 278–288.

Butler, A. C., Chapman, J. E., Forman, E. M., & Beck, A. T. (2006). The empirical status of cognitive-behavioral therapy: A review of meta-analyses. *Clinical Psychology Review, 26,* 17–31.

Centers for Disease Control and Prevention (CDC). (2001). Drug use, HIV, and the criminal justice system. Retrieved from http://www.cdc.gov/idu/facts/criminaljusticeFactsheet.pdf

Cotton, N. S. (1979). The familial incidence of alcoholism: A review. *Journal of Studies on Alcohol, 40,* 89–116.

Dakwar, E., & Levin, F.R. (2009). The emerging role of meditation in addressing psychiatric illness, with a focus on substance use disorders. *Harvard Review of Psychiatry, 17*, 254–267.

Davies, R., & Cameron, J. (2010). Self-identified occupational competencies, limitation and priorities for change in the occupational lives of people with drug misuse problems. *British Journal of Occupational Therapy, 73*(6), 251–260.

de Shazer, S. (1985). The death of resistance. *Family Process, 23*, 79–93.

Dunton, W. R. (1921). *Occupational therapy: A manual for nurses.* Philadelphia: Saunders.

Emrick, C. (2004). Alcoholics anonymous and other mutual aid groups. In N. Heather & T. Stockwell (Eds.), *The essential handbook of treatment and prevention of alcohol problems* (pp. 177–192). Chichester, UK: John Wiley & Sons.

Fidler, G. S., & Fidler, J. W. (1978). Doing and becoming: purposeful action and self-actualization. *The American Journal of Occupation Therapy, 32*(5), 305–310.

Gagne, C., White, W., & Anthony, W. A. (2007). Recovery: A common vision for the fields of mental health and addictions. *Psychiatric Rehabilitation Journal, 31*, 32–37.

Galanter, M., & Kleber, H. D. (2008). *The American Psychiatric Publishing textbook of substance abuse treatment.* Arlington, VA: American Psychiatric Publishing.

Goodwin, D. W., Schulsinger, F., Moller, N., Hermansen, L., Winokur, G., & Guze, S. B. (1974) Drinking problems in adopted and nonadopted sons of alcoholics. *Archives of General Psychiatry, 31*, 164–169.

Gorman, D. M. (2001). Developmental processes. In N. Heather, T. J. Peters, & T. Stockwell (Eds.), *International handbook of alcohol dependence and problems* (pp. 339–356). Chichester, UK: John Wiley & Sons.

Griffiths, S. (2008). The experience of creative activity as a treatment medium. *Journal of Mental Health, 17*(1),49–63.

Harwood, H. (2000). *Updating estimates of the economic costs of alcohol abuse in the United States: Estimates, update methods, and data report.* Prepared by the Lewin Group for the National Institute on Alcohol Abuse and Alcoholism. Retrieved from http://pubs.niaaa.nih.gov/publications/economic-2000/

Hasin, D. S., & Grant, B. F. (1995). AA and other help-seeking for alcohol problems: Former drinkers in the U.S. general population. *Journal of Substance Abuse, 7*, 281–292.

Hester, R. K. (1995). Behavioral self-control training. In R. K. Hester and W. R. Miller (Eds.), *Handbook of alcoholism treatment approaches: Effective alternatives* (2nd ed., pp. 148–159). Boston: Allyn and Bacon.

Hester, R. K., & Miller, W. R. (Eds.). (1995). *Handbook of alcoholism treatment approaches:Effective alternatives* (2nd ed.). Boston, MA: Allyn & Bacon.

Howe, M. C., Weaver, C. T., & Dulay, J. (1981). The development of a work-oriented day center program. *The American Journal of Occupational Therapy, 35*, 711–718.

Iveson, C. (2002). Solution-focused brief therapy. *Advances in Psychiatric Treatment, 8*(2), 149–157. Retrieved from http://apt.rcpsych.org/cgi/reprint/8/2/149

Jackson, J., Carlson, M., Mandel, D., Zemke, R., & Clark, F. (1998). Occupational in lifestyle redesign: The well elderly study occupational therapy program. *American Journal of Occupational Therapy, 52*, 326–336.

Kielhofner, G., Mallinson, T., Crawford, C., Nowak, M., Rigby, M., Henry, A., et al. (2004). *The Occupational Performance History Interview (OPHI-II), (Version 2.1).* Chicago, IL: Model of Human Occupation Clearinghouse. User's manual available from http://www.moho.uic.edu/assess/ophi%202.1.html

Kishline, A. (1996). *Moderate drinking: The moderation management guide for people who want to reduce their drinking.* New York, NY: Crown.

Korb, K. L., Azok, S., & Leutenberg, E. A. (1989). *Life management skills.* Beachwood, OH: Wellness Reproductions.

Law, M., Baptiste, S., Carswell, A., McColl, A., Polatajko, H., & Pollock, N. (2005). *The Canadian Occupational Performance Measure* (4th ed.). Ottawa, Ontario: Canadian Occupational Therapy Association.

Law, M., Cooper, B., Strong, S., Stewart, D., Rigby, P., & Lets, L. (1996). The person-environment-occupational model: A transactive approach to occupational performance. *Canadian Journal of Occupational Therapy, 63,* 9–23.

Leshner, A. I. (2001). Addiction is a brain disease. *Issues in Science and Technology Online.* Retrieved from http://www.issues.org/17.3/leshner.htm

Lowinson, J. H., Ruiz, P., Millman, R. B., & Langrod, J. G. (Eds.) (2005). *Substance abuse: A comprehensive textbook* (4th ed.). Philadelphia, PA: Lippincott Williams & Wilkins.

Marlatt, G. A., & Tapart, S. F. (1993). Harm reduction: Reducing the risks of addictive behaviors. In J. S. Baer, G. A. Marlatt, & R. J. McMahon (Eds.), *Addictive behaviors across the life span: Prevention, treatment and policy issues.* Newbury Park, CA: Sage.

Miller, W. R., Zweben, A., DiClemente, C. C., & Rychtarik, R. G. (1992). *Motivational enhancement therapy (MET): A clinical research guide for therapists treating individuals with alcohol abuse and dependence* (DHHS Publication N. ADM 92-1894). Washington, DC: U. S. Government Printing Office.

Moore-Corner, R. A., Kielhofner, G., & Olson, L. (1998). *Work Environment Impact Scale (WEIS), Version 2.0.* Chicago, IL: Model of Human Occupation Clearinghouse. User's manual available from http://www.moho.uic.edu/assess/weis.html

Morgenstern, J., Blanchard, K. A., Morgan, T. J., Labouvie, E., & Hayaki, J. (2001). Testing the effectiveness of cognitive-behavioral treatment for substance abuse in a community setting: Within treatment and posttreatment findings. *Journal of Consulting and Clinical Psychology, 69,* 1007–1017.

Moss, H. B., Chen, C. M., & Yi, H. (2007). Subtypes of alcohol dependency in a nationally representative sample. *Drug and Alcohol Dependence, 91,* 149–158.

Moyers, P. A. (1997). Occupational meanings and spirituality: The quest for sobriety. *American Journal of Occupational Therapy, 51*(3), 207–214. doi: 10.5014/51.3.207.

Moyers, P. A., & Stoffel, V. C. (1999). Alcohol dependence in a client with a work-related injury. *American Journal of Occupational Therapy, 53,* 640–645.

Moyers, P. A. & Stoffel, V. C. (2001). Community-based approaches for substance-use disorders. In M. E. Scaffa (Ed.). *Occupational therapy in community-based practice settings* (pp. 319–342). Philadelphia, PA: F.A. Davis.

Najavits, L. M., Liese, B. S., & Harned, M. S. (2005). Cognitive and behavioral therapies. In J. H. Lowinson, P. Ruiz, R. B. Millman, & J. G. Langrod (Eds.), *Substance abuse: A comprehensive textbook* (4th ed., pp. 723–732). Philadelphia, PA: Lippincott Williams & Wilkins.

National Alliance on Mental Illness (NAMI). (2003). Cognitive-behavioral therapy. Retrieved from http://www.nami.org/Template.cfm?Section5About_Treatments_and_Supports&template5/Content Management/ContentDisplay.cfm&ContentID57952

National Institute on Alcohol Abuse and Alcoholism (NIAAA). (n.d.). Rethinking drinking:Alcohol and your health. Retrieved from http://rethinkingdrinking.niaaa.nih.gov/default.asp

Oakley, F., Kielhofner, G., Barris, R., & Reichler, R. (1986). The role checklist: Development and empirical assessment of reliability. *Occupational Therapy Journal of Research, 6,* 151–170. Accessible version of the Role Checklist available from: Frances Oakley, MS, OTR, FAOTA. FOakley @cc.nih.gov

Office of National Drug Control Policy. (2004). *The economic costs of drug abuse in the United States: 1992–2002.* Washington, DC: Executive Office of the President (Publication No. 207303).

Ouimette, P. C., Finney, J. W., & Moos, R. H. (1997). Twelve-step and cognitive-behavioral treatment for substance abuse: A comparison of treatment effectiveness. *Journal of Consulting and Clinical Psychology, 65,* 230–240.

Parkinson, S., Forsyth, K., & Kielhofner, G. (2006). *The model of human occupation screening tool (MOHOST),* version 2.0. Chicago, IL: Model of Human Occupation Clearinghouse. User's manual available from: http://www.moho.uic.edu/assess/mohost.html

Parks, G. A., Marlatt, G. A., & Anderson, B. K. (2004). Cognitive-behavioral alcohol treatment. In N. Heather & T. Stockwell (Eds.), *The essential handbook of treatment and prevention of alcohol problems* (pp. 70–86). Chichester, UK: John Wiley & Sons.

Peloquin, S. M. (1994). Moral treatment: How a caring practice lost its rationale. *American Journal of Occupational Therapy, 48,* 167–173.

Rapp, R. C., Siegal, H. A., & Fisher, J. H. (1992) *A strengths-based model of case management/ advocacy: Adapting a mental health model to practice work with persons who have substance abuse problems* (pp. 79–91). In DHHS Publication No. (ADM) 92-1946, Alcohol, Drug Abuse, and Mental Health Administration, 401 pp. Retrieved from http://www.scan.uk.net/docstore/ Progress_and_Issues_in_Case_Management_NIDA_Research_Monograph_127b.pdf#page=86

Reynolds, F. (2000). Managing depression through needlecraft creative activities: A qualitative study. *The Arts in Psychotherapy, 27*(2), 107–114.

Rotgers, F. (2003). Cognitive-behavioral theories of substance abuse. In F. Rotgers, J. Morgenstern, & S. T. Walters (Eds.), *Treating substance abuse: Theory and technique.* (2nd ed., pp. 166–189). New York, NY: Guilford Press.

Stoffel, V. C. (1994). Occupational therapist's role in treating substance abuse. *Hospital and Community Psychiatry, 45,* 21–22.

Stoffel, V. C., & Moyers, P. A. (1997). *Occupational therapy practice guidelines for substance use disorders.* Bethesda, MD: The American Occupational Therapy Association.

Stoffel, V. C., & Moyers, P. A. (2004). An evidence-based and occupational perspective of interventions for persons with substance-use disorders. *American Journal of Occupational Therapy, 58,* 570–586.

Substance Abuse and Mental Health Services Administration (SAMHSA). (2010). *Results from the 2009 National Survey on Drug Use and Health: Volume I. Summary of National Findings* (Office of Applied Studies, NSDUH Series H-38A, HHS Publication No. SMA 10-4586 Findings). Rockville, MD.

Sundsteigen, B., Eklund, K., & Dahlin-Ivanoff, S. (2009). Patients' experience of groups in outpatient mental health services and its significance for daily occupations. *Scandinavian Journal of Occupational Therapy, 16,* 172–180.

Thompson, M., & Blair, S. (1998). Creative arts in occupational therapy: ancient history or contemporary practice? *Occupational Therapy International, 5*(1), 48–64.

U.S. Department of Health and Human Services, National Institutes of Health, National Institute of Drug Abuse, (2008a). *Understanding drug abuse and addiction.* Retrieved from http://drugabuse .gov/infofacts/understand.html

U.S. Department of Health and Human Services, National Institutes of Health, National Institute of Drug Abuse, (2008b). *A cognitive behavioral approach: Treating cocaine addiction.* Retrieved from http://www.drugabuse.gov/drugpages/treatment.html

Vaux, C. L. (1929). Habit training. *Occupational Therapy and Rehabilitation, 8,* 327–329.

Venes, D. (Ed.). (2009). *Taber's cyclopedic medical dictionary* (Vol. 21). Philadelphia, PA: F. A. Davis.

Wallace, J. (1987). Children of alcoholics: A population at risk. *Alcoholism Treatment Quarterly, 43,* 13–30.

Wallace, J. (2003). Theory of 12-step oriented treatment. In F. Rotgers, J. Morgenstern, & S. T. Walters, (Eds.), *Treating substance abuse: Theory and technique* (2nd ed., pp. 9–30). New York, NY: Guilford Press.

Webster, D., & Schwartzerg, S. L. (1992). Patients' perception of curative factors in occupational therapy groups. *Occupational Therapy Mental Health, 12*, 3–24.

Wells, E. A., Peterson, P. L., Gainey, R. R., Hawkins, J. D., & Catalano, R. F. (1994). Outpatient treatment for cocaine abuse: A controlled comparison of relapse prevention and twelve-step approaches. *American Journal of Drug and Alcohol Abuse, 21*(1), 1–17.

White, S., Meade, S. A., & Hadar, L. (2007). OT cognitive adaptation: An intervention in time management for persons with co-occurring conditions. *OT Practice, 12*(10), 9–14.

World Health Organization. (n.d.). Health topics: Substance abuse. Retrieved from http://www.who .int/topics/substance_abuse/en/

SUGGESTED RESOURCES

Alcoholic Anonymous Website: http://www.aa.org/lang/en/subpage.cfm?page=1

Asher, I. E. (Editor). (2007). *Occupational therapy assessment tools: An annotated index* (3rd ed.). Bethesda, MD: AOTA Press.

Baum, C., & Dunn, W. (2005). *Measuring occupational performance: supporting best practice in occupational therapy* (2nd ed.). Thorofare, NJ: Slack.

Health Ink & Vitality Communications. (2011). CAGE assessment (Alcohol Abuse). Retrieved from https://www.merck.healthinkonline.com/merckTools/AssessMerckSourceCAGE.asp

Hemphill-Pearson, B. J. (Ed.). (2007). *Assessments in occupational therapy mental health: An integrated approach* (2nd ed.). Thorofare, NJ: Slack.

National Institute on Alcohol and Abuse and Alcoholism Website: http://www.niaaa.nih.gov/Pages/ default.aspx

National Institute on Drug Abuse Web site: http://drugabuse.gov/NIDAHome.html

Substance Abuse and Mental Health Services Administration Website: http://www.samhsa.gov/

U.S. Department of Health and Human Services, Public Health Service, Substance Abuse and Mental Health Services Administration, Center for Substance Abuse Treatment. *Brief Interventions and Brief Therapies for Substance Abuse.* Retrieved from http://www.ncbi.nlm.nih.gov/books/ NBK14512/

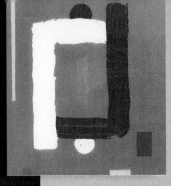

Chapter 25

Occupational Therapy in the Military: Working with Service Members in Combat and at Home

Robinette J. Amaker, PhD, OTR/L, CHT, FAOTA
Anne Pas Burke, EdD, OTR/L, FAOTA
Cecilia Najera, MOT, OTR, CPT, SP
Mary Vining Radomski, PhD, OTR/L, FAOTA

■ KEY TERMS

animal-assisted therapies/activities (AAT/AAA)

area of operations (AO)

concussion/mild traumatic brain injury (c/mTBI)

combat operational stress control (COSC)

combat operational stress reactions (COSR)

compassion fatigue

dissociation

dual agency

far forward

Glasgow Coma Scale (GCS)

local dining facility (DFAC)

Mayor's Cell

Military Acute Concussion Evaluation (MACE)

morale, welfare, and recreation (MWR)

OT BCT c/mTBI Reconditioning Program

prevention teams

Private First Class (PFC)

restoration program

second impact syndrome

Sergeant First Class (SFC)

service member (SM)

specialist (SPC)

treatment box

unit ministry teams (UMTs)

warrior

CHAPTER OUTLINE

Introduction
Working in the Field
    United States Army Combat Stress Control Units
    Restoration/Prevention
    Occupational Performance of a Service Member
    Occupational Therapy Role in U.S. Army Combat Stress Control Units
    Animal-Assisted Therapy in Theater
    Disaster Response
    Disaster: Recognizing the Value of Teamwork
    Disaster and Engagement in Occupation
    Disaster and the Health Care Providers' Role in Self-Care
Rehabilitation of Traumatic Brain Injury
    Concussion/Mild Traumatic Brain Injury (c/mTBI)
    Natural History of c/mTBI
    Effects of Recurrent Concussion
    c/mTBI in a Military Context
    Mechanism of Injury
    c/mTBI and Stress Disorders
    Occupational Therapy After c/mTBI Within a Military Context
    Occupational-Performance Problems of Service Members with c/mTBI
    Occupational Therapy Assessment and Intervention Across the Continuum of Care
    Occupational Therapy Interventions
Treating Warriors at Home: Acute Stress Reactions
    The Warrior Ethos
    Occupational Roles and Dual Agency
    Co-Existing Disorders
    Interdisciplinary Approach
    Communicating Occupational Therapy
    Promoting Occupational Therapy
    Intervention for the Practitioner
Summary

INTRODUCTION

This chapter focuses on three aspects of work with **service members (SMs)**, or warriors, in the military. The wars in Iraq and Afghanistan have necessitated occupational therapy involvement in all aspects of the military, from treatment of acute stress disorder in the theater and at home, with intervention that focuses on two conditions that now occur more in higher numbers in the military versus the general population, that is, traumatic brain injury (TBI) and post-traumatic stress disorder (PTSD). Because of the complexity of disorders as a result of combat, an interdisciplinary team approach is necessary and occupational therapists are important members of the team. It is ironically fitting that occupational therapists have figured prominently in military treatment because occupational therapists, particularly those who focus on mental health, originated in the military. This chapter begins with work in combat stress units in the theater and then moves on to treatment of TBI and stress disorders. The first section detailing occupational therapy's mission on combat stress reduction teams gives the reader a background and context to the conditions that SMs encounter while completing their missions. It gives context to the next sections on TBI and stress disorders. It also gives context to the complex and co-occurring disorders that present for treatment, and to the complex roles and mission of occupational therapists in the military.

WORKING IN THE FIELD
United States Army Combat Stress Control Units

The mission of **combat operational stress control (COSC)** units is to manage and minimize adverse effects experienced by SMs in combat or operational environments (see Figure 25-1); these experiences are collectively referred to as **combat operational stress reactions (COSR)** (Department of the Army, 2006). Deployed COSC clinics are organized as either detachment-sized units or company-sized units. "Detachment-sized COSC units can possess anywhere from approximately 25 to 45 personnel. Company-sized units may be twice that size" (Moore & Reger, 2007). These units are made up of teams of mental health professionals: psychiatrists, psychologists, social workers, occupational therapists, psychiatric nurses, as well as mental health specialists and occupational therapy assistants. Most recently, **unit ministry teams (UMTs)** have been added as members of the unit. These UMTs, composed of a chaplain and a chaplain's assistant, are charged with the primary mission of providing spiritual services to members of the unit and, as needed, to outlying units.

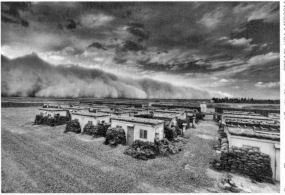

Source: Photo courtesy of Cecilia Najera, CPT MIL USA MEDCOM BAMC

FIGURE 25-1. A Sandstorm in the Field

Restoration/Prevention

In addition to the individual roles of each profession in the COSC, roles are further expanded as members are sectioned into either prevention or restoration teams. **Restoration programs** vary depending on the operational environment but are typically 3-day programs designed for SMs experiencing COSR. The SMs are screened for appropriateness upon their initial visit to the COSC unit. The program is designed to replenish the physiological status of the SM and to restore confidence in his/her ability to function in his/her SM role. This is accomplished by offering a therapeutic experience in a structured military environment in order to maintain the SM's military identity. A typical schedule will provide therapeutic classes and sessions but may also include physical training or weapons maintenance activities that are typically conducted in military units.

Prevention teams generally consist of two to three members whose primary mission is to overcome the stigma of mental health by developing positive relationships with its neighboring units and commanders, so that, in times of need, the COSC is trusted to treat its SMs and/or to respond to crises. Instead of SMs coming to the COSC clinic as in the restoration program, the prevention team goes out to meet with SMs in their **area of operations (AO)**. Prevention teams offer local support via coping skills classes, command consultation, or help-in-place as requested. In this type of role, the prevention team is essentially always working; for example, encounters at the **local dining facility (DFAC)** or at the gym offer the opportunities for interaction and for camaraderie with other units.

Occupational Performance of a Service Member

Service members' occupational performance can be adversely affected by the stress of combat and other military operations. Wartime missions allow the SM to do what he or she was trained to do and to put into practice the principles taught in school. In contrast with peacetime, war gives the SM the opportunity to engage in his/her primary occupation. While many find this fulfilling, other occupations may become impaired as a result of operational stressors. Service members are apart from families and friends for more than 6 months at one time and many have been away for over 15 months. This distance greatly impacts an SM's role as a spouse, parent, caregiver, friend, and son or daughter. These roles become blurred and many times lead to feelings of anxiety and depression. In addition, the lack of leisure activities or of time to self greatly impairs an SM's occupational performance. Although U.S. Army installations throughout Iraq and Afghanistan have **morale, welfare, and recreation (MWR)** facilities, activities offered may be limited and may not include activities that the SM engaged in at home. For example, an SM may have enjoyed mountain bike riding, skiing, or surfing while at home but no such activities are available in the deployed setting. Furthermore, many combat troops who reside in more remote locations, do not have access to MWR opportunities as others do.

Habits and routines also become impaired as missions and convoys are unpredictable, causing the need to fluctuate between day and night taskings. In addition to a variation in sleep routines, there may also be variations in personal hygiene routines. For example, many places require female and male SMs to share bathrooms; to accommodate for this, some installations have hour shifts for male and female use. In addition, SMs are required to be in uniform at all times and to carry their weapons with them during recreational activities and/or during personal hygiene. The inability to "break away" from the military in deployed times also becomes taxing on an SM. These operational stressors are often more taxing on SMs than physical stressors. Lang, Thomas, Bliese, and Adler (2007) found that psychological strain, when compared to physical strain, was a significant mediator of the job demands-performance relationship. Similarly, it is not surprising that many SMs seen at COSC clinics have impaired occupations as a result of operational stressors versus combat stressors (Deahl, Srinivasan, Jones, Thomas, Neblett, & Jolly, 2000).

Occupational Therapy Role in U.S. Army Combat Stress Control Units

Occupational therapists have a unique role in U.S. Army COSC units. "While other professions on the COSC team concentrate on psychiatric pathology and the remission of that pathology, in contrast the occupational therapist addresses occupational performance, regardless of pathology" (Gerardi & Newton, 2004). The occupational therapist recognizes the importance of occupation, roles, habits, and routines and provides treatment that attempts to restore these within the limits of the environment. In deployed settings, the occupational therapist in a COSC unit is first an SM but also a mental health practitioner with an occupational perspective. Being an SM first is important to recognize in a combat environment as it reminds the practitioner that he/she should be prepared to react to any attack. The practitioner should be well-rehearsed in soldiering skills as is expected in the SMs whom he/she treats.

In management of COSR, the occupational therapist will focus on an SM's occupational profile and formulate a treatment plan accordingly. This may mean encouraging the SM to explore recreational activities that are available in their setting. If a favorite pastime is not offered at MWR center, the SM is guided into starting one. A few real-life examples include a yoga enthusiast who started a yoga club and invited other interested SMs to participate or a female SM who started a dance class offered twice a week. Often times, 5K runs were organized for SMs on a monthly basis. At the COSC clinic, for normalization of habits and routines, SMs were instructed on breathing exercises to include guided imagery and muscle tense-release exercises. These exercises were termed "combat breathing" and were taught in ways that SMs could understand, for example, relating breathing exercises for relaxation with breathing during target practice. Relaxed breathing can effectively improve your aim in target practice by steadying the hand and therefore can also improve occupational performance during times of stress. Service members were also educated on the importance of developing habits and routines to the extent possible for their environments. The limitations of deployed environments challenge occupational therapists' creativity when creating a client-focused treatment plan. Supportive counseling often times occurred while the SM was engaged in occupation, for example, during a workout at the gym, or while cleaning his/her weapon, or performing preventive maintenance checks and services (PMCS) on a vehicle.

The COSC unit is often embedded with other units, allowing COSC staff to be seen eating, exercising, and working as their clients do. This set-up can be advantageous for the therapist, enabling daily interaction with clients and offering the opportunity to relate to the client's situation. Military health care providers, especially in mental health, may be perceived as not part of the "fighting force." This perception can be detrimental in developing rapport with clients. Co-location with other units gives health care providers the chance to work together as warriors with other SMs. It is important for the occupational therapist in a COSC unit to remember that he/she is an SM first and will perform the duties of an SM in addition to the duties of a therapist; this will not only aid with mission readiness but also help with developing a positive bond with other units.

Animal-Assisted Therapy in Theater

In December 2007, a new program was initiated by Army occupational therapists to include therapy dogs in COSC units. The intention of this program was to complement the job of the therapists by utilizing a highly skilled dog to achieve therapeutic goals. The dogs, **Sergeant First Class (SFC)** Boe and SFC Budge, were a donation from America's Vet Dogs, a subsidiary of Guide Dogs of America (see Figure 25-2).

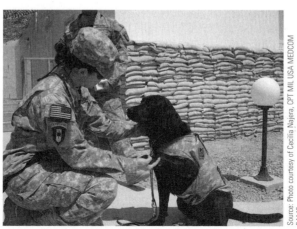

Source: Photo courtesy of Cecilia Najera, CPT MIL USA MEDCOM BAMC

FIGURE 25-2. SFC Boe on Duty in Iraq

Therapy dogs are trained to provide individuals a pleasurable interaction via **animal-assisted therapy (AAT)** or **animal-assisted activities (AAA)**. According to the Delta Society (2011):

> AAA provide opportunities for motivational, educational, recreational, and or therapeutic benefits to enhance quality of life. AAAs are delivered in a variety of environments by specially-trained professionals, paraprofessionals, and/or volunteers, in association with animals that meet specific criteria. AAT is goal-directed intervention in which an animal that meets specific criteria is an integral part of the treatment process. AAT is directed and/or delivered by a health/human service provider working within the scope of practice of his/her profession. AAT is designed to promote improvement in human physical, social, emotional, and/or cognitive functioning. AAT is provided in a variety of settings and may be group or individual in nature. This process is documented and evaluated.

SFC Budge and SFC Boe joined the 85th COSC unit during its last 3 months in Iraq. The dogs remained in theater with the replacing unit, the 528th COSC unit. At that time, it was determined that the dog's role would fit best in the unit's prevention team. The dogs were a tremendous success by allowing the handlers to be more approachable. Normally, the prevention team introduces themselves to SMs and commanders, explaining their services and offering support. In contrast, with the dogs in hand, the prevention team found that they were often approached first. Inquiries about the dog's purpose and role in a combat environment opened the door for handlers/occupational therapists to introduce COSC services. During this initial conversation, SMs often relayed memories or stories about their own pets back home or about the loss of a beloved pet. These conversations tended to digress into conversations about home front concerns or about the recent loss of a comrade. Furthermore, the SMs would engage in AAA, by kneeling down to the dog, petting the dog, or simply allowing the dog to kiss him/her. "I haven't been kissed by anyone in 9 months," an SM once exclaimed, "this feels good."

As members of the prevention teams, SFC Budge and SFC Boe, who traveled throughout northern Iraq, quickly became the most popular SMs in the area. It was not surprising to have SMs enter the doors of the COSC unit requesting a visit with the therapy dog. In fact, the COSC team quickly had to enforce "dog visiting hours" to ensure the dog had adequate time to rest. In addition to an increase in visits to the COSC unit, the prevention team—especially the therapy dogs—were invited to neighboring unit functions such as barbeques and promotion and re-enlistment ceremonies. Attending these events is vital for COSC prevention teams to build strong bonds with the SMs they serve.

CASE ILLUSTRATION

AAA—SFC Boe's Teddy Bear

Specialist (SPC) Brown was a helicopter mechanic in a Combat Aviation Brigade (CAB) unit. His commander was concerned about his behavior: He was frequently arguing with other unit members, not completing his duties, and was consistently late to his job. Fellow SMs also noted that he was neglecting his personal hygiene. The prevention team, an occupational therapist, mental health technician, and a therapy dog frequently visited the unit providing conflict resolution and stress management instruction. SPC Brown was particularly fond of the therapy dog, SFC Boe, and asked if he could visit her. He managed to visit her several times a week. During the SM's interactions with the dog, the therapist was able to have lengthy discussions with him and discovered that he was particularly frustrated with his lack of purpose in his job. He thoroughly enjoyed being a mechanic but found that instead of serving as a mechanic, he was doing other tasks he felt were unrelated.

During one of his visits, SPC Brown noted that SFC Boe's favorite toy, a brown teddy bear, was becoming severely tattered (its head was hanging by a thread and a leg and arm had already been dismembered). SPC Brown was concerned that SFC Boe would be unhappy without her favorite toy. He offered to fix the bear and the therapist agreed to let him take the bear. Within 30 minutes, the SM returned, eyes beaming with pride; he said "I fixed it." He tossed the bear toward SFC Boe, who caught it in her mouth and pranced joyfully around the room.

Discussion

The therapist took this opportunity to convey to the SM how activities that may seem unrelated to the mission can have a positive impact. For example, sewing up the teddy bear made SFC Boe happy, who in turn brought laughter to the other SMs present while she played. Although not as evident, tasks that SPC Brown has that are not directly related to his occupation also positively contribute to the mission readiness of the CAB unit. In addition there is also metaphoric and symbolic meaning in taking care of and "patching up" a toy.

Disaster Response

On a large U.S. military compound strategically stationed in the heart of Iraq during Operation Iraq Freedom, disaster struck in a place where many SMs found refuge. A U.S. Army SM released fire on fellow SMs in a COSC clinic, ultimately ending the lives of two military health care providers and three U.S. Army SMs. For the first time in the history of the U.S. Army, a COSC unit experienced a traumatic event within its own entity.

CASE ILLUSTRATION

AAT—Physical Training and Mission Readiness

Service members are required to adhere to physical health and training standards in order to meet mission needs. If an SM is overweight or cannot pass the Army physical fitness test (APFT), he/she may be barred from promotion, re-enlistment, or enlistment extension. Due to the lack in routines and predicted schedules while deployed, physical training and healthy diets are not always easy to maintain. **Private First Class (PFC)** Jones was a young SM due for promotion who was frustrated with his inability to pass the running portion of the APFT. He was being followed by the COSC team for feelings of depression related to being away from his newlywed wife. He often visited with the therapy dog, SFC Boe, as she reminded him of his dog back home. During one of the conversations, the therapist mentioned how

SFC Boe had also gained a few pounds because SMs were sneaking dog treats to her. The therapist asked him if he would be willing to run with her to help her lose weight. PFC Jones straightened up and said he would be honored to help her lose weight. He developed a morning routine to run with the therapy dog at least 3 times/week, under the supervision of the occupational therapist. Within 3 months, the PFC Jones increased his mileage time and was able to pass the APFT.

Discussion

PFC Jones' feelings of depression decreased his drive to exercise despite his desire to become promoted. The occupational therapist utilized the therapy dog as a motivational tool to encourage the SM to stick to an exercise routine.

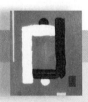

CASE ILLUSTRATION

Responding to Disaster—In Times of War, Everyone Is Susceptible

"There's been an incident. We don't have all the details but a soldier opened fire at a Combat Stress Control clinic and killed several soldiers, including two of their providers. . . . I need you to go there tonight." It must have taken me a

full minute to fully understand the words my Commander spoke. By then, I had been in Iraq almost 14 months and had become accustomed to urgent calls reporting traumatic events. As an occupational therapist in charge of a combat stress control prevention team, it was my responsibility to make contact with units that were impacted by such events. My team supported units by conducting traumatic event managements (TEMs), an organized but informal method of giving soldiers directly involved in a critical incident the opportunity to process through the event. At the end of each TEM, our team remains with the unit, as needed, offering supportive counseling to those who request it. As I neared the end of my 15-month deployment, I had become fairly confident in my reactions and responses to critical incidents. This time was different. Although not part of my own unit, I was familiar with the clinic and the people involved. In fact, I had toured their facility just months before and visited with the providers.

Goosebumps crept through my body as I looked about the old Iraqi building where I worked and lived. I thought about the psychiatrist and psychiatric nurse's office resting just behind the front door and about our psychologist's office sitting on the opposite end, and of all our soldiers in the waiting room. It was an early afternoon and our doors, as always, were open, welcoming any soldier needing support or guidance. "What if it had been us," I pondered.

Discussion

Military health care providers who are stationed in a strategic location, despite being in a combat environment, may become complacent with the relatively safe environment when compared with other SMs who travel often or are more frequently exposed to combat. The above scenario serves as a reminder that we are all vulnerable and should be prepared to react when attacked.

Disaster: Recognizing the Value of Teamwork

Becoming affiliated with local organizations prior to a disaster increases one's credibility and facilitates involvement when a disaster occurs (Scaffa et al., 2006). Disasters cannot be predicted but preparing for them allows communities to respond most effectively. Just as one must habituate himself/herself with emergency evacuation routes, one must also be familiarized with available resources and develop rapport with key members of the community. Many health care professionals are eager to help; however, an overwhelming amount of responders can cause chaos and disorganization, and thus, unintentionally inflict more stress on affected personnel. To prevent this, teamwork and role clarification are necessary. Occupational therapists are at an advantage in recognizing the importance of role clarification for health care professionals who respond to emergency and disaster. If possible, prior to beginning the response process, each member of the team should know exactly his/her role and purpose in the team. This process will minimize confusion and duplication of services. "Dividing and conquering" may prove to be most efficient when large numbers are affected.

CASE ILLUSTRATION

Responding to Disaster—The Importance of Networking

During my tour, I was fortunate to travel to different military installations throughout Iraq. The preferred mode of travel was flight, whether it is via a Blackhawk UH-60, Chinook CH-47, or C-17. A few times, I traveled via vehicle convoy. This allowed me to make relations with fellow flight units and with transportation units. Because flights were unpredictable and often times there were sandstorms, it was not rare to be stranded in another installation for a few days and even for weeks at a time. Months prior to the shooting incident, I found myself delayed at that same installation. Thanks to the skills I learned as a COSC prevention officer, and because I was there for so long, I was able to make many relations within the community to include key personnel from the **Mayor's Cell**, the Red Cross, and the local COSC. The Mayor's Cell is ultimately responsible for the base life support, force protection and infrastructure. Over 14,000 soldiers reside near the site of the incident (FCNL 2009). In order to cover such an expansive location our team of four decided to split into teams of two to reach out to as many personnel as we could.

Our original team consisted of one occupational therapist, a psychologist, a psychiatric nurse, and a mental health specialist.

Discussion

These relationships proved to be valuable. The day of the incident I managed to get a flight out that same night and to find accommodations for my team, despite the report that no rooms were available due to other events. My previous encounter with the local COSC proved even more advantageous. I arrived to find that many other personnel had also responded to the crisis, and although they were also eager to help, they did not have a rapport with the unit, who reportedly felt overwhelmed by the tremendous response. Due to the familiarity many soldiers had with me, and due to the similarity of our roles as COSC health care providers, my team was asked to stay. To facilitate our involvement as first responders, the Mayor's Cell not only assisted us with sleeping arrangements but also provided our team with a vehicle so that we could reach out to all who were affected.

Disaster and Engagement in Occupation

According to the Occupational Therapy Practice Framework (American Occupational Therapy Association [AOTA], 2008), engaging in occupation structures everyday life and contributes to health and well-being. For occupational therapists to complete the evaluation process, they must begin with determining the client's occupational profile. An occupational profile is the collection of a client's history, patterns of daily living, interests, values, and needs. In the previous case studies, the client is the collective experience of the members of the affected combat stress control unit. The therapist must determine the organization's overall interests, goals, and priorities. Because the Army occupational therapist related to the client as a soldier, as a deployed member of a COSC unit, and as a health care provider, determining the needs of the client and gathering information was relatively simple. Aside from mourning the loss of two of its members, the client's concerns related to returning to its occupation as a combat stress control clinic with health care providers in support of soldiers in their region. This outcome requires resumption and fulfillment of the client's habits, routines, rituals, and roles. In order to help the client reestablish its lost sense of control, the therapist aids in constructive activity to help the client move beyond shock and denial. This may require the client to engage in play, vigorous physical activity, or valued leisure occupations in order for survivors to get a quick respite from recurring thoughts, worries, and concerns about the future (Scaffa et al., 2006). For example, the day after the incident, members of the COSC unit volunteered in organizing a barbeque by planning various games and activities and acquiring the food for the event. This event allowed the members to gather and process through the events as well as to honor the loss of their fellow comrades. In addition, many members continued physical activity and invited several of their members to participate in morning runs. The runs proved therapeutic for some soldiers as it gave them the opportunity to exchange thoughts and feelings concerning the series of events while at the same time fulfilling their physical needs.

Disaster and the Health Care Providers' Role in Self-Care

Numerous accounts and news stories have reported on the assistance received by the victims of disaster; however, few have discussed the impression this leaves on those who responded and provided assistance. An article detailing first responders for Hurricane Katrina in 2005 depicted facility staff struggling with their own personal losses while providing daily assistance to their clients (Oakley, Caswell, & Parks, 2008). Another article goes on to state that although "many health care professionals encourage their patients to engage in healthy practices, the same professionals are not always likely to heed their advice" (Calderon-Abbo, Kronenberg, Many, & Ososfsky, 2008). Occupational therapy interventions are activity-based; furthermore, the activity a person is engaged in must be meaningful to the individual. Similarly, the therapist should recognize his/her occupational profile and make time to fulfill those interests and roles. At the most basic level, basic hygiene such as healthy eating, sleeping, and exercise habits should be incorporated into the daily life of a health care provider (Calderon-Abbo et al., 2008). See Figure 25-3 for one of the author's practicing these habits.

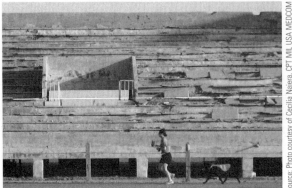

FIGURE 25-3. The Author "Practicing What She Preaches" with SFC Boe

Occupational therapy support of soldiers affected by combat stress is not new; in fact, the development of the OT profession was influenced by the success of reconstruction aides during the first World War (Gutman, 1995). The role of the occupational therapist is to evaluate a soldier's occupational performance and to implement interventions to enhance performance. By focusing on function and using occupation as their primary therapeutic medium, occupational therapists bring a unique perspective to the treatment of soldiers affected by COSR and play a key role in returning soldiers to effective functioning as a member of an Army unit. Similarly, it is essential for occupational therapists to follow their own philosophy and engage in meaningful occupation, especially during times of disaster where stress is magnified and outlets are minimal.

CASE ILLUSTRATION

Practicing What We Preach

Shortly after our team was briefed on the event, we discussed possible challenges and ways to approach the situation. In reality, we did not know what to expect. We knew the circumstances would be taxing and that we would have to practice self-care for our own personal sanity. Our stay lasted nearly a week and every day started early and ended late, leaving us with extreme physical and emotional fatigue.

Despite our exhaustion, we made an effort to meet at the end of every day to share our experiences, to vent, and to process through our own emotions. Although the days were long, we made time to decompress, to eat three times a day, and to sleep at least 6 hours each night. We also made time to call our families waiting for us back home, as events such as these magnify the longing to be reunited with loved ones.

REHABILITATION OF TRAUMATIC BRAIN INJURY

The wars in Iraq and Afghanistan—Operation Iraqi Freedom (OIF) and Operation Enduring Freedom (OEF)—have drawn attention to the short- and potentially long-term consequences of **concussion/mild traumatic brain injury (c/mTBI)**. Symptoms of c/mTBI may have immediate implications for warriors' safe return to duty (Helmick, Parkinson, Chandler, & Warden, 2007) and, in some cases, veterans' longer term ability to successfully reestablish social relationships and resume productive activities upon discharge from military service (Stålnacke, 2007). Occupational therapists have important contributions to rehabilitation after c/mTBI because of its potential impact on personal, vocational, and social functioning.

Occupational therapists have played mission-essential roles in the U.S. Military and Veteran Affairs for more than 75 years. As members of the Army Medical Specialist Corps, occupational therapists contribute to the Corps mission by applying their unique skills to "deliver leading edge health services to our Warriors and Military Families; maximize performance,[and] foster healthy and resilient people" (retrieved from https://amsc.amedd.army.mil/). This commitment to the health and well-being of active duty soldiers, reservists, National Guard, and veterans has helped to maintain troop levels, return soldiers to duty, and optimize recovery and reintegration outcomes—including that of psychosocial functioning.

This section of the chapter describes c/mTBI, its consequences for SMs, and how occupational therapists contribute to rehabilitation and reintegration efforts across an eight-level continuum of care.

Concussion/Mild Traumatic Brain Injury (c/mTBI)

While the rehabilitation community at-large has no singular definition, the Defense and Veterans Brain Injury Center (DVBIC) (2006) defines c/mTBI as "... an injury to the brain resulting from an external force and/or acceleration/deceleration mechanism from an event such as a blast, fall, direct impact, or motor vehicle accident (MVA) which causes an alteration in mental status typically resulting in the temporally related onset of symptoms such as headache, nausea and vomiting, dizziness/balance problems, fatigue, insomnia/sleep disturbances, drowsiness, sensitivity to light/noise, blurred vision, difficulty remembering, and/or difficulty concentrating" (p. 2). A TBI is characterized as mild if the individual experiences a loss of consciousness for 30 minutes or less and/or post-traumatic amnesia for 24 hours or less, and/or a **Glasgow Coma Scale (GCS)** (Teasdale & Jennett, 1974) score of 13 or greater immediately after the event (Kay et al., 1993).

Natural History of c/mTBI

Much of what is understood about c/mTBI stems from research conducted on concussed athletes. This literature suggests that a c/mTBI can be thought of as having two possible phases postinjury: acute-recovery and postconcussion syndrome (PCS).

Acute Recovery

Individuals who sustain c/mTBI typically become symptomatic at the time of incident (McCrea, 2008). Initial symptoms often include headache, dizziness, nausea and vomiting, sleep disturbances, sensitivity to noise and light, slowed thinking and reaction time, memory problems, and attention difficulties (McCrea et al., 2003). During the acute phase of recovery, symptoms are thought to be explained by a short-term neurometabolic process that renders neurons temporarily dysfunctional but not destroyed (McCrea, 2008). Based on studies with athletes, the majority of people with c/mTBI can be expected to fully recover within seven days (McCrea). While headaches may linger for a year or longer (Ruff, Riechers, & Ruff, 2010), c/mTBI symptoms typically resolve within 3 months of injury (Ruff, 2005). Similarly, vision disturbances often occur with combat-related c/mTBI with symptoms that may continue beyond the acute recovery phase (Goodrich, Kirby, Cockerham, Ingalla, & Lew, 2007).

Postconcussion Syndrome

While most people fully recover from c/mTBI, experts estimate that between 3% to 20% of those with c/mTBI experience symptoms that persist and impact the individual's ability to function in daily life (Alves, Colohn, OLeary, Rimel, & Jane, 1986; Edna & Cappelen, 1987; McCrea, 2008; Ponsford et al., 2000; Ruff, Camenzuli, & Mueller, 1996). Those who present with persistent problems 3 months postinjury may have PCS (Mittenberg & Strauman, 2000; Ruff, 2005).

A person with possible PCS has a history of head injury and, at 3 months postinjury, experiences symptoms in at least three of the following categories: headache, dizziness, malaise, fatigue, noise intolerance; irritability, depression, anxiety, emotional lability; subjective concentration, memory, or intellectual disabilities without neuropsychological evidence or marked impairment; insomnia; reduced alcohol tolerance; preoccupation with above symptoms and fear of brain damage (Mittenberg & Strauman, 2000). There is no agreed-upon explanation for these difficulties. Some experts suggest that microscopic brain damage explains (in part) the physical, cognitive, and emotional sequelae of c/mTBI (Cohen et al., 2007). It also may be that symptoms persisting beyond several days or weeks may be attributable to factors other than the c/mTBI, including psychosocial factors such as unstable relationships and a lack of social support systems (Carroll et al., 2004). For example, Montgomery (1995) proposed a multifactor explanation for PCS in which cognitive inefficiencies, distractions from physical symptoms, and situational stressors interact to compound the challenges presented by the c/mTBI. The vicious cycle is exacerbated as the person puts forth extra effort to perform everyday activities and becomes alarmed by inefficiencies and errors in performing premorbidly mundane tasks. The resultant hypersensitivity to error and anxiety mix with misattributions regarding the root cause of deficient performance, further sabotaging self-confidence and subsequent performance (Montgomery, 1995).

Effects of Recurrent Concussion

People who experience repeat c/mTBI over a relatively short period of time (days, weeks, or months) are at risk for potentially serious problems. In rare instances, **second impact syndrome** occurs if a second c/mTBI occurs during the acute recovery period from a first injury—the results of which may cause death or severe disability (Lew, Thomander, Chew, & Bleiberg, 2007). Additionally, people who experience multiple concussive events are at risk for later life cognitive decline. Guskiewicz and colleagues (2005) reported that retired professional football players with a history of three or more c/mTBI had a fivefold prevalence of mild cognitive impairment compared to retirees without a history of concussion.

c/mTBI in a Military Context

While estimates vary, it is clear that large numbers of SMs have experienced c/mTBI in OEF/OIF. The Department of Defense (DoD) reports that 202,281 SMs sustained a TBI between the years 2000 and through the end of 2010 (DoD Numbers for Traumatic Brain Injury accessed 4/1/2011 from http://www.dvbic.org/TBI-Numbers.aspx), most of which may be characterized as c/mTBI. Part of the challenge in obtaining accurate incidence estimates lies in the fact that c/mTBI is difficult to diagnose or identify. Symptoms may initially present themselves as a brief alteration of consciousness (AOC) or behavioral changes (Warden, 2006) and often there is no way of identifying the c/mTBI that is concurrent with more dire diagnoses such as limb loss, burns, spinal cord injury, or fractures. Some SMs with c/mTBI do not report symptoms until later in their medical care (especially if they suffer concomitant life-threatening injuries) or after deployment. In their postdeployment screening study, Terrio and colleagues (2009) reported that for some SMs, memory problems and irritability were first identified after the acute phase, possibly when they were faced with challenging novel tasks and/or feedback from loved ones. Finally, estimates of c/mTBI are difficult to determine because many SMs appear to incur more than one c/mTBI during their deployment. For example, the 115 patients identified from the March–September 2004 Navy-Marine Corps Combat Trauma Registry received approximately 200 TBI-related diagnoses (Galarneau, Woodruff, Dye, Mohrle, & Wade, 2008). This may be explained by the fact that many SMs have multiple blast exposures during deployment. Also, sometimes SMs under report as they do not want to admit to blast exposure or that symptoms they may be experiencing could be a c/mTBI as they want to remain with their unit, rather than seek care.

Mechanism of Injury

Blast exposures (explosions involving improvised explosive devices [IED]) are the most frequent causes of c/mTBI in OEF/OIF (Polusny et al., 2011). IEDs are often hidden along the road, within walls, or placed in small confined buildings. When detonated, the explosion sends both physical matter and blast waves that travel for hundreds of yards at speeds up to 1,600 feet per second. These blast waves occur in multiple phases with varying injury noted at each phase (DePalma, Burris, Champion, & Hodgson, 2005). The primary phase refers to direct exposure to over pressurized air waves. This may cause diffuse axonal injury and a coup-counter-coup type injury. During the secondary blast phase, the SM may be impacted by debris (e.g., tree limbs, rocks, sand, gravel) that follows the air waves and causes penetrating or non-penetrating wounds. The tertiary blast is when the individual is thrown or displaced and hits his or her head on a stationary object, and the quaternary blast injury consists of burns or inhalation of toxic fumes. As mentioned earlier, many warriors are exposed to multiple blasts and symptoms may or may not be apparent after the first exposure. Furthermore, some SMs may be reluctant to report symptoms of c/mTBI for fear of being separated from their unit (Polusny et al., 2011). The minimal neuronal damage that occurs with a single blast is compounded and symptoms may emerge as exposure proximity and frequency increase. In addition to c/mTBI, blast injuries may result in orthopedic and burn injuries and contribute to the development of PTSD.

c/mTBI and Stress Disorders

As mentioned earlier, the research literature based on civilian c/mTBI has largely informed current understanding and rehabilitation practices for SM with c/mTBI. However, the setting in which the trauma occurs distinguishes civilian and military populations, with most military c/mTBI occurring in combat operations that may involve witnessing atrocities (Sareen et al., 2007). This puts SMs with c/mTBI at risk for PTSD. In fact, experts estimate that 33% to 39% of SMs with c/mTBI also screen positive for PTSD (Carlson et al., 2009). This dual-diagnosis and overlapping symptomatology (see Table 25-1) appears to be particularly troublesome in terms of diagnosing

TABLE 25-1. Overlapping Symptoms of PTSD and c/mTBI

PTSD Symptoms	Symptoms of Both PTSD and c/mTBI	c/mTBI Symptoms
■ Re-experiencing the traumatic event (intrusive memories, nightmares) ■ Avoidance of thoughts and feelings that serve as reminders of the event; emotional numbing	■ Disordered sleep ■ Difficulty concentrating ■ Memory problems ■ Slowed processing speed ■ Feeling overwhelmed ■ Irritability ■ Anxiety ■ Depression	■ Headache ■ Visual disturbance (e.g., photophobia, convergence disorder) ■ Dizziness and vestibular dysfunction

Based on information from Goodrich et al., 2007; Hoffer, Gottshall, Moore, Balough, & Wester, 2004; and Kennedy et al., 2007.

both these conditions and the long-term implications for personal and psychosocial functioning (Polusny et al., 2011).

In summary, it is clear that many SMs experience a confusing constellation of symptoms associated with c/mTBI, PCS, or PTSD. Therapists appreciate that SM's symptoms may have dual or even multiple underlying causes, especially when symptoms continue for more than 3 months postinjury.

Occupational Therapy After c/mTBI Within a Military Context

As in civilian practice, rehabilitation after c/mTBI may involve a multidisciplinary team including occupational and physical therapists, speech-language pathologists, physicians, neuropsychologists, and counseling psychologists. The scope of practice of the various professionals may vary based on state licensure and practice setting. However, across all practice settings, occupational therapists provide services based on the individual SM's unique set of circumstances, goals, and functional performance problems, rather than based solely on diagnosis (Radomski, Davidson, Voydetich, & Erickson, 2009). Additionally, occupational therapists communicate an optimistic expectation for warriors' full recovery. As suggested by Ruff (2005), ". . . clinicians must avoid fostering the belief that the 'brain damage' subsequent to concussion always leads to permanent deficits" (p. 16).

Occupational-Performance Problems of Service Members with c/mTBI

The previous discussion underscores the fact that SMs with c/mTBI present with a number of symptoms and problems when referred to occupational therapy. In the acute setting, SMs may experience headache, dizziness, nausea and vomiting, sleep disturbances, sensitivity to noise and light, slowed thinking and reaction time, memory problems, irritability, depression, and visual changes (Carroll et al., 2004). These deficits have significant implications for deployed SMs. For example, visual disturbances will impact an SM's ability to see the enemy, identify possible IEDs hidden within the brush, read maps, and drive safely and effectively in a war zone. Dizziness may hamper use of weapons, negotiating difficult terrain, and tolerating position changes. Decreased processing and reaction time place SMs and their comrades at risk when quick decisions must be made.

On the home front, persistent symptoms associated with c/mTBI or PCS often lead to long-term activity limitations and social participation restrictions. The long-term disability often associated with c/mTBI may lead to anxiety, stress, depression, and social issues (Ponsford, 2005), especially if concomitant with other injuries. Activities such as returning to work or school may be challenging or impossible depending on the extent of symptoms. Returning to roles such as a spouse or parent presents challenges as irritability and decreased frustration tolerance impact relationships.

Cognitive inefficiencies, such as problems with attention and memory, make seemingly easy daily tasks like medication management a challenge (Steadman-Pare, Colantonio, Ratcliff, Chase, & Vernich, 2001). Finally, SMs with PTSD and c/mTBI are at risk for postdeployment depression, problematic drinking, and somatic complaints that have significant implications for social and occupational functioning.

Occupational Therapy Assessment and Intervention Across the Continuum of Care

In a military context, eight levels of care have been defined to describe medical and rehabilitation resources across the continuum of care—in combat theater through return to community. An SM may enter the rehabilitation system at any one of the eight levels or "ports of entry" and may enter and exit the Levels of Care multiple times throughout his or her lifetime.

In Combat Theater: Levels I to III

Level I: Buddy Aid to Battalion Aid Station (BAS). At this level of care, the combat medic initiates the **Military Acute Concussion Evaluation (MACE)** and neurologic screen to determine if the SM displays symptoms or red flags consistent with a diagnosis of c/mTBI. The combat medic may rest the SM in place or recommend to a supervising physician evacuating the SM to the Level II c/mTBI Reconditioning Center or Level III for neurologic evaluation. Army occupational therapists and occupational therapy technicians train the combat medics in the appropriate execution and interpretation of the MACE and neurological screen at this level.

Level II: c/mTBI Brigade Combat Team. This team includes an occupational therapist, occupational therapy technician, primary care physician, psychologist or social worker, and a physical therapist. In general, physical and cognitive rest is recommended until SMs with c/mTBI are symptom-free and then a stepwise progression of activity, with regression of intensity of activity with any symptom return (McCrory et al., 2005).

The **OT BCT c/mTBI Reconditioning Program**[1] is designed to conduct **far forward** (close to the point of injury) treatment of c/mTBI and other biopsychosocial conditions in a multidisciplinary outpatient setting at the BCT level. The program's primary function is maximizing far forward return to duty of SMs affected by c/mTBI and other biopsychosocial conditions by offering a continuous 1- to 21-day program for all SMs who meet the Joint Theater Trauma System Clinical Practice Guidelines (JTTSCPGs) dated 2010. The program maintains 24-hour operations and offers education and treatment in a structured setting focused on sleep, education,

---

[1] We acknowledge contributions of the original developers of the OT-PT c/mTBI Guidance document: Maggie Weightman, PT, PhD; Leslie Freeman Davidson, PhD, OTR/L; Marilyn Rodgers, MS, PT, MAJ; and Robyn Bolgla, MS, PT, CTRS.

balance and cognitive training, concentration exercises, problem solving, adaptive stress reactions, and resiliency. Treating the SM close to the point of injury speeds recovery by initiating treatment without delay; reassuring and educating early so the SM knows what to expect; and return to duty early so the SM can remain a valued, productive member of his/her unit and complete the mission.

Army occupational therapists evaluate SMs with c/mTBI with the MACE and neurological screen, as well as the cranial nerve screen and other occupational performance measures as needed per SM. Service members with c/mTBI need information about their condition early on and throughout their recovery. In fact, patients who receive one-on-one education with a therapist about their symptoms and instructions about the acute phase of recovery demonstrated fewer symptoms and shorter symptom duration than those who received a written handout with this information (Mittenberg, Tremont, Zielinski, Fichera, & Rayls, 1996). Therefore, provision of education regarding c/mTBI is an important component of occupational therapy services in theater.

Once SMs are asymptomatic and are ready to return to duty, occupational therapists evaluate SMs with an exertional test consisting of a short ride on a stationary bicycle to a precalculated target heart rate, followed by five push-ups. The purpose of the exertional testing is to see if symptoms such as headache or dizziness return once the SM is exerted. If exertional testing does not cause symptoms to return, the occupational therapist recommends to the primary physician that the SM is returned to duty. If symptoms do return, the SM remains in the BCT program until they are asymptomatic and they are re-tested.

If SMs have been in a Concussion Care Center for greater than 72 hours, they also complete a military performance assessment that consists of a 20-minute walk broken up into 5-minute increments while wearing the military combat uniform, combat boots, Improved Outer Tactical Vest (IOTV), and combat helmet. The first 5 minutes consists of a warm-up and the SM recites the phonetic alphabet (Alpha, Bravo, Charlie, etc.) as a dual task, which is necessary for executive function and performing the dual task with mobility tests safety and attentional capacity (McCulloch, Buxton, Hackney, & Lowers, 2010). At the end of the first 5 minutes, the SM is asked to "take a knee" (bend down so one foot is on the ground and one knee is on the ground) and touch their nose to their knee of the leg whereby the foot is on the ground. The purpose for touching their nose to their knee is to see if they have any increased symptoms. The next 5-minute walk is at a faster pace to get the heart rate up a little faster, again checking to see if symptoms return. The third 5 minutes consists of walking over and under obstacles such as logs, curbs, and turning corners, and the last 5 minutes is a cool down. If there are no symptoms, the SM removes the gear (IOTV and helmet) and rests for 10 minutes, and then performs a slow 5-minute jog to determine if percussion from bouncing increases the symptoms. If at any time during the military performance assessment the symptoms return, the test is terminated and the SM returns to the center for 24 hours before they are re-tested. They are only re-tested when asymptomatic. If they are asymptomatic following testing, the occupational therapist recommends to the physician that the SM be returned to duty.

Level III: OT c/mTBI Program at the Theater Hospital. The Level III c/mTBI program team complement is the same as the Level II with the addition of a neurologist and neuropsychologist and access to computerized tomography (CT) scan. Similar to the Level II, occupational therapists identify and address symptoms of c/mTBI for SMs remaining in theater. An SM is referred to the Level III when more comprehensive services are needed, or if the SM is not recovering at the Level II and the occupational therapist feels the SM would benefit from care at the Level III. The goal at the Level III is to return the SMs to duty as well, so once they are asymptomatic, exertional testing is done, and if symptoms do not return, they are returned to duty. If symptoms do return, they either remain in the program until asymptomatic and are re-tested, or they are evacuated to the Level IV.

Level IV: Evacuation Center (Landstuhl Regional Medical Center [LRAMC]). Occupational therapists may begin therapy plans of care during the relatively short episode of care at LRAMC before injured SMs are evacuated to CONUS (Continental United States). Therapists continue to evaluate and treat c/mTBI symptoms, address functional limitations and concomitant impairments, provide education about c/mTBI, and work with the medical team to identify c/mTBI.

Levels V to VIII: Single-Service and/or Interdisciplinary Rehabilitation Programming. Once SMs return to CONUS, they may receive occupational therapy services at Levels V, VI, VII, and/or VIII. These levels of care are defined as follows:

> Level V: Military medical treatment facility (MTF)—inpatient and outpatient
>
> Level VI: Inpatient rehabilitation (non-MTF, such as Veterans Affairs Medical Center and community partner facilities)
>
> Level VII: Outpatient rehabilitation (non-MTF, such as Veterans Affairs Medical Center and community partner facilities)
>
> Level VIII: Lifetime care (as Veterans Affairs Medical Center, a community partner hospital or outpatient facility)

In general, at Levels V to VIII, occupational therapists respond to a wide array of performance problems associated with c/mTBI and/or PTSD by providing education, addressing vision and cognitive inefficiencies, and by helping SM re-engage with work/duty, personal, and social tasks that are important to them. Each of these areas will be briefly summarized. (Note that in some settings, occupational therapists also address vestibular issues, which will not be addressed here.)

Occupational Therapy Interventions

Patient Education

In addition to patient education during the acute phase of recovery, SMs with c/mTBI benefit from patient education during Levels V to VIII to help them understand and manage potentially persistent cognitive inefficiencies. Occupational therapists teach SMs about normal human information processing and emphasize how a myriad of personal and situational factors (such as stress and fatigue) can contribute to intermittent cognitive failures at a given point in time (Montgomery, 1995). In addition to preventing misattribution of cognitive inefficiencies to brain damage, education paves the way for the development and employment of compensatory cognitive strategies.

Vision Problems

Occupational therapists perform vision screens in order to identify unrecognized visual deficits that interfere with daily life so that SMs can be referred for diagnostic evaluations with vision specialists such as optometrists (Bryan, 2004). To that end, occupational therapists use symptom checklists, observe functional performance, and screen vision function in a number of key areas (such as acuity, convergence, accommodation, visual fields, and scanning). (See Scheiman, Scheiman, and Whittaker [2006] for excellent discussions of occupational therapy vision screening.) This role is critical because undetected vision problems may confound rehabilitation efforts after c/mTBI. Occupational therapists provide vision treatment under the supervision of a vision specialist and also help SMs make habit and environmental modifications to optimize their safety and functioning.

Cognitive Problems

Occupational therapists also play key roles in assessing and treating the cognitive inefficiencies experienced by many SMs with c/mTBI. The primary purpose of cognitive assessment from an occupational therapy perspective is to identify (and ultimately address) possible cognitive barriers to functioning, not to diagnose neuropsychological impairment. Occupational therapists confine their assessments to those that have been standardized on individuals with c/mTBI and to structured observations of functioning, particularly the performance of complex tasks. For example, cognitive assessments that are relevant to and appropriate for SMs with c/mTBI include the following:

- Behavioral Assessment of Dysexecutive Syndrome (Wilson, Alderman, Burgess, Emslie, & Evans, 1997; Wilson, Evans, Emslie, & Alderman, 1998)
- Cognistat (Kiernan, Mueller, Langston, & Van Dyke, 1987)
- Contextual Memory Test (Toglia, 1993)
- Rivermead Behavioral Memory Test (Wilson, Cockburn, & Baddeley, 1985; Wilson, Cockburn, Baddeley, & Hiorns, 1989)
- Test of Everyday Attention (Robertson, Ward, Ridgeway, & Nimmo-Smith, 1996)

It is widely accepted that there is little empirical research to specifically guide cognitive intervention for prolonged cognitive symptoms associated with c/mTBI because the cognitive rehabilitation literature is based on studies involving subjects with moderate to severe TBI. However, in accord with the results of systematic reviews conducted by Cicerone and colleagues (2000, 2005), occupational therapists help SMs with c/mTBI by teaching them to use an array of compensatory strategies to manage problems with memory and attention.

Performing Personal, Work/Duty, and Social Tasks

As is the case in all areas of occupational therapy practice, occupational therapy practitioners address the personal, work/duty, and social problems that may accompany a c/mTBI. Structured interviews such as the Canadian Occupational Performance Measure (Law et al., 2005) have been used with persons with c/mTBI (Trombly, Radomski, & Davis, 1998; Trombly, Radomski, Trexel, & Burnett-Smith, 2002) and helps the occupational therapist focus intervention around the everyday problems of most concern to the SMs. For example, occupational therapists help SMs implement new strategies for improving their effectiveness in work/duty roles, parenting, home management, and driving through skill development and implementation.

Military occupational therapists utilize evidence-based evaluations and treatments whenever possible for c/mTBI. In deployed, rehabilitative, and community settings, occupational therapists use a holistic approach to address SMs' multifaceted needs after c/mTBI to advance their recovery and reintegration. Research is scant on acute c/mTBI, particularly in regard to activity needs, demands, and how soon activity should be introduced after a c/mTBI. Deployed occupational therapists are beginning to research c/mTBI, but much more research needs to be done in this environment, as well as in sports concussion. Also, traditional treatments may not be effective or appropriate because concomitant psychosocial problems oftentimes overlay a c/mTBI, or the environment may not be conducive due to the war effort.

TREATING WARRIORS AT HOME: ACUTE STRESS REACTIONS
The Warrior Ethos

Traditional military creeds contain statements of conduct, commitment, and cultural values. In light of the wars in Iraq and Afghanistan, the U.S. Department of Defense needed to revisit training of personnel for twenty-first century combat operations. Although traditional creeds still exist, a push for a more comprehensive, joint-service "ethos of war" began in the 1990s, became operational in 2003, and is now incorporated into all aspects of military training (Buckingham, 1999; Gregg, 2006). The term **warrior** is intended to instill basic values of courage, honor, and commitment, as well as a sense that being an SM sailor, airman, or Marine is more than a job, more than a career, but is a calling, an identity, and a way of life.

For a moment, put yourself into the body and mind of a military SM, transformed into "warrior." There's endless drilling, exhausting practice, rehearsal after rehearsal carving procedures into memory so actions will become automatic. To a warrior, survival means believing the training you receive works. Training procedures and their underlying rules are meant to protect, control chaos, and are essential to mission and survival. From a mental health perspective, the warrior ethos provides a deep sense of belonging, a reliable support structure, a personal identity, life role, and a consistent ethical framework for making decisions.

Training is the core of combat and deployment resiliency and most of the time it works. But when something goes wrong, warriors often believe it is their personal fault, not the fault of training or some other unexpected, extraordinary circumstance. Mild psychological impairment due to combat or deployment stress is treated with psychological first aid on-site, but if symptoms or decreased psychological functioning grossly impairs the warrior role, the warrior is likely to be removed from duty. When the warrior identity is suspended or surrendered because of needing physical or mental health care, or even because a tour of combat due has ended, there is often a profound sense of loss. Sometimes the realities of the battlefield falls short of the ideals of the warrior ethos that can lead to psychological issues such as anger, substance abuse, relationship problems, or self-harm.

Occupational Roles and Dual Agency

Occupational therapists are dual agents in military health care settings. The term **"dual agency"** is frequently used in the areas of real estate in discussions of an agents' ethical conduct—do they represent the needs of buyer, seller, or both? In health care, patients sometimes have issues with "dual insurance" when they have more than one policy, and the insuring companies dispute over which company will take responsibility for what procedure or cost. In military health care settings with active-duty warrior patients, occupational therapists are dual agents because of their responsibility to the military mission as well as the patient.

The Occupational Therapy Practice Framework (AOTA, 2008) considers life roles in all areas of occupational performance and contexts, including the role of occupational therapist. Occupational therapists are empathetic and caring people (as recently stated in the president's address to the AOTA 2011 conference, OTs are nice. and their education is typically client-centered from the very beginning [Clark, 2011]). Dual agency is challenging because an occupational therapist may automatically put patient or client needs first but perhaps the military mission is primary. For example, a patient's main occupational therapy goal is getting "fixed" and returning to duty as soon as possible. The therapist designs an evidence-based treatment program and is confident it will work. Despite an optimistic therapy outcome, however, the interdisciplinary team decides to remove the patient from active duty because the prolonged process of rehabilitation does not fit with the immediate military mission needs. Therefore the client-centered value of occupational therapy may conflict with the other role of the military occupational therapists and interventions must be considered from these distinct perspectives because it is a shift in perspective for the therapists' occupational role of clinician. Also, it is a shift in perspective relating to values that has to be reconciled by the occupational therapist.

Acute Military Psychiatry

There are three other important differences between and military and civilian acute psychiatric settings. First, according to the *DSM-IV-TR* (American Psychiatric Association [APA], 2000), a military setting is likely to have a larger proportion of patients diagnosed with adjustment or anxiety disorders on the Axis I diagnosis. Many civilian health insurances will not cover inpatient treatment when adjustment or anxiety disorders are non-psychotic or non–life-threatening. Ready access to firearms, explosives, and intelligence information quickly brings a person's uncertain psychological capacity to the organization's attention; therefore, a person exhibiting acute stress in a military setting may be hospitalized more readily. Second, the majority of military patients admitted to acute psychiatry are between the ages of 18 and 25, the prime age-range for a first psychotic break in schizophrenia or bipolar disorders. The age factor is important because research in neuroscience continues to show that brain circuitry, notably the prefrontal cortex, is not fully developed until at least the mid-20s (Massachusetts Institute of Technology, 2011). A recent multisite study of military personnel with Iraq or Afghanistan deployments highlights the third difference: There are a higher proportion of persons with co-occurring psychiatric and closed TBIs than is observed in the civilian population (Zatzick et al., 2010). These three factors generate a unique and complex patient population. Diagnostic clarification, stabilization and safety, as well as decisions regarding a warrior's military work abilities dictate the course of treatment.

Co-Existing Disorders

Since the beginning of the wars in Iraq and Afghanistan, diagnostic clarification in psychiatry has become increasing complex. The Defense Center of Excellence for Psychological Health and Traumatic Brain Injury and its component centers reflect extensive efforts to address the complex psychological health needs of returning warriors (http://www.dcoe.health.mil) as do the Veterans Administration/Department of Defense (VA/DoD) Evidence-Based Clinical Practice Guidelines (U.S. Department of Veteran Affairs, 2001, 2008, 2009a, 2009b, 2010a, 2010b). Co-existing disorders add to the complexity of health conditions and can confuse treatment priorities. For example, wounded warriors may present for care and have symptoms suggestive of mood, cognitive, psychotic, sleep, anxiety, substance abuse, pain, and/or personality disorders. Because these symptoms are common to many types of health issues, and diagnostic tests are currently not able to determine exact cause or etiology to each symptom, it can be difficult to pinpoint exactly where treatment should begin. Leaders in military psychological health have suggested these complex health conditions be perceived as person-centered "syndromes" rather than medical "symptoms" (Gever & Jasmer, 2008; Hoge, 2010a, 2010b). Recommendations for treatment and care of co-existing disorders have taken on a biopsychosocial approach very similar to the person-centered focus on occupational performance that has always guided occupational therapy.

The VA/DoD practice guidelines encourage health practitioners to view treatment interventions within the context of a person's individual circumstances rather than a microcosm of illness or disease; they are an important move away from traditional medicine's fragmented system of symptom reduction. In a fragmented system, for instance, a patient having trouble sleeping through the night could receive different diagnoses from different providers, such as a neurologist who suspects mild TBI or a psychologist who suspects PTSD.

While complex psychiatric diagnoses are found in most acute care settings, the military setting tends to have a greater number of patients with PTSD related to combat exposures than civilian settings. The role of occupational therapy on the interdisciplinary team is significant because while hospitalized, a person's performance in areas of occupation still occurs naturally within its context. It is the occupational therapy practitioner who can identify subtle performance deficits that often elude formal testing, an important factor for diagnostic clarification as well as medical retirement and disability compensation.

Occupational therapists need a good working knowledge of psychiatric and personality disorders, TBIs, PCSs, substance abuse, and somatic syndromes in an acute military psychiatry setting because of overlapping symptoms in occupational performance. For a good discussion of coexisting symptoms and diagnostic issues for the military population, see Gever, and Jasmer (2008), Hoge (2010a, 2010b), and VA/DoD Practice Guidelines (U.S. Department of Veteran Affairs, 2001, 2008, 2009a, 2009b, 2010a, 2010b).

Interdisciplinary Approach

In a discussion of survey results of 2,525 U.S. Army infantry warriors who recently returned from deployment, Hoge et al. (2008) concluded that complex, coexisting conditions require an interdisciplinary approach to diagnosis and treatment. The interdisciplinary approach was recommended by Hoge et al. because the current health system focuses on symptom reduction that has potential to lead to fragmented medical care. In a fragmented system, for example, a patient with difficulty sleeping through the night could receive different diagnoses from different providers such as a neurologist who suspects mild TBI or a psychologist who suspects PTSD. Among other recommendations from the Hoge et al. study was educating warriors so that they understand their symptoms and, thus, normalize their condition. Normalization of illness and disability has always been a core belief of occupational therapy and education is an intervention in the Occupational Therapy Practice Framework (AOTA, 2008). But how are occupational therapy principles and beliefs communicated to patients and interdisciplinary providers in a fast-paced setting with frequent staff and patient turnover?

Communicating Occupational Therapy

A practical way to educate patients and providers is to give deep thought to the occupational therapy "fit" within a work setting. How do therapists promote their work? How do therapists encourage patients to be active participants when treatment occupations are everyday activities and may not seem as important as a high-tech procedure? How can patients who are facing major life transitions "buy into" occupational therapy when the process of grieving and loss has not yet begun? How does occupational therapy "work" if treatment is limited to only a few sessions? The answers to these questions are easier if therapists reframe the occupational therapy process in the acute care setting: time restrictions; overworked clinicians who develop short attention spans so they can leave work on time; complex patients in crisis with limited cognition; frequent meetings; group sessions that use activities that are difficult for patients and clinicians to differentiate; and the expectation that everything will be documented. These questions will be answered by using examples from an acute psychiatry military hospital setting.

Promoting Occupational Therapy

Language

Have a description of occupational therapy in all materials used in the setting, and develop a consistent language to describe services. The following example corresponds with the types of occupational therapy interventions described in the second edition of the practice framework (AOTA, 2008): (a) preparatory methods, (b) purposeful activity, and (c) occupation-based intervention (p. 653). This simple framework provides consistency and is useful when describing individual or group interventions. Occupational therapy offers three types of groups and individual sessions as shown in Table 25-2.

Routine Group Observation and Documentation

Expressive activities (purposeful activity) occur frequently in acute care. Documentation needs to provide information unique to occupational therapy and be visually appealing to overworked clinicians. An organized procedure and system can make daily documentation informative and efficient. The Occupational Therapy Task Observation Scale (OTTOS©) (Margolis, Harrison, Robinson, & Jayaram, 1996) has been successful for documentation purposes and has good interrater reliability (.92). Each numerical rating has a verbal description that can be used in an accompanying

TABLE 25-2. Consistent Language to Describe Groups and Individual Sessions

Sensory-Motor Activities help you discover ways to deal with behaviors, thoughts, and emotions by regulating your "senses." Movement, relaxation, and visualization activities help you learn to connect your thoughts and feelings to control unwanted symptoms. (based on preparatory methods [AOTA, 2008]).

Expressive Activities help to increase awareness of how you "do things" in your daily routine. Hands-on experiences help you practice and improve awareness of your choices, decisions, and behaviors. Personal coping patterns can be identified and improved (based on purposeful activity [AOTA, 2008]).

Life-Skill Activities help with your identified goals after leaving the hospital and include vocational planning, healthy lifestyle management, and using strategies to manage and adapt your personal stressors (based on occupation-based intervention [AOTA, 2008]).

© Cengage Learning 2013

narrative summary to elaborate on a particular performance skill strength or deficit if needed. The OTTOS© version used in this setting has four numerical descriptors.

The OTTOS© is also very useful for teaching occupational therapy students and interns observations skills in a group setting. In reframing treatment for purposes of documentation, functional task behaviors can be viewed in the same way another therapist may consider changes in joint movement. A simple spreadsheet is used to track the specific task behaviors of interest. A graph is pasted into the electronic medical record and multiple sessions can be compared as shown in Figure 25-5.

Another way to help educate patients and increase meaningful participation, a "pre-group checklist," based on OTTOS© categories can be used (see Figure 25-6). Patients are given the checklist at the beginning of the treatment session, engage in the occupation, and refer back to it during a postgroup summary that is guided by the therapist.

Evaluation. The evaluations and assessments used in acute military psychiatry setting are typical to those found in many behavioral health facilities where occupational therapists' practice: The Canadian Occupational Performance Measure (Law et al., 2005); The Cognistat (http://www.cognistat.com); The Allen Cognitive Level Screen (Allen et al., 2006); Items from The Allen Diagnostic Module (Earhart, 2006); The LOTCA (Katz, Itzkovich, Averbuch, & Elazar, 1989); and Weekly Calendar Planning Activity (Toglia, 2010).

Methods similar to those described in the group documentation and observation section may be developed to report results. Therapists can obtain permission from the developer of the tool to use a summary form or request permission to use a modification as part of the medical record. Most facilities have documentation committees that approve the use of special forms. The documentation committee described in the sample facility was agreeable to specialized forms because they

1. Engagement	5. Independence
0 = Does not participate 3 = Requires repeated prompting, quickly loses interest 7 = Participates without prompting, sustains interest 10 = Eager to participate, engrossed in task	0 = Constant assistance or reassurance with no effort 3 = Requires assistance or reassurance on a repeated basis to continue with task 7 = Requires only occasional assistance or reassurance 10 = No assistance or reassurance necessary
2. Coordination	6. Initiative
0 = Unable to manipulate tools and materials 3 = Slow, awkward, drops tools and materials; decreased precision 7 = Handles tools and materials with occasional lapses, precision or awkwardness 10 = Precise with movement, handles tools with ease	0 = Makes no effort to proceed, prompts or cues have no effect 3 = Proceeds only with much prompting or cuing 7 = Proceeds with only occasional prompts or cues 10 = No assistance or reassurance necessary
3. Follows Directions	7. Decision Making
0 = Fails to follow verbal directions or demonstrations, fails to mimic 3 = Follows one-step verbal directions or mimics a simple demonstration 7 = Needs reminders or directions repeated only for multistep tasks 10 = Follows multistep instructions successfully without assistance	0 = Does not make decisions 3 = Chooses between two options only with prompting 7 = Chooses among multiple options with minimal assistance 10 = Makes decisions independently
4. Quality of Work	8. Concentration
0 = Disorganized, no attention to details, random execution 3 = Excessive usage of materials or major errors, poor attention to details 7 = Minor errors, most details correct, adequate use of materials and work space 10 = Organized, details perfect, work planned carefully, no errors	0 = Less than 30 seconds 3 = Attends to task work 10 minutes 7 = Attends to task for 35 minutes; re-attends after distraction 10 = Attends throughout tasks, re-attends to task after external interruptions and divides attention as necessary

FIGURE 25-4. The Occupational Therapy Task Observation Scale

9. Frustration Tolerance

0 = Immediately frustrated with task demands, stops task, refuses to resume even with encouragement

3 = Repeatedly frustrated resulting in cessation of task, requires specific instructions on frustration techniques

7 = Attempts to manage frustration using at least one technique; frustration only occasionally interferes with task, interruption is brief

10 = Independently tolerates and manages frustration without task interruptions

10. Problem Solving

0 = Unable to identify problem or respond even if prompted

3 = Requires directions in each state of problem-solving process

7 = Requires intermittent prompting to solve problems

10 = Recognizes solutions necessary to accomplish task and proceeds independently

11. Grooming and Hygiene

0 = Malodorous, unclean, unwashed, or grossly inappropriate grooming or attire

3 = Disheveled, unkempt or the attire inappropriate to the situation

7 = Mildly disheveled, clothing appropriate

10 = Neatly dressed and groomed, attire appropriate to the situation

12. Activity Level

0 = Pace too fast or slow to proceed with task despite repeated intervention

3 = Attempted to adjust to pace of task that required repeated directions

7 = Requires occasional cues to adjust to the pace of task

10 = Pace does not impede task performance

13. Expression

0 = Body and facial expression incongruent to setting, expression bizarre or flat attracting negative attention

3 = Body language or facial expressions are rarely congruent to situation

7 = Intermittently full range of facial and body expression that is congruent in response to situation

10 = Full range of expressions that is completely congruent to the environment

14. Cooperation

0 = Refuses to participate, no response to encouragement or limits

3 = Requires firm limits and or frequent redirections: difficulty sharing space and materials

7 = Needs occasional reminders concerning group expectations: shares materials when asked, tolerates proximity of others

10 = Complies with group expectations, no limits are needed to comply, spontaneously shares space and materials

15. Socialization

0 = No appropriate interactions with others

3 = Rare appropriate interaction despite constant intervention

7 = Appropriate interactions with others with occasional cues required

10 = Appropriate conversation interactions with others without therapist interventions

FIGURE 25-4. The Occupational Therapy Task Observation Scale (*Continued*)

Source: Margolis, R., Harrison, S., Robinson, H., & Jayaram, G. (1996). Occupational Therapy Task Observation Scale (OTTOS): A rapid method for rating task group function of psychiatric patients. *American Journal of Occupational Therapy*, 50 (5), 382. Reprinted with permission.

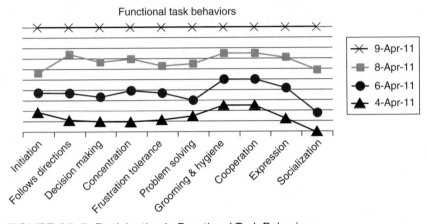

FIGURE 25-5. Participation in Functional Task Behaviors

Graph based on the OTTOS©

reduced the overall amount space used by a single provider in the medical record. Specialized forms or summary sheets are very useful for discussing evaluation results with patients, caretakers, and discharge providers.

Treatment Box. Constructing a **treatment box** can be a valuable on-the-go item to help accomplish a variety of needs. The treatment box that has been used in the sample military psychiatry setting has been a time-saver and method of generating interest in occupational therapy. For the treatment box to work however, occupational therapists must be skilled in the therapeutic use of self as described by Mosey (1996): "the use of oneself in such a way that one becomes an effective tool in the evaluation and intervention process" (p. 199). The following case study demonstrates "treatment buy-in" though cognitive reframing (Barrett & Rappaport, 2011) using a simple illustration of emotions (B. L. Porter, personal communication, November, 2010)

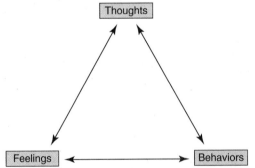

FIGURE 25-6. Pre-Group Checklist. Thoughts, Feelings, and Behaviors: Making Emotions Tangible

© Cengage Learning 2013

illustrated in Private R's initial meeting with his occupational therapist. Of note, although the U.S. military has a better understanding of acute stress since the wars in Iraq and Afghanistan and has taken measures to educate warriors, warriors' stigmas regarding mental health services continues to exist (Wright et al., 2009), therefore, treatment buy-in is occasionally needed.

CASE ILLUSTRATION

Evaluation of Private R.—Acute Stress Disorder

"Last week I was fighting a war and now I'm sitting here with a lady holding a box of crap?" Private R said as he sat stiffly with his muscular, tattooed, arms folded tightly. He shook his head from side-to-side, facial expressions in disbelief. "What happened?" he asked, "I can't really be here, I mean here in a mental ward, I'm not crazy!" The therapist placed her clear box on the table. It contained a variety of objects: a small, incomplete model car sat just below the clear lid. Several completed beaded key chains from the Allen Diagnostic Module (Earhart, 2006) were visible from the side. The Allen Cognitive Level (ACLS) Screen (Allen et al., 2006) was at one end, needles tucked away. At the other end was a small wooden medallion with outlined letters spelling "U.S. Army." The bottom contained papers including a scoring sheet and rating cards for the Canadian Occupational Performance Measure (Law et al. 2005), a Self-Directed Search assessment booklet (Holland, 1994), Toglia's (2010) weekly calendar planning activity, a summary describing the meaning of the ACLS scores, a pencil, and

two sheets of blank copy paper. "What could YOU do for me?" Private R said as he starred at the box. "You have no idea what I'm talking about, you're clueless." "You're right," the therapist said softly. "I really don't know what it was like, I haven't been there, but I know pain, I know anger and sadness, and I know outrage when something bad happens, it's not fair, and I know it's really hard when everything seems out-of-control."

Private R sat up and looked at the occupational therapist, still angry but with a softer facial expression. He watched quietly as the therapist opened the box and took out a pencil and blank sheet of paper. "Look," she said as she drew a triangle on the paper, "this is how we see it." At the top of the triangle she wrote the word "thoughts" In the bottom left corner she wrote "feelings," and then wrote "behaviors" in the bottom right. She said: "Right now it's difficult to separate these three things" as she drew arrows to show a connection among the three words. "Which word is the most difficult for you right now?" Private R pointed to "thoughts" and shook his head "No," "It's not right, just not right." Private R drifted off and seemed be somewhere else, a blank look in his eyes. "Private R, it's going to be OK," everything is going to be OK, just be here with us right now" said the therapist. "Private R, look at me," she continued. His eyes lost their glazed appearance as he slowly looked at the therapist. "I want you to come to my groups," she said. "You don't have to do anything, I just want you there." "You know, I'm really glad you're safe now even if you don't want to be here." She continued: "I'll look for you at 10:00, and don't laugh at me if I ask you to do something that looks really silly—I'm bringing out the arts and crafts today, I want you keep an open mind." Private R's mouth indicated the beginning of a smile as he rose up to leave.

A week before his first meeting with the occupational therapist, Private R had held a gun to his head. According to the medical record, he didn't say anything, just stood silently with the gun and was fortunately tackled to the ground safely. Two weeks earlier Private R's girlfriend sent him an email informing him that she was pregnant; the father was a high school friend of his. Three weeks before he held a gun to his head, Private R witnessed the death of his battle-buddy—the medical record described how he was covered with his friend's blood after an improvised explosive device (IED) detonated. The record also said he was very close to the blast and should be evaluated for possible TBI. Private R was 20 years old and had spent the past 13 months in a combat zone. He had no memory of holding the gun, a clear suicidal gesture. Private R was diagnosed with acute stress disorder (ASD) and rule-out diffuse axonal injury. He reported episodes of "feelings like things weren't real," a symptom of **dissociation** where the mind blocks out aspects of consciousness to avoid thinking about the traumatic event. Dissociation affects memory, sense of reality, and sense of identity or self (APA, 2000).

Private R's immediate, multidisciplinary treatment goal was to prevent his ASD from turning into PTSD. Short-term occupational therapy goals consisted of preparatory methods to build activity tolerance, with rapid progression to purposeful activity (AOTA, 2008). Private R was matched with the unit's sensory-motor and expressive group interventions—both available in the "Functional Task Behavior" group. Donated arts and crafts kits are very popular and requested frequently. Private R's short-term goals were:

- To strengthen ability to participate in a daily routine, Private R will attend at least 30 minutes of (2) 50-minute occupational therapy sessions within two days of hospitalization;
- Private R will select an activity with maximum of three, familiar, problem-solving steps and state his plan for organization, following directions, and concentration with moderate assist within (2) sessions.
- Private R will complete the "pre-group checklist" and identify personal task-related obstacles by occupational therapy session #3.

■ With moderate assist, Private R will be able to identify at least one task-related coping strategy that allowed him to continue working on activity by occupational therapy session #4.

Discussion

Private R met his short-term occupational therapy goals. The routine, structure, and predictability of treatment groups, especially the expressive group, combined with medications and the stability of the inpatient setting all contributed to his reduction in acute stress disorder symptoms. He remained on the unit for eight more days. Daily occupational therapy documentation showed patterns of difficulties with concentration, problem solving, and frustration tolerance if his activities contained more than three unfamiliar steps. He also continued to have difficulty understanding abstract concepts discussed in the occupational therapy life skills group that he attended. Private R was transferred to a traumatic brain evaluation program and pending medical discharge from the military.

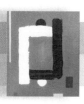

CASE ILLUSTRATION

Sergeant J

The trip from combat to inpatient psychiatry is likely to involve temporary changeovers or "stops" before arriving to the hospital. One wounded warrior described the four-day journey to get to the hospital because of unanticipated delays: "at each stop, coming to this place, I felt more like a loser . . . I'm flying around while they're still there [combat zone] without me . . . I need to get back to them." J is a 26-year-old male with six years of service in the U.S. Army Reserves. He was part of a tanker team patrolling Iraq early in the war at a time when infrastructures, including transportation routes were largely undeveloped. Part of Sergeant J's duties included radio communication every 15 seconds with tanks positioned forward and behind his own. Sergeant J's radio communication was momentarily interrupted when the lead sergeant needed to make an emergency announcement warning anticipating trouble ahead. Sergeant J missed one series of communications because of the announcement— about 30 seconds. He returned to the radio but was unable to reach the following tank. After several frantic attempts to reach the tank without getting a response, he knew something was very wrong. Tragedy had struck; the tank behind his hit a bank and overturned, trapping the warriors inside.

Sergeant J told the occupational therapist: "It was my fault . . . I was on the radio with my sergeant, he was saying we were about to be hit . . . I was out of communication . . . I didn't warn them . . . it's my fault." Sergeant J then buried his head in his hands as he described the sounds of yelling, banging, and knocking coming from the overturned tank as his crew did everything possible to rescue the people who were trapped. "We couldn't do anything, we were helpless, they were helpless, and then it just stopped," he whispered, "we didn't hear anything, and it was silent, just silent, just silent and dead." He told the occupational therapist: "Every time I close my eyes, I hear the knocking . . . I can't sleep . . . I don't deserve to sleep." It was a very tragic accident, and in reality, there was no way Sergeant J or anyone else could have predicted that the tank would overturn.

Sergeant J spotted the beaded key chains in the clear box brought by the occupational therapist and said that he had something similar in his personal belongings. The therapist helped retrieve the bracelet. It was macramé-styled and made from the 550 cord material commonly used in military missions. The bracelet was secured with a button from an army field uniform. "This was made on the back of a tank; we made these during downtime when we were bored," Sergeant J said as his eyes filled with tears.

Sergeant J agreed to complete an Allen Cognitive Level Screen and had a score of 5.0. The therapist provided a summary of results and discussed six areas of occupation most important to the role of warrior. A week later, he completed a keychain from the Allen Diagnostic Module and obtained a score of 5.4, and following discussion of his anxiety symptoms said he was ready for a scheduled field trip to a busy museum. Sergeant J had not been out in a nonmilitary community setting since arriving back in the United States.

Although the tank accident happened four months prior to arriving at the hospital, Sergeant J had ignored the changes in his daily routine such as difficulty sleeping more than two hours at a time, and intrusive, disturbing thoughts throughout the day which he said made him feel "like offing myself to get rid of them." He said he couldn't understand why the thoughts wouldn't go away despite telling himself to "get over it." It hadn't occurred to him to seek help because he believed "things happen" and "its part of the job." He added "I wasn't psycho or anything like that." The occupational therapist quietly listened. She intentionally avoided phases such as "You'll feel better after a good night's sleep," and let Sergeant J take the lead in the conversation, as he felt comfortable, at his own pace. She stated, "I am so sorry that happened; you must be exhausted after all that."

Sergeant J and his therapist discussed what he would like to accomplish while being in the hospital. He stated he wanted to "stop jumping at everything" (increased startle reflex)" and "just be comfortable being back here," as he had just spent 15 months in a combat zone. Although he said that he "not comfortable talking about himself in groups," he was encouraged to attend all meetings and groups sessions so that he could remain awake during the day, as one of his interdisciplinary team goals was to improve sleep hygiene. While discussing sleep/wake cycles and their affect on returning from a deployment, the occupational therapist described the 7:00 am yoga group she held daily. Specifically, she told him that many people gain a sense of control by regulating their feelings through breath and body movement by using a stress relief-type of beginning yoga, because learning how to recognize and control feelings is a cognitive-behavioral and a self-regulation approach that, according to research, "works."

Sergeant J attended morning yoga sessions without difficulty, but was initially isolative and sat alone with his back to the wall during expressive and life skills sessions held during the duty day. He was able to remain awake, but rarely talked to other patients or staff unless approached. Craft activities were scheduled for the third day of Sergeant J's expressive group. The occupational therapist placed several cut pieces of the 550 cord that were within the allowed length of the inpatient unit. She casually placed them next to a shoe box full of beads on her craft cart, but did not intentionally draw Sergeant KJ's attention to their presence. Fifteen minutes into the session, Sergeant J approached the therapist, pointed to the cords, and asked, "Who does that belong to?" "No one," said the therapist, "you can have it if you want." Sergeant J sat with his back to the wall, but by session's end, he independently, silently, completed a corded bracelet similar to the sample he shared two days earlier.

Following the expressive activity group, Sergeant J agreed to complete a Gecko key chain, part of the Allen Diagnostic Module: Bead-Kit II, and scored a 5.4. The therapist discussed an afternoon life skills group where specific coping skills are practiced in preparation for a field trip the patients took each week, along with the concept of exposure therapy, another evidence-based cognitive-behavioral approach. Sergeant J didn't say anything, but shook his head "yes," attended the life skills group, but did not actively participate. The next day, prior to the field trip, Sergeant J said he would like to attend the museum trip and stated, "I'm cool with it; I haven't been on United States soil outside of a military base since we landed." He was cleared for attendance by his psychiatrist along with 11 other patients, and during the brief safety and coping skills session prior to the trip, Sergeant J said he would use his "breathing" if needed.

The museum was unexpectedly crowded that day, Sergeant J stated he was "fine" before entering, but after 10 minutes he dropped to the ground and began "wave breathing" as learned in the morning yoga group. Within 30 seconds a security guard approached the group and another patient told the guard: "He's fine sir, just got back from Iraq, first time out," the guard nodded this head "OK," and remained with the group for the next three minutes, when Sergeant J got up from the floor and asked: "What's everyone looking at; isn't this what I'm supposed to do?"

Sergeant J continued to make slow but steady progress in his overall treatment. He was upset that his treatment team would "even consider a medical board." The next week he was transferred to an outpatient trauma program based on the recovery model. The last we heard Sergeant J was allowed to remain on active duty military service but with a restriction:

He was not allowed to be deployed into combat for one year.

Discussion

Sergeant J experienced slow but steady progress aided by an empathic therapeutic use of self, traditional individual occupational therapy interventions with craft activities, group intervention using expressive modalities and cognitive-behavioral stress reduction, and practice in the community.

Intervention for the Practitioner

Often when treating trauma, the treating therapists will experience similar, though less intense, symptoms of their clients. This experience is named as **compassion fatigue**. Caregiver's compassion fatigue is real and occupational therapists, with their focus on occupation and "doing" may have a tendency to ignore the symptoms. Compassion fatigue is an area of recent interest among persons working with military combat veterans—today's wounded warriors. Hayes (2009), in a study of compassion fatigue, identified seven areas of personal and professional functioning with potential to deteriorate when caregivers' experience compassion fatigue. Similar to the areas of occupation, caregivers can have some of the same difficulties as the people they treat. This is an area that is increasing being recognized and acknowledged within organizations that work with trauma survivors. One of the editors of this text experienced compassion fatigue before it was identified while working with women who were victims of severe physical and sexual abuse, including ritualized abuse, beginning at an early age and sustained for a length of time. Symptoms included intrusive thoughts and images of abuse, depressed mood, and increased vigilance, in addition to coming to grips with the recognition that evil may exist in the world. Alleviation of the symptoms occurs by acknowledging what is occurring, recognizing that it arises from working with trauma victims, and expressing oneself with others who experience the condition. For example, those occupational therapists working with the wounded warrior population on the inpatient psychiatric unit, developed a very successful informal lunch group where compassion fatigue is regularly and openly discussed.

SUMMARY

This chapter detailed the problems, evaluation, and treatment of service members (SMs) in the combat areas of operations and warriors at home in acute psychiatric units. Due to the wars in Afghanistan and Iraq, occupational therapists in the military are treating a variety of injuries, most prominently acute stress reactions, traumatic brain injuries (TBIs), and post-traumatic stress disorder (PTSD). They are on the cutting edge of treatment for responding to disasters, and injuries that have not heretofore been addressed (mild TBI and concussions), as well as responding at the scene of the injury rather than an evacuated area. Military occupational therapists use both traditional (craft, balance in daily living activities) and more recent treatment interventions (animal-assisted therapy), and the best examples of therapeutic use of self in carrying out their military mission. They treat what can only be considered mind and body, a true example of treating the whole person. Occupational therapists also identify a syndrome, compassion fatigue, which may affect all therapists who work with trauma survivors. Most likely as a result of the military occupational therapists new treatments and interventions will be identified and researched in the occupational therapy literature.

REVIEW QUESTIONS

1. A traumatic brain injury (TBI) is characterized as mild if the individual experiences a loss of consciousness for how many minutes? How long for post-traumatic amnesia?

2. A person with postconcussion syndrome will likely suffer from what symptoms that could affect day-to-day functional abilities?

3. Animal-assisted therapy (AAT) is a goal-directed intervention led by a health/human provider working within the scope of his/her practice. What are possible goals an occupational therapist in a COSC unit would use for AAT in a combat environment?

4. In a COSC unit, describe the difference between a restoration program and a prevention program. How would each program benefit from having an occupational therapist?

5. In many specialty treatment areas, occupational therapists obtain additional training or certifications in current, evidenced-based methods to enhance their use of occupation. In psychosocial practice, what are two of the current, evidence-based communication methods that add to the effectiveness of using occupation as therapy?

REFERENCES

Allen, C. K., Austin, S. L., David, S. K., Earhart, C. A., McCraith, D. B., & Riska-Williams, L. (2006). *Manual for the Allen cognitive level screen-5 (ACLS-5) and large Allen cognitive level screen-5 (LACLS-5)*. Camarillo, CA: ACLS & LACLS Committee.

Alves, W., Colohn, A., OLeary, T., Rimel, R., & Jane, J. (1986). Understanding posttraumatic symptoms after minor head injury. *Journal of Head Trauma Rehabilitation, 1,* 1–12.

American Occupational Therapy Association (AOTA). (2008). Occupational therapy practice framework: Domain and process (2nd ed.). *American Journal of Occupational Therapy, 62,* 625–683.

American Psychiatric Association (APA). (2000). *Diagnostic and statistical manual* (4th ed., text rev.). Washington, DC: Author.

Barrett, J. G., & Rappaport, N. (2011). Keeping it real: Overcoming resistance in adolescent males mandated into treatment. *Adolescent Psychiatry, 1,* 28–34. Retrieved from http://www.bentham science.com/aps/sample/aps1-1/7-Barrett_APS.pdf

Bryan, V. L. (2004). Management of residual physical deficits. In M. J. Ashley & D. K. Krych (Eds.), *Traumatic brain injury rehabilitative treatment and case management* (pp. 455–508). Boca Raton, FL: CRC Press.

Buckingham, D. W. (1999). *The warrior ethos.* Newport, RI: Naval War College. Retrieved from http://www.dtic.mil/cgi-bin/GetTRDoc?AD=ADA366676&Location=U2&doc=GetTRDoc.pdf

Calderon-Abbo, J., Kronenberg, M., Many, M., & Ososfsky, H. J. (2008). Fostering healthcare providers' post-traumatic growth in disaster areas: Proposed additional core competencies in trauma-impact management. *The American Journal of the Medical Sciences, 336*(2), 208–214.

Carlson, K., Kehle, S. M., Meis, L., Greer, N., MacDonald, R., Rutks, I., et al. (2009). The assessment and treatment of individuals with history of traumatic brain injury and post-traumatic stress disorder: A systematic review of the evidence. Evidence report/technology assessment prepared by the Minneapolis Veterans Affairs Medical Center, Minnesota Evidence Synthesis Program, Center for Chronic Disease Outcomes Research. Minneapolis: Minnesota. Retrieved from http://www.hsrd.research.va.gov/publications/esp/TBI-PTSD-2009.pdf

Carroll, L. J., Cassidy, J. D., Peloso, P. M., Borg, J., von Holst, H., Holm, L., et al. (2004). Prognosis for mild traumatic brain injury: Results of the WHO Collaborative Center Task Force on Mild Traumatic Brain Injury. *Journal of Rehabilitative Medicine, 43,* 84–105.

Cicerone, K. D., Dahlberg, C., Kalmar, K., Langenbahn, D. M., Malec, J. F., Bergquist, T. F., et al. (2000). Evidence-based cognitive rehabilitation: Recommendations for clinical practice. *Archives of Physical Medicine and Rehabilitation, 81,* 1596–1615.

Cicerone, K. D., Dahlberg, C., Malec, J. F., Langenbahn, D. M., Felicetti, T., Kneipp, et al. (2005). Evidence-based cognitive rehabilitation: Updated review of literature from 1998 through 2002. *Archives of Physical Medicine and Rehabilitation, 86,* 1681–1692.

Clark, F. (2011). High-definition occupational therapy's competitive edge: Personal excellence is the key. *American Journal of Occupational Therapy, 65*(6), 616–622. doi: 10.5014/ajot.2011.656001

Cohen, B. A., Inglese, M., Rusinek, H., Babb, J. S., Grossman, R. I., & Gonen, O. (2007). Proton MR spectroscopy and MRI-volumetry in mild traumatic brain injury. *American Journal of Neuroradiology, 28*(5), 907–913.

Deahl, M., Srinivasan, M., Jones, N., Thomas, J., Neblett, C., & Jolly, A. (2000). Preventing psychological trauma in service members: the role of operational stress training and psychological debriefing. *British Journal of Medical Psychology, 73*(Pt 1), 77–85.

Defense and Veterans Brain Injury Center (DVBIC) (2006). *DVBIC working group on the acute management of mild traumatic brain injury in military operational settings: Clinical practice guideline and recommendations.* Silver Springs, MD: Author.

The Delta Society (2009). *Animal-Assisted Activities/Therapy 101.* Retrieved from http://www.deltasociety.org/Page.aspx?pid=317.

DePalma, R. G., Burris, D. G., Champion, H. R., & Hodgson, M. J. (2005). Blast injuries. *The New England Journal of Medicine, 352,* 1335–1342.

Department of the Army. (2006). *Combat operational stress control; Field manual*, (No. 4-02.51 [FM 8–51]). Washington, DC: Author

Earhart, C. A. (2006*). Allen diagnostic modules: Manual* (2nd ed.). Colchester, CT: S & S Worldwide.

Edna, T. H., & Cappelen, J. (1987). Late postconcussional symptoms in traumatic head injury: An analysis of the frequency and risk factors. *Acta Neurochirurgica, 86*, 12–17.

Friends Committee on National Legislation. (2009). *If the US is ultimately leaving Iraq, why is The military building permanent bases?* Retrieved from http://www.fcnl.org/iraq/bases_text.htm

Galarneau, M. R., Woodruff, S. I., Dye, J. L., Mohrle, C. R., & Wade, A. L. (2008). Traumatic brain injury during Operation Iraqi Freedom: findings from the United States Navy-Marine Corps Combat Trauma Registry. *Journal of Neurosurgery, 108*, 950–957.

Gerardi, S. M., & Newton, S. M. (2004). The role of the occupational therapist in CSC (combat stress control) operations. *U.S. Army Medical Department Journal*, 20–27.

Gever, J., & Jasmer, R. (2008). *Posttraumatic stress often a sequel to Iraq war.* (Peer commentary on the article). Mild traumatic brain injury in U.S. military returning from Iraq by Hoge et al.). Retrieved from http://www.medpagetoday.com/Psychiatry/AnxietyStress/8152

Goodrich, G. L., Kirby, J., Cockerham, G., Ingalla, S. P., & Lew, H. L. (2007). Visual function in patients of a polytrauma rehabilitation center: A descriptive study. *Journal of Rehabilitation Research & Development, 44*, 929–936.

Gregg, S. C. (2006). *Developing warrior ethos: The making of a humble hero.* A Research Report Submitted to the Faculty In Partial Fulfillment of the Graduation Requirements. Maxwell Air Force Base, Alabama. Retrieved from https://www.afresearch.org/skins/rims/display.aspx?

Guskiewicz, K. M., Marshall, S. W., Bailes, J., McCrea, M., Cantu, R. C., Randolph, D., et al. (2005). Association between recurrent concussion and late-life cognitive impairment in retired professional football players. *Neurosurgery 5*, 719–726.

Gutman, S. A. (1995). Influence of the U.S. military and occupational therapy reconstruction Aides in World War I on the development of occupational therapy. *American Journal of Occupational Therapy, 49*(3), 256–262.

Hayes, M. J. (2009). *Compassion fatigue in the military caregiver.* Carlisle Barracks, PA: U.S. Army War College. Retrieved from http://www.dtic.mil/cgi-bin/GetTRDoc?Location=U2&doc

Helmick, K. M., Parkinson, G. W., Chandler, L. A., & Warden, D. L. (2007). Mild traumatic brain injury in wartime. *Federal Practitioner*, October, 58–65.

Hoffer, M. E., Gottshall, K. R., Moore R., Balough B. J., & Wester D. (2004). Characterizing and treating dizziness after mild head trauma. *Otology & Neurology, 25*, 135–138.

Hoge, C. W. (2010a). *Once a warrior always a warrior: Navigating the transition from combat to home including combat stress, PTSD, and mTBI.* Guilford, CT: GPP Life.

Hoge, C. W. (2010b). *PBS's 'This emotional life': Once a warrior always a warrior.* Retrieved from http://www.huffingtonpost.com/charles-hoge/post-traumatic-stress-dis_b_590583.html

Hoge, C. W., McGurk, D., Thomas, J. L., Cox, A. L., Engel, C. C., & Castro, C. A. (2008). Mild traumatic brain injury in U.S. military returning from Iraq. *New England Journal of Medicine, 358*, 453–463. Retrieved from http://www.nejm.org/doi/full/10.1056/NEJMoa072972

Holland, J. L. (1994). *The Self-directed search.* Odessa, FL: Psychological Assessment Resources.

Kay, T., Harrington, D.E., Adams, R., Anderson, T., Berrol, S., Cicerone, K., et al. (1993). Definition of mild traumatic brain injury. *Journal of Head Trauma Rehabilitation, 8*, 86–87.

Katz N., Itzkovich M., Averbuch S., Elazar B (1989). Loewenstein Occupational Therapy Cognitive Assessment (LOTCA) battery for brain-injured patients: reliability and validity. *American Journal of Occupational Therapy, 43*, 3, 184–92.

Kennedy, J. E., Jaffee, M. S., Leskin, G A., Stokes, J. W., Leal, F. O., & Fitzpatrick, P. J. (2007). Posttraumatic stress disorder and posttraumatic stress disorder-like symptoms and mild traumatic brain injury. *Journal of Rehabilitation Research & Development, 44*, 7. Accession Number: 205032975. Retrieved from http://www.biomedsearch.com/article/Posttraumatic-stress-disorder-posttraumatic-like/205032975.html

Kiernan R. J., Mueller, J., Langston, J. W., & Van Dyke, C. (1987). The Neurobehavioral Cognitive Status Examination: A brief but differentiated approach to cognitive assessment. *Annals of Internal Medicine, 107*, 481–485.

Lang, J., Thomas, J. L., Bliese, P. D., & Adler, A. B. (2007). Job Demands and Job Performance: The mediating effect of psychological and physical strain and the moderating effect of role clarity. *Journal of Occupational Health Psychology, 12*(2),116–124. doi: 10.1037/1076–8998.12.2.116

Law, M., Baptiste, S., Carswell, A., McColl, M. A., Polatajko, J., & Pollock, N. (2005). *Canadian occupational performance measure (COPM).*, Ontario: CAOT Publications ACE.

Lew, H. L., Thomander, D., Chew, K. T. L., & Bleiberg, J. (2007). Review of sports-related concussion: Potential for application in military settings. *Journal of Rehabilitation Research & Development, 44*, 963–974.

Margolis, R., Harrison, S. A., Robinson, H. J., & Jayaram, G. (1996). Occupational therapy task observation scale (OTTOS): A rapid method for rating task group function of psychiatric patients. *American Journal of Occupational Therapy, 50*(5), 380–385.

Massachusetts Institute of Technology. (2011). *Young adult development project.* Retrieved from http://hrweb.mit.edu/worklife/youngadult/index.html

McCrea, M. A. (2008). *Mild traumatic brain injury and post concussion syndrome.* New York: Oxford University Press.

McCrea, M., Guskiewicz, K. M., Marshall, S. W., Barr, W., Randolph, C., Cantu, R. C., et al. (2003). Acute effects and recovery time following concussion in collegiate football players, *Journal of the American Medical Association, 290*, 2556–2563.

McCrory, P., Johnston, K., Meeuwisse, W., Aubry, M., Cantu, R., Dvorak, J., et al. (2005). Summary and agreement statement of the 2nd International Conference on Concussion in sport. *British Journal of Sports Medicine, 39*, 196–204.

McCulloch, K., Buxton, E., Hackney, J., & Lowers, S. (2010). Balance, attention and dual-task performance during walking after brain injury: Associations with falls history. *Journal of Head Trauma Rehabilitation, 25*, 155–163.

Mittenberg, W., & Strauman, S. (2000). Diagnosis of mild head injury and the postconcussion syndrome. *Journal of Head Trauma Rehabilitation, 15*, 783–791.

Mittenberg, W., Tremont, G., Zielinski, R. E., Fichera, S., & Rayls, K. R. (1996). Cognitive-behavioral prevention of post-concussion syndrome. *Archives of Clinical Neuropsychology, 11*, 139–145.

Montgomery, G. K. (1995). A multi-factor account of disability after brain injury: Implications for neuropsychological counseling. *Brain Injury, 9*, 453–469.

Moore, B. A., & Reger, G. M. (2007). Historical and contemporary perspectives of combat stress and the army combat stress control team. In C. R. Figley & W. P. Nash (Eds.), *Combat stress injury: Theory, research, and management* (pp. 161–181). New York: Routledge.

Mosey, A. (1996). *Psychosocial components of occupational therapy.* Lippincott Williams & Wilkins.

Oakley, F., Caswell, S., & Parks, R. (2008). The Issue Is — Occupational therapists' role on U.S. Army and U.S. Public Health Service Commissioned Corps Disaster Mental Health Response Teams. *American Journal of Occupational Therapy, 62*, 361–364.

Polusny, M. A., Kehle, S. M., Nelson, N. W., Erbes, C. R., Arbisi, P. A., & Thuras, P. (2011). Longitudinal effects of mild traumatic brain injury and posttraumatic stress disorder comorbidity on postdeployment outcomes in National Guard soldiers deployed to Iraq. *Archives of General Psychiatry, 68*, 79–89.

Ponsford, J. (2005). Rehabilitation interventions after mild head injury. *Current Opinion in Neurology,* *18,* 692–697.

Ponsford, J., Willmott, C., Rothwell, A., Cameron, P., Kelly, A. M., Nelms, R., et al. (2000). Factors influencing outcome following mild traumatic brain injury in adults. *Journal of the International Neuropsychological Society, 6,* 568–579.

Radomski, M. V., Davidson, L., Voydetich, D., & Erickson, M. W. (2009). Occupational therapy for service members with mild traumatic brain injury. *American Journal of Occupational Therapy, 64,* 646–655.

Robertson, I. H., Ward, T., Ridgeway, V., & Nimmo-Smith, I. (1996). The structure of normal human attention: The Test of Everyday Attention. *Journal of the International Neuropsychological Society, 2,* 525–534.

Ruff, R. (2005). Two decades of advances in understanding of mild traumatic brain injury. *The Journal of Head Trauma Rehabilitation, 20,* 5–18.

Ruff, R., Camenzuli, L., & Mueller, J. (1996). Miserable minority: Emotional factors that influence the outcome of mild traumatic brain injury. *Brain Injury, 10,* 551–565.

Ruff, R. L., Riechers, R. G., & Ruff, S. S. (2010). Relationships between mild traumatic brain injury sustained in combat and post-traumatic stress disorder. *F1000 Medical Reports, 2,* 64. Retrieved from doi: 10.3410/M2-64)

Sareen, J., Cox, B. J., Afifi, T. O., Stein, M. B., Belik, S. L., Meadows, G., et al. (2007). Combat and peace-keeping operations in relation to prevalence of mental disorders and perceived need for mental health care: Findings from a large representative sample of military personnel. *Archives of General Psychiatry, 64,* 843–852.

Scaffa, M., Gerardi, S., Herzberg, G., & McColl, M. (2006). The role of occupational therapy in disaster preparedness, response, and recovery. *American Journal of Occupational Therapy, 60,* 642–649.

Scheiman, M., Scheiman, M., & Whittaker, S. G. (2006). *Low vision rehabilitation: A practical guide for occupational therapists.* Thorofare, NJ: Slack.

Stålnacke, B. M. (2007). Community integration, social support and life satisfaction in relation to symptoms three years after mild traumatic brain injury. *Brain Injury, 21*(9), 933–942.

Steadman-Pare, D., Colantonio, A., Ratcliff, G., Chase, S., & Vernich, L. (2001). Factors associated with perceived quality of life many years after traumatic brain injury. *The Journal of Head Trauma Rehabilitation, 16*(4), 330–342.

Teasdale, G., & Jennett, B. (1974). Assessment of coma and impaired consciousness: A practical scale. *Lancet, 2,* 81–84.

Terrio, H., Brenner, L A., Ivins, B. J., Cho, J. M., Helmick, K., Schwab, K., Scally, K., Bretthauer, R., & Warden, D. (2009). Traumatic Brain Injury Screening: Preliminary findings in a US Army Brigade Combat Team. *Journal of Head Trauma Rehabilitation, 24*(1), 14–23. doi.: 10.1097/HTR.0b013e31819581d8

Toglia, J. P. (1993). *The contextual memory test.* Tucson: Therapy Skill Builders.

Toglia, J. (2010). *Weekly calendar planning activity.* Unpublished manuscript, Graduate Occupational Therapy Program, Mercy College, Dobbs Ferry, N.Y.

Trombly, C. A., Radomski, M. V., & Davis, E. S. (1998). Achievement of self-identified goals by adults with traumatic brain injury: Phase I. *American Journal of Occupational Therapy, 52,* 810–818.

Trombly, C. A., Radomski, M. V., Trexel, C., & Burnett-Smith, S. E. (2002). Achievement of self-identified goals by adults with traumatic brain injury: Phase II. *American Journal of Occupational Therapy, 56,* 489–498.

U.S. Department of Veterans Affairs, U.S. Department of Defense. (2001). VA/DOD Clinical practice guideline for management medically unexplained symptoms: Chronic pain and fatigue. Retrieved from http://www.healthquality.va.gov/mus/mus_fulltext.pdf

U.S. Department of Veterans Affairs, U.S. Department of Defense. (2008). VA/DOD Clinical practice guideline for management of major depressive disorder (MDD). http://www.healthquality.va.gov/MDD_FULL_3c.pdf

U.S. Department of Veterans Affairs, U.S. Department of Defense. (2009a). VA/DOD Clinical practice guideline for management of bipolar disorder in adults. Retrieved from http://www.healthquality.va.gov/bipolar/bd_305_full.pdf

U.S. Department of Veterans Affairs, U.S. Department of Defense. (2009b). VA/DOD Clinical practice guideline for management of concussion/mild traumatic brain injury. Retrieved from http://www.healthquality.va.gov/management_of_concussion_mtbi.asp

U.S. Department of Veterans Affairs, U.S. Department of Defense. (2010a). VA/DOD Clinical practice guideline for management of opioid therapy for chronic pain. Retrieved from http://www.healthquality.va.gov/COT_312_Full-er.pdf

U.S. Department of Veterans Affairs, U.S. Department of Defense. (2010b). VA/DOD Clinical practice guideline for management of post-traumatic stress: Update 2010. Retrieved from http://www.healthquality.va.gov/PTSD-FULL-2010c.pdf

Warden, D. (2006). Military TBI During the Iraq and Afghanistan Wars. *Journal of Head Trauma Rehabilitation, 21,5*, 398–402.

Wilson, B. A., Cockburn, J., & Baddeley, A. (1985). *The Rivermead Behavioral Memory Test*. Reading, UK: Thames Valley Test. Gaylord, MI: National Rehabilitation Services.

Wilson, B. A., Cockburn, J., Baddeley, A., & Hiorns, R. (1989). The development and validation of a test battery for detecting and monitoring everyday memory problems. *Journal of Clinical and Experimental Neuropsychology, 11*, 855–870.

Wilson, B. A., Evans, J. J., Alderman, N., Burgess, P. W., Emslie, H. (1997). Behavioural assessment of the dysexecutive function. In P. Rabbitt (Ed.) *Methodology of frontal and executive function*, pp. 232–243, Taylor and Francis e-Library, 2005. Accessed at www.eBookstore.tandf.co.uk

Wilson, B. A., Evans, J. J., Emslie, H., & Alderman, N. (1998). The development of an ecologically valid test for assessing patients with a dysexecutive syndrome. *Neuropsychological Rehabilitation, 8*, 213–228.

Wright, K. M., Cabera, O. A., Bliese, P. D., Adler, A. B., Hoge, C. W., & Castro, C. A. (2009). Stigma and barriers to care in soldiers postcombat. *Psychological Services, 6*, 108–116. Retrieved from doi: 10.1037/a0012620

Zatzick, D. F., Rivara, F. P., Jorkovich, M.D., Hoge, C. W., Wang, J., Fan, M. Y., et al. (2010). Multisite investigation of traumatic brain injuries, posttraumatic stress disorder, and self-reported health and cognitive impairments. *Archives of General Psychiatry, 67*, 1291–1300. Retrieved from DOI: 10.1001/archgenpsychiatry.2010.158

SUGGESTED RESOURCES

Books and Publications

Scifers, J. R. (2008). *Special tests for neurologic examination*. Thorofare, NJ: Slack.

Websites

America's Vet Dogs: http://www.vetdogs.org

The Defense and Veterans Brain Injury Center: http://www.dvbic.org/

The Defense Centers of Excellence for Psychological Health: http://www.dcoe.health.mil/

The Defense and Veterans Brain Injury Center Public Service Announcement: http://www.dcoe.health.mil/Content/MediaRoom/Media/74.wmv

Brainline: http://www.brainline.org/

Motivational Interviewing: http://www.motivationalinterview.org

VA/DOD Clinical Practice Guideline–Bi-Polar Disorder in Adults: http://www.healthquality.va.gov/bipolar/bd_305_full.pdf

VA/DOD Clinical Practice Guidelines–Concussion/Mild traumatic brain injury: http://www.healthquality.va.gov/management_of_concussion_mtbi.asp

VA/DOD Clinical Practice Guideline–Major Depressive Disorder: http://www.healthquality.va.gov/MDD_FULL_3c.pdf

VA/DOD Clinical Practice Guideline–Post-Traumatic Stress, Update 2010: http://www.healthquality.va.gov/PTSD-FULL-2010c.pdf

VA/DOD Clinical Practice Guideline–Management of Medically Unexplained Symptoms: Chronic Pain and Fatigue: http://www.healthquality.va.gov/mus/mus_fulltext.pdf

VA/DOD Clinical Practice Guideline–Management of Opioid Therapy for Chronic Pain: http://www.healthquality.va.gov/COT_312_Full-er.pdf

VA/DOD Clinical Practice Guideline–Management of Post Traumatic Stress: http://www.healthquality.va.gov/PTSD-FULL-2010c.pdf

Yoga and Stress Relief–Good DVD for many physical and psychological issues: http://www.bodywisdommedia.com

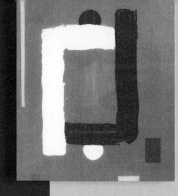

Chapter 26

Fieldwork Supervision in the Mental Health Setting

Patricia Crist, PhD, OTR, PC, FAOTA
Elizabeth Cara, PhD, OTR/L, MFT

KEY TERMS

clinical reasoning
coaching
eclectic
fieldwork education
intrapersonal

reflection
relationship
supervision
transformative learning

CHAPTER OUTLINE

Introduction
Role of the Fieldwork Educator or Supervisor in Mental Health
Transformative Learning
Dimensions of Fieldwork Education and Supervision
    The Supervisor and the Supervisor–Supervisee Relationship
    Supervisee Responsibilities
Clinical Reasoning and Reflection
Theoretical Foundations of Supervision
    Psychoanalytic or Psychodynamic Supervision
    Humanistic or Person-Centered Supervision
    Cognitive-Behavioral Supervision
    Developmental Approaches to Supervision
Practical Models and Methods of Supervision
    Occupational Therapy Supervision from a Developmental/Cognitive Perspective
    Counseling Psychology Model
Situational Supervision[1]

---

[1]This section of the chapter was published, in part, in *OT Advance* (Crist, 2007a, 2007b, 2007c, 2007d).

Coaching During Supervision[2]
    Fieldwork Instruction, Supervision, or Coaching
Maximizing Learning—Benefiting from Supervision
Trends and Recommendations
Summary

INTRODUCTION

This chapter focuses on the fieldwork experience and primarily the process of **supervision** during fieldwork as the interpersonal communication between fieldwork educator and student can be viewed from psychosocial and behavioral aspects. Because it emphasizes the fieldwork experience, a discussion of how to supervise other employees in the mental health setting is not included. However, since the chapter delineates useful models and practical approaches, the information should also be useful for general supervision and, especially, any fieldwork setting that addresses mental health, behavioral health, and/or psychosocial factors influencing the engagement. Effective fieldwork supervision is a multifaceted process adapted to specific supervisory situations and fieldwork contexts. This chapter provides a variety of interpersonal approaches to supervision. The reader is encouraged to study more broadly elsewhere to fully understand fieldwork education.

Mandated through the educational standards, all fieldwork settings are to reflect psychosocial approaches integrated into the development of client-centered, meaningful, occupation-based outcomes (American Council for Occupational Therapy Education, 2006a, 2006b). Thus, this chapter provides a guide to supervision in mental health settings but also approaches to supervision addressing general psychosocial practice evident in practice.

Figure 26-1 shows testimony by two fieldwork students, Tianna and Marisa (see Figure 26-2), who completed fieldwork in a mental health setting and supports the importance of effective supervision in facilitating their learning and professional development as practitioners.

While one can see the positive benefit from completing fieldwork in a mental health setting, the influence of this experience on their perceived competence to more fully address "whole person" needs is evident as well as the importance of integrating psychosocial approaches into practice

The purpose of **fieldwork education** is for students to acquire entry-level practice competencies in applying the occupational therapy process using evidence-based interventions to meet the occupational needs of diverse populations (American Occupational Therapy Association [AOTA], 2009a, p. 393). The student engages in a series of fieldwork education experiences that are designed to be developmental in nature by providing the opportunity to integrate academic knowledge with applied skills at progressively higher levels of performance and responsibility (Privott, 1998b). Typically, this

---

[2]This section of the chapter was published, in part, in *OT Advance* (Crist, 2010a, 2010b).

During the summer of 2009 we had the extraordinary experience of participating in a mental health internship in rural Trinity County, California. During this time we worked closely with Trinity County Behavioral Health and Alcohol and Other Drugs staff to introduce and provide education about the value of occupational therapy (OT) in mental health practice. We worked in a variety of settings within the county including a senior center, 2 clubhouses, and juvenile hall, in addition to our 1:1 sessions with behavioral health clients. We researched and identified types of groups that would be successful and beneficial within a rural county, such as arts and crafts, job skills, and health and wellness groups. We developed outlines for the groups, led these groups, and taught clients how to lead groups, thus allowing them to be sustained after our internship was completed. We assisted case managers in learning to use the Canadian Occupational Performance Measure (COPM) to establish more client-centered care plans and provided suggestions for home program development for clients. We had the opportunity to participate in staff meetings and advocate for our clients from an OT perspective.

At the end of the internship, we were able to present to the staff a binder full of occupational therapy resources including group outlines, handouts, and journal articles supporting occupational therapy practice in mental health. This internship allowed us to see the unique mindset and skills occupational therapy brings to a mental health setting with a focus on recovery; we developed an occupational profile on each person on our caseload incorporating their wants, needs, and expectations into client-centered goals that would maximize their functional independence. With this information we were able to grade groups to encourage contributions from all individuals who wished to participate. As occupational therapy interns we emphasized the importance of adding an activity component to groups in order to incorporate multiple ways of learning for our clients.

While our internship required self-initiative, we could not have done it without amazing guidance from our supervisor. Our supervision took place in the form of meetings, consultations, and receiving recommendations about whom to communicate with in order to implement our ideas. It required honest, open communication with our supervisor about our strengths and weaknesses as occupational therapy interns and the steps we needed to take in order to improve. We were provided with mentorship and invaluable learning opportunities regarding program development, collaborating with different professionals, and articulating the values and beliefs of OT to a variety of populations.

Whether or not someone eventually practices in a mental health setting, an internship in this field paves the way for a strong psychosocial core in any area of practice. As a result of our internship, even when working in physical disabilities, we recognize the need to constantly assess areas such as coping strategies, leisure pursuits, social participation, self-esteem, sleep hygiene, and self regulation, to name a few. Our internship was an incredible learning experience, which solidified the need to incorporate the authentic core values of occupational therapy into our treatments. With the tendency within hospitals and skilled nursing settings to conform to the medical model, a mental health internship has provided the opportunity to develop the skills to truly see a person as a "whole" and implement treatments that support our client's physical and psychosocial needs. This experience has made us the occupational therapy practitioners we are today: empathetic, passionate, and hopeful with the clients with whom we work.

FIGURE 26-1. Testimony from Fieldwork Students

Source: Courtesy of Tianna L. Russell and Marisa Moore

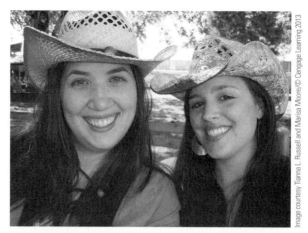

FIGURE 26-2. Tianna and Marisa During Their Fieldwork

development means that over a given fieldwork experience, the student is expected to move from direct, one-on-one supervision to less direct dependent on the competency of the student, the severity and safety demands of the clients, and the requirements for supervision in the setting. With the goal of entry-level education being preparation as a generalist practitioner, fieldwork education is organized to provide a broad exposure to the practice models and contexts where occupational therapy is practiced or emerging (American Council for Occupational Therapy Education, 2006a, 2006b). The occupational therapy or occupational therapy assistant student is able to test firsthand what was learned in school and to refine skills while interacting with clients and staff under the "supervision of qualified personnel." In Level II fieldwork, the qualified personnel must be an occupational therapy practitioner with at least one year of experience after initial certification and who meets all regulations governing practice. The occupational therapist must supervise the student a minimum of 8 hours per week if the student's day-to-day supervisor is not an occupational therapy practitioner. The person responsible for the day-to-day training is considered a fieldwork educator (also known as a clinical educator, fieldwork supervisor, or student supervisor). In this chapter the terms are used interchangeably. All designate the person responsible for the day-to-day supervision of the student (as opposed to the person who may be the on-site fieldwork coordinator and has primarily administrative duties). On campus, the individual who oversees the fieldwork education processes for the academic program is designated the academic fieldwork coordinator (American Council for Occupational Therapy Education, 2006a, 2006b).

ROLE OF THE FIELDWORK EDUCATOR OR SUPERVISOR IN MENTAL HEALTH

Regardless of setting, the fieldwork supervisor has multiple roles:

- Maintaining a contract with the academic setting and communicating with the academic fieldwork supervisor

- Facilitating the development of clinical competence through skill and knowledge development, particularly the clinical reasoning process
- Facilitating professional growth in attitude and performance in the supervisee
- Shepherding the supervisee through a training process that includes standards, expectations, and evaluation
- Introducing the supervisee to the people and culture of the department and the overall setting
- Being a role model of a professional and clinically competent occupational therapist
- Being alert to the differences and conflicts that may arise in the supervisory relationship

Perhaps, the most important emphasis in occupational therapy is on the supervisor's role of *educator* in the fieldwork setting. Accordingly, the role and approach of the supervisor educator dictate the important task of teaching clinical reasoning, discussed in the next section, along with the roles of manager, teacher, mentor, guide, and coach. The last role is important specifically in a mental health setting, where therapists emphasize being sensitive to the nuances of interpersonal relationships and often urge clients to be aware of emotions that may arise. In this edition, coaching is added to this chapter as the AOTA's *Blueprint for Entry-level Education* (AOTA, 2010a) delineates **coaching** as a skill at the person-centered factor level to provide psychological support in mental health and other areas of practice. Coaching, as an emerging practice skill, addresses concepts integral to the supervisory relationship such as fieldwork student motivation, self-efficacy, self-esteem, empowerment, and coping.

This chapter cannot prepare the practitioner for all aspects of being a fieldwork educator as the topic is broad and complex. However, in alignment with this publication, this chapter will focus on two areas: first, relevant fieldwork education supervisory approaches for supervisor–supervisee interaction with specific attention to frameworks applicable to psychosocial practice and, second, behavioral or mental health contexts or interpersonal communication including psychoanalytic, humanistic, behavioral, and developmental supervisory approaches.

Overarching this chapter will be the **transformative learning** approach that advocates for reflective practices to encourage students to go beyond a mere accumulation of facts and skills during fieldwork. Transformative learning blended with specific approaches to supervision provide a context for "best practices" during fieldwork supervision (AOTA, 2009c; Rose & Best, 2005). Counseling psychology's developmental stages, a cognitive development, and a situational leadership model each will be presented as options for building the supervisor–supervisee relationship. Knowing the counseling psychology developmental stages may enable the supervisor to better understand and to validate the student's emotions and behavior as they relate to the stages and critical issues. The supervisor and student can both learn and anticipate the ebb and flow of the fieldwork experience. Knowing the cognitive developmental model may enable the supervisor to design specific interventions and to use specific language in the supervision process. Student familiarity with the cognitive developmental stages can promote reflection on current and other options for responding to fieldwork challenges. Knowing situational leadership will provide a model to select a supervisory approach that matches the student's motivation and competence to learn and/or engage in specific fieldwork activities to facilitate learning. Knowing the various dimensions of supervision that have been researched in other literature will enable fieldwork educators to expand their repertoire of skills, understand students' needs and behaviors, and tailor the supervisory relationship and expectations to each individual student. *Students will find this information useful for self-reflection to improve their current interpersonal communication with supervisors and clients.*[3]

Tapping into academic programs in occupational therapy and the American Occupational Therapy Association, the reader will find many resources that address the transition to the fieldwork educator role as well as aspects of program administration, educational approaches, and student evaluation processes, all critical aspects of fieldwork education delivery but beyond the scope of this chapter. As noted earlier, this chapter limits its focus to supervision and primarily discusses the supervisor–supervisee relationship.

The American Occupational Therapy Association defines supervision as:

> a cooperative process in which two or more people participate in a joint effort to establish, maintain, and/or elevate a level of competence and performance. Within the scope of occupational therapy practice, supervision is aimed at ensuring the safe and effective delivery of occupational therapy services and fostering professional competence and development. (AOTA, 2005, p. 1)

Competence is the ability of the fieldwork student as a supervisee to perform the job responsibilities effectively. Supervision fosters growth and development; assures appropriate utilization of training and potential; encourages creativity and innovation; and provides guidance, support, encouragement, and respect while working toward a goal (AOTA, 1994, p. 1045).

This chapter will discuss, for those new to the role, the supervisory tools needed to assume the role of fieldwork educator and ways in which the process can be made smoother for individuals in both the educator and student supervisee positions. In an attempt to offer a comprehensive view of student supervision, different models that address particular aspects of the supervision process in occupational therapy and other fields will be presented. Hopefully, supervisors and supervisees can adapt this broad view for their specific experience and mental health setting.

In 2006, the American Occupational Therapy Association declared a vision to be achieved by the profession's 100th anniversary in 2017. This statement affirms that:

> We envision that occupational therapy is a powerful, widely recognized, science-driven, and evidence-based profession with a globally connected and diverse workforce meeting society's occupational needs. (AOTA, 2007)

---

[3]All italicized material in this chapter is material that is specifically directed to fieldwork students.

This vision represents our long-standing public commitment to service excellence. This road to excellence is paved in general, through quality supervision during fieldwork education, and, specifically, through fieldwork focusing on psychosocial and/or mental health aspects, as noted in AOTA's *Specialized Knowledge and Skills of Occupational Therapy Educators of the Future* (AOTA, 2009b). In this document, the attributes of five roles are advocated for all future occupational therapy practitioners who serve as educators, including fieldwork educators, to support the achievement of the *2017 Centennial Vision* (AOTA, 2007). For professional development purposes, the document provides a useful guide for each of the five attributes for the practitioner to aspire to demonstrate at the novice, intermediate, and advanced levels. For this chapter, it is useful to consider each of the five and then extrapolate the implications for supervision for this chapter as discussed in Table 26-1.

Fieldwork students are called to observe how one's supervisor puts these into action as well as consider foundational skills to develop now for later expansion. For instance, review your portfolio with your fieldwork educator regarding your career aspirations including documenting current fieldwork activities.

TRANSFORMATIVE LEARNING

Transformative learning is a contemporary approach to adult learners that has been strongly advocated as a viable approach to learning during fieldwork (AOTA, 2009c; Mezirow, 2000; Rose & Best, 2005). Transformative learning process encourages students to go beyond mere accumulation of factual knowledge to actual self-authorship of application by both the fieldwork educator and student. At the beginning of this chapter, Tianna and Marisa provided an excellent example of transformative learning. Examples related to mental health fieldwork and psychosocial practice are included in Table 26-2.

Supervisors should facilitate students to engage in this self-examination process when fieldwork problems arise and encourage students to change their perspective on a practice issue. Later in this chapter, situational leadership and coaching will be presented as approaches to supervision; both of these are student-centered, collaborative approaches lending themselves to encourage transformational learning in both the fieldwork educator and student as they engage the transformational learning process.

Further, all mental health-related supervision should target the profession's expectations specific to the specialized knowledge and skills for entry-level occupational therapy practice in the promotion of mental health and the prevention and intervention of mental health problems, including mental illness stated in the AOTA statement *Specialized Knowledge and Skills in Mental Health Promotion, Prevention, and Intervention in Occupational Therapy Practice* (AOTA, 2010b).

In occupational therapy as well as other professions, supervision is a valuable aspect for fieldwork education and professional development. The fieldwork experience is also important because it may influence graduates' selection of the field in

TABLE 26-1. Specialized Knowledge and Skills for OT Educators and Their Implications for Fieldwork Education

Specialized Knowledge and Skills for OT Educators of the Future (AOTA, 2009b)	Relationship to Supervision as a Fieldwork Educator
Innovator/Visionary: Someone who embraces new directions is forward-thinking, projecting into the future. This person thinks outside of the traditional confines of the profession to predict and propose how to meet future societal needs. A visionary can see past traditional boundaries to new possibilities at all levels of personal and societal life.	Expose students to emerging areas of practice in their context. Encourage student to envision innovative contexts and approaches to practice. Create a collaborative transformative fieldwork environment.[1]
Scholar/Explorer: A scholar/explorer is someone who seeks, uses, and produces knowledge and effectively disseminates new findings to internal and external audiences. These individuals use a critical, theoretically grounded, and systematic approach in their scholarly endeavors to produce outcomes that inform and address societal needs.	Model the integration of evidence into everyday practice decisions. Provide ongoing practice-scholar[2] activities to demonstrate site-specific practice outcomes.
Leader: Someone who analyzes past, present, and future trends and develops solutions to problems or strategies for taking advantage of opportunities by collaborating, inspiring, and influencing people to create a desired future.	Provide supervision that matches the student's readiness for practice competence. Discuss opportunities for servant leadership and emerging application of the profession's values and philosophy. Ensures student's alliance with the unique philosophy of practice in occupational therapy as a contributing participant in the health care system.
Integrator: Someone who seeks and finds divergent information, perceives meaningful relationships, and makes connections through analysis to create a new, more coherent understanding.	Modify supervision to serve the profession and its vision through partnership building. Facilitate a collaborative, resourceful, adult-learning model between supervisor and student.
Mentor: A trusted role model who inspires, encourages, influences, challenges, and facilitates the growth and development of others' goals and aspirations. This involves a collaborative process that may be between peers, colleagues, experienced and inexperienced individuals, practitioners and academicians, and others. The mentor may function in various roles such as educator, tutor, coach, counselor, encourager, consultant, etc.	Encourage students to acquire portfolio evidence and establish, if not extend, their professional network for entry-level practice and beyond.

[1] AOTA (2009c)
[2] Crist, Muñoz, Hansen, Benson, & Provident (2005)

© Cengage Learning 2013

which they are going to practice as well as where one is first employed (Andersen & Simhoni, 2002; Christie, Joyce, & Moeller, 1985). In most health professions, supervision is mandated and is recognized as a learning situation. A good **relationship** between the supervisor and supervisee is valued or, indeed essential, and the emphasis is on the role, rather than the techniques, of the supervisor (Christie et al., 1985; Gillfillan, 2001; Loganbill, Hardy, & Delworth, 1982; Noelle, 2003). Despite these

TABLE 26-2. Mental Health Fieldwork and Psychosocial Examples of Transformative Learning

Transformative Learning Processes	Mental Health Fieldwork Examples	Psychosocial Practice Examples
Gathering understanding of the context for practice.	Delineate the differences between occupational therapy in hospital-based versus community-based mental health settings.	Contrast the roles of occupational therapy, social work, and psychology in addressing psychological distress in the skilled nursing facility.
Critically reflecting on the current demands.	Create options for mental health occupational therapy in emerging settings for underserved populations, such as AIDS, autism, eating disorders, etc.	Provide intervention options for depression that may accompany response to recent physical trauma or illness diagnosis.
Evaluating existing beliefs and associated emotional reactions.	Explore your reactions to the lack of service funding for mental health from public and professional perspectives.	What degree of response to psychosocial concerns does an occupational therapy practitioner have in physical disability?
Exploring alternative assumptions that are present.	Applying personal and public perspectives: Are Asperger's, alcoholism, and substance abuse better served classified as a mental or physical health problem?	How does anxiety regarding a repeat heart attack or stroke contribute to motivation when trying to re-engage activity in a client?
Transforming an existing frame of reference into a new perspective including related performance habits and attitudes that are a better fit than prior ways to act, perform, or demonstrate practice competence.	Consider the advantages and challenges of changing the occupational performance intervention process in mental health from medical to empowerment paradigms.	Expand services for individuals dealing with the late effect functional limitations resulting from cancer interventions that occurred 10–15 years ago.

© Cengage Learning 2013

common assumptions, until recently, little formal training has been given prior to promoting someone to the role of fieldwork supervisor, and yet, it was expected that:

- Fieldwork education will be a somewhat smooth process.
- The supervisor will successfully guide the process.
- The supervisee will successfully become a competent occupational therapist.
- Quality occupational therapy will be promoted.
- Professional development of the involved individuals will be enhanced.

The student is expected to be motivated to learn and achieve entry-level competence in the setting. Prior to fieldwork, a student should review their mental health preparation (knowledge and skills) and during their orientation period, identify knowledge and skills bringing to the fieldwork placement along with a list of their goals for the fieldwork that reflects both translating classroom learning into practice but also how mental health can support their future practice. For instance, working with families is central to school-based practice. Noting that competence in working with family dynamics is important, what is available for student learning related to the psychosocial factors working with family systems?

Now with the voluntary certificate program for fieldwork educators (FWECP) a mechanism is in place to develop the knowledge and skills requisite to being an effective fieldwork educator (AOTA, 2009c). In fact, the topic of supervision is one of four major content modules in the AOTA certificate program process including also: administration, education, and evaluation. Certainly, other professions and private continuing education firms recognize that adequate preparation of competent, ethical, clinical supervisors for mental health or behavioral health is essential and provide workshops. While targeted to mental health students, they do not reflect the specific educational or professional needs of OT students nor contemporary processes or standards accepted and promoted within the profession.

Regardless of professional development approach to become a fieldwork supervisor, the intent must always be to become aware of one's personal style of supervision and be able to adapt supervision in response to observed student performance. To be an excellent practitioner is not sufficient in fieldwork education; one must embrace the educator role foremost to be an effective fieldwork supervisor and pursue relevant professional development activities (Crist, 2000).

DIMENSIONS OF FIELDWORK EDUCATION AND SUPERVISION

Supervision is an aspect of education or training that includes four elements: the supervisor, the supervisee, the relationship, and the context or environment (Frum & Opacich, 1987; Loganbill et al., 1982). Within the mental health arena specifically, supervision is "an intensive, interpersonal focused, one-to-one relationship in which one person is designated to facilitate the development of therapeutic competence in the other person . . . [It is] a master apprentice approach" (Loganbill et al., 1982, p. 4). Thus, approaches to supervision are as important to mental health fieldwork as understanding sensory processing in pediatrics or motor learning is in physical disabilities.

The Supervisor and the Supervisor–Supervisee Relationship

The supervisor assumes responsibility for the supervisee's client caseload and is responsible not only for the supervised person's development into a professional in clinical practice, but also for the outcome of client interventions. Bradley and Gould (2001) have suggested that the primary role of the supervisor is to teach the student and therefore, the primary commitment should be to the student while monitoring the client's welfare. Therefore, the supervisor assumes multiple roles (Munroe, 1988), serving as a coach, model, guide, teacher, organizer, and clinician all in one. The personality, roles, styles, and skills of the supervisor are dimensions that have been researched and are considered important to the supervision process (Bradley & Gould, 2001; Sumerall et al., 1998; Vidlak, 2002).

Christie, Joyce, and Moeller (1985), provided the long-standing study of supervisory approaches that promoted fieldwork student development and contributed to student's later professional decision making. The following were identified as effective strategies for supervisors:

Supervisor attributes

- Supervisory expectations clarified from outset of fieldwork
- Knowledge of theory and best practices
- Demonstrates enthusiasm and passion for occupational therapy
- Models ethical and professional behaviors
- Able to assess student learning needs
- Values differences
- Awareness of own strength and limitations
- Conveys supportive, caring attitude
- Listens when talks with student
- Open and honest with student including the use of self-disclosure

Supervisor–supervisee relationship attributes

- Teaches practical skills as needed
- Accessible for student inquiry and discussions
- Provides timely and constructive feedback
- Establishes a collaborative relationship with the student
- Fosters independence and autonomy
- Encourages student to explore ideas and considers alternative actions

The lower half of this list identifies preferences desired by students during supervision.

Useful skills and values that are necessary in the fieldwork educator for the specific task of supervision particularly in mental health environments are useful to consider when supervising students around psychosocial aspects of practice:

- Ability to facilitate the supervisory relationship and implement a supervisory plan (Campbell, 2006)
- Purposively listening (Gillfillan, 2001) more than talking (Fleck, 2001)
- Positive regard (Bradley & Gould, 2001)
- Build, trust, rapport, and mutuality (Campbell, 2006)
- Warmth and genuineness
- Emotional neutrality (Gillfillan, 2001)

- Tolerant, open, and accepting (Campbell, 2006)
- Interpersonal sensitivity (Nelson & Friedlander, 2001)
- Supportiveness, particularly in the early stages of fieldwork II (Ramos-Sanchez et al., 2002) or in fieldwork I (Cara, 2000; Sumerall et al., 1998)
- Self-awareness and the capacity for self-reflection
- Self-disclosure and the capacity to know when to self-disclose (Noelle, 2003)
- Ethics, particularly keeping confidentiality (Ladany, Lehrman-Waterman, Molinaro, & Wolgast, 1999)
- Guidance in difficult cases or clinical dilemmas (Shanfield, Hetherly, & Matthews, 2001)
- Integrity and ruthless honesty
- Sympathy for the student process and personal concerns (Shanfield et al., 2001)
- Provision of adequate time and attention to the supervisee (Trant, 2001)
- Ability to "own conflicts" and to resolve conflicts (Nelson & Friedlander, 2001)
- Ability to at least understand, if not work with, different perspectives (Ladany et al., 1999)

However, supervision is a transactional relationship between the supervisor and supervisee. Both bring responsibilities, ideas, and issues to share supervision for mutual consideration by both parties as well as the client.

Supervisee Responsibilities

Campbell (2006) outlined additional responsibilities of the supervisee related to supervision specific to counseling-type settings:

- *Adhere to ethical standards.*
- *Seek to become the best practitioner possible.*
- *Engage in supervision including preparation and participation.*
- *Follow rules of confidentiality.*
- *Avoid dual relationships with clients.*
- *Seek supervision immediately if a crisis occurs.*
- *Honestly report mistakes.*
- *Proactively identifies areas of bias or lack of competence.*
- *Submit accurate documentation according to facility procedures and in a timely manner.*
- *Be open to supervisory feedback, recommendations, and supervision.*
- *Accept referral to outside professional, if deemed appropriate to resolve individual issues contributing to fieldwork performance limitations.*
- *Provide supervisor with honest feedback about the quality of supervision.*

Supervision is deeper and more productive when both participants are student centered and reflective.

CLINICAL REASONING AND REFLECTION

Beginning in the 1990s, with the attention to Donald Schön's (1987) work on facilitating reflective practitioners, a myriad of theories related to the development of **clinical reasoning** in practitioners evolved within the profession of which a full review is beyond the intent of this chapter. However, the roots of this discussion fostered interest of the importance of **reflection** in practice as studies demonstrated that encouraging reflection and critical reasoning led to more profound learning by the student than other approaches (Cohn, 1989; Neistadt, 1996). Reflection on the therapeutic relationship improves the supervisee's experience (Peyton, 2002). Now, educational standards in occupational therapy as well as the role of the fieldwork educator are encouraged to include reflection on practice as part of ongoing supervisory practices. Likely, fieldwork educators who model reflection-in-action encourage students to do likewise. Encouraging student reflection as a part of all supervisory processes supports transformational learning that leads to self-direction and motivation for life-long learning.

THEORETICAL FOUNDATIONS OF SUPERVISION

Traditional psychotherapy professions have presented models for supervision that have been based in their theoretical orientation. However, concepts of supervision have an **eclectic** background, having been developed from various professions and theories (Bradley & Gould, 2001). Occupational therapy has also adopted ideas of supervision from various professions and theories. Concepts also have emerged in a trial-and-error way from the actual training of therapists. Each field has maintained a specific emphasis. Keeping with the theme of this publication, fieldwork supervision foundational theories emanating from psychosocial frameworks are the psychoanalytic, humanistic, behavioral, and developmental approaches in mental and behavioral health carry over into supervisory approaches today

Psychoanalytic or Psychodynamic Supervision

The concept of supervision began to develop in the 1920s with the acceptance of psychoanalysis. Psychoanalysis, or psychoanalytic therapy, goes much further than other theoretical practices in emphasizing the **intrapersonal** aspects of training and supervision. In fact, the dynamics of supervision and therapy are considered a rich process akin to an artistic weaving in which students learn how the process of therapy is intertwined with an individual's personality and tendencies to respond. A perspective from this theory that sheds light on the occupational therapy supervisory process is that of the supervisor as a master who joins the student therapist in a rite of passage and a form of parallel process, akin to that a client experiences (Meerloo et al., 1952; Hora, 1957). The purpose of supervision is for "the supervisee to learn through the process how to understand the dynamics of resolving relational conflicts between the supervisor and supervisee for work with future clients" (Bernard & Goodyear, 2004, p. 78).

Supervision using this approach does not recognize a developmental approach to learning. However, from psychodynamic supervision, interest grew among professionals to evolve other supervisory approaches to promote personal growth through the supervisory relationship (humanism), supervision focused on supervisee attainment of competence or productivity (cognitive-behavior), or growth-facilitating supervisory approaches (developmental).

Humanistic or Person-Centered Supervision

"Facilitative" supervision (Leddick & Bernard, 1980) was originally addressed by Carl Rogers, who discussed a program of experiences that gave trainees an opportunity to model the empathy and unconditional positive regard of the therapist/supervisor. Facilitative conditions such as genuineness, empathy, and warmth were central in the supervisory relationship (Bernard & Goodyear, 2004). Also, the successful supervisor had "profound trust that the supervisee has the ability to grow and explore both the therapy situation and the self" (p. 79). The supervisor was to provide a model of behavior so that supervisees could learn by example. The assumption was that the supervisor would be an excellent therapist/counselor. Later research was contradictory regarding which methods (modeling, personal growth, or didactic training) were more useful and whether the supervisory relationship was similar to, or different from, the counseling relationship.

Occupational therapy supervision is similar to humanistic supervision in that occupational therapy supervisors traditionally emphasize role modeling, mentoring, and positive reassurance.

Cognitive-Behavioral Supervision

Behavioral therapy stresses learning theory and focuses on observable behavior. Cognitive therapy stresses modifying cognitive processes, particularly "self-talk." Each evolved independently of the other. Over time the blending led to assumptions that both adaptive and maladaptive behaviors were maintained through consequences (Bernard & Goodyear, 2004). Trainees learn behaviors from skilled therapists through role modeling and coaching with skill acquisition and generalization being the primary goal of supervision. They learn goal setting—identifying and selecting appropriate learning techniques—in behavioral terms. That is, supervision includes instruction in various behavioral techniques.

Occupational therapy supervision is similar to cognitive-behavioral therapy supervision in the sense that traditional supervision stresses instruction in techniques, goal setting, and "self-talk" clarity related to performance and recognizes the supervisor role as that of a trainer.

Developmental Approaches to Supervision

Developmental models of supervision assume that development proceeds in a chronological, hierarchical, and sequential pattern and usually focus on cognition, intellectual, or relationship-building variables. Development proceeds through identifiable stages, each stage of learning increases in complexity, and each stage must be experienced prior to further development in the next stage (Bernard & Goodyear, 2004). A knowledge of developmental levels aids in designing and fostering learning experiences specific to each stage.

Being grounded in developmental philosophies as a profession, writings can be found in occupational therapy that promote a hierarchical growth and development approach to supervisory practices in psychosocial practice and/or mental health settings.

In this chapter, the models presented have philosophical roots, even cross-pollination between these four approaches to supervision today: psychodynamic, humanism, cognitive-behavior, and developmental groundwork. A newly emerging supervisory philosophy that may become a stand-alone, fifth approach is transformational supervision, which will be introduced later in this chapter.

PRACTICAL MODELS AND METHODS OF SUPERVISION

A useful developmental approach for supervision has been conceptualized in occupational therapy, although currently the psychology literature on supervision emphasizes dimensions of supervision that can fit broadly into the categorizations (discussed above) of the supervisor, the supervisee, the supervisory relationship, and the environment. That is, different aspects of the supervision process are explored, such as the supervisor–supervisee relationship and its impact on client treatment; the effect of the supervisor's personality, such as attractiveness or sensitivity, or of the supervisory style, such as supportive or directive on the process of supervision (Crist, 2007a, 2007b, 2007c, 2007d; Sumerall et al., 1998) and on the progress of the supervisee; how events in the supervision process or the personality characteristics of the supervisor influence the supervisee; or the willingness of the supervisee to disclose an accurate picture of his or her work and how this accuracy influences the supervision and the client treatment.

Although dimensions of supervision have been emphasized, many supervisors may find models of supervision as helpful guides in understanding the process that fieldwork students may go through. No one model may fit with a fieldwork educator or with a given fieldwork supervision situation. Thus, two models are presented for consideration. These models may guide how supervisors think about their students' skills, how they might talk about clients and cases, the timing of specific interventions in supervision, and the expectations they may have of their fieldwork students. The models also may be a guide for students to become aware of intrapersonal issues they may encounter in their fieldwork experience.

Occupational Therapy Supervision from a Developmental/Cognitive Perspective

Schwartz (1984) proposed a method of supervision based on a synthesis of developmental (meaning that skills and knowledge are acquired in a sequential and hierarchical manner) models of interpersonal style that are correlated with learning experiences. Her model emphasizes the supervisor (importance of the approach) and supervisee (particularly cognitive and personality style). Behavior that is typical of occupational therapy students in fieldwork, as well as student perceptions of the learning process and suggestions for supervisory interventions, are briefly described for each descriptive level, termed conscientious, explorer, and achiever.

Once the supervisor has gained some understanding of students' behavior or a reasonable expectation of what their behavior may mean, he or she can then plan and implement specific approaches. The supervisor's role is that of model and evaluator and involves teaching, counseling, and instruction. The student's role is to learn through doing and by analyzing and critiquing his or her behavior within the supervisory sessions.

Analysis of Cognitive Levels and Interventions

The developmental levels are posited as guides and not as rigid classifications. An individual does not always fit neatly into one level, particularly since this represents a combination of areas of development. However, the developmental model suggests patterns of learning and, therefore, clear methods of clinical supervision. (The levels noted are most typical of supervisees. It is assumed that knowledge in previous levels has been acquired by the time individuals begin fieldwork.)

Conscientious. Conscientious students usually obey rules without questioning because they wish to belong to a group and to gain approval from peers and authority figures. They have limited self-awareness and find it difficult to entertain many solutions to a problem, so they may personalize criticism. This group views the supervisor as the expert, which means that students do not realize or trust their own ability to elicit solutions. They will need assurance and an understanding of the separation of personal from professional worth. Structured questioning should elicit successful problem solving, and follow-up assignments should be given.

Explorer. In the explorer group, thinking becomes more complex. The individual is able to see more possibilities and alternatives, and self-reflective ability increases. There is a conflict between wanting to stand out yet not wanting to stand outside the group. Although thinking is more complex, beliefs are stated in a dogmatic way. Explorers may fail to incorporate feedback with which they do not agree, and they may challenge the rules. The supervisor should engage in comparing the student's own view with the professional judgment of others. The explorer group consists of students who are developing their own problem-solving techniques, which means that a discussion of alternative solutions may ensue. The discussion should be limited and not provide so much information as to overwhelm supervisees.

Achiever. Achievers are able to accept and utilize multiple strategies. Students are able to follow standards of performance in an individualistic way yet may still be hypercritical. The achiever group can define problems and solutions; therefore, an approach that will critique and analyze the solutions is useful. An analytical discussion of why and how solutions were arrived at can be useful. Also indicated is instruction in how new information can be accommodated or assimilated with previous knowledge.

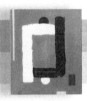

CASE ILLUSTRATION

Darren, Cordelia, and Tabetha—The Developmental Stages

Darren and Cordelia had started their internship at the same time. They came from the same school, where they had been friends and worked on group projects together. As fieldwork students, they were joined by Tabetha, a student from a different school. Darren was a conscientious student. He was quiet and rarely asked questions, but he listened intently to his supervisor and took notes during the supervisory sessions. He initially observed his supervisor's treatment. After each session, his supervisor carefully broke down her treatment in a step-by-step fashion and, for each step, explained what she was doing and why. She regularly provided Darren with a list of questions

posed as treatment hypotheses regarding the treatment sessions. Darren then would return to the next session and discuss his understanding of the hypotheses. His supervisor provided specific answers regarding his hypotheses, reassured him that his reasoning was sound, and thanked him for his earnest work.

Cordelia preferred to try out treatment right away. She was an explorer who was more comfortable discussing alternatives in which she was involved. Her supervisor began a treatment and invited Cordelia to assist. She then pointed out one or two steps she had observed and elicited alternative ways of treatment from Cordelia.

Tabetha was an achiever, who also preferred to experience treatment right away. In fact, she had arrived early to observe treatment before the formal internship began. In supervisory sessions, she reported what she had learned from her observations and what she might add to the treatment. She then reported how the treatment session had turned out, what her strengths and weaknesses were, what she might change, and the reasons why the session had turned out the way it had. She requested permission to do a research project that she had been thinking about before starting the internship. Darren, Cordelia, and Tabetha eventually designed their own peer supervision group.

Discussion

Although the interns were at different developmental levels, their supervisors were able to incorporate their levels of learning into the supervisory process. Moreover, the three were eventually able to help each other in the learning process.

Counseling Psychology Model

This model mainly addresses the supervisee and explains the process he or she may go through. It also emphasizes the relationship's ability to help the student progress successfully through the learning process. The model is explained briefly here because: training in occupational therapy supervision is based on it (Frum & Opacich, 1987); it is the model most cited in the supervision process literature; and it specifically focuses on affect and the emotional process that may occur in supervision.

The counseling psychology model was influenced by the developmental stage theorists (primarily Erik Erikson and Margaret Mahler). Both indicate optimism and trust in the adaptive capacities of human beings, and both encourage the emergence of qualities such as competence and a sense of personal and professional identity. Erikson discusses "potential crises," meaning periods of vulnerability and heightened potential. The supervisor can be aware of these crises in the supervisee's development and make appropriate interventions. In Erikson's developmental model, identity is central in development. The training process is one in which the central task of the student is to acquire a professional identity. Mahler emphasizes separation and autonomy. The supervisee not only is learning how to disengage from those on whom he or she has relied, such as teachers and classes, but is also learning how to become independent in thinking and behavior. The counseling psychology is a three-stage model of stagnation, confusion, and integration with key issues for each stage (Loganbill et al., 1982). It appears that students pass through and revisit different stages in the supervisory process. Moreover, they must grapple and struggle with the themes in each stage before reaching an emotional understanding that allows them to progress to the next stage. You will recognize some of the behavior, styles, and thinking as similar to the occupational therapy model.

Stage 1—Stagnation

In the stage of stagnation, the beginning supervisee is usually unaware, naively, of any difficulties or important issues in supervision. For the more experienced student, this is characterized more by feeling stuck or experiencing blind spots. Usually there is a naive sense of security and stability, and there may be some simplistic, black-and-white thinking or inability to define the nuances of interventions. The student may not be particularly insightful regarding his or her skills in practice. Typically, supervisees overestimate their skills or, conversely, believe that they have none or have not learned enough to prepare them for this endeavor.

Attitudes toward the world and environment can be characterized by very narrow and/or rigid thinking. With the more experienced student, this may be confined to a specific issue in practice. Usually, thinking is linear and uncreative and problem solving is narrow. Often the supervisee may accurately recognize problems in practice but offer a solution that is too narrow to be realistic.

Attitudes toward the self are usually characterized by a low self-concept and dependency on the supervisor as the source of new learning or by a lack of awareness leading to a false sense of well-being that is not based on actual behavior. Usually the attitude toward the supervisor is one of idealizing him or her as an omniscient and omnipotent figure or being indifferent to the supervisor and considering him or her somewhat irrelevant. Although this stage may seem somewhat negative by the supervisor, it can be characterized as one in which the supervisee is passively learning and constituting an identity that will aid in the next, turbulent stages.

Implications for Practice. This is a difficult stage for the supervisor (and obviously the supervisee), who should resist the temptation to give the supervisee too much early independence and responsibility. This stage demands an explanation of the intricacies of practice without too many demands for advanced knowledge. The supervisor should provide reassurance and understanding concerning the student's positive interventions. To cope with a defiant attitude, the supervisor must understand and tolerate both the tendency to idealize and to be indifferent. In other words, supervisors should enjoy being admired and not deny their knowledge. They must tolerate indifference and not personalize behavior.

Stage 2—Confusion

Stage 2 is one of confusion. This represents a marked shift from the first stage, which can occur abruptly or gradually. It is often marked by instability; erratic fluctuations in emotions, thoughts, and practice; confusion; and, sometimes, conflict. The supervisee no longer is guided by, or guarded about, beliefs about the self, others, and solutions. His or her attitude toward treatment or the setting is less characterized by rigid thinking, though solutions to problems seem inadequate and may be impossible. However, the supervisee will recognize that something is amiss.

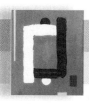

CASE ILLUSTRATION

Darren, Cordelia, and Tabetha—Stage 1, Stagnation

After the initial two weeks, Darren and Tabetha showed indications that they were in the stagnation stage, though they expressed it differently. Darren wanted to continue to observe and discuss treatment and planned interventions that were just like his supervisor's. He felt that he could never know as much as his supervisor and he wondered if he could pass the internship. Tabetha asked if she could have her own caseload and did not think that she needed more than weekly supervision. She was not sure whether her supervisor really provided the best interventions.

Generally, the attitude toward the self reflects the basis of this stage. Supervisees' attitudes fluctuate between a sense of self as inadequate and incompetent and a sense of being expert and able. The supervisee may know that she or he possesses some valuable skills or competencies yet be unsure that the skills will be useful in the context of practice. Students are also unsure whether their competencies are perceived by others.

Due to confusion and still-narrow thinking, the supervisee may continue to look to the supervisor for answers; however, the student will recognize that the supervisor does not have all the answers. Anger and disappointment may result. The supervisee may still idealize the supervisor and think he or she is deliberately withholding answers, or the supervisor may be viewed as incompetent or inadequate. Perhaps this is the source of the apparent contradiction in students' report that they perceive supervisors poorly while at the same time labeling their overall experience as good. Obviously, this stage may be difficult for the supervisor as well as the supervisee.

Implications for Practice. The supervisor must recognize and understand the particular stage and the emotions that characterize it and not take any display of disappointment or anger personally. Naming the problem and emotions and being able to discuss them in a non-defensive way will go a long way toward helping a student move through this stage.

The supervisor should validate a realistic portrayal of the student and resist joining in the erratic self-evaluation. It is important to resist the temptation to overvalue yet nevertheless maintain a realistic, reassuring viewpoint of the supervisee as an occupational therapist. The value of this stage is in giving up former rigid, narrow beliefs and experiencing the opportunity to gain new ideas, perspectives, and skills. It is important for the supervisor to:

- Remain objective.
- Remain unperturbed by the panic or turbulence that the supervisee may be experiencing.
- Be able to recognize and verbalize what is happening for the supervisee.

The supervisor can help the student remain aware that out of confusion come knowledge and learning.

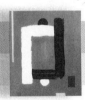

CASE ILLUSTRATION

Darren, Cordelia, and Tabetha— Stage 2, Confusion

After about five weeks, just prior to her midterm evaluation, Cordelia, who was usually talkative, became quiet and almost surly. She failed to attend two supervision sessions, claiming that her clients needed that treatment time. She revealed to Darren and Tabetha that she was not sure if any treatment in mental health was valuable or whether people really did get better. She was disappointed in her supervision and thought that her supervisor might be "testing" her before the midterm evaluation. A client who was paranoid and who, she believed, did not like her, stopped coming to Cordelia's vocational group. Cordelia began to feel better after her supervisor explained how students might feel at that stage and emphasized that her concerns were normal. She also became more aware of how her attitude affected her behavior with clients.

Stage 3—Integration

Stage 3 is characterized by integration, cognitive understanding, flexibility, and personal stability. The supervisee grasps and understands important issues for supervision. Usually supervisees can realistically assess their strengths and weakness without interference from their emotions and are able to grasp what skills need to be polished and integrated in treatment.

The supervisees' attitude toward the environment is less rigid and idealistic or extreme, and they now have a cognitive understanding of the therapeutic situation. There is acceptance and a sense of direction for the future. An individual's attitude toward the self is characterized by a more realistic view and an acceptance of both strengths and weakness. There is a sense of confidence that growth will continue, and the attitude toward the supervisor also becomes more realistic. The supervisor is now seen as a person who has strengths and weakness. The student is able to take more responsibility for the supervisory sessions and agenda, usually becoming more independent of the supervisor at this stage. This is a stable period with much flexibility and potential for further growth.

Implications for Practice. The supervisee can take much more responsibility for supervision, treatment, and learning. There is a consolidation and probably less need for structured supervision. The supervisor, while still providing feedback, can enlist the supervisee in reviewing what is important in treatment, what he or she has learned, and what can still be developed.

Themes in the Stages

Within these stages, certain themes, or issues, of competence, emotional awareness, autonomy, identity, and respect for individual differences for beginning professionals may appear. The issues may not necessarily appear in sequential order, and they tend to continually resurface.

CASE ILLUSTRATION

Darren, Cordelia, and Tabetha—Stage 3, Integration

In their peer supervision group held prior to their last weeks of the internship, Darren, Cordelia, and Tabetha discussed what they had learned and what they hoped for the future. They realized that their final project, in which they had developed a community outreach group that would be taken over by clients, was valued and desired by both staff and clients. They felt proud that they had been able to contribute.

The interns realized that although they were not sure whether they were advanced enough to work independently in mental health, they had acquired some good skills. They began to understand how their responses, attitudes, and behavior could affect clients; Cordelia had particularly learned this during stage 2. They appreciated what they had learned from their supervisor and other staff and were also able to differentiate what they could do best and less well. They realized that working in mental health is like an interesting dance between client and therapist; if they each listened to different music they would be unable to follow each other, but when they were hearing the same tune, treatment progressed more easily. They felt secure in their knowledge and identity as occupational therapists, and they had some ideas about the similarities and differences in their own and other mental health professions.

Competence. Competence means the ability to use skills and knowledge to carry out an appropriate treatment plan.

In the case illustration, Darren, Cordelia, and Tabetha displayed issues of competence in each stage. Darren was most questioning of his ability in stage 1, Cordelia felt frustrated in stage 2, and all three had realistically integrated their skills and knowledge during stage 3.

Emotional Awareness. Emotional awareness is important in the psychosocial arena because it relates to an ability to be aware of how one affects, and is affected by, client responses, behavior, and style. This awareness of personal reactions and attitudes toward a client is particularly useful for formulating impressions and directing interventions in the psychiatric arena.

While in stage 2, Cordelia had been most unaware of her feelings. After reassurance from her supervisor, however, she became able to accept them. In stage 3, she still wondered whether her feelings were important but was able to acknowledge and discuss with her supervisor concerns regarding her behavior toward clients.

Autonomy. Students may have the sense that they are merely a reflection of all the books they have read, and the theories and teachers they have experienced. They may doubt that they can be effective. Supervisees may have a shaky self-concept and difficulty thinking of themselves as responsible occupational therapists.

Darren initially displayed this issue in stage 1. However, by the middle of the fieldwork period he had become more confident in his ability to work independently. He thanked his supervisor for gently facilitating his independence through her concrete interventions and suggestions.

Identity. The theme of identity may appear as the student struggles to assume a theoretical identity or discern which theory works best. The supervisee may be caught in a conflict of learning one theory while practicing with therapists who use another.

In the Case Illustration, Darren and Cordelia had learned a specific theory for mental health treatment. They were able to use it throughout the treatment, and were pleased that their supervisor followed the same theory. Tabetha had not learned a specific theory for mental health treatment and initially felt skeptical about having to follow one. However, she gradually came to appreciate its use in the mental health setting. Her final project discussed the theory more in depth.

Individual Biases. The theme of individual biases arises because of the negative stereotypes associated with many people with mental disabilities and because of the fear, on the part of society in general, of those stereotypes. Particularly in mental health, one must separate out behaviors that are maladaptive and need change from aspects of the person, which need to be respected.

All three students initially were fearful of people with mental disabilities; specifically, they secretly believed them to be unpredictably violent, hopeless, and, maybe, lacking in discipline. They were able to discuss these attitudes with their supervisor, who tolerated the attitudes while at the same time questioning them. The students were shocked when they saw some of the symptoms of the different mental disorders about which they had read. At the same time, they were aware of how the people with whom they worked had thoughts, hopes, desires, dreams, frustrations, and struggles with many of the same issues as they had. Darren, Cordelia, and Tabetha finished their fieldwork with a new sense of respect for the clients' struggles to cope with their disorders and abilities to do many things independently in spite of the disorders.

SITUATIONAL SUPERVISION[4]

Fieldwork education is composed of two critical supervisory ingredients to promote student development leading to entry-level competence in a fieldwork setting: the selected fieldwork learning tasks and the supervisory approach to facilitate student professional growth. The fieldwork educator designs and implements the learning experience through identification of resources and experiences available through her program. However, the important task is to match the desired learning and skill development expectations with student capabilities. This is the foundation for delivering a student-centered educational experience. Situational Leadership (SL) is a widely used professional development model that facilitates student supervision by matching the learning task to the individual student's capabilities and "readiness for learning." The basis of the model is that every supervisory experience is balancing the expectations for fieldwork learning that the fieldwork educator has selected between three critical components: task behavior (directive behavior), supportive behavior (relational behavior), and the developmental level (maturity) of the learner derived from their amount of competence in the specific situation and commitment to demonstrate the desired performance (Ledlow & Coppola, 2011). Competence is the degree of knowledge and or skills that have been acquired. Commitment is a combination of motivation and confidence. Using situational supervision, the fieldwork educator will note that students will differ on their competence and commitment dependent on the selected fieldwork task.

Supervision begins with analyzing the supervisee's capabilities for each desired situation. Effective supervision is not the result of a consistent supervisory style, as many models purport, but the outcome of intentional decision making that is flexible and responsive to the learning in each situation. For instance, a student may be very familiar with using adapted feeding utensils (self-confidence and interest in doing) but may be unfamiliar with feeding and swallowing protocols (questioning ability and

---

[4]This section of the chapter was published, in part, in *OT Advance* (Crist, 2007a, 2007b, 2007c, 2007d).

TABLE 26-3. Relationship of Competence, Commitment, and Student Behaviors in Situational Learning

Student Scenario		Observed Student Behaviors During Fieldwork Education
Competence	**Commitment**	
High	High	Justifiably confident, self-reliant, autonomous, inspired, inspires others.
Moderate	Variable	Capable, self-critical, insecure, cautious, bored, contributing
Low	Low	Overwhelmed, confused, frustrated, still learning, flashes of competence
Low	High	Inexperienced, curious, hopeful, optimistic, unskilled, they may not know what they do not know!

Based on Blanchard, Zigarmi, & Zigarmi (2003)

hesitant to try for fear of harming the patient). Situational Leadership encourages the supervisor to consider four different hierarchically organized, student scenarios to analyze the student's observed behaviors in relationship to your assigned student expectation (see Table 26-3).

One can see that many students begin fieldwork overall or a new task exemplifying behaviors from the last two sections. Also, SL outlines both positive and negative behaviors that a student can demonstrate in each area. Sometimes, the awareness of their lack of competence makes them hesitant to attempt the task; other times, they are not motivated to perform through disinterest in either the current assignment or in acquiring a skill. Also a supervisee may have low commitment because the fieldwork educator has not given them sufficient information to understand the relative importance of a fieldwork task. Effective fieldwork supervision reflects corresponding the student's abilities with the current, desired learning outcomes or specific performance expectations. For example, during the first three weeks of fieldwork, one student might have excellent mental health knowledge and skills (pre-fieldwork competence) but knows that he or she does not want to practice in a mental health setting so shows minimal self-direction or interest during fieldwork (low commitment). Another student is motivated to become skillful in mental health practice as he or she recognizes the importance of psychosocial factors in their future goal to do home-health care (high commitment). However, successful intervention strategies with adolescents who have abused drugs are not observed as the student enthusiastically and randomly selects different interventions trying to see if one will work (low competence).

As supervisor, your goal is to move the student to a desired level of competence, in each task, which usually means either reinforcing the current level of student performance as the uppermost you expect during fieldwork or using the student's behaviors to move her or him into more independent performance or improved skill performance.

Having discussed this model with many fieldwork educators, the most important focus during supervision must be on the fieldwork student's task competence. Student motivation can vary and support or deter from desired learning, but the supervisor's determination of student competence is essential to protect and maximize patient care while limiting professional risks and liability.

However, to promote student fieldwork engagement, the fieldwork educator has to assess the student's readiness for performance per Table 26-3, then select an appropriate supervisory approach. Second, an effective supervisor in this model can use anyone of these approaches effectively at anytime. In situational leadership, this is called having style flexibility, which is a highly desirable trait as supervisees engage in performance at all four levels and best practices, indicate the supervisor must be ready to match their style to the supervisee to maximize the supervisory outcomes. As the arrow indicates in Table 26-4 the most fundamental approach is directing; the

TABLE 26-4. Situational Leadership Supervision, Supervisor Approaches and Styles

Observed Student Fieldwork Task Behavior	Supervisory Style	Recommended Supervisory Approaches
High competence with high commitment	Delegate	Self-direction accepted.
		Ask for input.
		Encourage supervising and mentoring others.
Moderate to high competence with variable commitment	Participating and Supporting	Facilitate joint problem solving.
		Encourage outside of task performance.
		Expect accurate self-assessment of strengths and weaknesses.
		Support student-initiated professional development plans.
Low to some competence with low commitment	Selling and Coaching	Assist with task organization and delivery.
		Use competence to reinforce learning tasks more fully.
		Encourage during task performance.
		Support what student knows, teach parts not known.
		Explain why desired performance is important.
		Inquire about student awareness of weaknesses and follow with suggestion action steps to remedy.
Low competence with high commitment	Directing	Establish goals and monitor outcomes.
		State clear performance expectations.
		Teach.
		Tell and model performance first.

Based on Blanchard et al. (2003)

most sophisticated is student performance requiring delegation in this hierarchical model.

Student "readiness" to engage in a specific skill or refine it is when she or he is not only able but also willing to participate in and complete certain tasks.

Here are some recommendations from professional experiences to assist in using situational leadership in the fieldwork supervision context:

- Always assume that supervision needs to start at the Directing Level with each new major fieldwork learning task. If the student shows task competence, then you can move quickly to Selling and Coaching and higher. With this strategy, you will be taking a positive approach to supervision, and you will avoid eroding his existing competence by having to point to his performance ineffectiveness or inability to initiate supervision. Most fieldwork educators want to start at the Participating and Supporting level and, frankly, students most frequently desire this level of supervision. However, when a student cannot perform a desired fieldwork task for whatever reason, the fieldwork educator must move down to Selling and Coaching and even Directing to support student learning.

- Acknowledge that in a 6–12 week experience, the primary goal is to be at the Participating and Supporting level of supervision in tasks that are central or primary to the given fieldwork placement. Seldom will a fieldwork educator be able to use the Delegate level.

- Years of discussion with students have indicated that students most often want their fieldwork educator to be their "friend, first and foremost." While understandable, friendship is not the cornerstone of effective supervision. In fact, a fieldwork educator who engages in a friend relationship with a student during fieldwork more often than not finds herself or himself being ineffective as an educator, particularly if a student begins to have difficulty with performance.

- Remember that you will see "backsliding" in student distress. Distress may be a new fieldwork learning situation and/or context, including ones that are familiar but may have a new twist or two. As a fieldwork educator, gently nudging from a lower level of supervision using reminders of performance in similar situations may allow a student to quickly ground and move forward.

- Using your skill in activity analysis, separate fieldwork learning and related performance into core or essential performance tasks and then create a list of options when a student has acquired the core entry-level competences. These options can be used as a reward or even given to students to choose in order to shape their own learning experiences. Students learn where to focus their attention and, if they are motivated and acquire these core skills, there is a benefit of additional learning available.

- Flexibility in supervisory style is central in order to match the learning situation with student readiness to perform. If a supervisory approach is not working, reconsider what student characteristic you are observing. More often than not, you can easily rectify the mismatch by adapting your approach.

CASE ILLUSTRATION

Darren, Cordelia, and Tabetha in Situational Supervision

Early descriptions of Darren, Cordelia and Tabetha's fieldwork performance using developmental stages can be reviewed in relationship to situational supervision. Each student was expected to lead four community participation groups for young adults with dual diagnoses who were transitioning from a residential facility to minimally supervised group homes.

Darren was described as a conscientious student. He was quiet and rarely asked questions, but he listened intently to his supervisor and took notes during the supervisory sessions. He initially observed his supervisor's group sessions. After each session, his supervisor carefully broke down her treatment in a step-by-step fashion and, for each step, explained what she was doing and why. She regularly provided Darren with a list of questions posed as treatment hypotheses regarding the treatment sessions. Darren then would return to the next session and discuss his understanding of the hypotheses. His supervisor provided specific answers regarding his hypotheses, reassured him that his reasoning was sound, and thanked him for his earnest work.

Darren is a student who has low competence but appears committed. Rightfully, his supervisor matched her developmental supervisory style to his need and used directing.

Cordelia preferred to try out treatment right away. She was an explorer, who was more comfortable discussing alternatives for meaningful community participation activities in which she was involved. Her supervisor began a treatment and invited Cordelia to assist. She then pointed out one or two steps she had observed and elicited alternative ways of treatment from Cordelia.

Cordelia exemplifies the student who is gaining competence and chooses a variety of approaches because she is not quite sure which one is better. Her supervisor is wise in using the selling and coaching supervisory approach to support her learning in the situations described. Cordelia though is beginning to show signs of the participating and supporting style by wanting to look at alternatives. If her foundation in an intervention is evident, then alternatives are good. However, if not then the supervisor may want to continue to coach and sell to strengthen

Cordelia's knowledge and application of the fundamentals before moving forward.

Tabetha was an achiever, who also preferred to experience treatment right away. In fact, she had arrived early to observe a community meeting before the formal internship began. Later, in supervisory sessions, she reported what she had learned from her observations and what she might add to the treatment. She then reported how the treatment session had turned out, what her strengths and weaknesses were, what she might change, and the reasons why the session had turned out the way it had. She requested permission to do a research project that she had been thinking about before starting the internship.

Tabetha builds upon a foundation and needs more shaping. Her competence is evident for the most part, in given situations. Her supervisor should select a participating and supporting style of supervision to facilitate Tabetha furthering her self-reliance. Her request for research shows her desire to generalize her skills to others areas. Her supervisor might start to encourage Tabetha to further grow by asking her to supervise a fieldwork level I student in interventions that she feels competent herself.

Remember in using situational supervision that in any given day, any given situation, the novelty or experience with a given task may vary for a supervisee and as a result the fieldwork educator must engage style flexibility to match the need. For instance, Cordelia might have the first opportunity ever to lead a therapeutic group learning social skills at your site, other than role-playing with her peers on campus, and the supervisor may need to be more directive to support her in this new fieldwork performance area.

Discussion

Darren, Tabetha, and Cordelia's experience can be explained by developmental models as well as from a situational learning perspective.

COACHING DURING SUPERVISION[5]

Fieldwork educators have long embraced two major approaches to working with students: teaching and supervision. Coaching, an emerging area of service delivery, affords a third alternative to engaging fieldwork students in their professional development process. In situational leadership or supervision, coaching is a supervisory style. However, coaching is evolving into a specific approach to interaction to assist with growth and development in the recipient. Coaching is a transformational approach that includes individualized consideration, intellectual stimulation, and performance expectations. Definitions of coaching are:

> . . . a transformative process for personal and professional awareness, discovery and growth. (International Association of Coaching)

---

[5]This section of the chapter was published, in part, in *OT Advance* (Crist, 2010a, 2010b).

. . . partnering with clients in a thought-provoking and creative process that inspires them to maximize their personal and professional potential. Through coaching, clients deepen their learning, improve their performance and enhance their quality of life (International Coaching Federation Standards of Ethical Conduct)

Coaches talk about forrwarding an individual's action toward a stated goal. Coaching is complementary to supervision as it also advocates to challenge and support individuals to achieve professional and personal goals (Campbell, 2006).

Coaching, according to AOTA's *Blueprint for Entry-level Education* (AOTA, 2010a, p. 188), is "a person-centered factor for psychological support or impact on performance, participation and well-being" to engage the concepts of "motivation, self-efficacy, self-esteem, self-concept, and identity. Coaching is future skill-development focused but emphasizes personal empowerment through guided self-reflection using powerful questions from a coach.

Fieldwork Instruction, Supervision, or Coaching

Fieldwork instruction or education focuses on identifying students' incoming knowledge and skills from their academic preparation. Fieldwork educators identify the students' learning needs so as to enhance entry-level practice knowledge. The fieldwork educator primarily uses methods instructional in approach. The educator considers specific learning objectives for the task at hand, providing learning experiences, strategies and resources to grade student progression in skill development toward entry-level practice competence.

The benefit of this approach is that students are learning new information and skills they had not previously acquired. Students will frequently sense that instructional fieldwork activities are intended to benefit them as learners. *Teaching-learning* is the focus.

Fieldwork supervision is a specific professional relationship in which a fieldwork supervisor provides a guided, apprentice-like experience. The supervisor is initially more directive and sets performance expectations and boundaries. With shaping, mentoring and/or supporting, the supervisor becomes less directive as the student demonstrates the expected behaviors.

The benefit of this approach is that students increase their ability to be independently competent in the fieldwork setting. Progress through fieldwork supervision is measured in terms of demonstrated new skills and acquired performance standards in given fieldwork situations or tasks. *Supervision-performance* is the focus.

Fieldwork coaching is when a fieldwork educator helps a student find a better solution to a fieldwork challenge or a different way of thinking or acting in response to a fieldwork situation. The fieldwork coach is more a facilitator; the student identifies what he or she wants to learn from the experience or which competencies he or she wants to improve.

The major difference between supervision and coaching is that in coaching the supervisee holds the goal and the energy for professional development. Both the supervisor and supervisee are committed to helping the student make powerful changes within a reciprocal supervisory relationship.

Coaching is beneficial when the student has self-selected specific professional goals and several options are plausible or have value in being considered. The coach helps the student consider these options and then challenges through homework and other fieldwork activities to try out new skills and then reflect on what was learned.

The benefit of this approach is that students are taught to be self-regulating and self-directed. Progress in fieldwork coaching is measured in terms of the student's reported feelings of professional fulfillment, empowerment, and self as an entry-level practitioner. Students frequently sense that the primary reason for coached fieldwork activities is to ensure that they deem themselves competent for practice in a variety of situations. *Coaching-self-efficacy* is the focus.

Whitmore (2009), in *Coaching for Performance*, concentrates on growing human potential. He notes that the essence of creating awareness and responsibility in another individual begins with artful questioning. A fieldwork education supervisor who raises questions, rather than just than telling his or her student what needs to be done, promotes self-direction, enhanced competence, and independent thinking.

The only time when telling or directing is mandated is when the student is engaging in action that is unsafe or might do harm. Yet the great temptation of a fieldwork educator is to direct when a student is simply considering practice choices that are ill-informed.

Whitmore's transformative guidelines on coaching for performance begin with making the fieldwork educator aware of her or his own supervising style; she or he can then select one that best serves the desired outcome for student learning. As the goal of fieldwork education is to help students link classroom information with practice through using knowledge, the tendency is to ask why questions. "Why would Plan A work better than B?" Why questions do promote analytical thinking based on prior learning; but they can also produce an undercurrent of doubt in students as to whether they have enough or the right knowledge. This leads to defensiveness or self-doubt.

Whitmore says that what, when, who, how much, and how many are better barometers because they seek to clarify, quantify, and/or gather facts as the basis for choosing responsible actions.

Inquiry beginning with these types of questions initiates an environment of collaboration or shared responsibility for the fieldwork student's learning and underpins the development of professional self-efficacy.

Fieldwork educators have more practice skills than students. Couple this with the time constraints in everyday practice, and the tendency is to simply tell a student what needs to be done. In *Coaching for Performance*, Whitmore (2009) advocates that using probing questions will initiate deeper reflection on the application of knowledge than just having the student report facts. Supervisors are to encourage students to provide detail about their reasoning or planned actions.

Performance coaching is good supervision and encourages students to lead the discussion. The following coaching skills are beneficial during fieldwork supervision:

- Provide probing question asked to encourage self-exploration of alternatives and reflections on potential actions
- Use these as homework that students can use to prepare in advance so that the students have time to think through their responses over time instead being requested to use on-the-spot replies or reactions, the latter of which is testing factual knowledge, not reasoning.
- Give a probing question at the end of each supervisory session or the day before as a form of homework

Asking good questions is not as easy as it sounds. With reflective practice, the skill can become a "best practice" for fieldwork supervision.

CASE ILLUSTRATION

Darren, Cordelia, and Tabetha each will benefit from coaching if the questions are modified to encourage reflection on their current skill set, build upon their individual strengths and empower them for future action. For instance, in the earlier example using community participation groups, Darren might be asked about how he would break down the steps to delivering an intervention instead of the supervisor providing the steps. Cordelia would benefit from reflective questions such as "Comparing two approaches to promote risk-taking to engage in community activities related to leisure, what do you feel the client would be more responsive to sustaining after discharge?"Or another might be: "What are the challenges you feel in doing this intervention on your own?" Tabetha's supervisor should use powerful questioning around creating new thinking, such as "What do you want to learn to do with your psychosocial learning and skills from this site when you get your 'dream-job' in school-based practice? Give me some ideas"

Discussion

Darren, Tabetha, and Cordelia's experience and behaviors were discussed from a supervisory coaching perspective.

MAXIMIZING LEARNING—BENEFITING FROM SUPERVISION

As a fieldwork student, you can use different ways of learning to maximize your experience and to benefit most from supervision beyond the list of supervisee responsibilities identified early in this chapter. Ways of maximizing learning during fieldwork are listed in Table 26-5 and elaborated in the following sections of this chapter.

Most individuals about to embark into fieldwork are excited, apprehensive, and willing to do all that they can to maximize the experience. Often the tendency is to find more academic texts or technical material to read. While seeking out information is always a good idea, certain information can be more useful for the fieldwork experience in mental health. Specifically, any texts that are personal stories or narratives that could broaden an understanding of people, of people with mental disabilities, or of oneself will help maximize the experience.

From the perspective of a supervisee, the models discussed in this chapter can help her or him be proactive in facilitating their fieldwork supervision experience by reflecting on their own development and supervisory needs and initiating discussion with their fieldwork educator as soon as possible to arrive at a collaborative supervisory plan regarding fieldwork expectations. For instance, knowledge of

TABLE 26-5. Guidelines for Maximizing Learning During Fieldwork

Emotional	Intellectual	Interpersonal	Professional
Read narratives and personal stories of mental illness or access them online at websites such as YouTube.	Review mental health course notes and texts.	Ask for help regarding how to address challenging client behaviors or situations.	Take initiative to self-direct learning.
Anticipate emotional issues and stages that are unique to mental health practice such as undetected stigma in the student.		Communicate expectations responsibly in supervision such as documentation, intervention planning, and implementation and confidentiality.	Become familiar with setting through engaging a thorough, structured orientation program at the beginning.
Know your learning style.	Plan a progressive program of involvement according to your learning style.	Discuss learning style in supervision.	Time management—plan a daily schedule and routine and use time effectively and flexibly.
Self-reflection.	Consider evidence-based literature and how relates to current fieldwork realities.	Remain open and genuine and communicate with awareness.	Schedule regular supervision time.
Recognize when the work setting touches off personal issues.		Communicate in supervision or with other staff when the work setting influences personal issues.	Communicate in supervision when the work setting influences personal issues.

the cognitive-behavioral levels or emotional stages, many which will be encountered, and understanding of the issues that might be most pertinent to yourself can help in anticipating potential personal "snags" in the process. Alerting the supervisor in advance to problems or anxieties with fieldwork expectations that might arise will help both the supervisor and supervisee to flow through troublesome spots.

Knowing oneself as a supervisee will assist in maximizing a successful fieldwork experience. However, expressing your supervisory needs in a direct, honest, and genuine manner with the ability to be self-reflective is also essential. In general, the more aware, open, and willing an individual is to communicate responsibly, the more the fieldwork and supervisory relationship will develop smoothly and the fewer problems will arise. With self-awareness and responsible communication, conflicts and disagreements can be avoided or resolved with mutual satisfaction. The four identified barriers for adult participation in learning to consider are:

- Situational barriers (depending person's situation at a given time).
- Institutional barriers (all practices and procedures that discourage adults from participation).
- Dispositional barriers (person's attitude about self and learning).
- Informational barriers (person is not aware of educational activities available) (Merriam & Caffarella, 1991).

Furthermore, with conflict the fieldwork educator in collaboration with their student should reflect on the reason that the problem is present by reducing barriers to full engagement in fieldwork. Consider the source of the barrier and how to reduce it to support the supervisee to learn or better yet, engage the supervisee in a transformational session focused on helping them reflect on options to reduce barriers that are preventing their learning. Thus, they have a life-long professional skill to draw upon.

TRENDS AND RECOMMENDATIONS

In the 1980s, specific models for mental health fieldwork were identified and advocated (Kolodner, Wiener, & Frum, 1989). Stanley (1996) called for mental health fieldwork to enhance awareness of this practice specialty and as motivator to choose this practice. This call-out has not been quenched. Mental health fieldwork and focus on psychosocial practices in occupational therapy has been shown to bring positive change in occupational therapy students' attitudes toward the practice area, particularly around stigma issues such as fear of people with mental illness and moving a focus on deficits to one more of enabling (Beltran, Scanlan, Hancock, & Luckett, 2007). Now, with focus on behavioral health, concerns about violence, bullying (children and workplace) and ever-increasing rates for depression, and the role of occupational therapy in mental health and psychosocial practice approaches, we are called to "walk-the-talk" regarding implementing fully the value regarding addressing whole person concerns versus interventions focused on a deficit, functional limitation, or preparatory skills for occupational engagement.

Approaches to engaging the relationship between the fieldwork educator and student are expanding beyond supervision primarily into recognition of a greater variety of opportunities, all needed to respond effectively to expanding, diversifying changes in mental health practice and society. To ensure the achievement of the *AOTA Centennial Vision* (AOTA, 2007) by 2017 and educate practitioners with readiness to engage fully in opportunities, the supervisor–supervisee relationship will be further acknowledged and differentiated into individualized approaches to target the specific professional development needs related to entry-level practice. According to literature, within and outside the profession related to clinical education, the following approaches will likely be instituted and all become integral to the outcomes from fieldwork education:

Coaching	Courageous questioning providing transformational experiences to allow the student to reach their highest agenda; the student possesses the professional development 'self-cure' that is 'teased-out' by the coach recipient empowered with self-efficacy.
Collaboration	Working more as partners on a task or project where both the fieldwork educator and student contribute to mutually agreed upon goals or activities using shared problem solving. Most often, collaboration is initiated by the fieldwork educator.
Consultation	Providing expert recommendations or advice to the student who can choose to take it or leave it; the fieldwork educator as consultant is expert and knows what needs to be done; student informed on how/what to consider but the actual choice of action remains with the student.
Counseling	Addressing the student's problematic, psychological behaviors, thoughts or feelings that distract from being able to engage therapeutic use of self (Bernard & Goodyear, 2004).[6]
Leading	Assisting the student to achieve goal-directed behaviors to achieve system-wide or organizationally selected vision, mission, values and/or goals (Ledlow & Coppola, 2011).

---

[6]Most fieldwork educators will refer students to outside counseling or therapy because education and counseling are polar opposites, creating confusion in the relationship and possibly even a conflict of interest. Caution cannot be overstated as frequently counseling or therapy gets enmeshed if not concealed by the student's response to the fieldwork educator's therapeutic engagement versus supervisory and educational expectations. If the following is observed from the student, then referral to counseling is frequently your better response to avoid role confusion or what is called dual purpose supervision in counseling psychology:

- Deteriorating work performance attributed to internal distress or external stressors
- Trouble coping with life routines or unwell more frequently than expected
- Student approaches supervisor and requests assistance (Rose & Best, 2005)

Mentoring	A transformational approach that takes the student mentee "under the supervisor's wing" to personally help with successful professional career trajectory (Ledlow & Coppola, 2011); serves psychosocial functions (role modeling, acceptance and confirmation, advice and guidance) and career functions (sponsorship, guidance, and advocacy; exposure and visibility; instruction and information; protection; providing challenging or "plum" assignments; access to resources) (Rose & Best, 2005; Taylor & Neimeyer, 2009).
Supervision	An intervention provided by the fieldwork educator, as a more senior member of a profession for a more junior member, the student through a relationship that is evaluative and extends over time. The simultaneous purposes are to: enhance the professional functioning of the student, monitor the quality of professionals services offered to the clients served, and serve as a gatekeeper for those who enter the profession (Bernard & Goodyear, 2004, p. 8).
Teaching	Reliance on a specific curriculum with educational goals and objectives that are universally applied to all learners using teaching-learning principles and approaches.
Therapy	Is a deficit-oriented approach where the problem is diagnosed and remediated; fieldwork educator is expert and diagnoses the problem and selects best approach to remediate; the student is healed, cured, or assisted/adapted (in chronic conditions).[7]
Training	Teaching a new skill set in order to enhance performance or expand knowledge using either a didactic or experiential approach; the instructor defines what the learner needs to know; the recipient is educated and prepared to do specific actions.

At this time, supervisors should clearly articulate which supervisory approach they are utilizing, at any given point in time, to support student performance as well as to avoid confusion in expectations, interaction, and desired performance outcomes.

Various trends in the psychological literature of the past five years indicate directions for occupational therapy fieldwork and research into fieldwork. Primary attention has been paid to the roles of the supervisor and supervisee. The role of the fieldwork educator indicates that students prefer the skills of support, warmth, genuineness, integrity, ethical behavior, mentoring, and ability to own and resolve conflicts (Bradley & Gould, 2001; Shanfield et al., 2001; Taylor & Neimeyer, 2009). The literature suggests that fieldwork educators can learn these facilitative skills

---

[7]See previous note.

in a variety of ways through classes, conferences, clinical councils, or purchasing consultation (Vidlak, 2002).

More attention has been paid to students' experiences in supervision related to their setting. A study has shown that clinical supervision differs based on the characteristics of the setting more so than the quality of the supervision (Smith, 2006). The role of the fieldwork student indicates that students who can be more reflective can develop advanced skills and trust in their own experiences as a guide to delivering occupational therapy (Peyton, 2002). Positive outcomes indicate that there is a role for emotion (Foullette & Batten, 2000; Hahn, 2001), the expression of emotion (Yourman, 2003), and self-disclosure in the supervision relationship (Ladany & Walker, 2003). Reflection is central to transformational learning and occupational therapy is embracing this skill with increasing intensity as discussed in this chapter. Fieldwork processes and the supervisor–supervisee relationship are central to modeling and reinforcing the use of reflection as a life-long skill supporting effective clinical reasoning.

Unfortunately, there are many more articles documenting negative supervisory experiences (Greer, 2002; Gross, 2005; Ladany et al., 1999; Nelson & Friedlander, 2001; Nelson, Gray, Friedlander, Ladany & Walker, 2001; Ramos-Sanchez et al., 2002; Trant, 2001). In some cases the experiences were harmful to students. One study in occupational therapy has indicated that negative experiences also happen in fieldwork (Lew, Cara, & Richardson, 2007).

Fewer studies have explored experimental programs for supervision; however, some innovations suggest programs that might be established in occupational therapy. For example, supervision groups (Altfeld, 1999; Oegren, Apelman, & Klawitter, 2001) and use of video supervision (Sorlie, Gammon, Bergvik, & Sexton, 1999) appeared successful. Also, a one-session introduction to supervision appeared helpful for residents (Whitman, 2001) and a three-hour training for practicum students appeared to increase self-efficacy and decrease anxiety (Cara, 2000).

Certainly as using evidence is to practice, practice competence is rapidly escalating as a focal point as well. Fieldwork education is a primary mechanism for ensuring competence in practice and will be at the cornerstone of many discussions in the future. At some point, occupational therapy, like many other health professions have already done, will have to clearly articulate the specific practice competency outcomes in fieldwork and ultimately the set of uniform or core competencies that every new entry-level occupational therapy practitioner will have acquired in order to be certified, licensed, and/or qualified to practice. This will also clarify our service to the public and, ultimately, help define, if not elevate, occupational therapy in mental health.

Most important, occupational therapy professionals have spent the past decade elevating the attention to fieldwork education and plans are to continue (AOTA, 2006). The need for well-trained fieldwork educators is evident (Crist, 2000; Lipsitt, 2009). The single most promising development is the voluntary AOTA Fieldwork Educator Certificate Program (FWECP) (AOTA, 2009c). Social networking, such as the AOTA fieldwork educator listserve is rapidly connecting fellow fieldwork educators for mutual support. The profession can never have enough opportunities to assist practitioners with role development and networking as fieldwork educators especially related to specialized settings such as mental health!

SUMMARY

Supervision is valued in most health professions, particularly mental health settings. Supervisors and supervisees often have different expectations of supervision. Students look more for instruction, while supervisors emphasize the interaction and relationship. The goal of the supervisee is often to learn techniques. The supervisor's goal is to help an individual become a professional.

There are four components influencing supervision: the supervisor, the supervisee, the relationship and the interaction of the two, and the environment or setting. Supervision is a dynamic process among these components. Theoretical models of supervision have been developed from the psychoanalytic, behavioral, humanistic, and developmental schools. Supervision usually involves an eclectic blend of techniques from all of these models. An occupational therapy developmental model emphasizes the supervisee and supervisor components. A counseling psychology model emphasizes the process the supervisee goes through and the supervisory relationship. Situational supervision provides a student-centered approach advocating for supervisor style flexibility once the student's readiness (competence and commitment) to perform a specific fieldwork task or activity has been determined. Coaching provides a strategy where students are empowered to self-direct aspects of their performance and professional development. Reflection continues to expand as a key skill with never more importance than in the psychosocial practices in occupational therapy. Thus, the transformational approach of coaching will enrich the supervisor–supervisee relationship and ready the student with contemporary practice skills. The transition to the role of supervisor is supported by a variety of experiences. Supervisors can develop a variety of skills, roles, and tasks to become an effective fieldwork educator as well as competent practitioner.

REVIEW QUESTIONS

1. Reflect on your prior experiences with supervisors. What did they do or say to make you feel motivated, competent, self-efficacious, empowered, and/or able to problem solve on your own? What did they do that eroded or set back your self-perspective in each of these areas? How does this experience inform your own supervisory skills?
2. Delineate how mental health fieldwork can assist with later practice competencies related to psychosocial factors in occupational therapy practice for other settings.

3. Develop a personal statement or checklist of your professional responsibilities and behaviors to be a competent, committed fieldwork student or fieldwork educator in mental health. Identify three to five requests for the type of supervision or supervisor–supervisee relationship that you believe will help during fieldwork. How will you share it with your future fieldwork educator(s) or students?

4. Compare and contrast the supervisory approaches of counseling psychology situational supervision, and coaching regarding strengths and challenges in helping students become proficient in mental health practice. What opportunities does fieldwork education provide to contribute to the expansion of psychosocial practice or mental health towards the 2017 *AOTA Centennial Vision* (AOTA, 2007)? Consider the fieldwork educator, the fieldwork student, their mutual relationship, and the context during the time the fieldwork actually occurs.

5. Explain the importance of reflection in psychosocial practice and application of reflection during the supervisor–student relationship. Of the three students in the examples and case studies, with whom are you most similar, and why? What are experiences that might be easy and those that might be difficult for you during your fieldwork experience?

REFERENCES

Altfeld, D. A. (1999). An experiential group model for psychotherapy supervision. *International Journal of Group Psychotherapy, 49*(2), 237–254.

American Council for Occupational Therapy Education. (2006a). *Accreditation Standards for a Master's-degree-level Educational Program for the Occupational Therapist.* Bethesda, MD: American Occupational Therapy Association.

American Council for Occupational Therapy Education. (2006b). *Accreditation Standards for an Educational Program for the Occupational Therapy Assistant.* Bethesda, MD: American Occupational Therapy Association.

American Occupational Therapy Association (AOTA). (1994). Guide for supervision of occupational therapy personnel. *American Journal of Occupational Therapy, 48*(11), 1045–1046.

American Occupational Therapy Association (AOTA). (2005). *Model state regulation for supervision, roles and responsibilities during the delivery of occupational therapy services.* Bethesda, MD: Author.

American Occupational Therapy Association (AOTA). (2006). *Ad hoc committee to explore and develop resources for OT fieldwork educators.* Bethesda, MD: Author.

American Occupational Therapy Association (AOTA). (2007). AOTA's Centennial Vision and executive summary. *American Journal of Occupational Therapy, 61*(6), 613–614.

American Occupational Therapy Association (AOTA). (2009a). Occupational therapy fieldwork education: Value and purpose. In *The reference manual of the official documents of the American Occupational Therapy Association* (pp. 393–394). Bethesda, MD: American Occupational Therapy Association.

American Occupational Therapy Association (AOTA). (2009b). Specialized knowledge and skills of occupational therapy educators of the future (Official document). *American Journal of Occupational Therapy, 63*(6), 804–818.

American Occupational Therapy Association (AOTA). (2009c). *AOTA fieldwork Educator Certificate Program (FWECP)*. Bethesda, MD: Author.

American Occupational Therapy Association (AOTA). (2010a). Blueprint for Entry-Level Education. *American Journal of Occupational Therapy, 64*(1), 186–203.

American Occupational Therapy Association (AOTA). (2010b). Specialized knowledge and skills in mental health promotion, prevention, and intervention in occupational therapy practice. *American Journal of Occupational Therapy, 64*(6), 313–326.

Andersen, S. O., & Simhoni, O. (2002). Fieldwork: A road to employment. *Occupational Therapy in Health Care, 16*(1), 37–43.

Beltran, R. O., Scanlan, J. N., Hancock, N., & Luckett, T. (2007). The effect of first year mental health fieldwork on attitudes of occupational therapy students towards people with mental illness. *Australian Occupational Therapy Journal, 54*(1), 42–48.

Bernard, J. M., & Goodyear, R. K. (2004). *Fundamentals of clinical supervision*. Boston, MA: Pearson Education.

Blanchard, K., Zigarmi, P., & Zigarmi, D. (2003). *Overview of situational leadership: Workshop*. Escondido, CA: The Ken Blanchard Companies.

Bradley, L., & Gould, L. J. (2001). Psychotherapy-based models of counselor supervision. In L. Bradley & N. Ladany (Eds.), *Counselor supervision: Principles, process, and practice* (pp. 147–180). New York: Brunner-Routledge.

Campbell, J. M. (2006). *Essentials of clinical supervision*. Hoboken, NJ: Wiley.

Cara, E. D. (2000). *The effects of a prepracticum educational module on self-efficacy, self-esteem, anxiety, and performance*. Unpublished doctoral dissertation, The Fielding Institute, Santa Barbara, CA.

Christie, B. A., Joyce, P., & Moeller, P. L. (1985). Fieldwork experience, Part II: The supervisor's dilemma. *American Journal of Occupational Therapy, 39*(10), 675–681.

Cohn, E. S. (1989). Fieldwork education: Shaping a foundation for clinical reasoning. A. *American Journal of Occupational Therapy, 43*(4), 240–244.

Crist, P. (2000). Understanding the role of the fieldwork educator in occupational therapy education. In S. Merrill & P. A. Crist (Eds.), *Meeting the fieldwork challenge*. Bethesda, MD: American Occupational Therapy Association.

Crist, P. (2007a). Match supervision to the student: Part I. *Advance for Occupational Therapy Practitioners, 23*(14), 6.

Crist, P. (2007b). Match supervision to the student: Part II. *Advance for Occupational Therapy Practitioners, 23*(14), 6.

Crist, P. (2007c). Match supervision to the student: Part III. *Advance for Occupational Therapy Practitioners, 23*(17), 8.

Crist, P. (2007d). Match supervision to the student: Part IV. *Advance for Occupational Therapy Practitioners, 23*(21), 10.

Crist, P. (2010a). Coaching for fieldwork performance. *Advance for Occupational Therapy Practitioners, 26*(23), 8.

Crist, P. (2010b). Fieldwork instruction, supervision and coaching. *Advance for Occupational Therapy Practitioners, 26*(15), 11.

Crist, P., Muñoz, J. P., Hansen, A. M. W., Benson, J., & Provident, I. (2005). The Practice-Scholar Program: An academic-practice partnership to promote the scholarship of "best practices." *Occupational Therapy in Health Care, 19*(1/2), 71–93.

Fleck, S. (2001). Fifty-five years of supervision. In R. Balsam (Ed.), *Psychodynamic psychotherapy: The supervisory process* (pp. 3–23). Madison, CT: International Universities Press.

Foullette, V., & Batten, S. (2000). The role of emotion in psychotherapy supervision: A contextual behavioral analysis. *Cognitive and Behavioral Practice, 7*(3), 306–312.

Frum, D., & Opacich, K. (1987). *Supervision: Development of therapeutic competence*. Bethesda, MD: American Occupational Therapy Association.

Gillfillan, S. (2001). On teaching the role of neutrality in listening within the era of managed care. In R. Balsam (Ed.), *Psychodynamic psychotherapy: The supervisory process* (pp. 229–247). Madison, CT: International Universities Press.

Greer, J. A. (2002). There to turn for help: Responses to inadequate clinical supervision. *Clinical Supervisor, 21*(1), 135–143.

Gross, S. M. (2005). Student perspectives in clinical and counseling psychology practicum. *Professional Psychology: Research and Practice, 36*(3), 299–306

Hahn, W. K. (2001). The experience of shame in psychotherapy supervision. *Psychotherapy: Theory, Research, Practice, and Training. 38*(3), 272–282.

Hora, T. (1957). Contribution to the phenomenology of the supervisory process. *American Journal of Psychotherapy, 11*, 769–773.

International Coaching Federation Standards of Ethical Conduct. Retrieved from http://www.coachfederation.org/ethics/

International Association of Coaching. Retrieved from http://www.certifiedcoach.org/

Kolodner, E., Wiener, W., & Frum, D. (1989). *Models for mental health fieldwork.* Bethesda, MD: American Occupational Therapy Association.

Ladany, N., Lehrman-Waterman, D., Molinaro, M., & Wolgast, B. (1999). Psychotherapy supervisor ethical practices: Adherence to guidelines, the supervisory working alliance, and supervisee satisfaction. *Counseling Psychologist, 27*(3), 443–475.

Ladany, N., & Walker, J. (2003). Supervision self disclosure: Balancing the uncontrollable narcissist with the indomitable altruist. *Journal of Clinical Psychology, 59*(5), 611–621.

Leddick, G., & Bernard, J. (1980). The history of supervision: A critical review. *Counselor Education and Supervision, 19*(3), 187–196.

Ledlow, G. R., & Coppola, M. N. (2011). *Leadership for the health professional: therapy, skills and application.* Sudbury, MA: Jones & Bartlett Learning.

Lew, N., Cara, E., & Richardson, P. (2007). When fieldwork takes a detour. *Occupational Therapy in Health Care*, 21, 1-2105-122.

Lipsitt, R. (2009). *Occupational therapy level II fieldwork: Effectiveness in preparing students for entry-level practice in a rehabilitation setting.* Unpublished dissertation: Temple University, Philadelphia.

Loganbill, C. R., Hardy, E. V., & Delworth, U. (1982). Supervision: A conceptual model. *Counseling Psychologist, 10*(1), 3–42.

Meerloo, J. A. (1952). Some psychological processes in supervision of therapists. *American Journal of Psychotherapy, 6*, 467–470.

Merriam, S., & Caffarella, R. (1991). *Learning in Adulthood* (pp. 86–90), San Francisco: Jossey-Bass.

Mezirow, J. (2000). Learning as transformation: Critical perspectives on a theory in progress. In J. Mezirow & Associates (Eds.), *Learning to think like an adult: Core concepts of transformation theory* (pp. 3–34). San Francisco: Jossey-Bass.

Munroe, H. (1988). Modes of operation in clinical supervision: How clinical supervisors perceive themselves. *British Journal of Occupational Therapy, 51*(10), 338–343.

Neistadt, M. (1996). Teaching strategies for the development of clinical reasoning. *American Journal of Occupational Therapy, 50*(8), 676–684.

Nelson, M. L., & Friedlander, M. L. (2001) A close look at conflictual supervisory relationships: The trainee's perspective. *Journal of Counseling Psychology, 48*(4), 384–395.

Nelson, M. L., Gray, L. A., Friedlander, M. L., Ladany, N., & Walker, J. A. (2001). Toward relationship-centered supervision: Reply to Veach (2001) and Ellis (2001). *Journal of Counseling Psychology, 48*(4), 407–409.

Noelle, M. (2003). Self-report in supervision: Positive and negative slants. *Clinical Supervisor, 21*(1), 125–134.

Oegren, M. L., Apelman, A., & Klawitter, M. (2001). The group in psychotherapy supervision. *Clinical Supervisor, 20*(2), 147–175.

Peyton, E. A. (2002). Reflecting on the therapeutic relationship: A qualitative study of trainees' experiences in learning a relational treatment modality. *Dissertation Abstracts International, 63*(6B), 3020 (UMI AAI3056998).

Privott, C. R. (1998). *The fieldwork anthology: A classic research and practice collection.* Bethesda, MD: American Occupational Therapy Association.

Ramos-Sanchez, L., Esnil, E., Goodwin, A., Riggs, S., Touster, L. O., Wright, L. K., et al. (2002). Negative supervisory events: Effects on supervision and supervisory alliance. *Professional Psychology: Research and Practice, 33*(2), 197–202.

Rose, M., & Best, D. (2005). *Transforming practice through clinical education, professional supervision and mentoring.* Edinburgh, England: Elsevier.

Schön, D. (1987). *Educating the reflective practitioner: How professionals think in action.* San Francisco: Jossey-Bass.

Schwartz, K. B. (1984). An approach to supervision of occupational therapy students. *American Journal of Occupational Therapy, 38*(6), 393–397.

Shanfield, S. B., Hetherly, V. V., & Matthews, K. L. (2001). Excellent supervision: The residents' perspective. *Journal of Psychotherapy, Practice, and Research, 10*(1), 23–27.

Smith, V. (2006). A study of the perception of occupational therapy students after completing fieldwork level II clinical training in the United States on supervision characteristics. Unpublished Dissertation: University of Tennessee.

Sorlie, T., Gammon, D., Bergvik, S., & Sexton, H. (1999). Psychotherapy supervision face to face and by videoconferencing: A comparative study. *British Journal of Psychotherapy, 15*(4), 452–462.

Stanley, P. (1996). Mental health: An endangered occupational therapy specialty. *American Journal of Occupational Therapy, 50*(1), 65–68.

Sumerall, S. W., Barke, C. R., Timmons, P. L., Oehlert, M. E., Lopez, S. J., & Trent, D. D. (1998). The adaptive counseling and therapy model and supervision of mental health care. *Clinical supervisor, 17*(2), 171–176.

Taylor, J. M., & Neimeyer, G. J. (2009). Graduate school mentoring in clinical, counseling & experimental academic training programs. *Counseling Psychology Quarterly, 22*(2), 257–266.

Trant, R. P. (2001). Elements and outcome of school psychologist internship supervision: A retrospective study. *Dissertation Abstracts International 61*(9–A), 3477.

Vidlak, N. W. (2002). Identifying important factors in supervisor development: An examination of supervisor experience, training, and attributes. *ETD collection for University of Nebraska–Lincoln.* Paper AAI3055295. Retrieved from http://digitalcommons.unl.edu/dissertations/AAI3055295

Whitman, S. M. (2001). Teaching residents to use supervision effectively. *Academic Psychiatry, 25*(3), 143–147.

Whitmore, J. (2009). *Coaching for performance.* Boston, MA: Nicholas Braeley Publications.

Yourman, D. B. (2003). Trainee disclosure in psychotherapy supervision: The impact of shame. *Journal of Clinical Psychology, 59*(5), 601–609.

SUGGESTED RESOURCES

Amerantes, J. (1994). *Supervisory styles of practicing occupational therapists.* Unpublished manuscript, San Jose State University, San Jose, CA.

Cara, E. (1994, May). *Ways of supervision: The Learning Styles Inventory.* Workshop presented at the San Jose State University Fieldwork Council.

Cara, E., & Schwartz, K. (1992, October). *Reflections on clinical supervision: What works, what doesn't.* Workshop presented at the Occupational Therapy Association of California, Los Angeles.

Cohn, E., & Frum, D. (1988). Fieldwork supervision: More education is warranted. *American Journal of Occupational Therapy, 42*(5), 325–327.

Kasar, J., & Clark, E. N. (2000). *Developing professional behaviors.* Thorofare, NJ: Slack.

Lewin, J. E., & Reed, C. A. (1998). *Creative problem solving in occupational therapy.* Philadelphia: Lippincott.

Mitchell, M., & Kampfe, C. (1990). Coping strategies used by occupational therapy students during fieldwork: An exploratory study. *American Journal of Occupational Therapy, 44*(6), 543–549.

Palladino, J., & Jeffries, R. N. (2000). *The occupational therapy manual for assessing professional skills.* Philadelphia: F. A. Davis.

Scott, S., Wells, S., & Hanebrink, S. (1997). *Educating college students with disabilities: What academic fieldwork coordinators need to know.* Bethesda, MD: American Occupational Therapy Association.

Sladyk, K. (2002). *The successful occupational therapy fieldwork student.* Thorofare, NJ: Slack.

Stafford, E. (1986). Relationship between occupational therapy student learning styles and clinic performance. *American Journal of Occupational Therapy, 40*(1), 34–39.

Swinehart, S., & Meyers, S. (1993). Level I fieldwork: Creating a positive experience. *American Journal of Occupational Therapy, 47*(1), 68–73.

Wells, S. A., & Hanebrink, S. (1998). *A guide to reasonable accommodations for occupational therapy practitioners with disabilities: Fieldwork to employment.* Bethesda, MD: American Occupational Therapy Association.

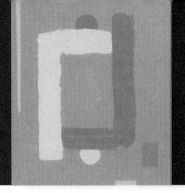

12-step programs Treatment programs for addiction based on principles of Alcoholics Anonymous. 12-step programs have been called a biopsychosocialspiritual model because they address interactive biological, psychological, social, and spiritual causative factors of addiction.

A

Abstract thinking The ability to critically reason using analytical methods to infer relationships between differing ideas and to filter irrelevant data from relevant data.

Acting out The expression of thoughts and feelings through maladaptive behavior instead of recognizing and verbalizing those ideas.

Activity group One whose content focuses on activity, emphasizes occupation, and addresses occupational performance components or skills to aid in occupational performance.

Acute pain A temporary pain that begins suddenly and is felt sharply that lasts no longer than months.

Adaptation Adjustment to one's disability.

Addiction Abnormal physical and/or psychological dependence on a substance or activity despite negative consequences on one's health.

Adjudication The legal proceeding in which a final judgment is made based on evidence presented, from the first hearing of evidence to final pronouncement and sentencing.

Adjustment In the context of this book it means adjustment to life with a physical disability.

Advocacy An act of an individual or group whose aim is to influence public policy and the allocation of resources within political, economic, and social systems and institutions. Acts of advocacy might include media campaigns, writing letters to people/institutions of influence, producing research, writing letters to editors, blogging about an issue, and lobbying to legislators.

Affect A freely provided and unconditional liking for another person as an individual, without demands or expectations on that person's behavior.

Affect regulation Abilities of infants and children to organize their emotions and develop self-regulating patterns of behavior.

Affective instability Marked shifts from baseline mood to depression, irritability, or anxiety.

Aging in place Intervention theory that promotes allowing aging individuals to live in the environment they are most comfortable and familiar with and for the best care possible to be provided in this location.

Allopathic Refers to the tradition of medicine practiced in the West.

Americans with Disabilities Act (1990) A U.S. federal law that provides for equal access and opportunity to all qualified individuals with disabilities in the areas of employment (Title I), equal access to public services (Title II), physical access to public facilities and transportation (Title III), and communications (Title IV) (EEOC, U.S. Department of Justice, 1991).

Animal-Assisted Therapies/Activities (AAT/AAA) A goal-directed intervention in which an animal that meets specific criteria is an integral part of the treatment process. AAT is designed to promote improvement in human physical, social, emotional, and/or cognitive functioning.

Anosognosia Refers to a cognitive impairment of persons with frontal lobe damage that inhibits them from recognizing deficits in cognition, perception, or mobility.

Applied Behavioral Analysis (ABA) A systematic model that strives to objectively measure, evaluate, and influence socially important human behavior that is extensively used with people who have intellectual and developmental disabilities or dementia. It needs further research due to criticisms about its outcomes.

Area of Operations (AO) An operational area defined by the joint force commander for land and naval forces. Areas of operation do not typically encompass the entire operational area of the joint force commander, but should be large enough for component commanders to accomplish their missions and protect their forces.

Army Physical Fitness Test (APFT) A physical fitness test that soldiers are required to take at least twice per year. There are three events that are measured: push-ups, sit-ups, and a timed two-mile run. Soldiers are required to score a minimum of 60 points on each event.

Assertive Community Treatment (ACT)   A form of "full-support" therapy that is characterized by small caseloads, a multidisciplinary team rather than single case manager responsibility, 24-hour coverage, time-unlimited service, significant provision of *in vivo* outreach, and direct skill training.

Assessment   A process involving the selection and application of a range of informal and standardized methods (interview, observation, questionnaires, dynamic assessment, and document review) to collect information from relevant sources.

Attachment behaviors   Any form of behavior that results in a person attaining or maintaining proximity to some other clearly identified individual who is conceived of as better able to cope with the world.

Attachment patterns   Characteristic ways of responding and relating to others based on early relationship bonds.

Attachment styles   Individual differences or patterns and behaviors that occur when there are consistent patterns of adequate, good-enough parenting or when there are patterns of inconsistent, inadequate, or insufficient parenting.

Autogenic training   A relaxation program that teaches people to respond physically and mentally to their own verbal commands.

Ayurvedic   The traditional medical practices of India.

B

Benzodiazapines   A group of medications that act as sedatives and are commonly used for treatment of anxiety.

Biopsychosocial focus   The theoretical paradigm that aims to provide the most comprehensive understanding of the development of normal and abnormal behavior by exploring the interaction among biological, psychological, and social influences on behavior.

Biopsychosocialspiritual model   A model that explains the development of addiction as an interaction among biological, psychological, social, and spiritual factors. 12-step programs are an example of a biopsychosocialspiritual model.

Board and care   A non-medical community-based residential facility or home that provides structured activities, meals, and supervision. Licensing and staffing requirements vary by state or region.

Brain plasticity   "The ability of the nervous system to change." The brain is much more changeable than formerly considered. Neurons grow and change throughout the lifespan in reaction to new experiences.

C

Carer   Any person involved in a relationship with another person, usually volunteer or unpaid, and can include family members, friends, and neighbors.

Chronic pain   Pain that endures beyond a time frame that would be considered part of a healing process or acute injury stage. Chronic pain may be caused by any number of variables, including, but not limited to nerve damage from a congenital issue, injury, illness, or medication, muscle abnormalities from immobility, illness, or lack of physical activity.

Client-centered approach   An approach to providing occupational therapy that recognizes the autonomy of the person receiving services as well as the need for client choice in making decisions regarding occupational needs. This approach emphasizes respect for the client and builds on the strengths clients bring to the occupational therapy encounter.

Clinical reasoning   Refers to forms of reasoning or rational thinking that the occupational therapist uses to always guide methods and interpersonal strategies used in practice in collaboration with the client. A thinking process that allows practitioners to use reflection, evidence, and judgment to evaluate ideas and make decisions related to practice.

c/mTBI   "... an injury to the brain resulting from an external force and/or acceleration/deceleration mechanism from an event such as a blast, fall, direct impact, or motor vehicle accident (MVA) which causes an alteration in mental status typically resulting in the temporally related onset of symptoms such as headache, nausea and vomiting, dizziness/balance problems, fatigue, insomnia/sleep disturbances, drowsiness, sensitivity to light/noise, blurred vision, difficulty remembering, and/or difficulty concentrating."

Coaching   Providing psychological support, e.g., motivation, empowerment, coping, to another individual at the person-centered factor level.

Co-existing disorders   Complex health needs and complex mental health disorders exist in one person, particularly returning wounded warriors, that make occupational therapy particularly important to assessment.

Cognitive-Behavioral Therapy (CBT)   A family of treatment approaches that includes rational behavior therapy, cognitive therapy, and dialectic behavior therapy. These approaches are based on the premise that disordered thoughts cause disordered feelings and behaviors.

Cognitive Behavioral Treatment (CBT) A branch of psychology treatment that combines elements of behaviorism and cognitive therapy that is currently one of the most popular forms of treatment and many intervention strategies are borrowed from this approach.

Cognitive deficits A broad range of impairments, including but not limited to actual intelligence. In schizophrenia, the common cognitive deficits include poor judgment and reasoning, impulsivity, limited ability to abstract, and delayed processing time.

Collaborative service delivery model A service delivery model that includes working with a variety of professionals while utilizing a team approach to determine and deliver services.

Combat Operational Stress Control (COSC) Leader actions and responsibilities to promote resilience and psychological health in military units and individuals, including families, exposed to the stress of combat or other military operations.

Combat Operational Stress Reactions (COSR) The expected and predictable emotional, intellectual, physical, and/or behavioral reactions of service members who have been exposed to stressful events in war or military operations other than war. Combat stress reactions vary in quality and severity as a function of operational conditions, such as intensity, duration, rules of engagement, leadership, effective communication, unit morale, unit cohesion, and perceived importance of the mission.

Community support team Support given by many members of a community to a client with serious and persistent mental illness.

Compassion fatigue The term refers to a physical or emotional fatigue the therapists experience when treating trauma. The experience could be similar to the symptoms of their client, though is less intense.

Comorbidity The term used to recognize co-existing health conditions regardless of the order of onset. Co-morbidity may designate the presence of two or more psychiatric diagnoses, or physical conditions, or a combination of both.

Compliance Complying with the actions or demands of others. Within a medical perspective, the term is used to denote the act of following a prescribed course of treatment. However, within a personal recovery perspective, it is often viewed as coercion because of the lack of collaboration in the decision-making process.

Compulsions Repetitive and deliberate actions intended to diminish obsessions.

Confabulation A behavioral reaction to memory loss in which the client fills in memory gaps with inappropriate words or fabricated details, often in great detail.

Consistency The routine, reliable aspects of treatment that develop trust and reliance in the human and nonhuman environment.

Coping strategies Strategies developed alone or through professional intervention that enable a disabled person to better cope with his or her circumstances.

Corrections The aspect of the criminal justice system that provides incarceration for those convicted for crimes, designed to punish, rehabilitate, or some combination, and includes the parole and probation period, as well as the administrative system charged with implementing and overseeing all activities.

Cortisol A hormone responsible for regulating stress.

Criminal justice An extensive system involving administration and enforcement of the laws governing criminal behavior including law enforcement, the courts, correctional facilities, parole, and probation of those charged with illegal behavior.

Critically Appraised Topics (CATs) A brief summary of the search and critical appraisal of the best available research evidence on a focused clinical topic.

Culture-bound syndrome Manifestations of mental illness unique to a particular cultural group.

Curative occupations A course designed to educate institution attendants in occupations for those with mental illness.

Cyclothymia A *DSM-IV* diagnosis that includes symptoms of mania, but is considered less severe than bipolar disorder.

D

DALYs Abbreviation for "disability-adjusted life years," which is the total number of years lost to illness, disability, or premature death within a population.

Decompensation When an individual experiences a regression in the progress made in recovery from a mental illness as evidenced by the return of clinical symptoms and an exacerbation of the disorder.

Delirium An acute confusional state accompanied by agitation, with a quick onset and fluctuating levels of alertness.

Delphi study A research method that is an iterative process collecting the judgments of experts. It is a sequential method of obtaining data and feedback at different junctions thus distilling the judgment of the experts.

Dementia A medical condition of deteriorated mentality often accompanied by emotional apathy and identified by the presence of multiple cognitive defects.

Demotivational syndrome Lack of interest and apathy toward previous occupations or events often resulting from frontal lobe damage.

Depersonalization Feelings of unreality.

Depression A pervasive and sustained emotional state.

Derealization Feeling of being detached from one's surroundings.

Detachment The dispatch of a military unit, such as troops or ships, from a larger body for a special duty or mission.

DFAC Dining facility in a military combat zone.

Diagnosis The result of a process of elimination in which a disorder is identified by meeting very specific criteria, including demographic information such as age, as well as range, severity, and duration of symptoms.

Dialectical Behavioral Therapy (DBT) A manualized or structured, uniform popular intervention method with some outcomes-related research, which has emerged within cognitive behavioral approaches and is used with people with borderline personality disorder or other disorders in which there is impulsive and self-injurious behavior such as self-cutting.

Diffuse axonal injury An injury resulting from the tearing and shearing of the axons of the nerve fibers throughout the brain due to the bouncing of the brain within the skull. The injury is not visible through brain imaging.

Dimensions A hierarchy of lower-order personality traits that are organized into higher-orders categories such as neuroeroticism or extraversion.

Disinhibition A condition resulting from frontal lobe damage causing a client to lose the ability to filter or screen behavior, often resulting in inappropriate language or actions.

Dissociation Where the mind blocks out aspects of consciousness to avoid thinking about a traumatic event; affects memory, sense of reality, and sense of identity or self (APA, 2000).

Diurnal system System responsible for regulating sleeping and waking.

Dual agency The role of an occupational therapist serving soldiers and wounded warriors is both to clients and to the primary military mission.

Dynamic A way of interacting between or among people; generally applied to a pattern of relating that is not explicitly or consciously acknowledged.

Dynamic assessment An assessment process that is not limited to the identification of deficits or what the person can achieve, but also the extent to which performance can be improved. Dynamic assessment focuses on individual variations in function under different circumstances rather than comparing the person to normative data or a criterion reference.

Dysfunction A deficit in the ability to perform tasks. It is often a result of effects of symptoms but there is not always a direct correlation. Occupational therapists view these deficits in a function/dysfunction continuum in the realm of occupational performance that includes work, leisure, and self-care activities.

Dysthymia A *DSM-IV* diagnosis that includes symptoms of major depression, but is considered less severe than major depression.

E

Eclectic Combining, sometimes synthesizing, information or practice approaches from a variety of sources including, but not limited to evidence, theories, frames of reference, expert modeling, prior experiences, and so on. Used to refer to theorists and practitioners who do not adhere to any one system of beliefs, but who select and utilize what they consider to be the best elements of many different theories in their attempts to understand and treat aberrant behavior and psychological dysfunction.

Education Acquisition of the knowledge, attitude, and skills in a given content area, such as, practice competencies related to the occupational therapy process.

Ego-syntonic Not disturbing to the ego; generally applied to disordered traits or patterns that would usually be disturbing.

Elder abuse The physical, emotional, or sexual abuse of the elderly in their own home or in nursing care facilities.

Electroconvulsive Therapy (ECT) A form of treatment for mental disorders, particularly depression, by the induction of unconsciousness and convulsions through the use of electric current applied to the brain.

Environmental contexts Describes the influences from a variety of environmental factors including cultural, social, physical, temporal, personal, virtual, and institutional that have an impact on occupation, occupational engagement, and occupational performance.

Epistemology A branch of philosophy concerned with knowledge, including the nature of knowledge, how knowledge is produced, the relationship of knowledge to truth and beliefs, and the validity of knowledge claims.

Ethology The study of primates in their environments and how they are influenced by their environment.

Evaluation A component of a broader assessment process. Data is collected to inform judgments about amount, degrees or levels of a specific construct, component or characteristic (e.g., level of independence) or to make a judgment about the degree to which an intervention has achieved the planned outcomes for a person or a group of people. Evaluation usually requires data to be collected at two time points in order to measure change over time. Evaluation may involve the translation of observations to numerical scores.

Evidence-based practice An approach to intervention that involves integrating a systematic analysis of the existing literature with the client's personal narrative and experience and the specific expertise of the practitioner.

Evolutionary theory "[S]pecies-specific system behaviours that lead to certain predictable outcomes, at least one of which contributes to reproductive fitness" (Cassidy, 2008, p. 5).

Executive function The ability to connect the intellectual functions of abstraction, reasoning, judgment, and analysis with current actions. People with deficits in executive function have difficulty in planning, organizing, and strategizing.

Extrapyramidal Symptoms (EPS) A set of possible neurological side effects most often associated with psychotropic medication. Commons symptoms associated with EPS include extreme restlessness and involuntary muscle movements.

F

Far forward Service members are treated close to the point of injury (far forward), rather than evacuating them out of the war zone as in past conflicts.

Fieldwork education AOTA mandated developmental experiences for students to integrate academic knowledge with practice skills.

Feng-Shui A Chinese art form that is concerned with how energies of the environment interact with individuals and their dwellings.

G

Generalization Using the same cognitive and functional skills in a variety of different environments.

Geriatric Branch of medicine that deals with the problem and diseases of old age.

Glasgow Coma Scale (GCS) A general assessment of neurological status often used in the hospital emergency departments or trauma centers to characterize severity of traumatic brain injury. It uses a 15-point system to test motor, eye-opening, and verbal capabilities (a higher score suggests less severe injury).

Goal setting An active collaboration and negotiation between the recipient of services and the therapist to develop agreed upon goals of intervention.

Group Two or more people who have a consciousness that they are a group. An intentional gathering of people for the purpose of change.

Group content Activity carried out in the group; what is said in the group. It can be verbal or nonverbal.

Group dynamics The forces that influence the relationships of members and influence the group outcome.

Group norms Standards, either implicit or explicit, verbalized or unstated, that are often developed by a group leader or based on group interaction.

Group process How the work of a group is carried out, including how participants relate to each other, who talks to whom, how tasks are accomplished and how decisions are made, and how therapy is undertaken; patterns or stages that groups usually go through.

Group protocol A description of a group, including its purpose, goals, content, structure, logistics, who would and would not benefit by participation in it, and referral process.

Group structure The way in which the activity is presented; the directions, procedures, techniques, and time arrangements; and the way in which membership is organized.

H

Habit training The development of cultural, personal, and occupational habits in the client with mental illness.

"Hardwired" An expression originating in computer science that designates an innate biological structure.

Harm reduction A therapeutic approach to addiction that views any changes leading to reduced usage as positive and healthy. If terminating usage is deemed unlikely, small steps are introduced to reduce usage and harm to physical, mental, and social functioning.

Health care disparities Differences in health outcomes, burden of disability or disease, or access to health care between different groups of people within countries and between countries.

Hoarding The acquisition of possessions and the inability to discard them, even if others deem the items worthless. Hoarding is considered to be compulsive or pathologic when the practice causes significant distress and impairs one's ability to perform basic activities of daily living or function in a work or community setting.

HPA effect   Early stress and developmental trauma influences the hypothalamic-pituitary-adrenal (HPA) system that is responsible for regulating an individual's stress response.

I

In vivo   A Latin term referring to any treatment or intervention that occurs within a client's natural environment ("in real life"), rather than in the artificial or simulated environment of a hospital, clinic, or laboratory setting.

Individual Placement and Support (IPS) model   A model of employment services where the individual is placed in a job of that client's choice, then provides intensive supports, including on-the-job training and ongoing assessment in the actual workplace context for as long as the client needs it.

Initiation   Refers to the ability to begin an activity at an appropriate time to accomplish a goal.

Institutionalized   The term originally referred to the placement of an individual in some form of treatment center, often against one's will. The term has also come to mean a set of passive or dependent behaviors that result from long-term placement.

Intentional Relationship Model   A conceptual practice model that explains how therapists can promote occupational engagement through an interpersonal reasoning process that involves choosing the appropriate mode of communication.

Intercultural Development Continuum (IDC)   A developmental continuum to understand how people tend to think and feel about diversity, progressing from a lesser to a more complex perception and experience of cultural differences.

Interdisciplinary   An approach to treatment that includes different disciplines that understand the specific role of each in collaboration with the team.

Internal working models   Internal working models are mental representations of self and other in past interactions that allow predicting future experience.

International Classification of Functioning, Disability, and Health (ICF)   A global classification system published by The World Health Organization (WHO) that is based on components of health and helps the occupational therapist understand the complexity of having a disability (WHO, 2001).

Interpretation   A therapeutic technique of putting words to behavior enabling the child to express feelings with words, which is more often appropriate than other means such as aggression or acting out.

Intersubjective process   A condition where the occupational therapist is more reflective, self-aware, and insightful in the therapeutic process because he or she is aware or the process between the therapist and client where each is affected by the other's subjective meanings and this interplay in turn affects the therapeutic process.

Intrapersonal   Denotes a person's internal, psychological process.

J

Job coach   A person providing a service whereby assistance is given in any or all of the phases of the supported employment (SE) approach, for example, skills training, job modifications, employee/employer interventions, and ongoing support.

K

KAWA Model   A theoretical framework as well as a practice tool to examine one's life circumstances through the metaphorical representation of the cross section of a river (Japanese word for river is *kawa*).

Knowledge   Principles and facts gained through classroom instruction.

L

Latency age   Between the ages of approximately 5 to 12 years. In Freudian theory, the stage when both sexual and aggressive drives and impulses are latent, or hidden and subdued.

Learning   Acquisition of new or adaptation of existing knowledge, which is the foundation for reflecting on facts, behaviors, and skills or synthesizing information from multiple sources.

Least restrictive environment   Environment with the optimum balance of individual freedoms and supervision where the client can function.

Life satisfaction   A person's satisfaction with the circumstances of her or his life. Life satisfaction is not necessarily correlated with the severity of a disability.

Lifestyle redesign   An approach utilized in occupational therapy to help clients make life changes that are healthy, meaningful, and satisfying. It was originally designed specifically for the well elderly but the approach is now used with a variety of populations.

Lived experience The preferred term to designate a first-hand account of a person's life. It is most commonly used in reference to people with mental illness or members of other disenfranchised groups. The term derives from a phenomenological research perspective, which strives to understand the personal and subjective view of an individual's life experiences.

Living Skills Development Group A group designed to help members develop mastery in basic and instrumental activities of daily living.

Lobotomy A surgical procedure introduced in the 1930s in which the nerve fibers connecting the frontal lobes to the thalamus were severed. It was thought to relieve some symptoms of mental disorders but permanently disabled people and is now banned.

M

Mania A mood that is elevated, expansive, or irritable. Associated symptoms are hyperactivity, pressured speech, flight of ideas, diminished need for sleep, grandiosity, distractibility, short attention span, and extremely poor judgment in interpersonal and social areas.

Maternal sensitivity Measurement of the caregiver response to children's signals.

Mayor's Cell A Mayor's Cell is responsible for all service members and civilians residing in a military compound in an operational area. It is responsible for base life support, force protection, and infrastructure.

Medicare A U.S. government-sponsored health care payment program, primarily for those over 65 years of age.

Melancholia As an emotional symptom, it is detachment, alienation, sadness, apathy, and dejection. Formerly used as a clinical term to describe the mental disorder of depression.

Mentalization A method that focuses on individual's capacities to understand their own and others' mental states in an attachment context (valued relationship).

Mentor A wise and trusted counselor, instructor, guide, coach, or advisor.

Meta-analysis A systematic method of combining and statistically analyzing data from several independent studies of the same intervention to calculate the overall effect of the intervention.

Milieu treatment A treatment approach that sets rules and expectations for the entire community as they interact together and originally all staff, whether health professionals or maintenance people, were trained in how to respond in a similar manner to the community.

Military Acute Concussion Evaluation (MACE) A neurologic screen to determine if the service member displays symptoms or red flags consistent with a diagnosis of c/mTBI.

Mindfulness A mental state of being aware of one's sensations, thoughts, bodily states, consciousness, and the environment, while also being accepting, open, and curious (Hofmann et al., 2010).

Model of Human Occupation A conceptual practice model that explains how occupation is motivated, patterned, and performed. Understanding these aspects of occupation is important in terms of therapeutic reasoning, choice of assessments, and treatment planning.

Monochronic (M-time) View of time as linear, as a commodity, and as something that can be saved or lost.

Mood An emotional state that usually colors one's whole psychological life.

Moral treatment A system of treatment for those with mental illness consisting of humanitarian and therapeutic approaches to illness and characterized by kindness and respect for the client.

Morale, Welfare, and Recreation (MWR) A network of support and leisure services designed for use by service members (active, Reserve, and Guard), their families, civilian employees, military retirees, and other eligible participants.

Motivational interviewing An evidence-based, person-centered counseling approach that uses nondirective, reflective listening.

Moxibustion An alternative medical practice from Asia employing cauterization and counter-irritation to treat disease.

N

Negative symptoms Absent or decreased emotional and behavioral repertoire. Includes flat affect, alogia (poverty of speech), avolition (poor initiation of activities and/or inability to sustain goal-directed activities), and anhedonia or hypohedonia (inability or decreased ability to experience pleasure).

Neurasthenia Term used by psychiatrists to refer to nervous conditions such as hysteria, hypochondria, depression, compulsive behavior, and anxiety.

Neuroplasticity The ability of the brain to reorganize alternate neuronal pathways to compensate for damaged areas.

Non-didactic developmental guidance A method that assumes caregivers are those best to use information about their child considering the relationship and emotions between the caregiver and parent.

Nondirective play group A play group that allows children to gravitate to and engage in the play occupations of their own choosing without the direction or suggestions for participation from the group leader.

O

Obsessions Persistent thoughts and images that are experienced as intrusive and unwanted.

Occupation-based interventions Refers to the use of occupation as a treatment modality and emphasizes occupations that are meaningful and pertinent to the client's daily life and goals for living.

Occupation-Based Self-Determination (OBSD) Derived from two models, one of self-determination and one occupation-based, refers to the opportunity for clients to be the primary agent in autonomously choosing occupations that are satisfying and maintain quality of life while using a plan, act, evaluate strategy.

Occupational alienation A social condition that deprives an individual or group of the experiences of meaningful and enriching engagement in occupations leading to alienation from the community.

Occupational apartheid The restriction or denial of access to meaningful occupations through the segregation of groups' based on their status in society.

Occupational deprivation A social condition, experienced by an individual or a group, with prolonged exclusion from meaningful and/or necessary occupations. Situations of occupational deprivation may include refugeeism, sex-role stereotyping, over or underemployment, incarceration, and geographic isolation.

Occupational enrichment The provision of environmental supports, resources, tools, and opportunities for a person or persons to engage in healthful and sociocultrally appropriate activities, usually provided in environments deprived of these resources.

Occupational health The balance of physical, mental, and social well-being derived through healthy work, household management, leisure, childcare, and other activities that are socially valued and individually meaningful.

Occupational imbalance The social condition of being occupied too little or too much of the time to engage in meaningful and necessary occupations.

Occupational justice The right of an individual or group to engage in occupations that are meaningful and enriching. Occupational justice describes the rights of individuals or groups to exert autonomy through choice in participation and engagement in occupations that are in the typical range of occupations within the community and of significant value to the group or individual.

Occupational marginalization A social condition that does not allow for individual choice and control in decision making of daily activities, occupations, and events.

Occupational profile Profile intended to provide an understanding of the client's occupational history and experiences, patterns of daily living, interests, values, and needs.

Occupational prognosis Predictions of the person's likely response to occupational therapy intervention and the degree to which identified contextual facilitators and barriers may impact progress toward achieving the person's desired outcomes.

Occupational restriction Context where an individual's choice of occupations is severely restricted and controlled by others.

Offender A person convicted of breaking a public law.

Ongoing assessment Monitoring how the client reacts and responds to interventions and engaging the client in review of progress toward goals at regular points throughout the process.

Ontology A branch of philosophy concerned with the meaning of existence and being in the world.

OT BCT mTBI Reconditioning Program In combat theaters designed to conduct far forward treatment of c/mTBI and other biopsychosocial conditions in a multidisciplinary outpatient setting at the BCT level.

Outcome The measured or observed consequence of an action. Outcomes may refer to a client's *desired outcome;* the *predetermined outcomes* that a service is expected to deliver, as described in a service level agreement or commissioning contract; the *negotiated outcome* between a client and therapist, as articulated in a goal; and the *actual outcome* which is the measured effects of a specific intervention or the effects of a multidisciplinary or interagency management plan for the client.

Outcome measure A measurement designed to evaluate change over time in order to establish whether the intervention has achieved the anticipated outcome.

P

PACE Model A model developed by Daniel Hughes (2006), which advocates an approach by those working with foster children that is playful, accepting, curious, and empathic.

Paradigm shift A significant change in the beliefs, values, and practices of a society.

Parallel task group A group that is structured by each client having his or her own project, which encourages work in a specific spot, focuses attention on a personal project, and provides opportunities for sharing and social interaction.

Participation Engaging in everyday activities and occupations that individuals want and need to do.

Perseveration Refers to the inability to disengage from an activity and reengage in other activities.

Personality Style of relating, coping, behaving, thinking, and feeling. A concept that represents a network of traits that persist over a lifetime.

Personhood skills Skills that depend on personal traits acquired through a combination of temperament and experience.

Polychronic (P-time) Cyclical and unscheduled time, typically a natural rhythm where several things can happen at once and is not controlled by human beings.

Polyculturalism State of identifying oneself as a member of several different cultural backgrounds.

Positive Behavioral Interventions and Supports (PBIS) A decision-making framework used in public schools that utilizes evidence-based practices to improve academic and behavior outcomes for all students.

Positive regard A freely provided and unconditional liking for another person as an individual, without demands or expectations on that person's behavior.

Positive symptoms The active symptoms of psychotic disorders, including delusions and hallucinations as well as disorganized speech and behavior.

Post-traumatic amnesia Short- or long-term memory deficits resulting from concussion or other brain trauma.

Power struggles Engaging with youth in struggles for power and control. This can cause role confusion for the therapist and the youth, and encourages youth to perpetuate negative, challenging behaviors. Alternatively, providing choices gives the adolescent the opportunity to have a sense of control and the ability to express autonomy in an acceptable, positive manner.

Prevention teams In combat areas of operation, generally consist of two to three members whose primary mission is to overcome the stigma of mental health by developing positive relationships with its neighboring units and commanders.

Prevocational services Offered to clients prior to returning to or obtaining work and based on tasks and skills needed for work, a program can target deficits and symptoms associated with failure to succeed in workplace integration.

Prisonization A phenomenon in which an incarcerated offender gradually adopts the norms of institutional life into habits, cognition, emotions, and actions.

Private First Class (PFC) A military rank.

Proxemics An aspect of culture that refers to people's use and comfort with personal and social space.

Psychiatric or psychosocial rehabilitation The use of various interdisciplinary interventions aimed at restoring function and role performance. The goal is to assist people with severe mental disabilities to function at their highest potential, in their environment of choice, with the least amount of professional support necessary.

Psychoanalysis A major theory and method considering unconscious processes and sexuality founded by Sigmund Freud at the turn of the 20th century that became a popular psychological treatment in Europe and the United States.

Psychobiological A major theory and approach proposed by Adolph Meyer at the turn of the 20th century that considered both "nature and nurture," that one's performance and occupational history were as important as biological and neurological information.

Psychodynamic Aspect of a therapeutic process in which change is brought about primarily by talking and reflecting on one's thoughts and actions, and by a therapist's or group leader's interpretations. It assumes an unconscious process.

Psychoeducational Aspect of a therapeutic process in which change is brought about by learning or through education, usually about a psychological topic. There is a clear objective to teach specific information or techniques.

Psychogenic Originating in the mind or in mental or emotional conflict.

Psychopathology From the Greek, meaning "the study of mind or brain disease," refers to the study and classification of symptoms; can characterize a condition as a mental disorder.

Psychopharmacology The science of how drugs effect psychomotor behavior and emotional states.

Psychosis Significant impairment of reality testing and daily functioning due to the presence of positive symptoms.

Psychotropic A descriptor for an agent, usually a prescribed drug, that directly affects the actions of the brain.

Q

Quality of life A term difficult to define in the medical literature but generally meaning a concept broader than health or disease and consisting of such characteristics as good mobility, social relations, self-esteem, independent living, and other daily living factors.

R

Rancho Los Amigos Levels of Cognitive Functioning A common rating scale used to assist an interdisciplinary assessment and treatment team in determining a client's cognitive, behavioral, and functional status following brain injury.

Recidivism Relapse by a former offender to criminal behavior that is usually measured as arrest, conviction, or incarceration for a new crime within three years of release or parole.

Recovery model "Recovery is described as a deeply personal, unique process of changing one's attitudes, values, feelings, goals, skills, and/or roles." (Anthony, 1993, p. 11)

Reactive attachment disorder A *DSM* disorder either inhibited, or withdrawn and unable to form attachments with any one person, or disinhibited, or forming attachments with any person indiscriminately regardless of attachment history.

Redirection A verbal tactic that adds to the structure of therapy by refocusing the child on the assigned or current activity in which the child is participating and providing cues as to appropriate involvement or behavior.

Reentry The term applied to the transition from incarceration to community-living for offenders upon release from their prison, jail, or community corrections sentence.

Referential thinking A belief that an individual is the cause or reason for someone else's thoughts, feelings or behavior in the absence of evidence.

Reflection Introspection of ideas and prior outcomes to either improve or guide clinical reasoning to facilitate "best practices" with current or future practice experiences.

Relationship Connection between two individuals that is facilitated by their context, roles, or common interests of shared goals.

Reliability The dependability and accuracy of assessment scales.

Reproductive or inclusive fitness Behavior that assures that one's genes will survive.

Resiliency A quality of a person; hardiness, strength, or being quick to recover.

Restoration programs Typically three-day programs designed for service members experiencing combat operational stress reactions (COSR).

Role acquisition frame of reference A frame of reference used in occupational therapy concerned with the learning of social roles required of the individual in an expected environment.

S

School mental health movement Refers to an increased focus on providing the full continuum of mental health services to students in general and special education including mental health promotion, early intervention, prevention, and treatment. This movement emphasizes an approach involving the family, school, and community working in partnership for wellness.

Second impact syndrome Occurs if a second c/mTBI occurs during the acute recovery period from a first injury.

Secure base functions The ability to feel secure (affect regulation) in the context of protection (including psychological availability) in a relationship.

Self-concept The mental image one has of oneself.

Self-Development Group A group that targets the capacity for self-discovery, -management, and -expression through exploration of personal factors in the context of an occupation-based theme.

Self-efficacy Belief that oneself can overcome barriers or problems in spite of obstacles.

Self-mutilation Intentional, non-suicidal self-inflicted wounds to one's own body, often done with sharp objects. These individuals frequently have difficulty expressing their emotions appropriately and directly, and use self-mutilation/cutting as a maladaptive coping skill for expression of difficult or problematic feelings.

Sensory Overresponsive Type (SOR) A newer term for sensory defensive individuals and refers to hypersensitivity and sensory defensiveness.

Sergeant First Class (SFC) A noncommissioned rank in the U.S. Army that is above staff sergeant and below master sergeant.

Seriously and Persistently Mentally Ill (SMI) Persons suffering the most severe forms of mental or physical disorder.

Service Member (SM) A member of the U.S. armed forces, active duty Soldiers, Reservists, National Guard, Sailors, Airmen, Marines, and Veterans.

Shared decision making The practice of collaboration between a recipient of mental health services and one or more members of the professional service team. Shared decisions include all aspects of services including course of treatment, medications, information sharing, and long-term planning.

Solution-Focused Brief Therapy (SFBT) A therapeutic approach that focuses on using clients' strengths to gather resources for goal achievement. Attention is focused on envisioning goals, and directing resources to that end. SFBT is a form of cognitive behavioral therapy.

Somatic Physical concerns.

Specialist (SPC) An enlisted rank in the U.S Army corresponding to the grade of corporal.

Splitting A psychoanalytic concept, considered a defense, that causes an individual to perceive people as either all good or all bad and be unable to acknowledge both negative and positive features in one person. Resulting behavior may correlate with destabilizing relationships among staff members.

Standardized In order to be considered standardized a test should: identify the population for whom the test was developed; provide a clear, systematic procedure for test administration including guidelines for observing behavior or asking questions; outline how information collected should be recorded in terms of fixed categories or a numerical scale; explain how information collected should be interpreted; and provide details of research related to the test's psychometric properties.

Strange Situation A formal research method to research situations where infants and toddlers were separated from their caregivers, then reunited with them.

Strategies Refers to the tangible tools that are often readily identified or observed in practice. Strategies are used interchangeably in this text with techniques. Strategies or techniques include the tangible tools that are often readily identified or observed in practice and also abstract abilities the person uses to fulfill the plan, or apply the methods, such as the style, finesse, capacity, craftsmanship, approach, or resourcefulness of the therapist.

Structure Providing a form and design for treatment.

Style Inclination to use the same adaptive strategies in various situations. A stable, consistent approach to attending, perceiving, and thinking. Cognitive style or orientation. Distinctive categorization of action that is individual to the person or a collection of characteristics or traits.

Substance abuse Abnormal and harmful pattern of use of a psychoactive substance.

Suicide When an individual chooses to end his or her own life, frequently as a result of ongoing depression, other mental health disorders, and/or psychosocial stressors. A major preventable public health problem, it is a leading cause of death of young people aged 15 to 24 years of age.

Supervision A process in which two or more people make a joint effort to promote, establish, maintain, and/or elevate a level of performance and service. The act of overseeing the application of knowledge in a clinical setting and providing guidance through instruction.

Supported Employment (SE) An approach grounded in psychiatric/psychosocial rehabilitation that assists a person to choose, get, and keep a job. It is often referred to as the Choose, Get, Keep approach.

Symptom A subjective experience of the individual, such as what he or she may feel, do, or think. It is different from a sign, which is the objective finding of a medical practitioner.

Systematic reviews The process of systematically searching, analyzing, and synthesizing all eligible research on a specified topic in order to answer a research question with the goal of minimizing bias and providing more reliable findings to guide clinical decision making.

T

Techniques Refers to the tangible tools that are often readily identified or observed in practice. *Techniques* is used interchangeably in this text with the term strategies. *Strategies* or techniques include the tangible tools that are often readily identified or observed in practice and also abstract abilities the person uses to fulfill the plan, or apply the methods, such as the style, finesse, capacity, craftsmanship, approach, or resourcefulness of the therapist.

Telepsychiatry A form of telemedicine. The technology used to provide an array of services including medication management, diagnosis, and assessment, as well as individual and group therapy. It is most widely used in rural and other underserved areas but is gaining in popularity throughout the world.

Therapeutic competencies Essential skills to support occupational therapy practitioners in their respective practices.

Three-tiered intervention approach An approach based on the idea that 80% of students can benefit from universal instruction, 15% need more specific and targeted interventions, and 5% of students need intensive, specialized instruction.

Time-out An intervention technique that results in behavioral changes and increases the child's understanding of her role in a situation by removing the young person from a problematic situation to a specific area.

TM/CAM Traditional medicine (TM) means the approach to medicine primarily practiced within one's own culture while complementary and alternative medicine (CAM) is typically viewed as health care techniques and treatments not compatible with Western medical practices.

Traits Distinguishing characteristics of one's personal nature. A person can respond to a particular situation in a particular way. When the response occurs in a variety of situations it becomes a habit. A group of response habits that form a repetitive way of psychological functioning or relating to the environment can be classified as a trait.

Transformative learning Going beyond mere accumulation of factual knowledge to actual reflection and re-evaluation of knowledge, beliefs and behaviors that leads to self-authorship and new action or application options.

Translational research/science Research that transfers knowledge obtained through basic science research into its application in clinical or community settings with the goal of improving the health of populations.

Treatment box A container that can be used by occupational therapy practitioners "on-the-go" to generate interest in occupational therapy. It contains all intervention items including but not limited to crafts, forms and worksheets, flyers or signs, client-goals, and assessment results.

Treatment buy-in A term commonly used in behavioral health and refers to the patient's commitment to change.

U

Unit ministry teams A chaplain and chaplain's assistant added to the military's combat operational stress control (COSC) unit team.

Universal design The design of products and environments usable by all people without the use of adaptation or specialized design.

Universal Design for Learning (UDL) The development of curriculum and teaching strategies that gives all individuals equal opportunities to learn. UDL provides a guide for creating instructional goals, methods, materials, and assessments that work for everyone and incorporate flexible approaches that can be customized and adjusted for individual needs.

V

Validity A term used in standardized tests to report the degree to which the test measures what the test is designed to measure and corresponds accurately to actual performance.

Vasodilatation Expansion of the blood vessels especially small arteries.

W

Well elderly Healthy and active older persons.

Warrior Intended to instill basic values of courage, honor, and commitment, as well as a sense that being a soldier, sailor, airman, or Marine is more than a job, more than a career, but is a calling, an identity, and a way of life.

Workload vs. caseload Terminology to describe time allocation of a school-based occupational therapy role. The workload approach promotes job descriptions for occupational therapists being determined by a collaborative service delivery model that is performed within the contexts of natural environments. A caseload approach operates from the viewpoint that the therapist's time is spent serving individual students in a one to one, often out of context, setting.

Work programming The focused application of occupational therapy principles, knowledge, and skills to assist people to work productively and resume culturally valued roles in their community. The term *work* is any productive activity, paid or nonpaid, that is valued and seen as contributing to the community.

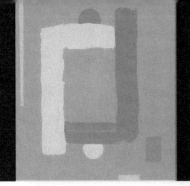

INDEX

A

Abstract thinking, impairment after brain injury, 560
Abuse and neglect
  attachment and, 359–364
    adoption, 360–361
    developmentally disabled children, 363–364
    foster care and institutionalization, 359–360
    middle childhood, 361–363
    neglect, 360
    parental abuse, 360
    reactive attachment disorder, 359
    secure base functions, 361–362
  elder abuse, 490–491
  HPA effect, 358–359
Acceptance
  defined, 54
  on the Intercultural Developmental Continuum, 54
Achiever students, 936
Acquired amputation
  phantom limb, 527
  phantom limb pain, 577
  psychosocial impact of, 526–527
  psychosocial issues, assessments, and interventions, 520
Acquisition frames of reference, 812–813
Acting out, 386
Action processes, 661
Action research, 87–88
Activity
  action processes, 661
  ADL. See Activity of daily living (ADL)
  categories, 662–663
  characteristics, 663–664
  configuration, 283, 298
  form and structure, 660
  groups, 677, 692–693
  occupation vs., 119
  outcome, 661
  properties, 660–661
  realistic and symbolic meaning, 661–662
  therapeutic use of, 659–660

Activity of daily living (ADL)
  activity groups, 693
  adolescent presenting problems, 433
  criminal justice, 727
  evaluations, 213
  groups, 697
  life satisfaction and quality of life, 518
Acute onset of disabling conditions, 514–516
  chronic disorders with acute onset, 523–530
    acquired amputation, 526–527
    cerebrovascular accident, 529–530
    overview, 523
    spinal cord injury, 523–526
    stroke, 529–530
    traumatic brain injury, 527–528
  disruption, 515
  enduring the self, 515–516
  striving to regain self, 516
  vigilance, 514–515
Acute pain, 574–576
Acute stress disorder, 268–269, 907–909
Adaptation, 510–516
  acute onset of disabling conditions, 514–516
  chronic disabling conditions, 510–514
  coping strategies, 510
  defined, 54
  factors, 518–519
  on the Intercultural Developmental Continuum, 54
  life satisfaction, 514
Addiction. See also Substance abuse
  as choice, habit, or disease, 843–844
  costs of, 842–843
  defined, 842
  risk factors, 843–844
  12-step programs, 844–848
ADHD. See Attention deficit hyperacticity disorder (ADHD)
Adjudication, 718–719, 720
Adjustment to life with physical disability, 504
ADL. See Activity of daily living (ADL)

Adler, Alfred, 146
Administration on Aging statistics, 474, 490
Adolescent and Adult Sensory Profile, 460
Adolescent mental health, Ch. 13
  bullying, 442–444
  case illustration, 465–468
  cultural effects on, 430–431
  disorders, 431–432
  eating disorders, 440–442
    interventions, 441–442
    treatment for, 440–441
  economic effects on, 430–431
  etiology of mental health or illness, 429–431
  evaluation, 460–461
  intervention, 461–468
    arts and crafts, 462–463
    case illustration, 465–468
    creative expression, 464–465
    games, 445, 463
    overview, 461–462
    resources for facilitating groups, 463–465
  presenting problems, 433–434
  psychopharmacology, 448
  rewards of working with adolescents, 469
  school violence, 442–444
  self-mutilation, 438–440
    causes of, 439
    defined, 438
    occupational therapy interventions, 439–440
    symptoms, 438
  settings and programs, 450–459
    evidence-based programs, 457–459
    group vs. individual services, 456
    implementing programs, 459–460
    inpatient programs, 451
    outpatient therapy, 452–454
    partial hospitalization, 451–452
    school-based programs, 455–457
    traditional settings, 451

Adolescent mental health, Ch. 13 (Cont.)
  suicide, 435–438
    contract for safety, 437
    frequency of occurrence, 435
    ideation, 436
    intent, 436
    occupational therapy, 437–438
    plan, 436
    prevention programs, 436–437
    risk factors, 435–436
  treatment
    eating disorders, 440–441
    limit setting, 444–445
    medications/
      psychopharmacology, 448
    power struggles, 445–446
    structure and consistency, 444
    team approach, 447–448
    therapeutic environment, 447
    therapeutic use of self, 446–447
Adolescent/Adult Sensory Profile
    Assessment, 33
Adoption and attachment theory,
    360–361
Adoption studies for genetic factors in
    psychopathology, 142
Adrenocorticotropin (ACTH), 141
Adult mental health. See Older adult
    mental health
Adult Sensory Profile, 211–212, 324
Advising, 647
Advocacy, 13, 655, 775–776
Affect
    affective disorder, bipolar illness, 229
    affective disorders, 223
    affective instability, 318
    causes of, 180
    defined, 180, 222
    depression, 181
    flat affect, 180
    flattening or blunting, 203
    lability, 181
    regulation, 357–359
Aggression following brain
    injury, 562
Aggression Replacement Training
    (ART), 458
Aging adults. See Older adult mental
    health
Aging in place, 489, 490
Agitation following brain injury, 562
Agoraphobia, 266
Agreeableness, 316
AIDS, 119
Ainsworth, Mary, 347, 351–354, 356
Alcohol abuse. See also Substance
    abuse
  Alcohol Severity Index, 851
  Alcoholics Anonymous, 862, 867

"at risk" or "heavy" drinking
    criteria, 842
  costs of, 842–843
  dependence on alcohol, 842
  "low risk" drinking criteria, 842
  physical changes due to, 844–845
  psychological changes due to, 845
  risk factors, 843
  social changes due to, 845
  spirituality, 845
  traumatic brain injury and, 549
  12-step programs, 844–848
  used with depression and bipolar
    episodes, 234
Alcohol and Drug Abuse (ADA) Center,
    861–868
  demographics of women, 862
  groups, 864–867
  hope, 862
  insidiousness of dependence, 861
  living skills, 867–868
  occupational therapy programming,
    862–864
  programming, 862
  self-discovery, 861
  student participation, 868
Allen Cognitive Levels (ACL) screening,
    33, 818, 903
Allen Diagnostic Module, 903
Alliances, work, 814–815
  community allies, 815
  internal allies, 815
Allopathic medicine, 42
Alogia, 203
Alzheimer's disease
  Alzheimer's Disease International,
    485, 492
  clinical course of, 481
  diagnosis, 480, 482
  frequency of occurrence, 480
American Occupational Therapy
    Association (AOTA)
  AOTA/FAST Research Project,
    442–443
  Blueprint for Entry-level Education,
    924, 949
  Centennial Vision, 70–71, 954–955
  children's mental health issues, 422
  core values, 41
  culture, defined, 41
  environment and culture, 29
  evidence related related to
    occupational therapy in
    criminal justice, 745–751
  Fieldwork Educator Certificate
    Program, 929, 956
  fieldwork supervision, 925–926
  founding of, 103
  intervention research, 69

  norms, 610
  Occupational Therapy Research
    Agenda, 71
  OTPF. See Occupational Therapy
    Practice Framework (OTPF)
  quality of life assessment, 485
  school mental health movement, 775
  Specialized Knowledge and Skills
    in Mental Health Promotion,
    Prevention, and Intervention in
    Occupational Therapy
    Practice, 926
  Specialized Knowledge and Skills of
    Occupational Therapy Educators
    of the Future, 926
  2017 Centennial Vision, 926
American Occupational Therapy
    Foundation (AOTF)
  intervention research, 69
  Occupational Therapy Research
    Agenda, 71
American Psychiatric Association
    (APA), DSM. See Diagnostic and
    Statistical Manual (DSM)
American Psychological Association
    (APA), 633
Americans with Disabilities Act, 814
Amnesia
  from acute stress disorder, 269
  post-traumatic amnesia, 544
Amputation. See Acquired amputation
Anatomical aberrations, 139
Anhedonia, 203
Animals used in occupational therapy
  animal-assisted activities, 882
  animal-assisted therapy, 881–883
  military applications, 881–883
  purpose of, 31
  therapy dogs, 882–883
Anorexia Nervosa, 440. See also Eating
    disorders
Anosognosia, 559
Anthony, William, 8
Anticipatory anxiety, 262
Antisocial personality disorder, 320–
    321, 326
Anxiety disorders, Ch. 9
  acute stress disorder, 268–269
  in adolescents, 432
  agoraphobia, 266
  anxiety, defined, 259
  assertiveness and social skills
    training, 287–290
  community mobility and
    reentry, 288
  craft and art activities, 289–290
  expressive activities, 288–290
  journal and diary writing,
    288–289

assessment, 278–280
derealization, 266
description, 261–263
  acute anxiety, 262
  anticipatory anxiety, 262
  anxiety, 262
  chronic anxiety, 262
  clinical anxiety, 262, 263
  free-floating anxiety, 262
  symptoms, 264
  trait anxiety, 262
due to general medical
  condition, 269
frequency of occurrence, 259
functional behavioral training,
  290–292
  education and lifestyle
    alterations, 290–291
  rational-cognitive approaches, 291
  time management, 291–292
functioning, impact on, 263–265
generalized anxiety disorder, 269
obsessive-compulsive disorders,
  267–268. See also Obsessive-
  compulsive disorder (OCD)
in older adults, 476
panic attack, 266
panic disorder/agoraphobia, 266
post-traumatic stress disorder, 268.
    See also Post-traumatic stress
    disorder
relaxation training
  autogenic training, 287
  breathing exercises, 285–286
  progressive muscle relaxation, 286
  visualization, 286–287
separation anxiety disorder, 388
settings for encounters, 260–261
  acute inpatient, 260
  home care, 260–261
  outpatient, 260
social phobia, 267
specific phobia, 266–267
substance-induced anxiety
  disorder, 269
symptoms, 259–260, 264
treatment for, 269–277
  biofeedback, 276
  cognitive-behavioral treatment,
    272–273
  counseling, 272
  exposure and response
    prevention, 275–276
  eye movement desensitization
    and reprocessing, 276–277
  imaginal exposure, 274
  interoceptive desensitization, 275
  interpersonal skills training, 277
  meditation, 276
  mindfulness, 273–274
  occupational therapy, 277–278
  psychopharmacology, 270–272
  self-management techniques,
    277–278
  systematic desensitization, 275
  virtual exposure, 274
  in vivo exposure therapy, 274
treatment interventions, 280–298
  assertiveness and social skills
    training, 287–290
  case illustration, 293–302
  functional behavioral training,
    290–292
  relaxation training, 282–287
  sensory modulation
    interventions, 292–298
AOTA. See American Occupational
    Therapy Association (AOTA)
AOTF. See American Occupational
    Therapy Foundation (AOTF)
Applied behavioral analysis (ABA), 150,
  151–152
Appraisals, 154–155
Area of operations, 879
Arequipa Sanatorium pottery, 110
Arthritis, 576
Arts and crafts as occupational therapy
  during the 1940s and 1950s, 114
  for adolescents, 462–463
  for anxiety disorders, 289–290
  clay, 114
  commercial viability, 109–110
  creative expression, 464–465
  development of, 103–105
  furniture making, 101
  group protocols, 702
  pottery, 110
  remunerative permanent
    occupation, 110
  textiles, 102
  for wounded soldiers, 109–110
Assertive community treatment
  (ACT), 827
Assertiveness and social skills training,
  287–290
  community mobility and
    reentry, 288
  craft and art activities, 289–290
  expressive activities, 288–290
  journal and diary writing, 288–289
Assessment. See also Evaluation
  criminal justice intervention,
    726–727, 732–735
  descriptive assessment, 626–628
  desired outcomes, 604–605
  discriminative assessment, 627, 628
  evaluative assessment, 627, 628–629
  goal setting, 607–609
  key concepts, 603–615
Kinetic Self-Image Assessment, 406
military context, 894–896
on-going, 622
overview, 601–603
personality disorders, 323–324
predictive assessment, 627
process of, 615–624
  complexity of assessment, 623–624
  confidentiality, 615, 617
  occupational diagnosis, 618–622
  occupational profile, 617–618
  occupational prognosis, 622
  on-going assessment, 622
  organizational framework, 616
  outcome measurement, 623
  problem formulation, 618
  timing, 617
  "top-down" or "bottom-up"
    approach, 617
purposes of, 625–636
  clinical purposes, 627
  criteria for test selection, 625, 626
  discriminative assessment, 628
  dynamic assessment, 635–636
  evaluative assessment, 628–629
  observation data, 630–631
  proxy report, 631–635
  self-report, 629–630
  sources of information, 629–635
  underlying driver, 625
qualitative and quantitative data,
  603–604
relationship to evaluation and
  outcome measurement, 605
school setting, 793
standardized tests, 609–615
  design of the test, 613
  reliability, 610, 611, 613–614
  validity, 610, 612, 614–615
substance abuse, 851–853
tasks, 601–602
terminology, 604
vocational programming, 815–826
  case illustration, 825–826
  characteristics of models for
    positive vocational
    outcomes, 824
  Occupational Profile Worksheet,
    819, 820–823
  pre-employment placement,
    816–817
  pre-employment treatment,
    815–816
  Program for Assertive
    Community Treatment,
    818–819
  purpose of assessment, 818
  tests, 818–819

Assessment of Life Habits
  (LIFE-H), 324
Assessment of Motor Process Skills
  (AMPS), 211, 603, 631
Assessments and Communication of
  Interaction Skills (ACIS), 212
Assumptions
  balance of occupation, 83
  checking of, 83, 84
  numbers and experience, 86–87
  occupation and health
    relationship, 83
  occupation and meaning, 80
  privileged triad, 83
  in research, 80, 83
Asylums
  early facilities, 100
  furniture making in, 101
  Gardner State Colony, 102
  Lunatic Asylum, 100
  moral treatment, 100–105, 116
  Sheppard Enoch Pratt Asylum,
    101–102
  textiles made in, 102
Ataque de nervious, 43–44
Attachment theory, Ch. 11
  abuse and neglect, 359–364
    adoption, 360–361
    developmentally disabled
      children, 363–364
    foster care and
      institutionalization, 359–360
    middle childhood, 361–363
    neglect, 360
    parental abuse, 360
    reactive attachment disorder, 359
    secure base functions, 361–362
  affect regulation, 357–359
    HPA effect, 358–359
    interpersonal neurobiology, 358
  attachment behaviors, 348
  attachment styles, 354
  clinical programs, 364–366
    catching-up, 366
    child-parent psychotherapy, 365
    circle of security, 366
    leiden programs, 366
    Minding the Baby program, 366
    therapeutic tasks, 364–365
    UCLA family development
      program, 366
    video-feedback intervention, 365
  cross-cultural studies, 356–357
  defined, 348
  description, 147–148
  evidence-base, 351–354
  family relationships and, 344–345
  history of, 345–348
  internal working models, 350–351

occupational therapy, 366–378
  application of, 369
  case illustrations, 369–378
  non-didactic developmental
    guidance, 367
  PACE model, 369
  relationship-centered care, 368
  roles, 374
  strategies, 374
  support and advocacy, 367
  patterns of, 354–355
  phases of, 349–350
  psychotherapy practice and, 148
  Strange Situation, 347, 351–354
Attention deficit hyperactivity disorder
  (ADHD)
  in adolescents, 432
  adult issues, 386
  characteristics, 387
  subtypes, 387
  symptoms, 388–389
Attributions, 155
Atypical features, 226
Autism, 363–364
Autogenic training, 284, 287
Autonomy, 654, 942
Avoidant personality disorder,
  321–322, 326
Avolition, 203
Axis I and II disorders, 315
Ayurvedic medicine, 42

B

Back pain, 577
Backsliding of students, 946
Bandura, Albert, 154
Bar and bas mitzvahs, 431
Barton, George, 110
Bayley Developmental Scale, 363
Beck, Aaron, 154–155
Beck Depression Inventory (BDI), 234
Beck's Hopelessness Scale, 614
Behavior after brain injury, 560,
    562–564
  agitation and aggression, 562
  case illustration, 563–564
  demotivational syndrome, 563
  disinhibition, 562
  emotional responses, inappropriate,
    563–564
  hypersexual behaviors, 562
Behavioral interventions
  exposure and response prevention,
    275–276
  imaginal exposure, 274
  interoceptive desensitization, 275
  systematic desensitization, 275

virtual exposure, 274
in vivo exposure therapy, 274
Behavioral perspective in mental
    health practice, 150–153
  applied behavioral analysis, 150,
    151–152
  occupational therapy applications,
    152–153
  overview, 150–151
  terms, 151
Behaviorism, 150
Behavioural Assessment of
    Dysexecutive Syndrome, 897
Beliefs, 156
Benzodiazapines, 270
Bias, 41–42, 942–943
Bierer, Joshua, 112
Big Five Factors, 234
Big Three Factors, 234
Binge-eating disorder, 440. See also
    Eating disorders
Biochemical factors, 139–141
Biofeedback, 276
Biological perspective of mental health
    practice, 136–144
  biochemical factors, 139–141
  brain, 137–139
  brain plasticity, 143
  genetic factors, 141–142
  hormonal factors, 141
  occupational therapy applications,
    143–144
  overview, 136–137
  psychopathology causal factors,
    139–143
Biopsychosocial focus, 129, 172
Biopsychosocial model, 847
Biopsychosocial-spiritual model,
    844–845
Bipolar disorder
  in adolescents, 432
  bipolar I, 225
  bipolar II, 225
  bipolar III, 229
  brain evolutionary theory, 230
  in children, 386
  cyclothymia, 223
  etiologic theories of causes, 228–229
  in older adults, 477
  in prisons, 722
  recurrent affective disorders, 229
  soft bipolar spectrum, 229
  symptoms, 223, 225
  treatment, 235–238, 248
Board and care facilities, 5
Body functions, 504
Body language, 48
Body structures, 504
Bonder, B., 121

Borderline personality disorder
    case illustrations, 314, 332–334
    defined, 317–318
    Freudian programs, 148
    symptoms, 320–321
    treatment, 326
Bowlby, John, 345–347, 351–354
Brain
    Brain Injury Association of
        America, 542
    brain-derived neurotropic
        factor, 235
    CVA. See Cerebrovascular
        accident (CVA)
    evolutionary theory
        bipolar disorders, 230
        depression, 230
        psychotic disorders, 230
    functional brain anatomy, 544, 545
    lobes, 137–139
    lobotomy, 112, 115
    memory. See Memory
    neuroplasticity, 544
    neurotransmitter dysfunction,
        139–141
    plasticity, 143
    psychopathology causal factors, 139
    scans, 143–144
    schizophrenia and, 196, 197
    structures, 137
    TBI. See Traumatic brain
        injury (TBI)
Breathing exercises, 285–286
British Association of Occupational
    Therapists, 629
Budgeting, 40
Built environment, 30–31
Bulimia Nervosa, 440. See also Eating
    disorders
Bullying, 442–444, 775

C

California Occupational Preference
    Survey, 819
Calming rooms, 695
Canadian Association of Occupational
    Therapists, 625
Canadian Model of Occupational
    Performance and Engagement
    (CMOP-E), 624
Canadian Model of Occupational
    Performance (CMOP), 32, 776
Canadian Occupational Performance
    Measure (COPM)
    adolescent evaluation, 460
    assessment complexity, 625–626
    assessment of older people, 629

criminal justice use of, 758
    interview format, 212
    military occupational therapy
        evaluation, 903
    for occupational assessment and
        evaluation, 603
    psychosocial practice in the 1980s
        and 1990s, 118
    recovery, 18
    substance abuse evaluation, 852
    therapeutic competencies, 730–731
    traumatic brain injury, 556
Cancer and pain management, 576
Carers, 633–635
Carers Assessment of Difficulties Index
    (CADI), 634
Carers Assessment of Managing Index
    (CAMI), 634
Carers Assessment of Satisfactions
    Index (CASI), 634
Caring for our Family–Family
    Connections, 458
Case illustrations
    adolescent mental health or illness,
        449–450, 452–454, 457, 459–460,
        465–468
    anxiety disorders, 293–302
    attachment theory, 346, 350, 355,
        369–378
    children's mental health
        acting out, 395
        family-based therapy, 417–418
        games, 413–414
        Kinetic Self-Image Assessment,
            407–408
        reactive attachment disorder,
            389–391
        school-based programs,
            404–405
        therapeutic use of self, 400
    criminal justice, 717–718, 755–756,
        757–758, 764–765
    culture, 47, 49–50, 52–53
    environment, 36–37, 39
    fieldwork supervision
        counseling psychology model
            stages, 939, 940, 941
        developmental stages, 936–937
        instruction, 951
        situational supervision, 947–948
    goal setting, 607–609
    groups, 677–678, 683–685, 688,
        704–705
    interpersonal strategies, 646–647,
        650–651, 663–664, 665–667
    military occupational therapy,
        883–886, 888, 907–912
    mood disorders, 239–240, 241–243,
        248–251

older adult mental health,
        478–479, 484, 485–486,
        488–491, 495
    pain management, 584–586,
        591–592
    personality disorders, 314, 323,
        332–334
    physical disability and psychosocial
        issues
        chronic disabling conditions, 513
        chronic disorders with acute
            onset, 524, 525–526
        concept of self, 508
        life satisfaction, 517, 519
        Parkinson's disease, 531
        spina bifida, 534
        stroke, 529–530
    psychosocial occupational
        therapy in the school setting,
        785–786
    recovery perspectives, 7, 8–9, 11,
        12–13, 21, 23–24
    schizophrenia, 202–203, 204, 207
    school psychosocial occupational
        therapy, 778–779, 780–781,
        790–791, 795–797, 799–801
    substance abuse, 854, 855–856
    symptoms, diagnosis, and
        dysfunction, 167–168, 170
    traumatic brain injury, 549, 561,
        563–564, 566
    vocational programming, 825–826,
        827–829, 833–835
Case-specific empathy, 657–658
Catatonia, 183, 226
Catechol-O-methyltransferase
    (COMT), 197
CBT. See Cognitive-behavioral
    therapy (CBT)
Central pain syndrome, 576
Cerebral palsy
    psychosocial impact of, 532–533
    psychosocial issues, assessments,
        and interventions, 522
    social isolation and rejection caused
        by, 510–511
Cerebrovascular accident (CVA)
    affect disturbances, 180
    psychosocial impact of, 529–530
    psychosocial issues, assessments,
        and interventions, 521
    stroke, 529–530, 576
Chaining, defined, 151
Child and Adolescent Functional
    Assessment Scale (CAFAS),
    406, 460
Child Behavior Checklist, 460–461
Child Occupational Self-Assessment
    (COSA), 406, 581

Children
  and attachment. *See* Attachment
    theory
  child psychiatry, 119
  child-parent psychotherapy, 365
  mental health. *See* Children, mental
    health of
  with mental health disabilities,
    784–786
Children, mental health of, Ch. 12
  acting out, 386
  ADHD, 386, 387, 388–389
  adolescents. *See* Adolescent mental
    health
  bipolar disorder, 386–387
  communication disorders, 387
  current trends and
    recommendations, 421–422
  depression, 386
  disruptive behavior disorders, 387
  DSM-IV-TR diagnoses, 386–393
  eating disorders, 387–388
  elimination disorders, 388
  emerging areas of practice, 416–420
    foster care direct service, 419
    foster care expert witness, 418–419
    foster care occupational therapy,
      416–418
    home-based occupational
      therapy, 419–420
  fetal alcohol spectrum disorders, 392
  learning disorders, 387
  mental retardation, 386, 387
  motor skills disorder, 387
  overview, 385–386
  pervasive developmental
    disorders, 387
  program implementation, 405–415
    evaluation and assessment,
      406–408
    games, 409–415
    overview, 405–406
    play interventions, 408–409
  psychiatric intervention
    situations, 392
  reactive attachment disorder,
    388–389. *See also* Attachment
    theory
  selective mutism, 388
  separation anxiety disorder, 388
  settings and programs, 402–405
    overview, 402
    partial hospitalization, 405
    school-based programs, 402–405
  tic disorders, 388
  Tourette's, 386, 388
  treatment
    family involvement, 400–401
    group rules, 394
    interpretation, 397
    limit setting, 398–399
    medications, 401–402
    structure and consistency,
      393–397
    team approach, 400–401
    therapeutic use of self, 399–400
    therapy tips, 395
    time-out, 397–398
Choose-Get-Keep, 816
Chronic anxiety, 262
Chronic congenital nonprogressive
  disorders, 532–534
  cerebral palsy, 532–533
  spina bifida, 533–534
Chronic disabling conditions
  accepting changes, 514
  adapting to, 510–514
  appreciation of altered physical
    condition, 511–512
  identity goals, 512–513
  life satisfaction, 514
  reappraisals, 511
  struggling against, 512
  struggling with, 512
Chronic headaches, 578
Chronic pain, 574–576
Chronic post-surgical pain (CPSP), 577
Circle of security, 366
Circumstantiality, 177
Clanging, 177
Classical conditioning, defined, 151
Client-centered therapy approach, 781
Client-driven challenges, 656–657
Clinical anxiety, 262, 263
Clinical Dementia Rating (CFR)
  Scale, 628
Clinical reasoning, 652–655, 932
Clinics. *See* Institutions and clinics
Coaching
  Coaching for Performance, 950–951
  defined, 924, 948–949, 954
  fieldwork education, 954
  purpose of, 649
  during supervision, 948–952
Cochrane Collaboration Project, 198
Code words, 398
Cofabulation, 183
Cognistat, 897, 903
Cognition after brain injury, 557–560
  abstract thinking impairment, 560
  anosognosia, 559
  attention deficits, 557–558
  case illustration, 561
  executive function impairment, 560
  generalization of skills, 560
  information processing
    impairment, 559
  initiation impairment, 559
    memory impairment, 558–559
    orientation impairment, 557
    perseveration, 559
Cognitive deficits of schizophrenia, 193
Cognitive perspective in mental health
  practice, 153–156
  appraisals, 154–155
  attributions, 155
  beliefs, 156
  expectations, 154
  occupational therapy
    applications, 156
  overview, 153
Cognitive restructuring, 153
Cognitive triad, 155
Cognitive-behavioral therapy (CBT)
  for anxiety disorders, 272–273
  behavioral perspective in mental
    health practice, 150–151, 152
  for depression, 235
  Emotional Processing Theory, 272
  for mood disorders, 243
  for substance abuse, 844, 846–848
  supervision, 933–934, 935–937
Collaboration
  attachment therapy, 372–374
  fieldwork education, 954
  partnership research priorities, 69
  for recovery, 20–22
  research orientation in practice,
    73–74
  schizophrenia treatment, 206–210
    defined, 206
    goal attainment, 206–208
    psychotropic medication,
      208–210
  service delivery model, 799
Collectivistic culture, 506
Columbine High School shooting,
  402, 443
Combat operational stress control. *See*
  United States Army Combat
  Stress Control (COSC) units
Combat operational stress reaction
  (COSR), 878
CommonGround, 184, 186
Communication. *See also* Language
  body language, 48
  criminal justice skills, 736–740
  cross-cultural guidelines, 46
  culture and, 46–50
  disorders in children, 387
  gestures, 48
  of group leaders, 690, 691
  groups, 698
  of military occupational therapy, 902
  nonverbal, 48
  theoretically based, 173
  therapist and client challenges, 48, 49

Community
    alliances, 815
    case illustration, 47
    employment
        applying skills, 830
        competitive, integrated,
            828–829
        interventions, 830–831
        transitional, 817
    environment, 40–41
    groups, 696
    intervention roles, 13, 14–15
    mobility and reentry training, 288
    school involvement. See
        Community-based practice in
        schools
    stigma, 40
    support team, 814
Community-based practice in schools,
        781–801
    children with mental health
        disabilities, 784–786
    evaluation of psychosocial issues,
        787–791
    positive behavioral interventions
        and supports, 782
    Response to Intervention,
        781–782
    three-tiered approach, 781–784,
        796–797
    universal design for learning, 782
Comorbidity, 174
Compassion fatigue, 912
Competence, 654, 942
Complementary and alternative
        medicine (TM/CAM), 42–43
Complete State Model of Mental Health
    human scale research agenda, 92
    illustration, 70
    occupational therapy research, 69
    purpose of, 71
The Complete State Model of Mental
        Health, 175
Complex regional pain syndrome
        (CRPS), 577–578
Compliance with prescribed
        medication, 184
Compulsions
    defined, 183
    description, 267
    OCD. See Obsessive-compulsive
        disorder (OCD)
Concept of self
    after acquired amputation, 527
    after brain injury, 565–566
    after traumatic brain injury, 528
    physical disability and, 507–510
Concerns to recovery, 19–20
Concreteness, 177

Concussion
    postconcussion syndrome, 891
    second impact syndrome, 891
Concussion/mild traumatic brain
        injury (c/mTBI), 889. See also
        Traumatic brain injury (TBI)
Conditioned response, 151
Conduct disorder, 432
Confabulation, 558
Confrontation, 649
Confusion stage in the counseling
        psychology model, 938–940
Congenital nonprogressive disorders,
        532–534
    cerebral palsy, 532–533
    spina bifida, 533–534
Conscientious students, 935
Conscientiousness, 316
Conscious, defined, 145
Consultation, 654–655, 954
Contextual empathy, 657–658
Contextual factors, 504
Contextual Memory Test (CMT),
        636, 897
Contract for safety, 437
Coping strategies, 506, 510, 565
COPM. See Canadian Occupational
        Performance Measure (COPM)
Cortisol, 358–359
COSC. See United States Army Combat
        Stress Control (COSC) units
Cost benefit of occupational therapy,
        69–71
Counseling
    for anxiety disorders, 272
    fieldwork education, 954
    fieldwork supervision, 937–943
        confusion, 938–940
        integration, 940–941
        stagnation, 938, 939
        themes in the stages, 941–943
    by peers, 13, 14–15
    vocational programming, 826–829
Crafts. See Arts and crafts as therapy
Creative expression, 464–465
Criminal justice, Ch. 21
    adjudication, 718–719, 720
    corrections, 718
    crime as occupation, 761–762
    criminal thinking, 758–761
    evaluation, assessment, and
        intervention, 726–727, 728–729
    health care in the system, 721–722
    IADL, 728–729
    international perspectives, 722–724
    mental health in, 722–724
    occupational deprivation, 716
    occupational health, 763
    occupational justice, 716

occupational justice and injustice,
        725–726
occupational perspective of crime,
        762–763
occupational therapy, 724–725
occupational therapy intervention,
        744–754
    employment assessment and
        intervention, 752–754
    evidence for practice, 744–751
occupation-based self-
        determination, 727, 729–730
offenders with mental health
        conditions, 717
overview, 716
prisonization and errors in critical
        thinking, 754–758
recidivism, 716, 763
reentry into the community,
        763–765
scope of, 719–720
sexuality in correctional settings,
        742–744
slang terms, 736–739
stages of offender involvement,
        718–719, 720
therapeutic competencies, 730–742
    communication skills, 736–740
    defined, 730
    environmental assessment,
        730–731
    interpersonal skills, 736–740
    models of practice and
        assessments, 732–735
    models of practice and practice
        knowledge base, 731–732
    professional and ethical
        behavior, 740
    risk assessment, 730–731
    tools and materials, 740–742
    "three strikes" laws, 721
Criterion-referenced test, 610
Critical thinking, prisonization and
        errors in, 754–758
Critically Appraised Topics (CATs), 65
Culture, Ch. 2
    adolescent mental health or illness
        and, 430–431
    attachment theory and, 356–357
    bar and bas mitzvahs, 431
    case illustration, 47, 49–50, 52–53
    collectivistic, 506
    communication, 46–50
    core values, 41
    culture-bound syndrome, 43–44
    defined, 41
    ethnicity, 44–45
    gender, 119, 204–205
    health care and, 42–43

Culture, Ch. 2 (Cont.)
ideal routine, 506–507
identification, 44–45
individualistic, 506
institutional environment, 39–40
Intercultural Developmental
Continuum, 54, 55
language, 45–46
mental health and, 43–44
multiculturalism, 45
occupational therapy and, 53–56
occupational therapy bias, 41–42
occupational therapy issues, 119
personality disorders and,
318–319
physical disability and, 504–505
polyculturalism, 44–45
proxemics, 50
psychosocial issues in the school
setting, 788
race or ethnicity, 44–45
rites of passage, 430–431
routines, 507
self-concept, 507
social relationships, 50–51
time sense, 51–53
values, 50–51
Curative occupations, 107–108
Cutting. See Self-mutilation
CVA. See Cerebrovascular
accident (CVA)
Cyberbullying, 775
Cyclothymia, 223, 432

D

DBT. See Dialectical behavioral
therapy (DBT)
Declaration of Alma Ata, 77
Decompensation, 431, 433
Defense and Veterans Brain Injury
Center (DVBIC), 889
Defense Center of Excellence for
Psychological Health and
Traumatic Brain Injury, 900
Defense mechanism
defined, 145
ego defense mechanisms, 146
Delirium, 481–482
Delphi study, 67
Delusions
defined, 176
paranoid, 200
schizophrenia, 199–200
thought and, 176
Dementia
assessment, 619–620
causes of, 480

Clinical Dementia Rating (CFR)
Scale, 628
defined, 480
dementia praecox, 193. See also
Schizophrenia
diagnostic statement, 619–620, 621
in older adults, 478–479
symptoms, 476, 480
vascular dementia, 480
Demotivational syndrome, 563
Denial
defined, 54, 146
on the Intercultural Developmental
Continuum, 54
Department of Defense, 900–901
Dependent personality disorder,
321–322, 326
Depersonalization, 264, 269
Depression
acquired amputation and, 526
adolescent, 433
brain evolutionary theory, 230
case illustration, 239, 241–242,
248–250
in children, 386
chronic pain and, 578
defined, 222
depressive disorders
dysthymia, 223
symptoms, 223
electroconvulsive therapy, 112
etiologic theories of causes, 228–229
evaluation, 234
group protocol, 705–708
involuntary defeat strategies,
230–231
major depression
in adolescents, 432
episodes, 223
frequency of occurrence, 226–227
in prisons, 722
symptoms, 223, 224–225, 232–233
mania, 181
obsessive-compulsive disorders
and, 234
in older adults, 476–477, 478,
482, 493
panic, 234
symptoms, 181
treatment, 235–238, 244–247, 248
Derealization, 264, 266, 269
Descriptive assessment, 626–628
Developmental groups, 693–694
Developmental models of supervision,
934, 935–937
Developmentally disabled children and
attachment, 363–364
Devereux Workshops, 109
Diagnosis, 168–175

case illustration, 167–168, 170
classification, 171
client attitudes, 170
clinical terminology, 167
controversy, 168–171
DSM. See Diagnostic and Statistical
Manual (DSM)
language, 169
process, evolution of, 174–175
Diagnostic and Statistical
Manual (DSM)
biopsychosocial approach,
172–173
DSM-5, 174, 175
DSM-III, 174
DSM-IV, 174–175
DSM-IV Axis II (SCID-II), 324
DSM-IV-TR
acute military psychiatry, 900
adolescent mental health or
illness, 431–432
anxiety disorders, 261–262,
265–269
eating disorders, 440
intent of, 174
mental health of children,
386–393
mood disorders, 222–223
offender mental health, 722
reactive attachment disorder, 359
DSM-IV-TR personality disorders,
314–316
Axis I, 315
Axis II, 315
classifications, 319
clusters, 319, 326
dimensions, 315, 316
history of, 111
purpose of, 171–172
theories, 172–173
Diagnostic Interview for Borderline
Patients-Revised (CIB-R), 324
Diagnostic statement, 619–620, 621
Dialectical behavioral therapy (DBT)
behavioral perspective in mental
health practice, 150–151, 153
for personality disorders, 328–329
Diary writing, 288–289
Diet and schizophrenia, 198
Diffuse axonal injury, 544
Dimensions of personality
disorders, 315
Directive groups, 694
Disability
defined, 505–506
disability-adjusted life years
(DALYs), 63
physical. See Physical disability and
psychosocial issues

Disaster, military
  engagement in occupation, 886–887
  healthcare providers' role in
    self-care, 887–888
  response, 883–885
  teamwork, the value of, 885–886
Discriminative assessment, 627, 628
Disinhibition, 562
Disorders, defined, 224. *See also specific disorder*
Displacement, defined, 146
Dissociation, 908
Dissociative identity disorder, 193
Distemporality, 201–202
Diurnal system, 359
Dix, Dorothea, 100
Documentation of outcomes, 703–704
Dopamine
  biochemical factor in psychological
    disorders, 139
  research on, 140
  schizophrenia and, 197, 209
Down syndrome and attachment,
    363–364
Drama therapy, 674
Drug abuse. *See also* Substance abuse
  costs of, 842–843
  dependence, 842
  drug addiction, defined, 843
  Narcotics Anonymous, 844, 862
  physical changes due to, 844–845
  psychological changes due to, 845
  social changes due to, 845
  spirituality, 845
  12-step programs, 844–848
Drugs
  for ADHD, 388
  for adolescent mental illness, 448
  for anxiety disorders, 270–272
  asenapine for schizophrenia,
    197, 208
  benzodiazapines, 270
  beta-blockers, 272
  for bipolar disorders, 235
  as cause of mood disorders, 227
  for children's mental conditions,
    401–402
  chloral hydrate, 112
  chlorpromazine, 112–113
  for chronic pain, 578–579
  Clozapine, 209–210, 235
  CommonGround, 184, 186
  compliance with prescribed
    medication regimes, 184
  dementia and, 479
  for depression, 235
  experimentation and
    schizophrenia, 194
  extrapyramidal symptoms, 209

interventions for medication
    management, 185
  monoamine oxidase inhibitors,
    270–271
  morphine, 112
  phenobarbital, 112
  psychopharmacology. *See*
    Psychopharmacology
  psychotropic drugs, 184–186
    CommonGround, 184, 186
    compliance, 184
    interventions, 185
    for schizophrenia, 208–210
    side effects, 183
    use in the 1980s and
      1990s, 120
    Wellness Recovery Action
      Plan, 184
  rational polypharmacy, 235
  reactive attachment disorder, 388
  schizophrenia, 209–210
  serpasil, 115
  side effects, 113
  SSRIs, 270, 326
  substance-induced anxiety
    disorder, 269
  thorazine, 115
  twentieth century treatment, 112
*DSM. See Diagnostic and Statistical
    Manual (DSM)*
Dual agency, 899–900
Dunton, William Rush,
    103–105, 110
Dynamic, 397
Dynamic assessment, 635–636
Dysarthria, 178
Dysfunction
  case illustration, 167–168
  clinical terminology, 167
Dysthymia, 223, 432

E

Eating disorders
  in adolescents, 432, 440–442
  Anorexia Nervosa, 440
  binge-eating disorder, 440
  Bulimia Nervosa, 440
  in children, 387–388
  interventions for adolescents,
    441–442
  treatment for, 440–441
Echolalia, 177
Eclectic approach for mental health
    intervention, 129–130
Eclectic background of
    supervision, 932
Ecology of Human Performance, 118

Economics
  adolescent mental health or illness
    and, 430
  high school dropout rates, 430
ECT. *See* Electroconvulsive
    therapy (ECT)
Education
  alterations, 290–291
  educator in fieldwork setting, 924
  fieldwork education, 921, 923. *See
    also* Fieldwork supervision
  groups, 698
  purpose of, 655
Effects and indicators, 604
Ego
  defined, 145
  ego-syntonic feeling, 313
Elder abuse, 490–491
Electroconvulsive therapy (ECT)
  for bipolar disorders, 237
  case illustration, 5
  for depression, 235–236
  history of use, 112
  procedure for delivery of, 237
  side effects, 237–238
  use during the 1940s and 1950s, 115
Elimination disorders, 388
Ellis, Albert, 156
Emotional awareness, 942
Emotional freezing, 319
Emotional Processing Theory, 272
Emotionally congruent, 587
Emotionally Unstable Personality
    Disorder, 317–318
Empathy
  case-specific, 657–658
  contextual, 657–658
  defined, 133
  intersubjectivity, 658–659
  occupational therapy method, 654,
    657–659
Employment. *See also* Vocational
    programming
  accommodations, 832
  employer involvement, 831–832
  in-house jobs, 817
  job coach, 829
  sheltered, 817, 828
  supported, 814, 833–835
  transitional, 817, 827–828
  volunteer, 827
Employment Development
    Department, 830
Encouragement, 647, 648, 654
Energy and motoric response, 183
Environment, Ch. 2
  for adolescent therapy, 447
  analysis and adaptation, 34
  assessment, 33–34

Environment, Ch. 2 (Cont.)
  built environment, 30
  case illustration, 36–37, 39
  community, 40–41
  criminal justice, assessment,
      730–731
  defined, 29
  environmental or task-driven
      challenges, 656–657
  Feng-Shui, 30
  health impact, 29
  home, 40–41
  home-based occupational therapy,
      419–420
  institutional and clinic, 36–40
  internal, 331–332
  intervention, 33–34
  mental health treatment, 34–36
  natural (animals and plants), 30–31
  occupational therapy conceptual
      models, 32–33
  for older adults, 488–491
  physical environment of the school
      community, 789
  school contexts, 775
  universal design, 29–30
Episodes, 223–224
  hypomanic episode, 224
  major depressive episode, 223
  manic episode, 224
  mixed episode, 224
Epistemology, 75
Erhhardt Developmental Prehension
      Assessment (EDPA), 406
Erikson, Erik, 147
Ethics
  criminal justice occupational
      therapist, 740
  of research, 83, 85
    reflexivity, 85
    representation of others, 85
    transparency, 85
Ethnicity, 44–45. See also Culture
Ethology, 345
Ethridge's Pre-vocational Evaluation of
      Rehabilitation Potential, 818
Evaluation. See also Assessment
  adolescent programs, 460–461
  anxiety disorders, 278–280
  children's mental health programs,
      406–408
  criminal justice intervention,
      726–727
  Function Questionnaire, 281, 296
  of groups, 703–704
  key concepts, 603–615
  Kinetic Self-Image Assessment,
      407–408, 460
  older adult mental health, 482–486

of pain, 579–582
process of, 615–624
  complexity of assessment,
      623–624
  confidentiality, 615, 617
  occupational diagnosis, 618–622
  occupational profile, 617–618
  occupational prognosis, 622
  on-going assessment, 622
  organizational framework, 616
  outcome measurement, 623
  problem formulation, 618
  timing, 617
  "top-down" or "bottom-up"
      approach, 617
relationship to assessment and
      outcome measurement, 605
role checklist, 278, 279–280, 294–295
for schizophrenia, 210–212
self-assessment of activities, 283
standardized tests, 609–615
  design of the test, 613
  reliability, 610, 611, 613–614
  validity, 610, 612, 614–615
  terminology, 604
Evaluative assessment, 627, 628–629
Evidence gathering for research, 18
Evidence-based practice, 64–66
  for adolescents, 457–459
  defined, 64
  hierarchy of evidence, 64–65
  resources, 65–66
Evolution
  attachment theory, 345–346
  brain
    bipolar disorders, 230
    depression, 230
    psychotic disorders, 230
  diagnosis process, 174–175
  mood disorders, 230
  psychosocial occupational therapy,
      113–121
    1920s and 1930s, 113–114
    1940s and 1950s, 114–115
    1960s and 1970s, 115–118
    1980s and 1990s, 118–121
Executive function, 176, 560
Executive Function Performance Test
      (EFPT), 211, 635–636
Expectations, 154
Expert witness for a foster care agency,
      418–419
Explicit methods of psychosocial
      interventions, 664–667
Ex-PLISSIT model, 743
Explorer students, 936
Exposure and response prevention
      (ERP), 275–276
Expressive activities, 288–290

    craft and art activities, 289–290
    journal and diary writing, 288–289
Expressive/projective group, 697
Externalizing, 433–434
Extinction of behaviors, 151
Extrapyramidal symptoms (EPS), 209
Extraversion, 316
Eye movement desensitization and
      reprocessing (EMDR), 276–277

F

FACE Core Assessment and Outcomes
      Package for Mental Health
      Services, 602
FACE Risk Profile, 628
Families and Schools Together,
      442–443
Family
  attachment. See Attachment theory
  dynamics after brain injury, 566
  intervention roles, 13, 14–15
  involvement in children's therapy,
      400–401
  parent-child activity group, 415
  support the mentally ill members, 6
Family Focused Therapy (FFT), 236
Feng-Shui, 30
Fetal alcohol spectrum disorders
      (FASD), 392
Fibromyalgia, 577, 584–586
Fidler, Gail, 114, 117, 148–149
Fieldwork Educator Certificate
      Program (FWECP), 929, 956
Fieldwork supervision, Ch. 26
  clinical reasoning, 932
  coaching during supervision,
      948–951
  dimensions of fieldwork, 929–932
    supervisee responsibilities,
        931–932
    supervisor/supervisee
        relationship, 929–931
  educator knowledge and skills, 927
  educator or supervisor roles,
      923–926
  fieldwork education, 921, 923
  maximizing learning, 952–953
  models and methods, 934–943
    counseling psychology model,
        937–943
    developmental/cognitive
        perspective, 935–937
  reflection, 932
  situational supervision, 943–948
  student testimony, 921, 922
  supervision, defined, 955
  theoretical foundations, 932–934

cognitive-behavioral supervision, 933–934
developmental approaches, 934
eclectic background, 932
humanistic or person-centered supervision, 933
intrapersonal aspects, 932
psychoanalytic supervision, 932–933
psychodynamic supervision, 932–933
transformative learning, 924, 926–929
trends and recommendations, 953–957
Fit for purpose, 85–86
Flashbacks, 268
Flat affect, 180
Food substances and schizophrenia, 198
Foster care
attachment theory and, 359–360
direct therapy services, 419
expert witness, 418–419
occupational therapy services, 416
participatory research in program development, 89–90
Fountain House, 812
Frankl, Victor, 133–134
Free-floating anxiety, 262
Freezing, 319
Freud, Sigmund
borderline personality disorder programs, 148
neo-Freudian theories, 146–147
psychoanalysis, 144–145
theory of cause of psychological problems, 111
Function Questionnaire, 281, 296
Functional behavioral training, 290

G

Gamblers Anonymous, 844
Games
as adolescent therapy, 445, 463
"Game of Life", 445
as therapy for children, 408, 411
Gamma-aminobutyric acid (GABA), 139, 140
Gardner State Colony, 102
Gender. See also Culture
occupational therapy issues, 119
schizophrenia prognosis, 204–205
Generalization, 560
Generalized anxiety disorder (GAD), 269
Genetic factors in psychopathology, 141–142

Genuineness, 133
Geriatric Depression Scale, 482
Geriatrics, 474. See also Older adult mental health
Gestures, 48
Glasgow Coma Scale (GCS), 547, 548, 889
Global Deterioration Scale, 480, 481
Global Mental Health Initiative (GMHI), 67–68
Glutamate
biochemical factor in psychological disorders, 139, 140
schizophrenia and, 197, 209
Goals
Goal Attainment Scaling (GAS), 629, 703–704
goal-setting
desired outcomes, 607
occupational diagnosis, 622
schizophrenia treatment, 206–208
SMART, 607, 622
for student intervention, 298–299, 796–797
Good-Enough-Harris Draw-A-Person test, 406
Grading the activity, 290
Grand Challenges in Global Mental Health Initiative (GMHI), 67–68
Groups
activity group, 677, 692–693
ADA House interventions, 864–867
for adolescent therapy, 456
advantages of, 673–674
characteristics, 672–673
content and structure, 676
defined, 672
documentation, 703–704
dynamics, 676
group work, 212–213
history of group therapy, 674–675
interpersonal strategies, 665–667
involvement in children's therapy, 400–401
leader, 689–692
communication skills, 690, 691
leadership styles, 689–691
personhood skills, 690, 691–692
roles, 689–691
life skills, 702, 863
limitations of, 674
mindfulness, 695
models, 675–676
mutual help, 135
nondirective play group, 409
norms, 673
observation and documentation, 902–912

occupational therapy groups, 692–698
activity, 692–693
ADL, 697
communication, 698
community, 696
developmental, 693–694
directive, 694
education, 698
expressive/projective, 697
IADL, 697
leisure, 698
neurodevelopmental, 694
physical contexts, 698
psychoeducational, 696
self-help, 135, 696
sensory intervention, 694–695
spiritual, 698
task, 693
thematic, 697
vocational, 698
outcome, 703–704
parallel task group, 396
parent-child activity group, 415
for personality disorder treatment, 332
play groups, 409–415
problems in groups, 685–689
hostility, 687–689
leadership style and manner of interacting, 689
monopolizing, 687
nonparticipation, 686
overview, 686
process, 672, 677–678
protocol, 672, 701–703, 705–708
roles and functions, 681–685
self-development, 863, 864
stages and patterns, 679–681
final stage, 680–681
initial, 679, 681
overview, 679
transition, 679–680, 681
working, 680, 681
starting a group, 699–701, 704–705
structure, 672
task-oriented, 117
teams
in adolescent therapy, 447–448
in children's therapy, 400–401
therapy rules, 394

H

Habits
concept of self, 507–508
habit training, 106–108
Hall, Herbert James, 108–111

Hallucinations
  defined, 178
  functional deficits, 179–180
  patterns, 178–179
  of schizophrenia, 202
  senses involved, 178
Hamilton Rating Scale for Depression
  (HRSD), 234
Hardwired behaviors, 313
Harm reduction, 847–848
Head injury. *See* Traumatic brain
  injury (TBI)
Headaches, 578
Health care
  allopathic, 42
  ayurvedic, 42
  in the criminal justice system,
    721–722
  culture and, 42–43
  disparities in criminal justice, 726
  moxibustion, 43
  TM/CAM, 42–43
Hierarchy of needs, 131
Hippocrates, 222
Histrionic personality disorder,
  320–321, 326
Hoarding, 176
Holland's Self-Directed Search
  (SDS-R), 752
Home
  environment, 40–41
  home-based occupational therapy,
    419–420
  money management, 40
Homelessness, 120, 121
Hormonal imbalance, 139, 141
Horney, Karen, 147
Hospital Anxiety and Depression Scale
  (HAD), 278
Hospitalization for mentally ill
  children, 405
Hostility, 687–689
HPA effect, 358–359
Human Scale Development, 91–92,
  131, 134
Human scale research, 91–92
Humanistic perspective of mental
  health practice, 130–136
  development of, 130–134
  occupational therapy applications,
    134–136
  overview, 130
  social context, 134
  supervision, 933
Huntington's disease
  psychosocial impact of, 531–532
  psychosocial issues, assessments,
    and interventions, 522
  symptoms, 139

Hypermanic, 239–240
Hypnosis, 144–145
Hypohedonia, 203
Hypomanic episode, 224

I

IADL. *See* Instrumental activities of
  daily living (IADL)
ICD-10. See International Classification
  of Diseases (ICD-10)
ICF. *See* International Classification
  of Functioning, Disability, and
  Health (ICF)
Ideation, 436
Identity, 942
Illusions, 180
Imaginal exposure, 274
Impairment Related Work Expense
  (IRWE), 829–830
Implicit methods of psychosocial
  interventions, 664–667
In vivo assessment, 483
In vivo exposure therapy, 274, 483
Inattention, 203
Inclusive fitness, 349
Independent Living Skills Assessment
  (ILS), 211
Independent living skills training
  (ILST), 518
Individual biases, 942–943
Individual Placement and Support
  (IPS) model, 816
Individualistic culture, 506
INECO Frontal Screening
  Test, 482
Infections as cause of
  psychopathology, 139
In-house jobs, 817
Initial Play Interview, 406
Initiation impairment after brain
  injury, 559
Insane, treatment before the twentieth
  century, 100–103
Institutions and clinics
  for adolescent mental illness,
    451–452
  for children, 405
  deinstitutionalization in the
    1960s, 812
  deinstitutionalization of
    patients, 120
  environment, 36–40
    advantages of therapeutic
      environment, 38
    case illustration, 36–37
    ethnic and cultural diversity,
      39–40

    negative environments, 36
    sensory stimulation, 37–38
  institutionalization and attachment
    theory, 359–360
  institutionalized, 5
  for schizophrenia, 195
Instrumental activities of daily
  living (IADL)
  activity groups, 693
  criminal justice, 727
  in forensic settings and OT
    interventions, 728–729
  groups, 697
  life satisfaction and quality
    of life, 518
Integration stage in the counseling
  psychology model, 940
Intellectualization, defined, 146
Intent of suicide, 436
Intentional Relationship Model (IRM),
  575–576, 587–592, 658
Intercultural Developmental
  Continuum (IDC), 54, 55
*Intercultural Developmental
  Inventory*, 54
Internal allies, 815
Internal self, 331–332
Internal working models, 350–351
Internalizing, 433
*International Classification of Diseases
  (ICD-10)*
  anxiety disorders, 261–262
  clinical picture, 319–323
  cultural controversy, 318–319
  diagnostic classification, 171
  personality disorders, 317–318
International Classification of
  Functioning, Disability, and
  Health (ICF)
  biopsychosocial model of human
    functioning and disability, 623
  children's mental health
    disabilities, 785
  information included, 171
  for occupational assessment, 617
  occupational therapist use of,
    504–505
  overview, 172
  purpose of, 503
Internet. *See* Technology; Web sites
Interoceptive desensitization, 275
Interpersonal modes applied to clients
  with pain-related disorder, 588
Interpersonal neurobiology, 358
Interpersonal skills
  criminal justice, 736–740
  training, 277
Interpersonal Social Rhythm Therapy
  (IPSRT), 236

Interpersonal strategies, Ch. 19
  advice, 647–649
  coaching, 649
  confrontation, 649
  encouragement, 647, 648
  fluid nature of, 645
  genuineness and authenticity, 645
  interpretation, 650–651
  limit setting, 646–647
  metaphors, 651
  overview, 644–645
  reality testing, 652
  reframing, 649–650
  techniques, defined, 644
  validation, 645–646, 648
Interpersonal therapy (IPT), for
    depression, 235
Interpersonal treatment approach,
    327–328
Interpretation, 397, 650–651
Intersubjectivity, 658–659
Intrapersonal aspects of training and
    supervision, 932
Inventory of Interpersonal Problems–
    Personality Disorder Scales
    (IIP–PD), 324
Involuntary defeat strategies,
    230–231

J

Jacobs Prevocational Skills
    Assessment, 819
Job coach, 829
Joint Theater Trauma System
    Clinical Practice Guidelines
    (JTTSCPGs), 894
Journal writing, 288–289
Jung, Carl, 146
Justice and Mental health Collaborative
    Project, 726

K

KAWA Model
  background, 42
  conceptual models, 32
  elements, 32
  for schizophrenia evaluation, 212
Kidner, Thomas, 110
Kinetic Self-Image Assessment, 406,
    407–408, 460
Knox Play Scale, 409
Kohlman Evaluation of Living Skills
    (KELS), 211
Kraepelin, Emil, 111

L

Labeling, 168–170
Lability, 181
Language. *See also* Communication
  criminal justice insider language,
      736–739
  culture and, 45–46
  labeling, 168–170
  politically correct, 46
  promoting occupational therapy,
      902, 903
  psychopathology, 177–178
  schizophrenia symptoms, 199
  speech patterns associated with
      mental illness, 177
Latency age of children, 410
Leading in fieldwork education, 954
Learning. *See* Fieldwork supervision
Learning disorders, 387
Least restrictive environment for
    therapy services, 35
Leiden programs, 366
Leisure, personality disorder and,
    329–330
Leisure group, 698
Life Management Skills, 865, 866
Life satisfaction
  client contributions to, 518
  defined, 517
  physical disabilities and, 514
Life skills
  ADL. *See* Activity of daily
      living (ADL)
  classes, 857–859
  groups, 702
  IADL. *See* Instrumental activities of
      daily living (IADL)
Lifestyle alterations, 290–291
Lifestyle redesign, 496, 863
Limit setting
  for adolescents, 444–445
  for children, 398–399
  defined, 398
  interpersonal strategies, 646–647
Lived experience, 4
Living skills at the ADA House,
    867–868
Living Skills Development
    Group, 863
Lobotomy, 112, 115
Local dining facility (DFAC), 879
Local-global research links, 90–91
Loosening of associations, 177
LOTCA, 903
Loving Intervention for Family
    Enrichment (LIFE), 458
Lower back pain, 577

M

Madhouses, 100
Magnification, 155
Major depression. *See also* Depression
  in adolescents, 432
  episodes, 223
  frequency of occurrence, 226–227
  in prisons, 722
  symptoms, 223, 224–225, 232–233
Managed care, 120–121, 135
Mania
  background of term, 222
  case illustration, 239–240, 242–243
  defined, 181, 222
  evaluation, 234
  manic episode, 224
  symptoms, 231–232
  treatment, 242–243, 246, 247
Maslow, Abraham, 131, 134
Maternal sensitivity, 363
Matrix of Needs and Satisfiers,
    131, 132
Max-Neef, Manfred, 131, 134
Mayers Lifestyle Questionnaire,
    626, 628
Mayor's Cell, 886
Meaning, defined, 134
Medical conditions as cause of anxiety
    disorders, 269
Medical model of diagnosis
    and treatment, 811–812
Medicare, 475
Medicine. *See* Health care
Meditation, 276
Melancholia
  background of term, 222
  description, 226
Memory
  after brain injury, 558–559
  amygdala and, 359
  confabulation, 558
  long term, 181
  prospective memory, 182–183
  short term, 181
  types of, 181–182
Mental health care
  culture and, 43–44
  environments, 34–36
  least restrictive environment, 35
  managed care, 120–121, 135
  mapping resources, 67
  roles of professionals, 19–23
    collaborative relationships,
        20–22
    occupational therapy used in
        recovery, 22–24
    resistance and concerns, 19–20

Mental health practice, Ch. 5
  behavioral perspective, 150–153
    applied behavioral analysis, 150, 151–152
    occupational therapy applications, 152–153
    overview, 150–151
    terms, 151
  biological perspective, 136–144
    biochemical factors, 139–141
    brain, 137–139
    brain plasticity, 143
    genetic factors, 141–142
    hormonal factors, 141
    occupational therapy applications, 143–144
    overview, 136–137
    psychopathology causal factors, 139–143
  biopsychosocial focus, 129
  cognitive perspective, 153–156
    appraisals, 154–155
    attributions, 155
    beliefs, 156
    expectations, 154
    occupational therapy applications, 156
    overview, 153
  eclectic approach, 129–130
  humanistic perspective, 130–136
    development of, 130–134
    occupational therapy applications, 134–136
    overview, 130
    social context, 134
  psychodynamic perspective, 144–150
    attachment theory, 147–148
    contemporary theories, 147–148
    ego defense mechanisms, 146
    neo-Freudian theories, 146–147
    object relations, 148
    occupational therapy applications, 148–150
    overview, 144–145
    psychoanalytic concepts, 145–146
    terms, 145
    two-person concept, 147
Mental health research. See Research
Mental illness
  burden of, 63–64
  descriptions, 6–7
  twentieth century treatment, 111–113
Mental retardation, 386, 387
Mentoring in fieldwork education, 955
Meta-analysis, 65
Metaphors, 651

Methodological position of research, 85–87
  fit for purpose, 85–86
  numbers and experience, 86–87
Methodology, 75
Meyer, Adolph, 105–106
Michigan Alcoholism Screening Test-Geriatric Version (MAST-G), 482
Middlesex Elderly Assessment of Mental State (MEAMS), 613
Milestones Outreach Service Team (MOST), 13, 14–15
Milieu treatment, 150
Military occupational therapy, Ch. 25
  CONUS, 896
  in the field
    animal-assisted therapy, 881–883
    disaster response, 883–885
    engagement in occupation, 886–887
    healthcare providers' role in self-care, 887–888
    service member occupational performance, 879–880
    teamwork, 885–886
    U.S. Army COSC units, 878, 880–881
  home treatment, 898–912
    acute military psychiatry, 900
    co-existing disorders, 900–901
    dual agency, 899–900
    interdisciplinary approach, 901–902
    occupational therapy, 902–912
    practitioner intervention, 912
  improvised explosive device (IED), 891–892
  Military Acute Concussion Evaluation (MACE), 894, 895
  occupational therapy, 902–912
    cognitive problems, 897–898
    communicating, 902
    group observation and documentation, 902–912
    language, 902
    patient education, 897
    performance of tasks, 898
    practitioner intervention, 912
    promoting, 902–912
    vision problems, 897
  Operation Enduring Freedom, 889
  Operation Iraqi Freedom, 889
  Private First Class (PFC), 884
  Sergeant First Class (SFC), 881
  service members, 877
  specialist (SPC), 883

traumatic brain injury rehabilitation, 889–898
  acute recovery, 890
  assessment and intervention, 894–896
  defined, 889
  mechanism of injury, 891–892
  military context, 891, 893
  occupational therapy interventions, 897–898
  occupational-performance problems, 893–894
  postconcussion syndrome, 890
  recurrent concussion, 891
  stress disorders and, 892–893
traumatic brain injury, second impact syndrome, 891
unit ministry teams, 878
warrior, defined, 898–899
Millon Clinical Multiaxial Inventory–III (MCMI–III), 324
Milwaukee Evaluation of Daily Living Skills (MEDLS), 211
Mindfulness, defined, 273, 653
Mindfulness groups, 695
Mindfulness-based cognitive therapy, 155, 273–274
Minding the Baby (MTB) program, 366
Minimization
  defined, 54
  on the Intercultural Developmental Continuum, 54
Minnesota Multiphasic Personality Inventory (MMPI-2), 324
Mixed episode, 224
Model of Human Occupation (MOHO)
  assessment complexity, 624
  conceptual models, 32
  Occupation-Based Self-Determination, 727
  for pain assessment, 580
  pain management and, 575–576
  psychosocial practice in the 1980s and 1990s, 118–119
  school-based programs, 776
  self-report assessment, 630
  use in pain treatment, 582–586
Model of Human Occupation Screening Tool (MOHOST)
  pain management, 580–581, 584–585
  substance abuse evaluation, 852
Model of Occupational Therapy Clearing House, 406
Modeling, defined, 151
MOHO. See Model of Human Occupation (MOHO)
Money management, 40, 829–830

Monoamine oxidase inhibitors (MAOIs), 270–271
Monochronic (M-time), 52
Monopolizing behavior, 687
Mood continuum, 238, 240
Mood disorders
  in adolescents, 432
  affect, 222. *See also* Affect
  causes and occurrence, 227–231
    cycling, 227
    etiologic theories, 228–229
    evolutionary theory, 230
    involuntary defeat strategies, 230–231
    medications, 227
    physical diseases, 227
    soft bipolar spectrum, 229
    temperament, 227, 229
  clinical picture, 231–233
  depression, 222. *See also* Depression
  diagnostic criteria, 222–226
    bipolar disorders, 225
    disorders, 224–225
    episodes, 223–224
    hypomanic episode, 224
    major depressive disorder, 224–225
    major depressive episode, 223
    manic episode, 224
    mixed episode, 224
    mood disturbances, 222–223
    specifiers, 226
  evaluation, 234
  frequency of occurrence, 226–227
  management, 235–238
  mania, 222
  melancholia, 222
  psychopathology, 140
  treatment and intervention, 238–251
    case illustration, 239–240, 241–243, 248–251
    interpersonal approach, 240–241, 242
    mood continuum, 238, 240
    person-to-person interventions, 243–247
    system interventions, 248
Moral treatment
  arts and crafts movement, 103–105
  defined, 100
  demise of, 102–103
  environment improvements, 101–102
  history of, 100–101
  humanistic principles, 120
  philosophy of, 101
  therapy in the 1960s and 1970s, 116

Morale, welfare, and recreation (MWR) facilities, 879
Morris, William, 103–104
Mosey's survey of task skills, 818
MOST (Milestones Outreach Service Team), 13, 14–15
Motivation, 652–655
Motor skills disorder, 387
Moxibustion, 43
M-time, 52
Multiculturalism, 45
Multiple personality disorder, 119, 193
Multiple sclerosis, 522
Music as occupational therapy, 114
Mutual help groups, 135
Myelomeningocele. *See* Spina bifida

N

Narcissistic personality disorder, 320–321, 326
Narcotics Anonymous, 844, 862, 867
National Health and Nutritional Examination Survey, 784
National Institute of Mental Health (NIMH)
  research priorities, 68
  schizophrenia statistics, 193
  suicide risk factors, 435–436
  translational science, 68
National Institute on Alcohol Abuse and Alcoholism (NIAAA), 842
National Pain Care Policy Act, 574
National Registry of Evidence-based Programs and Practices (NREPP), 457–458, 459
National Society for the Promotion of Occupational Therapy (NSPOT), 103
National Standards for Culturally and Linguistically Appropriate Services in Health Care (CLAS), 39
Natural environment, 30–31
Nature vs. nurture, 429
Negative reinforcement, 151
Negative symptoms for schizophrenia assessment scale, 203
  case illustration, 204
  for diagnosis, 198–199
Neglect. *See* Abuse and neglect
Neo-Freudian theories, 146–147
Neologism, 177
NEO-Personality Inventory-Revised (NEO-PI-R), 324
Neurasthenia, 108–111
Neurodevelopmental groups, 694
Neuropeptides and schizophrenia, 197

Neuroplasticity of the brain, 544
Neuroticism, 316
Neurotransmitter dysfunction
  as cause of psychological disorders, 139–140
  psychopharmacology, 140–141
  schizophrenia and, 197
  substances being studied, 139–140
  types of problems, 140
NIAAA (National Institute on Alcohol Abuse and Alcoholism), 842
NIMH. *See* National Institute of Mental Health (NIMH)
Non-didactic developmental guidance, 367
Nondirective play group, 409
Norepinephrine, 139, 140
Norms
  defined, 610
  of groups, 673
  norm-referenced test, 610
NREPP (National Registry of Evidence-based Programs and Practices), 457–458, 459

O

Object relations, 148
Observational assessment, 630–631
Obsessive-compulsive disorder (OCD)
  depression and, 234
  description, 267–268
  hoarding, 176
  rational-cognitive intervention, 291
  symptoms, 321–322
  thought and, 176
  treatment, 326
Occupation
  activity vs., 119
  balance of, 83
  health and, 83
  meaning and, 80
  privileged triad, 83
Occupational alienation, 725
Occupational apartheid, 725
Occupational Circumstances Assessment Interview Rating Scale (OCAIRS), 324, 630
Occupational deprivation, 716, 790
Occupational diagnosis, 618–622
  "best guess", 619
  diagnostic reasoning vs. medical diagnosis, 619
  diagnostic statement, 619–620, 621
Occupational enrichment, 725
Occupational health, 763–764
Occupational imbalance, 725
Occupational injustice, 725

Occupational justice, 33, 716, 777–778
Occupational Performance History
    Interview (OPHI), 118
Occupational Performance History
    Interview-II (OPHI-II)
    interview format, 212
    pain management, 580
    self-report, 630
    substance abuse evaluation, 852
Occupational profile, 617–618
Occupational Profile Worksheet, 819,
    820–823
Occupational prognosis, 622
Occupational restriction, 725–726
Occupational Self Assessment (OSA)
    for pain management, 581, 586
    self-report assessment, 630
    substance abuse evaluation, 853
    use with schizophrenia, 212
Occupational therapy
    adolescent suicide prevention,
        437–438
    aims of intervention, 620, 622
    attachment and, 366–378
        application of, 369
        case illustrations, 369–378
        non-didactic developmental
            guidance, 367
        PACE model, 369
        relationship-centered care, 368
        roles, 374
        strategies, 374
        support and advocacy, 367
    behaviorism applications, 152–153
    biases, 41–42
    biological perspective applications,
        143–144
    cognitive perspective
        applications, 156
    collaborative relationships, 22–24
    conceptual models, 32–33
    in criminal justice, 724–725, 744–754
    culturally competent practice, 53–56
    evidence-based practice, 64–66
    humanistic perspective applications,
        134–136
    least restrictive environment for, 35
    methods, 652–667
        activity analysis, 660–662
        activity categorization, 662–664
        clinical reasoning and motivating,
            652–655
        empathy, 657–659
        implicit and explicit methods,
            664–667
        intersubjectivity, 658–659
        interventions, 655
        relationships, building and
            repairing, 656–657

    therapeutic use of activity and
        occupation, 659–660
    therapeutic use of self, 655–656
    for military personnel, 893–898
    older adult mental health, 486–496
        behavioral techniques and
            humanistic philosophy,
            492–495
        environmental support and
            adaptation, 488–491
        occupation, 486–488
        prevention and health
            maintenance, 495–496
    pain assessment, 579–582
        clinical interview, 579
        occupation-focused assessment,
            580–581
        standardized ratings and
            assessments, 581–582
    in pain management, 592–593
    for personality disorders,
        328–334
    psychodynamic perspective
        applications, 148–150
    psychosocial. See Psychosocial
        occupational therapy
    in recovery paradigm, 22–24
    research, 62–63
    research priorities, 69–74
        Complete State Model of Mental
            Health, 69, 70
        comprehensive scope, 71
        cost benefit, 69–71
        research orientation, 73–74
        role emergent research areas,
            71–73
    for schizophrenia, 210–214
    self-management techniques,
        277–278
    for self-mutilation, 439–440
    substance abuse, 849–861
        assessment, 851
        discontinuation of services, 856,
            860–861
        gathering the occupational
            profile, 855–856
        interventions, 853–854
        life skills class offerings,
            857–859
        screening and evaluation,
            852–853
        solution-focused brief
            therapy, 854
    traumatic brain injury, 550–557
    use of animals and plants, 31
    vocational programming
        assessment, 815–826
        forms of intervention, 826–835
        roles, 814

Occupational Therapy Practice
    Framework (OTPF)
    adaptation recommendations, 34
    anxiety disorders, 261
    attachment theory, 358, 368
    children's mental health
        disabilities, 785
    culture, defined, 41
    documentation of outcomes, 703
    dual agency, 899
    eating disorders, 441–442
    environment, defined, 29, 34
    humanistic principles
        application, 135
    ICF as reference, 171
    interpersonal strategies, 644, 652
    interventions, 655
    occupation structures, 886
    personality disorders, 311
    personhood skills, 691
    physical disabilities, 504–505
    psychosocial issues in the school
        setting, 787–791
    psychosocial practice in the 1980s
        and 1990s, 118
    reality testing, 652
    sensory intervention groups, 695
Occupational Therapy Research
    Agenda, 71
Occupational Therapy Task
    Observation Scale
    (OTTOS), 902
Occupational Therapy Training
    Program (OTTP), 458
Occupation-Based Self-Determination
    (OBSD), 727, 729–730, 752
Occupation-focused eco-sustainable
    community development
    (OESCD), 34
Occupations for older adults,
    486–488
OCD. See Obsessive-compulsive
    disorder (OCD)
Offenders with mental health
    conditions, 717. See also
    Criminal justice
Older adult mental health, Ch. 14
    assessment, 482–486
        case illustration, 484, 485–486
        occupational therapy, 482–483
        quality of life, 485–486
        screening tests, 482, 483
    demographics of aging, 474–475
    elder abuse, 490–491
    measuring change in mental
        health, 629
    Medicare, 475
    occupational therapy intervention,
        486–496

behavioral techniques and humanistic philosophy, 492–495

case illustration, 488

environmental support and adaptation, 488–491

occupation, 486–488

prevention and health maintenance, 495–496

psychiatric diagnosis, 475–482

  Alzheimer's disease, 480–481

  case illustration, 478–479

  delirium, 481–482

  dementia, 480–482

  frequency of occurrence, 476

  incidence of, 475–476

  symptoms, 476–478

somatic concerns, 476

well elderly, 475

104 Activities That Build: Self-Esteem, Teamwork, Communication, Anger Management, Self-Discovery, and Coping Skills, 463–464

1-2-3 Magic! Training Your Preschoolers and Preteens to Do What You Want, 399

On-going assessment, 622

Ontology, 75

Operant conditioning, 151

OPHI. *See* Occupational Performance History Interview (OPHI)

Oppositional defiant disorder, 432, 433

Orientation, 181, 182

Osteoarthritis, 576

OT BCT c/mTBI Reconditioning Program, 894–895

OTPF. *See* Occupational Therapy Practice Framework (OTPF)

Outcome

of activities, 661

documentation, 703–704

measurement

  client's desired outcomes, 604–605

  process of, 606

process of assessment, 623

relationship to assessment and evaluation, 605

studies, 18

substance abuse CBT and 12-step programs compared, 848

terminology, 604

short-, medium-, and long-term, 607, 608–609

terminology, 604

Overeaters Anonymous, 844

Overgeneralization, 155

P

PACE model, 369

Pain management, Ch. 17

acute pain, 574–576

assessment of pain, 579–582

  clinical interview, 579

  occupation-focused assessment, 580–581

  standardized ratings and assessments, 581–582

chronic pain, 574–576

examples of disorders causing pain, 576–579

  arthritis, 576

  cancer, 576

  central pain syndrome, 576

  chronic headaches, 578

  chronic post-surgical pain, 577

  complex regional pain syndrome, 577–578

  depression and chronic pain, 578

  fibromyalgia, 577, 584–586

  lower back pain, 577

  peripheral neuropathy, 576–577

  phantom pain, 577

  substance abuse and chronic pain, 578–579

Intentional Relationship Model, 587–592

Model of Human Occupation, 582–586

National Pain Care Policy Act, 574

overview, 574

placebo effects, 575

Panic attack, 266

Paradigm

defined, 74

qualitative research paradigm, 76

quantitative research paradigm, 76

research thinking, 74–75

shift, 19

Parallel task group, 396

Paranoid

delusions, 200

personality disorder, 320

treatment, 326

Parasuicide, 438

Parent Project, 458

Parenting and schizophrenia, 194

Parent-Teacher Play Questionnaire, 409

Parkinson's disease

psychosocial impact of, 530–531

psychosocial issues, assessments, and interventions, 522

Participation

nonparticipation in groups, 686

personality disorders and social participation, 331

school

  disparities in, 775

  occupational justice perspective, 777–779

  psychosocial well-being and, 779–781

Participatory Occupational Justice Framework, 34

Partnership research priorities, 69. *See also* Collaboration

Pediatric Volitional Questionnaire (PVQ), 406

Peer interventions, 11–16

case illustration, 12–13

community and family roles, 13, 14–15

counseling and teaching, 13

for depression, 236

fear of recovery, 12–13

purpose of, 11

Wellness Recovery Action Plan, 15–16

Perception and sensation, 178–181

affect, 180

defined, 178

depression, 181

hallucinations, 178–180

illusions, 180

liability, 181

Perceptual distortion of schizophrenia, 200–203

Peripheral neuropathy, 576–577

Perseveration, 177, 559

Personal context of psychosocial issues in the school setting, 788

Personality Assessment Schedule (PASI), 324

Personality disorders, Ch. 10

after brain injury, 565

antisocial, 320–322

assessment, 323–324

avoidant, 321–322

borderline, 320–322

dependent, 321–322

DSM-IV-TR disorders, 314–316

  Axis I, 315

  Axis II, 315

  classifications, 319

  clusters, 319, 326

  dimensions, 315, 316

ego-syntonic, 313

etiology of, 311–314

hardwired behaviors, 313

histrionic, 320–322

maladaptive personality patterns, 312–313

narcissistic, 320–322

Personality disorders, Ch. 10 (Cont.)
    obsessive-compulsive, 321–322
    occupational therapy intervention,
        328–334
        case illustration, 332–334
        groups, 332
        leisure, 329–330
        self-care, 331–332
        social participation, 331
        work, 330–331
    overview, 309–311
    paranoid, 320
    personality, defined, 311
    personality continuum, 311–314
    polarities, 312
    schizoid, 320
    schizotypal, 320
    splitting, 323
    theories of, 310–311
    traits, 311–312
    treatment
        interdisciplinary, 324–328
        interpersonal approach,
            327–328
        occupational therapy, 328–334
        psychopharmacology, 325–327
Person-centered supervision, 933
Person-Environment-Occupation
    (PEO) model, 624, 776
Personhood skills, 689, 690, 691–692
Pervasive developmental disorders, 387
Phantom pain, 577
Pharmacology. See
    Psychopharmacology
Phobias, 266–267. See also Anxiety
    disorders
Phobocs, 267–268
Physical contexts group, 698
Physical disability and psychosocial
    issues, Ch. 15
    adaptation, 510–516
        acute onset of disabling
            conditions, 514–516
        chronic disabling conditions,
            510–514
        coping strategies, 506, 510
        factors, 518–519
        life satisfaction, 514
    chronic congenital nonprogressive
        disorders, 532–534
        cerebral palsy, 532–533
        spina bifida, 533–534
    chronic disorders with acute onset,
        523–530
        acquired amputation, 526–527
        cerebrovascular accident,
            529–530
        overview, 523
        spinal cord injury, 523–526

    stroke, 529–530
    traumatic brain injury, 527–528
    classification of functioning,
        504–505
    concept of self, 507–510
    cultural factors, 505–507
    issues, assessments, and
        interventions, 519–523
    life satisfaction, 517–519
    progressive physical disorders,
        530–532
        Huntington's disease, 531–532
        Parkinson's disease, 530–531
    quality of life, 517–519
    societal factors, 505–507
Physical environment of the school
    community, 789
Pinel, Phillipe, 100–101
Placebo effects on pain, 575
Place-Then-Train, 816
Plan for Achieving Self-Support
    (PASS), 829
Plan for suicide, 436
Plants used in occupational therapy, 31
Play intervention for children, 408–415
    copper tooling projects, 412
    creative task groups, 411–412
    games
        as adolescent therapy, 445, 463
        "Game of Life", 445
        as therapy for children, 408, 411
    play group protocol, 410
    play groups, 409–415
    playroom or therapy area, 414
    skills development group protocol,
        412, 413
Polarization
    defined, 54
    on the Intercultural Developmental
        Continuum, 54
Politics
    political activities of daily living
        reasoning tool, 34
    politically correct cultural
        language, 46
    research and, 88–89
Polychronic (P-time), 52
Polyculturalism, 44–45
Positive behavioral interventions and
    supports (PBIS), 782
Positive regard, 131
Positive reinforcement, defined, 151
Positive symptoms of schizophrenia,
    193, 199–203
    case illustration, 202–203
    delusions, 199–200
    distemporality, 201–202
    hallucinations, 202
    overview, 193

    perceptual distortion, 200–202
    sensory deficits, 200–202
Positivism, 150
Posspartum onset, 226
Postconcussion syndrome, 890
Post-traumatic amnesia, 544
Post-traumatic stress disorder (PTSD)
    acquired amputation and,
        526–527
    in adolescents, 432
    after the World Trade Center attack,
        268, 274
    c/mTBI and, 892–893
    description, 268
    eye movement desensitization
        and reprocessing treatment,
        276–277
    flashbacks, 268
    PTSD Reaction Index, 460
    from school violence, 444
    from traumatic brain injury, 542
    triggers, 268
Pottery as occupational therapy, 110
Poverty
    burden of mental illness, 64
    time sense, 51–52
Power struggles, 445–446
Practitioner-driven challenges,
    656–657
Predictive assessment, 627
Premenstrual Dysphoric Disorder
    (PMDD), 229
Premorbid psychosocial factors,
    547–549
Preschool Play Scale-Revised
    (PPS-R), 409
Prevention teams for military
    personnel, 879
Pre-Vocational Evaluation of
    Rehabilitation Potential, 818
Prevocational services, 810
Principle of reinforcement, 151
Prisonization, 754–758
Problem formulation, 618
Problem solving, 826
Program for Assertive Community
    Treatment (PACT), 818–819
Progressive muscle relaxation, 286
Progressive physical disorders,
    530–532
    Huntington's disease, 531–532
    Parkinson's disease, 530–531
Projection, defined, 146
Projective group, 697
Proxemics, 50
Proxy report, 631–635
Psychiatric disorders after brain
    injury, 564
Psychiatric rehabilitation, 812–813

Psychoanalysis
  for bipolar disorders, 237
  concepts, 144–145
  description, 236–237
  history and philosophy, 111
  transference, 237
Psychoanalytic supervision, 932–933
Psychobiology, 105–106
Psychodrama, 674
Psychodynamic perspective in mental
    health practice, 144–150
  attachment theory, 147–148
  contemporary theories, 147–148
  ego defense mechanisms, 146
  neo-Freudian theories, 146–147
  object relations, 148
  occupational therapy applications,
    148–150
  overview, 144–145
  psychoanalytic concepts,
    145–146
  terms, 145
  two-person concept, 147
Psychodynamic supervision, 932–933
Psychodynamic theories, 147–148
Psychodynamic work in groups, 700
Psychoeducation as research
    reciprocity, 88–89
Psychoeducational groups, 696
Psychogenic, 290
Psychological needs, 654, 845
Psychomotor agitation, 232
Psychopathology, 139–143, 175–183
  biochemical factors, 139–141
  brain plasticity, 143
  energy and motoric response, 183
  executive function, 176
  genetic factors, 141–142
  hormonal factors, 141
  language, 177–178
  memory, 181–183
  orientation, 181, 182
  perception and sensation,
    178–181
    affect, 180
    defined, 178
    depression, 181
    hallucinations, 178–180
    illusions, 180
    liability, 181
  speech patterns, abnormal, 177
  thought, 176
Psychopharmacology
  for anxiety disorders, 270
  biochemistry, 140
  history of, 113
  for personality disorders, 325–327
  use in the 1980s and 1990s, 120
Psychosexual stage, 145

Psychosis
  in older adults, 477
  of schizophrenia, 193
Psychosocial issues
  after brain injury, 564–567
    altered self-concept, 565–566
    case illustration, 534
    coping mechanism
      impairment, 565
    family dynamics, impact on,
      566–567
    personality changes, 565
    psychiatric disorders, 564
    social pragmatic impairment, 565
  physical disability and. See Physical
    disability and psychosocial
    issues
  traumatic brain injury, 547–549
Psychosocial occupational therapy, Ch. 4
  evolution of, 113–121
    1920s and 1930s, 113–114
    1940s and 1950s, 114–115
    1960s and 1970s, 115–118
    1980s and 1990s, 118–121
  founding of occupational therapy,
    103–111
    background, 103
    Dunton, William Rush, 103–105
    Hall, Herbert James, 108–111
    Meyer, Adolph, 105–106
    Slagle, Eleanor Clarke, 107–108
  history of treatment of the insane,
    100–103
  twentieth century treatment of
    mental illness, 111–113
Psychosocial rehabilitation, 812–813
Psychoticism, 316
Psychotropic medications, 183
P-time, 52
PTSD. See Post-traumatic stress
    disorder (PTSD)

Q

Qualitative research paradigm, 76
Quality of life
  assessment, 485–486
  client contributions to, 518
  defined, 517
  with physical disability, 504
Quantitative research paradigm, 76

R

Race, 44–45. See also Culture
Rancho Los Amigos Levels of Cognitive
    Functioning, 550–556, 562

Rational-cognitive intervention, 291
Reaction formation, 146
Reactive attachment disorder (RAD)
  in adolescents, 452–454
  case illustration, 389–391
  causes, 389
  characteristics, 388
  symptoms, 359, 388–389
Realistic meaning of activities, 661–662
Reality testing, 652
Recidivism, 716, 763
Recovery
  Are You in Recovery Yourself?, 850
  components of, 17
  evaluation instruments, 852–853
  fear of, 12–13
  intervention. See Recovery-focused
    intervention
  model, 10
  movement, 19
  perspectives. See Recovery
    perspectives
  process vs. outcome, 17
  recovery from vs. recovery, 17
  Recovery Movement, 120
  resistance and concerns, 19–20
  scope of, 16–19
  substance abuse programs, 849–861
  traumatic brain injury, 890
Recovery perspectives, Ch. 1
  case illustration, 7, 8–9, 11, 12–13,
    21, 23–24
  definition of recovery, 8
  definitions, 16–19
  mental health professional roles, 19–22
    collaborative relationships, 20–22
    resistance and concerns, 19–20
  mental illness described, 6–7
  occupational therapy used in
    recovery, 22–24
  peer interventions and recovery-
    oriented support, 11–16
    community and family, 13
    counseling and teaching, 13–15
    Wellness Recovery Action Plan,
      15–16
  personal perspective, 4–16
  professional perspective, 16–24
  recovery
    defined, 7–9
    movement, 19
    as realistic goal, 10–11
    scope of, 16–19
  research and evidence, 17–19
Recovery-focused intervention, 183–188
  overview, 183
  psychotropic medication, 184–186
  shared decision making, 184
  technology and access, 186–188

Redirection, 393–394
Reentry to the community, 763
Referential thinking, 232
Reflection, 932
Reflex sympathetic dystrophy, 577–578
Reflexivity
    action research transforming
        practice, 82–83
    defined, 80
    outsider-insider, 81–82
    research ethics, 85
Reframing, 649–650
Regression, defined, 146
Rehabilitation
    psychiatric, 812–813
    psychosocial, 812–813
    from substance abuse, 860–861
Reilly, Mary, 117–118
Reinforcement
    negative, 151
    positive, 151
    principle of, 151
Relatedness, 654
Relational theory, defined, 147–148
Relationship of supervisor and
    supervisee, 927
Relationship-centered care, 368
Relationships, building and repairing,
    656–657
Relaxation training, 282–287
    activity configuration, 284, 298
    autogenic training, 284, 287
    breathing exercises, 285–286
    progressive muscle relaxation, 286
    visualization, 286–287
Reliability of tests, 610, 611,
    613–614
Remunerative permanent
    occupation, 110
Representation of others in
    research, 85
Repression, defined, 146
Reproductive fitness, 349
Research, Ch. 3
    action research, 87–88
    AOTA/FAST Research Project,
        442–443
    burden of mental illness, 63–64
    defined, 62
    evidence gathering, 18
    evidence-based practice, 64–66
    examples, learning from others,
        87–90
        locating knowledge construction,
            87–88
        participatory program
            development, 89–90
        psychoeducation as research
            reciprocity, 88–89

human scale research agenda, 91–92
local-global research links, 90–91
mental health priorities, 66–69
    grand challenges, 67–68
    intervention development, 68
    mapping resources, 67
    partnerships, 69
    translational science, 68
methodological position, 85–87
    fit for purpose, 85–86
    numbers and experience,
        86–87
    occupational therapist input,
        62–63
    occupational therapy priorities,
        69–74
        Complete State Model of Mental
            Health, 69, 70
        comprehensive scope, 71
        cost benefit, 69–71
        research orientation, 73–74
        role emergent research areas,
            71–73
outcome measures, 18
pet ownership, 31
recovery, 17–19
schizophrenia, 17–18
thinking in research, 74–85
    checking assumptions, 80, 83
    conventions, questioning of,
        79–80, 81–83
    epistemology, 75
    methodology, 75
    ontology, 75
    peripheral factors in research
        design, 78
    reflexivity, 80, 81–83
    ways of thinking, 74–79
translational research, 91
Research Centre for Occupation and
    Mental Health (RCOMH), 70
Residential programming, 867–868
Resiliency, 429, 437
Resistance to recovery, 19–20
Response to Intervention (RtI),
    781–782
Restoration programs for military
    personnel, 879
Rett's syndrome, 532
Revised Memory and Behavior
    Problem Checklist
    (RMBPC), 633
Rheumatoid arthritis, 576
Rite of passage, 430–431, 509
Rivermead Behavioral Memory
    Test, 897
Rogers, Carl, 131–133
Role Acquisition Frame of Reference,
    812–813

Role checklist
    anxiety disorder assessment, 278,
        279–280, 294–295
    substance abuse evaluation, 853
Role emergent research areas, 71–73
Ruskin, John, 103–104

S

SAMHSA (Substance Abuse and
    Mental Health Service
    Administration), 16, 457–458
Scale for Assessing Copying Skills,
    632–633
Schindler, V., 119
Schizoid personality disorder, 320, 326
Schizophrenia, Ch. 7
    in adolescents, 433
    collaborative treatment, 206–210
        defined, 206
        goal attainment, 206–208
        psychotropic medication,
            208–210
    deficit schizophrenia, 199
    diagnosis, 198–199
    etiology, 196–198
        brain function and, 196, 197
        causes of, 196–198
    genetic factors, 142
    myths, 193–196
        bad parenting, 194
        danger and violence, 195–196
        drug experimentation, 194
        institutionalization and
            disability, 195
        lack of motivation, 194
        low intelligence, 195
        rising incidence, 195
        split personality, 193
    negative symptoms
        assessment scale, 203
        case illustration, 204
        for diagnosis, 198–199
    nondeficit schizophrenia, 199
    occupational therapy intervention,
        210–214
        evaluation, 210–212
        formats, 201
        treatment, 212–214
    overview, 193
    positive symptoms, 199–203
        case illustration, 202–203
        delusions, 199–200
        distemporality, 201–202
        hallucinations, 202
        overview, 193
        perceptual distortion, 200–202
        sensory deficits, 200–202

in prisons, 722
prognosis, 204–206
psychopathology, 139, 140
research and evidence, 17–18
Schedule for Deficit Syndrome, 199
statistics, 193
symptoms, 193
treatment formats, 201
Schizotypal personality disorder, 320, 326
School
    advocacy, 775–776
    bullying, 775
    community-based practice, 781–801
        children with mental health disabilities, 784–786
        evaluation of psychosocial issues, 787–791
        positive behavioral interventions and supports, 782
        Response to Intervention, 781–782
        three-tiered approach, 781–784, 796–797
        universal design for learning, 782
    cyberbullying, 775
    participation
        disparities in, 775
        occupational justice perspective, 777–779
        psychosocial well-being and, 779–781
    psychosocial issues, actions to address, 801–803
    psychosocial issues, evaluation of, 787–791
        cultural, 788
        intervention service delivery methods, 798–801
        occupational therapy intervention, 791–797
        personal, 788
        physical, 789
        social, 789–791
        temporal, 788–789
        virtual, 788
    school mental health movement, 775
    school-based programs
        for adolescents, 455–457
        for children, 402–405
        students who benefit from mental health interventions, 779, 780
        violence in, 442–444
Second impact syndrome, 891
Secure base functions, 361
Seeking Safety program, 458–459
Selective abstraction, 155
Selective mutism, 388
Self-assessment of activities, 297

Self-care, personality disorder and, 331–332
Self-concept. See Concept of self
Self-Determination Model, 727
Self-Development Group, 863, 864
Self-efficacy, 461, 463
Self-Esteem and Life Skills (SEALS), 463–464
Self-help groups, 135, 696
Self-injurious behavior, 438
Self-management techniques, 277–278
Self-mutilation
    causes of, 439
    defined, 438
    occupational therapy intervention, 439–440
Self-report, 629–630
Self-wounding, 438
Sensorimotor-affective, 351
Sensory defensiveness, 292
Sensory deficits of schizophrenia, 200–203
Sensory intervention groups, 694–695
Sensory modulation interventions, 292–293, 694–695
Sensory overresponsive type (SOR), 292
Sensory processing, 178
Sensory-processing deficits, 178
Separation anxiety disorder, 388
Seriously and persistently mentally ill (SMI), 814
Serotonin
    biochemical factor in psychological disorders, 139
    personality disorders and, 326
    research on, 140
    schizophrenia and, 197
Service members, 877. See also Military occupational therapy
7-Minute Screen, 482
Sexual behavior
    after traumatic brain injury, 562
    criminal justice system, 742–744
    Ex-PLISSIT model, 743
    psychosexual stages, 145
Shaping, defined, 151
Shared decision making, 184
Sheltered employment, 817, 828
Shenjing shuairuo, 44
Sheppard Enoch Pratt Asylum, 101–102, 103
Shock therapy, 115. See also Electroconvulsive therapy (ECT)
Short Anxiety Screening Test, 482
Short-Form McGill Pain Questionnaire, 581–582
"Sicker and quicker", 421
Situational avoidance, 266

Situational Leadership, 943
Situational supervision, 943–948
Skinner, B. F., 150
Slagle, Eleanor Clarke, 33, 72, 107–108, 110
Sleep, psychotropic medication and, 183
SMART goal format, 607, 622
Social Anxiety disorder, 267
Social environment of the school community, 789–790, 792
Social issues
    after brain injury, 565
    in substance abuse, 845
Social networking, 886, 956–957
Social participation, personality disorder and, 331
Social phobia, 267
Social relationships, 50–51
Social Security Administration
    client practice of skills, 830
    Impairment Related Work Expense, 829
    Ticket to Work, 830
Social skills training. See Assertiveness and social skills training
Society and physical disabilities, 504–505. See also Culture
Solution-focused brief therapy (SFBT), 854
Somatic concerns, 476
South Africa, primary health care approach, 77
Specifiers, 226
Spina bifida
    psychosocial impact of, 533–534
    psychosocial issues, assessments, and interventions, 522
Spinal cord injury
    case illustration, 524, 525–526
    psychosocial impact of, 523–526
    psychosocial issues, assessments, and interventions, 520
Spiritual group, 698
Spirituality in 12-step programs, 845
Split personality, 193
Splitting, 323
Stagnation stage in the counseling psychology model, 938, 939
Standardized tests, 609–615
    design of the test, 613
    reliability, 610, 611, 613–614
    validity, 610, 612, 614–615
State/Trait Anxiety Inventory (STAI), 278
Statistics, 86
Stereotypy, 183
Stigma, 40
Strange Situation, 347, 351–354

Strategies, defined, 644. *See also* Interpersonal strategies
Stress disorders
  acute stress disorder, 268–269, 907–909
  c/mTBI and, 892–893
  COSC. *See* United States Army Combat Stress Control (COSC) units
  PTSD. *See* Post-traumatic stress disorder (PTSD)
Stroke, 529–530, 576
Strong Kids, 783
Structural Analysis of Social Behavior Intrex Questionnaire (SASB-IQ), 324
Structured Interview for DSM Personality Disorders-IV (SIDP-IV), 324
Structured Interview for the Five-Factor Model (SIFFM), 324
Student Behavior Survey (SBS), 633
Sublimation, defined, 146
Substance abuse, Ch. 24
  addiction, 843
  in adolescents, 432
  advice from clients and therapists, 869
  alcohol abuse. *See* Alcohol abuse
  as choice, habit, or disease, 843–844
  chronic pain and, 578–579
  costs of, 842–843
  defined, 842
  drug abuse. *See* Drug abuse
  Narcotics Anonymous, 844, 862, 867
  occupational therapy at the ADA Center, 861–868
    client perceptions of the challenge, 861–862
    group interventions, 864–867
    occupational therapy programming, 862–864
    programming, 862
    student participation, 868
    supportive residential programming, 867–868
  occupational therapy rationale, 849, 850–851
  occupation-based intervention, 849–861
    assessment, 851
    discontinuation of services, 856, 860–861
    gathering the occupational profile, 855–856
    interventions, 853–854
    life skills class offerings, 857–859
    screening and evaluation, 852–853

    solution-focused brief therapy, 854
  in older adults, 478
  overview, 841
  recovery
    Are You in Recovery Yourself?, 850
    evaluation instruments, 852–853
    programs, 849–861
  risk factors, 843–844
  scope of the problem, 842–843
  traumatic brain injury and, 549
  treatment, 844–848
    cognitive-behavioral therapy, 846–848
    12-step programs, 844–848
Substance Abuse and Mental Health Services Administration (SAMHSA), 16, 457–458
Substance-induced anxiety disorder, 269
Substance-related disorders of adolescents, 432
Suicide
  adolescents, 435–438
    contract for safety, 437
    frequency of occurrence, 435
    ideation, 436
    intent, 436
    occupational therapy, 437–438
    plan, 436
    prevention programs, 436–437
    risk factors, 435
  depression as cause of, 233
Sullivan, Harry Stack, 146–147, 148
Superego, defined, 145
Superficial-moderate self-mutilation, 438
Supervision. *See* Fieldwork supervision
Supported employment, 814, 833–835
Symbolic meaning of activities, 661–662
Symptoms
  case illustration, 167–168
  clinical terminology, 167
  negative symptoms for schizophrenia
    assessment scale, 203
    case illustration, 204
    for diagnosis, 198–199
  positive symptoms for schizophrenia, 199–203
    case illustration, 202–203
    delusions, 199–200
    distemporality, 201–202
    hallucinations, 202
    overview, 193
    perceptual distortion, 200–202
    sensory deficits, 200–202

Systematic desensitization, 275
Systematic reviews, 65

T

Taken-for-granted ways, 507
Tangentiality, 177
Task groups, 693
Task Management Strategies Index (TMSI), 634
Task-oriented group, 117
TBI. *See* Traumatic brain injury (TBI)
Teaching in fieldwork education, 955
Teams. *See also* Groups
  in adolescent therapy, 447–448
  in children's therapy, 400–401
Techniques, defined, 644. *See also* Interpersonal strategies
Technology
  CommonGround, 184, 186
  telepsychiatry, 186–188
  treatment information access, 186–188
Telepsychiatry, 186–188
Temperament and Character Inventory (TCI), 324
Temporal aspects of the school community, 788–789
Temporality, 51
Test of Everyday Attention, 897
Test of Grocery Shopping Skills, 211
Test of Playfulness (TOP), 409
Test of Visual Motor Skills (TVMS), 406
Tests. *See* Assessment; Evaluation
Thematic group, 697
Therapeutic community, 112, 447
Therapeutic competencies, 730–742
  communication skills, 736–740
  defined, 730
  environmental assessment, 730–731
  interpersonal skills, 736–740
  models of practice and assessments, 732–735
  models of practice and practice knowledge base, 731–732
  professional and ethical behavior, 740
  risk assessment, 730–731
  tools and materials, 740–742
Therapeutic use of activity and occupation, 659–660
Therapeutic use of self
  adolescent suicide prevention, 438
  adolescent therapy, 446–447
  for children's therapy, 399–400
  occupational therapy method, 655–656

personhood skills, 692
use during the 1940s and 1950s, 114
Therapy in fieldwork education, 955
Thinking in research, 74–85
   checking assumptions, 80, 83
   conventions, questioning of, 79–80,
     81–83
   epistemology, 75
   methodology, 75
   ontology, 75
   peripheral factors in research
     design, 78
   reflexivity, 80, 81–83
   ways of thinking, 74–79
Thought
   broadcasting, 200
   control, 200
   defined, 176
   delusions, 176
   insertion, 200
   obsession, 176
   withdrawal, 200
"Three strikes" laws, 721
Three-tiered intervention approach to
    academics, 781–784, 796–797
Thresholds, 812
Ticket to Work, 830
Tics, 183, 388
Time management training
   for anxiety disorders, 291–292
Time sense, 51–53
   case illustration, 52–53
   monochronic (M-time), 52
   polychronic (P-time), 52
   temporality, 51
Time-out, 397–398
TM/CAM (complementary and
    alternative medicine), 42–43
Tourette's disorder, 386, 388
Training in fieldwork education, 955
Traits of personality, 311–312
Transference, 237
Transformative learning, 924,
    926–929
Transitional employment, 817, 827–828
Translational developmental
    neuroscience, 68
Translational research, 91
Transparency of research, 85
Traumatic brain injury (TBI), Ch. 16
   behavioral sequelae, 560, 562–564
     agitation and aggression, 562
     demotivational syndrome, 563
     disinhibition, 562
     emotional responses,
      inappropriate, 563–564
     hypersexual behaviors, 562
   central pain syndrome, 576
   cognitive sequelae, 557–560

abstract thinking impairment, 560
   anosognosia, 559
   attention deficits, 557–558
   case illustration, 561
   executive function
    impairment, 560
   generalization of skills, 560
   information processing
    impairment, 559
   initiation impairment, 559
   memory impairment, 558–559
   orientation impairment, 557
   perseveration, 559
costs of, 542–543
defined, 542
diagnosis, 543–544
diffuse axonal injury, 544
etiology, 543–544
functional brain anatomy, 544, 545
Glasgow Coma Scale, 547, 548, 889
military occupational therapy,
    889–898
   acute recovery, 890
   assessment and intervention,
    894–896
   cognitive problems, 897–898
   defined, 889
   mechanism of injury, 891–892
   military context, 891, 893
   occupational therapy
    interventions, 897–898
   occupational-performance
    problems, 893–894
   patient education, 897
   performance of tasks, 898
   postconcussion syndrome, 890
   recurrent concussion, 891
   second impact syndrome, 891
   stress disorders and, 892–893
   vision problems, 897
neuroplasticity of the brain, 544
occupational therapy evaluation
    and intervention, 550–557
post-traumatic amnesia, 544
premorbid psychosocial factors,
    547–549
psychosocial impact of, 527–528
psychosocial issues, assessments,
    and interventions, 521
psychosocial sequelae, 564–567
   altered self-concept, 565–566
   case illustration, 534
   coping mechanism
    impairment, 565
   family dynamics, impact on,
    566–567
   personality changes, 565
   psychiatric disorders, 564
   social pragmatic impairment, 565

Rancho Los Amigos Levels of
    Cognitive Functioning,
    550–556, 562
recovery prognosis, 544, 547
types of, 546–547
Treatment box, 906–907
Trencín Statement on Prisons and
    Mental Health, 721–722
Triangulation, 631
Triggers, 268
Tucson shooting, 443
Tuke, Samuel, 130–131
12-step programs, 844–848
Twin studies for genetic factors in
    psychopathology, 142
Two-person concepts, 147–148

U

UCLA family development
    program, 366
Unconditional positive regard, 133
Unconditioned response (UCR),
    defined, 151
Unconscious, defined, 145
Unit ministry team (UMT), 878
United States Army Combat Stress
    Control (COSC) units
   animal-assisted therapy, 881–883
   mission of, 878
   occupational therapy roles,
    880–881
Universal design, 29–30, 782
U.S. Department of Health and Human
    Services, 843
Use of self, 587–592

V

Validation, 645–646, 648, 654
Validity of tests, 610, 612, 614–615
Valpar series, 818
Values, 50–51
Van Leit, B., 121
Vascular dementia, 480
Vasodilatation, 287
Veterans, arts and crafts occupational
    therapy for, 109–110
Veterans Administration, 900–901
Video-feedback Intervention to
    Promote Positive Parenting
    (VIPP), 365
Violence and schizophrenia, 195–196
Virginia Tech violence, 443
Virtual context of psychosocial issues
    in the school setting, 788
Virtual exposure, 274

Virus as cause of schizophrenia, 197–198
Visualization, 286–287
Vitamins and schizophrenia, 198
Vocational group, 698
Vocational programming, Ch. 23. *See also* Employment
  alliances, 814–815
    community allies, 815
    internal allies, 815
  assessment, 815–826
    case illustration, 825–826
    characteristics of models for positive vocational outcomes, 824
    Occupational Profile Worksheet, 819, 820–823
    pre-employment placement, 816–817
    pre-employment treatment, 815–816
    Program for Assertive Community Treatment, 818–819
    purpose of assessment, 818
    tests, 818–819
  collaboration levels, 810, 811
  community interventions, 830–831
  context of services, 832–833
  counseling, 826–829
  employer involvement, 831–832
  history of, 810–813
    acquisitional frames of reference, 813–814
    deinstitutionalization, 812
    medical model of diagnosis and treatment, 811–812
    prevocational services, 810
    rehabilitation, 812–813
    work programming, 810–811

money management skills, 529–830
occupational therapy
  assessment, 815–826
  forms of intervention, 826–835
  roles, 814
skills, community application of, 830
supported employment, 814, 833–835
Vocational Rehabilitation Act, 810
Vocational Rehabilitation Amendment, 810
Volitional Questionnaire (VQ), 631
Volunteer employment, 827

W

Warrior ethos, 898–899
Watanabe, Sandra, 116
Weaving, 506
Web sites, 65–66
Weekly Calendar Planning Activity, 903
Well elderly, 475
Wellness Recovery Action Plan (WRAP)
  description, 15–16
  for peer teaching, 13
  purpose of, 15–16, 184
WFOT. *See* World Federation of Occupational Therapy (WFOT)
WHO. *See* World Health Organization (WHO)
Willard and Spackman's 10th edition, 659
Woodside, H., 115–116
Work
  personality disorder and, 330–331
  programming, 810–811. *See also* Vocational programming

work therapy, 108–111
Work Environment Impact Scale (WEIS), 819, 853
Work Opportunity Tax Credit program, 754
Worker Role Interview (WRI), 581, 819
Working alliance, 327–328
Workload vs. caseload, 798–799
World Federation of Occupational Therapy (WFOT)
  culture, defined, 41
  Guiding Principles on Diversity and Culture, 41
World Health Organization (WHO)
  biopsychosocial approach, 623
  Declaration of Alma Ata, 77
  environment and culture, 29
  International Classification of Diseases (ICD-10), 171
  International Classification of Function, 171, 172
  International Classification of Functioning, 504
  mental health resources, 67
  quality of life assessment, 485
  schizophrenia prognosis, 204
  traumatic brain injury diagnosis, 543
  Trencín Statement on Prisons and Mental Health, 721–722
World Trade Center attack and PTSD, 268, 274
WRAP. *See* Wellness Recovery Action Plan (WRAP)

Y

Youth Self-Report, 460–461